OCCUPATIONAL DISORDERS OF THE LUNG

OCCUPATIONAL DISORDERS OF THE LUNG:
Recognition, Management, And Prevention

Edited by

David J. Hendrick, MSC, MD, FRCP, FFOM
Professor of Occupational Respiratory Medicine, University of Newcastle upon Tyne,
Department of Respiratory Medicine, Royal Victoria Infirmary,
Newcastle upon Tyne, UK

P. Sherwood Burge, MSC, MD, FRCP, FFOM, DIH
Professor of Occupational Medicine,
Birmingham University,
Birmingham, UK

William S. Beckett, MD, MPH
Professor, Enviromental Medicine and Medicine,
University of Rochester School of Medicine and Dentistry,
Rochester, NY, USA

Andrew Churg, MD
Professor, Department of Pathology,
University of British Columbia,
Vancouver, BC, Canada

Edinburgh • London • New York • Oxford • Philadelphia • St Louis • Sydney • Toronto

2002

WB Saunders

An imprint of Elsevier Science Limited

© Harcourt Publishers Limited 2002
© Elsevier Science Limited 2002. All rights reserved.

The right of David J. Hendrick, P. Sherwood Burge, William S. Beckett and Andrew Churg to be identified as authors of this work
has been asserted by them in accordance with the Copyright, Designs and Patents Act 1988

First published 2002
Reprinted 2002

ISBN 0 7020 2507 0

British Library Cataloguing in Publication Data
A catalogue record for this book is available from the British Library

Library of Congress Cataloging in Publication Data
A catalog record for this book is available from the Library of Congress

Drug Nomenclature
Directive 92/27/EEC requires use of the Recommended International Non-proprietary Name (rINN) for medicinal substances. In most cases
the British Approved Name (BAN) and rINN are identical but where they differ the rINN has been used with the old BAN in parentheses.

**There are two important exceptions: adrenaline and noradrenaline, where the BAN is used first followed by the new rINNS
(epinephrine and norepinephrine) in parentheses.**

Note
Medical knowledge is constantly changing. As new information becomes available, changes in treatment, procedures,
equipment and the use of drugs become necessary. The editors/authors/contributors and the publishers have taken care
to ensure that the information given in this text is accurate and up to date. However, readers are strongly advised to confirm
that the information, especially with regard to drug usage, complies with the latest legislation and standards of practice.

 your source for books,
journals and multimedia
in the health sciences
www.elsevierhealth.com

Printed and bound in the United Kingdom
Transferred to Digital Print 2010

The
publisher's
policy is to use
paper manufactured
from sustainable forests

Contents

Preface

"The flesh, alas, is wearied: and I have read all the books there are"

Stéphane Mallarmé

'I am struck, not so much by the diversity of testimony, as by the many-sidedness of truth'

An unknown Judge

We dedicate this book first to our families, who allowed us to produce it and so had their lives disrupted for several years; and secondly to our readers, who unwittingly provided the stimulus and whose sufferings are still to come. May any weariness they encounter be alleviated by discovering at least some of the truth.

List of contributors

Daniel E. Banks, MD
Professor and Chair
Department of Medicine
Louisiana State University School of Medicine
Shreveport, LA
USA

Paul D. Blanc, MD, MSPH
Professor of Medicine
Division of Occupational Medicine
University of California, San Francisco
San Francisco, CA
USA

Jeremy Beach, MD, FRCP, FFOM
Associate Professor
Department of Occupational Medicine
University of Alberta
Edmonton
Canada

William S. Beckett, MD, MPH
Professor, Enviromental Medicine and Medicine
University of Rochester School of Medicine and Dentistry
Rochester, NY
USA

Anne Brichet, MD
Cliniques des Maladies Respiratoires
Hôpital A. Calmette
Lille
France

P. Sherwood Burge, MSc, MD, FRCP, FFOM, DIH
Director, Occupational Lung Disease Unit
Birmingham Heartlands Hospital
Birmingham
UK

Aurelia Carosso, MD
Consultant Physician in Respiratory and
Occupational Medicine
Servizio di Allergologia-ASL4-TO
Dispensario d'Igiene Sociale
Torino
Italy

André Cartier, MD
Head, Chest Department
Hôpital du Sacré-Cœur de Montréal;
Professor of Clinical Medicine
University of Montreal
Montreal
Canada

David C. Christiani, MD, MPH, MS
Professor of Medicine,
Professor of Occupational Medicine and Epidemiology
Harvard School of Medicine and Public Health
Boston, MA
USA

Andrew Churg, MD
Professor
Department of Pathology
University of British Columbia
Vancouver, BC
Canada

Sue Copley, MBBS, MRCP, FRCR, MD
Consultant Radiologist
Department of Radiology
Hammersmith Hospital
London
UK

Yvon Cormier, MD
Professor of Medicine
Laval Hospital
Quebec
Canada

David Coultas, MD
Professor and Associate Chairman, Internal Medicine
The University of Florida Health Science Center
Jacksonville, FL
USA

Robert L. Cowie, MD, MSc, FCP(SA)
Professor of Medicine
Health Sciences Centre
Calgary, AB
Canada

Andrew D. Curran, BSc, PhD, CBiol, MIBiol
Health and Safety Laboratory and Co-Director
Sheffield Occupational and Environmental
Lung Injury Centre
Sheffield
UK

Gerald S. Davis, MD
Professor of Medicine
Pulmonary Disease and Critical Care Medicine
College of Medicine
University of Vermont
Burlington, VT
USA

Nicholas H. de Klerk, BSc, MSc, PhD
Head, Biostatistics and Genetic Epidemiology
Institute of Child Health Research
Adjunct Professor, Department of Public Health
University of Western Australia
Tuw Telethon Institute For Child Health Research
Subiaco
Australia

Paul De Vuyst, MD, PhD
Professor of Medicine
Chest Department
Erasme Hospital
Universite Libre de Bruxelles
Brussels
Belgium

Jean-Dominique Dewitte, MD
Professor of Medicine
Service de Pathologies professionelles
CHRU Morvan
Brest-Cedex
France

Sophie Desurmont, MD
Cliniques des Maladies Respiratoires
Hôpital A. Calmette
Lille
France

Thomas A. Dillard, MD
Professor of Medicine
Pulmonary/Critical Care Section
Medical College of Georgia
Augusta, GA
USA

David Fishwick, MB, ChB, FRCP, AFOM, MD
Senior Lecturer in Respiratory Medicine
University of Sheffield;
Co-Director, Sheffield Occupational and Environmental
Lung Injury Centre
Sheffield
UK

Paul F. G. Gannon, MD, MRCP(UK), MFOM
Occupational Physician
Medical Centre
Wilton Site
Middlesbrough
UK

Pierre Alain Gevenois, MD, PhD
Professor of Radiology
Department of Radiology
Erasme Hospital
Université Libre de Bruxelles
Brussels
Belgium

Michelle Ng Gong, MD
Instructor in Medicine
Department of Pulmonary and Critical Care Medicine
Massachusetts General Hospital
Boston, MA
USA

Tee L. Guidotti, MD, MPH, FRCPC, CCBOM, MFOM, FACP, FACOEM, FCPM
Professor of Occupational and Enviromental Medicine,
Pulmonary Medicine, and Epidemiology
Director, Division of Occupational Medicine and Toxicology
School of Medicine and Health Sciences
George Washington University Medical Center
Washington, DC
USA

David M. Hansell, MD, FRCP, FRCR
Professor of Thoracic Imaging
Royal Brompton Hospital
London
UK

David J. Hendrick, MSc, MD, FRCP, FFOM
Professor of Occupational Respiratory Medicine
University of Newcastle upon Tyne
Department of Respiratory Medicine
Royal Victoria Infirmary
Newcastle upon Tyne
UK

Douglas W. Henderson, MBBS, FRCPA, FRCPath
Professor of Pathology
Flinders University and
Head of the Department of Anatomical Pathology
Flinders Medical Centre
Adelaide
Australia

Martin Iversen, MD, PhD
Associate Professor of Medicine
Department of Respiratory Diseases
University Hospital of Aarhus
Aarhus
Denmark

Jouni J.K. Jaakkola, MD, DSc, PhD
Professor, Enviromental Health Program
The Nordic School of Public Health
Gothenburg
Sweden;
Head, Environmental Epidemiology Unit
University of Helsinki
Helsinki
Finland;
Adjunct Associate Professor
The Johns Hopkins University
Maryland, PA
USA

Maritta S. Jaakkola, MD, DSc
Consultant, Finnish Institute of Occupational Health
Helsinki
Finland

Y. C. Gary Lee, MBChB, FRACP
United States–New Zealand Fulbright Graduate Research Fellow
Department of Pulmonary Medicine
St. Thomas Hospital/Vanderbilt University
Nashville, TN
USA

Christophe Leroyer, MD, PhD
Professor of Medicine
Départment de Médecine Interne et Pneumologie
Hôpital de la Cavale Blanche
Brest-Cedex
France

James E. Lockey, MD, MS
Professor and Director
Division of Occupational and Environmental Health
Department of Enviromental Health
University of Cincinnati Medical Center
Cincinnati, OH
USA

Douglas W. Mapel, MD, MPH
Medical Director
Lovelace Scientific Resources
Albuquerque, NM
USA

Grant McMillan, QHP, MD, MSc, FRCP, FRCP(Glasg), FFOM, FIOSH
Consultant Adviser in Occupational Medicine and
Deputy to the Medical Director General (Naval)
Office of the Second Sea Lord
Victory Building
HMNB Portsmouth
UK

Sarah Meredith, MBBS, MSc
Senior Clinical Epidemiologist
MRC Clinical Trials Unit
London
UK

Richard E. Moon, MD, FACP, FCCP, FRCPC
Professor of Anesthesiology
Associate Professor of Medicine
Medical Director, Centre for Hyperbaric
Medicine and Environmental Physiology
Duke University Medical Center
Durham, NC
USA;
Medical Director, Divers Alert Network

Gianna Moscato, MD
Head of the Allergy and Immunology Department
Fondazione Salvatore Maugeri
Clinica del Lavoro e della Riabilitazione
IRCCS, Instituto Scientifico di Pavia
Pavia
Italy

A. William Musk, MBBS, MS, MD, FRACP, FCCP, FAFOM, MFOM
Clinical Professor of Medicine and Public Health
University of Western Australia
Pulmonary Department
Sir Charles Gardiner Hospital
Perth
Australia

Benoit Nemery, MD, PhD
Professor of Toxicology and Occupational Medicine
Laboratorium voor Pneumologie (Longtoxicologie)
Katholieke Universiteit Leuven
Leuven
Belgium

Henrik Nordman, MD, PhD
Professor
Finnish Institute for Occupational Health
Helsinki
Finland

Dennis Nowak, MD, PhD
Professor of Occupational Medicine
Ludwig-Maximilians-University
Institute for Occupational and Environmental Medicine
Munich
Germany

Edmund Ong, MBBS, MSc, FRCP, FRCPI, DTMH
Consultant Physician and Senior Lecturer
Department of Infection & Tropical Medicine
University of Newcastle Medical School
Newcastle Upon Tyne
UK

Wai-On Phoon, PhD
Professor in Occupational Health and Executive Chairman
Centre for Occupational and Environmental Health
University of Sydney
Sydney
Australia

Anthony C. Pickering, FRCP, FFOM, DIH
Professor of Occupational Medicine
Northwest Lung Centre
Wythenshawe Hospital
Manchester
UK

Katja Radon, PhD
Research Assistant
Ludwig-Maximilians-University
Institute for Occupational and Environmental Medicine
Munich
Germany

Alastair S. Robertson, MB, ChB, FRCP, FFOM
Consultant Occupational Physician
University Hospital Birmingham NHS Trust
Birmingham
UK

Canzio Romano, MD
Allergy and Respiratory Disease Unit
Department of Occupational Medicine
University of Turin
Turin
Italy

Robin Rudd, MA, MD, FRCP
Consultant Physician
St Bartholomew's Hospital
Barts and the London NHS Trust
London
UK

David A. Schwartz, MD, MPH
Professor of Medicine and Genetics
Director, Division of Pulmonary and Certical Care Medicine
Duke University Medical Center
Durham, NC
USA

Dennis Shusterman, MD, MPH
Associate Clinical Professor of Medicine
University of California, San Francisco
San Fransisco, CA
USA

Malcolm Sim, BMedSc, MBBS, MSc, Grad Dip Occ Hyg, PhD, FAFOM, FFOM, FAFPHM
Associate Professor in Occupational and Environmental Health
Department of Epidemiology and Preventive Medicine
Monash Medical School
Alfred Hospital
Prahran
Australia

Akshay Sood, MD, MPH, FACCP
Assistant Professor of Medicine
Pulmonary and Critical Care Division
Southern Illinois University School of Medicine
Springfield, IL
USA

Judy Sparer, MSCE, CIH
Lecturer in Medicine
Yale Occupational and Environmental Medicine Program
New Haven, CT
USA

Chris Stenton, BSc, FRCP, MFOM
Senior Lecturer in Medicine
Department of Respiratory Medicine
Royal Victoria Infirmary
Newcastle Upon Tyne
UK

Kjell Torén, MD, PhD
Associate Professor
Department of Occupational and Environmental Medicine
Sahlgrenska University Hospital
Gothenburg
Sweden

Mark J. Utell, MD
Professor of Medicine and Environmental Medicine
Director, Pulmonary/Critical Care and
Occupational Medicine Divisions
University of Rochester Medical Center
Rochester, NY
USA

Hans Weill, MD
Emeritus Professor of Medicine
Tulane University
New Orleans, LA
USA

Benoit Wallaert, MD
Clinique des Maladies Respiratoires
Hôpital A. Calmette
Lille
France

Susan R. Woskie, PhD, CIH
Professor
Department of Work Environment
University of Massachusetts Lowell
Lowell, MA
USA

That injurious inhalants, and their associated health effects, continue to be present in some workplaces, is very usefully chronicled in the reports from the UK Surveillance of Work-related & Occupational Respiratory Disease (SWORD). Although the enumerated diseases will at times have been the result of exposures many years ago, or over a period of many years, current exposures continue to result in workplace-related disease of the lungs and airways, particularly asthma and acute inhalation injuries.

As the editors emphasize in Chapter 1, the primary focus of the book is an examination of the changing features of occupational lung disease. While the primary focus on mineral dusts is being replaced by organic dusts and chemicals, unresolved issues remain regarding aspects of the classical pneumoconioses. A repeated theme indicates that much is still to be learned about these conditions. Such new knowledge is generated by research, whether in regard to unanswered questions in long recognized diseases or the discovery of newly documented exposure-related conditions.

Work-related airways effects (mainly asthma and chronic bronchitis) are now more prominent than alveolar/interstitial abnormalities, and while, for example, there are still cases of silicosis, asbestosis and chronic beryllium disease coming to medical attention for the first time, these are relatively few.

Disorders of the airways may be acute, single episodes, as with exposure to high level irritant inhalants, or recurrent, as with occupational asthma. The causal exposures are likely to be airborne sensitizers or irritant gases and chemical vapors. Not resolved is whether workers who develop occupational asthma do so because of the host characterization of underlying bronchial hyper-responsiveness, or whether this is acquired as a result of the exposure. Chronic progressive airways obstruction has resulted from some long term exposures, such as to cotton dust, where excess annual decline in airways function has been shown to occur, particularly in the presence of an across-shift bronchoconstrictor response and smoking.

The chronic conditions caused (or made worse) by workplace exposures now most often have decreased specificity – they are frequently disorders that are difficult to distinguish from the diseases of the lungs and airways seen in the general population. Both latency of clinical manifestations (a clinically silent period after exposure begins) and persistence of symptoms after exposure ceases can make the establishment of a causal nexus with the occupational exposure even more difficult.

Occupational carcinogenesis has assumed an increasingly important role, and often, non-occupational factors play an important part (e.g. cigarette smoking). The role of non-malignant tissue responses (inflammation and fibrosis) in mediating the cancer risk continues to be of substantial interest (e.g. asbestosis and lung cancer).

The contents of this volume reflect the wide range of occupational lung disorders. Improving diagnostic tools and methods for exposure characterization have provided important information regarding the changes in the distribution and character of the diseases, and in the workplace environment.

Much of what we know about occupational lung disease has come from epidemiologic studies of exposed workers, both current and past. These studies are best accomplished by interdisciplinary research units, with the results used by regulators in setting appropriate science-based exposure standards that will help to prevent or minimize these conditions. Since the mid-1960s, investigators and those who need to interpret the results of population studies have had the benefit of Sir Austin Bradford-Hill's criteria for determining a causal relationship between exposure and disease. Perhaps the most important of these criteria is the demonstration of dose dependency of the risk. It is the dose-response relationships which are most useful to those responsible for the setting of exposure standards. Although these studies are difficult to carry out – often because of limited resources and suboptimal cooperation from managers and workers – increasingly, research quality data can be collected as part of worker medical and exposure monitoring in suspect environments.

Along with the editors, I have concluded that there is a legitimate need for this book, as a result both of continuing cases of occupational lung diseases of the "past", and the appearance of new agents causing well-known respiratory illnesses, often with new exposure/disease relationships. For instance, a list of causes of occupational asthma compiled today would certainly not be up-to-date in a year or two. Also, there will undoubtedly continue to be new evidence presented of previously unrecognized lung carcinogens.

Finally, the editors and contributors constitute an impressive group of lung physicians and scientists who collectively have had a very broad range of clinical experience and research accomplishment in the field. This book will be an important part of the library of chest and occupational physicians.

Hans Weill

INTRODUCTION

1 | WHY THIS BOOK? HOW TO USE IT

David J. Hendrick, P. Sherwood Burge, William S. Beckett, and Andrew Churg

Contents

BACKGROUND

Diseases have causes and consequences. The precise etiology of lung diseases is better studied than in many branches of medicine, partly because the response of the lungs to external agents can be monitored (with imaging and lung function tests) with more precision than in many branches of medicine, and partly because most lung diseases arise from substances that are inhaled. These substances can be measured in the air we breathe, and causal dose–response relationships can be established as a result. There are huge variations in the incidence of lung diseases around the world, for instance asthma is more than 40 times as common in some countries than others, and has increased by more than 200% in the lifetime of most readers. Similar variations occur for lung cancer, chronic obstructive pulmonary disease (COPD), tuberculosis, and pneumonia. All of these diseases can be caused by exposures at work.

The contribution of the workplace environment to diseases of the lung consequently appears to be changing, particularly in industrially developed countries, and the editors believe the spectrum of occupational lung disease is changing also. Thus, disabling pneumoconiosis (the archetypal lung disease of occupational origin) and associated tuberculosis, will occur very rarely indeed in those who join the workforce today in Australasia, North America, and western Europe thanks to the identification of its various causes and the introduction of effective means of control. By contrast, in areas of the world such as China, South America, the Indian subcontinent, and some parts of southern Africa, where there is a rapid pace of industrialization and infrastructure development (the construction of roads, railways, tunnels, and mines), disabling pneumoconiosis may continue to be seen alongside the newer lung disorders of occupational origin like hard-metal alloy disease and nylon flock workers' disease.

The declining importance of the traditional causes of occupational lung disease does not mean that the workplace is no longer a focus of concern – its contribution to the burden of lung disease in general has merely become more subtle. Most of the common disabling diseases of the respiratory tract such as COPD, chronic bronchitis (chronic productive cough), asthma, and lung cancer appear to be consequences of both 'the environment' and susceptibility of the affected individual. This might be considered true for respiratory infections also, and it may prove to be true for many of the less common diseases which cause interstitial fibrosis or alveolar disruption. For most individuals some 25–30% of exposure to 'the environment' occurs at work, and for many the occupational environment is contaminated to some degree by respirable agents which are not generally met within the domestic, recreational, or outdoor environments. Although these agents may not induce diseases which are uniquely occupational, they may be contributory causes (like non-occupational agents) of the many respiratory disorders which now occur commonly in the population at large. Thus exposure to mineral or metal dusts appears to be a risk factor for the later development of 'idiopathic' pulmonary fibrosis.

A major emerging difficulty is consequently distinguishing in the affected individual, lung disease of occupational origin from that of non-occupational origin, and evaluating the relative importance of each in the population at large using epidemiologically-derived estimates of risk. Epidemiological investigation of chronic disease in the workplace is, however, notoriously difficult, as those with disabling disease generally stop working, leaving for study subjects who are relative resistant to the adverse effects of the occupational exposure (survival bias). Investigation sometimes shows that those with the highest cumulative exposures have the best lung function, either because they were selected for their above average health (the 'healthy worker effect'), or because their lack of susceptibility allowed them to keep working longer. Thus subjects entering the dustiest and most hazardous jobs may have better lung function at employment onset than those entering less risky employment. This poses major difficulty for the choice of suitable control subjects.

The difficulties are compounded by the probability that in many individual cases both occupational and non-occupational agents contribute to disease severity, and so there are formidable problems in quantifying their separate contributions. At present there is no clear indication whether in general separate environmental exposures exert their effects multiplicatively (interactively) or simply additively, and this question may come to be answered differently in different situations.

What then is the respiratory physician, occupational physician, or other health professional to do when confronted with common respiratory disorders if his/her patient works (or has worked) in occupational environments in which there are respirable dusts, fumes, vapors, or gases? Are these exposures likely to be relevant, and if so what should he or she do next? How is true occupational disease to be recognized and how is it to be managed? Would the patient really benefit from a job change or, often more important and more relevant, a job loss? The potential responsibilities of the consulted physician do not end there. When should he/she communicate with the patient's employer, and when is there a need to report to regulatory authorities? Finally, what level of concern should be generated by industrial managers and their safety officials, and by regulatory authorities; what practically can be done to prevent the problem in the future?

Change additionally brings opportunity and we, the editors, anticipate that current research in the basic mechanisms of occupational lung disease (particularly interstitial fibrosis and asthma) is likely to lead to effective therapeutic agents over the next few years. This will provide the stimulus to make specific and secure diagnoses, and to identify more precisely the exposure agents of relevance.

We have wrestled with these issues in our response to the publisher's invitation to produce this book. There are several excellent textbooks of occupational lung disease already, and we took the view that we could not add sufficiently to current encyclopedic knowledge about disease characterization, pathogenic mechanisms, epidemiological and economic importance, or historical background to justify a further text. Nor could we contribute usefully to describing in detail the nature, investigation, or management of those respiratory diseases which occur commonly in the population at large anyway. This is the province of textbooks of respiratory medicine. We concluded, however, that with some innovation there is merit in drawing attention to the changing nature of the contribution the occupational environment makes to lung disease, and to the particular difficulties this poses for those who find themselves responsible for patient care or the management of relevant industries.

We consequently offered the authors of the chapters concerned with specific clinical disorders (Chapters 4–23) a difficult task, namely to follow the philosophy that has been outlined, use a standardized text format, and to focus their chapters on the practical 'nuts and bolts' of the following:

- Recognizing when a given respiratory disorder is occupational in origin, whether partly or wholly.
- Managing its consequences in both the affected individual and his/her place of work.
- Preventing its occurrence in the future.

In the hope of producing practical guidance for the reader that is readily identified, we have structured the book using a number of sections, separating in particular chapters that are centered on specific disorders (whatever their causal agents or causal occupational environments) from complementary chapters that are centered on specific industries (irrespective of the nature of the associated exposures and disorders). Some overlap of text between different chapters is therefore inevitable, and some topics are necessarily duplicated, at least partially, by different authors (e.g. the chapters on pneumoconiosis include reference to mining, and that on mining refers partly to pneumoconiosis; the chapters on chemical injury to airways and parenchyma both show that toxicity at one site is often associated with relevant toxicity at the other; and several chapters describe the International Labour Office classification of chest radiographs and the classification of asbestos fibers).

We consider this helpful, since most users will dip into the book reading only a single chapter (or sections from it) on a particular occasion. The most relevant information is thus conveniently available even if duplicated elsewhere. Also inevitable is some variability in the use of certain terms (for example pneumoconiosis itself), since different customs exist between and within different countries, and there is not always a uniformly agreed standard definition. Whenever practical, such terms are defined so that the authors' use of them is clear.

For each individual chapter a brief contents list introduces the nature of the material that is covered, and, whenever appropriate, Summary Points provide the salient conclusions. In addition, for some chapters, boxes have been used to insert text on a special topic within the chapter that has been written by a separate (and identified) author(s). The English language is used in different countries with recognized variations. No one variation can be considered correct or incorrect, but we chose 'American' English to be the book style.

INTRODUCTORY CHAPTERS

In the first section (Chapters 1–3), the book's outline and purpose are described, perspective is provided from surveillance data of both clinical and epidemiologic aspects, and guidance is offered (with illustrative case examples) for obtaining critical exposure information from the occupational history.

DISORDERS OF THE AIRWAYS, PARENCHYMA, AND PLEURA

The respiratory disorders of occupational origin provide the focus for the second and main section of the book (Chapters 4–23). The starting point is the disorder itself, rather than any causal agent or industrial environment, and a rough anatomic/pathologic sequence is followed from disorders of the airways, through those of the lung parenchyma, to those of the pleura. A standard format is used so that the book's principal aims are met and readily identified:

- **BACKGROUND**
  Causes
  Epidemiology
  Prognosis
- **RECOGNITION**
  Clinical features
  Investigation
  Differential diagnosis
- **MANAGEMENT**
  Of the individual
  Of the workforce

- **PREVENTION**
  In the workplace
  National regulatory
  strategies
- **DIFFICULT CASE**
  History
  Issues
  Comment
- **SUMMARY POINTS**
  Recognition
  Management
  Prevention

We hope this standardized format will allow the reader to find readily the answers to specific and obvious questions. This assumes that answers are available and can be given, but this is not always the case, and authors were asked to identify issues associated with uncertainty or controversy. They were additionally asked to illustrate their chapters with a 'notable example of effective management or prevention' if a particularly notable experience of relevance has been recorded.

PARTICULAR INDUSTRIES

Some occupational settings are, of course, associated with more than one type of respiratory disorder, just as a particular disorder may arise in more than one occupational setting. This provides an alternative strategy for structuring a text on occupational lung disorders, and the editors recognize that for some readers on at least some occasions, the principal concern may be industry-oriented rather than disease-oriented. With Chapters 24–30 we have consequently included a section which reviews the spectrum of disorders that may be encountered in certain industries. Authors of these relatively shorter chapters were asked to avoid unnecessary repetition of information given by other contributors in the chapters focused on the disorders themselves, but to bring into perspective the special problems of recognizing and managing occupational lung disease in these particular settings.

DIFFICULT CASES

The editors also recognize the possible magnitude of the diagnostic and management difficulties in individual cases. While it is essential that textbooks provide a clear outline of the typical features of given disorders, in clinical practice atypical cases are common and textbooks may fail through limitations of volume to cover adequately all diagnostic and management permutations. Our response to this dilemma has been to commission within each clinical chapter (Chapters 4–30) the description of an illustrative difficult, but genuine, case which our contributors have come across in everyday practice. In some chapters two such cases have been included because they illustrate different but important points.

During the drafting stage of the book, we were able to distribute most of the Difficult Case material among all the contributors (and editors), together with specific questions addressing obvious diagnostic or management issues. An editorial analysis of the responses was then used as the starting point for the chapter's author to provide a concluding comment. Readers may consequently judge how 'experts' assessed these difficult but not uncommon clinical problems, and how close (or otherwise) a consensus was achieved.

SPECIALIZED DISCIPLINES

Four chapters (31–34) are devoted to the specialized disciplines of imaging (radiology), lung function measurement, occupational hygiene, and mineralogic analysis of lung tissue, thereby providing overviews for the roles these critical disciplines play in the recognition, management, or prevention of occupational lung disease. Many chapters make independent references to one or another of these disciplines, and some differences of opinion may be detected between the respective authors. This too is an inevitable (though 'healthy') occurrence for a multiauthored book.

LEGISLATIVE CONTROLS AND COMPENSATION

Legislative controls over occupational processes and associated exposures vary inevitably from country to country and depend greatly on government structure, practicability, and level of economic development. So too do procedures for compensation, a further unavoidable subject when a textbook addresses disorders of occupational origin. In this initial edition through Chapters 35–37, the editors have commissioned contributions to summarize the processes and procedures in three major global regions – North America; the Pacific, Far East, and Australasia; and Western Europe. Although necessarily limited in scope, particularly for the regions involving large variations in economic development and large numbers of countries (Asia and western Europe), the chapters provide a broad overview and useful parochial data.

SOURCES OF INFORMATION AND INVESTIGATION CENTERS

Chapters 38–40 are similarly based on the composite regions of North America; the Pacific, Far East, and Australasia; and Western Europe. Their purpose is to provide sources of information during a period of rapid and unceasing change. This section of the book attempts additionally to identify centers for special diagnostic tests that are not widely available. Although a textbook cannot hope to be fully up to date, the identified centers are likely to be able to provide advice for the most expedient currently available source. The editors would welcome further information for subsequent editions.

ABBREVIATIONS

We have encouraged the use of abbreviations, though recognize that some are in less common use than others. Since an unfamiliar abbreviation can be irksome, we have limited the overall use of abbreviations and have listed those that have been adopted at the end of the book in the hope that they can be 'translated' with a minimum of inconvenience.

2 SURVEILLANCE: CLINICAL AND EPIDEMIOLOGICAL PERSPECTIVES

Sarah Meredith and Paul D. Blanc

Contents

INTRODUCTION

Disease surveillance involves 'the continued watchfulness over the distribution and trends of incidence through the systematic collection, consolidation, and evaluation of morbidity and mortality reports and other relevant data' [1]. Modern concepts of surveillance stem from the work of William Farr of the Statistical Department of the General Register Office for England and Wales for much of the 19th century [2]. Through weekly, quarterly, annual, decennial, and special reports he drew attention to public health issues, such as mortality associated with unhygienic living conditions and excess deaths during influenza epidemics. Because of the public health importance of tuberculosis, lung disease has long been a focus of surveillance. In the 20th century, surveillance methods that were originally developed for the detection and control of infectious diseases were extended to non-communicable diseases, particularly those such as occupational respiratory diseases that are caused by hazards in the workplace or environment.

Disease surveillance is more than routine data collection; it is 'information for action' [3] and the methods used are characterized by practicality and rapidity rather than complete accuracy [4]. Although no country has a complete and comprehensive system of surveillance for occupational respiratory diseases, there are a number of data sources that provide insights of variable quality into the frequency and causes of many of the disorders. Analysis of surveillance data cannot be expected to provide all the answers to the epidemiology of occupational lung disorders, but in conjunction with industrial hygiene and toxicology, and the results of epidemiological investigations, both in the workplace and in the community, it can provide valuable information to help guide those concerned with the prevention and control of work-related diseases.

Surveillance data can also be of use to clinicians, providing them with information on the distribution and determinants of occupational diseases within the population that they serve. The quality of those data is, in turn, often dependent on clinicians for completeness and accuracy. It is therefore important that clinicians be aware of local surveillance systems so that they can make use of all available information when advising their patients and, at the same time, ensure that appropriate cases come to the attention of the relevent body.

This chapter is divided into two sections. In Section I, the main sources of information of relevance to the surveillance of occupational lung disorders are reviewed. In Section II, some of the insights into the distribution and determinants of selected occupational lung disorders derived from surveillance data are described.

SECTION I: SOURCES OF SURVEILLANCE INFORMATION

Overview

Surveillance information relevant to occupational lung disease can be derived from multiple sources. Each source type has specific advantages and its own particular limitations. The goal of the following section is not to catalog every potential source of surveillance data for work-related respiratory conditions, but rather to characterize such sources within several broad groupings based on shared attributes. In general, approaches to the surveillance of work-related respiratory conditions can be classified into three categories: (i) surveillance data that have been intentionally collected *as such* in order to monitor occupational lung diseases; (ii) occupational data not collected as part of a surveillance program *per se*, but which can be used for this purpose; and (iii) general health data from which information on respiratory conditions and occupation can be extracted.

Occupational lung disease data

Reporting schemes

Since the late 1980s, starting in the USA and in the UK, there have been attempts to adapt many of the features of communicable disease surveillance to occupational illness. In the USA this has taken the form of the Sentinel Event Notification System for Occupational Risks (SENSOR). SENSOR involves cooperation between state and federal authorities under the auspices of the National Institute for Occupational Safety and Health (NIOSH). A network of sentinel providers, using specific and detailed diagnostic criteria, report cases to a center where they are analyzed and from which investigation and intervention activities are coordinated [5]. The coordinating center is usually located in the state health department. The reporting of cases is closely linked to their further investigation, including surveys of the index patient's coworkers and environmental assessment of the workplace. Two occupational respiratory diseases have been the focus of SENSOR surveillance: silicosis and occupational asthma.

In the UK, there has been a less uniform and more rapid development of a number of different schemes over the past few years, based on voluntary and confidential reporting by clinicians. This development was first proposed by McDonald and Harrington in 1981 [6], who suggested that to be successful, such a network would require a coordinating center

which was respected for its independence, and reporters should be assured of confidentiality. For those reasons it was recommended that the coordination of such a network be independent of any governmental regulatory agency. The first of these voluntary reporting schemes to be developed on a national basis was SWORD, the Surveillance of Work-related and Occupational Respiratory Disease project [7]. Since 1989, occupational and respiratory physicians throughout the UK have been asked to report any newly diagnosed case of respiratory illness that they attribute to exposure at work. Although funded by the Health and Safety Executive, a government agency, SWORD has been based in academic departments of occupational medicine, and the identities of participants and any cases that they report are treated as confidential.

The SWORD model has also been used in other countries. In Canada, voluntary reporting of occupational respiratory disease by chest physicians was piloted for 1 year each in the provinces of British Columbia [8] and Quebec [9]. The Surveillance of work-related and Occupational Respiratory Diseases in South Africa (SORDSA), is an ambitious project that was begun in 1996, funded in part by the World Health Organization [10]. Like SWORD, occupational and respiratory specialists throughout the country are invited to participate by submitting monthly reports of new cases of occupational lung disease that they diagnose. Unlike SWORD, occupational health nurses participate in addition.

There are also voluntary reporting schemes for occupational asthma only. The first of these was 'Shield', based in the West Midlands region of England which, like SWORD, began in 1989 [11]. Shield differs from SWORD in that it includes reports from the local Medical Boarding Centre where claimants for compensation are assessed. Thus Shield is able to gauge the overlap with the compensation statistics while, through local contacts, it is also in a position to investigate clusters of cases. Groups in France [12] and the Piedmont area of Italy [13] have also recently implemented schemes for the voluntary reporting of occupational asthma.

The statistical value of reporting schemes depends on the level of physician participation, completeness of reporting, and accuracy of diagnosis. However, in epidemiological terms, surveillance is a descriptive hypothesis-generating activity, information from which may need to be tested. The reasonable assumption is that participating clinicians act responsibly and competently; to ask for proof of either diagnosis or attribution would negate the primary purpose of these schemes and probably bring them to a rapid end. Therefore, surveillance schemes need to include provision for selective quality control and further investigation to clarify causal relationships. Even so, there may be difficulties of interpretation, in particular in relation to completeness, validity, and bias.

Underreporting is inevitable as only a fraction of work-related disease will be seen by participating physicians. Patients may not seek medical attention, and, even if they do, they may not be seen by a specialist. Moreover, even if all patients were seen by specialists, underreporting would still occur, due to doctors forgetting to report, and because not all relevant clinicians participate. Provided that underreporting is evenly distributed across diagnostic, occupational, gender, and age groups, the relative risks in the various groups of interest would be accurate and informative, although disease frequency would be underestimated overall. However, underreporting is unlikely to be evenly distributed: some groups seek medical attention more than others, some physicians may be more likely to recognize occupational disease than others, and for some diagnoses it may be impossible to attribute disease in an individual to a particular cause.

While cases reported by specialists are likely to have been diagnosed fairly accurately, there remain difficulties of incomplete recognition. With information on exposure based on history, and more than one possible cause for a disease, it may be difficult to make a causal attribution in an individual case. Thus for lung cancer many occupational causes are well established, but because the vast majority of cases occur in smokers, the synergistic or additive contribution of occupational exposures may be overlooked. As a result, occupational lung cancer tends to be seriously underascertained in all reporting schemes, whereas mesothelioma is nearly always attributed to asbestos, however remote the exposure history. Diagnosis and reporting may be sensitive to changes in fashion and to reports in the medical literature. For example, between 1989 and 1991 there were only three cases of asthma attributed to latex reported to SWORD, but over the next 6 years, as the relationship became more widely known, the estimated number of cases rose to 100 [13a].

Voluntary reporting schemes require continual stimulation of participants to maintain their interest and thus their active participation. In return for reporting, SWORD participants receive information in the form of monthly and quarterly digests and become part of an informal network through which they can make specific enquiries about reported cases and make contact with other clinicians with similar interests. Even with such incentives, loss of interest leading to decline in numbers of reports is inevitable. Therefore modifications and strategies to maintain interest are required; unfortunately, these may make time trends difficult to interpret.

Despite these difficulties, the schemes summarized above have demonstrated the feasibility and potential for surveillance based on clinical reports, and have provided a better picture than was previously available of the scope and burden of occupational illness. While voluntary reporting schemes undoubtedly underestimate disease frequency, the relative importance of different diseases and exposures are made clearer. However, results must be interpreted with caution, and with due consideration for the potential inaccuracies.

Occupational lung disease registries

Registries for occupational lung diseases may be comprehensive or disease-specific. The oldest and most comprehensive occupational disease registry is in Finland. Since 1964, the Finnish Registry of Occupational Diseases (FROD) has been maintained by the Institute of Occupational Health in Helsinki [14]. Registered cases come from three sources: (i) reports from provincial medical officers to whom physicians have been required by law since 1974 to report all cases of occupational disease they diagnose; (ii) claims made of insurance companies; (iii) cases diagnosed at the Institute of Occupational Health.

All employees must be covered by insurance and compensation for a confirmed occupational disease is relatively comprehensive; it includes cost of treatment and retraining as well as a pension [15]. There are, therefore, fewer disincentives for people whose health has been adversely affected by their job to come forward than in many other countries. In the Finnish system the diagnosis and causal link is usually well established. For example, most cases of occupational asthma are confirmed by inhalation challenge tests or serial respiratory function tests at and away from work.

Insurance for self-employed people is voluntary, however, and only a minority are covered. The self-employed are therefore probably underrepresented in the Finnish disease register. The main exception is self-employed farmers, who have been eligible for compensation since a change in the law in 1982. This had a substantial impact on both the number and type of case registered, especially for occupational asthma [16].

Disease-specific registries represent a highly focused example of surveillance, in which an attempt is made to identify all incident cases of a specified condition. The best example of this type of focused surveillance within the occupational arena is the US national beryllium lung disease registry that has been maintained for many years [17]. One advantage of the disease registry approach is that is allows for standardized collection of clinical data, including review of pathologic specimens. Disease registry data can supply important information on the natural history of disease (including survival patterns) and emerging sources of exposure. Although the beryllium disease registry was focused on a single, predominantly occupational disease, other registries include important subsets of work-related illness. The most relevant of these are cancer registries, which provide a major source of information on incident cases of mesothelioma, the bulk of which are likely to be due to past occupational asbestos exposure [18]. Cancer registry data have also been used as a surveillance tool in the estimation of work-related lung cancer incidence, although this often requires supplemental occupational data collection. Similar to the model of the cancer registry, a regional registry of interstitial lung disease was recently initiated in the state of New Mexico, which may also yield work-related surveillance data [19].

In the early 1970s, the American Medical Association initiated a 'Registry on Adverse reactions Due to Occupational Exposures' which was intended to be a general reporting scheme for illnesses rather than limited to specific diseases or discrete groups of conditions. This program was not continued, but in its initial report of 459 cases (based on 17 801 contact forms mailed out to potential physician reporters), 24% of the cases were respiratory in nature [20]. More recently, an international registry for acute toxic inhalation injuries has been proposed, although no data from this project have yet been reported [21].

Immunologic surveillance

Targeted occupational respiratory surveillance need not be limited to clinical case detection and reporting. Returning to the example of beryllium workers, occupational surveillance can be based on evidence of sensitization within a specified labor force using the lymphocyte transformation assay [22]. A more familiar example of surveillance for preclinical disease would be routine tuberculin testing of healthcare workers [23]. In addition to directing individual case follow-up, such surveillance schemes yield data that allow incidence estimation, risk assessment, and outbreak investigations. Another approach relevant to infectious occupational lung disease is serologic surveillance, for example for Q-fever among sheep-exposed animal handlers or laboratory workers [24]. Allergic diseases may also be amenable to immunologic surveillance, for example specific IgE or skin reactivity to amylase among bakers or to natural latex among healthcare workers [25,26].

Spirometric and radiographic surveillance

In many countries, occupational health standards for a variety of dusty trades call for periodic health examinations including spirometry and chest radiographs [27]. Frequently, these data are collected but never analyzed on a cohort or population basis for surveillance purposes. One exception to this has been among coal workers. In both the United States and in the United Kingdom, surveillance lung function and radiographic data have been analyzed to study trends over time in the incidence and prevalence of work-related lung disease [28–30]. To a lesser extent, similar surveillance analyses have been carried out among other underground miners and cotton textile workers based on periodic health-screening data. Many selected occupational cohorts have been assessed spirometrically, but this is typically performed in the context of a single, cross-sectional study rather than ongoing surveillance.

Mandatory systems

In direct contrast to disease-specific registers, general occupational disease surveillance programs include respiratory conditions as only one group among a wide range of illnesses and injuries. These surveillance programs represent an attempt to monitor occupational diseases overall and do not focus on occupational lung diseases specifically. One of the most intensively exploited of these programs in the USA has been the California 'Doctor's First Report' (DFR) system [31]. This surveillance system is based on legally mandated physician reporting for all occupational illnesses and injuries. Cases are required to be reported when first seen for treatment, but not on subsequent visits. The system is linked to insurance payment when such coverage is sought through the workers' compensation scheme. Only a fraction of the cases reported are illnesses as opposed to injuries, and respiratory conditions represent a minority of the illnesses.

The advantages of a mandatory reporting physician-based surveillance program such as the DFR derives from its inherent cross-industry, cross-occupation base. Incidence rates by occupation and industry (using statewide employment data) can be estimated. Rates for respiratory disease can be compared with other disease groups (for example, skin conditions). A clear disadvantage of insurance-driven physician reporting is that there are multiple incentives for underreporting, especially when reporting may lead to increases in insurance premiums. Self-employed workers and federal employees represent important exclusions from the DFR. Beyond these limitations, the most important disadvantage of mandatory physician reporting is that of fragmentary occupational exposure data. One approach to such limitations can be the use of initial surveillance reports as a source of index case identification, supplemented by detailed follow-up information ascertained systematically through the administration of structured questionnaires. This has been used with the California DFR system to confirm cases of occupational asthma under the guidelines of the NIOSH SENSOR program described earlier [32].

A number of other broad-based occupational illness and injury surveillance programs include occupational lung diseases within their scope. In addition to California, several other states in the USA have mandated the reporting by physicians of certain conditions that include occupational diseases [33]. Michigan has been a leader in state-based, active surveillance for occupational lung disease in the USA [34]. Most states that do require reporting take a limited approach, designating specific reportable diseases rather than generalizing that any disease considered work-related should be reported. The specific diseases listed typically include the pneumoconioses, for example, but often do not specify work-related asthma as an occupational disease mandated for reporting.

In the United States, the Department of Labor Statistics analyzes data from Occupational Safety and Health Administration-required workplace logs of illness and injury (OSHA 200 logs). This active surveillance system is designed to track temporal incidence trends and compare rates among groups on a national basis. Theoretically, these logs include respiratory illness, but for practical purposes, chronic occupational lung disease is unlikely to be recognized and entered into logs, which are geared largely to acute traumatic injury and, even in this area, are prone to underreporting [35].

In the UK, RIDDOR (the Reporting of Injuries, Diseases, and Dangerous Occurrences Regulations) was introduced in 1985 to supplement the disablement statistics and to improve surveillance of a range of occupational disorders. Under RIDDOR, an employer who has been informed by a doctor in writing that an employee has one of a number of specified conditions is supposed to report details to the Health and Safety Executive [36]. Follow-up by the authorities has resulted in investigation and improved control of hazards in some workplaces [37]. As a means of occupational disease surveillance, however, it has not proven successful, because very few cases are reported. Between 1986 and 1992, for example, an average of 62 cases per year of occupational asthma were reported under RIDDOR, compared to 200–300 state benefit awards each year for occupational asthma disablement [38].

Other occupational data

Workers' compensation

Although they are not designed for this purpose, other databases that include occupational disorders

can be exploited for surveillance purposes. Workers' compensation insurance data comprise the most straightforward example of this. The data are typically collected for the purposes of processing claims and making (or denying) awards. The purpose is not primarily to estimate incidence (although this is done for actuarial purposes in rate setting, by using the data to predict the likelihood of injury so that insurance premiums reflect risk) nor to track changing patterns of disease. None the less, workers' compensation data can provide a wealth of information on occupational lung diseases that can be used for surveillance purposes [39]. This can include diagnostic mix, industry and occupation-specific data, and demographics. Importantly, insurance claims data typically include information on healthcare charges which can be used to assess the economic impact of diseases as a surveillance measure. In many countries, workers' compensation statistics are the principal source of surveillance information. Their main advantages are that they are readily available and are based on confirmed cases of occupational disease, often using standardized diagnostic criteria. Thus they provide reliable *minimum* estimates for the numbers of people affected by occupational diseases.

The potential shortcomings of insurance compensation data are severalfold. First, when data are limited to 'accepted' claims, emerging illnesses may not appear until there is widespread acknowledgement of work-related causality. Second, diseases with long latency, such as work-related lung cancer, are more likely to go uncompensated (and may even be precluded under certain systems, although this is less common that it was in the past). Third, workers' compensation systems with highly restrictive criteria will tend to magnify the effect of both of the limitations noted above. This is especially so when pre-designated 'lists' of illness or exposures are eligible for compensation (a common practice in countries other than the USA). Fourth, there may be difficulty in interpreting trends over time if the recognized lists of diseases, exposures, or occupations change. This is a problem for UK statistics where, for example, the list of agents recognized as causes of occupational asthma has been changed three times. With each change, the numbers of awards increased [38]. Chronic bronchitis and emphysema were made prescribed diseases for coal miners for the first time in 1993, resulting in the approval of more than 4000 new claims the following year [38].

In addition, the relative value of awards and a variety of social and financial incentives and disincentives may influence whether or not claims are made. The introduction in 1986 of the '14 per cent rule' in the UK whereby for most diseases compensation was only provided if the extent of disability was assessed at 14% or more, not only reduced the number of awards, but also the number of claimants [38]. These problems are compounded by limitations due to workers' compensation employee exclusions (the self-employed) or underrepresentation (migrant workers). In the USA, public employees are often covered by separate systems [40]; this is less of an issue in countries with single national workers' compensation schemes.

Where the workers' compensation system is static, however, analyses of claims data *over time* for recognized conditions within consistently insurance-covered occupational groups should be comparable. For example, in assessing the relative trends in compensated asthma among bakers over a ten-year period, the absolute incidence may be underestimated, but the relative error should be consistent. Indeed, work-related asthma has been a particular focus of workers' compensation insurance claim-based surveillance in the USA, Canada, and Europe [41–43].

Exposure databases

Just as insurance claims for work-related illness can be exploited for surveillance purposes, so too may exposure data be analyzed with the goal of surveillance. By and large, such data sources have been relatively underutilized, even though they can be particularly relevant to occupational lung disease. One exception has been the analysis of pooled industrial hygiene data collected by United States OSHA, including the systematic assessment of measured silica exposure levels relative to permissible exposure limits [44–46].

Other examples of exposure-based surveillance in the USA have been the National Occupational Hazard Survey and the National Occupational Exposure Survey conducted by NIOSH in the 1970s and 1980s, respectively [47]. These surveys used walk-through inspections without industrial hygiene exposure measurements, and made qualitative assessments of the dustiness of working environments relevant to lung disease.

General health data

Mortality

There is a long tradition of using health statistics to draw surveillance inferences related to occupational diseases in general, and work-related lung diseases in particular. When population-based mortality statistics based on death records first began to be collected and analyzed in Great Britain, ecological inferences were made regarding respiratory conditions among the laboring classes [48,49]. Some of these analyses were quite detailed at the occupa-

tional level. Later, in the United States, private insurance company mortality experience was used for similar analyses of job-specific death rates, especially for tuberculosis [50].

The introduction of the International Classification of Diseases (ICD) provided a standard classification scheme for disease coding which facilitated such analyses by allowing for identification of conditions that are occupational by definition, such as asbestosis or silicosis. In addition, ICD-9 provides for supplemental coding of external causes of injury, which can further serve to link an occupational etiology to disease codes.

In the United States and elsewhere, death certificates (as opposed to insurance records) are notoriously unreliable in terms of occupational information [51–54]. One approach used to address this has been to supplement death certificate data with occupational information from other sources, for example, gathered by interviewing surviving family members or extracting information from city residence directories. Outside the United States, linkage of death statistics to social insurance databases containing occupational information is far less restricted, facilitating surveillance applications of mortality data. For example, Canadian investigators were able to link persons who received workers' compensation for occupational asthma in Ontario to death records, thus estimating mortality rates among those with work-related asthma [55]. The Scandinavian countries have the greatest experience linking occupation (through census surveys) to death records, with a particular emphasis on work associations with cancer mortality, including lung cancer [56].

Once occupation has been ascertained, the application of mortality data to surveillance purposes can be based on traditional epidemiological estimates of excess deaths compared to expected proportions or frequencies. An alternative approach to outcomes-based surveillance has evolved, known as 'sentinel health event' monitoring [57]. In this approach, certain disease-occupation dyads are presumed to be work-related until proven otherwise. For example, lung cancers among topside coke oven workers, smelters, uranium miners, asbestos workers, and chemists have been proposed as work-related sentinel health events [58].

One important use of mortality data for occupational disease surveillance that does not require person-specific occupational information is 'mapping' of disease-specific death rates, to make regional comparisons of incidence ratios. This kind of mapping allows broad ecological inferences to be made, for example, high rates of mesothelioma deaths in shipbuilding coastal areas or higher than expected death rates from obstructive lung disease in mining regions. Both the US National Cancer Institute and the National Institute for Occupational Safety and Health have published 'atlases' based on such mortality analyses [59,60].

Morbidity (including hospital discharges)

The approach applied to death certificates can also be used for morbidity data. For example, hospital discharge data can be exploited to estimate rates of work-related illnesses. For respiratory conditions, this approach has been used to estimate population-based rates for the pneumoconioses, extrinsic alveolitis (hypersensitivity pneumonitis), and respiratory illness from chemical inhalation (including chemical bronchitis and pulmonary edema) [61–64]. This approach may be fairly reliable for some of these conditions, such as coal workers' pneumoconiosis, but be a less effective strategy for others, such as extrinsic alveolitis [65,66]. Hospital discharge data can also be exploited using the sentinel health event approach, although this requires information on occupation, which is often lacking in hospital records [67]. At least one study has investigated possible work-related lung cancer in hospital discharge data using this approach [68].

Linkage approaches can also be used to exploit outpatient claims for the purposes of occupational lung disease surveillance. In Manitoba, this was done by linking occupational data from Census Canada to medical encounters for treatment of asthma and obstructive lung disease [69]. US data restrictions on divulging personal identifiers by and large preclude such approaches, although within 'proprietary' data sets this may become more possible. Using this approach, a joint union–management study in the auto industry was able to link occupational data with sick leave claims for acute respiratory illness, but such examples are uncommon [70].

Poison control

Poison control centers provide consulting services for the treatment of poisoning and drug overdose. Their main focus is the ingestion of drugs or other toxins, largely intentional among adults and inadvertent among children. None the less, an important subgroup of exposures are occupational and, among those, inhalations form the largest group. Poison center records provide an important source of information on such cases.

In the USA, there is direct public access to poison control centers, although healthcare providers also utilize the services. Internationally, many poison control centers are only accessible by healthcare professionals, although this varies. Whether or not there is public access, poison control center advice is not dependent on workers' compensation or other insurance eligibility criteria, which makes these data particularly useful for surveillance. Standardized databases are becoming widely used for poison control in which occupational cases are identified and the nature and route of the exposure are specified.

Approximately 4–5% of all adult poison control center consultations are for occupational exposures [71–78]. Inhalation exposures are far more frequently reported among occupational cases compared to other poison center cases, for which ingestion is the predominant exposure route. Because exposure by inhalation dominates occupational cases reported to poison control centers, useful surveillance inferences, for example on pesticide poisoning, can be made without subdividing the data by route of exposure [79,80]. Poison control center data are particularly important in the surveillance of certain inhalants, such as carbon monoxide and cyanide. In addition, novel toxin-related respiratory syndromes are likely to be reported to poison control centers as 'sentinel health events'. Poison control center cases can also be used for follow-up studies, for example, investigation of irritant inhalations and their sequelae [81,82].

Health surveys

Surveys of both general health and respiratory health present important opportunities for surveillance. General health surveys conducted using population-based sampling provide prevalence estimates for respiratory conditions, and may include data on occupation and industry. At times more detailed information is assessed, such as in the 1988 Occupational Supplement to the US Health Interview Survey which included specific questions on physician diagnosed work-related asthma among a list of conditions [83]. Another example is the US Social Security Disability Survey, which solicited subject reports of work relatedness for health conditions, including respiratory disease [84]. In the UK, the 1990 and 1995 Labour Force Surveys included questions on work-related illness in the preceding 12 months, from which prevalence estimates have been derived [85,86]. Surveys which are repeated periodically allow for surveillance of prevalence over time; those that follow the same subjects longitudinally also provide incidence estimates.

In addition to general health surveys, there have been a number of population-based respiratory health studies that can also be exploited for surveillance purposes. Longitudinal studies, including the Tucson and Six Cities studies, have provided important information on occupational risk factors for lung disease which can be used to estimate the prevalence of such conditions [87,88]. More recently, the European Community Respiratory Health Survey has provided information on the prevalence of work-related respiratory symptoms in several different countries [89].

SECTION II: DISEASE-SPECIFIC SURVEILLANCE ESTIMATES

Overview

The preceding section highlighted the variety of different potential sources of surveillance data relevant to occupational respiratory disorders. In the following section, we summarize the insights that these surveillance data have provided for asthma, acute inhalation injury, malignant mesothelioma, cancer of the lung, and pneumoconiosis. In these summaries, we emphasize a surveillance-based perspective, highlighting changing patterns of disease incidence and prevalence while underscoring the emergence of newly appreciated risk factors or the diminution of previously prominent ones.

Distribution and trends

Trends should be interpreted with caution since they may be affected by changes to the data collection methods or in the inclusion/exclusion criteria of the surveillance system. None the less, there are a few trends that are consistent among different populations. Over the course of the past fifty years, there has been a decline in the incidence and mortality of some of the 'traditional' occupational lung diseases, such as coal workers' pneumoconiosis and silicosis both in Great Britain and the United States [40,86].

The incidence and mortality of asbestos-related disease has continued to increase, mainly reflecting exposures during the 1940s to 1970s, although its incidence is predicted to decline in most parts of the world in the near future. Byssinosis, which in the past was one of the more common occupational diseases, is now rarely diagnosed in the USA or the UK, with a shift in textile production to other countries. During the 1980s in the UK, byssinosis incidence declined from 132 new cases diagnosed by the Special Medical Boards (state compensation) in 1982 to 15 in 1989. In the USA, however, where byssinosis surveillance is based on deaths, a similar decline has yet to be seen [90]. Field studies done elsewhere, for example China, suggest that byssinosis remains common worldwide [91]. Unfortunately, national surveillance data for occupational lung disease in most developing countries simply do not exist.

Analysis of reports to the voluntary surveillance schemes that include the full range of occupational respiratory diseases provide a picture of the relative frequency of the different diagnostic categories, as recognized by respiratory and occupational specialists in those countries (Table 2.1). In the UK, although the diseases with a long latent period (such as pneumoconiosis and malignancies) continue to predominate, asthma has become the single most common diagnosis [7,92–97]. This is even more apparent in data from the Canadian surveillance schemes [8,9]. A very different picture emerges from the South African data, where pneumoconiosis is by far the most frequently diagnosed disease [98]. Of the remainder in South Africa, the largest group is work-related tuberculosis (10.1%), including 6.9% with both tuberculosis and pneumoconiosis.

Table 2.1 Distribution of cases reported to voluntary reporting schemes by diagnosis

	UK	Canada		South Africa
	SWORD 1990–1998 [7,91–97]	BC* 1991 [8]	Quebec ProPulse 1992–1993 [9]	SORDSA 1996–1999 [98]
Number of cases	26984	246	453	4049
Disease category				
Asthma	29%	50%	63%	8%
Inhalation accident	9%	1%	5%	8%
Bronchitis and emphysema	2%	4%	1%	4%
Infectious disease	2%	0%	0%	10%
Pneumoconiosis	10%	18%	10%	61%
Non-malignant pleural disease	20%	5%	6%	3%
Mesothelioma	19%	12%	4%	1%
Lung cancer	3%	3%	2%	1%
Other	6%	6%	10%	4%
All disease combined	100%	100%	100%	100%

* BC, British Columbia.

Asthma

Diagnostic issues

The frequency with which occupational asthma occurs in a population depends in part on how the disease is defined and on the diagnostic criteria employed. Although most would agree with Newman Taylor's definition of occupational asthma as variable airways narrowing causally related to exposure in the working environment to airborne dust, gases, vapors or fumes [99], some limit the diagnosis to new-onset asthma, while others include work-related exacerbations of non-occupational asthma. There is also variation over the labeling of asthmatic symptoms due to exposure to a respiratory irritant, such as occurs in the reactive airways dysfunction syndrome, or RADS [100].

The SENSOR definition of occupational asthma encompasses both work-related exacerbations of pre-existing asthma and RADS; detailed diagnostic criteria for case reports are specified [101]. Other voluntary reporting schemes mainly focus on asthma *caused* by exposures at work and are less specific in their diagnostic criteria. SWORD, for example, asks physicians to report cases of asthma as they are diagnosed if the physician believes that, more likely than not, the condition was caused by an occupational exposure. Cases of RADS are included, but may be reported as inhalation accidents instead of asthma [102]. German statistics for occupational asthma are derived from compensated cases, which include rhinitis and chronic obstructive airways disease with asthma, but require an allergic etiology

and cessation of exposure before acceptance [43]. In Sweden, a register is maintained of all claims made for compensation for occupational diseases, whether or not compensation is awarded [103].

Estimates of incidence

There is considerable variation in the estimated incidence of occupational asthma based on the available sources of surveillance data (Fig. 2.1), which probably has as much to do with the biases and limitations of the schemes in question as with the underlying rate of disease occurrence. Estimates range from an average of five cases of occupational asthma per million working population identified by Massachusetts SENSOR each year [104] to 175 in Finland [14].

It is most unlikely that any of these estimates is strictly accurate. Even the Finnish Register, which is probably the most complete, excludes the uninsured, in particular many self-employed people for whom insurance is voluntary. There has been a steady rise in numbers of new cases of occupational asthma reported to the Finnish Register of Occupational Diseases (FROD) each year from 80 in 1976 [14], equivalent to a rate of 36 per million working population, to 423 in 1995, which represents a rate of 205 per million [106]. Much of the increase is due to the inclusion since 1982 of farmers in the compensation system [16]; in the period 1990–1995, half the cases registered by the FROD were in farmers.

The extent to which the voluntary reporting schemes provide accurate estimates of disease incidence depends upon the extent to which the targeted

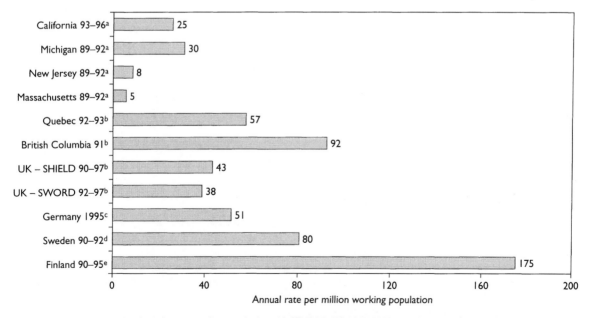

Fig. 2.1 Rates of occupational asthma from surveillance schemes. (a) SENSOR [32,104]. (b) Voluntary reporting schemes [7–9, 92–96, 105]. (c) Compensation statistics, includes rhinitis and chronic obstructive airways disease as well as asthma [43]. (d) Compensation claimants [103]. (e) FROD [106].

participants have access to the relevant patient group, the diagnostic accuracy of the reporters, and the level of their participation. The emphasis of SENSOR is on identification of potentially hazardous sentinel cases for the purpose of investigation and preventive intervention in the workplace, rather than obtaining an epidemiological overview of the distribution and determinants of disease in the population [5]. The estimation of disease frequency is not one of the aims of the SENSOR program, and, using capture–recapture techniques, Henneberger and coworkers have estimated that the average annual incidence for Michigan SENSOR should be 58–204 per million for 1988–1995 instead of the rate of 27 per million reported [104].

Comparison of successful new claims for occupational asthma from the province of Quebec between 1986 and 1988 with cases diagnosed in special surveys suggests that only about a quarter of cases that occurred were recognized in claims [107]. When reports to ProPulse, the province-wide voluntary surveillance scheme, were compared to compensation data, there were twice as many cases in one year that were judged highly likely to be related to work as there were cases compensated by the Workers' Compensation Board [9].

Agents

The distribution of commonly suspected causes of occupational asthma from Finland's FROD, the six voluntary reporting schemes, and the SENSOR programs in Michigan and New Jersey, demonstrates both striking similarities and differences (Table 2.2). The differences are probably largely due to variation among the regions in the types of industries, working practices, and the level of environmental protection found in the workplace. For example, over

half of the cases in British Columbia were attributed to wood dust, no doubt reflecting both the regional importance of the wood industry and the allergenic properties of western red cedar [8]. This compares to 2–6% occupational asthma caused by wood dust in European countries. Some of the variation may be spurious, however, due to differences in the sources of reports and the application of diagnostic criteria. For example, most cases from Finland were due to either animal allergens or flour and grain, compared with 3% from Michigan and New Jersey. The inclusion of self-employed farmers in the Finnish compensation system in 1982 resulted in a huge increase in cases due to animal epithelia, flours and grain, with little change in the numbers of cases attributed to other agents [16]. In the USA, farmers typically fall outside workers' compensation reporting and are unlikely to be well captured by SENSOR surveillance.

The proportion of cases attributed to isocyanates is very similar (16–20%) in most surveillance schemes apart from Finland (Table 2.2). In the UK, Canada, France and the USA, isocyanates are the most commonly reported cause of occupational asthma. There is evidence from both compensation statistics [86] and from SWORD that the incidence of isocyanate asthma is declining in the UK [13a], although it remains the single most common cause there as well.

The cross-country comparisons for other, smaller categories of agents are also interesting. The proportions of asthma attributed to aldehydes (formaldehyde and glutaraldehyde), glues and resins, and welding fume are similar in all case series in which they were specifically identified. The 'other' category varies in size from 19% in Finland to 65% in SENSOR (Table 2.2). Of particular note are the proportions attributed to coolant/oil mists in Michigan

Table 2.2 Distribution of suspected agents as a percentage of total cases of occupational asthma

Suspected agent	Finland, FROD 1991–1992 [15,109]	UK, SWORD 1989–1997 [13a]	West Midlands UK, Shield 1989–1991 [108]	British Columbia, Canada 1991 [8]	Quebec, Canada, ProPulse 1992–1993 [9]	France, ONAP 1996 [12]	Michigan and New Jersey, SENSOR 1988–1992 (110)	South Africa, SORDSA 1996–1998[a]
Animal allergens	41	9	2	3	10	1[b]	1	1
Flour and grain	25	8	10	4	14	20	2	12
Wood dust	2	5	6	47	11	4	1	0
Isocyanates	4	16	20	16	17	16	19	20
Aldehydes	2	5	2	NS	NS	7	5	1
Glues and resins	2	7	5	NS	NS	3	5	8
Welding fume	4	2	2	3	6	?	2	4
Other	19	47	53	27	41	49	65	54

[a] Esterhuizen, personal communication
[b] Laboratory animals only
NS, not stated.

and New Jersey (9.9%) [110] and in the West Midlands of England (6.5%) [108], and the proportions attributed to latex and platinum salts in South Africa (24% and 12% respectively of reported cases) (Esterhuizen, personal communication).

Occupation

Data from surveillance schemes have provided useful information on the risk of occupational asthma associated with different occupations. The most robust estimates are based on SWORD data, by virtue of the large number of reported cases. However, due to incomplete ascertainment, these should be regarded as minimum estimates, and the relative risks are of greater interest than the absolute values (Table 2.3). The majority of cases and most of the high-risk occupations are in manufacturing industries.

Comparison of occupation-specific rates between countries is complicated by differences in classifica-tion of occupations and industries, but Sweden and Finland use the same Nordic occupation classification. Interestingly, despite the fact that the overall rates from the Finnish data are approximately twice the rates of self-reported occupational asthma in Sweden, the occupation-specific rates are similar at the level of the broad occupational group (one-digit code) in both countries [103,106]. The higher overall rate in Finland is due almost entirely to the much higher rate associated with agricultural work, as noted previously.

Sex and age

In analyzes of SWORD cases, the rate of occupational asthma in working men was found to be almost twice the rate for women; however this was due to gender differences in occupations [111]. Similar increased risks for men were found in the rates of self-reported work-related asthma in England and Wales [85] and in Quebec [9]. In Sweden, however, the rate for men was only slightly higher than for women [103], and in Finland, there was no difference between men and women [106].

Analysis of cases reported to SWORD has consistently shown an apparent increase in risk of occupational asthma with age, particularly in men: in 1992–1997 estimated rates for men were 30 per million employed aged 16–29 years, 43 per million aged 30–44 years and 53 per million in those 45 years or more [13a]. This trend could not be explained by differences in occupation by age; indeed adjustment for occupation made the age gradient steeper in both sexes. Comparable age gradients were found in the self-reported cases in Sweden [103] and to a lesser extent in Quebec [9].

While the apparent increase in incidence with age may be real, it is also possible that it may be due to socioeconomic factors that affect an individual's likelihood of seeking medical attention. For example, a young person with work-related symptoms may simply change jobs, whereas an older person may look for compensation and early retirement or may wish, despite symptoms, to stay in a job in which he/she is experienced and secure. However, the susceptibility to respiratory sensitization may increase with age, perhaps because of previous exposures or behavioral factors such as smoking. In support of this argument, in the Barcelona soybean asthma outbreaks, older age was found to be an independent risk factor for disease [112].

Table 2.3 Estimated annual rate and relative risk of occupational asthma in the UK in selected high-risk occupations, SWORD 1992–1997 [13a]

Occupational set	Rate per million	95% CI	RR[a]
Coach and other spray painters	1464	968–2173	38.5
Bakers	951	618–1415	25.0
Chemical processors	573	357–898	15.1
Metal treatment workers	567	345–907	14.9
Plastics workers	380	220–635	10.0
Food processor (excluding bakers)	280	171–441	7.4
Welding, soldering and electronic assembly	266	181–389	7.0
Laboratory technicians and assistants	207	150–297	5.4
Wood workers	139	82–221	3.7
Other non-metal/electrical processing/making/repairing	132	83–176	3.5
Assembly and packing	74	44–122	1.9
Farmers and farm hands	68	34–123	1.8
Nurses	62	40–96	1.6
Other metal/electrical processing/making/repairing	59	44–78	1.6
All occupations	38	34–41	1.0

[a]Relative risk compared to the average annual rate of 38 per million.

Acute inhalation injury

Although occupational asthma is the acute respiratory condition that has been most extensively studied using surveillance data, these data also provide insights into other less common conditions, in particular acute inhalation injuries. Nine per cent of cases reported to SWORD are inhalation accidents. A study of cases in 1990–1993 showed that the occupations with both the largest proportion of cases and the highest rates were chemical processors (15% of cases; 164 per million per year), and engineers and metal workers (31% of cases; 45 per million per year) [113]. This study also found that these accidents resulted in considerable morbidity. In 26% of cases the subject had symptoms that persisted for 1 month or more, and at follow-up more than 1 year after the incident, 23% of these (6% of all cases) were considered by the reporting physician to have asthma or RADS [102]. Those who had inhaled a known sensitizing agent were the most likely to have developed asthma.

RADS as a separate category of asthma following acute inhalation of an irritant has proved to be an important component of SENSOR cases, ranging from 6% in California to 31% in New Jersey [101]. As was stated earlier, inhalation of agents at work are common among poison control center consultations, most of which involve respiratory symptoms.

Diseases of long latency

The main diseases in this group are pneumoconiosis, lung cancer, mesothelioma, and benign pleural disease. Although in the past coal workers' pneumoconiosis and silicosis predominated in Europe and North America, the majority of newly presenting cases of pneumoconiosis are now due to asbestos exposure. Industrial use of asbestos became widespread during the Second World War and world consumption peaked in the 1970s. Population surveys from northern Europe suggest that in some regions as much as a third of the adult male population has had occupational exposure to asbestos, with the construction industry accounting for much of that exposure. In North America and western Europe, exposure has declined since the 1960s and 1970s; however in eastern Europe and in the countries of the former Soviet Union, consumption did not start to decline significantly until the 1990s [114].

For diseases with a long latent period, it may be difficult to find appropriate denominators for the estimation of rates and therefore proportional mortality ratios, based on the occupation listed on the death certificate, are often used to identify high-risk occupations [115]. Although a useful method for epidemiological investigation, death certificates normally give the individual's last occupation, which may not be relevant for the exposure that led to death. Based on SWORD reports from 1989 to 1991 and using population estimates by occupation for men aged 15–54 from the 1961 UK census, rates of the long latency diseases have been estimated [7]. As has been said before, the rates will be underestimated because of incomplete reporting, but provide a more direct assessment of the relative risk for different occupational groups (Table 2.4).

Mesothelioma

Mesothelioma is one of the most easily identified occupational respiratory diseases, as it is very rare in

Table 2.4 Incidence of diseases of long latency in men from reports to SWORD 1989–1991, based on 1961 census data (7)

Occupation	Total cases	Lung cancer (%)	Mesothelioma (%)	Pneumoconiosis (%)	Non-malignant pleural disease (%)	Rate per million per year all types
Miners and quarrymen	350	3	2	89	6	281
Gas, coke and chemicals makers	43	5	30	23	42	100
Glass and ceramics makers	27	4	4	56	37	103
Electrical, electronics and power station workers	201	4	42	15	38	130
Carpenters, joiners and woodworkers	123	3	46	11	40	109
Other manufacturers	181	5	30	34	31	49
Engineers and foundry workers	605	5	30	24	41	84
Construction workers	451	4	22	35	39	323
Painters and decorators	31	10	32	19	39	21
Transport and communications	76	5	51	11	33	21
Shipyard and dock workers	324	5	44	14	37	753
Warehousemen and packers	20	10	40	13	40	18
Other	98	6	55	13	29	7
Occupation not stated/inadequately described	70	9	33	20	39	–
Total	2600	5	30	30	34	67

populations with little asbestos exposure (1–2 per million/yr [116]). Because it is associated with high short-term mortality, surveillance of incidence can be estimated effectively through cancer registries and death certificates. Since the level of risk depends on the type of asbestos, dose, and time since first exposure [114], the incidence of mesothelioma varies considerably [117]. In most cancer registries, the incidence in women is close to the 'background rate', but in North America and in western European countries the rates for men are 5–10-fold greater than those for women. Thus the discrepancy in rates between men and women provides an estimate of the contribution of occupational exposure to disease incidence.

Mesothelioma incidence has increased dramatically since the 1960s, especially among men, reflecting exposures some 30–40 years previously, although improved diagnostic accuracy may account for some of the increase. Analysis of incidence by birth cohort and age group has yielded extrapolations of the epidemic curve as a specific application of these surveillance data. It was estimated that the peak in the United States would occur at about the year 2000, with approximately 3000 cases per year [18]. The peaks in Great Britain and France are predicted to be later, in 2020 [118] and 2020–2060 [119], respectively. At its peak, there may be an estimated 2700 to 3300 deaths per year in men in Great Britain, with a predicted lifetime risk of 1.3% for men born in 1943–1948 [118]. In Finland, the peak incidence was initially predicted to occur in 2010, but more recent evidence suggests that it may be somewhat earlier [120].

Coggon [115] estimated from proportional mortality ratios by occupation that there were some 600 mesothelioma deaths each year in Great Britain in the 1990s due to occupational asbestos exposure. This estimate is consistent with that based on reports to the SWORD project between 1992 and 1998 (mean of 668 cases per year) [7,92–97], which suggests that for malignant mesothelioma at least, reports to SWORD may provide fairly accurate estimates of incidence.

Lung cancer

Asbestos exposure is the most common occupational cause of lung cancer, although other exposures, such as ionizing radiation, polycyclic aromatic hydrocarbons, chromates, nickel, and arsenic are associated with increased occupational risk [115]. In individual cases, however, concomitant cigarette smoking complicates the attribution to occupational exposures. Occupational cohort studies suggest that at least as many cases of lung cancer are attributable to asbestos exposure in a population as there are cases of mesothelioma [116], but both voluntary reporting schemes and compensation data include far fewer cases; thus surveillance data provide little insight into occupational lung cancer. Less biased information is available from linkage of census records and cancer registrations, such as has been done in the Nordic countries [56]. However, confounding due to tobacco exposure complicates interpretation of the data; the highest rates of lung cancer in men were found to be in waiters and tobacco workers, although miners and quarriers were also at increased risk.

Because of the complex interactions between smoking and asbestos on the risk of lung cancer [114] both exposures must be considered when predicting trends in disease incidence. With the decline in both prevalence of smoking and asbestos exposure, it is probable that the incidence of occupational lung cancer will fall in western Europe and North America. There is, however, cause for greater concern in other parts of the world, in particular in eastern Europe and the countries of the former Soviet Union, where cigarette consumption is increasing and asbestos use is greater than elsewhere [114].

Pneumoconiosis

Whether measured by incidence or mortality, there has been a dramatic reduction in pneumoconiosis due to coal and silica exposure in the latter half of the 20th century and a rise in cases of asbestosis in western Europe and North America. In 1992, the age adjusted mortality rate for coal workers' pneumoconiosis in the USA was 4.4 per million compared to 2.9 for asbestosis and 0.77 for silicosis [90]. In Great Britain, the number of new cases of asbestosis diagnosed by the Special Medical Boards now exceeds those attributed to coal (Fig. 2.2) [86]. The construction industry accounted for 44% of the asbestosis deaths in the USA in 1985–1992 [90], and was associated with the highest incidence of disease in the UK (see Table 2.4).

CONCLUSIONS

Occupational lung disease surveillance provides useful tools with which to gauge the absolute and relative importance of a wide variety of work-related respiratory conditions. For certain diseases, ongoing surveillance provides a basis for primary or secondary prevention for the individual worker by guiding interventions on a case-by-case basis. This can include, for example, the institution of tuberculosis prophylaxis, substitution of latex gloves, or removal from further exposure. Beyond the individual level, effective surveillance of occupational diseases can be helpful to both healthcare providers and others concerned with the protection of workers by allowing the monitoring of prevalence and incidence trends, the identification of new health risks, and the assessment of impact of control strategies.

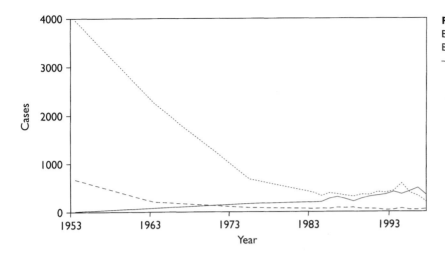

Fig. 2.2 Pneumoconiosis cases in Great Britain diagnosed by Special Medical Boards, 1953–1997 [85,121]. -------, Coal; ———, asbestos; – – – –, other.

SUMMARY POINTS

- Useful information on the distribution and determinants of occupational lung disorders can be derived from a variety of sources.
- Surveillance data are rarely complete, therefore relative distributions are more dependable than absolute incidence estimates.
- Variation in estimates for occupational lung disease incidence and prevalence derived from surveillance data is probably mainly due to differences in the completeness of the surveillance systems, differences in case definition, and regional differences in exposure hazards.

- Occupational asthma surveillance has been most effective through targeted reporting schemes.
- Reporting schemes provide limited information on occupational lung cancers, because it is difficult to attribute individual cases to occupational exposures when there is a history of tobacco smoking.
- Mesothelioma incidence can be monitored using cancer registry data and death records as surveillance tools.
- Surveillance for acute inhalation illness can utilize poison control center reporting.

REFERENCES

1. Langmuir AD. The surveillance of communicable diseases of national importance. *N Engl J Med* 1963; 268: 182–192.
2. Langmuir AD. William Farr: founder of modern concepts of surveillance. *Int J Epidemiol* 1976; 5: 13–18.
3. World Health Organization. *Report of the technical discussions at the Twenty-First World Health Assembly on 'National and Global Surveillance of Communicable Diseases', 18 May 1968.* A21. Geneva: WHO, 1968.
4. Last JM. *A Dictionary of Epidemiology.* Oxford: Oxford University Press, 1988.
5. Baker EL. Sentinel Event Notification System for Occupational Risks (SENSOR): the concept. *Am J Public Health* 1989; 79 (Suppl). 18–20.
6. McDonald JC, Harrington JM. Early detection of occupational hazards. *J Soc Occup Med* 1981; 31: 93–98.
7. Meredith SK, McDonald JC. Work-related respiratory disease in the United Kingdom 1989–1992: report on the SWORD project. *Occup Med* 1994; 44: 183–189.
8. Contreras GR, Rousseau R, Chan-Yeung M. Occupational respiratory diseases in British Columbia, Canada in 1991. *Occup Environ Med* 1994; 51: 710–712.
9. Provencher S, Labrèche FP, de Guire L. Physician based surveillance system for occupational respiratory diseases: the experience of ProPulse, Québec, Canada. *Occup Environ Med* 1997; 54: 272–276.

10. Hnizdo E, Rees D. Surveillance of occupational diseases – where does SORDSA fit in? *Occup Health SA* 1997; 3: 26–31.
11. Gannon PFG, Burge PS. A preliminary report of a surveillance scheme of occupational asthma in the West Midlands. *Br J Ind Med* 1991; 48: 579–582.
12. Ameille J, Calastreng-Crinquand A, Kopfersmitt MC *et al.* Incidence of occupational asthma in France in 1996. In: Chiyotani K, Hosoda Y, Aizawa Y, eds. *Advances in the Prevention of Occupational Respiratory Diseases*, pp. 430–433. Amsterdam: Elsevier Science, 1998.
13. Bena A, d'Errico A, Mirabelli D. A system for the active surveillance of occupational bronchial asthma: the results of two years of activity of the PriOR program. *Medicina del Lavoro* 1999; 90: 556–571.
13a. McDonald JC, Keynes HL, Meredith SK. Reported incidence of occupational asthma in the United Kingdom, 1989–97. *Occup Environ Med* 2000; 57: 823–829.
14. Keskinen H, Alanko K, Saarinen L. Occupational asthma in Finland. *Clin Allergy* 1978; 8: 569–579.
15. Meredith S, Nordman H. Occupational asthma: measures of frequency from four countries. *Thorax* 1996; 51: 435–440.
16. Karjalainen A, Keskinen H, Nordman H, Kurppa K. Trends in occupational asthma in Finland 1978–97. *Eur Respir J* 1998; 12(Suppl 29): 76S.

17. Sprince NL, Kazemi H. US Beryllium case registry through 1977. *Environ Res* 1980; 21: 44–47.

18. Price B. Analysis of current trends in United States mesothelioma incidence. *Am J Epidemiol* 1997; 145: 211–218.

19. Coultas DB, Hughes MP. Accuracy of mortality data for interstitial lung diseases in New Mexico, USA. *Thorax* 1996; 51: 717–720.

20. Deichman WB. Progress report: AMA registry on adverse reactions due to occupational exposures. *J Occup Med* 1971; 13: 577–580.

21. Guidoti TL. An international registry for toxic inhalation and pulmonary edema: notes from a work in progress. *Int Arch Occup Environ Health* 1996; 68: 380–386.

22. Kreiss K, Newman LS, Mroz MM, Campbell PA. Screening blood test identifies subclinical beryllium disease. *J Occup Med* 1989; 31: 603–608.

23. Fennelly KP. Occupational tuberculosis in the era of drug resistance and AIDS. *Semin Respir Crit Care Med* 1999; 20: 559–568.

24. Thomas DR, Treweek L, Salmon RL et al. The risk of acquiring Q-fever on farms: a seroepidemiological study. *Occup Environ Med* 1995; 52: 644–647.

25. Smith TA, Wastell Smith P. Respiratory symptoms and sensitization in bread and cake bakers. *Occup Med* 1998; 48: 321–328.

26. Liss GM, Sussman, GL. Latex sensitization: occupational versus general population prevalence rates. *Am J Ind Med* 1999; 35: 196–200.

27. American Thoracic Society. Surveillance for respiratory hazards in the occupational setting. *Am Rev Respir Dis* 1982; 126: 952–956.

28. Althouse RB. Ten years' experience with the coal workers' health surveillance program, 1970–1981. *MMWR* 1985; 34(1SS): 33S–37SS.

29. Goodwin S, Attfield M. Temporal trends in coal workers' pneumoconiosis prevalence. Validating the National Coal Study results. *J Occup Environ Med* 1998; 40: 1065–1071.

30. Soutar CA, Maclaren WM, Annis R, Melville AW. Quantitative relations between exposure to respirable coalmine dust and coalworkers' simple pneumoconiosis in men who have worked as miners but left the coal industry. *Br J Ind Med* 1986; 43: 29–36.

31. Division of Labor Statistics and Research, State of California. *Occupational disease in California 1988.* South San Francisco, CA: Division of Labor Statistics and Research, 1990.

32. Reinisch F, Cussler S, Harrison R. Occupational asthma surveillance in California 1993–1996. *Am J Respir Crit Care Med* 1998; 157: A882.

33. Freund E, Seligman PJ, Chorba TL et al. Mandatory reporting of occupational diseases by clinicians. *JAMA* 1989; 262: 3041–3044.

34. Rosenman KD, Reilly MJ. Asbestos-related X-ray changes in foundry workers. *Am J Ind Med* 1998; 34: 197–201.

35. Seligman PJ, Sieber WK, Pedersen DH et al. Compliance with OSHA record-keeping requirements. *Am J Public Health* 1988; 78: 1218–1219.

36. Health and Safety Executive. *A Guide to the Reporting of Injuries, Diseases and Dangerous Occurrences Regulations HS(R)23.* London: HMSO, 1985.

37. Carter JT. There's a lot of it about? *Br J Ind Med* 1991; 48: 289–291.

38. Health and Safety Commission. *Health and Safety Statistics 1995/96.* HSE Books, 1996.

39. Goldsmith DF. Uses of workers' compensation data in epidemiology research. *Occup Med* 1998; 13: 389–415.

40. Division of Respiratory Disease Studies, National Institute for Occupational Safety and Health (CDC). *Work-related lung disease surveillance report 1994.* DHHS (NIOSH) 94–120. Cincinnati, OH: National Institute for Occupational Safety and Health, 1994.

41. Kleinman GD, Cant SM. Occupational disease surveillance in Washington. *J Occup Med* 1978; 20: 750–754.

42. Chatkin JM, Tarlo SM, Liss G et al. The outcome of asthma related to workplace irritant exposures. A comparison of irritant-induced asthma and irritant aggravation of asthma. *Chest* 1999; 116: 1780–1785.

43. Baur X, Degens P, Weber K. Occupational obstructive diseases in Germany. *Am J Ind Med* 1998; 33: 454–462.

44. Froines JR, Dellenbaugh CA, Wegman DH. Occupational health surveillance: a means to identify work-related risks. *Am J Public Health* 1986; 76: 1089–1096.

45. Froines JR, Wegman DH, Dellenbaugh CA. An approach to the characterization of silica exposure in US industry. *Am J Ind Med* 1986; 10: 345–361.

46. Linch KD, Miller WE, Althouse RB et al. Surveillance of respirable crystalline silica dust using OSHA compliance data (1979–1995). *Am J Ind Med* 1998; 34: 547–558.

47. Seta JA, Sudain DS. Trends of a decade – a perspective on occupational hazard surveillance, 1970–1983. *MMWR* 1985; 34(2SS): 15SS–24SS.

48. Thackrah CT. *The Effects of Arts, Trades, and Professions, and of Civic States and Habits of Living, on Health and Longevity,* 2nd edn. London: Longman, 1832.

49. Richardson BW. *Health and Occupation.* London: Society for Promoting Christian Knowledge, 1879.

50. Dublin LI. *Causes of death by occupation. Occupational mortality experience of the Metropolitan Life Insurance Company, Industrial Department, 1911–1913.* US Department of Labor, Bureau of Labor Statistics, No 207. Washington DC: US Government Printing Office, 1917.

51. Buechley R, Dunn JE, Linden G, Breslow L. Death certificate statement of occupation: its usefulness in comparing mortalities. *Public Health Rep* 1956; 71: 1105–1011.

52. Frazier TM, Wegman DH. Exploring the use of death certificates as a component of an occupational health surveillance system. *Am J Public Health* 1979; 69: 718–720.

53. CDC. Use of death certificates for surveillance of work-related illnesses – New Hampshire. *MMWR* 1986; 35: 537–540.

54. Schade WJ, Swanson GM. Comparison of death certificate occupation and industry with lifetime occupational histories obtained by interview; variations in the accuracy of death certificate entries. *Am J Ind Med* 1988; 14: 121–126.

55. Liss GM, Tarlo SM, Bank D et al. Preliminary report of mortality among workers compensated for work-related asthma. *Am J Ind Med* 1999; 35: 465–471.

56. Andersen A, Barlow L, Engeland A et al. Work-related cancer in the Nordic countries. *Scand J Work Environ Health* 1999; 25(Suppl 2): 1–116.

57. Rutstein DD, Mullan RJ, Frazier TM *et al.* Sentinel health events (occupational): a basis for physician surveillance. *Am J Public Health* 1983; 73: 1054–1062.

58. Landrigan PJ, Baker DB. The recognition and control of occupational disease. *JAMA* 1991; 266: 676–680.

59. Mason TJ, McKay FW, Hoover R *et al. Atlas of cancer mortality for US Counties 1950–69.* DHEW Publication No (NIH) 75–780. Washington, DC: US Department of Health Education and Welfare, 1975.

60. Kim JH. *Atlas of respiratory disease mortality, United States: 1982–1993.* DHHS (NIOSH) 98–157. Cincinnati, OH: National Institute for Occupational Safety and Health, 1998.

61. Windau J, Rosenman K, Anderson H *et al.* The identification of occupational lung disease from hospital discharge data. *J Occup Med* 1991; 33: 1060–1066.

62. Reilly MJ, Rosenman KD. Use of hospital discharge data for surveillance of chemical-related respiratory disease. *Arch Environ Health* 1995; 50: 26–30.

63. Kipen HM, Gelperin K, Tepper A, Stanbury M. Acute occupational respiratory disease in hospital discharge data. *Am J Ind Med* 1991; 19: 637–642.

64. Kusiak RA, Liss GM, Gailitis MM. Cor pulmonale and pneumoconiotic lung disease: an investigation using hospital discharge data. *Am J Ind Med* 1993; 24: 161–173.

65. Liss GM, Kusiak RA, Gailitis MM. Hospital records: an underutilized source of information regarding occupational diseases and exposures. *Am J Ind Med* 1997; 31: 100–106.

66. Kipen HM, Tepper A, Rosenman K, Weinrib D. Limitations of hospital discharge diagnoses for surveillance of extrinsic allergic alveolitis. *Am J Ind Med* 1990; 17: 701–709.

67. Brancati FL, Hodgson MJ, Karpf M. Occupational exposures and diseases among medical inpatients. Prevalence, association, and recognition. *J Occup Med* 1993; 35: 161–165.

68. Balmes J, Rempel D, Alexander M *et al.* Hospital records as a data source for occupational disease surveillance: a feasibility study. *Am J Ind Med* 1992; 21: 341–351.

69. Kraut A, Walld R, Mustard C. Prevalence of physician-diagnosed asthma by occupational groupings in Manitoba, Canada. *Am J Ind Med* 1997; 32: 275–282.

70. Park RM, Krebs JM, Mirer FE. Occupational disease surveillance using disability insurance at an automotive tamping and assembly complex. *J Occup Environ Med* 1996; 38: 1111–1123.

71. Litovitz TL, Smilkstein M, Felberg L *et al.* 1996 annual report of the American Association of Poison Control Centers Toxic Exposure Surveillance System. *Am J Emerg Med* 1997; 15: 447–500.

72. Litovitz T, Oderda G, White JD, Sheridan MJ. Occupational and environmental exposures reported to poison centers. *Am J Public Health* 1993; 83: 739–743.

73. Bresnitz EA. Poison control center follow-up of occupational disease. *Am J Public Health* 1990; 80: 711–712.

74. Blanc PD, Olson KR. Occupationally related illness reported to a regional poison control center. *Am J Public Health* 1986; 76: 1303–1307.

75. Bonfiglio JF, Clark CS, Sigell LT *et al.* Poison centers: a resource for occupational health services. *Vet Hum Toxicol* 1988; 30: 569–572.

76. Yang CC, Wu JF, Ong HC *et al.* Taiwan National Poison Center: epidemiologic data 1985–1993. *Clin Toxicol* 1996; 34: 651–663.

77. Lam de Cort W, Sangster B. Acute intoxications during work. *Vet Hum Toxicol* 1988; 30: 9–11.

78. Hinnen U, Hotz P, Gossweiler B *et al.* Surveillance of occupational illness through a national poison control center: an approach to reach small scale enterprises? *Int Arch Occup Environ Health* 1994; 66: 117–123.

79. Olson DK, Sax L, Gunderson P, Sioris L. Pesticide poisoning surveillance through regional poison control centers. *Am J Public Health* 1991; 81: 750–753.

80. Richmond D. *Pesticide exposure and information calls handled by the Los Angeles County Medical Association regional poison information center June, 1986.* HS-1395. Sacramento, CA: California Department of Food and Agriculture, Division of Pesticide Management Branch, 1987.

81. Blanc PD, Galbo M, Hiatt P, Olson KR. Morbidity following acute irritant inhalation in a population-based study. *JAMA* 1991; 266: 664–669.

82. Blanc PD, Galbo M, Hiatt P *et al.* Symptoms, lung function and airway responsiveness following irritant inhalation. *Chest* 1993; 103: 1699–1705.

83. National Center for Health Statistics. *National Health Interview Survey, 1988. Occupational health public data tape.* Bethesda, MD: National Center for Health Statistics, 1992.

84. Blanc P. Occupational asthma in a national disability survey. *Chest* 1987; 92: 613–617.

85. Hodgson JT, Jones JR, Elliott RC, Osman J. *Self-reported work-related illness.* Research Paper 33. HSE Books, 1993.

86. Health and Safety Commission. *Health and Safety Statistics 1997/98.* HSE Books, 1998.

87. Leibowitz MD. Occupational exposures in relation to symptomatology and lung function in a community population. *Environ Res* 1977; 14: 59–67.

88. Korn RJ, Dockery DW, Spizer FE *et al.* Occupational exposures and chronic respiratory symptoms. *Am Rev Respir Dis* 1987; 136: 298–304.

89. Kogevinas M, Antó JM, Sunyer J *et al.* Occupational asthma in Europe and other industrialized area: a population-based study. *Lancet* 1999; 353: 1750–1754.

90. Division of Respiratory Disease Studies, National Institute for Occupational Safety and Health (CDC). *Work-related lung disease surveillance report 1996.* DHHS (NIOSH) 96–134. Cincinnati, OH: National Institute for Occupational Safety and Health, 1996.

91. Christiani DC, Eisen EA, Wegman DH *et al.* Respiratory disease in cotton textile workers in the People's Republic of China. I. Respiratory symptoms. *Scand J Work Environ Health* 1986; 12: 40–45.

92. Sallie BA, Ross DJ, Meredith SK, McDonald JC. SWORD '93: surveillance of work-related and occupational respiratory disease in the UK. *Occup Med* 1994; 44: 177–182.

93. Ross DJ, Sallie BA, McDonald JC. SWORD '94: surveillance of work-related and occupational respiratory disease in the UK. *Occup Med* 1995; 45: 175–178.

94. Keynes HL, Ross DJ, McDonald JC. SWORD '95: surveillance of work-related and occupational respiratory disease in the UK. *Occup Med* 1996; 46: 379–381.

95. Ross DJ, Keynes HL, McDonald JC. SWORD '96: surveillance of work-related and occupational respiratory disease in the UK. *Occup Med* 1997; 47: 377–381.

96. Ross DJ, Keynes HL, McDonald JC. SWORD '97: surveillance of work-related and occupational respiratory disease in the UK. *Occup Med* 1998; 48: 481–485.

97. Meyer JD, Holt DL, Cherry NM, McDonald JC. SWORD '98: surveillance of work-related and occupational respiratory disease in the UK. *Occup Med* 1999; 48: 485–489.

98. Esterhuizen T. *SORDSA News*, October–December 1999, Vol 3, No 3.

99. Newman Taylor AJ. Occupational asthma. *Thorax* 1980; 35: 241–245.

100. Bernstein IL, Bernstein DI, Chan-Yeung M, Malo JL. Definition and classification of asthma. In: Bernstein IL, Chan-Yeung M, Malo JL, Bernstein DI, eds. *Asthma in the Workplace*, pp. 1–4. New York: Marcel Dekker, 1993.

101. Jajosky RAR, Harrison R, Reinisch F *et al.* Surveillance of work-related asthma in selected US States using surveillance guidelines for state health departments – California, Massachusetts, Michigan, and New Jersey, 1993–1995. *MMWR* 1999; 48(SS-3): 1–20.

102. Ross DJ, McDonald JC. Asthma following inhalation accidents reported to the SWORD project. *Ann Occup Hyg* 1996; 40: 645–650.

103. Torén K. Self-reported rate of occupational asthma in Sweden 1990–2. *Occup Environ Med* 1996; 53: 757–761.

104. Henneberger PK, Kreiss K, Rosenman KD *et al.* An evaluation of the incidence of work-related asthma in the United States. *Int J Occup Environ Health* 1999; 5: 1–8.

105. Di Stefano F, Siriruttanapruk S, McCoach J, Burge PS. The incidence of occupational asthma in the West Midlands (UK) from the Shield surveillance scheme. *Eur Respir J* 1998; 12(Suppl 28): 30S.

106. Karjalainen A, Keskinen H, Nordman H, Kurppa K. Incidence of reported occupational asthma in Finland 1990–95. In: Chiyotani K, Hosoda Y, Aizawa Y, eds. *Advances in the Prevention of Occupational Respiratory Diseases*, pp. 434–438. Amsterdam: Elsevier Science, 1998.

107. Lagier F, Cartier A, Malo JL. Statistiques médico-légales sur l'asthme professionnel au Québec de 1986–1988. *Rev Mal Respir* 1990; 7: 337–341.

108. Gannon PFG, Burge PS. The Shield scheme in the West Midlands Region, United Kingdom. *Br J Ind Med* 1993; 50: 791–796.

109. Reijula K, Patterson R. Occupational allergies in Finland 1981–91. *Allergy Proc* 1994; 15: 163–168.

110. Reilly MJ, Rosenman KD, Watt FC *et al.* Surveillance for occupational asthma – Michigan and New Jersey, 1988–1992. *CDC-MMWR* 1994; 43: 9–17.

111. Meredith SK. Reported incidence of occupational asthma in the United Kingdom, 1989–90. *J Epidemiol Comm Health* 1993; 47: 459–463.

112. Sunyer J, Antó JM, Sabria J *et al.* Risk factors of soybean epidemic asthma. *Am Rev Respir Dis* 1992; 145: 1098–1102.

113. Sallie B, McDonald C. Inhalation accidents reported to the SWORD surveillance project 1990–1993. *Ann Occup Hyg* 1996; 40: 211–221.

114. Albin M, Magnani C, Krstev S *et al.* Asbestos and cancer: and overview of current trends in Europe. *Environ Health Persp* 1999; 107(Suppl 2): 289–298.

115. Coggon D. Occupational cancer in the United Kingdom. *Environ Health Persp* 1999; 107(Suppl 2): 239–244.

116. McDonald JC, McDonald AD. Epidemiology of mesothelioma. In: *Mineral Fibers and Health*. Lidell D, Miller K, eds. Boca Raton: CRC Press, 1991.

117. Parkin DM, Whelan SL, Ferlay J *et al. Cancer Incidence in Five Continents*, Vol VII. IARC Scientific Publication No 143. Lyon: International Agency for Research on Cancer, 1997.

118. Peto J, Hodgson J Mattews F, Jones J. Continuing increase in mesothelioma mortality in Britain. *Lancet* 1995; 345: 535–539.

119. Ilg AGS, Bignon J, Valleron AJ. Estimation of the past and future burden of mortality from mesothelioma in France. *Occup Environ Med* 1998; 55: 760–763.

120. Karjalainen A, Pukkala E, Mattson K, Tammilehto L. Trends in mesothelioma incidence and occupational mesotheliomas in Finland in 1960–1995. *Scand J Work Environ Health* 1997; 23: 266–270.

121. Jones DJ. Prescribed respiratory diseases in the 1990s. *Respir Med* 1992; 86: 283–287.

3 HOW TO TAKE AN OCCUPATIONAL EXPOSURE HISTORY RELEVANT TO LUNG DISEASE

P. Sherwood Burge

INTRODUCTION

An occupational exposure history is fundamental in assessing the respiratory risks of a worker, and in helping to establish a diagnosis of occupational lung disease. Two broad types can be distinguished, which are relevant respectively to two different groups of disorder:

- Disorders of long latency for which the cumulative level of exposure is critical.
- Disorders of short latency for which the timing of symptom onset is critical.

For the first group of disorders, examples of which are the pneumoconioses and lung cancer, the primary aims are to identify a putative causal agent and assess the approximate cumulative level of exposure. This comes from the product of the estimated average airborne concentration during work and the period of exposure. The clinician can then evaluate whether it provides a plausible explanation for the disorder under review.

For the second group of disorders, for which examples are toxic and allergic diseases such as the reactive airways dysfunction syndrome and hypersensitivity pneumonitis (extrinsic allergic alveolitis), the aim to identify a plausible etiological agent is centered more on the timing of exposure. Whether this occurred at a particular time is more crucial than cumulative exposure dose.

ASSESSING CUMULATIVE EXPOSURE

Exposure may start in infancy related to environmental exposure or materials bought home on adults' clothes. This is best documented for asbestos where cases of mesothelioma have arisen entirely from asbestos brought home on the working clothes of adults – occasionally only for the purpose of washing. For mesothelioma, therefore, enquiries should be made of all adults who were living in the home when the patient was a child, of their jobs, and of any potential source of occupational or domestic exposure to asbestos. In some situations asbestos exposure may come from the environment because of geological outcropping of asbestos-containing rock. This particularly occurs with tremolite and anthophyllite in certain well-recognized areas (Table 3.1).

The occupational history should then include every job since starting work, with the start and stop dates, names and addresses of employers, and descriptions of the occupational tasks. The aim is to make an assessment of the agents to which the individual patient is likely to have been exposed and also the likely extent of the exposure. It is often helpful to ask for a completed form outlining the occupational history in advance of a clinic visit. If there is difficulty with dates, it is often useful to associate jobs with important more readily remembered events (e.g. special birthdays, military service, marriages,

Table 3.1 Sources of environmental asbestos (or asbestos-like) fibers related to plaque prevalence and mesothelioma incidence

Country	Fiber	Plaques (%)	Mesothelioma/million/year	
Turkey	Erionite (a zeolite)	65	High	Farmers
	Tremolite	1–25	High	White wash
	Amosite	2–7	High	Around mine
Greece	Tremolite			
Metsovo		47	280	White wash
Macedonia		24	High	
Corsica	Tremolite	41	High	Population
Finland	Anthophyllite	6.5–9	Not increased	
Bulgaria	Anthophyllite and tremolite	F 2.8 M 5.6	Not increased	Tobacco growers
Austria	Tremolite	5.3	Not increased	Vineyards
South Africa	Amosite and crocidolite	2.5–6.6	High	Around mine

retirements, and major national or global catastrophes). Unexplained gaps may signal periods (perhaps in prison) which the individual prefers to forget.

TIMING OF EXPOSURE

Some occupational diseases first provoke symptoms at the time of relevant exposure, or at least within a matter of hours. These include acute toxic reactions and hypersensitivity disorders such as asthma and allergic alveolitis. The latter additionally require an interval between first exposure and disease onset, during which sensitization develops. This is usually a matter of months, though may be as little as weeks or days, or as much as several years. With the disorders resulting from the slow accumulation of mineral dusts (e.g. the pneumoconioses associated with coal, silica, and asbestos, lung cancer, berylliosis, and cadmium-induced emphysema), the period of latency between exposure onset and disease onset characteristically extends for many years.

DOSE

Some diseases are associated only with high levels of exposure. This particularly applies to asbestosis, coal miners' pneumoconiosis, byssinosis, and occupational chronic obstructive pulmonary disease (COPD). Conversely, some diseases may be induced following quite low cumulative levels of exposure such as occupational asthma, berylliosis, mesothelioma, and asbestos-related benign pleural disease. Occupational asthma may develop when exposure

levels are well within the regulatory limits, which are rarely designed to prevent sensitization. Once sensitization has occurred, asthma exacerbations may occur following surprisingly small exposures, such as contact with a work colleague outside the workplace.

SPECIATION

This is the name given to a particular physical form of a substance, often a chemical. In several occupational situations, some forms give rise to disease whereas others do not. Good examples include nickel and chrome and the induction of lung cancer. The risk does not lie with refined metallic nickel and chromium, but with sulfide ores and primary smelting in the case of nickel, and with the reactive hexavalent form in the case of chromium. The main sources of hexavalent chromium are in primary refining, pigment manufacture, welding, and electroplating.

Platinum salts are prominent among the most potent causes of occupational asthma, but not all platinum salts are asthmagenic. Figure 3.1 shows the results of 20 years' surveillance of workers in a platinum refinery, separating those exposed to ammonium hexachlorplatinate in the refining process, those exposed to tetramine platinum dichloride in a catalyst manufacturing process on the same site, and those exposed to both [1]. There was no sensitization in those exposed to the tetramine platinum dichloride but substantial sensitization in those exposed to ammonium hexachlorplatinate.

Coal miners' pneumoconiosis is much more common in workers exposed to high-grade carbon coals than coals of lower grade. Similarly, asbestos fiber type has a profound influence on the risks for

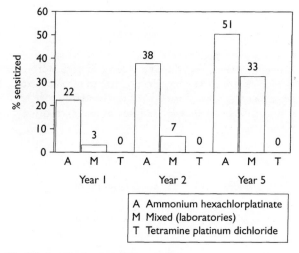

Fig. 3.1 Sensitization in a platinum refinery.

asbestos-induced disease. It appears likely that serpentine fibers (i.e. the curved ones of white asbestos, chrysotile) uncontaminated with amphibole fibers (the straight ones) pose little risk for mesothelioma or benign pleural disease compared with blue or brown amphibole asbestos (crocidolite, amosite), though in high cumulative doses may still cause asbestosis and lung cancer. Unfortunately some chrysotile deposits are contaminated with the amphibole, tremolite, thereby blurring this distinction. Furthermore, in many countries where asbestos has been imported there has been extensive mixing of the different fiber types before use. The occupational history may not, consequently, be able to distinguish serpentine asbestos from amphibole asbestos.

ALTERNATIVE/ADDITIONAL SOURCES OF EXPOSURE

It is occasionally important to evaluate alternative sources of potentially relevant exposure, since some workers are engaged in second (and perhaps more hazardous) jobs in addition to their main job, or they encounter hazardous exposures in the course of travel or domestic/recreational activity. Such exposures may not be admitted readily, particularly if encountered illegally or without tax declaration.

ADJUVANTS AND PROTECTIVES

Some diseases occur more readily when an adjuvant is present, for instance smoking enhances the risk of lung cancer due to asbestos, radon, and chrome. It also enhances the risk of sensitization to a number of agents causing occupational asthma, particularly platinum salts, laboratory animals, acid anhydrides,

and soya and green coffee beans, and it may enhance the effect of silica in causing occupational COPD. Other irritants, such as chlorine in platinum refineries and amines in soldering fluxes containing colophony, are thought to influence adversely the risk of occupational asthma in certain settings. There is also some evidence that simian virus 40 is implicated in the induction of some mesotheliomas.

Curiously, smoking appears to exert a protective effect against allergic alveolitis, and may similarly reduce the risk in some varieties of occupational asthma (e.g. that due to western red cedar). Although not strictly relevant to occupational lung disease, it additionally reduces the risk of pulmonary sarcoidosis, implying a broader inhibitory influence on immunologic responsiveness. Interference with the presentation of antigen by alveolar macrophages has been cited as a possible explanation.

Respiratory protective devices offer a more fundamental means of interfering with the presentation to the lungs of hazardous aerosols or gases, and the use of such equipment needs to be assessed during the occupational history, together with details concerning its maintenance and effectiveness. A crude but useful means of evaluation is to ask whether distinctive odors and tastes can still be detected during use.

EXPOSURE AT THE TIME OF DISEASE PRESENTATION

For diseases due to toxicity or sensitization, the occupational history should concentrate on exposures at the time of first symptoms and during the preceding 12–24 hours. With certain toxic agents the preceding few days (or even weeks to months, see Chapter 12) may also be relevant. There is a need to identify all toxic (or allergenic) agents present in the workplace to which the individual might be exposed. Relevant exposures are often indirect; for instance in electronics factories exposure to soldering flux fume (colophony) is often as high for those working beside solderers as for the solderers themselves.

It may also be important to identify previous exposures, since an apparent reaction on first exposure implies a toxic or irritant cause. Such a reaction may, however, be an effect of allergy and of sensitization following a previous symptomless period of exposure, and it may reflect an unusually heavy exposure – perhaps accidental. It may also be important to investigate the physical nature of the exposure, for instance the particle size (is it respirable?) and the temperature if the agent is heated. The one will influence the likelihood of the agent entering the lungs, and the other the chemical nature of any heat-degradation products.

ILLUSTRATIVE CASES

The following real cases pose common questions. They illustrate some of the problems that may be encountered in eliciting an occupational exposure history.

Case 1

Is this joiner at increased risk for asbestos-related disease, and if so which?

Apprentice joiner	1947–1952
Airforce airframe mechanic	1952–1955
Joiner and shopfitter	1955–1997
Retired sick	1997

His father made ball bearings; his mother (a housewife) did not wash her husband's overalls; there were no other adults in the childhood home.

- He occasionally sawed asbestos sheets by hand in his workshop to put above lights in cabinets.
- He had demolished the furnishings of about 30 shops including ceiling tiles of unknown content.
- He had repaired asbestos sheeting that backed on vitreolite glass in a chemist's shop seven times.

This case illustrates the difficulty in making a quantitative assessment of asbestos exposure. It is unlikely that the type of asbestos will be known by the individual. However, amosite and crocidolite were widely used for insulation in ceiling tiles in his neighborhood, and workers involved in demolition were often heavily exposed. His exposures were relatively short-lived and the cumulative level is unlikely to lead to asbestosis or lung cancer. There is a sufficient period of latency, and probably sufficient exposure, for him to develop mesothelioma or benign pleural disease, and in fact he did die from mesothelioma.

In situations like this, it is often helpful to measure asbestos fibers in bronchoalveolar fluid or lung tissue. In this particular case lung tissue was obtained at autopsy. Table 3.2 shows the results of scanning electron microscopic fiber counts. The amosite fiber count of over 1 million per gram of dried lung suggests from the reference values of the examining laboratory that there had been a clinically significant level of amosite exposure. There are substantial differences in the reference ranges for asbestos fiber counts depending on the

Table 3.2 Lung fiber count (scanning electron microscopy) per gram of dried lung

Fibre	Millions of fibers/g
Total	6.89
Crocidolite (blue)	0.33
Tremolite	0.08
Amosite (brown)	1.88
Chrysotile (white)	0
Anthophyllite	0
Mullite	4.6

laboratory and method, but some standardization has been developed in Europe [2]. The fiber count supports the opinion that this mesothelioma was due to asbestos exposure. Obtaining fiber counts from the same laboratory helps the clinician refine his/her estimates of exposure based on the history.

Case 2

What are the main risks of respiratory disease for this doctor?

Building laborer, Kuruman, South Africa	1962–1963
Microbiology technician, South Africa	1963 (2 months)
Medical school, London	1963–1969
Junior doctor (general medicine and infectious diseases)	1969–1975
Lecturer (clinical immunology)	1975–1980
Chest physician	1980–now

The main risk will be of tuberculosis, particularly while working in a microbiology laboratory in South Africa in the 1960s and as a respiratory physician for many years (see Chapter 16). The risk of tuberculosis, at least in the UK, is about double that of social class and race-matched workers outside the healthcare sector, despite the use of BCG vaccination [3]. The risk in the unvaccinated is about threefold higher. Respiratory physicians are also commonly exposed to latex and glutaraldehyde, both common causes of occupational asthma. Building laborers particularly around Kuruman in South Africa would have been exposed to crocidolite asbestos which was mined in the local hills.

Case 3

This lady has airflow obstruction and wonders whether she has byssinosis.

Chemist shop assistant	1959 (6 months)
Shoe machinist	1959–1961
Cotton winder (twilight shift)	1967–1969
Office cleaner	1969–1974
Cotton winder	1974–1978
Shoe machinist	1978–1984
Table hand (gluing shoes)	1984–1996
Sorter (clothes manufacture)	1996–1999

Working in cotton mills as a winder raises the possibility of byssinosis. This is a disease of high exposure over a long period of time. Exposure is usually measured as total dust less fly. The risk of byssinosis is thought to be <5% when the total exposure is 40–80 [mg/m^3] yr, and <1% at <28 [mg/m^3] yr. Table 3.3 illustrates low, average, and high levels of exposures in UK cotton mills. Taking the worst case scenario (a waste cotton mill), the

Table 3.3 Typical personal exposures to cotton less fly (mg/m³)

	Exposure conditions		
	Best	Average	Waste mill
Carding	0.8	5	75
Winding	0.1	1	2.5
Spinning	0.4	3	? 40

cumulative exposure would be 15 [mg/m³] yr. This is well below the level at which there is a 1% risk of byssinosis. Byssinosis is therefore an unlikely cause for her airflow obstruction. Shoe manufacturers are exposed to a number of agents capable of causing asthma including: isocyanates from molded soles; colophony in hot melted adhesives; latex, acrylics, and epoxy curing agents in adhesives; casein used in leather treatment; and, perhaps, leather dust itself.

Case 4

This man worked for much of his life in an iron foundry. What is the main respiratory hazard to which he will have been exposed, and for which diseases does this pose some risk?

Wheelbarrow assembly	1963–1969
Iron casting shakeout, by hand (foundry)	1969–1972
Foundry shakeout, mechanical bed operator	1972–1998

For many years he removed iron castings from molds which were made of silica sand. He would probably have sustained exposure also to the heated derivatives of silica (tridymite and crystobalite). If unprotected, he would now be at some risk of silicosis, tuberculosis, and possibly lung cancer. Respirable silica exposure can also lead to occupational COPD, systemic vasculitis, focal glomerulonephritis and renal tubular dysfunction, and (in huge doses) acute alveolar proteinosis (very unlikely from the above history). If the casting contained cores (inserts in the mold of greater robustness than the external shell that leave hollow volumes in the casting, e.g. for an engine block), the core binding resins could pose a risk for occupational asthma. The cold box system contains the isocyanate MDI (diphenylmethane diisocyanate), the hot box system phenol formaldehyde or furanes.

Case 5

This 62-year-old lady developed asthma in 1998. What is the most likely cause, and to which other diseases might this pose some risk?

Turner of bolts (dry)	1951–1953
Warehouse packer	1953–1969
Gas welder	1969–1975
Packer of electronics	1975–1977
Gas welder	1977–1978
Stellite welder of car valves (depositing cobalt powder onto valve stems)	1978–1999

She had had exposure to welding fumes which are implicated in chronic bronchitis and occasionally in asthma but had no symptoms at the time. Her symptoms began while she worked as a stellite welder. Stellite contains cobalt and is a potent cause of asthma. It may also cause a number of other diseases including giant cell interstitial pneumonitis (hard metal disease), contact dermatitis, cardiomyopathy, polycythemia and goiter.

REFERENCES

1. Linnett PJ, Hughes EG. 20 years of medical surveillance on exposure to allergenic and non-allergenic platinum compounds: the importance of chemical speciation. *Occ Environ Med* 1999; 56: 191–196.

2. De Vuyst P, Karjalainen A, Dumortier P *et al.* Guidelines for mineral fibre analyses in biological samples: report of the ERS Working Group. European Respiratory Society. *Eur Respir J* 1998; 11(6): 1416–1426.

3. Meredith SK, Watson JM, Citron KM *et al.* Are healthcare workers in England and Wales at increased risk of tuberculosis? *BMJ* 1996; 313(7056): 522–552.

DISORDERS OF THE AIRWAYS, PARENCHYMA, AND PLEURA

4 ASTHMA

David J. Hendrick and P. Sherwood Burge

BACKGROUND

Although disabling respiratory symptoms attributable to a variety of occupational settings have been recognized for centuries, particularly through the pioneering work of Ramazzini and Paracelsus, it was not until the 20th century that investigatory techniques acquired the sophistication to distinguish respiratory disorders arising primarily in the airways from those arising primarily in the lung parenchyma. The definition of asthma, the elucidation of its clinical characteristics and pathogenic mechanisms, and the evolution of strategies for its recognition, management, and prevention have been comparatively recent events. The realization that asthma may arise as a direct consequence of inhaled occupational agents has been the focus of particular attention over the last two to three decades, and most current knowledge has been obtained during this period.

Definitions

Asthma is a disease of the intrathoracic airways which is characterized, and often defined, by (1) its means of clinical expression (diffuse airway obstruction which varies in degree over time within the affected individual), and (2) its underlying pathogenic basis (a state of enhanced airway responsiveness). There is an inherent tendency for the bronchi to constrict in response to what may be a wide variety of stimuli, both specific and non-specific.

Occupational asthma is asthma caused by exposure to agents encountered primarily (and usually exclusively) in the working environment. Two distinct mechanisms are recognized, though the precise pathogenic pathways have yet to be clarified. For the first, which accounts for the great majority of cases, hypersensitivity mechanisms appear responsible; for the second, acute toxicity is the initiating event, generally a consequence of industrial accidents involving respiratory exposure to toxic chemicals.

Asthma is, of course, a common disorder in the population at large, and individuals with preexisting asthma (or previous asthma) are probably at increased risk of developing worsening asthma (or recurrent asthma) through either of these mechanisms as a consequence of new exposures in the workplace. The choice of a suitable diagnostic label for this situation has provoked controversy; in effect the individual then has occupational asthma as well as non-occupational asthma (or previous non-occupational asthma). The consequences may be equally great as in those with no preexisting asthma.

When new regulations were enacted in the UK for state compensation (Department of Health and Social Security Act 1975), occupational asthma was defined as 'asthma whose primary cause is a sensitizing agent inhaled at work'. The descriptive text added that 'there is usually a preliminary period ranging from days to years before the onset of symptoms, which occur during the working week and often remit during absence from work. Removal from exposure to the sensitizing agent may lead to remission of asthma, although sensitization can be permanent'. Before the introduction of this legislation, state compensation was already payable for respiratory disease arising from industrial accidents, and so the later recognition that asthma could also arise as a consequence of accidents and the inhalation of toxic agents did not require any further revision of the state compensation laws.

Some like to place qualifications on the diagnosis of occupational asthma. For example, supporting evidence of hypersensitivity may be required from specific immunoglobulin E (IgE) antibody responses, in contrast to hypersensitivity being presumed. Presumption is common if there is an initial asymptomatic latency period before the development of asthma without any apparent increase in occupational exposure level, the level itself having no obvious adverse effect in other asthmatic subjects.

A further issue is that of worsening asthmatic symptoms when an individual with preexisting asthma becomes exposed to airborne irritants in the workplace, such as noxious gases or fumes, smoke, or cold dry air. If a similar effect is to be expected in any asthmatic subject, the effect can be considered 'non-specific'; the exposure is not likely to cause asthma nor to worsen airway responsiveness, and so is not a true cause of occupational asthma. The phenomenon is commonly identified as work-aggravated asthma. It is important to distinguish asthma that is in some way 'work-related' (asthma of any cause which is more symptomatic in the workplace) from asthma that is specifically 'occupational' (asthma caused by an agent encountered at work).

Clinical expression

It is important to realize that airway responsiveness varies in level from subject to subject over a considerable range, and that it can be quantified throughout the population at large. Its distribution (like that of blood pressure and most biologic parameters) is unimodal, and it follows the common biologic pattern of a 'bell-shaped' curve. The tail in which responsiveness is most marked gives rise to asthma, just as the tail in which blood pressure is most marked gives rise to the adverse effects of hypertension, but the adjacent segment implies vulnerability and the opposite tail implies comparative impunity. It is misleading, therefore, to think of asthmatic subjects and non-asthmatic subjects being fundamentally different because of the present or absence of airway hyperresponsiveness; the issue, rather, is whether an individual's level of airway responsiveness is sufficiently high to make

clinically meaningful bronchoconstriction likely when there are appropriate extrinsic or intrinsic provoking stimuli.

Whether the resulting degree of bronchoconstriction is perceived to be distressing (or is perceived at all), depends not only on the level of airway responsiveness, the degree of sensitization, and the strength of provocative stimuli, but on psychological factors within the affected individual. This additional modifying influence adds an important further level of complexity and variability, since at all levels of asthmatic severity as defined physiologically, there will be a wide spectrum of perceived disability. This is particularly so in asthma of occupational origin because of resentment, even anger, over the possible liability and negligence of a third party (the employer), and because of the possibility of compensation.

Furthermore, longstanding asthma (particularly that of severe degree) is commonly associated with airway obstruction which has a lost or reduced capability for reversal. Thus obstruction may become increasingly fixed; as it progresses it may come to simulate physiologically chronic obstructive pulmonary disease (COPD). Indeed some describe asthma as one of the causes of COPD.

Mechanisms

Clear differences in the patterns of evolution make it useful to distinguish occupational asthma arising through presumed hypersensitivity pathways from that arising more obviously through toxic mechanisms. For both, individual susceptibility plays an important role since in general only a minority of similarly exposed workers actually develop disease.

Hypersensitivity

For some 90–95% of all cases of occupational asthma there is a latent ('sensitizing') period of exposure to everyday concentrations of the inducing agent in the workplace which appears to have no adverse clinical effect in either the affected subject or fellow workmates sharing the same occupational environment. This latency may extend for weeks to years, but is often less than 2 years. In exceptional cases it may be as short as a few days but there are many incidences where longer latent intervals are recorded; for instance, in a prospective flour and bakery study, the mean latency for apparent new incident cases was 8.8 years with most starting after more than 5 years exposure [1]. Once sensitization has occurred, ongoing exposures at similar concentrations predictably cause asthmatic reactions and increases in the background level of airway responsiveness.

Although much is known concerning the precise mechanisms underlying asthma of allergic origin in general, many of the occupational agents that cause asthma are reactive chemicals of low molecular weight against which immunologic mechanisms of hypersensitivity cannot readily be demonstrated. They are assumed to react with body proteins, thereby producing antigenic hapten–protein complexes, but convincing evidence for this has been shown only for a few. Furthermore, when antibody responses have been demonstrable, whether against hapten–protein conjugates or high-molecular-weight allergens of more natural origin, they have not always been closely correlated with disease. They may consequently be a reflection of exposure and subsequent immunization rather than of occupational asthma, but they nevertheless provide useful supporting evidence that immunologic hypersensitivity pathways, particularly those involving IgE, play a role in pathogenesis.

Toxicity

In 1985 it was reported that exposures causing acute, even life-threatening, toxicity of the lower respiratory tract could lead directly to asthma [2]. The exposures, in 10 subjects, involved a variety of irritant chemicals, fumes, and smoke, which were encountered in high concentration as a consequence of accidents or inadequate ventilation in confined environments. Symptoms began within a matter of minutes or hours and persisted for at least 3 months (and in most for more than a year). The authors noted that similar outcomes had been recorded previously following inhalation accidents involving industrial chemicals.

Many other reports have followed [3–5]. The causal agents have proved to be non-specific in that any agent with sufficient toxic potential which is inhaled in sufficient dose may induce asthma in this way. Airway obstruction is commonly a feature of the initial toxic response, especially to reactive agents of high or moderate solubility which tend to affect the airway mucosa more than the lung parenchyma. Wheezing and high levels of airway responsiveness become evident as the toxic response subsides, and the victim is left with asthma that persists for months or years, even indefinitely. The levels of exposure that produce such a response are necessarily accidental in nature, and most occur in working rather than domestic environments, simply because such agents are rarely used domestically in sufficient quantity.

In the initial report the phenomenon was called the reactive airways dysfunction syndrome (RADS). Although RADS is a commendably brief and useful term, it may disguise the fundamentally asthmatic nature of the disease. Perhaps as a consequence an alternative term, 'irritant-induced asthma', has become popular over recent years. This too may create a problem since irritancy implies a much less disruptive initial event, and it is not yet clear whether inflammatory insults of minor or mild degree have true asthmagenic potential. The issue is complicated because the preexisting level of airway responsiveness is likely to be of considerable relevance. Subjects who already have levels of airway responsiveness close to the asthmatic range may require a much lesser 'toxic' insult to develop asthma than subjects with more average levels. Furthermore, it is logical to ask whether repeated daily exposures to low (i.e. truly 'irritant') levels of a potentially toxic agent might produce the same cumulative effect over weeks, months, or years as would a single overwhelming and life-threatening exposure. Some evidence favoring such a cumulative mechanism has recently been published [5,6]. This might more logically be called 'irritant-induced asthma' or 'irritant asthma', but the pathogenic pathways may prove to be fundamentally the same as those underlying RADS. Until these issues are resolved, this unfortunate dilemma over nomenclature will remain.

The possibility that frequently repeated irritant exposures might cumulatively increase airway responsiveness by stepwise degrees, which are individually unrecognizable, to a level at which active asthma becomes likely would of course simulate the latent period of asthma arising through hypersensitivity mechanisms. Furthermore, once there is a high level of airway responsiveness, ongoing 'irritant' exposures could provoke asthmatic reactions, again simulating asthma of hypersensitivity origin. They should, however, provoke similar reactions in any asthmatic subject with a similar level of airway responsiveness, irrespective of any hypersensitivity, and this should allow 'irritant' and hypersensitivity pathways to be distinguished from each other. The issue illustrates the point that the precise mechanisms underlying many, if not most, cases of occupational asthma are yet to be fully clarified.

It has additionally been postulated that some cases of occupational asthma arise through what have been termed 'idiosyncratic' mechanisms (like, for example, the effect of aspirin, other non-steroidal anti-inflammatory drugs, and alcoholic beverages), or pharmacological mechanisms (perhaps beta-adrenergic blockade), but the evidence to date has not been fully persuasive, and at present only the hypersensitivity and toxic/irritant mechanisms are useful as a means of classification. The 'idiosyncratic' effect of aspirin appears actually to be pharmacologic in nature, and a consequence of cyclooxygenase inhibition and shunting in the lipoxygenase pathway.

Inducers and triggers

Some environmental agents may both increase the level of airway responsiveness (and so cause asthma) and provoke directly asthmatic reactions. By contrast others may differentially increase airway responsiveness without necessarily exerting much direct influence on bronchoconstriction (for example, ozone and viruses infecting the upper respiratory tract), or provoke asthmatic reactions without having any apparent adverse effect on airway responsiveness (for example, cold or dry air, and gases or dusts which are irritating in nature but not toxic). There may consequently be benefit in distinguishing the concept of *inducing* asthma (increasing airway responsiveness) from that of *triggering* asthmatic reactions, and hence of identifying whether particular environmental or occupational agents are asthma inducers, asthma triggers, or both. Alternative terms which have been used to the same purpose are 'inciters' and 'provokers', respectively.

In general, the inducers which exert their effects by presumed hypersensitivity mechanisms are also triggers, and the demonstration of both properties is helpful in confirming their etiological role in occupational asthma. However, many occupational agents have irritating but not inducing properties at the exposure levels generally encountered in the workplace, and so these commonly act non-specifically as asthma triggers in subjects who are already asthmatic, without being true inducers of occupational asthma. Some may nevertheless have the potential to induce asthma if inhaled in toxic doses through the mechanism underlying RADS.

Interactions

A more challenging concept than distinguishing the induction of occupational asthma from the triggering (or worsening) of asthmatic symptoms at work, is that either event could be the consequence of both occupational and non-occupational factors. Thus the level of airway responsiveness may, for example, rise to within the asthmatic range only because of the combined or interactive effects of domestic exposure to pet allergens, occupational exposure to an industrial asthma inducer, and an intercurrent viral infection. Furthermore, asthma arising through occupational factors (i.e. true occupational asthma) may produce its most obvious symptoms only when the affected worker encounters strong non-specific stimuli away from work (e.g. he plays football in cold environments). Conversely, asthma of non-occupational origin may be most troublesome at work if non-specific triggers are most prevalent there (e.g. exercise, cold air, irritant dusts/fumes).

Epidemiology

The available sources of data are reviewed in Chapter 2. The reported incidence of occupational asthma varies widely, depending on the criteria for entry to the respective registers. Estimates from statutory notification schemes, compensation registers, and voluntary surveillance schemes, as well as from general population surveys, suggest that 5–15% of asthma beginning in adult life is attributable to work. Many estimates center around 9%, implying that, when asthma arises for the first time in a working adult, the background odds favoring an occupational cause over a non-occupational cause are crudely of the order 1 in 10.

This is consistent in Britain with the not implausible assumption that asthma develops in 2–3% of the general adult population (i.e. a mean of 333–500 per million per year if adult life averages 60 years), and with the estimate from SWORD project data (Surveillance of Work-related and Occupational Respiratory Disease) that about 40 cases of occupational asthma arise in Britain each year per million employed workers (Chapter 2) [7–10]. The odds for an occupation cause versus a non-occupational cause (observed: expected) would be of the order 1 in 7–12 if 40 occupational cases are included among the 333–500 each year (1 in 8–12 if they are not).

Not all emerging cases of occupational asthma are identified by the SWORD project, and so the reported total may be an underestimate. There may also be a proportion of false-positive reports, since the diagnostic criteria behind each SWORD report are not strict. The reporting physician is simply asked to identify a case if he or she considers the diagnosis to be more likely than not. Diagnostic error is not, however, likely to lead to an exaggeration of the true total in Britain, and it has been suggested that the true incidence may be two- or even threefold greater than that suggested by SWORD. In Finland, for example, where the capture of incident cases is likely to be more complete and where diagnostic error is minimized by the extensive use of inhalation provocation tests, the figure is as high as 175 per million per year. However, much of this is a consequence of the high proportion of the population engaged in farming, and the great majority of reporting schemes discussed at length in Chapter 2 indicate a more conservative incidence of 25–100 per million per year.

The SWORD project has usefully considered in addition the incidence of reported new cases of occupational asthma within specific working groups in which there are identified and particular occupational exposures. For example, in spray painters, who generally use two-part isocyanate or epoxy-resin paints, the average incidence of occupational asthma from 1992 to 1997 was 1464 cases per million per year, some 38-fold more than the average incidence of occupational asthma among all employed workers. Thus, in the case of spray painters developing asthma in adult life, the background odds would favor an occupational cause over a coincidental cause. Knowledge of inducing agents within particular working environments and the average incidence of occupational asthma in such environments therefore provides an initial valuable step for estimating the probability of an occupational cause irrespective of the particular clinical features of an individual case. The latter then add further information which allows the clinician to estimate the relative probabilities, if full investigation of the individual proves to be impractical. Table 2.3 of Chapter 2 provides data for all occupational settings in which the relative risk for developing occupational asthma exceeds the average risk.

Causal agents and specific types

A very large number of agents have been reported as causes of occupational asthma, and many of them are included in Table 4.1. It is always difficult to know what degree of proof is required for listing. Sometimes the evidence for causation is immunologic, but cross-reacting antibodies occur which may lead to spurious attribution. Some of the evidence comes from workplace challenges where the complete constituents of the exposure are rarely known, and some comes from specific challenges in the laboratory which have not always been adequately controlled. Thus some asthmatic 'responses' might have occurred even without the challenge exposure, and some might have occurred in any asthmatic subject regardless of any prior occupational sensitization. Sometimes the evidence is epidemiological without specific identification of a causal agent, but where significant disease is strongly associated with the workplace environment. For the agents included in Table 4.1 there has been at least one published report; the evidence suggests the agent is a plausible cause of occupational asthma, but not necessarily a definite cause.

There are more biologic agents than low-molecular-weight chemicals on the list, as the arguments about irritancy/toxicity as opposed to sensitization pose less of a problem with biological agents.

Table 4.1 Reported causes of occupational asthma

Acid anhydrides
Benzophenone tetracarboxylic dianhydride
Cyclohexylphthalate (meat wrapper)
Diglycidyl ether bisphenol A
Dioctyl phthalate
Hexahydrophthalic anhydride
Himic anhydride
Maleic anhydride
Methyltetrachlorphthalic anhydride
Methyltetrahydrophthalic anhydride
Phthalic anhydride
Pyromellitic anhydride
Tetrachlorphthalic anhydride
Trimellitic anhydride

Adhesives
Acrylics
Alkyl cyanoacrylate
Cyanoacrylate
Ethylcyanoacrylate
Ethylene methacrylic acid copolymer
Hexapropylacrylate
Isobutylmethacrylate
Methylcyanoacrylate
Methylmethacrylate
Triethylenedimethylacrylate
Trihydroxymethylpropyltriacrylate

Isocyanates
HDI (hexamethylene diisocyanate)
NDI (naphthylene diisocyanate)
TDI (toluene diisocyanate)
TDI prepolymer
MDI (diphenylmethane diisocyanate)
MDI prepolymer
PPI (polymethylene polyphenylisocyanate)

Amines
4-Amino-4-metoxydiphenylamine
Chloramine
Diaminodiphenylmethane (in EPO60)
Dichloramine
Dimethyl ethanolamine
3-(Dimethylamino)propylamine (epoxy)
EPO 60 (polyamine, 4-4-diaminodiphenylmethane +
    isophoronediamine + tetraethylenepentamine)
Epoxy polyamide floor sealant (trimethyl-1,
    6-hexanediamine and isophorone diamine)
Ethylenediamine (drugs, color developer, plastics)
Isophoronediamine (floor sealant)
N-Methylmorpholine (polyurethane production)
Paraphenylene diamine (fur)
Piperazine
Triethylene tetramine
Trimethyl-1, 6-hexanediamine (floor sealant)

continued

Table 4.1 Reported causes of occupational asthma (*contd.*)

Animals (excluding birds and fish)
Astrakhan
Bats
  Black bat
  Red hairy bat
Bovine
  Caseine (leather spray)
  Cow dander
  Cow urine
  Lactalbumin (food aerosol)
  Serum albumin (laboratory)
  Suprarenal extract
  Testes extract
Cat
Deer
Fox
Frog brain (*Rana catesbieana*)
Fur (furrier)
Guinea pig
Horse
Ivory
Marten
Mink
Monkey
  Capuchin, Cotton-Top Tamarin
  Mastomys natualensis
Mouse
Pig
Rabbit
Rat
Reindeer
Sausage dust
Sheep (lamb)
Skunk
Tooth enamel
Wool dust

Arthropods
Antheraea (wild silk moth on wild silk)
Arrowhead scales, *Unapsis yanonensis* Kuwana (on
  mandarin oranges)
Blowfly (*Lucilia cuprina*)
Caddis fly
Calandra granaria (baker)
Callifora erythrocephala larvae (fish bait)
Carmine (*Coccus cactus*)
Chironomus larvae (fishfood)
Chironomus thumii thumii
Cricket (*Acheta domestica*)
Culex larvae (fishfood)
Daphnia (fishfood)
Dermestid beetle (Coleoptera) (museum curator)
Drosophila melanogaster
Echinodorus plasmosus larvae (mosquito larvae, fish bait)
Ephestia kuhniella (baker)
Galleria mellonella (beemoth, fish bait)
Honeybee (processor)
Hoya (sea squirt in oyster shuckers)
Lesser mealworm (*Alphitobius diaperinus* Panzer)

Locusta migratoria
Lucilia caesar (fish bait)
Marphysa sanguinea (marine worm, fishbait)
Mexican bean weevil (*Zabrotes subfasciatus* Boh)
Musca carnaria (fly)
Musca domestica maggot (fish bait)
Mushroom fly
New Mexico range moth (farmer, entomologist)
  (*Hemileuca oliviae* Cockerell)
Psychoda (sewage filter fly)
Schistocerca gregaria
Screw worm fly (*Chrysomya bezziana*) (pilot)
Sericin (silkworm) (hairdresser)
Shellac
Sitophilus granarius
Sitotroga cerealla (baker)
Tenebrio molitor
Tenebroides mauritanicus
Tribolium castaneum (baker)
Tussock moth (on Douglas fir)

Biotechnology
Aspergillus niger
Candida tropicalis
Methylomonas methanolica
Paecillomyces varioti
Pruteen

Birds
Chicken
  Egg protein
Duck
Pheasant
Turkey

Chemicals (other than acid anhydrides, adhesives,
amines, disinfectants/preservatives, irritants, and plastics)
Acids (hydrochloric, hydrofluoric, nitric, perchloric, or
  sulphuric)
Azodicarbonamide
Furanes (furfuryl alcohol); (coremaker)
Permanent wave solution
Persulphate (bleach)
Sodium iso-nonanoyl oxybenzene sulphonate (detergent)

Corals and sponges
Ancorina alata
Dysidea defigilis
Dysidea herbacea
Litophyton sp.
Lobophytum denticulatum
Phyllospongia sp.
Spongia sp.
Stellata conulosa

Crustacea, worms, etc.
Clam
Clams liver

continued

Table 4.1 Reported causes of occupational asthma (*contd.*)

Corals and sponges(*contd.*)
Eisenia foetida (fish bait) earthworm
King crab
Lobster
Marphysa sanguinea (fish bait)
Mussel
Oysters
   Styela plicata
   Styela clava
   Ciona intestinalis
Pearl shell
   Mother of pearl
Prawn unspecified
Prawn (*Nephrops norwegicus*)
Red soft coral (fisherman)
Sea snails (button maker)
Sea squirt (*Hoya*), Ascidiacea
Shrimp (brineshrimp, fishfood) (*Penaeus setifecus boding*)
Wate
Snow crab

Disinfectants and preservatives
Benzalkonium chloride
Chloramine T (sodium tosylchloramide)
Chlorhexidine, hexachlorophene
Chlorguanide
Denatonium benzoate (in methylated spirits, aftershave,
   gasoline, antifreeze, etc.)
Ethylene oxide
Formaldehyde
Glutaraldehyde
Isothiazolinones
Monochloramine (baker)
Phenylmercuric propionate (for laundry)
Sulphonechloramides, halazone
Tetrachlorisophthalonitrile (greenhouse fungicide)
Tributyl tin (fungicide)
X-ray developer

Drugs
Adrenocorticotrophic hormone (ACTH)
Adipic acid (binder)
Alginate
Alpha methyl dopa
Aminophylline
Amoxacillin
Ampicillin
Amprolium hydrochloride (poultry feed)
Benzodiazepine intermediate
Benzyl penicillin
Captafol (fungicide)
Carbochromine
Cefradine
Ceftazidime
Cephalexin disolvate
Cephalosporamic acid (7-amino)
Cimetidine
Clometocillin
Dichloramine

Enfluorane (anesthetist)
Ethylenediame
Fluorocarbons
Glycyl compound (salbutamol intermediate)
Gonadotrophin
Hydralazine
Hydroquinone
Insecticide (Mortein pressure pak)
Ipecacuanha
Isoniazid
Mercury (in amalgum?)
Methionine
Pancreatin (pharmacist)
Penicillamine (manufacturer)
6-Amino-penicillanic acid
Phenylglycine acid chloride (ampicillin sidechain)
Phosdrin (organophosphorus)
Piperazine
Pituitary snuff
Podophyllin
Potassium bromate (baker)
Psyllium (ispaghula)
Rose hips (in vitamin C)
Senna
Spiromycin
Sulphathiazole (leather impregnation spray)
Tetracycline
Virginiamycin

Dyes
Carmine Cochineal
Chicago acid
Cibachrome brilliant scarlet
Diazonium chloride (in copy paper)
Diazonium tetrafluoroborate
Drimaren brilliant blue
Drimaren brilliant yellow
Electro cardiogram G ink, methylene blue
Henna
Lanasol yellow 4G
Levafix marinblau
Levafix black
Levafix brilliant blue
Levafix brilliant yellow
Patent blau (triarylmethane dye, green)
Ramazol black GF
Ramazol brilliant orange FR
Ramazol brilliant yellow 4GL
Ramazol Gold Gelb (gold yellow) RNL
Ramazol marine blue BB
Ramazol Schwarz (black) B
Rifazol black GR
Rifazol orange 3R
Rifafix yellow 3RN

Fish
Cod
Cuttlefish

continued

Table 4.1 Reported causes of occupational asthma (*contd.*)

Fish (contd.)
Eel
Plaice
Salmon
Sardine
Tunny

Fuels and explosives
Boiler cleaners (vanadium pentoxide)
Diesel
Gasoline
Mesquit charcoal
Oil mists
Pulverized fuel ash
Tetrazine
Woodchips, fuel

Irritants
Chlorine
Sulfur dioxide
Histamine and methacholine
Hydrogen fluoride

Jointing agents
Aluminium tetrafluoride
Amine flux activators (non-corrosive electronic
   soldering)
Aminoethylethanolamine
Ammonium chloride
Colophony
Dicumyl peroxide (for polyethylene)
Phosphorus hexate (Acqua-core)
Polyether alcohol-polypropylene glycol
Tall oil
Zinc chloride

Metals
Aluminum fluoride
Chrome (welding)
   Ammonium bichromate
   Bichromate (cement)
   Zinc chromate
Cobalt (hard metal)
Manganese (miner)
Nickel
Palladium
Platinum
   Ammonium hexachlorplatinate
   Ammonium tetrachlorplatinite
   Chlorplatinic acid
Vanadium pentoxide
Zinc

Microorganisms
Alternaria (baker, wood trimmer)
Aphanocladium album (harvest asthma)
Aspergillus clavatus (malting)
Aspergillus flavus (mouldy weaving warps)
Aspergillus fumigatus (tobacco alveolitis)

Aspergillus glaucus (mushroom)
Aspergillus niger (biotechnology)
Aureobasidium pullulans (humidifier)
Bacillus subtilis
Botrytis cinerea (grapes)
Conisporum sp.
Cryptostroma corticale
Dental plaque
Dictyostelium discoideum
Didymella exitialis
Flavobacterium (humidifier)
Lycopodium powder (dental technician)
Merulius lacrymans
Mucor sp. (sawmill alveolitis)
Neurospora (plywood mold)
Oyster mushroom (*Pleurotus ostreatus, P. florida*)
Paecillomyces bacillosporus (harvest asthma)
Paecillomyces varioti
Penicillium casei (greenhouse, cheese)
Penicillium expansus
Penicillium frequentans (cork)
Penicillium nodatum (fruit mold)
Penicillium sp. (oak bark) (humidifier)
Rhizopus sp. (sawmill)
Saccharomonospora viridis (logger)
Scopulariopsis brevicaulis (tobacco mold)
Sewage sludge
Streptomyces albus (fertilizer)
Thermoactinomyces sacchari
Trichoderma koningii
Trichosporon cutaneum
Verticillium lecanii (harvest asthma)

Plants (excluding spices)
Allium cepa seed
Baby's breath (*Gypsophilia paniculata*)
Banana (cook)
Barley
Begonia pollen
Buckwheat (noodle cook)
Carob bean flour
Castor bean (*Ricinus communis*, Euphorbiacae)
   cinnaron and pacific
Castor oil
Celery
Chick pea
Chicory (*Cichorium intybus*)
Coconut oil
Cotton
Cyclamen pollen
Entada gigas (cocoon seeds strung for jewelry)
Epoxidized soybean oil (meat-wrapping labels)
Esparto grass (*Stipa tenacissima*) plasterer
Euphorbia fulgens Karw (florist)
Flax
   Linseed oil
Ginseng (Brazil), *Pfaffia paniculata*
Glomosa pollen

continued

Table 4.1 Reported causes of occupational asthma (*contd.*)

Plants (excluding spices) (*contd.*)
Gluten hydrolysate
Grape vine pollen
Grass pollen (technician)
Green coffee beans
Guar gum (insulator in rubber cables, paper additive, carpet dye adhesive)
Gum arabic (gum acacia)
Gum tragacanth
Hay
Henna
Karaya gum (Indian gum)
Latex
Lathyrus sativus flour
Lentil
Lily pollen
Limonium tataricum
Maiko (*Amorphophalus konjac* root)
Mercuralia annua pollen
Mushrooms
  Basidiomycete (*Pleurotus cornucopiae, Pleurotus florida, Pleurotus ostreatus*)
  Shiitake (*Lentinus edodes* spores, *Cortinellus shiitake* spores)
Narcissus
Oilseed rape
Peanut
Pectin
Phortensis bedulis
Pokeroot (pharmacist)
Potato
Potato riddler
Rape pollen
Refuse plant sorters
Rhubarb (pharmacist)
Rice
Rye
Seaweed
Sesame seed (baker)
Sisal hemp
Soya
Swiss chard
Strawberry (? pollen)
Sugar beet pollen
Sunflower pollen
Tamarind seed
Thatch (New Guinea)
Tea
  Dog rose
  Gruzyan
  Indian
  Sage
Tobacco
Vetch (*Vicia sativa*, legume crop)
Voacana africana seed (pharmaceutical)
Wheat flour

Plastics
Burning plastic (fireman)

Polyethylene
Polyvinyl chloride
Polyvinyl pyrrolidone (hair spray)

Spices
Caraway
Chilli
Cinnamon
Coriander
Curry
Garlic
Ginger
Juniper oil
Mace
Onion
Oregano (wild marjoram in pizza cook)
Paprika
Parsley

Storage mites
Acarus farris
Acarus siro
Dermatophagoides pteronyssinus (librarian)
Lepidoglyphus destructor
Northern fowl mite
Panonychus ulmi (Koch) (apple mite)
Pediculoides ventricosus (wheat mite)
Spider mite (*Tetranychus urticae* Koch)
Tyrophagus farinae (baker)
Tyrophagus longior
Tyrophagus putrescentae (Glycyphagus)

Woods
Abiruana
African zebrawood (microberlinia)
Ash
Beech
Boxwood (jeweler)
Cabreuva (*Myrocarpus fastigiatus* Fr. All.)
Californian redwood (*Sequoia semipervirens*)
Carbonless paper (alkylphenol novalac resin)
Cedar of Labanon (*Cedra lebani*)
Cedar, unspecified
Cinnamon (*Cinnamonum zeylanicum*)
Cocabolla (*Dalbergia retusa*, rosewood)
Congo hardwood
Cork
Danta or Kotibe (*Nesorgordonia papaverifera*)
Eastern white cedar (*Thuja occidentalis*)
Ebony (*Diospyros crassiflora*)
Ho (Mongolia hypoleuca sieb zucc)
Iroko
Kejaat (*Pterocarpus anglolensis*)
Koto
Latex
Mahogany
Makore
Mansonia (*Sterculiacea altissima*)

continued

Table 4.1 Reported causes of occupational asthma (*contd.*)

Woods (*contd.*)	Rimu (*Dacrydidium cupressinum*) (podocarpic acid)
Maple (bark mold)	Ryobu (*Clethara barbinervis*)
Mukali (*Aningeria robusta*)	South African boxwood (*Gonioma kamassi*)
Mulberry	Spindle tree (*Euonymus europaeus*)
Oak (bark mold)	Tanganyika aningre
Oak wood	Theater hat and mask
Obeche (African maple) ? *Triplochiton scleroxlon*,	Walnut, central American (*Juglans clanchana*)
Samba, Wawa	Weeping fig
Orangewood	Western red cedar (*Thuja plicata*)
Palisander (rosewood, *Dalbergia nigra*)	Zelkova tree (Japan)
Paper dust	
Pine	**Solvents**
Pine deodorant, turpentine	Perchlorethylene
Quillaja bark (soapbark, saponin)	Styrene
Ramin (*Gonystylus bancanus*)	

Aldehydes and other sterilizing agents [11]

Formaldehyde is widely used in industry, as an adhesive in wood products, and as a sterilizing agent; a series of reports has indited it as a cause of occupational asthma [12–14]. Much of the literature concerns the low levels of exposure that are present in buildings where particle board or insulating foam containing urea-formaldehyde resins have been used. The evidence for asthma from this source is unconvincing [15], but at higher levels of exposure a clear risk has been confirmed by inhalation challenge studies [13,16]. Reports of occupational asthma due to glutaraldehyde have shown a considerable increase in number over the last 10 years, and it is now one of the more commonly recognized causes, despite the very limited number of exposed workers [17]. Its main use is as a cold sterilizing agent, particularly suitable for endoscope sterilization. Lower levels of glutaraldehyde are present in radiographic dark room fumes [17], where occasional cases have been seen. Specific IgE antibodies to glutaraldehyde–albumin conjugates were found in 29% of cases in one study [18]. There is some cross-reactivity with formaldehyde in bronchial provocation testing [17]. Sensitization does not appear to be related to atopy or smoking. It is possible that the sterilizing activity of a chemical is associated with its ability to act as a sensitizer, as there are reports of chemically unrelated sterilizing agents causing occupational asthma, such as chlorhexidine, isothiazolinones, benzalkonium chloride, hexachlorophene, chloramine-T and even chlorine (chloramines being the sensitizing agent).

Aluminum potroom asthma [19]

Asthma has been recognized for many years in aluminum smelters [20], which may persist after exposure ceases [21]. This occupational environment has often not been included among listed causes of occupational asthma because of the coexisting exposures to hydrogen fluoride and sulfur dioxide, raising the possibility that the mechanism is primarily irritant. Similar exposures may occur in foundries where fluoride fluxes are used to clean molten aluminum. There is an association between the level of fluoride exposure and disease, with a fivefold excess risk when fluoride exposure is averaged above 0.8 mg/m^3 [22,23]. The incidence is more common in smokers but not in those with childhood allergy. It still remains unclear whether the primary cause is aluminum fluoride acting as a sensitizer or hydrogen fluoride acting as an irritant. Positive challenge tests to aluminum salts in aluminum welders favor sensitization [24], but both exposures may be relevant since, in platinum refineries, exposure to chlorine and concentrated acid is thought to enhance the probability of asthma from platinum salt exposure [20,22].

Antibiotics and other drugs

Some of the most severe cases of occupational asthma have occurred from the manufacture of drugs, particularly among workers involved in the mixing processes prior to tabletting, but there is a lack of epidemiological data. The sensitizing agent may be the drug itself or a constituent of the tablets such as the binding agent, gum acacia. There is substantial work with the biologic aperient, ispaghula (psyllium) [25], which may sensitize dispensers and nurses as well as those manufacturing the drug. Antibiotics are probably the most important drugs causing occupational asthma. Some workers develop anaphylactic reactions following inhalation of very low levels of airborne antibiotic, and a risk from subsequent therapeutic use has been demonstrated by oral challenge tests [26,27]. Other drugs causing occupational asthma are shown in Table 4.1.

Bakers' asthma

Bakers' asthma was first described by Bernardo Ramazzini in about 1700, and remains one of the most common causes of occupational asthma in societies where bread is the staple cereal food. Enzymes (particularly fungal amylase, hemicellulase, and xylanase) are commonly added to bread dough, though are not generally used in pastries. Recent work has shown a clear dose–response relationship between flour [28] and amylase [29] levels in air and subsequent sensitization to each, detected by finding positive skin prick tests or specific IgE antibodies, respectively. A positive skin prick test to wheat is uncommon in the general population. In one study from Germany it was present in about 11% of healthy bakers, 74% of bakers with rhinitis, and 94% of bakers with occupational asthma [30]. By contrast, in UK studies a large proportion of symptomatic workers with work-related respiratory symptoms had no detectable specific IgE [31]. Some exclude a diagnosis of bakers' asthma in these circumstances. The latent interval from first exposure to first symptom is often longer in bakers' asthma than in other types of occupational asthma, averaging 7.2 years in one study, with some cases occurring more than 20 years after first exposure [1]. Bakers' asthma is often preceded by occupational rhinitis. Atopy is a significant risk factor for amylase, and probably flour, sensitization [29]. There are cross-reacting antigens between different grains including wheat, rye, barley, and soya [32], and some shared antigens with grass pollen [33].

Colophony [34]

Colophony (rosin) is an extract of pine tree resin. When distilled, the distillate is turpentine and the residue colophony; tall oil and pine oil contain many of the same agents. Occupational asthma may occur when colophony is heated and inhaled; on rare occasions it can occur when colophony is in particulate form when being handled cold. Colophony is the principal constituent of electronic soldering flux, and most affected individuals have been electronics workers. Colophony may be encountered additionally in many other occupational settings [34,35]. Current evidence suggests that resin acids present in the fumes are the principal sensitizing agents. In high concentration the fumes can also be toxic to the respiratory mucosa, in common with other wood-derived respiratory sensitizers such as plicatic acid [36]. Epidemiological studies have shown that the degree of exposure is the most important determinant in the development of colophony asthma, which is also more common with smoking and atopy. Substitute fluxes without colophony are now

available, but anecdotal cases show that not all are without similar risk [37]. Studies of colophony asthma have been hampered by the lack of an *in vitro* test for detecting sensitization. Colophony conjugates are immunogenic in mice [38], but so far IgE antibodies have not been detected in man.

Cotton

The role of cotton dust is discussed separately in Box 4.1 Byssinosis.

Enzymes

Inhaled enzymes are a potent cause of occupational asthma [49,50]. Most affected workers come from the manufacture of biologic detergents containing alcalase and maxtalase, but sensitization has occurred in a many other situations. Alcalase used in the detergent industry caused an acute outbreak of occupational asthma shortly after the processes were started in 1968 [49]. Sensitization was shown to be more common in those who were highly exposed and atopic. The exact relationship between IgE antibodies and disease has not been formally studied in representative groups of workers. Sensitization has been all but eliminated following remedial action (stricter dust control, improved exhaust ventilation, enclosure of the plant, protective clothing, purchasing the enzyme in slurry not powder form, and subsequent encapsulation). Of the original highly exposed workers, nearly 80% of the atopic subjects developed IgE antibodies to the enzymes and 40% of the non-atopics. There have only been three further workers sensitized from jobs with potentially high exposures since 1974 in one factory studied [49].

Epoxy resins

Epoxy resins are formed from the cross linking of a resin (bisphenol A) with a hardening agent, either an acid anhydride which requires heat to complete the reaction, or a cold-curing system containing an amine such as triethylene tetramine. So far nearly all the cases of occupational asthma have resulted from the hardening agents, although much of the dermatitis and one report of asthma [51] relates to the basic resin. The exposure may be to the powdered material in those manufacturing chemicals or adding them to mixes, or to fumes during curing. The same curing agents are used in other resins, plasticizers, fire retardants, and during the synthesis of various dyes, perfumes, weedkillers, and organic acids. All these chemicals are irritants at high concentrations and can give rise to eye and nose irritation. The acid anhydrides are fairly common causes of occupational asthma and may sensitize up to 25% of exposed workers – as shown by skin prick tests or IgE antibody assays using acid anhydride–protein conjugates. Antibody responses to tetrachlorophthalic anhydride are more common in smokers than non-smokers [52], a feature of some other asthma-inducing agents including laboratory animals, green coffee beans, and platinum salts. Trimellitic anhydride may also give rise to a febrile reaction and, very rarely, pulmonary infiltrates with hemolytic anemia (Chapter 23).

Grain dust [53]

Workers exposed to grain dusts include farmers (particularly during harvesting), grain elevator workers, animal feed makers, millers, bakers, and other cooks. Respiratory problems vary along this production pathway. About 25% of all grain harvesters develop occupational asthma [54]. It is thought that molds from the grain are the major cause. During storage the grain may be contaminated by thermophilic organisms, endotoxin, grain storage mites, and weevils, any of which may be responsible for occupational asthma occurring in grain elevator workers. By the time flour is produced the grain itself is the major allergen, unless enzymes are added. In addition to asthma and rhinitis, occupational exposure may cause grain fever, chronic obstructive pulmonary disease, and extrinsic allergic alevolitis. Grain dust may activate both the classical and alternative complement pathways, and it causes a dose-dependent reduction in ventilatory function in exposed workers which is probably not immunologically mediated [55]. Occupational asthma may be associated with a neutrophilic rather than eosinophilic inflammation in the bronchi [56], and workers with large across-shift falls in FEV_1 (like those exposed to higher levels of endotoxin) may be those with accelerated longitudinal declines [57,58]. Occupational asthma attributable to IgE-mediated hypersensitivity does, nevertheless, occur in grain workers, particularly with grain of high moisture content in which grain storage mites are more readily found [59].

Isocyanates

Isocyanates are the cross linking agents with which polyurethanes are made. They are the most common cause of occupational asthma recognized in most compensation and surveillance schemes; they often lead to a severe asthma with incomplete recovery following reduction of [60] or removal from exposure [61–67]. Spray painters using two-part polyurethane paints are the group at highest risk, especially if painting is done in small automobile-repair shops. The isocyanate aerosol remains airborne for some time after spraying has stopped, a time when the worker often lifts the visor of his air-fed hood to inspect his work. Airborne isocyanates are sometimes present outside spray booths in paint-mixing areas, when touch-up spraying is done in the open shop, or when isocyanate-based body fillers are used. Isocyanates are a common cause of occupational asthma in situations where the etiologic agent is initially obscure [68].

Toluene diisocyanate (TDI) is volatile at room temperature. It is widely used in foam insulation, varnishes and paints, adhesives, surface coatings, and in the insulation around copper wires used in electronics, where it is liberated during soldering. It is being replaced in many settings by diphenylmethane diisocyanate (MDI), which is solid at room temperature but still causes occupational asthma when heated. This is a particular problem when MDI is used to make cores for castings in foundries. Hexamethylene diisocyanate (HDI) is the most volatile isocyanate. It was used in car and aeroplane spray paints, where it proved to be a potent sensitizing agent, and so is now largely replaced with HDI prepolymers. These are less volatile but still lead to sensitization, as the aerosol allows inhalation [69]. Other isocyanates are much less frequently used but may all cause occupational asthma. Despite the use of 'blocking' polymer formulations, cases of respiratory sensitization to isocyanates have continued to occur [70–72], some due to the polymer and some probably due to residual monomer.

Some workers become exquisitely sensitive to isocyanates so that they may react when outside the plant if walking downwind, or to material on colleagues' clothes or hair. Reactions have been induced during bronchial provocation testing to concentrations of TDI of less than 0.001 ppm. There is a possibility of clinical cross-reactivity between TDI and MDI, and even the chemically dissimilar HDI [73]. Delayed reactions and prolonged recovery times are quite common with isocyanate asthma. One longitudinal study of TDI asthma in polyurethane workers showed an incidence of 5% over 5 years from exposure to levels of around 0.02 ppm [74].

It is possible to quantify IgE antibodies to isocyanate conjugates, but only about 20% of subjects with occupational asthma have positive tests. The antibody half-life is short and the assays are often negative in those who have been removed from exposure [75]. Atopic workers are not at excess risk of developing isocyanate asthma, although those with preexisting asthma are [76].

Laboratory and other animals [77]

About one-third of all laboratory workers handling rats, mice, rabbits, guinea pigs, and hamsters develop some form of hypersensitivity reaction to them. Symptoms usually develop in the first few years of exposure. In one prospective study [78], 15% developed some sort of reaction during the first year of exposure, with 2% developing occupational asthma. Increased exposure levels are associated with increased rates of sensitization [79], the dose–response relationship being steeper for atopics than non-atopics [79], and [80] for smokers than non-smokers in some studies. In cross-sectional studies the prevalence of occupational asthma is often 4–10%. The main allergens are urinary proteins, with some derived from the pelt as well.

Exposure levels are highest when examining animals, are intermediate when cleaning cages, and are relatively low when weighing and dosing. Exposure levels also vary with the density of animals in the room, with the rate of air change produced by ambient ventilation, and the choice of litter [81]. Background levels in animal rooms are higher at night when rodents are active than during the daytime. Most workers with occupational asthma have specific IgE antibodies to urinary proteins but these are also found in a small proportion of symptomless individuals. Severe reactions can occur in sensitized workers from contact with antigen on laboratory workers' clothes. There is some evidence that immunotherapy is of benefit and that wearing full respiratory protection can reduce reactions in sensitized workers [78]. In Finland, cow dander is the most common cause of occupational asthma [82], which may be related to the way the animals are cared for in the long indoor winter feeding season. In other countries, there are more respiratory symptoms in farmers rearing pigs than cows [83].

Many arthropods can cause occupational asthma but locusts are particularly important as they are widely used in schools, universities, and research establishments. In one cross-sectional study, 26% of those handling locusts in a research center reported work-related wheeze and breathlessness [84]. The major antigen is contained within the peritrophic membrane which lines the mid- and hindgut, and is rapped around the fecal pellets. As with rodents, IgE antibodies to locust antigens are related to the development of occupational asthma and atopic workers are more susceptible. The major antigens have some cross-reactivity to house dust mite antigens. This has led to the finding of locust IgE antibodies in 20% of non-exposed people. The finding of specific IgE antibodies in an otherwise non-atopic individual correlates well with locust allergy. A more specific antigen with less cross-reactivity to *Dermatophagoides pteronyssinus* has now been prepared [85].

Latex

Latex allergy, mostly in healthcare workers, has shown a very steep rise in incidence in recent years. The use of natural rubber latex (NRL) gloves began early in the 1900s, it has increased with the rising awareness of acquired immunodeficiency syndrome (AIDS), and it has been associated with an increased frequency of allergic reactions. It soon became evident that allergy from rubber gloves may not only cause contact dermatitis, but can give rise to life-threatening asthma and anaphylaxis, with a number of deaths [86]. The prevalence of NRL sensitization amongst healthcare workers ranges from 3% to 22%, much of the variability being due to the use of non-standardized allergen extracts [87]; atopics are at increased risk.

There are only two studies in glove manufacturers: the prevalence of positive latex prick tests (>2 mm wheal) was 11% in Canada [88] (4.7% for wheal >3 mm) and 2% in various factories in Malaysia [89]. Both used non-standardized extracts. Sensitization appears much less common in areas where latex is produced, despite very high air levels; perhaps because sensitization is usually through the skin. In decreasing order the most common manifestations of latex allergy are urticaria, angioedema, rhinitis, asthma, and anaphylaxis. The main source of latex in air (causing asthma) is from disposable gloves, particularly if powdered with corn starch, as the latex binds to the starch. Latex levels in air are reduced, but not eliminated, by the use of powder-free gloves. The problems are much less prevalent in areas where latex gloves are washed and reused. Once sensitized, about 50% of affected individuals develop cross-reactions with fruits – particularly bananas, mangoes, kiwi fruit, walnuts, and avocados [90]. Sensitized workers should carry a warning of their sensitization; most of the deaths have occurred when latex gloves were used on them during operations, or latex balloons were inserted on catheters, etc. The disease is preventable by using non-latex gloves.

Platinum salts [91]

The complex salts of platinum are among the most highly allergenic substances encountered at work and may cause asthma, rhinitis, or dermatitis in at least one-third of relatively heavily exposed workers, (heavy exposure, 0.002 mg/m^3) [92]. The main sensitizing agents are ammonium hexachloroplatinate and tetrachloroplatinite [93]. Exposure to these compounds is principally found in the platinum-refining industry and in platinum scrap recovery. Platinum metal is not a sensitizing agent in the lungs and platinum salts without chloride-leaving ligands do not cause positive skin prick tests in sensitized workers [94]. The replacement of chloroplatinates by tetramine platinum dichloride in autocatalytic converters abolished sensitization in those making the converters; occupational asthma remained a problem in those manufacturing the tetramine platinum dichloride from chloroplatinates [95].

Platinum salts are unusual low-molecular-weight agents in that they induce immediate skin weal and flare reactions when used in an unconjugated form during skin prick testing. Suitable concentrations are 10^{-9} to 10^{-3} g/ml, the stronger solutions being used only if the more dilute ones produce no reaction. Most workers with occupational asthma from platinum salts have positive skin prick tests at the time of first symptoms, but there remain a few whose tests are negative when asthma develops [92]. Skin tests may also become negative shortly after exposure ceases. Positive skin tests are sometimes seen also in workers without symptoms. Once sensitization has occurred, highly sensitized workers may react to material on the clothes or hair of other workers outside the workplace. Spouses of workers have been sensitized at home by material brought home in a similar way [96]. Sensitization is quicker and more prevalent in atopic workers compared with non-atopic workers; however, cigarette smoking is an even greater risk factor [97]. Few sensitized workers can remain at work due to the extreme sensitivity that usually occurs. In UK practice, skin tests from routine 3-monthly surveillance are used to detect sensitized workers at the earliest opportunity; they are removed immediately from further exposure, most losing skin test reactivity quickly. Those with asthma make a more rapid and more complete recovery than occurs with other forms of occupational asthma [98,99].

Wood

Many wood dusts can cause occupational asthma. The most studied is western red cedar (*Thuja plicata*), the predominant problem occurring in sawmill workers in British Columbia where it is grown, and in workers of other parts of the world to which it is exported [100,101]. Cabinetmakers may also be exposed to varnishes and glues, isocyanate exposure being a particular problem in the northern Italian furniture industry. The standard woodworking adhesive contains urea–formaldehyde, which releases formaldehyde on heating; formaldehyde is a rare cause of occupational asthma. About 4.5% of western red cedar sawmill workers develop occupational asthma even when airborne dust concentrations are low (<1 mg/m³) [101]. The major allergen appears to be plicatic acid, which has a molecular weight of 400 and is probably acting as a hapten. However, only about 40% of affected workers have IgE antibodies to a plicatic acid–human serum albumin conjugate, and it may be that plicatic acid is not the only component from western red cedar that can cause asthma. Most affected workers experience conjunctivitis and rhinitis before the onset of asthma, which usually develops within the first 2 years of exposure. The rimu tree (*Dacrydium cupressinum*) in New Zealand may cause similar problems [102].

Although plicatic acid is able to activate the classical complement pathway, the bronchial pathology of western red cedar-induced asthma is similar to that seen in atopic asthma [103]. Atopy does not, however, appear to predispose to western red cedar asthma. In one study, smokers appeared to be less affected than non-smokers. There is a good follow-up study of exposed workers showing that many do not make a complete recovery following removal from exposure [100], and there is evidence that continued exposure in symptomatic workers leads to an accelerated longitudinal decline in FEV_1 [104].

Box 4.1 Byssinosis (Anthony C. Pickering)

Byssinosis is a form of lung disease associated with occupational exposures to vegetable dusts arising from the processing of cotton, flax, hemp, and to a limited degree sisal. It is one of the most studied and least understood forms of occupational lung disease. The first full description was published in 1845 by Mareska an Heyman: 'all the workers have told us that the dust bothered them much less on the last days of the week than on Monday or Tuesday'. Subsequently the disease was described and classified by Schilling and colleagues [39]. Recently new terminology has been introduced dividing byssinosis into 'acute' and 'chronic' forms.

Production of cotton
Cotton is a natural fiber derived from the cotton boll of the plant *Gossypium*. It was initially harvested by hand, allowing fibres of high quality to be picked. This was then succeeded by mechanical harvesting, which collects a considerable quantity of leaf and bract (the outer covering of the boll) in addition to the cotton fiber. It is believed that these biologically active contaminants are the source of the etiologic agent(s) that cause byssinosis. In the traditional method of cotton spinning, the bales of raw cotton were fed by hand into a bale breaker following which the cotton fiber was passed automatically into opening and scutching machines. These processes were designed to tease open the cotton fiber and to remove dust and debris. At the end of the process, the fibers were gently compressed into a blanket or lap. The laps were then transferred to carding machines where the fibers were carded to align them with each other. This converted the lap into a rope of parallel fibers known as a sliver. The sliver was then combed to remove shorter fibers and taken into draw frames, where it was blended with other slivers and drawn out into a narrower

continued

Box 4.1 Byssinosis (Anthony C. Pickering) (contd.)

product. The draw frame sliver was then converted on speedframes into a thinner *roving*, which was wound on to bobbins suitable for spinning. The spinning process applied a twist and attenuated the roving to produce the yarn. The early production processes of opening and carding were associated with the highest dust exposure levels and the highest prevalence of byssinosis.

Acute byssinosis

Acute byssinosis refers to the acute airway response which is seen in volunteers exposed to cotton dust for the first time. It has been well documented in artificial cardroom studies where approximately one-third of volunteers exposed to cotton dust for the first time have falls in ventilatory function which may exceed 30% [40]. This response may be related to the airway reactivity of the individual and may explain the high labor turnover observed in the cotton industry during the first year of employment [41].

Chronic byssinosis

This is the classical form of byssinosis and is characterized by a feeling of chest tightness and difficulty in breathing which the worker experiences as being most severe on the first day of the working week. The onset of symptoms occurs after exposure to cotton dust for many years and is unusual in workers exposed for less than 10 years. The onset of chest tightness over the working shift may occur either rapidly on starting work (60%) or be delayed, developing over the second half of the shift (40%), and possibly progressing into the evening after leaving the workplace. Workers perceived that their symptoms improved over the working week but were further exacerbated when cleaning took place at the end of the week.

This pattern of symptomatology generally, but not always, differentiates byssinosis from other forms of occupational asthma. Some workers exposed to cotton dust describe other symptoms including cough and wheeze, which may occur in the absence of chest tightness, and therefore technically do not fulfill the criteria for a diagnosis of byssinosis [42]. They are similar to those with byssinosis in terms of their demographic features and exposure histories, and it seems likely that they are suffering from the same disease process. Chronic bronchitis is more common in cotton workers than in the population at large, the effect of current exposure to cotton dust being at least as important as smoking [43].

Lung function changes have been demonstrated in byssinosis with cross-shift changes in forced expired volume in 1s (FEV_1) of 10–20%. The lowest mean measurements occur at the end of the working week but the largest cross-shift change occurs on the first working day, consistent with the severity of symptoms. Affected workers possibly become conditioned to lower levels of lung function as the week progresses [44]. In addition to lung function abnormalities, increased levels of airway responsiveness are demonstrable in byssinotics (78%) compared to asymptomatic workers (17%) [45]. The cross-shift lung function changes and the presence of increased airway reactivity are consistent with an asthmatic process. The cross-shift changes have additionally been related to an excess longitudinal decline in ventilatory function [46]. There are no specific pathologic features in byssinosis which differentiate it from the features of smoking-related airways disease except for the absence of evidence of pulmonary emphysema, which appears to be specifically related to cigarette smoking [47]. The prevalence of the disease in the UK and Europe has fallen progressively over the past 30 years from a level of 50% in workers engaged on the dustiest parts of the process to currently 3%. However, in developing countries, where cotton production is increasing, the prevalence rates remain high at 30–50% [42].

Recent studies in cotton textile workers have not revealed consistent excesses in overall mortality. In a prospective study, the overall and respiratory mortalities in the cohort were less than expected, but there was an excess mortality in workers with byssinosis [48].

The mechanisms of and the etiologic agents causing byssinosis remain obscure. While endotoxin derived from Gram-negative bacteria is thought to be the most likely cause, there are a number of other industries where exposure to organic dusts heavily contaminated with endotoxin occurs and symptoms of byssinosis are rarely seen. The prevention of chronic byssinosis relates to reducing dust exposure with appropriate enclosure and exhaust ventilation of the production process. As a result of prospective longitudinal studies of cotton spinning workers, levels of personal dust exposure which are not associated with the development of respiratory disease are now known. The current personal exposure limit in the UK is 2.5 mgm/m^3.

Prognosis

There is good evidence that continued exposure, once occupational asthma has developed, leads to a worse prognosis, and that early removal from exposure leads to a better prognosis. When exposure ceases within 6–12 months, full recovery is common though by no means certain. The prompt recognition that newly developed asthma is occupational in origin is consequently critical to an optimal prognosis since, without this, ongoing exposure may be prolonged and the brief window of opportunity for a cure may be lost.

In practice, many affected workers do not make a full recovery, and loss of employment is a major disincentive to removal from exposure in places where compensation is not focused on redeployment and retraining. There is evidence for reduced symptoms [21], improved lung function [105], improved airway responsiveness [21,62,106], reduced levels of specific IgE [107], and often reduced income [105,108,109] in those removed from exposure to the sensitizing agent. The proportion making a full recovery varies with different studies, most of which are based on subjects reaching referral centers. They may be the more severely affected. Current evidence suggests that any increase in FEV_1 reaches a peak within 12 months of removal from exposure, and that any improvement in airway responsiveness is complete within 24 months. However, there is some evidence for further recovery beyond this time [110]. These changes are often compounded by increased treatment in the early stages.

Factors consistently related to a poor prognosis are a longer period of exposure after symptoms first develop, a longer period from first exposure to first symptom, and more severe disease (or lower FEV_1) at presentation [63,100,111]. Some studies also show that a dual asthmatic reaction following specific challenge tests implies a worse prognosis than an isolated immediate or late reaction. Smoking and atopy do not generally affect prognosis [100,112]. There are insufficient studies to know whether specific agents are associated with a better prognosis than others. A follow-up of cases notified to SWORD showed a poor prognosis in the UK, with at least 75% of affected subjects remaining symptomatic whatever the causal agent [113]. With sensitization to platinum salts, however, a particularly good prognosis has been noted, possibly because the major source of data is a factory with 3-monthly surveillance, where workers are removed from exposure at the first sign of symptoms or positive skin prick tests to the platinum salts [114]. Similar workers from the USA and Germany, where relocation to reduced exposure rather than complete removal is usual, showed less complete recovery [99,115].

Once sensitization has occurred, it is likely to remain for life, even if exposure ceases completely. Reexposure on specific challenge after a long period usually results (at least initially) in asthmatic reactions of diminished strength, though sometimes an increase in airway responsiveness alone is observed [116,117]. It is likely that longer periods of reexposure would result uniformly in the reactivation of occupational asthma. A few workers have remained at work away from exposure, but became inadvertently reexposed, resulting in severe or even fatal attacks of asthma [118].

The reasons behind incomplete recovery are unclear. It is possible that in some cases there is continued exposure after leaving work (for instance to flour in bakers), or that cross-reacting antigens maintain symptoms (for instance, bananas with latex sensitization). In some cases the initial diagnosis may have been incorrect, or the wrong sensitizing agent was avoided. Some individuals develop sensitization to more than one unrelated occupation sensitizer, for instance, glutaraldehyde and latex, and unless all relevant causal agents are avoided, symptoms are likely to continue. It is also possible in some subjects that, once the mechanisms underlying asthma are activated, the process cannot be reversed.

Once susceptibility has been demonstrated to one occupational asthma inducer, there is likely to be an increased level of susceptibility to another, and this (whether justified or not) may contribute to the reluctance of a potential new employer to offer work. The prognosis from the viewpoint of future employment as opposed to future asthmatic disease may therefore be a gloomy one, and the majority of subjects in Britain who cease to be employed because of occupational asthma become permanently unemployed.

RECOGNITION

Occupational asthma is conveniently recognized from the diagnostic approach to two sequential but distinct questions:

1. Does the individual under review have asthma?
2. If asthma is confirmed, is it occupational in origin?

The early recognition of an occupational cause of asthma is of particular importance in view of the brief opportunity to effect a cure from prompt cessation of exposure. The fact that the majority of affected subjects are never able subsequently to obtain gainful employment emphasizes the potentially profound consequences of occupational asthma to both the affected worker and his/her family. Its economic consequences are of much wider concern, since it may require major and expensive adjustments to factories and manufacturing processes, which could render the product financially non-viable, to say nothing of the costs attending the compensation process. Asthma arising in an adult should always prompt consideration of the possibility that it is occupational in origin and, if this cannot reasonably be discarded by the primary care physician, referral for more expert advice should follow.

Clinical features

Occupational asthma is simply asthma for which the initiating cause happens to be known, and so its clinical features are not fundamentally different from those of asthma in general – wheezing, breathlessness, and chest tightness from bronchoconstriction, often with cough. These symptoms are episodic if the asthma is mild, but continuous though of varying degree if severe. They are a consequence of the underlying level of airway responsiveness and the outcome when triggering factors are superimposed. Some of these are endogenous (e.g. those resulting from sleep) and not always readily examined, but many are exogenous and of both non-specific (irritant) and specific (allergic or idiosyncratic) types. The degree of bronchoconstriction that results from such stimuli consequently depends on the respective levels of sensitization and airway responsiveness, and the strength of the stimulus [119,120].

With irritant stimuli this strength depends on the inherent potency of the agent and the exposure dose, and so the same outcome may result from lesser levels of airway responsiveness but stimuli of greater strength, or vice versa, and the same stimulant strength may result from an agent of lesser potency but higher dose. With allergic stimuli it is the degree of individual hypersensitivity that determines the relative potency of the allergen for the particular asthmatic subject, its dose again influencing further the overall strength of the stimulus. This is illustrated in Fig. 4.1.

History

Once asthma is induced, whether by occupational exposure or not, symptoms are likely to be provoked in non-occupational situations, if appropriate stimuli are encountered. This close clinical similarity between asthma of non-occupational origin and occupational asthma may obscure the true cause.

This is particularly so with occupational asthma arising via the RADS pathway, since there is no allergy to any occupational agent. Affected workers will respond no differently from workmates with non-occupational asthma if non-specific triggers are encountered in the working environment – providing the levels of airway responsiveness are of similar degree. The only difference in history lies with the initiating event, the accidental episode of toxicity at work. This is likely to have been severe, to have required emergency medical care, and to have affected fellow workers with comparable levels of exposure.

With occupational asthma arising through presumed hypersensitivity mechanisms, however, ongoing exposures to the inducing agent may produce very characteristic clinical patterns over and above the typical clinical picture of non-occupational asthma. If the inducing agent is one of high molecular weight (e.g. rodent urinary protein) and the subject has IgE antibodies to rodent urinary protein, immediate asthmatic reactions are likely once a presumed threshold level of exposure has occurred. These characteristically begin within a matter of minutes, rapidly reach a peak, resolve within 1–2 hours if there is no ongoing exposure, and are unassociated with any increase in airway responsiveness. A typical immediate reaction, observed following a laboratory-based inhalation provocation test, is illustrated in Fig. 4.2. The degree to which an IgE response is generated following repeated exposures to allergen is, like airway responsiveness, unimodal in distribution and the classification of individuals as atopic or non-atopic is somewhat artificial. As with

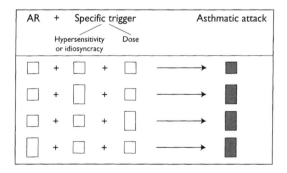

Fig. 4.1 Interrelationships between sensitization, exposure dose, and airway responsiveness. The level of airway responsiveness (AR), the degree of specific sensitization, and the magnitude of the exposure dose exert independent influences on the severity of any ensuing asthmatic reaction. If one is increased, but the others remain unchanged, a stronger reaction is to be expected, but if one increases while another decreases a reaction of similar strength may occur. Relative magnitudes are represented by box sizes.

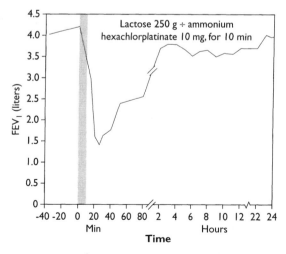

Fig. 4.2 A typical immediate reaction, observed following a laboratory-based inhalation provocation test with a powdered platinum salt. The dust mixture was tipped repeatedly between two trays. The asthmatic reaction began within a few minutes of exposure onset, reached its peak within 30 min of exposure ceasing, and largely resolved within 1–2 hours.

airway responsiveness, the issue is whether IgE responsiveness is sufficiently strong to make atopic disease likely. The greater the degree of IgE responsiveness, the more likely is an immediate asthmatic reaction to follow exposure.

In contrast to high-molecular-weight allergens, reactive chemicals of low molecular weight often produce late asthmatic reactions (Fig. 4.3). Again a threshold level of exposure must be assumed, following which there is no obvious adverse effect for a latent period of at least 1–2 hours, and often up to 4–10 hours. The onset is consequently indistinct and progression is often slow. The peak may not be reached for many hours, and the working shift may have been completed before any respiratory distress occurs. The relevance of the occupational environment may not, consequently, be readily evident. Spontaneous recovery usually requires many hours, sometimes days, and there is often sleep disturbance during the following night or nights. This is likely to be a consequence of an increase in the level of airway responsiveness which characteristically accompanies late reactions.

The increase in airway responsiveness can sometimes be detected before the late reaction becomes evident and, when (under experimental conditions) no treatment has been instituted, the dramatic phenomenon of recurrent nocturnal asthma over many days has occasionally been noted following a single exposure (Fig. 4.4). It is easy to accept that agents which cause late reactions are potential inducers of asthma, whereas this is not necessarily so for those that cause only immediate reactions (for example, exercise or the inhalation of cold/dry air). It may not be so easy, however, to recognize that worsening asthma from a provoker of a late reaction was a

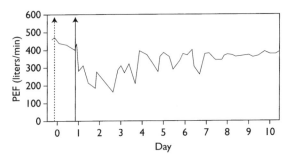

Fig. 4.4 Recurrent nocturnal asthma over many days following a single laboratory-based exposure to formaldehyde. Recurrent troughs of PEF occurred each night for 7 days following a single challenge exposure, before this pattern petered out. It is likely to have been a consequence of a temporary increase in airway responsiveness, and hence an exaggerated asthmatic circadian rhythm. ↑ (dashed), challenge onset – water; ↑, challenge onset – formalin 25% (8 min). The challenge fluid was 'painted' on board.

consequence of a particular exposure some hours earlier.

These differences between immediate and late asthmatic reactions are most evident under experimental conditions, particularly those associated with inhalation provocation tests in the laboratory. Under natural working conditions, such patterns are usually less obvious and of unknown importance, partly because there is often ongoing exposure to the relevant agent throughout the working shift. A further explanation is that both immediate and late reactions may be provoked (dual reactions), and with continued exposure following the onset of the immediate reaction it may not be obvious that two distinct patterns are occurring.

In practice, the patterns in affected workers exposed regularly to the relevant inducing agent are best elucidated with serial peak expiratory flow (PEF) measurements. They depend principally on the types of reaction, the speeds of recovery, and circadian rhythms.

- *Hourly patterns.* Immediate, late, or dual reactions are superimposed on normal diurnal variations such that immediate reactions are more commonly observed on afternoon shifts when the occupational exposure is superimposed on the declining part of the normal diurnal variation, and late reactions are more common on the morning shift. Most common for day-shift workers is the 'flat' pattern, where the normal rise in ventilatory function in the hours after waking is not seen on workdays, but is seen on days away from work.

- *Weekly patterns.* Weekly patterns relate most to the speed of recovery. If recovery is rapid and effectively complete by the following morning, each work day will result in equivalent

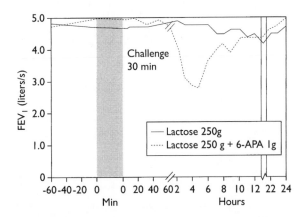

Fig. 4.3 A typical late asthmatic reaction, observed following a laboratory-based inhalation provocation test with powdered 6-amino-penicillanic acid (6-APA). The asthmatic reaction did not begin until 2 hours after exposure onset (1 hour after exposure ceased), did not reach its peak for 5–6 hours after exposure ceased, and did not resolve until 10 hours after exposure ceased.

deterioration and there will be rapid improvement on the first day away from work at a weekend. If recovery is incomplete by the following morning but is substantial within a 2–3-day period away from work, then symptoms become progressively severe day by day at work. Symptoms may then be present only at the end of the working week. Such progression of symptoms with daily exposure is the most common pattern seen, and probably relates to increasing levels of airway responsiveness with successive exposures. A few workers have symptoms that are maximal at the beginning of the working week, or in the middle of the working week, and improve despite continued exposures. These patterns are more common in a few specific situations such as exposure to cotton dust, contaminated humidifiers, and coolant oil aerosols. In all of these situations there is a substantial bioaerosol including endotoxin, when tolerance seems to develop with repeated exposures.

- *Long time interval patterns.* When recovery is not complete within 2–3 days away from work, repeated weeks of exposure may lead to progressive deterioration of asthma. Fortunately deterioration does not usually continue indefinitely, and a plateau is reached. At this stage, diurnal variation in peak flow may be reduced and improvements on days away from work minimal. On leaving work, however, some workers continue to improve for up to 6 weeks.

The major elements in the history that can be used to help recognize occupational asthma can be summarized as follows:

1. Does the individual under review have asthma?

- Are there suggestive symptoms of wheeze, breathlessness, chest tightness, cough?

- If so, are they episodic?

- If continuous rather than episodic, are they of varying severity?

- Are they common at night, or worse at night, thereby disturbing sleep?

- Are they triggered by exposure to common irritants (e.g. smoke, cold or dry air), exercise, and intercurrent viral infections of the upper respiratory tract?

- Are they triggered by exposure to common allergens (e.g. house dust, pets, pollens)?

- Are they quickly relieved by inhaled bronchodilators?

- Has any other medication been prescribed (i.e. one likely to control asthma or to cause it)?

2. If asthma is confirmed, is this occupational in origin?

- RADS pathway:
  - Was there an initiating episode of respiratory toxicity resulting from an exposure, usually accidental, at work?
  - Did asthmatic symptoms begin at that time or during the recovery period?

- Hypersensitivity pathway:
  - Did asthmatic symptoms begin (or, in an individual with preexisting asthma, worsen appreciably) following onset of the period of employment under review?
  - If so, what was the latent interval from first exposure to first symptom?
  - Are symptoms more troublesome on work days than rest days?
  - If so, is the timing consistent with early or late types of asthmatic reaction (or both)?
  - Are nocturnal symptoms more troublesome on workdays than rest days, and are there work-related recurrent nocturnal attacks?
  - Are symptoms associated with any particular job task, or exposure to any particular agent?
  - Were symptoms associated with any particular accidental exposures at work?
  - If so, what were the timing characteristics?
  - Are symptoms less troublesome on vacations than at other times?
  - Are symptoms more troublesome on returning to work after vacations?
  - Are nocturnal symptoms less troublesome on vacations than at other times?
  - Have fellow workers had similar symptoms, and do they associate these with the workplace?
  - Are there recognized asthma sensitizers in the workplace?
  - If so, is there any possibility of exposure to them?
  - If there are no recognized sensitizers, are there nevertheless exposures to any dust, fume, gas, or vapor?

Investigation

Clinical

The following summarize the clinical diagnostic approaches.

1. Does the individual under review have asthma?

- Spirometry   Airway obstruction which is substantially reduced by inhaled bronchodilator medication.

▪ Serial PEF	Increased diurnal variation.
▪ Airway responsiveness	Most useful if spirometry is normal but history suggests asthma. Best achieved with methacholine or histamine tests, but other pharmacologic constrictor agonists may be used, as may an exercise test.
▪ Atopy	Not necessary to diagnose asthma, but useful to assess whether common allergens are likely to be relevant if asthma is confirmed. Conveniently achieved with skin prick tests or serum IgE measurements.
▪ Imaging	Not necessary to diagnose asthma, but useful to exclude other diagnoses or asthmatic complications (e.g. pneumothorax, consolidation).

Most of these steps are readily achievable by the primary care physician, though the measurement of airway responsiveness would usually be left to a respiratory or occupational physician, or even to a referral center. If spirometry is not available to the primary care physician, the measurement of PEF may be sufficient to demonstrate clinically significant variability or improvement following the inhalation of a bronchodilator, but PEF alone does not allow an obstructive loss of ventilatory function to be distinguished from a restrictive loss. More important it is less sensitive to detecting suboptimal effort on behalf of the test subject.

If doubt remains over the presence or absence of asthma, a methacholine or histamine test provides the most satisfactory means of confirming the diagnosis. This assumes the test is carried out with properly calibrated equipment and established limits of repeatability. The result will consequently be in an asthmatic range, a non-asthmatic range, or an intermediate ('gray') range equivocal for active asthma. If exposure has ceased and symptoms have regressed at the time of evaluation, an individual with occupational asthma will not uncommonly show a level of airway responsiveness outside the asthmatic range. The quantification of airway responsiveness is considered in more detail in the chapter on lung function (Chapter 32).

2. If asthma is confirmed, is this occupational in origin?

▪ PEF monitoring	A convenient and popular procedure to assess whether occupational exposures trigger asthmatic reactions.
▪ Antibody tests	If available, demonstrate whether an immunologic response has been mounted to the relevant occupational sensitizer.
▪ Environmental characterization	Occasionally valuable to assess what occupational agents are respirable. Quantification of exposure levels will show whether excess levels are likely to have been encountered, thus increasing the probability of sensitization, though occupational asthma commonly develops when measured air levels are well within the exposure standards.
▪ Inhalation provocation tests	Generally require special laboratory facilities to reproduce under close experimental control the exposures of the working environment. Associated with some risk of provoking an undue asthmatic reaction, and so most suited to tertiary referral centers with appropriate expertize. If carried out with a suitable double-blind protocol, they provide the 'gold standard' for confirming whether or not: (1) a given test agent is an asthma inducer; and (2) a particular test subject is affected. Depending on the circumstances, a negative test may not exclude occupational asthma.

These investigations are appropriate only to the 'hypersensitivity' causal pathway of occupational asthma. Occupational asthma arising from the 'RADS' pathway can only be recognized from identifying the initiating toxic exposure. The history alone may be sufficient for this, but because this may be markedly distorted by the passage of time (and possibly grossly exaggerated), independent confirmation from contemporary medical records should be obtained. The critical points are that asthma did not exist previously (or if it did, its severity was clearly of a lesser order of magnitude), that the episode could plausibly have produced pulmonary toxicity, that similarly exposed fellow workers similarly developed toxic responses, that objective markers of toxicity were recorded within 24 hours, and that asthma was evident as the other toxic effects subsided.

PEF monitoring can generally be undertaken by the primary care physician as well as the respiratory or occupational physician, but interpretation of the data often requires experience unless the outcome is clearly negative. When there are no discrepant features, and when occupational asthma has already been detected in the particular working environment which is known to harbor a recognized asthma inducer, there is rarely any need for additional investigation if PEF monitoring gives a positive result, especially if the relevant antibody test is positive also.

When the outcome is less clear or is disputed, there may be a need for laboratory-based inhalation provocation tests. This level of investigation should be pursued if a novel cause of occupational asthma is strongly suspected, since without confirmation the need for job changes and plant/process modifications are more difficult to justify.

Peak flow monitoring

Serial PEF measurements provide the best method for the initial validation of occupational asthma, and for the confirmation of successful relocation away from exposure to the offending agents. They are best performed before attempts to control the asthma with drugs, but can also be used in subjects receiving regular asthma treatment.

- Teach the worker how to record PEF; if using a manual meter check ability to read to nearest 10 liters/min and ability to reach reproducibility within 20 liters/min.

- Record highest reading; if best two not within 20 liters/min, make more readings.

- Make readings approximately 2-hourly from waking to sleeping. For many workers the timings need to be adjusted to the work pattern. Readings can usually be made:
  - On waking
  - On arriving at work
  - During each work break
  - On leaving work
  - Mid-evening
  - On going to bed.

- Select a period of about 4 weeks during which there are days away from work. The analysis

depends on comparing days at work with days away from work. Rest days are very important; readings on rest days at similar times to those on workdays should be emphasized. Many workers tire of keeping readings over time; 4 weeks is optimal, but the exercise can be repeated later if the outcome is equivocal.

- Keep treatment constant throughout. The aim is to analyze changes in PEF in relation to work, not to show that asthma is controlled with treatment.

- Record each day:
  - Waking time
  - Time arriving at work
  - Time leaving work
  - Time going to bed
  - Any unusual exposures, changes in exposure, or respiratory infections.

- Check PEF measurement technique when the worker returns with the records.

- Plot record in a standard manner. OASYS (Occupational Asthma System) [121] provides plots of daily maximum, mean, and minimum PEF, which aid interpretation and are illustrated in Fig. 4.5. The subject was a school laboratory science technician preparing classes in chemistry, biochemistry, biology, and physics. There is improvement in PEF on each period away from work and deterioration on each period at work. There are, however, anomalous days when PEF is unchanged at work (e.g. 25 November) but deteriorates away from work (1 December). It transpired that the school had not been cleaned over the weekend of 23/24 November, and the technician's asthma was later shown by specific bronchial provocation testing to be due to the residue on the floor of the material used to clean it.

- Provide if possible a score for the probability of a work effect [122]. This is illustrated in Fig. 4.6a by the OASYS record of an automobile body assembly worker who had developed occupational asthma attributable to zinc fumes as a spot welder of the zinc coated bodies. This was confirmed by specific bronchial provocation testing with zinc sulfate. He was then relocated to work within the plant's assembly line, though away from further direct exposure, and the PEF record investigated the outcome. There is a small deterioration during Week 1 when he worked the morning shift, an improvement over the following weekend (particularly of the minimum), and a greater deterioration in Week 2 when he worked the night shift – possibly because an

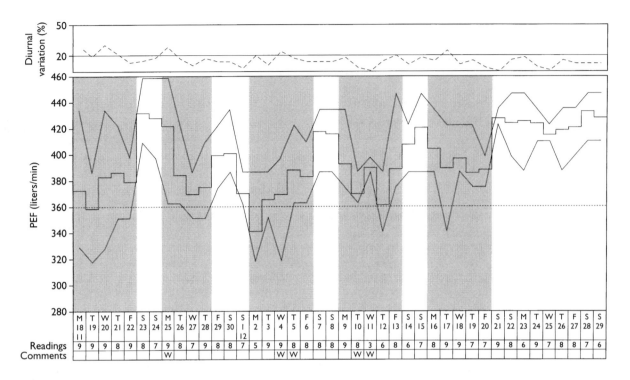

Fig. 4.5 Serial 2-hourly PEF measurements, waking to sleeping, for 6 weeks in a laboratory technician. Top panel: diurnal variation expressed as % predicted. Middle panel: daily maximum, mean, and minimum PEF. Bottom panel: date and numbers of PEF readings per day; W indicates days without a waking measurement. Dotted line: PEF, 359 represents the predicted PEF.

occupational effect was superimposed on a circadian effect or because the environmental conditions were less satisfactory at night. The plot additionally shows the OASYS scores for each work–rest–work and rest–work–rest complex. A score of 4 represents a definitely positive outcome confirming a work effect, and a score of 1 represents a definitely negative outcome without any suspicion of this. The overall weighted score is 3.21, implying an unequivocally positive result. He was then relocated once more, with no possibility of indirect ongoing exposure, and a final OASYS record (Fig. 4.6b) gave a negative result.

■ For equivocal records, repeat before, during, and after a 2-week period away from exposure (e.g. a vacation or period of sickness absence). The measurement of airway responsiveness can be added before and after the period off work (Fig. 4.7), but has not been shown to increase the sensitivity of the record. It may, however, increase the specificity, and so provide validation in workers who are thought to have kept unreliable readings.

Help is available for downloading record forms and OASYS support on occupationalasthma.com.

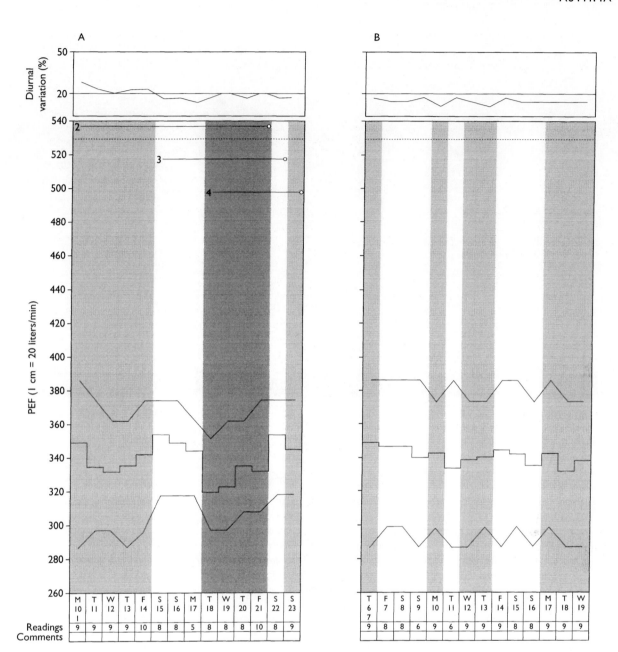

Fig. 4.6 (a) Serial 2-hourly PEF measurements, waking to sleeping, in an automobile assembly worker. The OASYS plot is displayed as in Fig. 4.5 but additionally includes scores (1–4) for each work–rest–work and rest–work–rest complex. (b) Serial 2-hourly PEF measurements in the subject of (a) after complete cessation of exposure to zinc fumes from spot welding. The OASYS plot is displayed as in (a), but no longer shows any work-related effect.

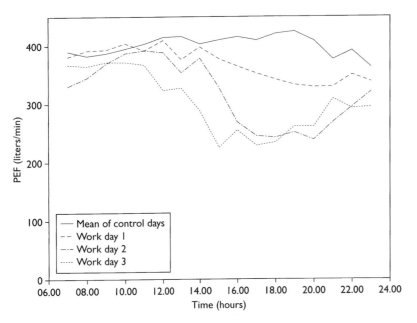

Fig. 4.7 PEF monitoring with PD_{20} measurement. With 3 successive days at work at an isothiazolinone manufacturing plant following an absence of 18 days, there were progressively stronger late asthmatic reactions, each beginning a little earlier. This pattern can be attributed to a steadily increasing level of airway responsiveness. Sequential PD_{20} measurements were: 115 μg (last day at work before study); 267 μg (10 days after ceasing work); 1107 μg (18 days after ceasing work); 110 μg (1 day after the 3-day study).

Box 4.2 Immunologic tests (Andrew D. Curran and David Fishwick)

Occupational asthma is a condition with an underlying immunologic basis. Complex interactions between cellular and humoral aspects of the immune system result in the clinical symptoms associated with the disease. Of particular importance are specific IgE antibodies (in serum or bound to mast cells) and specific T-lymphocytes; both may be measured in affected individuals, and both may aid in diagnosis.

IgE can be quantified as either total or specific immunoglobulin, and can be measured by either indirect or direct methods. The decision to measure IgE as an aid to diagnosis when occupational asthma is suspected assumes that the condition has an etiology based on Type I hypersensitivity. Whilst this may not always be true of occupational allergens, particularly those with a low molecular weight (e.g. colophony [123]), appropriately performed IgE antibody measurement is still the most important immunologic test available to suggest a cause and effect relationship in cases of occupational asthma.

Total IgE measurement

A range of standard assays are available to determine the concentration of total IgE in serum. Individuals who are atopic (as judged by high levels of specific IgE to common environmental allergens) usually have high levels of circulating total IgE. The 'normal' range for non-atopic individuals is 1–120 kU/liter, with a mean of 25 kU/liter. However, approximately one-third of atopic individuals have total IgE within the normal range. The only certainty with this approach, therefore, is that individuals with total IgE less than 25 kU/liter are not atopic, whereas individuals with total IgE greater than 400 kU/liter are atopic [124]. Furthermore, total IgE measurement does not enable the specific sensitivity of the individual to be determined, and

therefore it is of very little, if any, use in the investigation of occupational asthma.

Specific IgE measurement

Skin prick testing

Skin prick testing (SPT) does not measure specific IgE directly. It measures the wheal and flare response to locally administered allergen. This reaction results from the cross-linking of mast cell-bound specific IgE, releasing mediators such as histamine, leukotrienes, prostaglandins, and cytokines from tissue mast cells. The test comprises the application of a drop of allergen extract, usually in 50% glycerol, to the surface of the skin, which is impregnated by either lifting and puncturing the surface with a needle (modified skin prick test), or direct puncture (prick puncture test) using commercially available lances. Intradermal testing, where allergen is injected directly into the skin, may be used for less common allergens, or where titrations of allergen are to be performed. However, this technique should not be used outside a specialist center as it can lead to severe or life-threatening allergic reactions. Therefore, skin prick testing is the method of choice for commercially obtained, standard allergens.

When performing the test it is essential that a standard protocol is followed to ensure that the sensitivity and specificity of the results can be assured. In particular, it is important that measurement criteria are consistent since various methods of measurement can be used, for example, maximal wheal diameter or mean wheal diameter [(largest diameter + orthogonal diameter)/2]. In addition, appropriate controls should be used (histamine as a

continued

Box 4.2 Immunologic tests (Andrew D. Curran and David Fishwick) (contd.)

positive control, and diluent as a negative control), time of measurement following impregnation should be consistent, and results should be recorded in a standard format (e.g. using adhesive tape to record wheal size). It is important that some medications are avoided prior to testing as these may significantly depress the wheal and flare response (e.g. antihistamines).

The major difficulty with skin prick testing is obtaining allergen extracts that are well characterized and of suitable quality. For example, false-positive skin prick tests results have been reported in individuals tested with some commercial dog dander skin prick test solutions. Detailed analysis showed that the concentration of the major dog allergen (Can f1) in five commercial extracts varied from 3.8 μg/ml to 170 μg/ml. Furthermore, all these extracts also contained significant amounts of Der P1 (the major house dust mite allergen), which led to false-positive responses in patients sensitized to house dust mite [125]. There is also some evidence to suggest that the consistency of response is highly batch and operator dependent.

In conclusion, skin prick testing is ideal for well-characterized workplace allergen extracts, if a suitable standard protocol is used to perform the test.

Biochemical methods

The measurement of specific IgE in serum enables the determination of IgE antibodies which have been produced in response to workplace exposures, e.g. wheat flour or fungal α-amylase-specific IgE antibodies may be found in individuals with occupational asthma working in a bakery. Unlike skin prick testing, this approach measures allergen specific IgE directly.

Measurement of specific IgE can be achieved using a range of commercial kits, all of which require some technical knowledge and specialist equipment, e.g. RAST (Upjohn-Pharmacia), UNICAP (Upjohn-Pharmacia), AlaSTAT-RIA (Diagnostic Products Corp.), Chemiluminescent Assay (CLA), Magic Lite (ALK), Allergodip (Allergopharma). Essentially, all are based on the binding of serum IgE to workplace allergens immobilized on a solid matrix (beads, paper disks, etc). Detection of bound IgE is achieved with an anti-IgE polyclonal serum or monoclonal antibody tagged with a detecting reagent (e.g. radioisotope, fluorochrome, chromophore). Tests which use a monoclonal antibody detection system are more consistent in their measurement of bound specific antibody. The most common test used in the investigation of occupational asthma has been RAST (radioallergosorbent test), since it can be adapted for almost any workplace allergen. This adaptability has allowed successful demonstration of exposure–response relationships to be determined for a number of causes of occupational asthma. Results may be expressed as the RAST percent binding (% of total radiolabeled IgE bound to the disk), RAST score (RAST % binding of test/RAST % binding of negative control), RAST

class (relationship of the test serum to four or five reference serum dilutions), or modified RAST scoring (test results normalized against a single positive standard – 251 U/ml IgE – reacted with anti-IgE).

Low-molecular-weight chemicals are not recognized by the immune system unless they are first bound to a carrier protein, i.e. low-molecular-weight chemicals act as haptens. Therefore, an additional step is required in their analysis to attach the low-molecular-weight chemical to a suitable carrier protein (usually human serum albumin). These hapten–protein conjugates should be fully characterized prior to their use in a RAST to ensure that the chemical is attached covalently [126,127]. Therefore, there is an inherent assumption made when performing RAST for low-molecular-weight chemicals, that the hapten protein conjugate is appropriate and represents the *in vivo* events. This may not always be the case, and may account for the low sensitivity and specificity seen with RAST testing for some chemical sensitizers.

RAST inhibition may be used to confirm the binding seen in a RAST, and may also be used to identify cross-reactivity with other allergens (e.g. storage mites and house dust mite).

In summary, biochemical measurements are an ideal approach for most occupational allergens, as the test can be made bespoke for a particular workplace allergen. However, caution is advised in their use for assessing the immunologic response to some low-molecular-weight chemicals.

Cellular tests

Basophil degranulation

In vitro basophil degranulation has been used to determine sensitization to allergens. Again, a number of techniques have been employed. Essentially, all the tests measure the amount of histamine released from basophils obtained from whole blood. Advances have been made using flow cytometry (Basotest), but this approach does not provide a significant advantage over the measurement of IgE by simpler biochemical methods [128].

T-Cell markers

Whilst IgE measurement is useful for many occupational allergens, it is of limited use in workers exposed to many low-molecular-weight chemicals. For example, isocyanates can give false-positive results and glutaraldehyde can give false-negative results [127,129]. The reasons for these observations are not clear, but inappropriate measurement techniques for low-molecular-weight chemical specific IgE antibody may be responsible or the activation of non-IgE-dependent mechanisms [130].

An alternative approach has been to measure changes in the activation of T-cells both in peripheral blood and *in vitro* following challenge with suspected allergen. The

continued

Box 4.2 Immunologic tests (Andrew D. Curran and David Fishwick) (contd.)

technique most often used to detect these changes has been flow cytometry, which allows cells of a particular type to be identified and enumerated [131].

In vitro challenge studies have been performed in both atopic individuals [132] and individuals with occupational asthma [133]. In brief, isolated T-cells are challenged in vitro with the putative allergen (e.g. house dust mite or plicatic acid–human serum albumin conjugates). Individuals with documented clinical responses to the allergens showed increased reactivity of T-cells following in vitro challenge compared to control subjects, but the proportion of responding cells appeared to be lower in the subjects with occupational asthma compared to those with atopic asthma.

A sample of peripheral blood can also be used to determine the activation state of T-cells in vivo. Unlike the in vitro challenge system, this technique does not allow exposure response relationships to be identified, but it does give valuable information regarding the immunologic profile of exposed individuals. For example, an increase in activated helper T-cells has been shown in peripheral blood of asthmatics using flow cytometry to identify cells of the CD4CD25 phenotype [134,135]. Mapp et al. [136] emphasized the importance of the cellular response when considering the respiratory sequelae resulting from chemical exposure. Some of the findings in atopic asthmatic patients have been reproduced in patients with asthma induced by toluene diisocyanate and other occupational allergens [137,138].

Using flow cytometry, Curran et al. have shown differences in the immune cell profile between workers exposed to different respiratory hazards [139]. Specific cell types were measured in the peripheral blood of bakers exposed to wheat flour, who reported work-related

respiratory symptoms, and glass bottle manufacturers, reporting similar symptoms, but exposed to a range of irritant chemicals. The bakers showed activation of helper T-cells, consistent with mild to severe asthma, but the bottle workers showed a very different pattern – a significant reduction in total T-cells. Other studies have used flow cytometry of peripheral blood to identify cells involved in the etiology of the asthmatic response a few hours after allergen exposure in sensitized individuals. For example, the nature and extent of the T-cell response before, during, and after allergen challenge in subjects with atopic asthma has been characterized [140]. These studies have given a valuable insight into the cellular mechanisms responsible for both environmental and occupational respiratory disease, and may ultimately lead to diagnostic tests with increased sensitivity and specificity.

Sensitivity and specificity

It is important to know the sensitivity and specificity of the tests available, but these unfortunately vary with different exposure agents. In general, both sensitivity and specificity are good for both skin prick testing and biochemical methods for measuring specific IgE against high-molecular-weight allergens. When reviewing results it is important to consider the benchmark against which the test has been judged, since different authors use different approaches. In particular, IgE measurements to low-molecular-weight chemicals do not always show acceptable sensitivity and specificity. Table 4.2 lists reported sensitivity and specificity data from a number of published studies. It is difficult to compare data between studies, since each uses a different 'gold standard' for comparison, and many use a range of 'cut-off' values to determine a positive or negative

continued

Table 4.2 Sensitivity (Sens) and specificity (Spec) for IgE measurement techniques

	SPT		RAST		UNICAP		AlaSTAT-RIA		Allergodip		Ref
	Sens (%)	Spec (%)	Sens (%)	Spec (%)	Sens (%)	Spec (%)	Sens (%)	Spec (%)	Sens (%)	Spec (%)	
Latex	97	100			97.0	86.0	100.0	83.0			141
Atopy			80	92	86.0	94.0					142
Isocyanates			4	100							143
Isocyanates	26.4	100	14	99.7							144
Isocyanates			28	91							145
Various	75.8		75								
Alternaria	75.8		75								146
Occupational	74	89	57	86							147
Enzymes	100	93	62	96							148
Latex					79.5	90.2	73.8	91.7			149
Latex					91.5	70.5			85.1	75.0	150
Inhalant			93	89	89	91.0					151

Box 4.2 Immunologic tests (Andrew D. Curran and David Fishwick) (contd.)

response. Furthermore, the time interval between the date of collection of blood for analysis and the date of last exposure is important, but not always known or recorded.

In subjects with occupational asthma, Tee et al. showed that the sensitivity of RAST for isocyanate fell from 41% during exposure to 14% when blood was taken more than 30 days after exposure [75]. However, in general, the data do show reasonable concordance between skin prick testing and measurement of specific IgE antibodies for high-molecular-weight allergens.

What is the best approach?

The immunologic basis of occupational asthma is complex; indeed, different immune mechanisms may exist for high-molecular-weight chemicals and low-molecular-weight chemicals. Therefore, it is important to know the limitations of each technique when choosing the most effective immunologic approach. The problem is best viewed as completing a jigsaw. Some conditions require only a few pieces to see the complete picture, e.g. bakers' asthma, where a combination of appropriately performed skin prick testing or specific IgE determination to workplace encountered allergens (wheat flour, soya flour, oat flour, fungal α-amylase and other enzymes) in combination with atopic status determination is likely to give sufficient information to aid a diagnosis. For most low-molecular-weight allergens, more pieces of the jigsaw are required to make immunologic testing worthwhile; indeed, it could be argued that we do not at present have sufficient pieces to warrant immunologic tests for some low-molecular-weight sensitizers.

Box 4.3 Inhalation provocation tests (André Cartier and David J. Hendrick)

Specific inhalation challenges are considered by most investigators as the gold standard to confirm, in the individual patient, a diagnosis of occupational asthma arising through the pathway of hypersensitivity [153–155]. Originally carried out in the laboratory and aiming to mimic work exposure [156], they are now often conducted in the workplace. The tests are safe when performed under the close supervision of an experienced physician and with trained personnel, but when carried out in the laboratory should be limited to specialized centers where resuscitative measures are available. Exposure chambers in laboratories should be enclosed and the laboratory should be well ventilated to minimize exposure to staff. In most cases, the tests can be carried out on an outpatient basis.

Methods

Methodology is limited by practical issues, and what may be ideal is not always feasible. Different investigators have consequently developed different approaches and there is no uniformly adopted standard protocol. The basic principles of the methodology are, however, well developed [153–156]:

- Concurrent medication: this should be minimized since it may weaken or mask a positive outcome, though must be adequate to maintain asthma control.
- Challenge procedure: the administered stimulus should simulate that occurring in the workplace, but be controlled and safe.
- Monitoring tests: the outcome should be closely and adequately monitored.
- Control data: these are essential so that the effect of the challenge agent can be properly assessed.

- Patient safety: the test subject must be suitable and closely observed, and emergency treatment must be readily available, so that any adverse effect is quickly recognized and treated.
- Informed consent: the test subject should fully understand the principles and methodology. Written consent to participate is considered important in some countries.
- Ethical approval: if carried out for research purposes, the protocol and study should have ethical approval.

Medication

Drugs which prevent (or reduce) asthmatic reactions should be withheld before specific bronchial challenges according to standard recommendations, whenever this is possible [153]. Short-acting β2 agonists (oral and inhaled) and ipratropium bromide should be withheld for 8 hours while long-acting β2 agonists and leukotriene antagonists should be withheld for at least 72 hours. In most subjects, long-acting theophylline should be withheld for 48 hours (or 72 hours for once-daily preparations). In a few cases, such withdrawal is not possible without there being an unacceptable worsening of symptoms. In these circumstances challenge tests may not be feasible, though useful results are generally obtained if medication is reduced to the minimum level that maintains adequate asthma control, and this is taken at the same times and dose levels on both control days and challenge exposures days. If theophylline is used, there should be daily serum monitoring to ensure a uniform effect.

continued

Box 4.3 Inhalation provocation tests (André Cartier and David J. Hendrick) (contd.)

Corticosteroids (inhaled or oral), sodium cromoglycate, and nedocromil sodium should be continued (otherwise worsening asthma may be a consequence of their withdrawal rather than the challenge tests), but it may be useful to administer the full daily dose in the evenings throughout the period of investigation. Although the dose threshold of reactivity for the challenge agent may be increased by concurrent medication, it is not likely to mask completely a positive response in a sensitized subject.

Challenge procedure

The challenge exposures, and the test protocols, may be performed in the laboratory or in the workplace.

When performed in the laboratory, specific bronchial challenges can be conducted in several ways, depending on the nature of the agent (i.e. powder/dust, liquid, aerosol, or gas). With dust and powders, such as flour, psyllium, or red cedar sawdust, occupational exposure may be mimicked by pouring a sample from one tray to another [156] or by using a dust generator (Fig. 4.8) [157]. When the agent is

known to have high potency, the challenge sample can be diluted to a measured degree with an inert carrier, such as dried lactose powder. The dose may be conveniently increased sequentially by serial increases of the exposure period, and/or increasing the concentration of the challenge sample.

If the challenge agent is gaseous or volatile, a closed-circuit generating chamber [158,159] or a whole-body exposure chamber [160,161] becomes necessary, if only to protect laboratory personnel. Ideally a steady state is created with a dynamic adjustable equilibrium between generation, release, ventilation, and extraction, in which case long periods of occupational exposure can be simulated. In most cases, however, a standard format is used for generating the gas or vapour (eg mixing and hence activating the components of epoxy resins or polyurethane, or 'painting' the volatile agent on inert board) in a simple whole-body chamber in which the test subject remains for a measured brief period. Alternatively off-gassing vapours from an activation procedure can be

continued

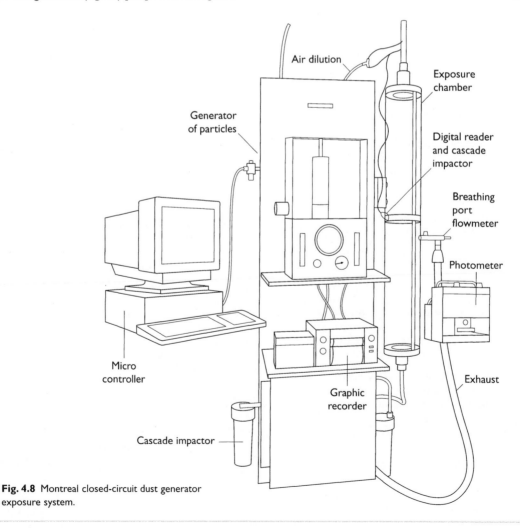

Fig. 4.8 Montreal closed-circuit dust generator exposure system.

Box 4.3 Inhalation provocation tests (André Cartier and David J. Hendrick) (*contd.*)

led into an inert 200 litre Tedlar bag [162]. The concentration of a specific challenge agent may then be adjusted by air dilution, thereby increasing precision of challenge delivery. Similarly, a challenge agent which is liquid or water soluble can be administered as an aerosol by conventional nebuliser in precise doses [163]. Other methods using dry powder inhalers have also been proposed but not used extensively [164,165].

Whenever possible, the level of exposure should be monitored so that inadvertently high levels are not produced, safety is maintained, and irritant reactions are avoided. This requires sophisticated monitoring equipment, however, particularly if 'real-time' analyzers are used to produce instant measurements. They are unfortunately beyond the means of many investigators.

Tests in the workplace are convenient and particularly useful when the relevant agent at work is unknown, when there are several recognized sensitizing agents of potential relevance, or when evidence of airway lability (active asthma) has been discordant from earlier monitoring of PEF and measurements of airway responsiveness. The worker is asked either to perform his/her usual tasks or to stay in his/her usual working environment as an observer. The duration of exposure may be increased in a stepwise fashion from day to day, but usually involves a whole day (or several days) before a test sequence can be considered 'negative'. Spirometry is monitored throughout the day as with laboratory-based tests [166]. Exposure to the challenge agent is, however, less well controlled than in the laboratory and it may be difficult to ensure that the subject is appropriately exposed to the relevant agent.

Test protocol

Before any challenges are administered, it is essential to obtain control data to ensure there is asthmatic stability and to provide a comparative baseline. With severe disease a period of observation is useful before any inhalation procedure, but for most test subjects control data can be acquired on the first study day following inhalation challenge with a 'control' agent (e.g. lactose powder, paint diluent, resin without activator, nebulized saline without solute, etc.) that is presented in the same way as the test agent [153,155].

Most challenges are administered in an 'open' fashion, the test subject knowing that exposure is taking place. This is inevitable for workplace challenges, and with laboratory challenges that mimic workplace tasks. When possible, investigators may prefer to administer seemingly identical challenges with control (dummy) agents so that the challenge procedure is blinded to the test subject and also the supervising physician [162,163,167]. This double-blinded approach adds considerable strength to the interpretation of the outcome, and is particularly useful when novel agents are being evaluated for their potential asthmagenic properties. If the challenge agent has distinctive odor or

taste, this may be masked or disguised by adding other odorous agents to the challenge exposure or by giving the test subject a cough lozenge or anesthetic pastille to suck.

For high-molecular-weight agents, for which positive skin tests can be elicited and for which an immediate reaction might be expected, the exposure period can be increased progressively at 10-min intervals (e.g. one breath, 10–15 s, 1 min, 2 min, 5 min, etc.) for up to 2 hours or until a 20% decrement in FEV_1 is detected from spirometry measurements [168]. If, however, the subject gives a history suggestive of an isolated late asthmatic reaction or the test agent is of low molecular weight (and more likely to be associated with isolated late responses), exposure increments should be administered on separate days. It may still be useful to administer each daily dose progressively by component increments to lessen the possibility of an undue immediate reaction (e.g. one breath, 15 s, 45 s and 2 min on the first day, up to 30 min on the second day, and 2 hours on a third day). The protocol may need to be modified at any point in light of the observations.

Measured exposure levels in the workplace provide a guide to what dose will be safe on the initial challenge day (perhaps 1/10 or 1/100 of that likely to be inhaled in the test subject's work area) [162,163]. Further guidance for the choice of starting dose can be taken from the measurement of airway responsiveness. The higher the level, the lower the starting dose for the challenge sequence.

Twofold increments from day to day can be considered safe, but 10-fold increments carry some hazard. A convenient compromise used by some investigators is √10-fold (i.e. 3.2-fold) [162,163,169]. This produces an incremental sequence of 1, 3.2, 10, 32, 100, ... dose units as the protocol advances, control days with dummy challenges being interspersed to maintain double blinding if this is required. A dose range as great as 1000-fold can therefore be accommodated in 7 days, excluding the control days. If no asthmatic reaction is observed, the sequence continues until a maximum dose is administered which exceeds (by 1 or 2 dose levels) that ever likely to be experienced at work. A negative outcome then makes the test agent an improbable cause of the test subject's asthma.

Monitoring tests

Although symptoms are highly relevant, the chief purpose of inhalation provocation tests is to provide objective evidence that exposure to the challenge agent causes an asthmatic reaction. A secondary purpose is to assess whether testing increases the level of airway responsiveness.

Spirometry should be followed at identical intervals on both control and challenge-agent days – ideally throughout the waking hours, but at least for 8 hours [153,170]. PEF may not be adequately reliable, as it may underestimate or overestimate the magnitude of any change [171–173].

continued

Box 4.3 Inhalation provocation tests (André Cartier and David J. Hendrick) (*contd.*)

Spirometry may give an additional benefit in providing permanent tracings to assess validity. Although there is some value in forced vital capacity (FVC) measurements and in the $FEV_1/FVC\%$, multiple expirations to residual volume may be uncomfortable and, in practice, FEV_1 measurements alone may be preferable, the forced expiratory maneuver being discontinued after 1 s. Following baseline assessment of FEV_1, FVC, and PEF, most investigators measure FEV_1 at about 10-min intervals for 1 hour after the end of the challenge exposure so that any immediate asthmatic reaction can be detected. Subsequent measurements (with or without FVC and PEF) are generally taken at hourly intervals so that any late reaction can be detected. It is important that baseline spirometry on each challenge exposure day should reproduce, whenever possible, that of the control day (i.e. $\pm$ 10%).

In parallel to daily spirometry measurements, airway responsiveness should be measured (usually from methacholine or histamine tests) before and after the sequence of challenge tests to assess whether an increased level has been induced.

While FEV_1 is the standard parameter used to assess airway calibre, measurement of airway resistance may be used also. Since these measurements are less reproducible, many consider them less reliable. Some investigators additionally measure lung volumes on the control day (total lung capacity, residual volume, and functional residual capacity) so that these can also be used to confirm airways obstruction (air-trapping, hyperinflation) following challenge with the test agent if reliability of FEV_1 maneuvers becomes questionable.

If there is no significant variation in FEV_1 on the last challenge day, and if airway responsiveness has not increased, there is no need for further exposure. If airway responsiveness is increased (PC_{20} or PD_{20} is decreased), however, without there being clear evidence of an asthmatic reaction, it may be useful to conduct a further challenge exposure at a higher dose level, as the test may then prove to be unequivocally positive [174].

The use of sputum induction to monitor airway inflammation has recently been proposed to identify the bronchial response to inhalation challenge, as this may be more sensitive than spirometry or airway responsiveness [175], but further studies are needed before its routine use can be recommended.

Outcomes

Many regard a fall in FEV_1 of 20% as 'significant'. Typical patterns of bronchial reactions have been described (Fig. 4.9) [156,168]. Immediate reactions are maximal

continued

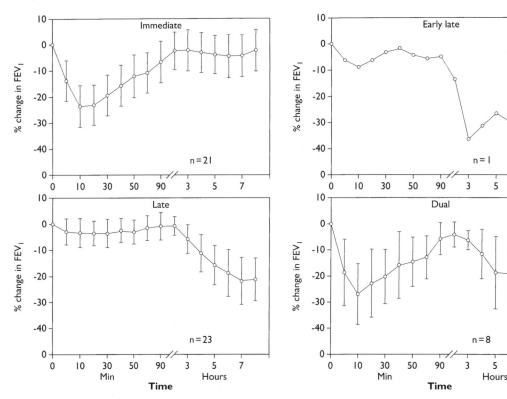

Fig. 4.9 Typical patterns of asthmatic reaction to provocation tests. Mean $\pm$ SD or individual values of the percent change in FEV_1 (on the ordinate) as a function of time since exposure (on the abscissa) for the four typical patterns of reactions. The numbers of individuals for each pattern are presented. Adapted from Perrin *et al.* [168]

Box 4.3 Inhalation provocation tests (André Cartier and David J. Hendrick) (*contd.*)

between 10 and 30 min after the exposure threshold is reached with complete recovery within 1–2 hours; although usually readily reversible by inhaled β2 agonists, they are the most dangerous as they can be severe and unpredictable, particularly in subjects for whom skin tests with the suspected agent are not possible. The risk is lessened by administering the challenge exposure in a progressive manner. Late reactions develop slowly over several hours. If accompanied by fever and general malaise, an additional alveolar response should be considered. They respond variably to inhaled β2 agonists, and the response may be of shorter duration than usual [176]. Dual reactions are a combination of early and late. A recurrent nocturnal asthma pattern (Fig. 4.4) has also been described and is likely related to an increase in the level of non-allergic airway responsiveness that is usual (and may be marked) with late asthmatic reactions [177,178].

Atypical patterns (Fig. 4.10) have also been described [168]. They include the progressive type (starting within minutes after the end of exposure and progressing over the next 7–8 hours), the square-waved reaction (with no recovery between the immediate and late components of the reaction), and finally the prolonged immediate type with slow recovery. They probably represent mixtures of immediate and late reactions of different strengths. Non-specific 'irritant' reactions are not well characterized, but falls in FEV$_1$ which recover spontaneously and rapidly within 10 or 20 min are suggestive of an irritant pattern.

It may be difficult, even impossible, to interpret results of specific bronchial challenges in subjects with marked variability of FEV$_1$, which stresses the importance of comparative control data of good quality. Some investigators have developed statistical methods to allow for this [170]. Control data are obtained over 3 days, and a minimum of three technically satisfactory FEV$_1$ measurements are obtained at each time point. This allows a 'lower 95% confidence band' of the mean hour by hour FEV$_1$ plot to be calculated from the pooled variance. Any breach of this by plots from subsequent test days, which persists for a minimum of 1 hour, is interpreted to indicate a significant late asthmatic reaction (Fig. 4.11).

An alternative approach is to measure the area over the curve of the FEV$_1$ time plot, extrapolating the mean baseline to provide the upper boundary. This gives a summary measure of the degree by which the FEV$_1$ subsequently remains below the mean baseline through the following hours of the surveillance period. Figure 4.12 shows a conventional FEV$_1$ plot following a nebulized challenge with the low-temperature bleach-activating agent SINOS (sodium iso-nonanoyl oxybenzene sulphonate): it illustrates how a 2–12-hour area decrement (AD) is calculated to provide a summary measure of a late asthmatic reaction, and it compares the AD following SINOS 32 μg with the ADs on 3 control days and their 95% and 99% confidence limits. The AD

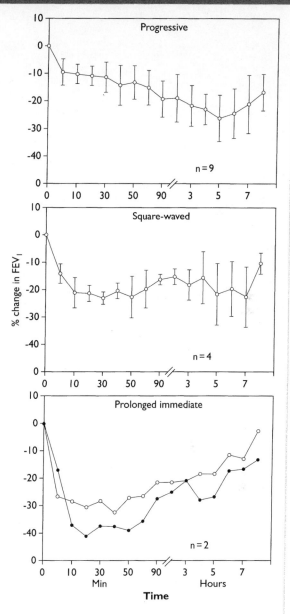

Fig. 4.10 Atypical patterns of asthmatic reaction to provocation tests. Mean ± SD or individual values of the percent change in FEV$_1$ (on the ordinate) as a function of time since exposure (on the abscissa) for the three atypical patterns of reactions. The numbers of individuals for each pattern are presented. Adapted from Perrin *et al.* [168]

summary measure can then be used to provide dose–response information and hence reaction thresholds, and (in rare circumstances) estimates of specific sensitivity (the slope). This is illustrated in Fig. 4.13 where the results from two studies are compared. One illustrates the outcome of serial challenges with increasing daily doses of SINOS and the other the outcome with the antibiotic

continued

Box 4.3 Inhalation provocation tests (André Cartier and David J. Hendrick) (contd.)

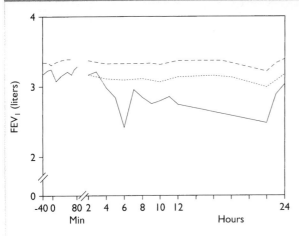

Fig. 4.11 Inhalation provocation test with nebulized ceftazidime. Upper plot: mean FEV$_1$ at each measurement point from 3 control days. Middle plot: the lower 95% confidence band for the control mean FEV$_1$. The lower confidence band is breached by the FEV$_1$ plot following ceftazidime challenge for well over 1 hour, indicating a significant decrement consistent with a late asthmatic reaction.

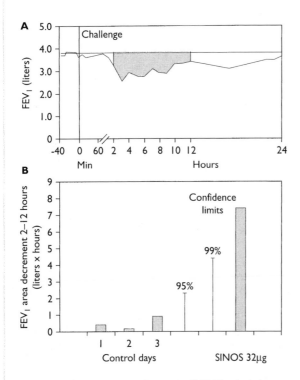

Fig. 4.12 (a) 2–12-hour area decrement (AD). The shaded area on the FEV$_1$ time plot defines the summary measure of area decrement 2–12 hours after challenge onset with nebulized SINOS 32 μg. The line demarcating the upper boundary is the mean of FEV$_1$ measurements during the period -40 to 0 min. (b) This is compared with the AD measurements on 3 control days and can be seen to exceed both their 95% and 99% confidence limits.

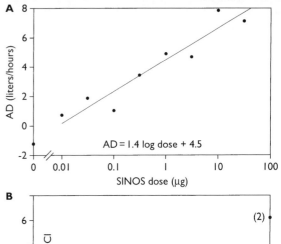

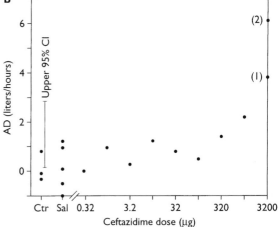

Fig. 4.13 Dose–response plots using AD as a summary measure for late asthmatic reactions. With SINOS (a) there is a linear relationship with increments in dose allowing specific sensitivity to be calculated by the slope of the dose–response plot, but with ceftazidime (b) there is a threshold below which no detectable reaction is seen. In view of the clear and strong response, no further doses of ceftazidime could be administered.

ceftazidime [169]. A negative value for the 2–12-hour FEV$_1$ AD indicates the mean FEV$_1$ increased rather than decreased compared with baseline.

A positive test confirms the diagnosis of occupational asthma, but a negative test may not satisfactorily exclude it. There may be a number of reasons for this apart from the acknowledged greater difficulty in proving a negative than a positive, and the possibility of a technical aberration in the testing procedure. It may be that the wrong test agent has been used or it has been used at an inappropriately low dose. Sometimes an antagonistic medication is used inadvertently. Workers who have not been exposed for several months may become 'desensitized' by the time of challenge testing [179], though in practice positive responses are commonly demonstrable for several years [117]. Diminished sensitivity may be suspected if there is an increase in

continued

airway responsiveness following the specific challenges but no apparent asthmatic reaction [174]. If, in such circumstances, a repeated challenge test at a greater dose level does not elicit a positive response, the test subject should then be returned to work. Only if regular monitoring of PEF and airway responsiveness over several weeks gives a negative outcome can the diagnosis of occupational asthma be excluded with reasonable confidence.

If the test system reproduces symptoms, but provokes no change in ventilatory function or airway responsiveness, the possibility of hyperventilation syndrome should be considered.

If the test agent is an important focus of attention as well as the test subject (a novel agent is suspected of causing occupational asthma), a negative outcome in one subject will obviously not provide much confidence that the agent has no sensitizing effect in others. If, by contrast, the test series produces a significant asthmatic reaction and a significant increase in airway responsiveness, the outcome has considerable diagnostic

strength, particularly if the outcome is shown to be reproducible and the test protocol is carried out in a double-blind manner.

Patient safety

The aim of inhalation challenge tests is to provoke asthmatic reactions and increase the pre-existing level of airway responsiveness. Although the former can be expected to resolve within a day or so, the latter may persist for several days or weeks. These tests consequently carry some risk, and need to be conducted with considerable care. Testing should not usually proceed unless, for example, the baseline FEV_1 is ≥ 2.0 liters and $\geq 60\%$ of predicted, or ≥ 1.5 liters and $\geq 70\%$ of predicted; close supervision is essential, and prompt treatment must be readily available. Otherwise the tests should be postponed in the hope that asthmatic control can be improved by adjusting medication. When such guidelines are followed, the benefit of challenge tests in removing diagnostic uncertainty fully justifies the small risks.

MANAGEMENT

It is critical that management responsibilities are recognized to extend beyond the care of the newly recognized affected worker, since fellow workers may be similarly affected, perhaps more severely. Furthermore, if the extent of the problem is not evaluated, appropriate environmental controls within the workplace or alternative and safer means of product manufacture may be delayed, resulting in other workers developing asthma needlessly.

Of the individual

Conventional medication

Asthma of any cause should be treated with conventional medication according to severity and need, and this applies fully to occupational asthma. In the case of occupational asthma arising via the RADS pathway there is no alternative option, since once asthma has arisen, nothing further can be done within the workplace to modify its course, assuming further episodes of pulmonary toxicity are prevented. There is an important caveat for occupational asthma arising via the hypersensitivity pathway, however. Effective pharmacological management might have the unfortunate effect of diminishing the stimulus for full investigation, and so might lessen the chances of asthma being recog-

nized to be occupational in origin when it arises first in adult life. This may have serious consequences, since the opportunity for cure might be lost if the diagnosis in the affected individual is delayed, and this in turn may lead to the persistence of the workplace hazard and to other workers becoming affected. The onus lies consequently with the physician who is initially consulted to consider whether there may be an occupational cause whenever asthma first arises (or appreciably worsens) in adult life.

Cessation/reduction of exposure

The particular advantage of asthma of occupational (and hypersensitivity) origin is that effective management may ensue from controlling ongoing exposure to the inducing agent alone. Prompt cessation of exposure can generally be expected to lead to improvement if not cure. The benefits are less following long periods of symptomatic exposure, but there is always some hope of improvement. Equally important is the probability of worsening severity if exposure continues at unmodified levels. There is consequently always some benefit in confirming the diagnosis, identifying the inducing agent, and introducing strategies for the future elimination or reduction of ongoing exposure.

The most favorable outcome is associated with complete cessation of exposure, and this should always be the goal. The ideal solution for both affected employee and employer is that the offending agent is removed from the workplace and a suitable safe substitute found. If this is not achievable, finding a new job with the same employer that excludes any possibility of further exposure is satisfactory for the individual if not for other members of the workforce. This secures continuing gainful employment for the affected employee, and limits the possible liability of the employer who might otherwise be responsible for appropriate compensation if further employment proves to be illusive. Such a solution will often require relocation to a different building, even a different site, and this may not always be available. The affected individual may, of course, find new and safe employment elsewhere. More commonly, employment elsewhere proves to be illusive.

When ongoing employment without ongoing exposure is not available, the option of compromise has to be considered. Can the current job be modified so as to minimize ongoing exposure, and are the risks involved acceptable? The dilemma here is that, for affected subjects (who necessarily show unusual degrees of susceptibility, otherwise all similarly exposed fellow workers would be affected), industrial hygiene improvements to the workplace or modifications to the manufacturing process may not be sufficient within the boundaries of reason and economic viability to provide an ongoing risk-free working environment. In general, such measures are driven by the need to minimize the risk for sensitization in workers who are unaffected, but the very nature of allergy is that, once the mechanisms are fully primed in affected workers, ongoing exposure at even trivial levels may still be hazardous. The affected worker may therefore find that his/her symptoms continue to be more troublesome during periods at work than on vacation, and that further modifications to the working environment are not practical.

Surveillance

When the compromise of continued employment with minimized levels of exposure is followed, it is essential that a comprehensive program of surveillance is established. Thus regular medical examinations are carried out so that the individual's medical history is reviewed, spirometry is measured, serial PEF measurements made, and the level of airway responsiveness is quantified. Assays of antibody levels, when available, may also be useful since a diminishing level would provide valuable evidence that exposure levels have indeed been reduced by a clinically meaningful degree. The employer should in any event have a regular surveillance program to monitor respirable levels of the inducing agent.

Standards of care and audit

The following standards of care for the management of occupational asthma provide a summary of management strategy, and a useful basis for audit. They are the guidelines approved by the 1998 World Asthma Meeting.

- Investigation should be undertaken while the worker is still exposed to the causal agent. This greatly aids diagnosis, allowing for the measurement of PEF, spirometry, and airway responsiveness in relation to work exposure. It also provides the highest chance of finding specific IgE to the causal agent (serological tests often become negative away from exposure), and it lessens the likelihood of those without occupational asthma losing their jobs unnecessarily. Such an approach is obviously unsuitable (and unnecessary) for workers with rare but catastrophic work-related reactions.

- The diagnosis should be supported by objective data. This may include specific IgE antibodies and the demonstration that exposure (either in the workplace or a challenge laboratory) is related to measured physiological changes in ventilatory function and/or airway responsiveness. A history alone is not sufficiently specific to risk jeopardizing employment.

- Exposure should cease within 12 months of the first work-related symptom. The prognosis is likely to be worsened if exposure continues for more than 12 months after the first symptom. It is preferable to relocate the worker earlier if possible.

- There should be continued worthwhile employment. Unemployment is bad for health and wealth. Many relocated workers leave interesting and skilled work, and are offered unrewarding and degrading employment. Unresolved work issues lead to increased psychological morbidity.

- A revised risk assessment should take place to remedy the cause and prevent further cases.

- The affected worker should be reassessed after 2 years to assess long-term disability. There is evidence that improvement can occur for at least 2 years after exposure ceases, spirometry improving before airway responsiveness.

Compensation

For many, the issues surrounding compensation cloud those of diagnosis and clinical management. The specific conditions of particular compensation schemes should not influence diagnostic or management strategies that are devised for purely clinical reasons, and appropriate management should be provided for the most likely diagnosis irrespective of the conditions relevant to compensation. When expert opinions are required for specific compensation schemes, a distinction may be inevitable between a clinical diagnosis of occupational asthma, and one that satisfies the requirements for compensation. For instance, in Germany, state compensation for occupational asthma requires evidence of sensitization – usually a positive skin prick test or specific IgE antibodies to the occupational agent. This probably explains why most asthma-inducing chemicals of low molecular weight do not appear on German compensation scheme reports. The exception is the recent introduction of a separate category for isocyanates. Some schemes have lists limiting the agents or jobs for which compensation is allowable, and most exclude the self-employed.

The aims of compensation should allow the removal of the affected worker from the causative agent as soon as possible, and maintenance of a resonable job and income. There is good evidence that the prognosis from the point of view of asthma is better with early removal, but in many countries there are severe employment and financial detriments to this approach. The best schemes use expert centers to make an accurate diagnosis, and then concentrate on redeployment to suitable jobs without exposure, with supported retraining when relocation is not possible. The less satisfactory schemes concentrate inappropriately on quantifying disability (the main problem for an affected worker is often not disability but the handicap of not being able to continue with his/her original job), and make little attempt to relocate the worker away from exposure or offer retraining.

Of the workforce

A major benefit of full investigation of occupational asthma in an affected individual is that a true hazard in the workplace is identified. Individual susceptibility plays an important role in the evolution of occupational asthma via the hypersensitivity pathway (but to a much lesser extent via the RADS pathway), and there will be occasions when only the most susceptible member of the workforce becomes affected – especially if the number of employees is small. In effect, different members will have different threshold levels for becoming sensitized. Present legislative limits are rarely set with sensitization as the outcome to be prevented, and have yet to make a significant impact on reducing the incidence of occupational asthma.

There is consequently an onus on any employer to evaluate the circumstances by which occupational asthma has arisen in any employee, and for this to be possible, there is an additional onus on the investigating physician to make the diagnosis and the investigatory results available. In many countries this requires the consent of the worker if the physician is not connected with the workplace, but in others legislative requirements require a report of such events irrespective of patient confidentiality.

Whatever mechanisms are in place for proper communication, the employer has a number of obvious responsibilities once a case of occupational asthma is confirmed amongst the workforce. The circumstances of exposure for the index case have to be established, and the particular inducing agent has to be identified. The exposure of the index case may be unique to the individual's job, necessitating modification of the tasks involved and the exposures associated with them. More likely, other workers will also be seen to be at risk, and so some form of survey will be needed to assess whether any have become affected. Once environmental controls have been introduced that eliminate (or minimize) exposure and lessen the risks for the future, there will additionally be a need for a regular surveillance program to check that any emergent cases in the future are identified as expeditiously as possible.

Suitable survey and surveillance programs have essentially the same components. Regular environmental sampling allows a check to be made on exposure levels and on compliance with regulatory limits, and regular antibody tests (when such are available) among the workforce allow both prevalence and titers to be kept under scrutiny. This provides an indirect, but clinical, method of assessing ongoing exposure. The minimum requirement for clinical surveillance is a record of current symptoms and ventilatory function, and these can be achieved readily with questionnaires and spirometry. When 'failures' are detected, the individual should be referred to a clinician with expertise in the diagnosis of occupational asthma. It is often appropriate to start investigations with serial measurements of PEF at this time.

PREVENTION

In the workplace

A basic principle of occupational health is that the workplace should be made safe for all employees, regardless of individual susceptibility. With immunologic hypersensitivity, however, the range of individual susceptibility may be wide and, when there is a major practical difficulty in reducing exposure to uniformly safe levels, a number of additional preventive approaches may necessary. Prevention depends most on recognizing when there is a potential hazard (is there a known asthma-inducer within the workplace?) and when an individual worker has become affected. In either circumstance there is an obligation on the employer to carry out a risk assessment. Subsequent action depends on the perceived level of risk.

Exposure control

The essence of prevention lies with controling exposure to a practical minimum. This is most commonly achieved by the tools of industrial hygiene, for example, containment/enclosure of the processes generating or releasing dust, vapors, or gases; ventilation; local exhaust extraction. The most effective method is the substitution of less hazardous ingredient materials, or the manufacture of the end-product in a less hazardous form (e.g. enzyme-containing detergents as pellets rather than powder). The use of respiratory protection equipment should be the last resort if potentially hazardous levels of exposure cannot be achieved otherwise, since their effectiveness depends critically on the compliance of the user. The topic is discussed more fully in Chapter 33.

Preemployment evaluation/selection

There is often pressure on the occupational physician to exclude workers at the time of a preemployment medical, who are thought to be at high risk. Those who are already asthmatic provide the most obvious example, but a past history of probable asthma, the presence of high atopic status, and current smoking are additional factors which may increase the risk for some types of occupational asthma. An example often quoted is the reduced incidence of occupational asthma among platinum refinery workers following the exclusion of atopic subjects, but it has been suggested that the exclusion of current smokers would be more effective [97]. The exclusion of atopic individuals from work in animal laboratories provides an additional example where this practice has been recommended. However, in neither of these situations was sensitization reduced to acceptable levels and many individuals who would never have developed occupational asthma were denied employment.

Environmental and IgE antibody monitoring

When the presence of airborne sensitizers within the working environment cannot be avoided, the risks can be limited by regular monitoring of exposure and antibody levels. By the former, any mechanical failures causing excessive release can be quickly identified and corrected. By the latter, only possible if an IgE antibody test is available, the relevant inducing agent is monitored biologically. An increasing prevalence of antibody-positive workers

(or an increasing titer in those with previously detected antibodies) indicates an unsatisfactory level of exposure, and the likelihood that new cases of occupational asthma will emerge. By contrast, a decreasing prevalence or a diminishing titer suggests that hygiene controls are being effective.

Clinical surveillance

Whenever a known asthma-inducer is recognized to be present within the working environment or an individual worker has been shown to be affected, a risk assessment identifies the nature of the preventive measures that are needed, and the extent to which exposed workers need to be subjected to regular medical surveillance. In addition to any monitoring of IgE antibody responses, the latter may usefully include:

- Questionnaires
- Spirometry or PEF measurements
- Measurement of airway responsiveness.

Clear written instructions to the workforce concerning the nature of occupational asthma, the relevant inducing agent(s) in the particular working environment, the principles underlying the surveillance program, and the need to seek advice from the employer's medical service or the employee's own primary care physician, if asthmatic symptoms arise, provide a final but equally important measure. It is sensible that all employees are required to sign a document indicating that they have read and understood the information and instructions provided.

When the evidence suggests an asthmatic hazard of low degree, a questionnaire with spirometry may reveal a low probability for the presence of unrecognized asthma, and the surveillance procedures may not need to be repeated for 1 year. This assumes that the workforce is familiar with the risks involved and will seek appropriate advice speedily if symptoms emerge, and that new employees will undergo the same procedures during the course of preemployment medical evaluations.

When the considered hazard is of greater concern, much closer surveillance will be necessary, particularly for the workers whose questionnaires or spirometry are not fully satisfactory, and who appear to have no antecedent evidence of asthma. For them, serial measurements of airway responsiveness may be very useful, since these may detect increasing levels before there is an obvious worsening of symptoms or a reduction of ventilatory function. When asthma-inducers of perceived high potency are involved, repeated evaluations as frequently as 3-monthly may be advisable, though the interval can be steadily lengthened for the individual if each evaluation proves to be satisfactory. Intervals should not exceed 1 year, however, otherwise the advantage of early detection may be lost. When antibody tests are available for the particular inducing agent, these may be an extremely useful surveillance tool, since they provide an independent clinical means of evaluating the effectiveness of the measures of exposure control of the relevant agent.

National regulatory strategies

A variety of regulations are used in different countries for preventing occupational asthma, but all depend on a similar strategies. First, exposure standards should be defined and enforced whenever the potential for occupational asthma is recognized. Second, incident cases once recognized should be reported to the government agency, whether local or national, that is responsible for maintaining safety within the workplace. This should lead to an inspection and to an assessment of whether any modifications are needed to the work environment or working practices. Ongoing surveillance may additionally be necessary to ensure that compliance is achieved and further cases do not arise.

The topic is discussed in more detail in Chapters 33 and 35–37.

DIFFICULT CASE

History

A 47-year-old guard was locked in the security compartment of his cash-carrying van for $1\frac{1}{2}$ hours while diesel fumes leaked into the inadequately ventilated environment. During this period, he developed dizziness, a tightness of the chest, hoarseness of the voice, and a dry discomfort of the nose, but was unable to call attention to his plight. He was weak on being released, felt faint, vomited three times, and had slight breathlessness. Wheezing was noted on arrival at a local hospital, where he was said to be comfortable and not cyanosed. The PaO_2 was 12.7 kPa (95 mmHg), the PCO_2 was 3.5 kPa (26 mmHg), and the pH was 7.45. The pulse was regular at 92/min, the blood pressure was recorded at 174/115, and both electrocardiogram and chest radiograph proved to be normal. No other specific treatment was given. No lung function measurements were carried out at the time, but the peak flow rate was measured at 275 litres/min 6 days later (predicted 500). The wheezing and breathlessness persisted, and he was evaluated in a referral center after 6 months.

He had been a pipe smoker since the age of 20 years, consuming $1\frac{1}{2}$ ounces of tobacco per week. He denied any previous respiratory symptoms suggestive of asthma, and his medical records with the family medical practice supported this claim. They were, however, very suggestive of asthma from the time of the incident in the security van. He reported regular nocturnal waking (usually twice each night) because of respiratory distress, and wheeziness with undue breathlessness for 2–3 hours each morning after rising. Asthmatic symptoms were additionally provoked readily by exercise and intercurrent respiratory infections.

Skin prick tests to assess atopy were unhelpful because they revealed dermatographism. Prebronchodilator spirometry gave 2.40/3.05, respectively 72% and 75% of the predicted values. Following bronchodilator inhalation, the values were 2.24/2.72. Airway responsiveness, measured by the Yan method, gave a PC20 of 0.08 μmol/ml (normal >8 μmol/ml), thereby indicating a high level of responsiveness.

Issues

The issues in this case center on whether the guard developed asthma through the acute toxicity pathway (i.e. RADS) as a consequence of his work and his entrapment in the security van, and on what action might usefully have been taken in the local hospital and the referral center.

Comment

There was uniform agreement among the book's contributors that this was a case of RADS, but the range of confidence with which the diagnosis was reached showed a wide range. Neither marked nor moderate respiratory toxicity was evident at the time of the initial hospital examination, the spirometric measurements at the time of the referral center evaluation were not clearly suggestive of airway obstruction, and there was no apparent response to the administration of a bronchodilator. There had additionally been a moderate consumption of tobacco. In the absence of clear objective evidence for asthma, there is some concern that his symptoms might have been influenced by compensation issues.

The book's contributors favored measurement of the carboxyhemoglobin level at the time of the initial hospital examination, which might have provided useful confirmation that a high level of toxic exposure had indeed occurred. Unlike petrol engines, however, an efficiently running diesel engine generally produces little carbon monoxide in its exhaust – providing it is not run in a confined environment with limited oxygen. They would also have recommended a fuller respiratory evaluation at that time, with the measurement of spirometry, gas transfer, and lung volumes to assess whether there was parenchymal disease and whether this was associated with increased or decreased lung volume; peak flow monitoring; and a reevaluation within 1–2 weeks. A minority additionally suggested computed tomography (CT) imaging or bronchoscopy with bronchoalveolar lavage so that preexisting emphysema could be distinguished from acute parenchymal inflammation. Most would also have measured the immediate effect of an inhaled bronchodilator, and would have prescribed inhaled corticosteroids along with bronchodilators until the reevaluation.

DIFFICULT CASE

History

At about the age of 38 years, a coal miner of 23 years experience began to notice mild undue breathlessness on exertion at work together with wheezing and mild chest tightness. He attributed this to the greater level of exertion required in the mine compared to that associated with his domestic activities. He also noted that abrupt changes in temperature provoked a dry cough. His symptoms slowly worsened, and he sought advice from his general practitioner after 3 years. He had smoked only briefly, admitting to no more than 1 pack year. A diagnosis of asthma was confirmed following a respiratory physician's evaluation, and he was treated with inhaled bronchodilator and corticosteroid medication. He found the bronchodilator to he helpful over the following hours, but considered that his asthma continued to worsen slowly up to the time of his retirement aged 50 years and his evaluation in a referral center for a further opinion the following year. By then no further provoking factors had become evident, and there were no obvious domestic exposures of possible relevance apart from dogs until he was aged 48 years.

During the course of his mining career he had worked predominantly at the face with exposure to coal dust, though had been a stone cutter for a cumulative period of 2–3 years. In addition he had spent 2–3 hours daily over a 6-year period 'roof-bolting', and for the following 9 years up to the time of his retirement he had been involved with roof-bolting work for about 5 hours each month. The roof-bolting procedure was carried out (necessarily) at the heads of developing (hence blind ending) tunnels, and he claimed that dust and gaseous emanations were less readily exhausted than from the remainder of the mine. As a consequence, all underground miners experienced some exposure to the easily recognized odorous products that diffused from roof bolting work into the mine as a whole.

He was one of a cluster of 21 miners and ex-miners who had sought state compensation for occupational asthma. All claimed to have first developed symptoms after starting work in coal mines, all had worked as roof-bolters, and several identified the polyester resin used to retain the roofing bolts as a possible cause of their symptoms. Fourteen were evaluated in the referral center, and eight showed convincing evidence of asthma for which the clinical histories suggested a probable occupational cause.

The roof-bolting process represents a major advance in mining technology since the late 1960s. Tunnel roof, wall, and floor stability is achieved by the perpendicular insertion of long (2–5 m) steel bolts through the various layers of surrounding rock and sediment, rather than by traditional steel arches. These inhibit local movement of one layer on another, thus producing rigidity and strength. Bore holes are drilled through coal into the rock strata and the bolts are fixed in position using resins of polyester and styrene, and the cross-linking chemical dibenzoyl peroxide. The resin components, separated in sealed capsules, are inserted into the bore holes first; capsule rupture, content mixing, and resin activation follow when the rotating bolt is forced into position. Many gaseous products are released during polymerization (though dibenzoyl peroxide

itself is not volatile), and a distinctive odor (chiefly from the styrene) is easily recognized. Styrene is, however, an improbable causal agent since it has only rarely been reported to induce occupational asthma despite widespread industrial use, often at high concentrations (≥100 ppm). Measured levels in coal mines have been substantially less (generally <1 ppm, and always <5 ppm). The local maximum exposure limit averaged over 8 hours is 100 ppm, and the short-term exposure limit averaged over 10 min is 250 ppm.

Issues

The first issue here is whether this man's asthma was truly occupational in origin and a consequence of his exposures to the volatile activation products of the roof-bolting resin. Since this resin system has not previously been identified as a cause of occupational asthma, a second and wider issue is whether additional investigation is required before it can be accepted as an asthma-inducer and before his compensation claim can be evaluated.

Comment

A small majority of the book's contributors considered that he had developed occupational asthma, but a substantial minority were uncertain, arguing that further investigation was needed to resolve the matter. Most suggested specific inhalation provocation tests in the laboratory, or peak flow monitoring at and away from the coal mine. He was, however, already retired, and his former employer was unwilling to allow any return to the working environment because of insurance/indemnity issues. Both his legal adviser and the employer nevertheless favored laboratory-based specific challenge tests, and eventually a study was arranged involving six asthmatic volunteer miners who had all worked with the roof-bolting resin. For this, the miner described was able to discontinue his regular inhaled medication without undue adverse effect.

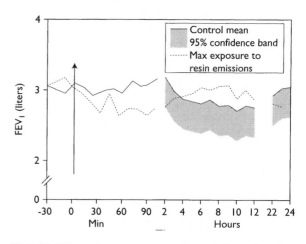

Fig. 4.14 FEV₁ measurements from maximum challenge dose of the second Difficult Case. The FEV₁ plot does not breach the lower 95% confidence boundary, indicating there has not been a statistically significant late decrement in ventilatory function.

The tests for each participant were conducted sequentially over several days in a double-blind placebo-controlled fashion, the 'dose' range (using off-gassing styrene as a marker) extending beyond the maximum likely to have been experienced occupationally during a single day's work. Immediately following resin activation, the volatile emissions were diluted with dry compressed air and directed into a 200-liter inert polyvinyl fluoride bag. The predetermined concentration for each test was achieved by further dilution under guidance from simultaneous sampling and the use of real-time analyzers. Their accuracy was confirmed later by equipment with greater precision. The challenge mixtures were inhaled from the bag in increasing dose on separate days, with dummy challenges (air alone) interspersed irregularly during the sequence so that neither test subject nor physician directly supervising the day's investigation knew the identity of the challenge agent. The series of tests were completed without any significant decrements in FEV_1 (Fig. 4.14) or significant increases in airway responsiveness in any subject, and so it was concluded that this resin system is not likely to have been the cause of asthma in these miners [160].

SUMMARY POINTS

Recognition

Does the individual under review have asthma?

- History of variable wheeze, shortness of breath, and chest tightness.
- Spirometry shows airway obstruction reversible with a bronchodilator.
- Serial PEF shows variability, and a typical asthmatic circadian rhythm.
- Airway responsiveness in asthmatic range.

If asthma is confirmed, is it occupational in origin?

- Symptoms worsen at work, and improve away from work (especially on vacation).
- PEF or spirometry worsens at work, and improves away (i.e. return-to-work provocation study).
- Airway responsiveness worsens in association with return-to-work provocation study.
- Environmental characterization shows a sensitizer in the workplace, perhaps at an excess level.
- IgE antibody assays show sensitization to relevant asthma-inducer.
- Laboratory-based inhalation provocation tests are positive.

Management

Of the individual

- Conventional medication (note: this might mask the recognition of occupational asthma induced by the hypersensitivity pathway).
- Cessation of exposure to inducing agent.
- If continued employment with minimized exposure, surveillance program to assess progress (questionnaire, spirometry, airway responsiveness, antibody titers).
- Compensation.

Of the workplace

- Identification of the inducing agent.
- Environmental characterization to establish exposure levels associated with various tasks and sites.
- Consider alternative production processes to avoid continuing use of the inducing agent.
- If use of the inducing agent cannot be avoided, environment hygiene improvements to minimize ongoing exposure levels.

- Surveillance program to monitor exposure levels and establish compliance with regulatory exposure controls.
- Surveillance of workforce (including antibody assays if available) to establish extent of problem with liaison with primary care physicians if indicated.
- Preparation of written essential information about occupational asthma for the workforce, including details of pertinent asthma-inducers, symptoms, the purpose of the surveillance program, and advice in the event of emerging symptoms of relevance.

Prevention

In the affected workplace

- Basic principle to provide safe working conditions for all employees regardless of susceptibility.
- Control relevant exposure levels:
  - Substitution of less hazardous ingredient materials
  - When relevant, manufacture end-product in less hazardous form
  - Containment/enclosure of manufacturing processes
  - Ventilation
  - Local exhaust extraction
  - Use of personal respiratory protection as last resort.
- Preemployment selection or job selection to exclude workers with greater susceptibility (e.g. atopics, smokers, and those with existing or earlier asthma) is not generally satisfactory.
- Environmental and specific IgE monitoring may aid the identification of unsatisfactory exposure levels.
- Clinical surveillance using questionnaires, PEF/spirometry, and measurements of airway responsiveness aids the identification of emergent cases at the earliest opportunity.
- Provision of clear written information and guidance to all members of the workforce limits ignorance and misunderstanding, and helps reduce unsatisfactory work practices.

National regulatory strategies

- Develop exposure/sensitization relationships and set standards to eliminate sensitization.
- Require formal reports of sentinel events so that inspections are triggered, safety is assessed, and (if necessary) the workplace environment is modified.

REFERENCES

1. Smith TA, Patton J. Health surveillance in milling, baking and other food manufacturing operations – five years' experience. *Occup Med* 1999; 49: 147–153.

2. Brooks SM, Weiss MA, Bernstein IL. Reactive airways dysfunction syndrome (RADS). Persistent asthma syndrome after high level irritant exposures. *Chest* 1985; 88: 376–384.

3. Kern DG. Outbreak of the reactive airways dysfunction syndrome after a spill of glacial acetic acid. *Am Rev Respir Dis* 1991; 144: 1058–1064.

4. Tarlo SM, Broder I. Irritant-induced occupational asthma. *Chest* 1989; 96: 297–300.

5. Alberts WM, do Pico GA. Reactive airways dysfunction syndrome. *Chest* 1996; 109: 1618–1626.

6. Kipen HM, Blume R, Hutt D. Asthma experience in an occupational and environmental medicine clinic. Low-dose reactive airways dysfunction syndrome. *J Occup Med* 1994; 36: 1133–1137.

7. Ross DJ, Keynes HL, McDonald JC. SWORD '96: surveillance of work-related and occupational respiratory disease in the UK. *Occup Med* 1997; 47: 377–381.

8. Ross DJ, Keynes HL, McDonald JC. SWORD '97: surveillance of work-related and occupational respiratory disease in the UK. *Occup Med* 1998; 48: 481–485.

9. Meyer JD, Holt DL, Cherry NM, McDonald JC. SWORD '98: surveillance of work-related and occupational respiratory disease in the UK. *Occup Med* 1999; 47: 485–489.

10. Newman Taylor A. Non-malignant disease. In: McDonald JC, ed. *Epidemiology of Work Related Diseases*, 2nd edn. London: BMJ Books, 1999.

11. Di Stefano F, Siriruttanapruk S, McCoach JS *et al.* Occupational asthma due to glutaraldehyde. *Monaldi Arch Chest Dis* 1998; 53: 50–55.

12. Hendrick DJ, Lane DJ. Formalin Asthma in hospital staff. *Br Med J* 1975; i: 607–608.

13. Burge PS, Harries MG, Lam WK *et al.* Occupational asthma due to formaldehyde. *Thorax* 1985; 40: 255–260.

14. Nordman H, Keskinen H, Tuppurainen M. Formaldehyde asthma – rare or overlooked? *J Allergy Clin Immunol* 1985; 75: 91–9.

15. Harving H, Korsgaard J, Dahl R. Low concentrations of formaldehyde in bronchial asthma: a study of exposure under controlled conditions. *Br Med J* 1986; 293: 310.

16. Hendrick DJ, Lane DJ. Occupational formalin asthma. *Br J Ind Med* 1977; 34: 11–18.

17. Gannon PF, Bright P, Campbell M *et al.* Occupational asthma due to glutaraldehyde and formaldehyde in endoscopy and x ray departments. Thorax 1995; 50: 156–159.

18. Di Stefano F, Siriruttanapruk S, McCoach J *et al.* Glutaraldehyde: an occupational hazard in the hospital setting. *Allergy* 1999; 54: 1105–1109.

19. Kongerud J, Boe J, Soyseth V *et al.* Aluminium potroom asthma: the Norwegian experience. *Eur Respir J* 1994; 7: 165–172.

20. Kongerud J, Soyseth V, Burge PS. Serial measurements of peak expiratory flow and responsiveness to methacholine in the diagnosis of aluminium potroom asthma. *Thorax* 1992; 47: 292–297.

21. Soyseth V, Kongerud J, Boe J *et al.* Bronchial responsiveness and work-related asthma in aluminium potroom workers: effect of removal from exposure. *Eur Respir J* 1992; 5: 829–833.

22. Kongerud J, Samuelsen SO. A longitudinal study of respiratory symptoms in aluminium potroom workers. *Am Rev Respir Dis* 1991; 144: 10–16.

23. Soyseth V, Kongerud J. Prevalence of respiratory disorders among aluminium potroom workers in relation to exposure to fluoride. *Br J Ind Med* 1992; 49: 125–130.

24. Vandenplas O, Delwiche JP, Vanbilsen ML *et al.* Occupational asthma caused by aluminium welding. *Eur Respir J* 1998; 11: 1182–1184.

25. Marks GB, Salome CM, Woolcock AJ. Asthma and allergy associated with occupational exposure to ispaghula and senna products in a pharmaceutical workforce. *Am Rev Respir Dis* 1991; 144: 1065–1069.

26. Coutts II, Dally MB, Newman Taylor AJ *et al.* Asthma in workers manufacturing cephalosporins. *Br Med J* 1981; 283: 950.

27. Davies RJ, Hendrick DJ, Pepys J. Asthma due to inhaled chemical agents: ampicillin, benzyl penicillin, 6 amino-penicillanic acid and related substances. *Clin Allergy* 1974; 4: 227–247.

28. Houba R, Heederik D, Doekes G. Wheat sensitization and work-related symptoms in the baking industry are preventable. An epidemiologic study. *Am J Respir Crit Care Med* 1998; 158: 1499–1503.

29. Houba R, Heederik DJ, Doekes G *et al.* Exposure–sensitization relationship for alpha-amylase allergens in the baking industry. *Am J Respir Crit Care Med* 1996; 154: 130–136.

30. Travers-Glass SA, Griffin P, Crook B. Bacterially contaminated oil mists in engineering works: a possible respiratory hazard. *Grana* 1991; 30: 404–406.

31. Smith TA, Smith PW. Respiratory symptoms and sensitization in bread and cake bakers. *Occup Med* 1998; 48: 321–328.

32. Sandiford CP, Tee RD, Newman Taylor AJ. Identification of crossreacting wheat, rye, barley and soya flour allergens using sera from individuals with wheat-induced asthma. *Clin Exp Allergy* 1995; 25: 340–349.

33. Sander I, Raulf-Heimsoth M, Duser M *et al.* Differentiation between cosensitization and cross-reactivity in wheat flour and grass pollen-sensitized subjects. *Int Arch Allergy Immunol* 1997; 112: 378–385.

34. Burge PS. Occupational asthma, rhinitis and alveolitis due to colophony. *Clin Immunol Allergy* 1984; 4: 55–82.

35. McCoach JS, Robertson AS, Burge PS *et al.*, eds. Floor cleaning materials as a cause of occupational asthma. *Indoor Air 99*, p. 5: 459–464. Watford: Building Research Establishment, 1999.

36. Ayars GH, Altman LC, Frazier CE *et al.* The toxicity of constituents of cedar and pine woods to pulmonary epithelium. *J Allergy Clin Immunol* 1989; 83: 610–618.

37. Convery RP, Ward RJ, Hendrick DJ. Occupational asthma due to a widely used soft solder flux not containing colophony. *Eur Respir J* 1997; 10: 238–240.

38. Cullen RT, Cherrie B, Soutar CA. Immune responses to colophony, an agent causing occupational asthma. *Thorax* 1992; 47: 1050–1055.

39. Schilling RSF, Hughes JPW, Dingwall-Fordyce I *et al.* An epidemiological study byssinosis among Lancashire cotton workers. *Br J Ind Med* 1995; 12: 217–227.

40. Castellan RM, Olenchock SA, Hankinson JL *et al.* Acute bronchoconstriction induced by cotton dust: dose related response to endotoxin and other dust factors. *Ann Intern Med* 1969; 101: 157–163.

41. Koskela R-S, Klockars M, Jarvinen E. Mortality and disability among cotton mill workers. *Br J Ind Med* 1991; 48: 143–144.

42. Niven RMcL, Pickering CAC. Byssinosis: a review. *Thorax* 1996; 51: 632–637.

43. Niven RMcL, Fletcher AM, Pickering CAC *et al.* Chronic bronchitis in textile workers. *Thorax* 1997; 52: 22–27.

44. Merchant JA, Halprin GM, Hudson AR *et al.* Evaluation before and after exposure – the pattern of physiological response to cotton dust. *Ann New York Acad Sci* 1974; 221: 38–43.

45. Fishwick D, Fletcher AM, Pickering CAC *et al.* Lung function, bronchial reactivity, atopic status and dust exposure in Lancashire mill operatives. *Am Rev Respir Dis* 1992; 145: 1103–1108.

46. Glindmeyer HW, Lefante JJ, Jones RN *et al.* Cotton dust and across-shift change in FEV1 as predictors of annual change in FEV1. *Am J Respir Crit Care Med* 1994; 149: 584–590.

47. Honeybourne D, Pickering CAC. Physiological evidence that emphysema is not a feature of byssinosis but is due to concomitant cigarette smoking. *Thorax* 1986; 41: 6–11.

48. Hodgson JT, Jones RD. Mortality of workers in the British cotton industry in 1968–1984. *Scand J Environ Health* 1990; 16: 113–120.

49. Juniper CP, How MJ, Goodwin BFJ *et al.* Bacillus subtillis enzymes: a 7 year clinical, epidemiological and immunological study of an industrial allergen. *J Soc Occup Med* 1977; 27: 3–12.

50. Baur X, Konig G, Bencze K *et al.* Clinical symptoms and results of skin test. RAST and bronchial provocation test in 33 papain workers. *Clin Allergy* 1982; 12: 9–17.

51. Kanerva L, Jolanki R, Tupasela O *et al.* Immediate and delayed allergy from epoxy resins based on diglycidyl ether of bisphenol A. *Scand J Work Environ Health* 1991; 17: 208–15.

52. Venables KM, Topping MD, Howe W *et al.* Interaction of smoking and atopy in producing specific IgE antibody against a hapten protein conjugate. *Br Med J* 1985; 290: 201–204.

53. Chan-Yeung M, Enarson D, Grzybowski S. Grain dust and respiratory health. *Can Med Assoc J* 1985; 133: 969–973.

54. Darke CS, Knowelden J, Lacey J. Respiratory disease of workers harvesting grain. *Thorax* 1976; 31: 294–302.

55. Chan-Yeung M, Dimich-Ward H, Enarson DA *et al.* Five cross-sectional studies of grain elevator workers. *Am J Epidemiol* 1992; 136: 1269–1279.

56. Park HS, Jung KS, Hwang SC *et al.* Neutrophil infiltration and release of IL-8 in airway mucosa from subjects with grain dust-induced occupational asthma. *Clin Exp Allergy* 1998; 28: 724–730.

57. Tabona M, Chan-Yeung M, Enarson D *et al.* Host factors affecting longitudinal decline in lung function among grain elevator workers. *Chest* 1984; 85: 782–786.

58. Post W, Heederik D, Houba R. Decline in lung function related to exposure and selection processes among workers in the grain processing and animal feed industry. *Occup Environ Med* 1998; 55: 349–355.

59. Revsbech P, Andersen G. Storage mite allergy among grain elevator workers. *Allergy* 1987; 42: 423–429.

60. Banks DE, Rando RJ, Barkman HW Jr. Persistence of toluene diisocyanate-induced asthma despite negligible workplace exposures. *Chest* 1990; 97: 121–125.

61. Lozewicz S, Asoufi BK, Hawkins R *et al.* Outcome of asthma induced by isocyanates. *Br J Dis Chest* 1987; 81: 14–22.

62. Pisati G, Baruffini A, Zedda S. Toluene diisocyanate induced asthma: outcome according to persistence or cessation of exposure. *Br J Ind Med* 1993; 50: 60–64.

63. Tarlo SM, Banks D, Liss G *et al.* Outcome determinants for isocyanate induced occupational asthma among compensation claimants. *Occup Environ Med* 1997; 54: 756–761.

64. Paggiaro PL, Vagaggini B, Bacci E *et al.* Prognosis of occupational asthma. *Eur Respir J* 1994; 7: 761–767.

65. Mapp CE, Corona PC, De Marzo N *et al.* Persistent asthma due to isocyanates. A follow up study on subjects with occupational asthma due to toluene diisocyanate (TDI). *Am Rev Respir Dis* 1988; 137: 1326–1329.

66. Paggiaro PL, Bacci E, Dente FL *et al.* Prognosis of occupational asthma induced by isocyanates. *Bull Eur Physiopathol Respir* 1988; 23: 565–569.

67. Adams WGF. Long-term effects on the health of men engaged in the manufacture of tolylene diisocyanate. *Br J Ind Med* 1975; 32: 72–78.

68. Venables KM, Dally MB, Burge PS *et al.* Occupational asthma in a steel coating plant. *Br J Ind Med* 1985; 42: 517–524.

69. Vu-Duc T, Huynh CK, Savolainen H. Do the isocyanate monomer standards still protect against attacks of occupational asthma? Should a standard including polyisocyanates be evolved? *Schweiz Med Wochensch* 1997; 48: 2000–2007.

70. Seguin P, Allard A, Cartier A *et al.* Prevalence of occupational asthma in spray painters exposed to several types of isocyanates, including polymethylene polyphenylisocyanate. *JOM* 1987; 29: 340–344.

71. Vandenplas O, Cartier A, Lesage J *et al.* Prepolymers of hexamethylene diisocyanate as a cause of occupational asthma. *J Allergy Clin Immunol* 1993; 91: 850–861.

72. Vandenplas O, Cartier A, Lesage J *et al.* Occupational asthma caused by a prepolymer but not the monomer of toluene diisocyanate (TDI). *J Allergy Clin Immunol* 1992; 89: 1183–1188.

73. O'Brien IM, Harries MG, Burge PS *et al.* Toluene di-isocyanate-induced asthma. I. Reactions to TDI, MDI, HDI and histamine. *Clin Allergy* 1979; 9: 1–6.

74. Butcher BT, Jones RN, O'Neil CE *et al.* Longitudinal study of workers employed in the manufacture of toluene-diisocyanate. *Am Rev Respir Dis* 1977; 116: 411–421.

75. Tee RD, Cullinan P, Welch J *et al.* Specific IgE to isocyanates: a useful diagnostic role in occupational asthma. *J Allergy Clin Immunol* 1998; 101: 7109–715.

76. Diem JE, Jones RN, Hendrick DJ *et al.* Five-year longitudinal study of workers employed in a new toluene diisocyanate manufacturing plant. *Am Rev Respir Dis* 1982; 126: 420–428.

77. Longbottom JL. Occupational allergy due to animal allergens. *Clin Immunol Allergy* 1984; 4: 19–36.

78. Botham PA, Davies GE, Teasdale EL. Allergy to laboratory animals: a prospective study of its incidence and the influence of atopy on its development. *Br J Ind Med* 1987; 44: 627–632.

79. Cullinan P, Lowson D, Nieuwenhuijsen MJ *et al.* Work related symptoms, sensitisation, and estimated exposure in workers not previously exposed to laboratory rats. *Occup Environ Med* 1994; 51: 589–592.

80. Heederik D, Venables KM, Malmberg P et al. Exposure–response relationships for work-related sensitization in workers exposed to rat urinary allergens: results from a pooled study. *J Allergy Clin Immunol* 1999; 103: 678–684.

81. Gordon S, Tee RD, Lowson D et al. Reduction of airborne allergenic urinary proteins from laboratory rats. *Br J Ind Med* 1992; 49: 416–422.

82. Ylonen J, Mantyjarvi R, Taivainen A et al. Comparison of the antigenic and allergenic properties of three types of bovine epithelial material. *Int Arch Allergy Immunol* 1992; 99: 112–117.

83. Iversen M, Dahl R, Korsgaard J et al. Respiratory symptoms in Danish farmers: an epidemiological study of risk factors. *Thorax* 1988; 43: 872–877.

84. Burge PS, Edge G, O'Brien LM et al. Occupational asthma in a research centre breeding locusts. *Clin Allergy* 1980; 10: 355–63.

85. Tee RD, Gordon DJ, Hawkins ER et al. Occupational allergy to locusts: an investigation of the sources of the allergen. *J Allergy Clin Immunol* 1988; 81: 517–25.

86. Axelsson IGK, Eriksson M, Wrangsjo K. Anaphylaxis and angioedema due to rubber allergy in children. *Acta Paediatr Scand* 1988; 77: 314–316.

87. Vandenplas O, Delwiche JP, Evrard G et al. Prevalence of occupational asthma due to latex among hospital personnel. *Am J Respir Crit Care Med* 1995; 151: 54–60.

88. Tarlo SM, Wong L, Roos J, Booth N. Occupational asthma caused by latex in a surgical glove manufacturing plant. *J Allergy Clin Immunol* 1990; 85: 626–631.

89. Azizah MR, Shahnaz M, Hasma H et al. Latex protein allergy: a prospective study of factory workers. *J Nat Rubb Res* 1996; 11: 240–246.

90. Moller M, Kayma M, Vieluf D et al. Determination and characterisation of cross-reacting allergens in latex, avocado, banana and kiwi fruit. *Allergy* 1998; 53: 289–296.

91. Pepys J. Occupational allergy due to platinum complex salts. *Clinics Immunol Allergy* 1984; 4: 131–158.

92. Calverley AE, Rees D, Dowdeswell RJ et al. Platinum salt sensitivity in refinery workers: incidence and effects of smoking and exposure. *Occup Environ Med* 1995; 52: 661–666.

93. Pepys J, Pickering CAC, Hughes EG. Asthma due to inhaled chemical agents – complex salts of platinum. *Clin Allergy* 1972; 2: 391–396.

94. Cleare MJ, Hughes EG, Jacoby B et al. Immediate (type 1) allergic responses to platinum compounds. *Clin Allergy* 1976; 6: 193–195.

95. Linnett PJ, Hughes EG. 20 years of medical surveillance on exposure to allergenic and non-allergenic platinum compounds: the importance of chemical speciation. *Occup Environ Med* 1999; 56: 191–196.

96. Newman Taylor AJ, Venables KM. Asthma related to occupation of spouse. *Practitioner* 1989; 233: 809–810.

97. Venables KM, Dally MB, Nunn AJ et al. Smoking and occupational allergy in workers in a platinum refinery. *Br Med J* 1989; 299: 939–942.

98. Baker DB, Gann PH, Brooks SM et al. Cross-sectional study of platinum salts sensitization among precious metals refinery workers. *Am J Ind Med* 1990; 18: 653–664.

99. Merget R, Schulte A, Gebler A et al. Outcome of occupational asthma due to platinum salts after transferral to low-exposure areas. *Int Arch Occup Environ Health* 1999; 72: 33–39.

100. Chan-Yeung M, MacLean L, Paggiaro PL. Follow-up study of 232 patients with occupational asthma caused by western red cedar (Thuja plicata). *J Allergy Clin Immunol* 1987; 79: 792–796.

101. Vedal S, Chan-Yeung M, Enarson D et al. Symptoms and pulmonary function in Western Red Cedar workers related to duration of employment and dust exposure. *Arch Environ Health* 1986; 41: 179–183.

102. Norrish AE, Beasley R, Hodgkinson EJ et al. A study of New Zealand wood workers: exposure to wood dust, respiratory symptoms, and suspected cases of occupational asthma. *New Zealand Med J* 1992; 105: 185–187.

103. Frew AJ, Chan H, Lam S et al. Bronchial inflammation in occupational asthma due to western red cedar. *Am J Respir Crit Care Med* 1995; 151: 340–344.

104. Lin FJ, Dimich-Ward H, Chan-Yeung M. Longitudinal decline in lung function in patients with occupational asthma due to western red cedar. *Occup Environ Med* 1996; 53: 753–756.

105. Gannon PF, Weir DC, Robertson AS et al. Health, employment, and financial outcomes in workers with occupational asthma. *Br J Ind Med* 1993; 50: 491–496.

106. Burge PS. Occupational asthma in electronics workers caused by colophony fumes: follow-up of affected workers. *Thorax* 1982; 37: 348–353.

107. Barker RD, Harris JM, Welch JA et al. Occupational asthma caused by tetrachlorophthalic anhydride: a 12-year follow-up. *J Allergy Clin Immunol* 1998; 101: 717–719.

108. Weir DC, Robertson AS, Jones S et al. The economic consequences of developing occupational asthma. *Thorax* 1987; 42: 209.

109. Ameille J, Pairon JC, Bayeux MC et al. Consequences of occupational asthma on employment and financial status: a follow-up study. *Eur Respir J* 1997; 10: 55–58.

110. Perfetti L, Cartier A, Ghezzo H et al. Follow-up of occupational asthma after removal from or diminution of exposure to the responsible agent: relevance of the length of the interval from cessation of exposure. *Chest* 1998; 114: 398–403.

111. Park HS, Nahm DH. Prognostic factors for toluene diisocyanate-induced occupational asthma after removal from exposure. *Clin Exp Allergy* 1997; 27: 1145–1150.

112. Cote J, Kennedy S, Chan-Yeung M. Outcome of patients with cedar asthma with continuous exposure. *Am Rev Respir Dis* 1990; 141: 373–376.

113. Ross DJ, McDonald JC. Health and employment after a diagnosis of occupational asthma: a descriptive study. *Occup Med* 1998; 48: 219–225.

114. Assoufi BK, Venables KM, Cook A et al. Outcome of occupational asthma due to platinum salts. *Thorax* 1996; 51(Suppl 3): A41.

115. Baker DB, Gann PH, Brooks SM et al. Cross-sectional study of platinum salts sensitization among precious metals refinery workers. *Am J Ind Med* 1990; 18: 653–64.

116. Butcher BT, O'Neil CE, Reed MA et al. Development and loss of toluene diisocyanate reactivity: immunologic, pharmacologic and provocation challenge studies. *J Allergy Clin Immunol* 1982; 70: 231–235.

117. Lemière C, Cartier A, Dolovich J et al. Outcome of specific bronchial responsiveness to occupational agents after removal from exposure. *Am J Respir Crit Care Med* 1996; 154: 329–333.

118. Carino M, Aliani M, Licitra C *et al.* Death due to asthma at workplace in a diphenylmethane diisocyanate-sensitized subject. *Respiration* 1997; 64: 111–113.

119. Bryant DH, Burns MW. The relationship between bronchial histamine reactivity and atopic state. *Clin Allergy* 1976; 6: 373–381.

120. Bryant DH, Burns MW. Bronchial histamine reactivity its relationship to the reactivity of the bronchi to allergens. *Clin Allergy* 1976; 6: 523–532.

121. Gannon PF, Newton DT, Belcher J *et al.* Development of OASYS-2: a system for the analysis of serial measurement of peak expiratory flow in workers with suspected occupational asthma. *Thorax* 1996; 51: 484–9.

122. Burge PS, Pantin CFA, Newton DT *et al.* Development of an expert system for the interpretation of serial peak expiratory flow measurements in the diagnosis of occupational asthma. *Occup Environ Med* 1999; 56: 758–764.

123. Elms J, Allan LJ, Pengelly I *et al.* Colophony: an in vitro model for the induction of sensitization. *Clin Exp Allergy* 2000; 30: 209–213.

124. Fifield R, Bird AG, Carter RH *et al.* Total IgE and allergen-specific IgE assays: guidelines for the provision of a laboratory service. *Ann Clin Biochem* 1987; 24: 232–245.

125. van der Veen MJ, Mulder M, Witteman AM *et al.* False-positive skin prick test responses to commercially available dog dander extracts caused by contamination with house dust mite (*Dermatophagoides pteronyssinus*) allergens. *J Allergy Clin Immunol* 1996; 98: 1028–1034.

126. Lucyznska CM, Topping MD. Specific IgE antibodies to reactive dye-albumin conjugates. *J Immunol Metho* 1986; 95: 177–186.

127. Curran AD, Burge PS, Wiley K. Clinical and immunologic evaluation of workers exposed to glutaraldehyde. *Allergy* 1996; 51: 826–832.

128. Paris-Kohler A, Demoly P, Persi L *et al.* In vitro diagnosis of cypress pollen allergen by using cytofluorimetric analysis of basophils (Basotest). *J Allergy Clin Immunol* 2000; 105: 339–345.

129. Butcher BT, Mapp CE, Fabbri LM. Bernstein IL, Chan Yeung M, Malo J, Bernstein DI, eds. Polyisocyanates and their pre-polymers. In: Asthma in the Workplace. New York: Marcel Dekker, 1993, pp. 415–438.

130. Elms J, Allan LJ, Pengelly D *et al.* Colophony: an in vitro model for the induction of sensitization. *Clin Exp Allergy* 2000; 30: 209–213.

131. Curran AD. Flow cytometry in the exploration of the physiopathology of occupational lung disease. *Occup Environ Med* 1999; 56: 742–747.

132. Chang JH, Chan H, Quirce S *et al.* In vitro T-lymphocyte response and house dust mite-induced bronchoconstriction. *J Allergy Clin Immunol* 1996; 98: 922–931.

133. Frew A, Chang JH, Chan H *et al.* T-lymphocyte responses to plicatic acid–human serum albumin conjugate in occupational asthma caused by western red cedar. *J Allergy Clin Immunol* 1998; 101: 841–847.

134. Corrigan CJ, Hartnell A, Kay AB. T-lymphocytes activation in acute severe asthma. *Lancet* 1988; 1: 1129–1132.

135. Robinson DS, Hamid Q, Bentley A *et al.* Activation of CD4+ T-cells, increased Th2 type cytokine mRNA expression and eosinophil recruitment in bronchoalveolar lavage after allergen inhalation in patients with atopic asthma. *J Allerg Clin Immunol* 1993; 92: 313–324.

136. Mapp CE, Saetta M, Maestrelli P *et al.* Mechanisms and pathology of occupational asthma. *Eur Respir J* 1994; 7: 544–554.

137. Finotto S, Fabbri LM, Rado V *et al.* Increase in numbers of CD8 positive lymphocytes and eosinophils in peripheral blood of subjects with late asthmatic reactions induced by toluene diisocyanate. *B J Ind Med* 1991; 48: 116–121.

138. Frew A, Chang JH, Chan H *et al.* T-lymphocyte responses to plicatic acid–human serum albumin conjugate in occupational asthma caused by western red cedar. *J Allergy Clin Immunol* 1998; 101: 841–847.

139. Curran AD, Gordon SB, Morice AH *et al.* Expression of lymphocyte cell surface markers in workers exposed to different respiratory hazards: biomarkers of occupational respiratory disease? *Biomarkers* 1997; 2: 367–371.

140. Lara-Marquez ML, Deykin A, Krinzman S *et al.* Analysis of T-cell activation after bronchial allergen challenge in patients with atopic asthma. *J Allergy Clin Immunol* 1998; 101: 699–708.

141. Ebo DG, Stevens WJ, Bridts CH, De Clerck LS. Latex specific IgE, skin testing and lymphocytes transformation to latex in latex allergy. *J Allergy Clin Immunol* 1997; 100:618–623.

142. Kam KL, Hsieh KH. Comparison of three in vitro assays for serum IgE with skin testing in asthmatic children. *Ann Allergy* 1994; 73:329–336.

143. Wass U, Belin L. Immunologic specificity of isocyanate-induced IgE antibodies in serum from 10 sensitised workers. *J Allergy Clin Immunol* 1989; 83:126–135.

144. Baur X, Dewair M, Fruhmann G. Detection of immunologically sensitised isocyanate workers by RAST and intracutaneous skin tests. *J Allergy Clin Immunol* 1984; 73:610–618.

145. Pastorello EA, Incorvaia C, Pravettoni V *et al.* A multicentre study on sensitivity and specificity of a new in vitro test for measurement of IgE antibodies. *Ann Allergy* 1991; 67;365-370.

146. Valencia M, Randazzo L, Tapias G, Granel C, Olive A. Allergy to Alternaria. II. Diagnostic comparison of skin-tests and RAST. *Allergol Immunopathol (Madr)* 1993; 21:84–87.

147. Rasanen L, Kuusisto P, Penttila M, Nieminen M, Savolainen J, Lehto M. Comparison of immunologic tests in the diagnosis of occupational asthmna and rhinitis. *Allergy* 1994; 49:342–347.

148. Merget R, Stollfuss J, Wiewrodt R *et al.* Diagnostic tests in enzyme allergy. *J Allery Clin Immunol* 1993; 92:264–277.

149. Ownby DR, Magera B, Williams PB. A blinded, multi-center evaluation of two commercial in vitro tests for latex-specific antibodies. *Ann Allergy Asthma Immunol* 2000; 84:193–196.

150. Niggemann B, Wahn U. A new dipstick test (Allergodip) for in vitro diagnosis of latex allergy: validation in patients with spina bifida. *Pediatr Allergy Immunol* 2000; 11:56–59.

151. Paganelli R, Ansotegui IJ, Sastre J *et al.* Specific IgE antibodies in the diagnosis of atopic disease. Clinical evaluation of a new in vitro test system, UniCAP, in six European allergy clinics. *Allergy* 1998; 53:763–768.

152. Chan-Yeung M, Malo JL. Occupational asthma. *Chest* 1987; 91: 130S–136S.

153. Cartier A, Bernstein IL, Burge PS *et al.* Guidelines for bronchoprovocation on the investigation of

occupational asthma. Report of the Subcommittee on Bronchoprovocation for Occupational Asthma. *J Allergy Clin Immunol* 1989; 84: 823–829.

154. EAACI. Guidelines for the diagnosis of occupational asthma. Subcommittee on 'Occupational Allergy' of the European Academy of Allergology and Clinical Immunology. *Clin Exp Allergy* 1992; 22: 103–108.

155. Cartier A, Malo JL. Occupational challenge tests. In: Bernstein IL, Chan-Yeung M, Malo JL, Bernstein DI, eds. *Asthma in the Workplace*, pp. 215–248. New York: Marcel Decker Inc. 1993.

156. Pepys J, Hutchcroft BJ. Bronchial provocation tests in etiologic diagnosis and analysis of asthma. *Am Rev Respir Dis* 1975; 112: 829–859.

157. Cloutier Y, Malo JL. Update on an exposure system for particles in the diagnosis of occupational asthma. *Eur Respir J* 1992; 5: 887–890.

158. Vandenplas O, Malo JL, Cartier A *et al.* Closed-circuit methodology for inhalation challenge tests with isocyanates. *Am Rev Respir Dis* 1992; 145: 582–587.

159. Lemière C, Cloutier Y, Perrault G *et al.* Closed-circuit apparatus for specific inhalation challenges with an occupational agent, formaldehyde, in vapor form. *Chest* 1996; 109: 1631–1635.

160. Banks DE, Tarlo SM, Masri F, Rando RJ, Weissman DN. Bronchoprovocation tests in the diagnosis of isocyanate-induced asthma. *Chest* 1996; 109: 1370–1379.

161. Sostrand P, Kongerud J, Eduard W *et al.* A test chamber for experimental hydrogen fluoride exposure in humans. *Am Ind Hyg Assoc J* 1997; 58: 521–525.

162. Convery R, Ward A, Ward R *et al.* Asthmagenicity of coal mine roof-bolting resins: an assessment using inhalation provocation tests. *Occup Med* 2000; 51: 100–106.

163. Stenton SC, Dennis JH, Walters EH *et al.* The asthmagenic properties of a newly developed detergent ingredient – sodium iso-nonanoyl oxybenzene sulphonate. *Br J Ind Med* 1990; 47: 405–10.

164. Lin FJ, Chen H, Chan-Yeung M. New method for an occupational dust challenge test. *Occup Environ Med* 1995; 52: 54–56.

165. Merget R, Heger M, Globisch A *et al.* Quantitative bronchial challenge tests with wheat flour dust administered by spinhaler: comparison with aqueous wheat flour extract inhalation. *J Allergy Clin Immunol* 1997; 100: 199–207.

166. Malo JL, Cartier A, Boulet LP. Occupational asthma in sawmills of Eastern Canada and United States. *J Allergy Clin Immunol* 1986; 78: 392–398.

167. Stenton SC, Beach JR, Dennis JH, Keaney NP *et al.* Glutaraldehyde, asthma and work – a cautionary tale. *Occup Med* 1994; 44: 95–98.

168. Perrin B, Cartier A, Ghezzo H *et al.* Reassessment of the temporal patterns of bronchial obstruction after exposure to occupational sensitizing agents. *J Allergy Clin Immunol* 1991; 87: 630–639.

169. Stenton SC, Dennis JH, Hendrick DJ. Occupational asthma caused by ceftazidime. *Eur Respir J* 1995; 8: 1421–1423.

170. Stenton SC, Avery AJ, Walters EH *et al.* Technical note: Statistical approaches to the identification of late asthmatic reactions. *Eur Respir J* 1994; 7: 806–812.

171. Bérubé D, Cartier A, L'Archevêque J *et al.* Comparison of peak expiratory flow rate and FEV1 in assessing bronchomotor tone after challenges with occupational sensitizers. *Chest* 1991; 99: 831–836.

172. Gautrin D, D'Aquino LC, Gagnon G *et al.* Comparison between peak expiratory flow rates (PEFR) and FEV_1 in the monitoring of asthmatic subjects at the outpatient clinic. *Chest* 1994; 106: 1419–1426.

173. Giannini D, Paggiaro PL, Moscato G *et al.* Comparison between peak expiratory flow and forced expiratory volume in one second (FEV1) during bronchoconstriction induced by different stimuli. *J Asthma* 1997; 34: 105–111.

174. Vandenplas O, Delwiche JP, Jamart J *et al.* Increase in non-specific bronchial hyperresponsiveness as an early marker of bronchial response to occupational agents during specific inhalation challenges. *Thorax* 1996; 51: 472–478.

175. Lemiere C, Pizzichini MM, Balkissoon R *et al.* Diagnosing occupational asthma: use of induced sputum. *Eur Respir J* 1999; 13: 482–488.

176. Malo JL, Ghezzo H, L'Archevêque J *et al.* Late asthmatic reactions to occupational sensitizing agents: frequency of changes in nonspecific bronchial responsiveness and of response to inhaled beta 2-adrenergic agent. *J Allergy Clin Immunol* 1990; 85: 834–842.

177. Zammit-Tabona M, Sherkin M, Kijek K *et al.* Asthma caused by diphenylmethane diisocyanate in foundry workers. Clinical, bronchial provocation, and immunologic studies. *Am Rev Respir Dis* 1983; 128: 226–230.

178. Cockcroft DW, Hoeppner VH, Werner GD. Recurrent nocturnal asthma after bronchoprovocation with Western Red Cedar sawdust: association with acute increase in non-allergic bronchial responsiveness. *Clin Allergy* 1984; 14: 61–68.

179. Cartier A, Malo JL, Forest F *et al.* Occupational asthma in snow crab-processing workers. *J Allergy Clin Immunol* 1984; 74: 261–269.

5 CHRONIC OBSTRUCTIVE PULMONARY DISEASE (COPD)

Chris Stenton

BACKGROUND

Definitions

Chronic obstructive pulmonary disease (COPD), often called 'chronic obstructive airway disease', is the commonest form of chronic lung disease in developed countries, affecting some 5–10% of their populations [1]. The term emphasizes the physiologic abnormality of long-standing, fixed, airflow obstruction rather than any specific pathologic process or etiology. It is not the result of a single disease process, being associated with chronic bronchitis, emphysema, bronchiolitis, and asthma, or any combination of these. The cause, or component causes, in an individual case cannot always be identified reliably during life or even defined with complete precision.

■ *Chronic bronchitis* is defined clinically as a productive cough which persists for several months over a period of at least 2 years. It is associated with hypertrophy of the mucous glands of the airways. It contributes little if anything to airflow obstruction and to increased mortality (though is strongly associated with both), and is best regarded as an independent disease process caused by a similar range of environmental agents.

■ *Emphysema* is defined pathologically as an increase in the size of alveolar air spaces because of destruction of the walls which initially separated them. The associated loss of structural, essentially elastic, support for the small airways allows them to collapse and become distorted, increases resistance to airflow, and increases trapping of gas within the lung on expiration. In addition, the loss of alveolar surface area leads to a reduction in oxygen-transfer capacity.

■ *Bronchiolitis* refers to inflammation and fibrosis in the walls of the distal bronchioles which narrow their lumina and increase airway resistance. Bronchiolitis and emphysema are usually seen together in smokers with COPD, and the extent to which one rather than the other is the main cause of the airflow obstruction is disputed.

■ *Asthma* is usually considered separately from other forms of COPD because in its early stages it can be distinguished by much greater variability of the airflow obstruction. With chronicity, however, airway remodeling occurs in a proportion of affected individuals. This is associated with the development of fixed airflow obstruction, though some degree of variability may persist.

In normal individuals, lung function is maximal by about the age of 20–25 years, remains constant until about 30 years, and deteriorates slowly after that [2]. Features of the ageing lung include a relative decrease in the amount of elastic tissue and an increase in the amount of collagen. These cause a variety of lung function changes which mimic those of COPD; there is a decrease in pulmonary elastic recoil and an increase in pulmonary compliance causing reduced expiratory airflow and gas trapping, and a decrease in oxygen-diffusing capacity [3]. The normal rate of decline of FEV_1 with age is approximately 25–30 ml per year but it is more rapid in those destined to develop COPD, and cigarette smokers for example have an average annual loss of FEV_1 which is 10–20 ml greater than that of non-smokers. The average effect in a population of smokers is small but there is a wide range of individual susceptibility. The majority of smokers show little excess longitudinal loss of ventilatory function and a minority of 10–15% become severely affected [4]. These individuals typically seek medical attention in their 6th or 7th decade when their reserves of ventilatory function have been sufficiently eroded for symptoms to develop during normal day-to-day activities. By then there is usually marked impairment of ventilatory function, but susceptible individuals can be detected much earlier by screening lung function tests.

COPD was first subjected to extensive medical investigation in the 1950s. Initial epidemiological research focused on the role of respiratory infections and urban pollution, but the dramatic importance of cigarette smoking was soon established and attention became diverted away from other possible etiologic agents. By the 1980s, the US Surgeon General reported that smoking and the inherited condition, α_1-antitrypsin deficiency, were the only conditions which had an established causal link with COPD [5]. More recently epidemiological investigations have reported an excess prevalence of COPD in a variety of industrial settings. Most reviewers now accept a causal occupational link [6–9], and the conditions experienced by workers in several industries over recent decades are considered by many to be of similar potency to cigarette smoking. However, the scientific evidence on which these conclusions are based is complex and considerable controversy remains [6,10–12].

Epidemiology

With most occupational diseases, an individual's condition can be attributed to his work because of the temporal pattern of symptoms (e.g. asthma or alveolitis), because the disease does not occur outside the occupational setting (e.g. pneumoconiosis), or because it is otherwise so uncommon that an occupational cause can usually be assumed (e.g. malignant mesothelioma). In contrast, occupational COPD has no characteristic clinical or other features which allow it to be distinguished from COPD caused by cigarette smoking, and it is not usually possible to establish a firm diagnosis in an individual. The importance of occupational exposures in a particular working population can only be identified by demonstrating that there is a greater prevalence of COPD than would be expected when smoking and other potential influences on lung function are taken into account. Unfortunately, this is not a simple process.

Selection bias

An individual's place of work is not governed by random events but by a series of influences which can confound epidemiological investigations. As a rule, those in work enjoy better health and have higher levels of lung function than the remainder of the population – the *healthy worker effect*. A study which demonstrates similar levels of lung function in working and control populations might thus mask a true adverse work-related effect. For similar reasons, the lung function of those in poorly paid or low prestige work might be lower than that of a control group employed in other work, since no alternative work is available despite poor lung function [13]. The work environment here might be associated with impaired function, but is not the cause of it. Also, individuals who are most able to tolerate an adverse working environment will tend to remain there longest and sustain the greatest cumulative levels of exposure, whereas those who are most severely affected will leave soonest. A study which includes only the current workforce might consequently fail to detect an occupational problem because of this *survivor effect*. In physically demanding jobs the level of lung function will determine (at least partly) how long work can continue, and so result in a positive correlation between exposure and lung function which might mask an adverse effect of the working environment. The actual outcome of an investigation will depend on the relative strengths of the two opposing effects.

Because of these difficulties in establishing suitable control populations, most major epidemiological investigations of occupational COPD have estimated the relative effects of different levels of exposure (both daily and cumulative) within the same working population. Multiple regression techniques are used to assess whether increasing levels of exposure are associated with increasing risk after adjustments are made for other factors of relevance. These require that for each individual some estimate is made of exposure to the agent under investigation, and that evaluations are made of all other factors which might influence lung function (covariates) such as age, height, weight, smoking, ethnic group, and the severity of any concomitant disease.

Measurement error

There are few industries in which detailed individual exposure measurements are collected routinely. Often these have to be estimated from data that are more readily available such as duration of work or job category. Neither of these is entirely satisfactory. Duration of work, for example, is often very closely associated with age leading to difficulty in separating the effects of the one from the other in regression analysis. Even when calculations are made of exposure for each individual, they are usually based on samples obtained from a small proportion of the workforce. They often require extrapolation backwards beyond the start of the study, and so the validity of the manipulations can be challenged [12]. Measurements obtained to monitor compliance with legal requirements can represent worst case rather than typical exposures and have sometimes been of questionable accuracy [14].

Accurately quantifying cigarette smoking poses a further difficulty because the estimates of individual workers are not always reliable. In one UK study it was concluded that up to 7% of smokers and ex-smokers had incorrectly described themselves as never-smokers [15], while in a US study of coal miners, 15% of participants described themselves as never-smokers despite records from earlier surveys which had documented them as smokers [11].

Confounding and interactions

The cumulative amount smoked, like the extent of occupational exposure, is often associated with age, again posing a difficulty separating the effects of one from the other. Those who smoke might also be those who best tolerate noxious occupational environments, implying that the effects of the occupational exposure might be different between smokers and non-smokers because smoking acts as a marker of differences in susceptibility. In one study of shipyard workers it was found that those in trades with high exposure to welding fume were twice as likely to smoke as those in low-exposure trades. This trend was already clearly established in school leavers at the time they applied for work in the same respective trades and before any occupational exposure began. Choosing to smoke was thus associated with choosing a career in a high fume-exposure trade, leading to potential confounding [16].

Socioeconomic status and education level are important determinants of respiratory health. The relevance of this to investigations of occupational COPD is illustrated by studies showing that while miners have an excess of respiratory symptoms, their wives similarly report more symptoms than the wives of other manual workers [17]. These effects might be mediated by an increased prevalence of childhood illness, exposure to passive smoking in childhood, housing quality, nutrition, and environmental exposures outside the workplace. For example, chronic exposure to low levels of nitrogen oxides, such as those found in homes with gas stoves, may lead to respiratory impairment, especially in children [18]. Studies of coal miners have identified very substantial differences in lung function between workers in different mines. As average dust exposures differ between mines, this geographic or 'mine effect' has the potential to confound the results of multicenter studies.

Individual susceptibility

Although it is recognized that there is a very wide range of individual susceptibility to developing COPD, no account can usually be taken of this in epidemiological investigations. It has been argued that whereas the small average effect of cigarette smoke on lung function is caused by a few severely affected individuals, occupational exposures affect a greater proportion of the population with each individual being only mildly affected [19]. It is difficult to demonstrate that this is not correct, but there is no particular reason why occupational exposures should act differently from cigarette smoke and the view is not widely accepted [8].

The inherited condition α_1-antitrypsin deficiency is strongly associated with the development of COPD but it is uncommon, being found in about 1–2% of affected individuals [20]. Other host factors such as atopy, airway hyperresponsiveness, and family history of respiratory disease have been shown to be associated COPD also, but they have not been considered in most studies of occupational COPD. Nor, generally, has asthma been taken into account, or a previous history of pneumonia or chest trauma [21]. There is considerable potential for the outcome of a given study to have explanations beyond those advanced by the investigators [21,22].

Cross-sectional vs longitudinal analysis

Cross-sectional analyses appear to overestimate the effect of age on FEV_1 compared with that demonstrated when the same population is followed longitudinally. For example, the studies of Rogan and Love (illustrated in Table 5.1) investigated samples of men from the same population group of coal miners, yet the cross-sectional analysis suggested a change in FEV_1 with age which was about 50%

Table 5.1 Estimated loss of FEV$_1$ (ml) attributable to 40 years exposure to coal mine dust at the current exposure limit (2 mg/m^3), smoking 20 cigarettes/day for 40 years, and ageing 40 years

	Reference	n	Dust	Smoking	Age
Cross-sectional studies					
Rogan, 1973	[23]	3581	125[a,b]	123[c]	1880
Soutar, 1986	[35]	4059	96[b]	536	1640
Attfield, 1992	[38]	7139	88[c]	408	1240
Seixas, 1993 (1972–5 survey)	[27]	977	2398	376	2060
Seixas, 1993 (1985–8 survey)	[27]	977	514	342	1692
Henneberger, 1996 (1969–75)	[28]	1915	43	423	1080
Henneberger, 1996 (1985–88)	[28]	1915	104	542	1520
Longitudinal studies					
Love, 1982	[24]	1677	182[d]	443[e]	1229[f]
Attfield, 1985	[39]	1161	204[g]	478	1322[f]
Seixas, 1993	[27]	977	–	421	1348[f]
Carta, 1996	[40]	909	123 to 608[h]	320	1221[f]
Henneberger, 1996	[28]	1915	6 to −160[i]	740[b]	1172[f]

a. Using revised exposure estimates reported in [26], mean of effect in smokers and non-smokers
b. Assuming average age of starting smoking at 17 years
c. Assuming a miner works for 1600 hours per year
d. Relates only to exposures encountered before follow-up period. No effect identified for current exposures
e. For average smoking. Amount not stated in paper
f. Derived from difference between initial and final FEV$_1$ minus losses attributable to smoking, dust exposure etc
g. Derived from coefficient for intersurvey dust concentration (P = 0.12). The only significant association was with years of exposure at the coal face during the survey
h. Not including a positive effect for exposures before the start of the study
i. Loss identified for exposures before start of study, indicates gain for exposures during study.

greater than that observed longitudinally [23,24]. Larger differences between the two types of analysis have been observed in other studies [25]. The explanation probably lies with the improving mean levels of ventilatory function of young adults in developed countries throughout the 20th century, which in turn are probably consequences of improvements in nutrition and infection control. Cross-sectional studies compare older individuals (reaching lesser maximum levels of lung function in their youths) with younger fitter individuals, and so overestimate the effect of ageing (Fig 5.1). This raises the possibility that other variables that are time-dependent, such as occupational exposure and amount smoked, might similarly be influenced by the method of analysis. Age is the variable measured with greatest precision in most studies, and the variability in the estimates of its effect on ventilatory function give some indication of the imprecision which is likely to be associated with the estimated effects of the other variables.

It is also possible that the method of regression analysis, which assumes a steady rate (i.e. linear) decline of lung function with exposure, is not the most appropriate for evaluating the adverse effects of occupational environments. There may, for example, be a greater effect in those who are exposed at a young age when the lungs are still maturing [23,26–29]. The

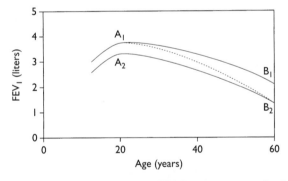

Fig. 5.1 Discrepant mean decline in FEV$_1$ from cross-sectional and longitudinal data. A$_1$–B$_1$ represents future true longitudinal decline for subjects currently aged 20 years. A$_2$–B$_2$ represents past longitudinal decline for subjects currently aged 60 years. A$_1$–B$_2$ represents apparent decline using cross-sectional data from subjects currently aged 20–60 years.

effect of age itself is not easily modeled in regression analyses. The annual rate of decline of FEV$_1$ is more rapid in older subjects and so fitting a simple linear model to a dataset overestimates lung function in middle age and underestimates it in the elderly [30].

Weight and weight change

Weight change is one potential source of confounding in studies of lung function for which adjustment is not usually made. Weight does not appear to be an important determinant of ventilatory function in cross-sectional studies, but weight gain due to increased fat deposition in middle age is associated with a marked reduction in FEV_1 and FVC in longitudinal studies [31,32]. The average effect of a 1-kg change in body mass is of similar magnitude to the average annual change of FEV_1 attributed to ageing. Confounding could arise because of the complex relationship between weight change, occupational status, and smoking. Stopping manual work and stopping smoking are both likely to lead to weight gain, sedentary work might be associated with lesser occupational exposures and more weight gain than manual work, and weight gain can be a consequence of rather than a cause of impaired lung function. The ability of weight change to confound the investigation of occupational exposures has been demonstrated in one study of welders [31].

It is clear that formidable difficulties have to be overcome before it can be concluded that a particular occupational environment can cause COPD, and it is a tribute to the extent of epidemiological investigation that some picture seems to be emerging. The remainder of this chapter aims to reflect the current consensus of opinion but it should be borne in mind that some experts remain sceptical about the extent to which the issues have been resolved.

Causes

Coal

Coal miners have probably been the most thoroughly investigated of all working groups because of the enormous numbers of workers previously employed in the industry, their political influence, and the early recognition of pneumoconiosis as a specific and easily identifiable occupational illness. Chronic bronchitis is common among coal miners with up to 45% of non-smoking workers reporting relevant symptoms [33]. Chronic bronchitis itself is unlikely to be the cause of significant breathlessness, but it provides convincing evidence that coal mine dust has one adverse effect on the airways, and so may have the potential to cause other airway effects. It is established that ventilatory function is impaired when pneumoconiosis is complicated by the development of progressive massive fibrosis and the associated distortion of lung architecture. There is, however, no correlation between the category of simple (i.e. uncomplicated) coal workers' pneumoconiosis and impairment of ventilatory function [23,34,35].

Some evidence suggesting an association between coal dust exposure and airflow obstruction comes from the structure of the coal macule – the pathological abnormality of simple pneumoconiosis. Coal macules develop around terminal bronchioles and are associated with centrilobular emphysema [36].

The significance of the emphysema so far as lung function is concerned has been disputed for some time [12], but a number of studies have now demonstrated that centrilobular emphysema is more common in miners than in control populations and is related to the dust content of the lungs [37].

Most epidemiological investigations of coal miners have suggested an adverse effect of coal mine dust on ventilatory function independent of simple pneumoconiosis. Estimates of the magnitude of this effect from several large studies are shown in Table 5.1 together with the estimated effects of cigarette smoking and ageing [23,24,27,28,35,38–40]. Those of ageing are broadly similar, with the cross-sectional studies predicting greater losses over 40 years than the longitudinal. Estimates of the average effect of smoking are also broadly similar, with the exception of the Rogan study in which a much lesser effect was noted. In contrast, the estimated effects of coal mine dust exposure were considerably more variable, ranging over almost two orders of magnitude. This probably reflects imprecision in the estimates of cumulative exposure in the individual miners together with confounding by the other variables which influence lung function, and may reflect differences in coal rank or incorporated contaminants.

Most studies have identified a greater effect of coal mine dust in younger compared with older miners [23,26–29]. Rogan and colleagues for example estimated that the magnitude of the effect of exposure on FEV_1 was almost four times greater at the age of 25 than at 64 [23]. Seixas and colleagues showed a marked exposure-related impairment of FEV_1 within 5 years of starting mining with some recovery over the next 10–14 years, and a lesser dose-related impairment at the end of their study period [27]. More experienced miners had less exposure-related impairment of FEV_1 both initially and at follow-up, suggesting a survivor benefit associated with lesser susceptibility [28]. This raises the possibility that younger workers with lung function which is not fully mature are at greater risk from exposure than others. There are, however, alternative explanations which include a survivor effect in the populations studied and a disproportionate effect of smoking in older subjects [8]. Some investigators have additionally suggested that smokers are at greater risk than non-smokers (Fig 5.2), but most have found no evidence of such an interaction.

It is not clear whether the dust-associated impairment of ventilatory function seen in coal miners is entirely due to airflow obstruction, as many studies have reported FEV_1 without vital capacity measurements. Others have reported a greater decrease in FVC associated with coal mine dust than is seen with cigarette smoking, and less reduction in FEV_1/FVC

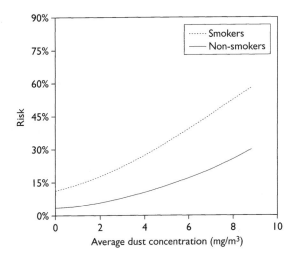

Fig. 5.2 Estimated risk of a deficit in FEV_1 of at least 942 ml after 35-year exposure to coal mine dust. The slope describing the relation between risk and exposure is steeper for smokers than non-smokers, indicating a positive interaction. Adapted from Soutar and Hurley [35].

ratio [28,35,38,40]. The effect of coal dust thus appears to be partly obstructive and partly restrictive. It has been suggested that this reflects the combined effects of emphysema and peribronchiolar fibrosis which can be found in the lungs of miners [35]. In cigarette smokers the dominant abnormality appears to be airflow obstruction, irrespective of occupational exposures, and that is the pattern which will most often be identified in symptomatic individuals [35].

The evidence of coal mining-induced COPD produces something of a paradox in relation to pneumoconiosis. It is recognized that there is a close correlation between the category of simple pneumoconiosis, cumulative dust exposure during work, and the amount of dust found in the lungs postmortem [41,42]. There is also an association between impaired ventilatory function and cumulative dust exposure, but there is no association between the category of simple pneumoconiosis and airflow obstruction. This could indicate either that the airflow obstruction of miners is primarily an airway disease and is independent of the emphysema which is associated with coal macules, or the particle size necessary to cause pneumoconiosis is different from that which causes airflow obstruction. The observation is, however, essentially unexplained.

Other mineral dusts

Several cross-sectional and longitudinal studies have demonstrated a relationship between dust exposure and airflow obstruction in hard rock miners exposed to silica [43,44]. Also, emphysema assessed quantitatively at autopsy has been shown to be related to years of exposure among men mining gold from siliceous rock, an effect which is independent of silicosis [45].

Pathologic studies have also identified bronchiolar abnormalities similar to those associated with cigarette smoking, and it is not clear whether it is these or emphysema which is the cause of the airflow obstruction [46]. There are close parallels with coal mine dust though the potency of silica in causing COPD appears to be approximately an order of magnitude greater than that of coal dust, paralleling its greater potency in causing pneumoconiosis [6].

Small airway inflammation and fibrosis is an early feature of asbestos exposure, and animal studies have shown a correlation between asbestos-induced increased airway wall thickness and reduced airflow [47,48]. A number of human studies have reported an excess prevalence of airflow obstruction, mostly using sensitive but imprecise measures of airflow at low long volumes, but there are no large studies of ventilatory function in asbestos-exposed populations and the clinical significance of these observations is uncertain [22].

Fume

Cadmium fume is encountered in the production of alloys and in other settings. It is associated with airflow obstruction, and with lung function and radiological evidence of emphysema [60]. Its potency in causing airflow obstruction appears to be 1 to 2 orders of magnitude greater than that of coal dust, regression analysis suggesting that 40 years exposure at 2 mg/ml would be associated with a decrement of FEV_1 of more than 5 litres.

A number of investigations of welders have demonstrated an excess prevalence of chronic bronchitis. Cotes and colleagues also demonstrated adverse effects on lung function in both cross-sectional and longitudinal studies [49,50]. The effect of fume exposure was of similar magnitude to that associated with smoking, and there appeared to be an interaction so that the combined effect of smoking and welding was more than additive. Welding is occasionally associated additionally with asthma, and a higher prevalence of airway hyperresponsiveness has been demonstrated in welding apprentices [16]. This raises the possibility that the COPD of welders could arise through a mechanism shared with asthma, at least in some welders.

Organic dusts and asthmagenic agents

Cotton dust was the first occupational agent to be recognized as a cause COPD, and from this the term 'Grade 3 byssinosis' arose. Cotton dust exposure is also associated with a productive cough and the immediate work-related symptoms and lung function abnormalities that are characteristic of occupational asthma [51]. Grain and wood dusts have been shown to cause a similar range of respiratory problems, i.e. chronic bronchitis, occupational asthma, cross-shift decrements in ventilatory function, and an accelerated longitudinal decline of FEV_1 [52,53]. There is evidence from both cotton and grain-exposed populations of a relationship between acute (across shift) changes and the subsequent longitudinal rate of change of ventilatory function [51,54]. This suggests, as with welding fume, that the asthmagenic and COPD-producing mechanisms of these organic dusts are related. The natural history of the COPD effect does, however, appear to be distinct from that of the fixed airflow obstruction which may develop late in the course of occupational asthma.

The accelerated longitudinal decline of ventilatory function in workers exposed to cotton, grain, and wood dust raises the possibility that other asthmagenic exposures might also contribute to the development of COPD. Support for this notion comes from a study of workers exposed to toluene diisocyanate, which is one of the most potent asthmagenic agents encountered in industrialized countries. Diem and colleagues demonstrated an excess mean annual loss of FEV_1 attributable to diisocyanate exposures (which averaged 2 ppb) of approximately 10 ml/year [55]. This was of similar magnitude to the effect of smoking in the same population, and to the effects seen in populations exposed to mineral dusts. It appeared to be distinct from occupational asthma since it was still evident when all recognized asthmatics were excluded from the analysis. These observations with diisocyanates have not been confirmed by all investigators, but they raise the question whether other occupational exposures to reactive chemical agents might be making a contribution to COPD, possibly even at levels which are within statutory control limits.

Other exposures

The term 'nuisance dust' is often used to describe exposures which are thought to be without adverse health effects. However, the demonstration that a wide variety of occupational exposures are associated with chronic bronchitis and COPD raises the issues of whether 'nuisance' is an appropriate term and whether all dust exposures have the potential to cause a productive cough and contribute to airflow obstruction. The marked difference in the potencies of coal, silica and cadmium suggests that there is some degree of agent specificity, but a broader effect of occupational dust exposures is supported by a number of general population studies. Bakke and colleagues showed that Norwegian workers exposed to high levels of airborne dust were 3.6 times more likely to have symptoms of asthma or COPD, and 1.4 times more likely to have impaired lung function than non-exposed workers, though the latter was not statistically significant [56]. Kaufmann and colleagues showed an association between FEV_1 decline over 12 years in middle-aged factory workers and their exposures to

Table 5.2 Some agents and exposures suspected of causing occupational COPD

Agent	References
Mineral dusts	
Asbestos	[48]
Carbon black	[70]
Ceramic fibers	[71]
Coal	[8,23,24]
Iron/steel dust	[32,57]
Silica/hard rock mining	[43,44]
Wollastoninte	[69]
Organic dusts	
Cotton	[51]
Grain	[52]
Wood	[53]
Gases/fume/chemicals	
Ammonia	[58]
Cadmium	[60]
Firefighting	[73]
Isocyanates	[55]
Sulfur dioxide(in paper mills)	[72]
Welding fume	[31]

This list is not comprehensive. The evidence relating to some agents derives from single studies and is not universally accepted.

dust, gases, and heat [57]. Krzyzanowski and colleagues reported that the effects of occupational dust exposure were approximately half of those attributable to current smoking [58]. These studies derive some strength from the incidental nature of their findings in that their primary focus was not on occupational exposures, but they relied on subjects' own descriptions of their occupational exposures and these might have been subject to recall and other biases. Agents suspected of causing or contributing to COPD are listed in Table 5.2.

Conclusions

The evidence in favor of a contribution from occupational exposures to COPD does not, therefore, derive from any single study, or even from studies of one particular working environment, and no single investigation has given an overwhelmingly convincing outcome. Rather, the evidence derives from the apparent consistency with which an excess prevalence of COPD has been reported in many different settings. The overall importance of occupational exposures is more difficult to determine. At one end of the spectrum, some authorities remain unconvinced that there is any important effect. At the other, it is possible that a wide variety of apparently unremarkable occupational exposures are as damaging to the airways as cigarette smoking.

Prognosis

COPD in susceptible individuals tends to progress so long as exposure to the causative agent or agents continues. In the case of cigarette smoke the accelerated rate of decline of lung function stops when smoking ceases. FEV_1, however, continues to decline at the normal rate of 25–30 ml/year and disablement may therefore continue to progress. With coal dust, the rate of decline of lung function has often been shown to be most closely related to earlier rather than current exposures suggesting that an adverse effect is likely to persist after the cessation of exposure. The same might be true with other mineral dusts that are retained in the lung and have ongoing biologic effects. For example, welding fume has been reported to cause accelerated longitudinal decline of ventilatory function after exposures ceased, but this might have been primarily a consequence of weight gain [31,50]. It might alternatively have been a consequence of iron retention in the lungs though siderosis, unlike coal workers' pneumoconiosis and silicosis, is generally considered to be 'benign'. There is little evidence about any ongoing effect of cotton dust or other agents which are unlikely to be retained in the lungs, but it is probable that their effects are similar to that of cigarette smoke and cease when exposures cease.

RECOGNITION

Clinical features

COPD has a wide spectrum of severity. The majority of affected individuals have mild disease which can be identified from lung function abnormalities but which causes no or few respiratory symptoms. The characteristic presenting feature in those who are more severely affected is progressive exertional breathlessness with an associated diminution of exercize capacity. There may be an accompanying productive cough with seasonal exacerbations, but these are not essential to establish the diagnosis. Features on physical examination may include overinflation and hyperresonance of the chest, pursed lip breathing, use of the accessory muscles of respiration, and diminution of the breath sounds with expiratory wheezing. Finger clubbing is not a feature.

Investigation

Lung function

The cardinal feature of COPD is fixed (i.e. irreversible) obstruction to forced expiratory airflow. This can be measured simply in most individuals from spirometry as a reduction in the FEV_1/VC ratio. Most commercially available spirometers measure FEV_1 and VC accurately, and good quality measurements depend more on the skill and training of the supervisor than on the choice of equipment. Guidelines set down by the European and American Thoracic Societies are described in Chapter 32. If there is no other cause of impaired ventilatory function, the degree of airflow obstruction is best quantified by the reduction in FEV_1 below the value predicted from reference equations which take into account the individual's age, gender, height, and ethnicity. In general the lower limits of the normal ranges for FEV_1 and FVC equate to about 80% of the predicted values [59].

Occasionally it is useful to inspect a flow–volume curve for evidence of convexity within the expiratory limb, as this can indicate reduced flow at low lung volumes. This is a feature of mild or early COPD, and reflects disease at bronchiolar level. However, indices derived from flow at low lung volumes, such as FEF_{50}, FEF_{75}, FEF_{75-85}, are all much less reproducible than FEV_1 and add little additional information in most established cases [59]. Quantifying the response to inhaled bronchodilators and/or oral corticosteroids is useful in distinguishing COPD from asthma, and in identifying a mixed picture.

A single measurement of lung function at around the lower end of the normal range can be difficult to interpret, and serial measurements are much more powerful in detecting early COPD. Even in the most severely affected individuals, the annual fall in FEV_1 is less than the variability of the measurement, and so it is usually necessary to obtain measurements over at least 5 years to obtain a clear picture of the rate of change. Annual declines of FEV_1 of more than 50 ml/year which cannot be attributed to weight gain suggest that an individual is at risk of developing severe COPD.

The resting diffusing capacity for carbon monoxide (D_LCO or T_LCO) is reduced in most individuals with COPD because there is accompanying emphysema. However, the correlation between the clinical severity of the disease and the reduction of D_LCO in individual patients is poor. The measurement can be useful additionally in distinguishing COPD from asthma, since the latter is associated with a normal or even supranormal D_LCO [3]. The reasons for this are not entirely clear.

Little is known whether COPD of occupational origin is caused primarily through an effect on the airways or by emphysema. If purely a disease of the airways (i.e. the result of bronchiolitis), then D_LCO might not be impaired to the same extent as with smoking-induced COPD, and the measurement could help quantify the relative contributions of the two exposures. Carta and colleagues showed that the reduction in FEV_1 in coal miners was paralleled by a reduction in $D_{L}CO$ [40]. Chronic low level exposures to cadmium has a similar effect [60] but there does not appear to be any association between impaired $D_{L}CO$ and duration of exposure to silica or to welding fume exposures [13,50]. No clear association has been demonstrated between cotton dust exposure during life and emphysema at autopsy [61], and it might be that some occupational agents are associated only with emphysema (e.g. fibrogenic dusts) and others only with airway disease. Some may be associated with both, as is tobacco smoke.

Imaging

The chest radiograph might show overinflation of the lungs or attenuation of lung markings, but in general radiology has little role in the diagnosis of COPD. Even with occupational exposures such as coal dust and welding fume, which are associated with interstitial radiologic abnormalities, there is no association between the presence of simple pneumoconiosis and COPD. The plain radiograph is invaluable, nevertheless, in helping to exclude alternative causes of respiratory disease. High-resolution computed tomography (CT) scanning is much more sensitive than the chest radiograph for detecting emphysema. It may also detect disease of the small airways, and help determine the relative importance of airway disease and emphysema. Basal predominance of emphysema and a pan acinar pattern may suggest α_1-antitrypsin deficiency.

Serology

Homozygous α_1-antitrypsin deficiency can be detected in 1–2% of all patients with COPD but the incidence is related negatively to the age of onset of symptoms, and 50% of patients presenting with severe disease before the age of 40 years are affected [20]. Screening younger patients with COPD by α_1-antitrypsin levels can help explain their susceptibility, and can allow specific therapy to be considered. It may additionally lead usefully to screening other family members, but the procedure is of very limited value in the occupational setting.

Attributing COPD to occupation

When an individual is found who has COPD, has never smoked, and has no other obvious lung disease, then the COPD can usually be attributed to relevant occupational exposures. Even so, unexplained airflow obstruction is occasionally found in middle-aged never-smokers, and chronic undiagnosed asthma sometimes presents with fixed airflow obstruction. The diagnostic difficulties are much greater in smokers who work in environments contaminated by dust or fume. If the two different exposures can each cause COPD, then in any affected individual it is unlikely that one is responsible and the other is entirely innocent. The issue is one of apportioning responsibility between the two. At present this problem is encountered principally by those involved in litigation or in establishing and administering compensation schemes. However, employers are likely to be faced with similar issues in the future as emphasis is placed on the early detection of COPD through periodic surveillance in the workplace, and on the prevention of severe disease.

It is first necessary to determine whether an employee's exposures had the potential to cause, or contribute to, the development of COPD. This has only been established with any reasonable degree of certainty for a few occupational environments (Table 5.2). However, given the wide variety of agents which have now been reported to be associated with COPD, it cannot be assumed that heavy occupational exposure to any inhaled substance is free from risk. The matter can only be resolved by epidemiological study, and by the reporting of consistent outcomes. Once there is some consensus as to the approximate average effect of a given level of cumulative exposure (and of any interaction with smoking or other factor), attribution in the individual case can be attempted. Any estimate that is produced will, however, be crude – and almost certainly a source of controversy.

For a smoker it is necessary to make some cumulative quantification of both smoking and occupational exposures (which may be multiple), if only into broad categories such as 'heavy', 'light,' or 'none'. It is then necessary to assume that the relative potency of their effects on the airways is constant and that individuals who are most susceptible to one are also most susceptible to any other. The relative potency of smoking and the occupational exposures must be determined from the epidemiological data if exposures are to one of the agents for which data such exists. Otherwise, an estimate must be made by analogy with or by extrapolation from existing data.

In the UK, the civil court case which determined the relative potencies of welding fume and smoking for legal purposes lasted 6 weeks, and the case which determined the issues relating to coal mine dust lasted 9 months [12,62], reflecting the complexities of the issues involved. The judgements took account of much scientific data and informed opinions on the matter, though in the setting of an adversarial courtroom rather than that of scientific consensus. Heavy welding-fume exposure in confined spaces with inadequate ventilation was considered half as potent as average smoking as a cause of

COPD, and exposure to coal mine dust sufficient to pose a risk of uncomplicated pneumoconiosis was considered equipotent to average smoking. Although such estimates were made as a consequence of particular litigious experiences in only two industries, it is unlikely that they have no relevance beyond coal mine dust and welding fume. The implication is that coal mine dust exposures which fall within current exposure standards for respirable 'nuisance' dusts (i.e. <5 mg/m^3) are almost equipotent to smoking. The effect of lower levels of exposure is likely to be proportionately less, but the effect of other occupational exposures might well be similar or of even greater magnitude.

MANAGEMENT

Of the individual

Exposure cessation

There is good evidence from cigarette smokers that stopping exposure is the single most important step in managing COPD. As impairment of lung function has been shown to be related to cumulative exposure with several occupational agents, preventing or reducing further occupational exposure in individuals with established disease is likely to be similarly important. At present, little attention is paid to this and most affected individuals stop work or change their job only when they become too disabled to continue. However, with increased awareness of occupational COPD, litigation, and the introduction of surveillance schemes, this situation is likely to change.

COPD has a wide spectrum of disease severity, and there is probably no threshold level of exposure to dusts and fumes which has no biologic effect. In most dusty industrial settings associated with COPD it may not be possible to prevent completely any degree of lung function impairment. If an employee is identified with significant disease then some estimate should be made of the extent to which it is due to the effects of smoking, and to the effects of occupational exposure. Future changes in lung function can then be predicted, and so some estimate can be made of the likely final severity of COPD if smoking and occupational exposure do or do not continue unchanged. In making such predictions it must be borne in mind that while the effect of cigarette smoke ceases when an individual stops smoking, this is not necessarily so with occupational exposures.

An acceptable degree of work-induced impairment of lung function needs to be established. To date there are no guidelines which address this but an appropriate degree of impairment might be the level of lung function found in fewer than 5% of the normal population, i.e. more than 1.65 standard deviations below an individual's predicted FEV$_1$ [63]. This equates to approximately 20% impairment. If it is estimated (from the rate of change of lung function and from the smoking history) that this might be exceeded if occupational exposures continue, then steps should be taken to limit those exposures.

Smoking cessation

It is possible that with some occupational agents there is a multiplicative interaction with smoking, and that there would be a disproportionate benefit from stopping either exposure. Some studies of coal miners have suggested such an effect but most have not [8,26]. There is little evidence of synergism between smoking and grain dust but such an effect has been reported with welding fume [50]. Because of its additional associations with other diseases it is likely that smoking cessation would make the greatest contribution to the health of most working populations, and every effort should be made to persuade individuals with COPD to stop smoking.

Medication

COPD patients are usually prescribed bronchodilator drugs (β$_2$-agonists, anticholinergics, or theophyllines) to improve symptoms and quality of life [64]. There is a range of bronchodilator responsiveness but in general the effect is small and much less than in asthma. The bronchodilator effect of β$_2$-agonists is approximately related to the logarithm of the dose and some patients appear to derive symptomatic benefit from large doses administered via a nebulizer [65]. The role of corticosteroids is controversial but inhaled corticosteroids have been shown in one study to reduce the exacerbation rate [66]. No pharmacologic treatment to date has been shown to alter the natural history of COPD or to prolong life. Supplemental oxygen has this effect when administered for at least 16 hours per day to hypoxic patients. Pulmonary rehabilitation programs improve exercise capacity and quality of life but have no significant effect on lung function [67].

Compensation

The development of compensation schemes for occupational COPD has generated considerable scientific and political conflict, and the schemes themselves have often created anomalies as a consequence of the difficulty in assessing disability and in distinguishing the effects of cigarette smoking. These can be illustrated by UK experience with coal mine dust.

COPD in coal miners was accepted as a compensable condition under the state Industrial Injuries Benefit scheme in 1992. The initial legislation provided compensation for any miner with COPD who had more than 20 years underground experience, at least Category 1 pneumoconiosis on the chest radiograph, and an FEV_1 of at least 1 liter below the predicted value. The requirement for an abnormal chest radiograph was included as an indication of sufficient exposure to make disability from coal exposure likely, but was not based on any epidemiological evidence that miners with normal radiographs are less likely to have impaired lung function than those with abnormal films. The qualifying duration of work and level of FEV_1 impairment were arbitrary. Perhaps because the prediction equations used were not equally applicable to men from all parts of the country, compensation rates varied considerably, and for oldest and shortest miners the target of 1 liter below the predicted value was almost incompatible with survival. No account was taken of cigarette smoking and so smokers were disproportionately compensated.

The legislation was revised in 1996 to remove the radiologic criterion, and to allow miners with an FEV_1 of less than 1 liter to receive compensation even if the measured value was within 1 liter of the predicted level. More recently, a further scheme was introduced following the civil litigation described above. Disability is apportioned according to the judgment that coal mine dust of a degree sufficient to pose a risk of pneumoconiosis is equipotent to average smoking in causing COPD. There is no requirement for an abnormal chest radiograph, or for any minimum period of employment. The scheme requires all applicants to be assessed by a respiratory physician and to undergo detailed lung function testing, and so is relatively expensive to administer. It requires the assumption to be made that individuals who are the most sensitive to cigarette smoke are also the most sensitive to occupational exposures, and that at any level of disability the contributions of smoking and work can be apportioned according to the degree of exposure to coal dust, cigarette smoke, or both.

COPD due to other occupational exposures is not recognized for state compensation in the UK. Welding fumes have been accepted by the courts to cause COPD and have been the subject of much civil litigation. It is likely that the effects of other exposures will be tested in the courts in the near future.

Of the workforce

If an employee is identified with probable occupational COPD which has not occurred as a result of a very marked individual susceptibility (e.g. α_1-antitrypsin deficiency), then it is likely that other workers are similarly affected. Steps should be taken to identify those workers, to limit further exposures

to the entire workforce, and to initiate surveillance of lung function.

PREVENTION

In the workplace

Worker selection

With the exception of α_1-antitrypsin deficiency there are no individual characteristics which identify individuals at sufficient risk for the development of COPD that have any value in screening prospective employees. Homozygous α_1-antitrypsin deficiency has a prevalence of approximately 1:3000 in Europeans and so routine screening at preemployment would be difficult to justify. However, any individual who is already known to have α_1-antitrypsin deficiency should avoid work in dusty jobs. Airway hyperresponsiveness, atopy, and family history all have some predictive value for the development of COPD, but this is insufficient to be of any practical value. Acute airway responses to cotton and grain dusts are associated with an accelerated decline of FEV_1 with ongoing exposures, which raises the possibility that some individuals at excess risk of disabling COPD could be identified from the extent of immediate bronchoconstriction to the occupational agent of relevance. This possibility awaits further experimental evidence.

Because cigarette smoking is a potent cause of COPD and might interact adversely with occupational agents, a case could be argued for the employment only of non-smokers in jobs posing such risk [68]. This might certainly protect the cynical employer from compensation claims, but it would run counter to the first principle of disease prevention – the elimination or reduction of hazardous exposure. Such a measure is most justified when the interactive effect is high and when necessary low levels of exposure can not readily be achieved by engineering controls. This situation does apply for some types of occupational asthma, for instance the refining of platinum, but is much less justifiably applied to COPD.

Exposure control

Occupational COPD should be a preventable disease if exposures to causative agents are carefully controled. At a time when occupational causes of COPD are barely recognized, it is not surprising that the necessary target concentrations for dust and fume control have yet to be established. In coal mining, for example, the control of dust exposure in Sardinia to approximately 1 mg/m^3 has been reported to be associated with a substantial persisting risk of COPD, though this level of control has been associated with a considerable reduction in the prevalence of pneumoconiosis. This may be largely a consequence of the current regulations being directed primarily at the prevention of the pneumoconiosis rather than COPD. Dust particles reaching the alveoli and contributing to the development of pneumoconiosis are largely in the range 0.5–5μm, and most dust sampling strategies quantify dust particles in this range. Larger particles may be more relevant to COPD. Until more specific and precise targets for dust control become available, attempts should be made to control workers' exposures to the lowest practical level, and possibly well below current levels for 'nuisance dust'.

Smoking cessation

Because of the additive (and possibly interactive) effects of smoking, the most effective preventive measure for occupational COPD is likely to arise from smoking cessation. While smoking may be usefully prohibited within the workplace, much greater benefit is likely to accrue from complete smoking cessation. A smoking ban in the workplace does, however, prevent involuntary passive smoking among non-smoking employees, and it helps create a no smoking culture that may help smoking employees to give up the habit.

Surveillance

Given that there is a wide range of individual susceptibility, that the risks of occupational COPD in many industries are unquantified, and that safe levels of exposure are unknown even in those industries with an established risk, surveillance schemes need to be considered. Spirometric measurements are inexpensive and relatively simple to perform. They can provide a reliable means of recognizing COPD and quantifying its severity. A single cross-sectional survey will allow those with established disease to be identified, but periodic spirometric measurements at 2–5-year intervals are necessary if newly evolving disease is to be identified at a stage before meaningful disability occurs. Thus workers with a rapid rate of decline of FEV_1 can be removed from further exposure, or provided with appropriate respiratory protection. Their identification should also trigger additional efforts to control exposure levels. If data from surveillance schemes are collated appropriately with estimates of exposure, the risk in the particular industry will be estimated more accurately. This will be enhanced if the surveillance schemes include unexposed 'controls' or at least workers with very low level exposures.

National regulatory strategies

There are few if any occupational exposure standards which have been specifically designed to prevent the development of COPD. Coal dust levels in mines are limited to 2 mg/m^3 of respirable dust in the UK and the USA with the aim of preventing the development of Category 2 simple pneumoconiosis. This level of control is likely to reduce the risk of COPD though it might not be sufficient to prevent it [40]. Silica levels are controlled more closely with a permitted exposure limit (PEL) in the USA of 0.1 mg/m^3, again to prevent the development of pneumoconiosis. The exposure standard for cotton dust of 0.2 mg/m^3 was established to protect against the acute effects of exposure on the assumption that this would in turn prevent the longer term development of COPD [61]. Other organic dusts with specific exposure standards include grain dust (4 mg/m^3) and some hard wood dusts (1 mg/m^3).

Potentially of greatest importance to COPD are exposure standards for 'nuisance dusts' or 'particulates not otherwise classified – agents which lack specific toxicity. The current exposure standard in the UK and the USA is 10 mg/m^3 for inhalable particles and 3 mg/m^3 for particles of respirable size. Because of the complexity of the mixture, welding fume has a lower exposure standard of 5 mg/m^3 for inhalable particulates. As the extent to which the development of COPD may be a generic property of any dust entering the airways rather than a specific property of the few agents which have been investigated, these standards will have to be kept under review as more information becomes available.

DIFFICULT CASE

History

A 40-year-old man presented (in 1995) with undue shortness of breath on exertion. He had noticed this over the preceding 3 years, particularly after walking 1–1½ miles or running more than 20 yards. He had been unemployed for 1 year, though previously from the age of 15 years had worked as a coal miner. The first 3 of his 24 years of mining were spent on general underground work, but for the following 15 years he was engaged at the coal face on work widening the ends to support supply tunnels. His last 6 years were spent driving new shafts. All these tasks were said to be 'dusty'.

He started smoking at the age of 16 and smoked 10 cigarettes daily until becoming unemployed. Consumption then increased to 15 daily. He was taking no regular medication.

There were no abnormalities on physical examination or on a plain chest radiograph. Lung function showed:

FEV$_1$ prebronchodilator	2.40 liters (63% predicted)
FEV$_1$ postbronchodilator	2.60 liters (69% predicted)
FVC prebronchodilator	3.55 liters (78% predicted
FVC postbronchodilator	3.63 liters (80% predicted)
FEV$_1$/FVC prebronchodilator	68%
FEV$_1$FVC postbronchodilator	72%
Total lung capacity	5.86 liters (87% predicted)
Residual volume	2.13 liters (112% predicted)
Transfer factor (D$_L$CO)	7.22 (69% predicted)
Transfer coefficient (KCO)	1.33 (83% predicted)
Arterial oxygen saturation (air)	99%
Expired carbon monoxide level	27 ppm

Issues

The chief diagnostic issues here are whether this former coal miner has developed COPD, and if so have his occupational exposures to coal mine dust contributed? If his occupational exposures are considered to have contributed, a further issue over management arises – should he be permitted to resume coal mining if employment became available?

Comment

The lung function tests show airflow obstruction with little response to bronchodilator, air trapping, and impaired gas transfer which are all typical features of COPD. The

book's contributors uniformly agreed with this diagnosis and considered the occupational exposures to coal mine dust had contributed. There was a wide spectrum of opinion, however, as to the magnitude of the occupational component. Estimates ranged from less than 10% to more than 75%. The point was made that his work driving tunnels and shafts may have involved additional exposure to silica, which may in turn have posed a greater hazard for COPD. A majority would have advised him against any return to coal mining exployment.

He worked mostly in the 1970s and 1980s when current hygiene standards were in place, and so his exposures were probably modest in comparison with those experienced by older miners, and the coal he worked was of moderate not high rank. His reported cigarette consumption was also modest and he thus appears to be an individual with a marked susceptibility to developing COPD. Were he to claim compensation under the UK Miners Compensation Scheme, his 24 years of relatively light mine dust exposure would probably be held to have caused approximately half as much airflow obstruction as his 23 years of smoking.

If he had entered adult life with average lung function, and if the previous rate of decline of lung function were to be maintained, his FEV$_1$ would fall to 1 liter by approximately the age of 60. It is clear that steps should be taken to reduce any further decline, and that he should be advised against any return to coal mining employment and to stop smoking.

SUMMARY POINTS

Recognition
- COPD is usually readily identified by spirometry.
- Serial measurements are particularly useful in identifying early disease.
- Occupational COPD can rarely be distinguished from non-occupational COPD in individuals.

Management
- Smoking cessation for all smokers.
- Reduce occupational exposures to prevent worsening.

Prevention
- Current exposure standards may not be sufficient to prevent the disease

REFERENCES

1. Strachan DP. Epidemiology: a British perspective. In: Calverley P, Pride N, eds. *Chronic Obstructive Pulmonary Disease*. London: Chapman and Hall, 1995.
2. Burrows B, Cline MG, Knudson RJ *et al.* A descriptive analysis of the growth and decline of the FVC and FEV$_1$. *Chest* 1983; 83: 717–724.
3. Gibson GJ. *Clinical Tests of Respiratory Function*. London: Chapman and Hall, 1996.
4. Fletcher CM, Peto R, Tinker C, Speizer F. *The Natural History of Chronic Bronchitis and Emphysema*. Oxford: Oxford University Press, 1976.
5. US Department of Health and Human Services. *The health consequences of smoking: cancer and chronic lung disease in the workplace. A report of the Surgeon General*. Rockville, MD: Office of Smoking and Health, 1985.
6. Oxman AD, Miur DC, Shannon HS *et al.* Occupational dust exposure and chronic obstructive pulmonary disease. A systematic review of the evidence. *Am Rev Respir Dis* 1993; 148: 38–48.

7. Becklake MR. Occupational exposures and chronic airways disease. In: Rom WN, ed. *Environmental and Occupational Medicine*, 3rd edn. Philadelphia: Lippincott Williams & Wilkins 1998.
8. Coggan D, Newman Taylor A. Coal mining and chronic obstructive pulmonary disease: a review of the evidence. *Thorax* 1998; 53: 398–407.
9. Hendrick DJ. Work and chronic airflow limitation. In: Baxter PJ, Adams PH, Aw T-C, Cockcroft A, Harrington JM, eds. *Hunter's Diseases of Occupations*, 9th edn. London: Edward Arnold, 2000.
10. Stenton SC, Hendrick DJ. Airflow obstruction and mining. *State Art Rev* 1993; 8: 155–170.
11. Lapp NL, Morgan WK, Zaldivar G. Airways obstruction, coal mining and disability. *Occup Environ Med* 1994; 51: 234–238.
12. Rudd R. Coal miners' respiratory disease litigation. *Thorax* 1998; 53: 337–40.
13. Cowie RL, Mabena SK. Silicosis, chronic airflow limitation, and chronic bronchitis in South African gold miners. *Am Rev Respir Dis* 1991; 143: 80–84.

14. Comptroller General of the United States. Report to Congress. *Improvements still needed in coal mine dust-sampling program and penalty assessment and collections* (RED-76-56). Washington, DC: Departments of the Interior and Health, Education and Welfare, 1975.

15. Wald NJ, Nanchahal K, Thompson SG, Cuckle HS. Does breathing other people's tobacco smoke cause lung cancer? *BMJ* 1986; 293: 1217–1221.

16. Beach JR, Dennis JH, Avery AJ et al. An epidemiological investigation of asthma in welders. *Am J Respir Crit Care Med* 1996; 154: 1394–1400.

17. Higgins ITT, Cochrane AL, Gilson JC, Wood CH. Population studies of chronic respiratory disease. *Br J Ind Med* 1959; 16: 255–267.

18. Melia RJW, Florey C, du Valtman DG, Swan AV. Association between gas cooking and respiratory disease in children. *Br Med J* 1977; 11: 149–152.

19. Morgan WKC. On dust, disability and death. *Am Rev Respir Dis* 1986; 134: 639–641.

20. Jones MC, Thomas GO. Alpha-1 antitrypsin deficiency and pulmonary emphysema. *Thorax* 1971; 26: 652–656.

21. Banks DE, Shaw AA, Lopez M, Wang M. Chest illness and the decline of FEV_1 in steelworkers. *J Occup Environ Med* 1999; 41: 1085–1090.

22. Wang M, Banks DE. Airways obstruction and occupational inorganic dust exposure. In: Banks DE, Parker JE, eds. *Occupational Lung Disease: an international perspective*. London: Chapman and Hall, 1988.

23. Rogan JM, Attfield MD, Jacobsen M et al. Role of dust in the working environment in development of chronic bronchitis in British coal miners. *Br J Ind Med* 1973; 30: 217–226.

24. Love RG, Miller BG. Longitudinal study of lung function in coal-miners. *Thorax* 1982; 37: 193–197.

25. Glindmeyer HW, Diem JE, Jones RN, Weill H. Noncomparability of longitudinally and cross-sectionally determined annual change in spirometry. *Am Rev Respir Dis* 1982; 125: 544–548.

26. Marine WM, Gurr D, Jacobsen M. Clinically important respiratory effects of dust exposure and smoking in British coal miners. *Am Rev Respir Dis* 1988; 137: 106–112.

27. Seixas NS, Rbins TG, Atfield MD et al. Longitudinal and cross sectional analyses of exposure to coal mine dust and pulmonary function in new miners. *Br J Ind Med* 1993; 50: 929–937.

28. Henneberger PK, Attfield MD. Coal mine dust and spirometry in experienced miners. *Am J Respir Crit Care Med* 1996; 153: 1560–1566.

29. Lewis S, Bennett J, Richards K, Britton J. A cross sectional study of the independent effect of occupation on lung function in British coal miners. *Thorax* 1996; 53: 125–128.

30. Ware JH, Weiss S. Statistical issues in longitudinal research on respiratory health. *Am J Respir Crit Care Med* 1996; 154: 212–216.

31. Chinn DJ, Cotes JE, Reed JW. Longitudinal effects of change in body mass on measurements of ventilatory capacity. *Thorax* 1996; 51: 699–704.

32. Wang ML, McCabe L, Hankinson JL et al. Longitudinal and cross-sectional analyses of lung function in steelworkers. *Am J Respir Crit Care Med* 1996; 153: 1907–1913.

33. Kibelstis JA, Morgan EJ, Reger R et al. Prevalence of bronchitis and respiratory obstruction in American bituminous coal miners. *Am Rev Respir Dis* 1973; 168: 886–893.

34. Higgins ITT, Oldham PD. Ventilatory capacity in miners. *Br J Ind Med* 1962; 19: 65–76.

35. Soutar CA, Hurley JF. Relation between dust exposure and lung function in miners and ex-miners. *Br J Ind Med* 1986; 43: 307–320.

36. Kleinerman J, Green FHY, Harley R et al. Pathology standards for coal workers' pneumoconiosis: Report of the Pneumoconiosis Committee of the College of American Pathologists to the National Institute for Occupational Safety and Health. *Arch Pathol Lab Med* 1979; 103: 375–432.

37. Ruckley VA, Gauld SJ, Chapman JS et al. Emphysema and dust exposure in a group of coal workers. *Am Rev Respir Dis* 1984; 129: 528–532.

38. Attfield MD, Hodous TK. Pulmonary function of US coal miners related to dust exposure estimates. *Am Rev Respir Dis* 1992; 145: 605–609.

39. Attfield MD. Longitudinal decline in FEV_1 in United States coal miners. *Thorax* 1985; 40: 132–137.

40. Carta P, Aru G, Barbieri MT et al. Dust exposure, respiratory symptoms, and longitudinal decline in lung function in young coal miners. *Occup Environ Med* 1996; 53: 312–319.

41. Rossiter CE. Relation of lung dust content to radiological changes in coal workers. *Ann NY Acad Sci* 1972; 200: 465–477.

42. Hurley JF, Burns J, Copland L et al. Coalworkers' simple pneumoconiosis and exposure to dust at 10 British coalmines. *Br J Ind Med* 1982; 39: 120–127.

43. Irwig LM, Rocks P. Lung function and respiratory symptoms in silicotic and non-silicotic gold miners. *Am Rev Respir Dis* 1978; 117: 429–435.

44. Hnizdo E. Loss of lung function associated with exposure to silica dust and with smoking and its relation to disability and mortality in South African gold miners. *Br J Ind Med* 1992; 49: 472–479.

45. Becklake MR, Irwig L, Kielkowski D et al. The predictors of emphysema in South African gold miners. *Am Rev Respir Dis* 1987; 135: 1234–1241.

46. Churg A, Wright JL, Wiggs B et al. Small airway disease and mineral dusts. *Am Rev Respir Dis* 1985; 131: 139–143.

47. Wright JL, Churg A. Morphology of small-airway lesions in patients with asbestos exposures. *Hum Pathol* 1984; 15: 68–74.

48. Begin R, Masse S, Sebastien P et al. Asbestos exposure and retention as determinants of airway disease and asbestos alveolitis. *Am Rev Respir Dis* 1986; 134: 1176–1181.

49. Cotes JE, Feinmann EL, Male VJ et al. Respiratory symptoms and in welders and caulker/burners. *Br J Ind Med* 1989; 46: 292–301.

50. Chinn DJ, Stevenson IC, Cotes JE. Longitudinal respiratory survey of shipyard workers: effect of trade and atopic status. *Br J Ind Med* 1990; 47: 83–90.

51. Glindmeyer HW, Lefante JJ, Jones RJ et al. Cotton dust and across-shift change in FEV_1 as predictors of annual change in FEV_1. *Am J Respir Crit Care Med* 1994; 149: 584–590.

52. Chan-Yeung M, Enarson DA, Kennedy SM. The impact of grain dust on respiratory health. *Am Rev Respir Dis* 1992; 145: 476–487.

53. Enarson D, Chan-Yeung M. Characterisation of health effects of wood dust exposure. *Am J Ind Med* 1990; 17: 33–38.

54. Becklake MR. Relationship of acute obstructive airway change to chronic (fixed) obstruction. *Thorax* 1995; 50 (Suppl): 516–521.

55. Diem JE, Jones RM, Hendrick DJ et al. Five-year longitudinal study of workers employed in a new toluene diisocyanate manufacturing plant. *Am Rev Respir Dis* 1982; 126: 420–428.

56. Bakke PS, Batse V, Hanoa R, Guisvik A. Prevalence of obstructive lung disease in a general population: relation to occupational title and exposure to some airborne agents. *Thorax* 1991; 46: 863–870.

57. Kauffmann B, Drouet D, Lellouch J, Brille D. Occupational exposure and 12-year spirometric changes among Paris area workers. *Br J Ind Med* 1982; 39: 221–232.

58. Krzyzanowski M, Jedrychowski W, Wysocki M. Occupational exposures and changes in pulmonary function over 13 years among residents of Cracow. *Br J Ind Med* 1988; 45: 747–754.

59. Pearson MG, Calverley PMA. Clinical and laboratory assessment. In: Calverley P, Pride N, eds. *Chronic Obstructive Pulmonary Disease*. London: Chapman and Hall, 1995.

60. Davidson AG, Fayers PM, Newman Taylor AJ et al. Cadmium fume inhalation and emphysema. *Lancet* 1988; i: 663–667.

61. Beck GJ, Schacter EN. The evidence for chronic lung disease in cotton textile workers. *Am Statistician* 1983; 37: 404–412.

62. Knox and others v Cammell Laird and others. Unreported Judgment, Liverpool Crown Court, 1990.

63. Froines JR. Occupational regulatory approaches. In: Harber P, Schenker MB, Balmes JR, eds. *Occupational and Environmental Respiratory Disease*. St Louis, MD: Mosby, 1996.

64. British Thoracic Society guidelines for the management of COPD. *Thorax* 1997; 52 (Suppl 5).

65. Newnham DM, Dhillon DP, Winter JH et al. Bronchodilator reversibility to low and high doses of terbutaline and ipratropium bromide in patients with chronic obstructive pulmonary disease. *Thorax* 1993; 48: 1151–1155.

66. Burge PS, Calverly PMA, Jones PW et al. Randomised, double blind, placebo controlled study of fluticasone propionate in patients with moderate to severe chronic obstructive pulmonary disease: the ISOLDE trial. *BMJ* 2000; 320: 1297–1303.

67. Lacasse Y, Wong E, Guyatt GH et al. Meta-analysis of respiratory rehabilitation in chronic obstructive pulmonary disease. *Lancet* 1996; 348: 1115–1119.

68. Seaton A. The new prescription: industrial injuries benefit for smokers? *Thorax* 1988; 53: 335–336.

69. Hanke W, Sepulveda MJ, Watson A et al. Respiratory morbidity in wollastonite miners. *Br J Ind Med* 1984; 41: 474–479.

70. Gardiner K, Trethowan W, Harrington MJ et al. Respiratory health effects of carbon black: a survey of European carbon black workers. *Br J Ind Med* 1993; 50: 1082–1096.

71. Trethowan WN, Burge PS, Rossiter CE et al. Study of the respiratory health of employees in seven European plants that manufacture ceramic fibres. *Occup Environ Med* 1995; 52: 97–104.

72. Henneberger PK, Ferris BG, Sheehe PR. Accidental gassing incidents and the pulmonary function of pulp mill workers. *Am Rev Respir Dis* 1993; 148: 63–67.

73. Sparrow D, Bosse R, Rosner B et al. The effect of occupational exposure on pulmonary function. *Am Rev Respir Dis* 1982; 125: 319–322.

6 TOXIC TRACHEITIS, BRONCHITIS, AND BRONCHIOLITIS

David A. Schwartz

BACKGROUND

Many fumes, gases, vapors, dusts, and other inhaled substances have potentially toxic effects that are manifested by pulmonary as well as extrapulmonary injury. Exposure to toxic aerosols, fumes, and gases may occur in industrial settings as well as in the home, in public places, and in other environments. The events in Bhopal, India, dramatically illustrate the potential consequences of acute exposure to toxic inhalants. In the workplace, toxic inhalants cause a variety of clinical problems ranging from mild irritation of the upper airways to non-cardiogenic pulmonary edema (adult respiratory distress syndrome [ARDS]) and death. Exposure to toxic inhalants presents problems in clinical management for the following reasons:

- Exposures occur at infrequent, unpredictable intervals.
- Exposures may involve large numbers of individuals.
- The causal toxic agent may not be known to the patient or physician.
- There is a broad range of acute clinical manifestations with varying times of onset.
- The chronic effects of acute exposures have not been clearly characterized.

Despite these problems, knowledge of the basic principles underlying these acute responses to lung injury allows the clinician to respond appropriately. This chapter focuses on the perspective of a clinician who is faced with a patient with respiratory problems following inhalant exposure to a noxious agent. Importantly, many of the exposures that can result in acute toxic injury to the upper airway, the conducting airways, and/or the parenchyma, may also result in subacute and chronic complications that can dramatically alter lung function. Such effects occur regularly in the clinical setting, though are poorly understood.

Thus toxic inhalant injury has different manifestations at different levels, and at each level the clinical effects may cover a wide spectrum. Some overlap is to be expected, of course, since vulnerability at one level is not likely to be associated with immunity at the next, and there are general principles of relevance at all levels. These general principles will be addressed first, followed by a more detailed discussion of the particular effects at each level. At the most distal level of the bronchioles, further overlap inevitably occurs with the parenchymal structures of the lung, and the effects there are reviewed further in Chapters 12 and 13.

Causes

Table 6.1 lists selected agents that can acutely cause lung injury. All agents on this list are capable of

Table 6.1 Selected chemicals known to cause acute pulmonary injury

Chemical	Properties and pulmonary sequelae
Gases	
Acetaldehyde	Strong oxidizer, upper airway irritant, delayed ARDS
Acrolein	Oxidizer, upper airway irritant, delayed ARDS
Ammonia	Alkali, water soluble, upper airway irritant
Boranes	Water-insoluble, upper airway irritant
Chlorine	Intermediate solubility, upper and lower airway irritant
Hydrogen chloride	Water-soluble, upper airway irritant
Hydrogen fluoride	Irritating odor, upper airway irritant, ARDS
Isocyanates	Reactive chemical, irritant, airway reactivity
Lithium hydride	Odorless, strong oxidizer, upper airway irritant
Oxide of nitrogen (NO, NO_2, N_2O_4)	Water-insoluble, pneumonitis, ARDS, bronchiolitis obliterans
Ozone	Water-insoluble, pneumonitis, ?ARDS
Phosgene	Water-insoluble, pneumonitis, ARDS
Sulfur dioxide	Water-soluble, pneumonitis, ARDS, bronchiolitis obliterans
Metals	
Antimony	Oxidizer, upper airway irritant
Cadmium	Odorless, pneumonitis, ARDS
Cobalt	Oxidizer, irritant, dyspnea
Manganese	Oxidizer, metal fume fever
Mercury	Odorless, pneumonitis, ARDS
Nickel	Musty odor, asthma, pneumonitis
Zinc	White aerosol, upper airway irritant, metal fume fever

causing toxic pneumonitis but more commonly result in airway edema and inflammation. Patients usually can recall the specific exposure or event that was associated with the onset of symptoms. In most cases, there is a clear temporal relationship between exposure and the onset of symptoms. However, with less-soluble agents, such as nitrogen dioxide and phosgene, the onset of symptoms may occur hours to days after the exposure. In addition, delayed or subacute complications (e.g. asthma, bronchitis, and bronchiolitis obliterans) may take days to weeks to develop. Thus, clinicians need to pursue an occupational and environmental history in cases of non-bacterial pneumonia, adult onset asthma or bronchitis, and all cases of bronchiolitis obliterans, and focus on relatively high exposures to the agents listed in Table 6.1.

Characteristics of toxic inhalants

Inhaled toxins exist in many forms and may be categorized by taking into account their physical properties. The initial pathologic responses to a harmful inhaled agent depend on a number of factors, including the concentration of the substance in the ambient air, its pH and relative water solubility, the presence of particles and their size, the duration of exposure, and whether the exposure occurs in an enclosed space or an area with adequate ventilation and free circulation of fresh air. In addition, an undetermined number of host factors, including age, smoking status, the presence of preexisting pulmonary or extrapulmonary disease, and the use of respirators or other protective breathing devices all impact upon an individual's susceptibility and response to the inhalation of a toxic substance [1,2].

Table 6.2 summarizes the water solubility of several common inhalants. The mass of gas dissolved by a given volume of liquid is proportional to the partial pressure of the gas in equilibrium with the solution [3]. The amount of a specific gas absorbed onto the respiratory epithelium is also dependent on the solubility of the gas in the airway lining fluid and the presence of other ions or molecules in the lining fluid (which decreases gas solubility) or molecules with which the gas readily reacts. For example sulfur dioxide reacts with the water in the airway lining fluid, and as the reaction proceeds the concentration of sulfur dioxide in solution decreases, thus increasing the driving pressure gradient for absorption of more sulfur dioxide. The solubility of gases in water can be described by the Henry constant; gases with low Henry constants have high solubility. Ammonia, with a Henry constant of 11, will be absorbed in the amount of 0.09 g/100 ml water at a partial pressure of 11.5 mmHg, while ozone, with a Henry constant of 20 283, will be absorbed in the amount of 0.0000493 g/100 ml water. Thus, under equivalent conditions, about 1800 times more ammonia will go into solution

Table 6.2 Water solubility and mechanisms of lung injury of gaseous respiratory irritants. After Schwartz [2]

Irritant gas	Water solubility	Mechanism of injury
Ammonia	High	Alkali burns
Chlorine	Intermediate	Acid burns, reactive oxygen species
Hydrogen chloride	High	Acid burns
Oxides of nitrogen	Low	Acid burns, reactive oxygen species
Ozone	Low	Reactive oxygen species
Phosgene	Low	Acid burns
Sulfur dioxide	High	Acid burns

than ozone. Under conditions of inhalation, this means ammonia will be taken up rapidly in the upper airways, and ozone will penetrate more readily to distal lung.

Inhaled gases with irritant effects manifest their actions at different anatomic locations in the respiratory system [1,2] (Tables 6.2 and 6.3). In general, substances that are highly water soluble, such as ammonia, sulfur dioxide, and hydrogen chloride cause immediate irritant injury to the upper airway. The acute effects of highly water-soluble irritants on the upper airway, exposed skin, and other mucous membranes often produce such unpleasant symptoms that exposed persons quickly leave the area of exposure, and avoid continued inhalation of the harmful toxins. In contrast, inhaled toxins that have low water solubility, such as phosgene, ozone, and oxides of nitrogen, often have little or no acute effect on the upper airway, and instead produce their toxic effects dominantly at the level of the terminal bronchiole and alveolus. Because agents of low water solubility do not produce immediately noticeable upper

airway irritation (except in episodes of massive acute exposure), exposed persons may inadvertently remain in the area, and thus increase their cumulative level of exposure. Agents that exhibit intermediate water solubility, such as chlorine, may exert their pathologic effects throughout the respiratory tract, and extreme exposure to any one of these irritants may result in similar diffuse effects. Furthermore, absorption on to particulate matter may also influence the level of involvement.

In addition to solubility, the size of inhaled particles is important in the pathogenesis of the toxic inhalation injury [1]. Aerosols can produce upper airway injury as well as parenchymal damage. The location and extent of injury depend on the size of the inhaled particles as well as the intensity of the exposure. Particles that are 5.0 μm or less in diameter have the ability to penetrate into the lower respiratory tract (conducting airways and alveoli), and often produce significant injury at the level of the terminal bronchioles and alveoli. Zinc chloride (hexite) particles, for example, have an average

Table 6.3 Pulmonary manifestations of toxic inhalation

Substance	Onset	Acute clinical manifestations		Chronic clinical manifestations		
		Upper airway irritation	Pneumonitis ARDS	Bronchiolitis obliterans, BOOP	Obstructive lung disease	RADS
Irritant gases						
Ammonia	Minutes	Severe	+	+	+	+
Chlorine	Minutes to hours	Moderate	+	−	+	+
Hydrogen chloride	Minutes	Severe	+	−	−	−
Oxides of nitrogen	Hours	Mild	+	+	+	+
Ozone	Minutes to hours	Mild	+	−	−	−
Phosgene	Hours	Mild	+	−	+	−
Sulfur dioxide	Minutes	Severe	+	+	+	+
Metals						
Cadmium	Hours	Mild	+	−	+	−
Mercury	Hours	Mild	+	+	−	−
Zinc chloride	Minutes	Mild	+	−	−	−
Zinc oxide	Hours	Mild	+	−	−	−

+, exposure reported to be associated with clinical entity; −, exposure as yet not reported to be associated with clinical entity.

diameter of 0.1 μm and it is estimated that up to 20% of the inhaled hexite reaches the bronchiolar level, with the remainder deposited in more proximal airways [4]. The particles themselves may have direct toxic effects, or they may serve simply as vehicles for adsorbed gaseous agents that are carried more distally into the lungs.

Irritants directly injure cells through non-immunologically mediated mechanisms of injury and inflammation. Cell injury involves the deposition or formation of an acid (chlorine, hydrogen chloride, oxides of nitrogen, phosgene, and sulfur dioxide), alkali (ammonia), or reactive oxygen species (ozone, oxides of nitrogen and possibly chlorine) [2,5]. The primary injury is localized in airway epithelial tissues, but extensive damage may also occur in subepithelial and alveolar regions. Acid injury results in coagulation of the underlying tissue, while acute injury due to alkali results in liquefaction of the mucosa and deep penetrating lesions in the airways. Reactive oxygen species include oxygen-derived metabolites (such as hydrogen peroxide and hydro-chlorous acid), and oxygen-derived free radicals (such as superoxide anions and hydroxyl radicals). Lipid peroxidation can directly injure cells and lead to elab-oration of inflammatory mediators that can perpetu-ate the initial damage [5]. Regardless of the initial mechanism, networks of proinflammatory cytokines may be subsequently activated. The resultant in-flammation may be important with regard to per-petuation of the acute injury as well as long-term sequelae. In addition, disruption and eventual repair of the airway epithelia may decrease the host's ability to defend against future inhaled infectious or irritant substances.

RECOGNITION

Clinical features

Initial attention should focus on the extent and pace of the lung injury. Dyspnea is the most common symptom following inhalation of irritant gases or aerosols, an aerosol being a dispersion in air of res-pirable particles or fluid droplets. It is essential to grade the degree of dyspnea (at rest, with minimal exertion, or with extensive exertion) to both establish a new baseline and also determine the extent of lung injury. The rate of change in dyspnea and specific signs of pulmonary disease are key features used to guide clinical management. Other symptoms include chest tightness and burning, a cough that may or may not be productive of sputum, and wheezing. Patients with dyspnea at rest and a cough with or without pink, frothy sputum should be assumed to

have extensive lung injury and are at high risk of developing (or having) ARDS. Other acute symptoms may suggest asthma and bronchial inflammation, or bronchitis.

Importantly, days to weeks after the exposure, individuals may first recognize symptoms of asthma, bronchitis, or even bronchiolitis obliterans. These subacute symptoms primarily develop from the delayed onset of airflow obstruction and include wheezing, dyspnea with exertion, and cough with - or without sputum production. Unlike the acute symptoms, the symptoms from these delayed complications may worsen over time.

The environmental or occupational history is important because the clinical presentation can be confused with other more common forms of asthma, bronchitis, pneumonia, or ARDS. However, in many cases in which symptoms develop acutely following exposure, the exposure history is clearly evident.

Physical signs

Acutely following the exposure, the clinician should assess the pace and extent of the lung injury. Given the potential life-threatening consequences of these exposures, the initial examination should be directed toward essential measures of cardiopulmonary function, such as gas exchange, pulmonary edema, and hemodynamic stability. In addition, if significant injury has occurred to the airway, signs of upper airway edema and stenosis along with generalized airflow obstruction may be present. Fever usually is not part of the initial clinical picture; however, it may be present when diffuse parenchymal injury has occurred. Thus, wheezing and rhonchi with patchy areas of rales are frequently observed. Because the onset of subacute airway and parenchymal disease can be insidious, the clinical evaluation should main-tain a relatively low threshold for pursuing these delayed complications.

Investigation

Immediately following exposure, the clinician should be concerned with gas exchange and the extent of the lung injury. Arterial blood gases (ABG) can ade-quately assess gas exchange, and the chest radi-ograph is helpful in determining the overall extent of the pulmonary injury. Because several chemicals, particularly the less-soluble ones, may have between 12 and 24 hours of delay between exposure and the full development of the lung injury, it is reasonable (and sometimes important) to observe patients for at least 12 hours following the exposure. Symptomatic patients should be hospitalized for a minimum of 24 hours, regardless of the results of the initial chest radiograph and ABG. In the first 24–48 hours following exposure, use of pulmonary function tests is not needed and the results may be misleading. However, several days to weeks following the exposure, pulmonary function tests can be used to identify problems with airflow obstruction, restrictive lung function, or abnormal gas exchange. Occasionally, an open lung biopsy is needed to establish the diagnosis of bronchiolitis obliterans in patients with patchy involvement of the lung parenchyma several months following the exposure.

The upper airway

Individuals exposed to irritants that injure the upper airway often have associated injury to exposed mucous membranes and skin. Clinical presentations include burns of exposed skin and corneas, rhinitis, conjunctivitis, tracheobronchitis, and oral mucositis. Persons exposed to upper airway irritants may experience burning sensations of the eyes, nasal passages and throat; profuse lacrimation and copious sputum production may also occur. Coughing and sneezing may be prominent symptoms. Upper airway injury from irritant inhalants is generally acute and self-limited. Life-threatening upper airway obstruction due to mucosal edema, large amounts of secretions and sloughed epithelial cells, or laryngospasm can occur in cases of massive acute exposure. Hoarseness or stridor may warn of impending airway compromise, and patients presenting with either of these physical findings must be carefully observed. They may require emergent management of acute upper airway obstruction.

The conducting airway

Inhaled irritants that penetrate to the conducting airways are capable of inducing immediate as well as long-lasting injury through a variety of mechanisms. The airway epithelium provides a barrier that protects inflammatory cells and submucosal structures (nerves, vessels, and muscle) from direct exposure to environmental agents. Disruption of the integrity of this protective barrier may result in edema, inflammation, direct smooth muscle contraction, and stimulation of neuronal afferent receptors. Moreover, this primary lesion in the airway epithelium can facilitate stimulation by subsequent agents that come in contact with the denudated epithelial surface.

The tight junction interface between epithelial cells appears to be the primary site of injury following exposure to a variety of gases and aerosols. Ozone [6] has also been shown to increase airway epithelial permeability. Thus, damage to the airway epithelium, particularly at tight junctions, renders the respiratory mucosa permeable to other inhaled substances (including microbial organisms), which are then able to penetrate the subepithelial mucosal region. These agents may directly interact with effector cells in subepithelial mucosa. Thus, they may have direct smooth muscle bronchoconstrictive effects, and they may also stimulate parasympathetic sensory afferent nerve endings, resulting in extensive bronchoconstriction [7].

Inhalation of irritant gases and aerosols may cause airway hyperresponsiveness by initiating a localized inflammatory response. Inhalation studies with allergens and specific environmental irritants have demonstrated that neutrophils and eosinophils are recruited within hours to the airway and alveolar surface, and this response has been shown to persist for at least 48 hours following this type of challenge [8]. Moreover, the number of mast cells, eosinophils, and airway epithelial cells obtained by bronchoalveolar lavage following an aerosol challenge has been found to correlate strongly with the degree of airway hyperreactivity in mild atopic asthmatics [9]. Inflammatory cells such as neutrophils appear to be critical elements in the development of airway hyperreactivity following exposure to ozone [10].

The inflammatory response in the epithelial and subepithelial regions can result in chronic remodeling of the underlying airway architecture. Striking pathologic changes, such as extensive collagen deposition beneath the epithelial basement membrane, eosinophil infiltration, and mast cell degranualtion, are seen in transbronchial biopsy specimens obtained from asthmatic persons following methacholine or allergen aerosol challenges [11]. Chronic bronchitis, an inflammatory state characterized by neutrophil infiltration, is strongly associated with airway hyperresponsiveness and has been demonstrated in animals following exposure to irritant gases [2].

Lower airway injury resulting from irritant toxin inhalation can be manifested as transient or long-lasting intrathoracic airflow obstruction, and has been reported following inhalation of ammonia [12], chlorine [13], ozone [14], and mixed gas exposures [15]. The precise mechanism of the obstruction is not clear, but likely involves one or more inflammatory mechanisms. Exposed individuals who are cigarette smokers or who have preexisting airway obstruction may be at increased risk for the persistence of toxin-induced airflow obstruction. Significant clinical manifestations of lower airway injury may not be initially recognizable, but may develop and worsen over the first 24–48 hours after exposure. Spirometry may initially be normal, but in some cases progressive airflow obstruction develops, and thus a case can be argued for obtaining baseline airflow indices and following the exposed individuals with spirometry over the first 24–48 hours after exposure.

Reactive airways dysfunction syndrome

The persistence of airway reactivity following acute exposure to respiratory irritants has been termed 'reactive airways dysfunction syndrome' (RADS) [16]. A variety of inhaled irritants have been associated with this syndrome, including sulfuric acid, glacial acetic acid, chlorine, ammonia, household cleaners, and smoke. Most often, the initial inhalation injury is due to a single, acute, high-intensity exposure. Symptoms of airflow obstruction, including cough, dyspnea, and wheezing, are reported immediately or several hours after the end of the exposure, and may persist for months to years. Previous exposure or sensitization to the toxic agent does not appear to be necessary, and individuals who develop RADS generally have no prior history of respiratory illness. Once established, RADS is associated (like any other case of active asthma) with persistent positive responses to methacholine challenge testing, even in the presence of normal pulmonary function tests. These indicate the presence of non-specific bronchial hyperreactivity, which may persist for months to years following the initial inhalation injury.

Bronchial biopsies of patients with RADS demonstrate an inflammatory response characterized by epithelial desquamation and mucous cell hyperplasia. The exact pathophysiology of RADS is unclear, but implicated mechanisms include altered neural tone and vagal reflexes, modified beta-adrenergic sympathetic tone, and the influence of a number of proinflammatory mediators. The direct irritant injury may expose and damage subepithelial irritant receptors. Subsequently, repair mechanisms that are not fully understood may result in alteration of the irritant receptor threshold and lead to airways hyperreactivity. Changes in epithelial permeability may also contribute to the resultant hyperreactivity.

Chronic obstructive pulmonary disease (COPD)

Previously healthy individuals who experience acute toxic inhalation may go on to develop clinical and pathologic features of chronic obstructive pulmonary disease (COPD). Inhaled irritants most often implicated in the development of chronic bronchitis and emphysema include chlorine [17] and sulfur dioxide [18]. However, definitive evidence that demonstrates a causal relationship between a toxic exposure and resultant chronic respiratory disease is at times difficult to elicit. This is often because of the frequent concomitant presence of potentially confounding factors, most prominently cigarette smoking, that independently increase any individual's risk for the development of COPD. Nevertheless, there is some evidence that acute exposure to a number of inhaled irritants may produce conditions in the conducting airways that lead to a complex interaction of inflammation, smooth muscle activity, and neuronal inputs that are involved in the creation and perpetuation of varying degrees of fixed and reversible airflow obstruction. The initial irritant insult to epithelial cells appears to be central to subsequent abnormal function and continuing injury processes that involve the epithelium as well as subepithelial structures. Repair of the acute injury may also contribute to resultant chronic airflow obstruction via scarring and other mechanical factors. Disruption of normal protective structures and mechanisms may also predispose exposed individuals to chronic pulmonary infections. In addition, damage to and destruction of functional alveoli may involve ongoing inflammatory and repair processes that have been initiated by the acute irritant exposure.

The development of irritant-induced COPD appears to be dependent on the intensity of the exposure. In addition, underlying host factors, including cigarette smoking and preexisting pulmonary disease may increase an individual's likelihood of developing or worsening COPD. It is extremely difficult to accurately assess the potential contribution of acute irritant inhalation to chronic lung disease in individuals who smoke cigarettes. Baseline measures of pulmonary function can help determine the presence of preexisting disease, but unfortunately this information is often unavailable, especially in cases of accidental acute exposure. Evaluation of possible irritant-induced COPD includes a thorough history, physical examination, radiographic evaluation, and objective measures of pulmonary function, including spirometry, measurement of lung volumes, determination of diffusing capacity, and assessment of gas exchange. The topic is discussed further in Chapter 5. Frequent measurement of spirometry may help identify progression, or regression, of the airflow abnormalities.

The bronchioles

Toxic agents that have relatively low water solubilities, such as phosgene, ozone and nitrogen oxides, produce most of their irritant damage distal to the upper airway, because inhalation does not typically result in upper airway irritation. In addition, massive acute inhalation of gases and aerosols that have intermediate (chlorine) or high water solubilities (ammonia, sulfur dioxide) can overwhelm the absorptive capacity of the upper airway and injure more distal structures. Damage may be particularly severe when particulates with adsorbed gases are inhaled and deposited in the distal airways. The clinical consequences of these injuries include diffuse bronchiolar inflammation and obstruction as well as alveolar filling (pulmonary edema). Atelectasis may result from destruction or disruption of the surfactant layer. Exposed individuals are also more susceptible to subsequent pulmonary infection.

Pulmonary parenchymal injury that results from inhalation of toxic substances runs the spectrum of acute lung injury. It includes pneumonitis, pulmonary edema, and ARDS, and may be complicated by life-threatening secondary infection. Pneumonitis is the most frequent parenchymal manifestation of inhalation injury. Clinical features include dyspnea, productive or dry cough, hypoxemia, mild restriction of ventilation, decreased alveolar gas diffusion, and diffuse bilateral infiltrates on the chest radiograph. Generally, pneumonitis caused by toxic inhalation is a self-limited process, with clinical improvement mirrored by rapid clearing of infiltrates seen on the chest X-ray.

Bronchiolitis obliterans

Bronchiolitis obliterans can occur as a late consequence of the inhalation of several toxins, the most prominant being ammonia, mercury, oxides of nitrogen, and sulfur dioxide [19–22]. High-intensity inhalation exposures causing acute pulmonary edema and ARDS may be followed by a relatively asymptomatic period of 1–3 weeks that is succeeded by the development of irreversible airflow obstruction. Early inspiratory crackles are a characteristic finding on physical examination. The appearance of the chest radiograph is variable, but tends to correlate with the degree of clinical severity. In mild cases chest radiographs appear normal, while in more severe cases there is hyperinflation. Infiltrates are generally absent. If computed tomography (CT) scans are obtained, the patchy nature of the bronchiolar abnormalities and the different degrees of severity are characterized by a mosaic pattern, particularly on expiration. Thus air is expelled through normal bronchioles, increasing attenuation, but it is trapped by severely obstructed bronchioles.

Pulmonary function tests typically demonstrate air trapping with an increased residual volume, and a mixed spirometric picture of airflow obstruction and ventilatory restriction. The histologic picture is characterized by the presence of granulation tissue plugs within the lumen of small airways and occasionally alveolar ducts, as well as by the destruction of small airways with obliterative fibrous scarring.

Bronchiolitis obliterans organizing pneumonia (BOOP)

A further delayed consequence of the inhalation of toxic substances is bronchiolitis obliterans organizing pneumonia (BOOP) [23,24]. Its clinical presentation is characterized by a persistent, non-productive cough, fever, sore throat, and malaise. Physical examination typically reveals late inspiratory crackles but no wheezes; many patients have no abnormalities on physical exam. The characteristic chest X-ray findings include bilateral, patchy, 'ground glass' densities which start as focal lesions but may coalesce with time. In contrast to patients with the less-extensive abnormalities of bronchiolitis obliterans alone, those with BOOP have a more dominant restrictive pattern of ventilatory impairment, and decreased diffusing capacity. The subject in further discussed in Chapter 12.

The histology of BOOP includes the presence of granulation tissue in the small airways and alveolar ducts, as in bronchiolitis obliterans. In addition, the granulation tissue extends into the alveoli and may result in interstitial scarring. This distinction between the histologic features of BOOP and those of 'pure' bronchiolitis obliterans (without organizing pneumonia) may reflect different host responses to similar inhaled toxins [23]. Examination of the granulation tissue plugs from patients with BOOP demonstrates temporal uniformity in a patchy distribution with the preservation of background architecture. Bronchoalveolar lavage fluid demonstrates a neutrophilic alveolitis; lymphocytes may also be prominent. These findings suggest that the pathologic process results from an initial insult (e.g. an inhaled toxin) with subsequent inflammatory and reparative processes.

MANAGEMENT

Of the individual

Immediate management involves prompt removal of the patient from the exposure, supportive care, and medical observation. The upper airway in particular must be carefully evaluated, since the most common life-threatening manifestation of acute inhalational injury is upper airway obstruction due to a combination of tissue edema, thick secretions, and laryngospasm. Provision of adequate supplemental oxygen is additionally necessary if there is evidence of hypoxemia. Inhaled racemic epinephrine (adrenaline) may be useful for patients with upper airway obstruction, but should not substitute for, or delay, emergency airway management by endotracheal intubation or tracheostomy if this becomes necessary. Corticosteroids have not been conclusively shown to influence the outcome, but have been suggested in cases with extensive upper airway edema.

Toxic substances that remain present on the skin or mucosal surfaces should be removed by irrigation with large amounts of water, and if the potential for toxic injury is recognized within the workplace, emergency showers should be provided at strategic sites.

In addition to the upper airway, the treating physician must also be aware that these injuries can result in acute bronchospasm and diffuse parenchymal injury. Treatment again is largely supportive, and involves use of inhaled bronchodilators and corticosteroids, supplemental oxygen, and possibly even mechanical ventilation. The use of parenteral corticosteroids has not been shown to be of significant benefit in the treatment of pneumonitis or ARDS and, in fact, may limit the effectiveness of reparative mechanisms in the lung. Given the delayed onset of ARDS, all patients with evidence of upper airway lesions or respiratory symptoms following the inhalation of toxic gases or aerosols should be observed in the hospital for at least 24 hours.

Treatment of RADS includes the use of inhaled corticosteroids to minimize inflammation in the acute phase, and ongoing conventional medication for asthma according to need. Despite aggressive initial treatment, many individuals with RADS will be left with persistent asthma, at least for a period of months. In some cases remission never occurs.

Although bronchiolitis obliterans may not respond, a 6-month trial of corticosteroids should be given. Bronchodilators may be efficacious in some symptomatic individuals, although clear-cut evidence of benefit is not available. Treatment of BOOP with corticosteroids often results in dramatic clinical improvement. Pulmonary function abnormalities may improve considerably, and in some cases there is a rapid return to normality. The radiographic abnormalities may also clear rapidly. Relapse is common, however, and such therapy is generally required for at least 6 months. Its duration should be guided by the rate and degree of the clinical response. A small proportion of patients with BOOP do not respond to corticosteroid therapy, and may develop progressive fibrosis.

Of the workforce

Inhalation injuries are a consequence of accidents. Members of the workforce who were neither involved nor affected, require no specific management, but they do need to be familiar with the risks and the principles of emergency treatment. These are addressed in the following section on prevention.

PREVENTION

In the workplace

Preventive measures should be taken to avoid the tragedies that are associated with acute inhalational injuries. In addition to limiting exposure through better industrial hygiene, and reducing the risk of accident through careful regular maintenance, prevention involves:

- Provision of a comprehensive Accident Plan, including:
  action to be taken by each individual
  clear identification of leadership responsibilities
  facilities for evacuation
  regular practice drills
- Education of workers at risk of exposure:
  nature of the risks
  principles of the Action Plan
  action expected of the individual worker
  action the individual worker can expect from other employees
- Provision of:
  emergency air supplying respirators (SCBA – self-contained breathing apparatus)
  oxygen
  showers at strategic sites
  cardiopulmonary resuscitation
- Availability of informed medical personnel to evaluate the exposed individuals.

National regulatory strategies

Most substances causing these conditions are regulated in the US by Permissible Exposure Limits (PELs), which restrict the maximum average 8-hour exposure, and by Short-Term (maximum) Exposure Limits (STELs). The latter allow brief periods of higher average exposure (15 minutes) providing the PEL is not exceeded when cumulative exposure is averaged over 8 hours. Where higher levels occur in the workplace, employers must provide respiratory protection equipment. The principles and details of regulatory strategies are discussed more fully in Chapter 33 and Chapters 35–37.

DIFFICULT CASE

History

A 21-year-old male with a non-significant past medical history was transferred to a hospital intensive care unit for management of an acute inhalation injury. Three days prior to the transfer, he had been exploring a cave with three friends. After entering from above, one of his friends left the cave and dropped a zinc chloride smoke bomb into it. This was not done maliciously, but was meant to be a practical joke. The patient spent about 10 minutes extracting himself and the other two individuals.

Immediately afterwards, he and his friends presented coughing to the emergency room of the local hospital. There was minimal sputum production and he had several episodes of emesis. He complained of shortness of breath, but arterial blood gases were normal (pH 7.44, P_{CO_2} 36 mmHg [4.8 kPa], P_{O_2} 114 mmHg [15.2 kPa]) as was an initial chest radiograph. He was hospitalized and continued to complain of dyspnea. Two days after the episode, his arterial oxygen tension breathing room air was noted to have fallen to 41 mmHg [5.5 kPa] without significant change in pH or P_{CO_2}. He was treated with 50% Fi_{O_2} by mask and oxygenation improved. A chest radiograph at that time showed a ground glass (acinar) pattern. He began treatment with intravenous methyl prednisolone, inhaled albuterol (salbutamol), and inhaled N-acetylcysteine, and because of his persistent respiratory problems was transferred to the intensive care unit.

Initial physical examination in the intensive care unit was characterized by an increased respiratory rate, no use of accessory muscles, and rales auscultated bilaterally. On 60% Fi_{O_2}, arterial blood gas analysis gave pH 7.39, P_{CO_2} 44 mmHg [5.8 kPa], P_{O_2} 86 mmHg [11.4 kPa]. Other laboratory values were normal, and his continuing cough was unproductive. There was slow improvement over the following 7 days during which he received intravenous methyl prednisolone and inhaled albuterol. However, 11 days after his initial injury his symptoms worsened and he required 100% Fi_{O_2} to maintain a normal oxygen saturation. Two days later he developed bilateral pneumothoraces. This resulted in arterial desaturation once more, and he required bilateral chest tube placement, endotracheal intubation, and mechanical ventilation with high Fi_{O_2} requirements. A normal pH was maintained with minimal ventilatory needs, and CT scanning showed diffuse ground glass opacification (Fig. 6.1).

The two friends who had been exposed to the fumes also suffered an inhalation injury but with a less severe clinical course.

Issues

This case posed a number of difficulties in both diagnosis and management. The first major issue is whether the zinc chloride smoke bomb was solely responsible for this young man's dramatic illness, or whether there were additional factors of relevance. A second major issue is the cause (or causes) of the deterioration on day 11. Finally, there is difficulty in predicting the outcome, and in particular the chances of survival.

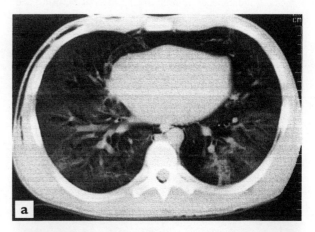

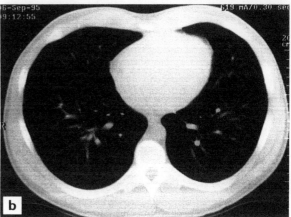

Fig. 6.1 Difficult Case: high-resolution CT scans. The scans were obtained 1 week (**a**) and 12 weeks (**b**) after the accident. They demonstrate extensive interstitial lung disease which resolved radiographically.

Comment

The book's contributors did attribute the initial respiratory disorder to the toxic products released from the smoke bomb. Its short latency essentially excluded the possibility that an infection acquired in the cave had played any role. A majority of contributors nevertheless considered that concomitant fungal exposure in the cave (most obviously to *Histoplasma*) may have contributed to the later clinical deterioration. Most prominent among a number of other identified possibilities for this were ARDS, bronchiolitis obliterans, nosocomial infection consequent to the steroid therapy, and atelectasis resulting from mucus retention. There was uniform agreement that the chances for survival hovered around 50%.

Zinc chloride ($ZnCl_2$, or hexite) is a major ingredient of smoke bombs [4,25]. Oxides and chlorides of zinc together with chlorine are formed by the ignition of hexachlorethane, zinc chloride and calcium chloride, and are produced by some of the smoke-generating devices used by the military, in firefighter training, and for the generation of special effects in the entertainment industry. Zinc chloride is a hygroscopic, caustic salt that forms hydrochloric acid and zinc oxychloride upon contact with water on mucous membranes and other surfaces. The severity of injury is related to the intensity of the exposure, and depends on both the duration of exposure and the concentration of zinc chloride in the smoke. Irritation and burning of the eyes, skin, and mucous membranes result. Zinc chloride is present in a fine particulate form with a reported average size of 0.1 μm. This makes it possible for relatively large amounts to penetrate into the lower respiratory tract, and as much as 20% may reach beyond the level of the respiratory bronchioles. The remainder settles throughout the tracheobronchial tree. There is thus diffuse lung injury, which is probably a consequence of hydrochloric acid formation [25].

Signs and symptoms of tracheobronchitis and pneumonitis are common following inhalation of smoke that contains zinc chloride. Initial chest radiographs can be normal, but can also show diffuse bilateral infiltrates that are consistent with pneumonitis. Hypoxemia may not be present initially, but can develop over a course of several days. Progression to ARDS following an initial period of clinical stabilization or partial resolution has been reported. Pneumothorax is a frequent complication of the acute lung injury due to subpleural emphysema.

The treatment of zinc chloride inhalation includes oxygen supplementation and mechanical ventilatory support with positive pressure if indicated. Corticosteroids have been used but it is unclear whether they significantly alter the clinical course. N-Acetylcysteine may minimize oxidant-induced lung injury, but it is not clear whether this influences the clinical outcome [4]. Exposed individuals who survive may have persistent ventilatory and diffusion defects.

The outcome in this particular case was very favorable. The patient required one further week of mechanical ventilation, during which the abnormalities of gas exchange resolved. The abnormalities on high-resolution CT resolved also, as did the abnormalities of pulmonary function (Table 6.4). Although there was a continuing non-productive cough for several months following the the inhalation injury, he did eventually returned to his normal activities and was virtually asymptomatic 6 months later.

Table 6.4 Difficult Case: serial lung function tests

	1 week	3 weeks	12 weeks
FVC	2.5 (54%)	3.2 (68%)	5.7 (119%)
FEV$_1$	2.2 (52%)	3.0 (69%)	4.7 (107%)
FEV$_1$/FVC	88%	75%	83%
TLC	3.6 (61%)	4.9 (82%)	6.9 (114%)
RV	1.1 (90%)	1.3 (106%)	1.2 (94%)
D$_L$CO	14 (44%)	19.1 (58%)	48.7 (141%)

The tests were obtained 1, 3, and 12 weeks after the accident. They demonstrate marked restrictive lung function and abnormal gas exchange, which resolved within 3 months.

SUMMARY POINTS

Recognition
- Inhalation exposure to a number of toxic substances produces a broad spectrum of reactions at different levels of the airway.
- Solubility and particle size play a critical role in determining the level at which the dominant effects are produced.
- The causal agent is often not known to the affected individual and the managing physician.

Management
- Treatment is generally supportive rather than specific.
- Awareness of the patterns of presentation and the potential consequences help guide initial and subsequent management.
- The clinical course is often unpredictable, and it is prudent to have a low threshold for hospitalization.

- Careful observation and frequent regular monitoring are essential if complications are to be recognized before they become critical.

Prevention
- Whenever there is a risk of toxic inhalation injury, a comprehensive Accident Plan should be drawn up outlining the action to be taken by each employee, identifying leadership responsibilities, and describing the facilities for evacuation.
- The Accident Plan should be subjected to practice drills.
- Employees should be informed of the nature of any risk, the principles of the Accident Plan, and the actions expected of them in the event of an inhalation accident.
- There should be provision for air supplying respirators, oxygen, showers, and cardiopulmonary resuscitation.
- Informed medical personnel should be promptly available.

REFERENCES

1. Kizer KW. Toxic inhalations. *Emerg Med Clin North Am* 1984; 2(3): 649–666.
2. Schwartz DA. Acute inhalational injury. *Occup Med* 1987; 2(2): 297–318.
3. Morgan M, Frank R. Uptake of pollutant gases in the respiratory system. In: Brain J, Proctor D, Reid L, eds. *Respiratory Defence Mechanisms.* Part I. New York: Marcel Dekker, 1977.
4. Hjortso E, Qvist J, Bud MI *et al.* ARDS after accidental inhalation of zinc chloride smoke. *Inten Care Med* 1988; 14(1): 17–24.

5. Barnes PJ. Reactive oxygen species and airway inflammation. *Free Rad Biol Med* 1990; 9(3): 235–243.

6. Menzel DB. Ozone: an overview of its toxicity in man and animals. *J Toxicol Environ Health* 1984; 13(2–3): 183–204.

7. Holgate ST, Beasely R, Twentymen OP. The pathogenesis and significance of bronchial hyperresponsiveness in airways disease. *Clin Sci* 1987; 73: 561–572.

8. Metzger WJ, Richerson HB, Worden K *et al.* Bronchoalveolar lavage of allergic asthmatic patients following allergen bronchoprovocation. *Chest* 1986; 89(4): 477–483.

9. Wardlaw AJ, Dunnette S, Gleich GJ *et al.* Eosinophils and mast cells in bronchoalveolar lavage in subjects with mild asthma: relationship to bronchial hyperreactivity. *Am Rev Respir Dis* 1988; 137: 62–69.

10. Fabbri LM, Aizawa H, Alpert SE *et al.* Airway hyperresponsiveness and changes in cell counts in bronchoalveolar lavage after ozone exposure in dogs. *Am Rev Respir Dis* 1984; 129(2): 288–291.

11. Beasley R, Roche WR, Roberts JA, Holgate ST. Cellular events in the bronchi in mild asthma and after bronchial provocation. *Am Rev Respir Dis* 1989; 139: 806–817.

12. Flury KE, Rogers R Dines DE, Rodarte JR, Case report. Airway obstruction due to inhalation of ammonia. *Mayo Clin Proc* 1983; 58: 389–393.

13. Schwartz D, Smith D, Lakshminarayan S. The pulmonary sequelae associated with accidental inhalation of chlorine gas. *Chest* 1990; 97: 820–825.

14. Kleinfeld M, Giel C. Clinical manifestations of ozone poisoning: report of a new source of exposure. *Am J Med Sci* 1956; 231: 638–643.

15. Cullinan P, Acquilla S, Ramana Dhara N. Respiratory morbidity 10 years after the Union Carbide Gas leak at Bhopal: a cross sectional survey. *BMJ* 1997; 314: 338–343.

16. Brooks SM, Weiss MA, Bernstein IL. Reactive airways dysfunction syndrome (RADS). Persistent asthma syndrome after high level irritant exposures. *Chest* 1985; 88(3): 376–384.

17. Moore BB, Sherman M. Chronic reactive airway disease following acute chlorine gas exposure in an asymptomatic atopic patient [see comments]. *Chest* 1991; 100(3): 855–856.

18. Charan NB, Myers CG, Lakshminarayan S, Spencer TM. Pulmonary injuries associated with acute sulfur dioxide inhalation. *Am Rev Respir Dis* 1979; 119(4): 555–560.

19. Galea M. Case report. Fatal sulfur dioxide inhalation. *Can Med Ass J* 1964; 91: 345–347.

20. Kanluen S, Gottlieb CA. A clinical pathologic study of four adult cases of acute mercury inhalation toxicity. *Arch Pathol Lab Med* 1991; 115(1): 56–60.

21. McAdams AJ, Krop S. Injury and death from red fuming nitric acid. *JAMA* 1955; 58: 1022–1024.

22. Price SK, Hughes JE, Morrison SC, Potgieter PD. Fatal ammonia inhalation. A case report with autopsy findings. *S Afr Med J* 1993; 64(24): 952–955.

23. Epler GR, Colby TV, McLoud TC *et al.* Bronchiolitis obliterans organizing pneumonia. *N Engl J Med* 1985; 312(3): 152–158.

24. Epler GR. Bronchiolitis obliterans organizing pneumonia: definition and clinical features. *Chest* 1992; 102(1 Suppl): 2S–6S.

25. Homma S, Jones R, Qvist J *et al.* Pulmonary vascular lesions in the adult respiratory distress syndrome caused by inhalation of zinc chloride smoke: a morphometric study. *Human Pathol* 1992; 23: 45–50.

7 SILICOSIS

Gerald S. Davis

BACKGROUND

Silica is a naturally occurring widely abundant mineral that forms the major component of most rocks and soil. Silicosis is a chronic diffuse interstitial fibronodular lung disease caused by long-term inhalation of dust containing free crystalline silica. Silicosis requires high-dose and usually prolonged silica inhalation, and does not develop with trivial exposure. The inhalation of silica is also associated with a variety of other adverse health effects that occur at lower doses than may be needed to produce silicosis, including chronic bronchitis (industrial bronchitis), chronic obstructive pulmonary disease (COPD), tuberculosis, scleroderma, and other rheumatologic conditions, and an increased risk for lung cancer.

Silicosis – the pneumoconiosis caused by crystalline silica – has become relatively uncommon in the industrialized nations of the world through aggressive measures to control airborne dust in the workplace. Thus clinicians in more developed countries will more frequently deal with chronic airway disease or lung cancer in a worker with low levels of silica exposure, or will be challenged by possible cases of silicosis that prove not to be. Silicosis remains a common and severe form of lung disease in developing nations where industrial hygiene measures have not achieved safe levels of mineral dust in the work-place. In these settings the emphasis should be placed on prevention, since little or no effective therapy is available for silicosis.

Mineralogy

Exposure to silica occurs by inhalation of dry mineral particles of respirable size (0.2–10 μm aerodynamic diameter). The element silicon (Si) is very abundant and widely distributed in nature, comprising approximately 25% of the earth's crust. Silicon is usually complexed with oxygen to form silica (SiO_2) or with other anions and oxygen to form various silicates. Silica occurs in several crystalline forms, and in amorphous non-crystalline forms as glass. Among the crystalline polymorphs, quartz is the most abundant, and is the form usually associated with human disease. Cristobalite and tridymite are less common, but more biologically active, and can cause disease with appropriate exposure. Stishovite and coesite appear to be less toxic. All of these crystalline forms have the same chemical formula, and all but stishovite assume the shape of a tetrahedron with four oxygen atoms shared by two silicon atoms. The exact dimensions and shape of the crystal lattice differ among the polymorphs, and may be related to their different fibrogenicities. The surface properties of the particles appear to be critical in conferring the biologic properties to crystalline silica.

Natural stones, such as beach sand or sandstone, may be almost pure crystalline silica, or may be a mixture of silica particles with other minerals and silicates as in granite, shale, or basalt. Working with these stones may liberate respirable particles of crystalline silica, and thus cause silicosis or other silica-related lung diseases. Amorphous silica that occurs as commercial or natural glass appears to be non-fibrogenic. Inhalation of glass particles or fibers appears to be relative harmless unless the dose is so large as to cause a non-specific irritant effect. Commercial glass is created by melting 'glass sand', pure crystalline silica, and allowing it to cool slowly. Amorphous non-crystalline forms of silica occur in nature as diatomaceous earth (the skeletons of marine organisms) and as vitreous silica or volcanic glass. The amorphous forms of silica are classified as nuisance dusts. High-temperature processes may convert non-crystalline materials into crystalline forms, including cristobalite. This sequence occurs in the mining and processing of diatomaceous earth and in certain applications of ceramic fibers.

Sources of exposure

Exposure to airborne particles of respirable silica can occur in numerous industries, avocations, and environments. These can be grouped broadly into trades where rock is drilled or removed from the earth (mining, quarrying), trades where silica-bearing stone is worked to produce other products (sculpting, cutting), jobs utilizing abrasives containing silica (tool grinding, sand blasting) or where abrasives are directed at a stone surface (building cleaning), and occupations where powdered silica is made or used as a raw material or additive in manufacture (glass, paint, plastics). Some of these specific industries are listed in Table 7.1. The critical elements in all of these trades are the free crystalline silica content of whatever dust aerosol may be generated, the concentration of particles in the air, and the duration of exposure (see exposure–response relations). The effects of the exposure will be modified by the health, susceptibility, and personal work habits of each individual.

RECOGNITION

The diagnosis of silicosis requires three elements: (1) a history of sufficient exposure to silica; (2) chest radiographic evidence of small opacities consistent with this disease; and (3) no other concomitant illness that mimics silicosis.

Table 7.1 Occupations with exposure to silica

Removal of stone
Hard rock mining
Tunnel drilling
Stone quarrying
Processing stone or sand
Stone crushing
Granite monument carving
Stone sculpting
Stone masonry
Abrasive use of silica or sand
Abrasive blasting
Foundry casting
Tool grinding
Knife sharpening
Production of fine silica powder
Silica flour production
Diatomaceous earth production
Utilization of sand or silica powder
Glass manufacture
Plastics manufacture
Paint manufacture
Pottery
Ceramic manufacture

History

The occupational history is the key to recognizing silicosis and to establishing the diagnosis. The symptoms of silicosis are non-specific and are common to many chronic respiratory diseases. Patients report cough and gradually progressive shortness of breath with exertion. The symptoms evolve slowly over years, and there is little variation from day to day. Most workers with clinically evident silicosis are 40 years of age or older, because of the long exposure required to cause illness and the slow progression of the disease. Cough and sputum production are frequent, and many workers have associated bronchitis. Since many workers exposed to silica also smoke tobacco, it may be very difficult to distinguish the symptoms of silicosis from those of COPD. It is important to record precisely the specific activities and the intensity of effort needed to produce dyspnea at the time of evaluation. Quantification of dyspnea using standard scales [1–4] or common repeated activities (climbing stairs, carrying tools) is helpful. This information may be essential in future determination of the degree of impairment and in monitoring the progression of the disease. A detailed current and past general medical history should also be obtained to identify diseases that could mimic silicosis or conditions that would contribute to the symptoms and the degree of impairment.

The work history is essential in establishing an appropriate exposure that may lead to silicosis. Years of exposure to airborne silica are usually required in order to produce this disease. Silicosis may progress long after exposure has ended because of the effects of the mineral retained in the lung. Thus it is critical to obtain a complete past work history, not merely a current exposure history; work as a miner 10 or 20 years before clinical presentation could be the key to the diagnosis. It is essential to record both the job title if known (e.g. boiler repairman) and the actual work performed (e.g. sand-blasting of boiler interiors). Many workers may know that they were employed in a dusty trade but have no knowledge of the mineral content of the airborne dust. The specific industry, name of the employer, materials used (with brand names if possible), and the dates of beginning and ending employment should all be recorded.

Physical signs

Crackles (rales) and scattered wheezes may be found on physical examination of the chest, but often auscultation is normal despite relatively advanced silicosis. Percussion and tactile fremitus are usually normal, as are other physical examination maneuvers. With advanced disease, emphysema or overdistension may surround zones of fibrosis leading to diminished breath sounds. Silicotic lesions within or adjacent to airway walls cause narrowing and prolonged expiration. Clubbing of the digits is rare in silicosis and, if present, suggests other diseases.

Clinical investigation

Lung function

Lung function abnormalities in silicosis are uncommon in early or simple silicosis. A mixed pattern of obstruction and reduction in lung volumes appears in workers with more advanced disease. This pattern may be confused with the abnormalities produced by COPD if the worker is or was a tobacco smoker. Progressive massive fibrosis produces severe restriction, loss of pulmonary compliance, and hypoxemia.

Radiology

The imaging appearances of silicosis are quite distinctive, and offer a specific diagnosis if a compatible exposure history is present. The characteristic abnormalities include a diffuse pattern of small rounded opacities, predominantly in the upper lobes of the lung, and enlargement of hilar and mediastinal lymph nodes with peripheral calcification. Specific categories and descriptions of radiographs that relate to silicosis are included in the classifica-

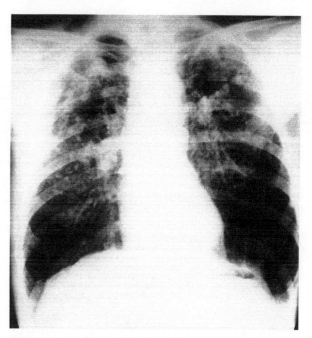

Fig. 7.1 Chest radiograph of a Barre, Vermont, granite cutter, employed for decades before the imposition of effective dust controls, shows small and medium rounded opacities in moderate profusion. The hilar lymph nodes are enlarged. The disease is predominantly in the upper lobes, and the hila show upward traction.

tion scheme developed by the International Labor Office and related groups [5,6]. This is described fully in Chapter 31.

Simple silicosis is manifest as diffuse rounded opacities (type p, profusion 1–2). More extensive disease involves enlargement in nodule size and increased numbers of them (types p–q, profusion 2–3), as shown in Fig. 7.1. Peripheral 'eggshell' calcification of the hilar nodes is quite characteristic of silicosis, though only a small proportion of chest radiographs in silicosis will demonstrate this. Infrequently, simple silicotic nodules in the lung parenchyma may calcify as well. With advanced disease, the discrete rounded opacities coalesce to form large irregular-shaped masses, as shown in Figure 7.2(a), thus the label of 'progressive massive fibrosis'. All of these abnormalities can be visualized much more clearly with high-resolution computed tomography (HRCT) of the chest, as illustrated in Figures 7.2b and c. This technique is recommended strongly for the assessment of patients with possible silicosis. Subpleural nodules that sometimes calcify are characteristic of silicosis, and may be quite prominent on computed tomograms even when they are not apparent on plain chest radiographs (see pathology, Figs 7.3 and 7.4). The degree of pulmonary function impairment is generally related to the severity of the radiographic abnormalities and to the computed tomographic findings [7].

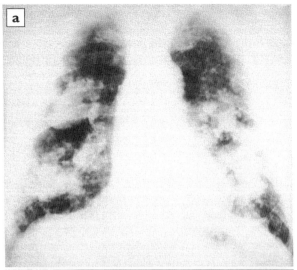

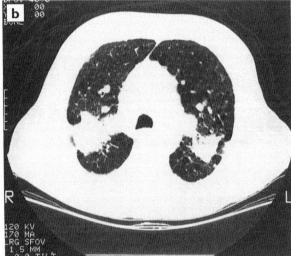

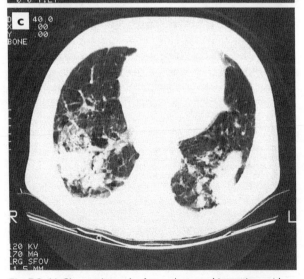

Fig. 7.2 (a) Chest radiograph of an underground iron miner with advanced silicosis and progressive massive fibrosis. Large conglomerate masses with surrounding areas of emphysema are evident. (b) Computed axial tomography scan at the level of the trachea shows bilateral masses and hilar node enlargement. (c) Scan through the lower lung zones shows conglomerate masses, subpleural nodules, and traction emphysema.

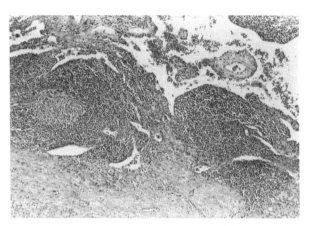

Fig. 7.3 The edge of large silicotic lesion shows dense collagen at the center (lower left side) surrounded by a macrophages and fibroblasts, then a layer of numerous lymphocytes and small mononuclear cells extending out into the alveolar interstitium.

Serology

Laboratory blood tests are non-specific and not particularly helpful in silicosis. Elevation of serum immunoglobulin levels, circulating immune complexes, rheumatoid factor, and antinuclear antibodies are sometimes observed [8–10]. It is not clear whether these diverse antibodies are related directly to the pathogenesis of tissue inflammation or are secondary phenomena that are the result of the disease. Non-specific polyclonal activation of humoral immunity appears to be common in silicosis. Other laboratory abnormalities are not found usually.

Pathology

Histopathology

The histopathology of silicosis is quite distinct, and usually offers a definitive diagnosis. The characteristic lesion of silicosis is the silicotic nodule, found in lung tissue, with surrounding fibrosis and other changes [11]. The typical silicotic nodule is composed of whorled collagen and reticulin centrally, with surrounding macrophages, fibroblasts, and lymphocytes. Fig. 7.3 illustrates these features. Nodules are located near or about the respiratory bronchiole. This localization may be the result of the site of dust depositing in the lung, since initial deposition is non-uniform and is concentrated at alveolar duct bifurcations [12,13] close to the respiratory bronchioles. The minimal lesion is a collection of macrophages with refractile dust particles concentrated within it. The developing silicotic nodule shows a distinct architecture centered around cells and dust. Large macrophages are abundant at the center and contain some dust.

As nodules enlarge, whorled concentric layers of collagen appear at the center of the lesions, as

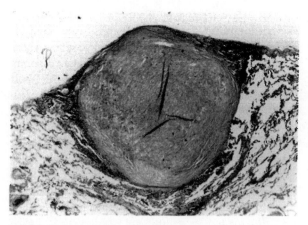

Fig. 7.4 A silicotic nodule at the pleural surface is composed of whorled collagen with a rim of inflammatory and mesenchymal cells.

shown in Fig. 7.4. Smaller macrophages and many lymphocytes surround the central cells, and dust may move to the periphery as the lesions enlarge. Epithelioid giant cells are a variable feature. Rarely, typical granulomata occur. Diffuse fibrosis extending outwards from the conglomerate silicotic masses can be seen with advanced disease. Perinodular emphysematous regions may coalesce to form macroscopic blebs, and can rupture causing a pneumothorax.

Tissues outside the lung parenchyma can be involved if inhaled particles are carried to remote sites by lymphatic or hematogenous routes, but without pulmonary nodules 'silicosis' should not be diagnosed. The hilar lymph nodes that drain lung tissue are virtually always involved, with typical silicotic nodules and abundant dust. Mediastinal lymph nodes are frequently involved, and sometimes supraclavicular nodes, as secondary lymphatic drainage sites. Dust may sometimes be carried outside the thorax as well. Dystrophic ossification occurs frequently in silicotic nodules, particularly in lymph nodes, producing the calcification seen on plain chest radiographs. With HRCT scanning, small flecks of calcium can often be found within parenchymal and subpleural nodules as well as within the hilar and mediastinal nodes.

Mineral analysis

Silica particles appear as birefringent crystalline material when lung tissue is examined under polarized light microscopy. The smallest particles, those less than 0.5 μm, may be very difficult to see, but larger particles and aggregates of small ones can usually be detected easily. Quartz produces a red tinge which may help distinguish it from the 'white polarization' of more brightly birefringent silicates. Cristobalite and the other polymorphs of silica are less birefringent and so may be difficult or impossible to detect.

Mixed silicates, talc, and other minerals are also birefringent under polarized light, and may be confused with silica if the environmental exposure history is not clear-cut. Special techniques of mineral analysis can be applied to lung tissue in order to determine the exact composition of the crystalline materials that are present. The simplest approach utilizes scanning electron microscopy (SEM) with back-scattered X-ray energy dispersive spectrometry. Paraffin-embedded lung tissue sections can be examined by SEM, electron-dense particles identified, and their relative composition of medium-to-high atomic number elements determined. Only Si would be recorded from particles of pure quartz, while Mg, Al, Fe, and other elements would be identified in mixed silicates, talc, or asbestos fibers. Dust samples recovered from the air can be subjected to a similar type of analysis. This approach has direct clinical utility for confirming the exact nature of an occupational or environmental exposure if it is in doubt.

Clinically significant silicosis that results in substantial functional impairment always involves exposure to large quantities of inhaled dust. Silica particles are always abundant in the lung tissue of such patients. If the diagnosis is in doubt and lung biopsy is obtained, the absence of abundant silica essentially excludes silicosis. The converse finding is more troublesome, because substantial numbers of birefringent mineral particles from mixed silicates or silica may be found in lung tissue or in bronchoalveolar lavage samples with little or no pathological response [14,15]. Thus the presence of the mineral confirms exposure but does not automatically establish that a clinically significant disease is present.

Larger specimens of lung tissue can be ashed and subjected to X-ray diffraction analysis for quantitative reporting of the amount of specific minerals present. This approach is very rarely needed for clinical diagnosis or industrial hygiene purposes, but may be useful for research programs.

Mechanisms

The pathogenic mechanisms that lead from the inhaled mineral particle to tissue injury, inflammation, fibrosis, and lung remodeling have recently been reviewed in detail [16]. The pathogenesis of silicosis focuses on interactions between lung cells and inhaled particles, and the secondary responses triggered by this interaction. At exposure levels encountered in most occupational settings, the resident alveolar macrophage appears to be the most important lung cell that interacts with silica. At higher workplace exposure levels for man, or in many of the exposures used to create silicosis in experimental animals, alveolar epithelial cells and possibly other mesenchymal cells may also interact directly with silica particles.

The interaction between silica and resident or recruited lung cells can result in several categories of events that are not mutually exclusive. The particles may be coated with alveolar lining lipids and proteins to render them less biologically active. The contact cell, particularly the macrophage, may ingest the particle and sequester it. The particle alone, or cells containing particles may be transported out of the lung by mucociliary clearance or relocated by interstitial lymphatics to lymph nodes or other sequestered sites. The cell in contact with silica particles may be damaged, rendered dysfunctional, killed, or directed to programmed cell death (apoptosis). The cell in contact with silica particles may be stimulated to produce cytokines and other biologic mediators that secondarily alter the function of other cells.

Workers in dusty trades may inhale large amounts of mineral particles. Black sputum expectorated by coal miners, and gray phlegm from granite workers, are hallmarks of these trades. The large visible particles are deposited in the nose and proximal airways, and are promptly removed by mucociliary clearance. The smaller particles (less than 5–10 µm) that are deposited in the alveoli may be cleared with reasonable efficiency, but a substantial fraction remains within the lung. These particles can remain in the alveolar spaces indefinitely, but many are translocated to peribronchial, subpleural, and interstitial pulmonary sites as well as intrathoracic lymphoid tissues [17,18]. Most of the clearance that will occur by direct mucociliary removal takes place immediately after inhalation, while translocation between the air space and the interstitium continues indefinitely [19]. An important aspect of silica toxicity is this persistence in tissue. Little or no silica is dissolved in tissue, in contrast to many other minerals, and it appears to remain biologically active for a very long time.

The biological response to silica appears to rest upon its crystalline nature, and the highly reactive surface radical groups associated with the crystalline rather than amorphous polymorphs. The reactivity of surface groups with biological materials, particularly internal or external cell membranes, may be the key element in toxicity. Quartz demonstrates abundant strongly reactive surface sites [20]. Cristobalite, the most biologically active isoform, contains the greatest number of these reactive groups [21].

Alveolar macrophages recovered from animals and human workers exposed to silica aerosols contain many particles but demonstrate normal viability, normal phagocytic function, and enhanced bacterial killing [12,22]. Although some macrophages may be injured or killed by silica, most appear to be stimulated. The macrophage responds to the ingestion of crystalline silica particles with activation and the release of a wide variety of cytokines and other reactants. These include oxidant radicals and enzymes that could injure nearby cells, chemoattractants that recruit inflammatory cells, cytokines that activate lymphocytes and other cells, growth factors that promote fibroblast and epithelial cell proliferation, and profibrotic factors that stimulate production of collagen and other matrix materials. Key mediators include chemokines [23], tumor necrosis factor-α (TNF-α), and interleukin-1 (IL1) [24–26], interferon-γ [27,28], fibronectin [29], platelet-derived growth factor (PDGF) [30–32], and transforming growth factor-β [33,34]. It is important not to oversimplify this scheme: multiple mechanisms may overlap; inflammatory pathways and mediators are often redundant; downregulatory and proinflammatory influences often coexist or compete simultaneously.

The silicotic nodule appears to be a paradigm for the mechanisms of chronic silicosis. Within this site, silica particles interact with macrophages, lymphocytes and neutrophils amplify the inflammatory environment, and fibroblasts proliferate and deposit excess connective tissue matrix material. The disease *in toto* could be viewed as the sum of many microscopic foci of injury, inflammation, and fibrosis evolving in parallel. These nodules may be at different sizes and stages of development in different locations. Finally, they merge or aggregate to form the large lesions of progressive massive fibrosis. The rate at which this process advances may be defined by a complex interaction between the type of silica, intensity of exposure, the duration of exposure, the genetic responsiveness of the host, and many other factors.

Environmental investigation

Atmospheric characterization

Assay of the air in the workplace for content of silica can be achieved through methods that capture airborne particles, determine their size and mass, enumerate the fraction that is respirable, and analyze their mineral composition. These techniques are applicable to periodic industrial hygiene surveys, and occasionally to the investigation of individual sites where a problem is suspected. These approaches are discussed later. Characterization of the workplace is rarely applicable for a single case of silicosis because of the expense and special techniques that are required, and because the workplace has usually changed extensively between the time most of the exposure occurred and disease became apparent.

Exposure–response relations

Silicosis obeys strict exposure–response relations. The most important factors that interact to influence the severity of silicosis are the intensity and duration of exposure to crystalline silica. The mineral isoform (quartz, cristobalite, tridymite), the proportion of the inhaled dust represented by silica, the percentage of particles of a size suitable for alveolar deposition (respirable fraction), the concentration of the dust in the air (number of particles or weight per unit volume), and the duration of exposure (work years) all interact to determine the prevalence, latency, and progression of silicosis. Other factors may be important, but play a lesser role. Simultaneous exposure to other occupational dusts or fumes and tobacco smoking may (theoretically) interfere with the efficient clearance of silica from the lung, or may produce independent lung diseases that compound the adverse effects of silica. Personal work habits, particularly disregard for safe work practices, increase risk substantially. Genetic susceptibility appears to play little if any role. Most workers will develop silicosis of similar extent under similar exposure conditions.

Diagnosis and clinical patterns

The diagnosis of silicosis is established on the basis of a compatible clinical picture with an appropriate exposure history. The physical findings are often minimal, and any pulmonary function abnormalities are non-specific. They demonstrate that lung disease is present and define its severity. A clear exposure history linked with a typical chest radiograph may be sufficient for both medical and compensation purposes, and most national compensation boards rely on this evidence alone. HRCT lung scans (commonly) or lung biopsy with tissue analysis (uncommonly) may be needed to establish a diagnosis if the clinical features are atypical or if the work exposure is inconclusive.

Silicosis virtually always requires prolonged exposure to substantial airborne quantities of respirable crystalline free silica. Most patients will be aware that they worked for many years in a dusty trade, although they may not know the exact mineral composition of the dust. In many industries silicosis is a well-known hazard, and workers will be aware that their lungs have become 'rocked up'. For some work environments, airborne dust measurements may be available and so will confirm or refute relevant levels of exposure. Exposure to crystalline free silica at or below nationally accepted standards

$(5–10 \mu g/m^3)$ appears to cause little or no radiographic silicosis in most or all industries.

Four clinical patterns of diffuse lung disease may be seen with silicosis: simple nodular silicosis, progressive massive fibrosis, accelerated silicosis, and acute silicosis or silicoproteinosis.

Simple silicosis is the pattern most commonly seen among workers at all ages, represented by a profusion of small rounded opacities throughout the lung fields. Hilar lymph nodes may be prominent, and calcification can be seen. Subtle radiographic changes may be the first manifestation of the disease. The radiograph may appear quite abnormal while symptoms are minimal and pulmonary function is well preserved. The nodules of simple silicosis are less than 1 cm in diameter. As silicosis progresses, the individual nodules enlarge and coalesce in a transition to progressive massive fibrosis.

Progressive massive fibrosis (PMF) occurs with pure silicosis and with coal workers' pneumoconiosis. Confluent nodules greater than 1 cm in diameter appear against a background of smaller nodules, as individual lesions conglomerate to form larger masses. Emphysema develops in lung tissue surrounding the coalescent masses as the conglomerates shrink through fibrosis. Calcification within the conglomerate masses and in hilar and mediastinal nodes is common with PMF. Substantial impairment of pulmonary function with marked dyspnea upon exertion, and then at rest, develop as PMF advances. Destruction of the pulmonary capillary bed leads to elevated pulmonary vascular resistance, and may produce cor pulmonale with heart failure. Progressive hypoxemia complicates this process. PMF may produce severe impairment, even death.

Accelerated silicosis is relatively rare, but can develop within 2–5 years with intense exposure to free silica [35–37]. Dyspnea is apparent early, and soon becomes disabling. The radiographic picture is of diffuse small irregular opacities or reticulonodular opacities, rather than the upper lobe nodular opacities typical of simple silicosis. Accelerated silicosis appears to be uniformly fatal within several years after the appearance of clinical signs.

Acute silicosis is a rare consequence of exposure to free silica at very high concentrations, usually in tunneling through hard rock, abrasive blasting with pure sand, or the use of finely divided silica powder [38–41]. Acute silicosis presents with rapidly progressive dyspnea and respiratory insufficiency. Radiographically, the appearance is that of a diffuse perihilar alveolar filling process with ground-glass opacities. Upon pathological examination, the alveolar spaces are filled with a lipid and proteinaceous exudate and cellular debris; damage to the epithelium is extensive. Thus, acute silicosis more closely mimics pulmonary alveolar proteinosis than it does interstitial fibrosis, and it is sometimes referred to as silicoproteinosis. Acute silicosis appears to be a uniformly fatal disease.

Differential diagnosis

A variety of lung diseases may mimic some of the features of silicosis, and it is essential to recognize the differences and similarities. Sarcoidosis, histoplasmosis, and other chronic fungal infections, tuberculosis in some forms, and pneumoconiosis resulting from mixed dust exposures can all resemble silicosis. Patients may be diagnosed and treated fruitlessly for these other conditions, while missing compensation for silicosis. More commonly, patients with some silica exposure history may be mistakenly diagnosed with silicosis and thereby miss effective therapy for other diseases.

Sarcoidosis shares many features with silicosis. Both are chronic granulomatous lung diseases dominated by mononuclear inflammation that follows a lymphocyte T_H1 phenotype and cytokine pattern. Both produce nodular lung disease and central thoracic lymph node enlargement. Both can cause small subpleural nodules evident on HRCT scan. In its advanced chronic form, sarcoidosis may produce coalescence of central masses and midzone fibrosis with compensatory emphysema involving the upper and lower lung zones. If longstanding, this type of sarcoidosis can cause calcification within hilar lymph nodes and even within granulomatous masses in the lung tissue. Thus advanced 'Stage IV' sarcoidosis can be difficult to distinguish from silicosis based on the plain chest radiograph alone.

Important differences will usually permit clear distinction between silicosis and sarcoidosis. The key distinction lies in the presence or lack of an extensive exposure to silica. The onset of sarcoidosis shows a peak incidence in patients aged 20–40 years, while silicosis is uncommon in patients younger than 40. Sarcoidosis commonly involves extrathoracic organ systems, with disease evident in the eyes, skin, liver, and lymph nodes outside of the thorax, while silicosis almost never does so. Within the chest, sarcoidosis is generally diffuse or patchy with a random distribution, while silicosis is generally symmetrical with an upper zone predominance. On HRCT scan, the nodular densities of sarcoidosis tend to follow an axillary distribution along airways and blood vessels, while silicosis is distributed more diffusely through the parenchyma. Sarcoidosis rarely, if ever, forms the large conglomerate masses that define PMF in silicosis.

Histoplasmosis could be mistaken for early or mild silicosis. The soil fungus *Histoplasma capsulatum* is endemic to the Ohio River and St Lawrence River valleys of North America and a few other regions. In its most common pattern, hystoplasmosis causes a mild respiratory illness followed by gradually healing lung parenchymal and thoracic lymph node lesions. This infection provokes a granulomatous tissue response that could be mistaken pathologically for silicosis in lung or lymph node tissue if mineral particles were not sought. The affected hilar and mediastinal lymph nodes following histoplasmosis may remain enlarged for life, and may form dystrophic calcifications. Small rounded nodules may be formed in the lung parenchyma, and also often contain calcifications. Thus, an older-aged resident from an endemic area might demonstrate some radiographic features that suggest silicosis. The other clinical syndromes caused by *H. capsulatum* infection, such as disseminated histoplasmosis, chronic cavitary infection, or fibrosing mediastinitis are not likely to cause confusion with silicosis.

Important differences between silicosis and histoplasmosis usually make the distinction between them straightforward. Histoplamosis typically produces a small number (1–10) of discrete, rounded, small pulmonary nodules of similar size, rather than the numerous variably sized and shaped rounded opacities of silicosis. The thoracic lymph nodes of histoplasmosis demonstrate central flecks of calcification rather than the peripheral rim of 'eggshell' calcification usually seen with silica. Histoplasmosis typically causes tiny lesions with calcification in the spleen and sometimes the liver that can be seen radiographically, while silicosis does not.

Prior infection with tuberculosis could cause confusion with silicosis, as both may produce thoracic lymph node enlargement with calcification, and both may cause parenchymal nodules or scars. The distinction can be made, however. The parenchymal lesions of healed tuberculosis usually appear as either single, dense, rounded nodules or apical scars, rather than the numerous, small, rounded opacities of silicosis. The latter may simulate those of miliary (and active) tuberculosis, but the rapidly obvious life-threatening nature of this disease is readily distinguished from silicosis. The enlarged thoracic nodes associated with non-miliary tuberculosis are usually unilateral, and the calcification is central, while silicotic nodes are usually bilateral with peripheral rims of calcification. These distinctions are limited to patients who do not have a history of silica exposure. Detecting and managing active tuberculosis in patients who also have silicosis is an important and difficult clinical problem, which is dealt with in more detail below.

Pneumoconiosis due to mixed dusts, coal, talc, or silicates other than SiO_2 may cause confusion with silicosis. In some instances, the disease may be true silicosis, attributable to the crystalline free silica in the inhaled dust mixture. Coal and talc are dealt with in detail elsewhere in this book (Chapters 8 and 10). Both may cause clinically significant pulmonary disease with many features that resemble silicosis. Mixed particulates that contain little or no silica are generally considered as 'nuisance dusts', and are thought to cause short-term bronchitis due to irritation but not diffuse pulmonary fibrosis. This topic is dealt with in detail in Chapter 10. Mixed dust exposures may result in low categories of radiographic abnormalities (1/0, 1/1) but usually do not produce either the central lymph-node enlargement or the clear-cut abnormalities of full-blown silicosis. Detailed information regarding the exact nature of the occupational exposure is the key to identifying the cause and the disease.

Other disorders from silica inhalation

Chronic bronchitis and COPD

Cough and sputum production associated with occupational exposure to dusts or fumes has been termed 'industrial bronchitis' [42]. It is common among worker groups with exposure to silica. It may be difficult to define the limits of industrial bronchitis precisely, since it is commonly associated with airway obstruction and produces similar symptoms to those of mild silicosis. The degree of airway obstruction is variable, posing the question whether productive cough and airway obstruction are both features of the same disorder or manifestations of two independent silica-induced disorders (chronic bronchitis and COPD). It can be detected epidemiologically in a cohort of silica-exposed workers who have no radiographic evidence of silicosis but who report respiratory symptoms. Industrial bronchitis has been identified among a variety of worker groups throughout the developing and industrialized nations of the world [43–48]. A metanalysis of 13 studies among coal and gold miners confirmed an excess of bronchitic symptoms and obstructive physiology, even among non-smokers [49]. There may be a synergistic effect between tobacco smoke and industrial pollutants in producing chronic bronchitis and airflow obstruction. Thus exposure to silica and other dusts at levels that appear not to cause overt silicosis can cause airway disease. The topic is discussed further in Chapters 5 and 29.

Tuberculosis

The association between tuberculosis and silicosis has been well known since the 19th century. Although

these two diseases were sometimes confused with one another, the advent of microbiological techniques to identify tubercle bacilli permitted their clear distinction [50]. It soon became apparent that they often coexisted, and that each influenced the course of the other. The combined disease is sometimes referred to as silicotuberculosis. The association between silicosis and increased susceptibility to tuberculosis has been demonstrated in hard-rock miners, coal miners, granite workers, and other industrial groups [51–53]. Workers with established silicosis appear to be more susceptible than the general population to developing active tuberculosis when exposed, and to a more chronic persistent form of tuberculosis once infected. It is not clear whether low levels of exposure to silica, without the development of overt silicosis, also predispose to tuberculosis. The rising rates of pneumoconiosis in developing countries as mining industries grow, coupled with the high prevalence of tuberculosis in those countries, focus public health attention on the issue of silicotuberculosis [54].

The radiographic changes are similar in both silicosis and tuberculosis, with progression of densities and infiltrates in upper lung zones; thus definitive diagnosis may be difficult. Tuberculosis with silicosis may be indolent and progress slowly, with few organisms shed, and barely positive sputum smears or cultures. Silicosis predisposes to infection with both typical *M. tuberculosis* and 'atypical' non-tuberculous mycobacteria. If mycobacteria are isolated from the sputum of a silica-exposed individual, the species and drug sensitivities must be confirmed. Patients with silicotuberculosis usually respond well to conventional antituberculous therapy in regards to clinical improvement and radiographic stabilization, but complete eradication of organisms may be very difficult. Reactivation following an apparent cure is common in silicotuberculosis, though in some occupational settings it may be a consequence of new infection from infected workmates. The topic is discussed further in Chapters 16, 17 and 29.

Scleroderma

Epidemiologic studies have revealed an excess prevalence of scleroderma (progressive systemic sclerosis) among workers exposed to silica in mining and stone-cutting trades [55–59]. The features of scleroderma appear to be the same as those seen in a non-occupational setting [60]. The association with scleroderma appears to be convincing for substantial silica exposure as well as overt silicosis [61].

An association between silica exposure and rheumatoid arthritis, systemic lupus erythematosus, and other connective tissue diseases is less compelling. Although some studies have suggested an increased prevalence of these systemic diseases in workers with silica exposure [62–64], other surveys have not [65]. The association appears to be strongest for workers with overt silicosis rather than silica exposure alone. The high prevalence of autoantibodies and elevated serum immunoglobulin concentrations in workers with silicosis who have no rheumatologic complaints [8] could lead to false diagnoses of connective tissue diseases. Individuals who have silicosis and develop rheumatoid arthritis may show large pulmonary nodules that undergo central necrosis, a picture known as 'Caplan's syndrome' (Chapter 8).

Lung cancer

Epidemiologic studies from around the world reveal an increased risk for lung cancer among workers exposed to silica [61,66,67]. Although the issue is complex, and reservations can be raised regarding the methodologies and populations of most studies, the balance of evidence favors this association. Crystalline silica has been classified as a human carcinogen by the International Agency for Research on Cancer (IARC) [68], and silica exposure as a factor that increases lung cancer risk has been recognized by international associations and experts [61,67,69]. However, some authors question this link [70–72]. The statistical problems of confounding variables, such as smoking, radon, or hydrocarbon exposure, and of selection bias in the detection of pneumo coniosis cases, has been emphasized [73].

Cohort mortality studies of miners with silica exposure in the USA, the UK, Scandinavia, China, Australia, and South Africa have revealed a significant increase in mortality due to lung cancer [74–80], with two- to fivefold increases in risk. Several of these studies adjusted for the effects of smoking. Radon exposure may be a further important variable for cancer risk in underground miners, and the independent effects of silica, smoking, and radon radiation (and how they might interact), have not been clearly defined.

Reports from Italy, Canada, Germany, Japan, and Indonesia have identified lung cancer with increased frequency among workers registered with silicosis [81–89]. The relative risk for lung cancer compared to the general population ranged from 1.3 to 6.9. These studies attempted to adjust for the effects of smoking, and still found a slight excess cancer mortality. In all series the dominant effect producing cancer appeared to be smoking. Worldwide, workers in granite [90,91], slate [92], diatomaceous earth [93,94], foundries [95], ceramic manufacture [96,97], potteries [98], and general dusty trades [94,99] have been observed to have a slightly increased lung cancer risk (Standardized Mortality Ratio [SMR] 1.4–2.0), with adjustment in many studies for smoking.

Conflicting results from different nations have been observed with some study designs. Silica exposure or silicosis was more frequent among lung cancer cases identified at autopsy than among matched case controls in Italy [100,101], but not in Holland [102] or South Africa [103]. A record linkage study tracked lung cancer among nearly 85 000 Scandinavian workers who were exposed to silica [104], and observed a slight overall increase in cancer risk for workers in foundries, ore mining, and stone cutting in two of the four countries. The effects of radon exposure for miners and smoking habits for all workers were considered important cofactors, but could not be analyzed statistically. Low levels of silica exposure, generally near or within national air quality standards, have shown cancer risk to increased slightly [94,105] or not at all [106,107].

The mechanisms by which silica promotes lung cancer, or potentiates tobacco smoke as a cause of cancer, are not clear. The mineral could act as a cocarcinogen inducing cancer, a cancer promoter stimulating growth of transformed cells, a passive means of carrying tobacco carcinogens into the lung or impairing their clearance, or could alter immune surveillance mechanisms resulting in a failure to eliminate malignant cells when they arise. More research will be needed to determine which of these possibilities are important.

The epidemiologic studies have generated comparable and mutually supportive conclusions, despite the differences of their methods and nations of origin. Exposure to high levels of silica dust (level and duration enough to cause overt silicosis in some workers) produces a two- to four-fold increased risk for lung cancer in tobacco smokers. This risk obtains for surface industry workers in granite sheds, foundries, and mills, as well as for underground miners, thus implicating a true effect of the mineral dust rather than an effect produced by radon daughters, trace elements, or other confounding carcinogens in the mine environment. It is likely that silica exposure sufficient to cause silicosis also increases the lung cancer risk among non-smokers. Whether silica exposure below a level sufficient to cause silicosis produces an increased cancer risk for workers who do not smoke tobacco requires more cases for greater statistical certainty. The effect of silica on enhancing lung cancer risk among smokers appears to be less than the risk for comparably exposed asbestos workers. Larger, ideally prospective, studies will be needed to determine whether silica exposure within regulated levels that are safe for silicosis still cause a significantly increased lung cancer risk. The topic is discussed further in Chapters 20 and 29.

MANAGEMENT

Of the individual

There is no specific conventional therapy for silicosis. Although a variety of therapeutic approaches have been tried, and some may provide help for severely diseased patients, no simple remedies can be offered. Theoretically, strategies for the treatment of excessive silica exposure could be based on the sequence of events that lead to lung injury, inflammation, and fibrosis. Both the endogenous responses of the lung to silica and the some of the medical treatments that have been devised for silicosis can be related to

these strategies, as summarized in Table 7.2. Many workers with abnormal chest radiographs and mild simple nodular silicosis experience few symptoms and mild impairment, while individuals with PMF are usually quite ill. Thus, treatments need not remove all dust or all reaction to it, but might still be useful if PMF could be prevented while simple silicosis still developed. As always, prevention is much more effective than treatment.

Therapeutic whole lung lavage has been employed as a technique for physically removing silica from the aveolar spaces (Box 7.1). This treatment has been directed primarily at workers who have received massive exposures, or who have already

Table 7.2 Theoretical strategies for reducing the effects of silica inhalation

Theoretical strategy	Endogenous lung response	Treatment Measure
Physically remove dust from the lung		Whole lung lavage
Enhance pulmonary transport mechanisms for dust removal	Mucous hypersecretion, cough	
Render the dust in the lung less toxic		Aluminum powder inhalation
Sequester the dust at harmless locations in the lung	Lymph node and subpleural nodule sequestration	
Reduce the inflammatory response to silica		Corticosteroid drugs
Decrease tissue fibrosis accompanying inflammation		?? Tetrandrine drugs??
Repair or replace damaged tissues		Lung transplantation

Box 7.1 Therapeutic whole lung lavage (William S. Beckett)

Although there are still no known effective therapies for silicosis, whole lung lavage (washing of the bronchi and alveoli to remove dust) has been proposed based on the rationale that lavage can remove from the lung several grams of dust, inflammatory cells, and soluble materials. This in turn might slow the progression of established silicosis. Whole lung lavage has been used successfully in the treatment of pulmonary alveolar proteinosis, a condition of unknown cause that resembles acute silicosis. It can be performed under general anesthesia in the operating room using a double lumen endotracheal tube to ventilate one lung while instilling serial volumes of saline warmed to body temperature into the other (e.g. as many as 10–20 liters of saline for each lung). In some cases both lungs have been lavaged serially in a single procedure. Manually inflating the lavaged lung with positive pressure may increase the yield of dust but may also increase risk for thoracic barotrauma [137].

The largest case series of whole lung lavage in pneumoconosis has been reported by Y.P. Liang [138] of the Rehabilitation Centre for Pneumoconiosis of the China National Coal Corporation (Beidaihe, China) in miners, both with silicosis and with coal workers'

pneumoconiosis. Under general anesthesia, each lung was lavaged 10 times with 1–2 liters of saline, with lavage of one lung taking approximately 1 hour. In some cases each lung was lavaged during a separate procedure, while in others both lungs were lavaged during a single period of general anesthesia. Approximately 1–3 g of total mineral dust can be removed from both lungs by such procedures, an amount much less than the total burden measured from autopsy examination of lungs with silicosis. Such case series have shown the feasibility of this approach as well as the efficacy in removing relatively large amounts of mineral dust as well as macrophages and fluid with increased concentration of cytokines.

Case series have demonstrated short-term improvement in chest symptoms after lavage, but controlled trials have not been performed that demonstrate short-term or long-term improvement in lung function, quality of life, or survival. Observers of these initial series have suggested that controlled trials are warranted. They have also suggested the possibility of using whole lung lavage as part of a multimodality treatment program for silicosis that might utilize newer experimental medications to attenuate the pulmonary inflammatory and fibrotic processes.

developed acute silicosis or silicoproteinosis. One case of mixed dust pneumoconiosis was treated in the USA with whole-lung lavage without change in pulmonary function [108]. Recent studies of coal miners in China have reported that several grams of dust can be removed from the lung in this fashion, but no objective improvement in lung function has been observed [109,110].

Several strategies have been developed in an attempt to render inhaled silica less toxic. Aluminum powder inhaled simultaneously with silica dust was tested in animal studies in the 1930s and 1940s, with less fibrosis apparent in animals that received the aluminum treatment [110]. It was believed that aluminum salts and/or aluminum oxide interacted with the reactive surface groups on silica particles and rendered them less toxic. These animal findings led to the inhalation of finely divided aluminum powder as a 'preventive' in human workers exposed to silica. A 4-year randomized controlled trial of aluminum powder inhalation in human pottery workers and miners was reported in 1956, but no objective beneficial results were detected [111]. Inhalation of 'MacIntyre powder' (finely divided aluminum and aluminum oxide) was used at some locations in Canadian mines from 1944 through 1979. Exposed and unexposed miners were evaluated recently for neurological impairment, and the miners who had received aluminum therapy proved to have impairment on cognitive testing [112]. A limited trial in China with aluminum citrate suggested benefit in reducing the radiographic progression of silicosis, but adverse effects were not evaluated in detail [113]. The effectiveness of aluminum lactate inhalation administered after the development of silicosis has been tested in sheep following intrabronchial silica instillation [114]. The sheep that received aluminum therapy showed less silicosis and accelerated clearance of silica from their lungs. Although animal results with aluminum treatment appear promising, aluminum toxicity may limit its application to man.

Corticosteroid treatment is directed primarily at reducing the inflammatory response to silica through its actions on lymphocytes, macrophages, and other cells. Although fibrosis dominates the tissues of advanced or complicated silicosis, substantial accumulations of lymphocytes and monocyte–macrophages are found as part of the silicotic nodule. These mononuclear cells are believed to be the directing force behind fibroblast proliferation and excessive collagen deposition. A beneficial result with steroid therapy, evidenced by radiographic and physiologic improvement, was reported for one patient with acute silicosis [115]. In India, a trial of daily prednisolone for 6 months was carried out among 34 stone-crushing workers with silicosis [116]. Pulmonary function and gas exchange

improved, and brochoalveolar lavage inflammatory cell numbers decreased, from the beginning to the end of the trial. The anecdotal experiences and this one trial suggest that steroids may sometimes be helpful in patients with rapidly progressive silicosis. It is not clear whether the improvement is maintained, whether progression of disease is delayed, or how long treatment must be continued in order to obtain benefit. Experiences with other anti-inflammatory or cytotoxic agents have not been reported.

Chinese researchers are engaged in the evaluation of tetrandrine and other agents derived from traditional Chinese medicine that appear to have activity in reducing silica-induced fibrosis in animal models and possibly in man [110,117,118]. Compounds directed at blocking the effects of cytokines from macrophages or lymphocytes could be useful in silicosis. Although promising in short-term animal studies, these approaches may be limited in man by the slow progression of the disease and its course over decades.

Lung transplantation is the ultimate extension of the lung repair strategy – the complete replacement of damaged tissue. Transplantation has become the final resort of therapy for many chronic diffuse diseases that are localized to the lung, and silicosis may be no exception. Lung transplantation for silicosis has been reported among case series of patients from many countries [119–123]. Lung transplantation is expensive, and access is severely limited by the availability of suitable organs. Most transplant programs limit therapy to younger patients, and severe silicosis is often not apparent until patients are in their 60s or 70s. This treatment should be considered for younger patients with severe impairment who show progressive disease.

General supportive care is the best that can be offered for many patients with chronic respiratory impairment due to silicosis. Pulmonary function and symptoms, rather than the appearance of the chest radiograph, should guide the assessment of severity. Useful treatment measures may include supplemental oxygen to maintain normal oxygen saturation, respiratory and limb muscle exercises to promote strength and endurance, bronchodilator medications if reversible airflow obstruction is present, and early antibiotic therapy for acute exacerbations. Smoking cessation is critical, if the patient has not already quit. A high level of vigilance for tuberculosis should be maintained, since new signs may be subtle and this treatable complication will lead to accelerated loss of lung function. The progression of silicosis is usually quite slow, thus elderly workers may be encouraged that their degree of impairment may not become too severe during their lifetime. For younger individuals with severe progressive disease, early referral for lung transplantation should be considered.

Of the workforce

Screening

Worker health screening for silicosis may be carried out by the industries which employ them, by government agencies charged with responsibility for occupational health, by State or Federal regulatory agencies, or by research institutions. The point is to identify other affected individuals or individuals at high risk, and to learn more about the silicosis risk in the particular working environment of the affected 'index' case. Screening programs may be 'cross-sectional', in which all workers are examined simultaneously at one point in time, or 'longitudinal', wherein a cohort of workers is examined repeatedly at periodic intervals. In most instances the screening efforts will include demographic information (age, work history), some form of respiratory symptom questionnaire, pulmonary function testing, and a chest radiograph. The air of the workplace may be sampled, as discussed below. Most screening is carried out by government agencies or by the larger companies operating mines, quarries, or production facilities.

The demographic information collected about each worker should include age, racial background (although little is known about the effects of race), and current and past smoking history. Detailed information should be recorded about the current job title and exact job description, as well as the length of time in the industry and previous job titles. This information is essential for relating health status to silica exposure.

Standardized respiratory symptom questionnaires have been carefully validated and responses can be compared with those of many other worker groups. Such general instruments include those by the British Medical Research Council, the United States National Institutes of Health with the American Thoracic Society, and the St George's Respiratory Questionnaire, or brief specialized instruments. Completing the questionnaire can be time consuming, and may require a skilled interviewer for workers who are poor readers. An abbreviated set of a few simple questions is used commonly. Questionnaires appear to be reasonably sensitive at detecting symptomatic and impaired workers, but are not specific for silicosis. A physical examination may or may not be included in a general worker health screening, but adds little to screening for silicosis. The physical signs of silicosis are few and non-specific, thus it may not be cost effective to include a physical examination in a survey aimed specifically at this disease.

Pulmonary function testing is a key part of worker screening for silicosis because these tests will offer objective numerical data for estimating the degree of any excess impairment attributable to work exposure, whether for individuals or specific worker cohorts. Forced expiratory spirometry is the standard test, with forced vital capacity (FVC), forced expired volume in 1 second (FEV_1), and the FEV_1/FVC ratio as the most robust variables. The importance of trained personnel administering the test, careful standardization of test procedures, frequent calibration of equipment, and appropriate selection of normal predicted values must be emphasized.

The conventional posteroanterior chest radiograph made at full inspiration is another essential element in screening for silicosis. Radiographic abnormalities often precede symptoms or pulmonary function impairment, thus radiology may be the most sensitive indicator of early disease. High-quality films meeting modern standards utilize a small focal spot, high kilovoltage generator source, and a film-screen combination offering a long gray scale. These conditions should be available at most hospital radiology facilities, but may be more difficult to achieve with mobile field units. The chest radiographs obtained from an industrial screening for pneumoconiosis usually are interpreted by those who have achieved certification as 'B readers' in the classification scheme developed by the International Labor Office and related groups (ILO-UICC) [5,6]. Specific categories and descriptions of radiographs that relate to silicosis are included in this ILO-UICC scheme, and films are reported using a standard nomenclature and form.

The information gathered from each element of the worker health screening effort must be collated into two types of reports: a summary report for each individual, and a comprehensive report of all workers surveyed. The individual report should list the name and demographic information, positive symptom responses, a summary of physical findings if an examination was performed, numerical data for pulmonary function with normative comparisons and interpretation, and a summary of the radiographic findings. Each worker should receive a copy of his or her report, perhaps in a simplified 'plain language' version. The comprehensive report for all workers should list statistical information about each group of data collected, and should include the proportion of workers falling into the abnormal range for each parameter. Ideally, the results of smokers and non-smokers should be compared; abnormalities in 'never-smokers' may be particularly hard to explain as due to causes other the work exposure. Worker groups with varying types of exposures within the industry should be compared if possible (e.g. grinders versus baggers). In rare instances, a 'control' group of non-exposed workers will be available for comparison from within or outside of the industry surveyed.

Carrying out industrial health screening as described above is time consuming, as each worker may need 1–3 hours or more to complete the survey process. Thus, industrial productivity may suffer as workers step away from their jobs for survey evaluation. The process can be costly, both in terms of the direct expenses for the medical tests and the wages (or time) lost from production. The time and expense must be balanced against the value of the information gained for each new testing element or questionnaire added to a survey.

Individual workers who report respiratory symptoms, demonstrate impaired pulmonary function, or show abnormal chest radiographs with patterns that suggest silicosis should be referred for individual health care evaluation to determine whether their lung disease is due to their current or previous occupational exposure, to cigarette smoking, or to some other cause or combination of causes. If they prove to have disease caused by silica, three actions seem appropriate: (1) they should be removed from any ongoing exposure; (2) they should be considered for worker compensation programs; and (3) their work environment should be surveyed carefully for air quality, safe work practices, and for other workers who may be impaired. The actions that might be taken based on the results of the survey of all workers are discussed below.

High risk

The identification of workers at high risk for silicosis could be based on either their job or their personal characteristics. The effects of genetic background on developing silicosis do not appear to be very great, although the issue has not been studied in detail. With high levels of exposure virtually all workers develop disease with similar features, as demonstrated by reports from Europe, the USA, South Africa, China, Southeast Asia, and Australia. It is possible that, with lower levels of exposure, individuals from one race or genetic background might be more susceptible to silicosis than another, but this difference has not been described. Thus one cannot identify workers at high risk based on their race or genetic background.

Cigarette smoking probably identifies workers at greater risk for industrial bronchitis and for lung cancer among those exposed to silica. Smoking does not appear to predict greater risk for radiographic silicosis. The presence of coexistent lung disease or other medical conditions could alter risk for silicosis

if the comorbid disease changes breathing patterns, lung clearance of inhaled particles, or other aspects of the body's response to silica. Caplan's syndrome in silica workers with rheumatoid arthritis may be an example of this phenomenon.

Workers at high risk can sometimes be identified based on their job within an industry. For example, custodial staff who sweep dust from the floor of a facility may have much greater exposure than production workers who use wet cutting or air-extraction devices at the point where dust is generated. Drillers at a mine face may experience much higher dust exposure than workers who transport the ore to the surface. The workers themselves often know who has the dustiest job. Individuals in these types of jobs should receive more frequent health screening and particular attention for education about safe work practices.

Workers at high risk can sometimes be identified by their personal work habits. The individuals who disregard safe work practices, who fail to wear mask respirators when specified, or who fail to adjust dust-extraction devices appropriately, are likely to be at excess risk of developing silicosis. This phenomenon may be demonstrated when the rare worker has obvious silicosis in an industry that passes all air quality surveys and has no other workers with mild or early disease. If an individual repeatedly ignores safe work practices despite education and warnings, there may be cause for dismissal.

PREVENTION

In the workplace

Hygiene surveys

Industrial hygiene surveys offer periodic assessment of the safety of a workplace in which airborne silica may be present. The survey should detect whether the conditions of the workplace meet air quality and industrial safety standards and whether optimum safe work practices are being followed.

Air quality is the key to workplace safety. Three aspects must be considered: the total quantity of dust per volume of air, the size distribution of the airborne particles, and the composition of the dust with regard to silica. The quantity may be determined in terms of the numbers of particles or their weight per unit volume of air (e.g. mppcf, millions of particles per cubic foot; mg/m³, milligrams of dust per cubic meter). Although large particles may be very visible in the air, it is the smaller particles that cause disease; particles with mass median aerodynamic diameters greater than approximately 5–10 µm do not reach the lower respiratory tract. The fraction of silica in the dust is a critical feature: sand used for glass manufacture or blasting may be virtually pure SiO_2; granite or mine rock may contain 10–25% silica, while coal may be 5–10% silica or less. Sampling and analytical techniques must address each of these aspects.

Sampling devices that collect and quantify airborne dust operate by entraining a high volume of air and trapping the particles on a filter or in a liquid, with or without selection of particles based on size. The air may be sampled at an open area within the workplace by a relatively large and complicated device (area sampler) or may be collected near the face of the worker by a device worn on the lapel (personal dust sampler). Area sampling is usually employed for regulatory purposes.

The first attempts to sample airborne dust and relate the results to health outcomes began in the 1920s. The Greenburg–Smith impinger, and its smaller field equivalent the 'midget impinger', were used from 1925 through the 1950s. These devices accelerated air through a nozzle into a liquid, and the number of particles in the liquid was then enumerated and expressed in terms of the volume of air entrained. The captured dust could be analyzed chemically for the silica fraction. Health effects and regulatory standards were expressed in terms of dust "millions of particles per cubic foot" (mppcf) of air. These devices did not discriminate particle size, thus large non-respirable particles were included in the count. Simple non-selective impingers are no longer in general use.

In the late 1960s sampling and regulatory standards began to be based on size-selective gravimetric techniques. The most widely used instrument is a cyclone device that operates at airflow rates of 1.7 or 2.0 liters/min, excludes particles larger than 10 μm, and captures the smaller particles on a 10-mm nylon membrane filter. The filter can then be weighed to express the airborne respirable particulates as mg/m^3, and the trapped mineral can be analyzed for silica content by X-ray diffraction, infrared analysis, or chemical methods. The results can then be expressed in terms of milligrams of respirable crystalline free silica per cubic meter of air.

Comprehensive industrial hygiene surveys should include multiple air samples taken when the work site is in full operation. Samples should be obtained at a variety of locations throughout the workplace and at several times throughout the working day or week. It is important to detect the problem sites with peak levels as well as the overall average air quality for the workplace. Regulatory standards (see below) are defined in terms of the average airborne dust concentration over a work day (8-hour time-weighted average) or the peak maximum exposure level. Different approaches might be taken depending on whether the purpose of the air quality sampling is to uncover the source of a known health problem or merely to meet the requirements of a scheduled survey. The topic is discussed further in Chapter 33.

Exposure control

A variety of measures to control and reduce silica exposure have been developed. Safe work practices with silica center on isolating workers from air with a high silica content, and on strategies for reducing the amount of respirable mineral in the air:

- Increase the airflow through the workplace.
- Replace dusty air with fresh air.
- Suppress dust by spraying water on the surface of rocks being drilled, cut, crushed, or polished.
- Position vacuum-hose air extractors at the point of contact between stone and tools.
- Substitute low-silica material (e.g. iron carbide) for high-silica material (e.g. sand) in abrasive blasting procedures (abrasive blasting can generate large amounts of airborne silica either from the abrasive, e.g. sand, or from the target material, e.g. a granite monument).

Several of these prevention approaches can be applied simultaneously in many workplaces. For example, in tunnels and mines efforts may include improved ventilation with outside air, filtration of recirculated air, and spraying water on drills and tunneling machines. In the granite industry the major problems occur in indoor sheds where the stone is cut and processed rather than in outdoor quarries. The air in the sheds is exchanged by large ceiling and window fans, sawing and polishing are done with water sprayed on the cutting surface to trap and wash away the dust particles, and vacuum-extractor hoses are positioned over power chisels and precision tools where cutting must be done dry. These combined measures have led to air quality within federal standards and a low-to-nil rate of detectable silicosis.

Strategies to isolate workers from high dust levels include containment booths, independent personal air sources, and various respiratory protective devices. For example, abrasive blasting to clean small items or to engrave stones can be performed in a sealed booth with workers outside using rubber gloves that extend into the booth. The highly contaminated air in the booth can be extracted and filtered directly to the outside of the building. Alternatively, independent personal air hoods cover the head and neck of the worker, and fresh air is pumped into the hood under positive pressure. Workers with independent air hoods can perform stationary tasks at sites with high ambient dust levels. Mask respirators are designed to fit closely over the nose and mouth, and to trap particles in high-efficiency filter cartridges as contaminated air is breathed in by the worker. A variety of federal guidelines specify the characteristics of these respirators, and the materials with which each may be used. Simple paper 'dust masks' are not sufficient to remove respirable silica particles from the air; they let in dust both through and around the mask.

These approaches to isolating the worker from contaminated air have many disadvantages compared to primarily cleaning the air or preventing the generation of airborne dust. The abrasive blasting booths may be difficult to work in, and a potential for air leakage occurs each time the booth is opened to exchange work pieces. The independent air source systems are cumbersome, heavy, and require connection to an outside or compressed air source. The personal respirator mask is close fitting and confining, making communication difficult; most workers find it hard to perform physically strenuous work that requires heavy breathing. These isolation strategies are quite suitable for tasks that do not require heavy exertion and only need be performed occasionally. It is very difficult for any worker to comply with scrupulous use of independent air sources or respirator masks all day, every day, week after week. Thus, these devices may fail in practice despite excellent operating characteristics in short-term use.

National regulatory strategies

Air quality standards for silica have been put forward by governmental, scientific, and advisory agencies in many countries. These standards attempt to define what is considered to be a reasonably safe level of airborne respirable silica particles, and thus both a goal for industries to strive for and a regulatory limit for governments to enforce. Although the absolute levels are generally similar, there are important disagreements about: (1) whether the same limits should be applicable in all industries; (2) whether the same levels that may be safe regarding silicosis are also safe with regards to COPD and lung cancer; and (3) whether the average level over a work week or transient peak levels are more important.

United States federal regulations were imposed for non-mining industrial workplaces under the authority of the Walsh–Healy Public Contracts Act of 1936. The initial regulations adopted in 1968–1970 by the Occupational Safety and Health Administration (OSHA) utilized the recommendations of the American Conference of Governmental Industrial Hygienists (ACGIH) [124], and defined the maximum permissible exposure limit (PEL) [125] as:

$$PEL = \frac{250}{\% \text{ quartz} + 5} \text{ mppcf}$$

or

$$PEL = \frac{10}{\% \text{ quartz} + 2} \text{ mg/m}^3$$

Thus, workers exposed to respirable size (<10 μm) stone dust particles composed of 25% quartz would have been considered safe at airborne total dust levels below 8.3 mppcf or 0.37 mg/m^3. In 1989 this standard was changed to define the limit solely in terms of the respirable crystalline free silica, and defined PELs of 0.1 mg/m^3 for α-quartz, and 0.05 mg/m^3 for cristobalite or tridymite. These values were calculated as a 'time-weighted average' (TWA) across an 8-hour work day. This rule was remanded by the US Circuit Court of Appeals in 1992, and the current standard has reverted to the equations listed above. The standard based on particle number is applied to marine industries. Similar but slightly different standards apply to coal mining, metal, and non-metal mining worksites. European and international regulatory and advisory groups have offered similar standards, and similar data to support them. The UK Health and Safety Executive (HSE) specifies a transient peak 'maximum exposure limit' (MEL) of 0.3 mg/m^3 [126].

There has been substantial controversy over whether the US quartz standard (0.1 mg/m^3) is adequate [61,127]. Graham and colleagues have presented extensive evidence from the Vermont granite industry showing dust levels at or below this level are not associated with clinical silicosis [90,128–130]. Other investigators have examined American miners [131–134], foundry workers [135], and other industries [136] and concluded that significant silicosis and an excess lung cancer risk may be occurring at levels of respirable silica between 0.05 mg/m^3 and 0.10 mg/m^3. The National Institute for Occupational Safety and Health (NIOSH) has recommended 0.05 mg/m^3 as the standard for quartz.

The air quality in a workplace may be tested voluntarily by management or may be examined by federal or state regulatory agencies. Government inspections may occur as part of a routine schedule of recurring evaluations, may be triggered by a complaint from workers, or may result from the detection of cases with potential occupational lung disease. The exact inspection process and level of detail may vary substantially depending on the industry, the inspecting agency, and whether it is routine or prompted by disease reports. If a significant deviation from the regulatory standards is detected, then remedial measures, fines, or even closure of the worksite may occur. Unfortunately, many potentially hazardous workplaces are never inspected. Both workers and employers may be poorly informed regarding the health hazards of silica and the effective measures that can be taken to reduce exposures and prevent disease.

While it may be debated whether the regulatory quartz standard is low enough, many industries and individual workers continue to be exposed to airborne silica at levels that are clearly above current standards and above safe limits. A composite estimate based on OSHA regulatory compliance inspections indicated that 1.3–1.9% of construction, foundry, and metal services workers were exposed to silica at 10 times the standard; 6% of stone industry workers were exposed to levels above the standard [136]. The problem is probably worst in small shops and businesses with few workers, scant resources for education, and at too small a scale to be a target for government inspections. The prevention of silicosis remains as much a problem of implementation and enforcement as of enlightened legislation.

DIFFICULT CASE

History

A 68-year-old man was referred for evaluation of progressive shortness of breath with exertion. He first noted slight dyspnea with intense effort about 5 years previously, with gradual worsening since that time. He began using home oxygen about 6 months prior to evaluation. He had no cough, no sputum production, and no wheezing. His past medical history was unremarkable, review of systems was negative except for right arm and shoulder arthritis, and his family history did not include any relatives with lung disease. He had smoked one pack of cigarettes per day from age 20 to 35, a total of 15 pack-years.

He had worked as a granite cutter in the Barre, Vermont, granite industry from age 22 until retirement at age 64, with total exposure for 42 years. He stated his retirement had not been prompted by respiratory symptoms, but because of soreness and numbness in his right arm ('cutters' hand') and his age. He had crafted, cut, and polished granite throughout his career, working in an indoor environment. He had worked in several different medium-sized sheds, some of which required respiratory protection. He believed that his industrial screening chest radiographs had been normal prior to retirement, and that he had tested negatively for tuberculosis.

He appeared lean, muscular, and healthy. There was a mild dorsal kyphosis, but full inspiration and normal percussive tone. High-pitched end-inspiratory crackles (fine rales) were heard over the lower half of both lung fields. No wheezing was evident. His cardiovascular examination was normal. His hands were large and roughened, with evidence of trauma and Heberden's nodes (osteoarthritis). He had prominent digital clubbing.

A conventional chest radiograph and subsequently an HRCT scan of the chest were obtained (Figs 7.5 and 7.6). Pulmonary function tests showed vital capacity and total lung capacity at the lower limits of normal, but with evidence from prior tests of a loss of 500 ml over 2 years. The FEV_1/FVC ratio was 121% of predicted. Gas transfer (D_LCO) was reduced to 33% of predicted. Hypoxia was evident at rest breathing room air, with PO_2 46 torr (6.1 kPa, O_2 saturation 86%).

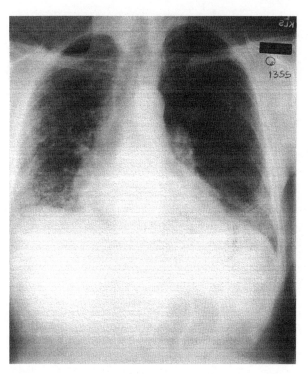

Fig. 7.5 Chest radiograph of Difficult Case, a 68-year-old granite cutter.

Issues

The chief issue here is whether this man's respiratory disease was fundamentally occupational in origin, and a consequence of his exposures to silica. If it was, what needs to be taken into account in assessing compensation; if not, what is the likely diagnosis, and what management should be offered?

Comment

The physical findings, the imaging investigations, and the lung function abnormalities (hypoxemia out of proportion to the restrictive impairment) all suggested diffuse interstitial

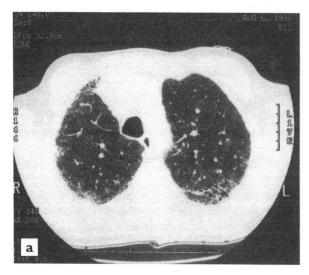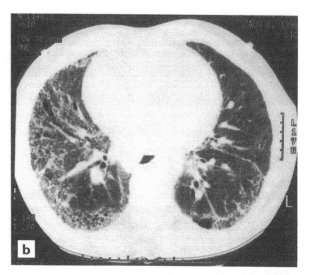

Fig. 7.6 High-resolution computed tomography (HRCT) scan of the Difficult Case, imaged through the upper lung zones (a) and through the lung bases (b).

lung disease, without evidence of airway obstruction. His respiratory disorder did not, therefore, appear to be related to smoking which he had given up long before.

The plain chest radiograph did not show rounded opacities, coalescent nodules, calcified nodules, hilar node enlargement, or nodal calcification and so was not typical of silicosis. The HRCT scan showed small irregular shadows throughout both lower lung zones, with a substantial degree of peripheral cystic formation (honeycomb changes), traction bronchiectasis, and sub-pleural fibrosis. These are the appearances of idiopathic pulmonary fibrosis (cryogenic fibrosing alveolitis), which was strongly suggested by the auscultatory crackles and the digital clubbing. A thoracoscopic lung biopsy was not considered necessary to confirm this diagnosis, but a possible future need for this was recognized.

The HRCT scan did, however, show a few small round calcified nodules (3–5 mm) in subpleural locations, and there was slight enlargement of several hilar and mediastinal lymph nodes with minor calcification. These additional findings are not specific, though are consistent with minimal simple nodular silicosis. Any contribution from silicosis to his respir-

atory disability was evidently negligible. The Barre, Vermont, granite industry has been surveyed frequently and studied in detail [128–130]. Virtually no cases of typical silicosis with disease of this magnitude had been found for more than 30 years, and none where exposure began after rigorous dust controls were instituted in the early 1940s.

He was offered anti-inflammatory/cytotoxic treatment for idiopathic pulmonary fibrosis, and selected azathioprine 125 mg per day and methylprednisolone 16 mg every other day. At reevaluation 4 months after beginning therapy, he reported a slight improvement in his exercise tolerance, and no adverse side-effects from his medications. After 1 year of therapy, he had noted definite improvement in effort-related dyspnea, and was working daily doing light carpentry in a family business. He continued to use oxygen at 3 litres/min for 24 hours/day, however, and serial measurements of lung function over the 20 months following treatment onset showed no clear evidence of improvement or deterioration. No adverse drug effects were noted.

This case illustrates that a suggestive occupational exposure history alone does not establish a diagnosis of

Table 7.3 Difficult case: pulmonary function tests

Time of observation	−24 months	Initial visit	Initial visit % pred	+4 months	+12 months	+20 months	+20 months % pred
FVC (L)	3.54	3.04	84 %	3.42	3.18	3.26	91 %
FEV$_1$(L)	2.99	2.54	101 %	2.67	2.51	2.62	106 %
FEV$_1$/FVC	0.85	0.84	121 %	0.78	0.79	0.8	117 %
TLC (L)	4.92	4.58	80 %	4.65	4.68	4.71	82 %
D$_L$CO (ml/min/mmHg)	10.80	7.92	33 %	8.49	7.74	8.13	34 %
pO$_2$ (rest, RA) (torr)		47				57	
O$_2$ saturation (rest, RA)		86%		92%	92%	89%	
Home O$_2$ therapy		3 L/min		3 L/min	3 L/min	3 L/min	
6 min walk distance				500 ft	560 ft	690 ft	
6 min walk O$_2$ Rx				5 L/min	5 L/min	3 L/min	

The data are presented as absolute values and, at two time points, as the percentage of age-height-related predicted values. L, liter; FVC, Forced Vital Capacity; FEV$_1$, Forced Expiratory Volume in 1 s; TLC, Total Lung Capacity; D$_L$CO, Diffusing Capacity for Carbon Monoxide (single breath); RA, room air.

occupational lung disease; the patient must have compatible clinical features as well. In this case all the clinical features pointed to a diagnosis of idiopathic pulmonary fibrosis rather than silicosis. Interstitial lung disease that is indistinguishable from idiopathic pulmonary fibrosis may complicate systemic sclerosis, and systemic sclerosis is occasionally a consequence of silica exposure. However, no evidence of scleroderma was ever noted in this patient. Some epidemiologic studies report a slightly increased odds ratio for prior work in dusty trades among patients with idiopathic pulmonary fibrosis compared to matched case controls [139–140].

SUMMARY POINTS

Recognition

- Exposure to respirable silicon dioxide (SiO_2) is associated with:
  - diffuse interstitial lung disease (silicosis)
  - industrial bronchitis and COPD
  - tuberculosis
  - lung cancer
  - scleroderma
- Silicosis is a chronic fibronodular diffuse interstitial lung disease caused by the inhalation of crystalline free silicon dioxide (SiO_2), occurring as α-quartz, cristobalite or tridymite.
  - Silicosis occurs in a wide variety of industries wherever sand or stone are cut, drilled, blasted, or added to other materials in such a way that very fine dust particles become airborne.
  - At risk are miners, drillers, foundry workers, stone cutters, abrasive blasters, metal workers, and many other groups
  - Silicosis requires prolonged exposure to airborne respirable particles of silica, and usually appears years after the exposure began.
  - The rapidity of development and the severity of silicosis are related directly to the intensity and duration of exposure.
- A diagnosis of silicosis is established by a compatible exposure history, typical radiographic findings, and the exclusion of other diseases that might cause similar abnormalities.
  - The chest radiograph and computed tomography scan show dense rounded opacities with upper lung zone predominance that may later coalesce

to form large conglomerate opacities, and enlargement of hilar and mediastinal lymph nodes often with (eggshell) calcification.
  - Pulmonary function testing shows a restrictive deficit, often with associated airflow obstruction.
  - Physical findings are few and non-specific.

Management

There is no specific treatment for this disease; the key to silicosis management is the prevention of exposure to high levels of airborne silica.

Prevention

- Workplace exposure to silica can be minimized by efficient air exchanges, vacuum extraction of air above cutting or drilling surfaces, spraying water on the contact surfaces of dust generation, and respiratory protective devices.
- Current or proposed air quality dust standards appear to be safe with regards to providing protection from classical silicosis in most industries.
  - The limits of respirable silica that provide safety from an excess risk of COPD and bronchogenic carcinoma, particularly in smokers, are not known.
  - Safe standards must be applied in developing nations, particularly through the production of inexpensive equipment for ventilation, air extraction, and the application of water to stone-cutting surfaces.
  - Vigorous application of the lessons learned over many centuries as well as new ideas and new technologies are needed to combat the lung diseases caused by silica.

REFERENCES

1. Mahler DA, Horowitz MB. Clinical evaluation of exertional dyspnea. *Clin Chest Med* 1994; 15: 259–269.
2. Eakin EG, Resnikoff PM, Prewitt LM *et al.* Validation of a new dyspnea measure: the UCSD Shortness of Breath Questionnaire. University of California, San Diego. *Chest* 1998; 113: 619–624.
3. Grant S, Aitchison T, Henderson E *et al.* A comparison of the reproducibility and the sensitivity to change of visual analogue scales, Borg scales, and Likert scales in normal subjects during submaximal exercise. *Chest* 1999; 116: 1208–1217.
4. Mahler DA, Harver A. Do you speak the language of dyspnea? *Chest* 2000; 117: 928–929.
5. The International Labor Office. Radiographs of the pneumoconioses – 1980. Washington, DC: ILO, 1980.
6. Classification of radiographs of the pneumoconioses. *Med Radiogr Photogr* 1981; 57: 1–17.
7. Begin R, Ostiguy G, Cantin A, Bergeron D. Lung function in silica-exposed workers. A relationship to disease severity assessed by CT scan. *Chest* 1988; 94: 539–545.
8. Doll NJ, Stankus RP, Hughes J *et al.* Immune complexes and autoantibodies in silicosis. *J Allergy Clin Immunol* 1981; 68: 281–285.
9. Karnik AB, Saiyed HN, Nigam SK. Humoral immunologic dysfunction in silicosis. *Indian Med Res Infect Dis* 1990; 92: 440–442.
10. Nagaoka T, Tabata M, Kobayashi K, Okada A. Studies on production of anticollagen antibodies in silicosis. *Environ Res* 1993; 60: 12–29.
11. Craighead JE, Kleinerman J, Abraham JL *et al.* Diseases associated with exposure to silica and nonfibrous silicate minerals. Silicosis and Silicate Disease Committee. *Arch Pathol Lab Med* 1988; 112: 673–720.

12. Brody AR, Roe MW, Evans JN, Davis GS. Deposition and translocation of inhaled silica in rats. Quantification of particle distribution, macrophage participation, and function. *Lab Invest* 1982; 47: 533–542.

13. Brody AR, Roe MW, Evans JN, Davis GS. Use of backscattered electron imaging to quantify the distribution of inhaled crystalline silica. *Scan Electron Microsc* 1980; 301–306.

14. Lapenas DJ, Davis GS, Gale PN, Brody AR. Mineral dusts as etiologic agents in pulmonary fibrosis: the diagnostic role of analytical scanning electron microscopy. *Am J Clin Pathol* 1982; 78: 701–706.

15. Christman JW, Emerson RJ, Hemenway DR et al. Effects of work exposure, retirement, and smoking on bronchoalveolar lavage measurements of lung dust in Vermont granite workers. *Am Rev Respir Dis* 1991; 144: 1307–1313.

16. Mossman BT, Churg A. Mechanisms in the pathogenesis of asbestosis and silicosis. *Am J Respir Crit Care Med* 1998; 157: 1666–1680.

17. Absher MP, Hemenway DR, Leslie KO et al. Intrathoracic distribution and transport of aerosolized silica in the rat. *Exp Lung Res* 1992; 18: 743–757.

18. Hemenway DR, Absher MP, Trombley L, Vacek PM. Comparative clearance of quartz and cristobalite from the lung. *Am Ind Hyg Assoc J* 1990; 51: 363–369.

19. Vacek PM, Hemenway DR, Absher MP, Goodwin GD. The translocation of inhaled silicon dioxide: an empirically derived compartmental model. *Fundam Appl Toxicol* 1991; 17: 614–626.

20. Fubini B, Giamello E, Volante M, Bolis V. Chemical functionalities at the silica surface determining its reactivity when inhaled. Formation and reactivity of surface radicals. *Toxicol Indust Health* 1990; 6: 571–598.

21. Fubini B, Bolis V, Cavenago A et al. Structural and induced heterogeneity at the surface of some SiO_2 polymorphs from the enthalpy of adsorption of various molecules. *Langmuir* 1993; 9: 2712–2720.

22. Christman JW, Emerson RJ, Graham WG, Davis GS. Mineral dust and cell recovery from the bronchoalveolar lavage of healthy Vermont granite workers. *Am Rev Respir Dis* 1985; 132: 393–399.

23. Driscoll KE, Lindenschmyd HRC, Maurer JK et al. Pulmonary response to silica or titanium dioxide: inflammatory cells, alveolar macrophage-derived cytokines, and histopathology. *Am J Respir Cell Mol Biol* 1990; 2: 381–390.

24. Piguet PF, Collart MA, Grau GE et al. Requirement of tumour necrosis factor for development of silica-induced pulmonary fibrosis. *Nature* 1990; 344: 245–247.

25. Mohr C, Gemsa D, Graebner C et al. Systemic macrophage stimulation in rats with silicosis: enhanced release of tumor necrosis factor-alpha from alveolar and peritoneal macrophages. *Am J Respir Cell Mol Biol* 1991; 5: 395–402.

26. Davis GS, Pfeiffer LM, Hemenway DR. Persistent over-expression of interleukin-1β and tumor necrosis factor-α in murine silicosis. *J Environ Pathol Toxicol Oncol* 1998; 17: 99–114.

27. Davis GS, Pfeiffer LM, Hemenway DR. Expansion of interferon-gamma-producing lung lymphocytes in mouse silicosis. *Am J Respir Cell Mol Biol* 1999; 20: 813–824.

28. Davis GS, Pfeiffer LM, Hemenway DR. Interferon-gamma production by specific lung lymphocyte phenotypes in silicosis in mice. *Am J Respir Cell Mol Biol* 2000; 22: 491–501.

29. Driscoll KE, Maurer JK, Lindenschmidt RC et al. Respiratory tract responses to dust: relationships between dust burden, lung injury, alveolar macrophage fibronectin release, and the development of pulmonary fibrosis. *Toxicol Appl Pharmacol* 1990; 106: 88–101.

30. Bauman MD, Jetten AM, Bonner JC et al. Secretion of a platelet-derived growth factor homologue by rat alveolar macrophages exposed to particulates in vitro. *Eur J Cell Biol* 1990; 51: 327–334.

31. Vanhee D, Gosset P, Wallaert B et al. Mechanisms of fibrosis in coal workers' pneumoconiosis. Increased production of platelet-derived growth factor, insulin-like growth factor type I, and transforming growth factor beta and relationship to disease severity. *Am J Respir Crit Care Med* 1994; 150: 1049–1055.

32. Liu JY, Morris GF, Lei WH et al. Rapid activation of PDGF-A and -B expression at sites of lung injury in asbestos-exposed rats. *Am J Respir Cell Mol Biol* 1997; 17: 129–140.

33. Williams AO, Flanders KC, Saffiotti U. Immunohistochemical localization of transforming growth factor-beta 1 in rats with experimental silicosis, alveolar type II hyperplasia, and lung cancer. *Am J Pathol* 1993; 142: 1831–1840.

34. Jagirdar J, Begin R, Dufresne A et al. Transforming growth factor-beta (TGF-beta) in silicosis. *Am J Respir Crit Care Med* 1996; 154: 1076–1081.

35. Ehrlich RI, Gerston KF, Lalloo UG. Accelerated silicosis in a foundry shotblaster. A case report. *S Afr Med J* 1988; 73: 128–130.

36. Seaton A, Legge JS, Henderson J, Kerr KM. Accelerated silicosis in Scottish stonemasons. *Lancet* 1991; 337: 341–344.

37. Banks DE, Morring KL, Boehlecke BA et al. Silicosis in silica flour workers. *Am Rev Respir Dis* 1981; 124: 445–450.

38. Chapman EM. Acute silicosis. *JAMA* 1932; 98: 1439–1441.

39. Buechner HA, Ansari A. Acute silicoproteinosis. *Dis Chest* 1969; 55: 174–177.

40. Suratt PM, Winn WC Jr, Brody AR et al. Acute silicosis in tombstone sandblasters. *Am Rev Respir Dis* 1977; 115: 521–529.

41. Dumontet C, Biron F, Vitrey D et al. Acute silicosis due to inhalation of a domestic product. *Am Rev Respir Dis* 1991; 143: 880–882.

42. Morgan WKC. Industrial bronchitis. *Br J Ind Med* 1978; 35: 285–291.

43. Ulmer WT. Chronic obstructive airway disease in pneumoconiosis in comparison to chronic obstructive airway disease in non-dust exposed workers. *Bull Physiopathol Respir (Nancy)* 1975; 11: 415–427.

44. Ulmer WT, Reichel G. Epidemiological problems of coal workers' bronchitis in comparison with the general population. *Ann NY Acad Sci* 1972; 200: 211–219.

45. Hnizdo E, Baskind E, Sluis-Cremer GK. Combined effect of silica dust exposure and tobacco smoking on the prevalence of respiratory impairments among gold miners. *Scand J Work Environ Health* 1990; 16: 411–422.

46. Holman CD, Psaila Savona P, Roberts M, McNulty JC. Determinants of chronic bronchitis and lung dysfunction in Western Australian gold miners. *Br J Ind Med* 1987; 44: 810–818.

47. Ng TP, Phoon WH, Lee HS *et al*. An epidemiological survey of respiratory morbidity among granite quarry workers in Singapore: chronic bronchitis and lung function impairment. *Ann Acad Med Singapore* 1992; 21: 312–317.

48. Rastogi SK, Gupta BN, Chandra H *et al*. A study of the prevalence of respiratory morbidity among agate workers. *Int Arch Occup Environ Health* 1991; 63: 21–26.

49. Oxman AD, Muir DC, Shannon HS *et al*. Occupational dust exposure and chronic obstructive pulmonary disease. A systematic overview of the evidence. *Am Rev Respir Dis* 1993; 148: 38–48.

50. Rosner D, Markowitz G. Consumption, silicosis, and the social construction of industrial disease. *Yale J Biol Med* 1991; 64: 481–498.

51. Snider DE. The relationship between tuberculosis and silicosis. *Am Rev Respir Dis* 1978; 118: 455–460.

52. Westerholm P, Ahlmark A, Maasing R, Segelberg I. Silicosis and risk of lung cancer or lung tuberculosis: a cohort study. *Environ Res* 1986; 41: 339–350.

53. Prowse K, Cavanagh P. Tuberculosis in the Potteries 1971–74. *Lancet* 1976; 2: 357–359.

54. van Sprundel MP. Pneumoconioses: the situation in developing countries. *Exp Lung Res* 1990; 16: 5–13.

55. Cowie RL. Silica-dust-exposed mine workers with scleroderma (systemic sclerosis). *Chest* 1987; 92: 260–262.

56. Cowie RL, Dansey RD. Features of systemic sclerosis (scleroderma) in South African goldminers. *S Afr Med J* 1990; 77: 400–402.

57. Haustein UF, Ziegler V, Herrmann K *et al*. Silica-induced scleroderma. *J Am Acad Dermatol* 1990; 22: 444–448.

58. Martin JR, Griffin M, Moore E *et al*. Systemic sclerosis (scleroderma) in two iron ore mines. *Occup Med (Lond.)* 1999; 49: 161–169.

59. Pelmear PI, Roos JO, Maehle WM. Occupationally-induced scleroderma. *J Occup Med* 1992; 34: 20–25.

60. Rustin MH, Bull HA, Ziegler V *et al*. Silica-associated systemic sclerosis is clinically, serologically and immunologically indistinguishable from idiopathic systemic sclerosis. *Br J Dermatol* 1990; 123: 725–734.

61. Beckett WC, Abraham JL, Becklake MR *et al*. Adverse effects of crystalline silica exposure. American Thoracic Society Statement. *Am J Respir Crit Care Med* 1997; 155: 761–765.

62. Klockars M, Koskela RS, Jarvinen E *et al*. Silica exposure and rheumatoid arthritis: a follow up study of granite workers 1940–81. *Br Med J (Clin Res Ed)* 1987; 294: 997–1000.

63. Rosenman KD, Zhu Z. Pneumoconiosis and associated medical conditions. *Am J Ind Med* 1995; 27: 107–113.

64. Rosenman KD, Moore-Fuller M, Reilly MJ. Connective tissue disease and silicosis. *Am J Ind Med* 1999; 35: 375–381.

65. Turner S, Cherry N. Rheumatoid arthritis in workers exposed to silica in the pottery industry. *Occup Environ Med* 2000; 57: 443–447.

66. Pairon JC, Brochard P, Jaurand MC, Bignon J. Silica and lung cancer: a controversial issue. *Eur Respir J* 1991; 4: 730–744.

67. Finkelstein MM. Silica, Silicosis, and lung cancer: a risk assessment. *Am J Ind Med* 2000; 38: 8–18.

68. International Agency for Research on Cancer. Silica and some silicates. *IARC Monogr Eval Carcinog Risk Chem Hum* 1987; 42: 39–143.

69. Donaldson K, Borm PJ. The quartz hazard: a variable entity. *Ann Occup Hyg* 1998; 42: 287–294.

70. Weill H, McDonald JC. Exposure to crystalline silica and risk of lung cancer: the epidemiological evidence. *Thorax* 1996; 51: 97–102.

71. McDonald C. Silica and lung cancer: hazard or risk. *Ann Occup Hyg* 2000; 44: 1–2.

72. Checkoway H, Franzblau A. Is silicosis required for silica-associated lung cancer? *Am J Ind Med* 2000; 37: 252–259.

73. Amandus HE, Shy C, Wing S *et al*. Silicosis and lung cancer in North Carolina dusty trades workers. *Am J Ind Med* 1991; 20: 57–70.

74. Amandus H, Costello J. Silicosis and lung cancer in US metal miners. *Arch Environ Health* 1991; 46: 82–89.

75. Hodgson JT, Jones RD. Mortality of a cohort of tin miners 1941–86 [published erratum appears in Br J Indust Med 1990; 47(12):846]. *Br J Ind Med* 1990; 47: 665–676.

76. Chen SY, Hayes RB, Liang SR *et al*. Mortality experience of haematite mine workers in China. *Br J Ind Med* 1990; 47: 175–181.

77. Chen J, McLaughlin JK, Zhang JY *et al*. Mortality among dust-exposed Chinese mine and pottery workers. *J Occup Med* 1992; 34: 311–316.

78. Hnizdo E, Sluis Cremer GK. Silica exposure, silicosis, and lung cancer: a mortality study of South African gold miners. *Br J Ind Med* 1991; 48: 53–60.

79. de Klerk NH, Musk AW. Silica, compensated silicosis, and lung cancer in Western Australian goldminers. *Occup Environ Med* 1998; 55: 243–248.

80. Cocco P, Rice CH, Chen JQ *et al*. Non-malignant respiratory diseases and lung cancer among Chinese workers exposed to silica. *J Occup Environ Med* 2000; 42: 639–644.

81. Carta P, Cocco PL, Casula D. Mortality from lung cancer among Sardinian patients with silicosis. *Br J Ind Med* 1991; 48: 122–129.

82. Chiyotani K, Saito K, Okubo T, Takahashi K. Lung cancer risk among pneumoconiosis patients in Japan, with special reference to silicotics. *IARC Sci Publ* 1990; 95–104.

83. Merlo F, Doria M, Fontana L *et al*. Mortality from specific causes among silicotic subjects: a historical prospective study. *IARC Sci Publ* 1990; 105–111.

84. Finkelstein M, Liss GM, Krammer F, Kusiak RA. Mortality among workers receiving compensation awards for silicosis in Ontario 1940–85. *Br J Ind Med* 1987; 44: 588–594.

85. Zambon P, Simonato L, Mastrangelo G *et al*. Mortality of workers compensated for silicosis during the period 1959–1963 in the Veneto region of Italy. *Scand J Work Environ Health* 1987; 13: 118–123.

86. Ng TP, Chan SL, Lee J. Mortality of a cohort of men in a silicosis register: further evidence of an association with lung cancer. *Am J Ind Med* 1990; 17: 163–171.

87. Bruske-Hohlfeld I, Mohner M, Pohlabeln H *et al*. Occupational lung cancer risk for men in Germany: results from a pooled case-control study. *Am J Epidemiol* 2000; 151: 384–395.

88. Finkelstein MM. Radiographic silicosis and lung cancer risk among workers in Ontario. *Am J Ind Medust* 1998; 34: 244–251.

89. de Klerk NH, Musk AW. Silica, compensated silicosis, and lung cancer in Western Australian goldminers. *Occup Environ Med* 1998; 55: 243–248.

90. Costello J, Graham WG. Vermont granite workers' mortality study. *Am J Ind Med* 1988; 13: 483–497.

91. Chia SE, Chia KS, Phoon WH, Lee HP. Silicosis and lung cancer among Chinese granite workers. *Scand J Work Environ Health* 1991; 17: 170–174.

92. Mehnert WH, Staneczek W, Mohner M *et al.* A mortality study of a cohort of slate quarry workers in the German Democratic Republic. *IARC Sci Publ* 1990; 55–64.

93. Checkoway H, Heyer NJ. Demers PA, Breslow NE. Mortality among workers in the diatomaceous earth industry. *Br J Ind Med* 1993; 50: 586–597.

94. Checkoway H, Hughes JM, Weill H *et al.* Crystalline silica exposure, radiological silicosis, and lung cancer mortality in diatomaceous earth industry workers. *Thorax* 1999; 54: 56–59.

95. Sherson D, Svane O, Lynge E. Cancer incidence among foundry workers in Denmark. *Arch Environ Health* 1991; 46: 75–81.

96. Tornling G, Hogstedt C, Westerholm P. Lung cancer incidence among Swedish ceramic workers with silicosis. *IARC Sci Publ* 1990; 113–119.

97. Meijers JM, Swaen GM, Slangen JJ. Mortality and lung cancer in ceramic workers in The Netherlands: preliminary results. *Am J Ind Med* 1996; 30: 26–30.

98. Cherry NM, Burgess GL, Turner S, McDonald JC. Crystalline silica and risk of lung cancer in the potteries. *Occup Environ Med* 1998; 55: 779–785.

99. Amandus HE, Castellan RM, Shy C *et al.* Reevaluation of silicosis and lung cancer in North Carolina dusty trades workers. *Am J Ind Med* 1992; 22: 147–153.

100. Lagorio S, Forastiere F, Michelozzi P *et al.* A case-referent study on lung cancer mortality among ceramic workers. *IARC Sci Publ* 1990; 21–28.

101. Hessel PA, Sluis Cremer GK, Hnizdo E. Silica exposure, silicosis, and lung cancer: a necropsy study. *Br J Ind Med* 1990; 47: 4–9.

102. Meijers JM, Swaen GM, van Vliet K, Borm PJ. Epidemiologic studies of inorganic dust-related lung diseases in The Netherlands. *Exp Lung Res* 1990; 16: 15–23.

103. Mastrangelo G, Zambon P, Simonato L, Rizzi P. A case-referent study investigating the relationship between exposure to silica dust and lung cancer. *Int Arch Occup Environ Health* 1988; 60: 299–302.

104. Lynge E, Kurppa K, Kristofersen L *et al.* Silica dust and lung cancer: results from the Nordic occupational mortality and cancer incidence registers. *J Natl Cancer Inst* 1986; 77: 883–889.

105. Amandus HE, Shy C, Castellan RM *et al.* Silicosis and lung cancer among workers in North Carolina dusty trades. *Scand J Work Environ Health* 1995; 21(suppl 2): 81–83.

106. Ulm K, Waschulzik B, Ehnes H *et al.* Silica dust and lung cancer in the German stone, quarrying, and ceramics industries: results of a case-control study. *Thorax* 1999; 54: 347–351.

107. Soutar CA, Robertson A, Miller BG *et al.* Epidemiological evidence on the carcinogenicity of silica: factors in scientific judgement. *Ann Occup Hyg* 2000; 44: 3–14.

108. Begin RO. Bronchoalveolar lavage in the pneumoconioses. Who needs it? *Chest* 1988; 94: 454–454.

109. Tan KX. Observation of the therapeutic effect of whole lung lavage on silicosis and other pneumoconiosis. *Chin J Ind Hyg Occup Med* 1990; 8: 220–222.

110. Banks DE, Cheng YH, Weber SL, Ma JK. Strategies for the treatment of pneumoconiosis. *Occup Med* 1993; 8: 205–232.

111. Kennedy MCS. Aluminium powder in the treatment of silicosis of pottery workers and pneumoconiosis of coal-miners. *Br J Ind Med* 1956; 13: 85–101.

112. Rifat SL, Eastwood MR, McLachlan DR, Corey PN. Effect of exposure of miners to aluminium powder. *Lancet* 1990; 336: 1162–1165.

113. Zou SQ, Liu H, Zhou YY *et al.* Preventive effect of aluminium citrate on silicosis. *Chin Med J (Eng)* 1990; 103: 173–176.

114. Begin R, Cantin A, Masse S *et al.* Aluminium inhalation in sheep silicosis. *Int J Exp Pathol* 1993; 74: 299–307.

115. Goodman GB, Kaplan PD, Stachura I *et al.* Acute silicosis responding to corticosteroid therapy. *Chest* 1992; 101: 366–370.

116. Sharma SK, Pande JN, Verma K. Effect of prednisolone treatment in chronic silicosis. *Am Rev Respir Dis* 1991; 143: 814–821.

117. Chen F, Sun S, Kuhn DC *et al.* Tetrandrine inhibits signal-induced NF-kappa B activation in rat alveolar macrophages. *Biochem Biophys Res Comm* 1997; 231: 99–102.

118. Chen F, Lu Y, Demers LM *et al.* Role of hydroxyl radical in silica-induced NF-kappa B activation in macrophages. *Ann Clin Lab Sci* 1998; 28: 1–13.

119. Dromer C, Velly JF, Jougon J *et al.* Long-term functional results after bilateral lung transplantation. Bordeaux Lung and Heart-Lung Transplant Group. *Ann Thorac Surg* 1993; 56: 68–73.

120. Roman A, Morell F, Astudillo J *et al.* Unilateral lung transplantation: the first 2 cases. Group of Lung Transplantation of the University General Hospital of the Vall d'Hebron. *Med Clin* 1993; 100: 380–383.

121. da Silva JP, Vila JH, Cascudo MM *et al.* The heart–lung transplant. Initial clinical experience. *Rev Port Cardiol* 1993; 12: 9, 51–55.

122. Lung Transplant Group. Single lung transplantation for end-stage silicosis: report of a case. *J Formos Med Assoc* 1992; 91: 926–932.

123. Metras D, Kreitmann B, Vaillant A *et al.* Heart and heart–lung transplantation 3 years' experience in Timone CHU (Marseilles 1985–1988). *Arch Mal Coeur Vaiss* 1990; 83: 209–215.

124. Documentation of the Threshold Limit Values and Biological Exposure Indices, 5 edn. Cincinnati, OH: American Conference of Government Industrial Hygienists, Inc., 1986.

125. Code of Federal Regulations. Labor. Title 29, Part 1000, 1989. 126.

126. Health and Safety Executive. *Respirable Crystalline Silica – Exposure Assessment Document.* Sudbury: HSE Books, 1999.

127. Markowitz G, Rosner D. The limits of thresholds: silica and the politics of science, 1935 to 1990. *Am J Public Health* 1995; 85: 253–262.

128. Graham WGB, O'Grady RV, Dubuc B. Pulmonary function loss in Vermont granite workers: a long-term follow-up and critical reappraisal. *Am Rev Respir Dis* 1981; 123: 26–28.

129. Graham WG, Ashikaga T, Hemenway D *et al.* Radiographic abnormalities in Vermont granite workers exposed to low levels of granite dust. *Chest* 1991; 100: 1507–1514.

130. Graham WG, Weaver S, Ashikaga T, O'Grady RV. Longitudinal pulmonary function losses in Vermont granite workers. A reevaluation. *Chest* 1994; 106: 125–130.

131. Villnave JM, Corn M, Francis M, Hall TA. Regulatory implications of airborne respirable free silica variability in underground coal mines. *Am Ind Hyg Ass J* 1991; 52: 107–112.

132. Kreiss K, Greenberg LM, Kogut SJ, *et al.* Hard-rock miming exposures affect smokers and nonsmokers differently. Results of a community prevalence study. *Am Rev Respir Dis* 1989; 139: 1487–1493.

133. Kreiss K, Zhen B. Risk of silicosis in a Colorado mining community. *Am J Ind Med* 1996; 30: 529–539.

134. Steenland K, Brown D. Silicosis among gold miners: exposure–response analyses and risk assessment. *Am J Public Health* 1995; 85: 1372–1377.

135. Rosenman KD, Reilly MJ, Rice C *et al.* Silicosis among foundry workers. Implication for the need to revise the OSHA standard. *Am J Epidemiol* 1996; 144: 890–900.

136. Linch KD, Miller WE, Althouse RB *et al.* Surveillance of respirable crystalline silica dust using OSHA compliance data (1979–1995). *Am J Ind Med* 1998; 34: 547–558.

137. Wilt JL, Banks DE, Weissman DN *et al.* Reduction of lung dust burden in pneumoconiosis by whole-lung lavage. *J Occupat Environ Med* 1996; 38: 619–624.

138. Liang WP, Sun Y, Chen CY. Clinical evaluation of massive whole lung lavage for treatment of coal workers pneumoconiosis. *He Bei: Liao Yang (J Hebei Convalescence)* 1992;1:1–9.

139. Hubbard R, Lewis S, Richards K, Johnston I, Britton J, Occupational exposure to metal or wood dust and aetiology of cryptogenic fibrosing alveolitis. *Lancet* 1996; 347: 284–289.

140. Baumgartner KB, Samet JM, Coultas DB, Stidley CA, Hunt WC, Colby TV *et al.* Occupational and environmental risk factors for idiopathic pulmonary fibrosis: a multicenter case-control study. Collaborating Centers. *Am J Epidemiol* 2000; 152: 307–315.

8 COAL WORKERS' PNEUMOCONIOSIS

Anne Brichet, Sophie Desurmont, and Benoit Wallaert

BACKGROUND

Definition

'Pneumoconiosis' is the term generally applied to interstitial disease of the lung resulting from chronic exposure to airborne mineral dust, its inhalation and deposition, and the tissue reaction of the host to its presence. Pneumoconiosis due to coal dust (and coal mine dust) is known as 'coal workers' pneumoconiosis' (CWP). It is one of three types of pneumoconiosis of major epidemiological importance, the other two being silicosis and asbestosis [1], which are described in Chapters 7 and 9, respectively. The pneumoconioses differ in a number of ways from the acute allergic and toxic interstitial diseases which are associated with exposure to organic dusts, principally because of their long latency periods (usually 10–20 years or more) between exposure onset and disease recognition.

Pneumoconiosis is generally first recognized from the plain chest radiograph, which is critical also in evaluating disease progression. The radiographic appearances are most usefully described by the coding system devised for standard films of pneumoconiosis under the auspices of the International Labour Office (ILO). In brief, small opacities (i.e. those <10 mm in diameter) within the lung fields are defined by their average shape, size, and profusion:

- Rounded (nodular)   *p*   for diameters ≤ 1.5 mm
           q   for diameters 1.5–3 mm
           r   for diameters 3–10 mm
- Irregular (reticular)   *s*   if fine
           t   if medium
           u   if coarse.

Profusion of these opacities is scored in four major categories defined by the standard films (0–3):

- Category 0   Small opacities absent or less profuse than in category 1
- Category 1   Small opacities present but few in number
- Category 2   Small opacities numerous
- Category 3   Small opacities very numerous and obscure the normal radiographic markings.

Each major category may be divided further into three minor categories, providing a range of 12 profusion subgroups, though readings at this level are associated with a good deal of interreader variability. Conglomeration, or coalescence, of these opacities to produce one or more opacities with diameters greater than 10 mm, defines a 'large' pneumoconiotic opacity and this in turn defines 'complicated' pneumoconiosis. If there is no such conglomeration, the pneumoconiosis is said to be 'simple' or 'uncomplicated'. Large shadows represent fibrotic conglomeration of smaller fibrotic lesions. A more detailed description of the appearances from imaging techniques is given in Chapter 31 along with details of the subclassification of large pneumoconiotic (A, B, C) shadows.

In clinical practice, simple CWP is characterized by small rounded opacities (micronodules) rather than small irregular opacities, though the latter may be seen in much lesser profusion. In some coal-mining communities, particularly among more distant generations, large opacities occurred quite frequently, and the term 'progressive massive fibrosis' (PMF) was in common use.

Nature of coal

Coal is not a mineral of uniform composition. Its nature and its potential to cause pneumoconiosis vary widely from mine to mine, and from coalfield to coalfield. It is graded by rank, which reflects its carbon content and thus combustibility, and may contain hazardous impurities, especially silica. Anthracite is coal of the highest rank, with a carbon content around 98%. Lower ranked coals, bituminous and subbituminous (i.e. softer coals), have carbon contents of 90–95%. The rank of coal has an influence on the risk of both simple and complicated CWP: the higher the rank, the greater the risk [2]. Thus, exposure–response relationships vary with coal rank, and there is an additional influence from the length of time the dust has been in the lung [3,4].

Silica contamination increases the pneumoconiosis risk meaningfully and, if this is in the form of quartz at a concentration of 15% or more, there is a high risk of rapidly progressive pneumoconiosis simulating silicosis itself. Local geographic variation consequently exerts considerable influence, and the risk of pneumoconiosis is particularly increased when coal seams are thin and separated by silica-containing rock [5]. Pneumoconiosis in some coal miners may consequently represent a mixed picture of CWP and silicosis.

Pneumoconiosis does, nevertheless, occur when coal dust exposure is encountered without any silica contamination, and it is clear that coal dust itself poses a significant hazard. Overall, coal rank and the degree of silica contamination are probably the principal factors that account for observed variability in risk between one coal mine and another.

Exposure sources

The underground miner, and especially the face worker, roof bolter, or tunnel driller, encounter the most obvious risk of inhaling hazardous amounts of dust, depending on how effective is the mine's ventilation and its method of dust suppression. A less obvious risk comes from the use of sand on rail tracks in some mines to increase friction and wheel-holding. This may be crushed to produce respirable silica, and silica may have contaminated the dusts that have been used in some mines to suppress the risk of fire or explosion.

In open-cast coal mines, dust levels rarely approach those in the confined environments of underground mines. However, drill operators and laborers who are not protected by working in enclosed machine cabins may nevertheless be exposed to high levels. In previous generations coal 'trimmers' in ships faced similar risks. They worked in the confined environment of the hold to distribute coal so that the ship was properly balanced and fit to set sail. Once coal has been burned in power stations, the residual dust (known as 'fly ash'), has a variable composition depending on the combustion process, the coal source, and the fly ash precipitation technique. Experimental studies suggest that fly ash has much lower toxicity with respect to inflammatory potential and fibrogenicity compared to coal mine dust or silica [6].

Epidemiology

CWP was first recognized in Scottish miners in 1830 [7]. For a long time, the pneumoconiosis of coal miners was thought to be silicosis. Hart and Aslett then proved that it could arise in coal miners exposed only to washed coal which was free of silica [8]. In 1936, the British Medical Research Council recognized the seriousness of CWP and established its Pneumoconiosis Research Unit. The Unit began an extensive epidemiological program in 1950 with the British National Coal Board, which is known as its Pneumoconiosis Field Research [9]. In parallel, considerable attention was given to coal miners' respiratory diseases in the USA, beginning with a pilot prevalence study of CWP conducted from 1962 to 1963 [10]. These and other studies led to important advances in measuring personal levels of exposure to respirable dust and in understanding the principles of dust control. These in turn helped clarify the nature of CWP [11].

Although mortality statistics for coal miners during the first half of the 20th century suggested a greater risk of premature death in coal miners than non-miners, much of this was a consequence of accidents, and less privileged living standards. Studies over the second half of the century have indicated no difference in mortality from the general population, though moderate differences remain between white collar and blue collar workers [12–14]. Since standardized mortality ratios (SMRs) for lung cancer and heart disease tend to be less for coal miners than the populations from which they arise because of a lesser consumption of tobacco, there may still be a minor occupational survival disadvantage resulting from non-malignant respiratory disease. This cannot be attributed to simple pneumoconiosis; it appears to be chiefly a consequence of airway disease, though complicated pneumoconiosis of advanced degree (now very rare) plays some role, since a raised SMR for this has been a consistent observation. Even so, mean life expectancy for coal miners with complicated pneumoconiosis extends into the eighth decade.

In recent decades the incidence of CWP has been declining in industrial countries owing to improved dust controls, though increased mechanization in the mid-1960s led in some to a temporary increase in dust levels. In parallel, through the period 1950–1980, the annual UK rate for the recognition of CWP for state compensation in current and retired miners decreased from about 7% to 1–2%. The overall prevalence of CWP, which reflects more distant exposure and earlier incidence, declined from about 13% to 5%, but there were substantial regional differences. Similar regional differences and similar declines have been noted in the USA and other countries. A prevalence study conducted from 1969 to 1971 showed that 46% of American coal miners in eastern states had simple CWP and 14% PMF [15]. By contrast in western miners, who worked a lower rank coal often from surface mines, 4.6% had simple CWP and none had PMF. By the late 1970s, the overall prevalence of CWP was estimated to be about 10% in the USA, and that of complicated CWP no more than 0.5%.

Prognosis

Simple CWP is not associated with premature mortality, but approximately 4% of deaths in coal miners are directly due to complicated pneumoconiosis [2,12]. Among 346 South Wales miners and ex-miners with category B or C complicated CWP, death was attributed to the pneumoconiosis in about one-third of cases [13]. In categories 1, 2, and 3 of simple CWP and category A of complicated CWP, life expectancy is the same as that among the general population without pneumoconiosis [14]. The rate of progression to PMF appears to be influenced chiefly by the age at which the miner begins

to show radiographic changes of CWP, the earlier the diagnosis, the more likely is there to be progression [16]. This in turn is likely to reflect individual susceptibility and the level of cumulative exposure [17].

RECOGNITION

Clinical features

Simple CWP and category A complicated CWP are not associated with respiratory symptoms. As in most populations engaged in manual work, breathlessness and cough in coal miners are usually a consequence of cigarette smoking. Coal miners, however, typically smoke less than other manual workers, yet show a greater prevalence of chronic productive cough irrespective of pneumoconiosis, and it has become clear that coal mine dust may itself cause chronic bronchitis and chronic obstructive pulmonary disease (COPD). This is discussed more fully in Chapter 5.

By contrast, complicated pneumoconiosis (PMF) at categories B and C may present with undue breathlessness and productive cough, the sputum being mucoid, mucopurulent, or discolored as if mixed with black ink (melanoptysis). This is the result of necrosis within the conglomerate, coal-containing lesions that characterize PMF. Progressive undue exertional dyspnea is usually the dominant symptom, but rarely there may be breathlessness at rest [2,18,19].

There are no specific abnormal physical signs in CWP, but when complicated CWP is very advanced, the signs of emphysema or fibrotic lobar shrinkage may be detected. Finger clubbing and fine inspiratory crackles are not features of the disease and, if these are present, another explanation should be sought [2,18–20]. Only in a small proportion of severe cases of complicated disease does CWP evolve to produce chronic respiratory failure and pulmonary heart disease (cor pulmonale). When this does occur, extensive and multifocal conglomerate lesions are to be expected, generally with emphysema and concomitant disabling chronic airway obstruction. Bronchopneumonia commonly follows [1].

Associated disorders

Irrespective of PMF, there are a number of other disorders with which CWP may be associated – most notably the autoimmune disorders rheumatoid disease and progressive systemic sclerosis. The latter, however, is more clearly associated with silicosis, and it is not clear whether it occurs with greater incidence than expected when there is occupational exposure to coal alone.

Caplan's syndrome

The association of pulmonary rheumatoid nodules with CWP is known as Caplan's syndrome [21]. The diagnosis is suggested by the association of coal dust exposure, rheumatoid arthritis, and multiple, well-defined, large, rounded opacities (nodules with diameter >10 mm) on the chest radiograph. Caplan *et al.* [21] showed that most subjects with these features have rheumatoid factor in the serum. Radiographically, the nodules may appear calcified or cavitary, and the differential diagnosis from tuberculosis can be difficult. The nodules are typically circular, 0.5–5 cm in diameter, and smooth in outline, though rarely completely homogeneous. Spontaneous disappearance is common, with or without initial cavitation, and new nodules commonly emerge in different locations. If the nodules become superimposed, suggesting conglomerate masses, PMF may be simulated, but often the radiological appearances of simple CWP are absent and there is a need to consider the possibility of primary lung tumor.

In some cases, the appearances of simple CWP or PMF have been present for years when additional changes develop in relation to the development of rheumatoid arthritis. There is no evident relationship between the severity of the rheumatoid disease and the extent of Caplan's syndrome. It is difficult to assess its prevalence because it is rare and there are difficulties in recognizing it. Pathologically, the Caplan (or rheumatoid) nodule is generally larger than the nodule of complicated CWP, smoother in outline, and distributed at random within the lung fields. Large opacities of complicated CWP more characteristically affect the upper zones. The Caplan nodule is also more likely to cavitate, thereby producing a concentric ring pattern, and so is also known as a necrobiotic nodule. Central necrosis is rare in nodules of CWP, though it may occur in conglomerate lesions. When it does the affected subject may expectorate coal-discolored sputum, so that 'melanoptysis' is produced.

Infections

CWP has also been linked with a number of specific infections, the most prominent of which historically has been tuberculosis. A prospective study of 53 753 coal miners in Spain during the period 1971 to 1985 showed an incidence of about 150 cases per 100 000 miners per year of confirmed pulmonary tuberculosis. The risk was three times greater than that for the general population of the same area [22]. Une and colleagues similarly found a high annual incidence of tuberculosis (81.6 per 100 000/year) in a coal mining district of Japan. The incidence was 58.1 in the surrounding region, and 46 throughout Japan [23]. In contrast to silicosis, however, CWP does not increase significantly the risk for infection with

Mycobacterium tuberculosis [18]. The association observed with coal mining (and hence CWP) in some countries appears to have been a consequence only of close contact during long hours of work in the confined mine environment.

Non-tuberculous mycobacteria, on the other hand, may infect lungs damaged by CWP and other types of pneumoconiosis with greater than usual frequency, and so CWP does appear to increase the risk for infection with opportunistic organisms. *M. avium* is probably the most important of these and is poorly sensitive to antibiotic agents. *M. kansasii* and *M. malmoense* may also be pathogenic in this setting, though are more readily eradicated with antimycobacterial agents. The development of mycobacterial infection in a patient with CWP may be symptomless, at least in its early course, and it may be difficult or impossible to distinguish radiographic evidence of it from PMF lesions, since both characteristically begin in the apices. It may similarly be difficult to attribute change in the radiographic appearances to advancing infection or progressive PMF. Experimental studies additionally suggest that mycobacterial infection is a factor which helps explain the progression from simple to complicated peumoconiosis [24,25].

Other opportunistic infections reported in association with CWP have included nocardiosis, sporotrichosis, and cryptococcosis; and *Aspergillus* species have been noted to colonize cavities in conglomerate lesions of complicated CWP [26].

Emphysema and bronchitis

A further association with complicated CWP, if manifested by bullous emphysema, is spontaneous pneumothorax, though this is not likely to occur with excess incidence in simple pneumoconiosis [1]. The advanced stages of complicated CWP are additionally associated with recurrent episodes of acute and subacute bronchitis, as well as a regular productive cough. Persistent productive cough is common in coal miners in the absence of CWP, however, as is airway obstruction, though both owe more to cigarette smoking than coal mine dust exposure. There is no evidence of a causal relationship between CWP and carcinoma of the lung, though there is strengthening evidence linking silica exposure with lung cancer (see Chapter 20) [27,28]. In practice coal miners smoke less heavily than other manual workers, as we have noted above, and lung cancer rates are diminished as a result.

Investigation

Lung function

Simple CWP and category A complicated CWP have no important effect on spirometric measures, when prior dust exposure and smoking habit are taken into account [29,30]. Thus, for the same degree of exposure or pack-year consumption, spirometry is not meaningfully diminished by CWP of categories 1–3 or A compared with category 0. However, working coal miners without complicated CWP of categories B or C tend to have minimally reduced spirometric values compared with non-exposed controls, probably because of coal dust-induced COPD [31]. Healthy worker selection bias might, of course, be expected to produce rather better results from spirometry among coal miners at the time of recruitment compared with control groups since coal mining requires more than average physical fitness, and survival bias might further mask any adverse occupational effect of coal mining work if investigators examine only miners who remain sufficiently fit to continue working.

Several studies have shown more subtle abnormalities of lung function in relation to the radiographic appearances, there being a mildly lower diffusing capacity (gas transfer) in association with p shadows than with q or r shadows [32]. Furthermore, the arterial oxygen tension may be slightly reduced at rest in simple CWP, especially in category p cases, though this tends to correct on effort and the abnormalities are minimal in miners who have never smoked [32]. This difference may be a consequence of a higher dust content within the lungs with p compared to q or r opacities.

In complicated CWP of categories B and C, lung function depends on the extend of the conglomerate lesions and the degree of associated emphysema. Studies of lung function in the more advanced stages of PMF have shown a mixed obstructive and restrictive pattern, with reduction in compliance and diffusing capacity if the effect of emphysema dominates [30]. This is usually the case, especially if the affected miner is a smoker. Ultimately, respiratory failure may occur. As with the probability of radiographic progression, ongoing change in pulmonary function in miners with CWP is most likely to occur in those who have had the most intense exposure to dust. The assessment of lung function is addressed more fully in Chapter 32.

Imaging

The radiographic pattern of simple CWP is typically one of small rounded opacities which appear first in the upper zones. The middle and lower zones become involved as the number of opacities increases. The nodules increase in profusion with increasing dust exposure, but a change in profusion after dust exposure has ceased is very unusual [6,19,33,34]. Calcification of the nodules may occur in 10–20% of cases.

Complicated pneumoconiosis is defined as a lesion of 1 cm or greater in longest diameter. Complicated

pneumoconiosis (PMF) is divided into categories A, B, and C based on the size of the large opacities:

- Category A   Greatest diameter ≥1 cm and <5 cm, or several opacities each greater than 1 cm, the sum of which <5 cm
- Category B   One or more opacities the diameter sum of which exceeds that of category A, but the area of which does not exceed that of the right upper lobe
- Category C   One or more opacities the area of which exceeds that of the right upper lobe.

The large opacities are usually predominant in the upper lobes, may be uni- or bilateral, and are symmetrically or asymmetrically distributed. The pattern of change in size is variable and unpredictable. Most PMF occurs on a background of simple pneumoconiosis, but this is not invariably so, and it may occur after dust exposure has ceased. Cavitation can develop within a PMF lesion, and occasionally there is a dense peripheral arc or rim at its lower pole which represents calcification. Dense calcification with the lesion is also seen sometimes. PMF is often associated with bullous emphysema [35] and fibrotic scarring leading to distortion of the lung, and shift of the trachea and mediastinum to the affected side [1]. Irregular, mainly basal, opacities may also be seen on standard radiographs. Cockroft [36] reported that they are associated pathologically with emphysema and to a lesser degree with diffuse interstitial fibrosis, though often both are present in combination. PMF can pose diagnostic difficulties. Large nodular opacities can be rheumatoid nodules of Caplan's syndrome, and lung cancer must be kept in mind [1]. 'Eggshell' calcification is uncommon in CWP but may occur in intrapulmonary, hilar, or mediastinal lymph nodes, possibly because of concomitant exposure to silica.

Pleural effusion is uncommon in CWP. Its presence may be related to an associated infection or an interaction with a systemic collagen vascular disease such as rheumatoid arthritis or progressive systemic sclerosis. More commonly it is unrelated.

In simple CWP, computed tomography (CT) shows parenchymal lesions which can be detected in miners with normal chest radiographs. There is thus greater sensitivity compared with plain radiographs in detecting simple CWP, but less obvious benefit for complicated pneumoconiosis [33]. There is a posterior and right-sided predominance in the upper zones; in miners with more severe involvement, micronodules are diffusely distributed through the lungs. Detection is dramatically influenced by CT technique, and a 10-mm collimation is considered best. Micronodules have been detected in the subpleural areas of 87% of coal miners with radiographic evidence of CWP (Fig. 8.1). Coalescence of these produces 'pseudoplaques'. However, isolated subpleural micronodules cannot be considered as an early sign of CWP because they may be observed among smokers and ex-smokers without coal mine dust exposure.

Large nodules are usually observed against a background of parenchymal micronodules and are generally associated with subpleural micronodules [37]. Two categories of lesions can be observed in PMF: lesions with irregular borders that are associated with disruption of the pulmonary parenchyma and lead to typical scar emphysema (Fig. 8.2), and lesions with regular borders that are unassociated with scar

emphysema [35]. When the lesions are larger than 4 cm in diameter, irregular areas of aseptic necrosis can be observed with or without cavitation (Fig. 8.3).

Computed tomography, particularly high-resolution images, may additionally distinguish other pathological processes whether they are related to CWP or not. Focal lung emphysema indicates distension of the bronchioles in association with macules and is considered an integral part of the lesions of CWP. Bullous changes around PMF lesions are referred to as paracicatricial or scar emphysema; non-bullous emphysematous lesions are defined as irregular emphysema [37] (Fig. 8.4). Lesions of diffuse pulmonary fibrosis can be detected on high-resolution CT as honeycombing or areas of ground-glass attenuation (Fig. 8.5). Two specific etiologies of fibrosis in coal miners should be considered: a direct effect of deposited coal or silica particles, or an indirect effect due to an association with scleroderma. It is impossible to distinguish lung fibrosis attributable to occupational ex-

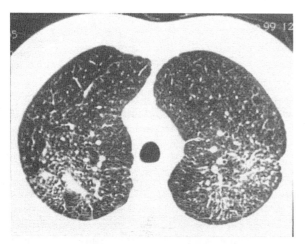

Fig. 8.1 High-resolution computed tomography (HRCT) scan obtained at the level of the upper lobes showing micronodules and nodules with a posterior predominance, and subpleural nodules.

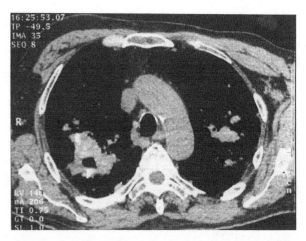

Fig. 8.3 CT scan showing conglomerate (PMF) shadows with necrosis and calcification.

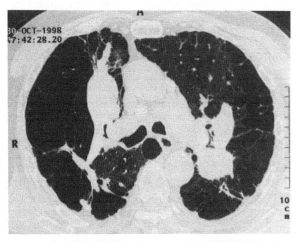

Fig. 8.2 HRCT scan showing bilateral masses consistent with progressive massive fibrosis. There is a background of micronodules associated with bullous changes around PMF lesions referred to as paracicatricial emphysema. There are calcified mediastinal lymph nodes.

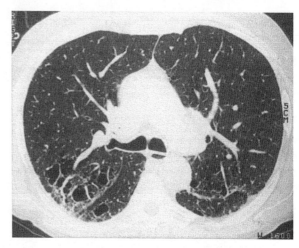

Fig. 8.4 HRCT scan showing small bullae and areas of low attenuation, without PMF lesions, defined as non-paracicatricial emphysema.

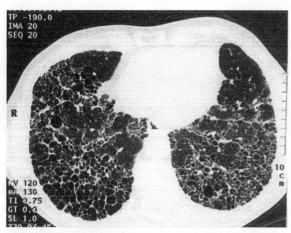

Fig. 8.5 HRCT scan obtained at the level of the lower lobes in a coal miner. It shows a bilateral microcystic honeycomb pattern, which is characteristic of scleroderma though may be observed in coal miners in northern France without scleroderma.

posure from fibrosis of non-occupational origin on the basis of CT appearances [37]. Eggshell calcification of hilar and mediastinal lymph nodes is an uncommon feature of CWP but may occur, as may punctuate or massive calcification of lymph nodes. Nodal enlargement can occur in all mediastinal sites [37].

Serological and immunological features

There are no specific biological markers of CWP. The blood differential cell count is normal, there is no systemic inflammatory response, and neither renal or hepatic function is modified.

A number of immunologic abnormalities are, however, well described in association with CWP. Lippmann and colleagues reported circulating antinuclear antibodies (ANA) among 34% of coal miners with radiographic opacities of pneumoconiosis, with a higher prevalence in anthracite miners (55%) compared with bituminous miners (21%) [38]. A lower overall prevalence was reported by Soutar and colleagues (17%), who showed that the prevalence was greater in PMF (27%) compared with simple CWP (9%) [39]. Rheumatoid factor has been observed in 4–10% of coal miners with radiographic opacities of pneumoconiosis [38,39]. Miners with CWP additionally have significantly raised levels of serum immunoglobulins IgA and IgG compared to nonminers [40,41]. Increased serum angiotensin-converting enzyme level has been observed in coal miners, whatever the classification of pneumoconiosis [42]. These immunologic features have no clinical significance and no diagnostic value in the absence of Caplan's syndrome. Constitutional differences may explain the variations in response to inhaled dust.

Bronchoalveolar lavage

The results of studies of bronchoalveolar lavage (BAL) in CWP have provoked controversy. While two

studies have demonstrated similar total and differential cell counts in miners compared with control subjects, and similar oxygen radical release, a third has shown a significant increase in cell numbers [1,43,44]. The latter was most marked in miners with PMF, and was evident after making allowances for smoking habits. There was no change in differential cell count, in contrast to a number of other interstitial disorders of the lung (e.g. sarcoidosis, chronic idiopathic interstitial pneumonia, hypersensitivity pneumonitis) in which an abnormal percentage of lymphocytes and/or neutrophils is usually present. Alveolar inflammatory cells from patients with simple CWP released spontaneously more superoxide anions than did those from control subjects [44]. Superoxide release by alveolar inflammatory cells from patients with PMF was dramatically increased when compared with both control subjects and miners with simple CWP, and, among the nonsmokers, those with PMF demonstrated significantly lower values of lung volumes and diffusing capacity than did those with simple pneumoconiosis. However, no correlation was found between these cellular characteristics of BAL and the pulmonary function abnormalities [44]. Superoxide and/or products of superoxide are capable of destroying many elements of the alveolar structure, and so this study supports the view that the alveolar macrophages may be responsible, at least in part, for lung injury in PMF by releasing increased amounts of superoxide anion.

Biopsy and histopathology

Surgical biopsy is very rarely required in the investigation of CWP, and most of the histological features have been learned from autopsy examinations. However, biopsy material (whether surgical, transbronchial, or from percutaneous fine needle aspiration) may be needed in special circumstances; for example, when there is uncertainty over the nature of conglomerate lesions in PMF (is lung cancer present?) or the nodular lesions in simple CWP (is disseminated mycobacterial infection or Kaposi's sarcoma present in a coal miner with AIDS?).

Radiographic simple CWP correlates with the presence of small (less than 1 cm) macular and nodular lesions on pathologic examination, whereas lesions larger than 1 cm on either radiographic or pathologic examination constitute complicated CWP, as has been described. The latter can include, in cases with Caplan's syndrome, pulmonary rheumatoid nodules [45,46].

On gross examination the pleural surfaces in patients with coal-dust exposure show an irregular pattern of bluish black pigmentation, often outlining the pleural lymphatics when dust exposure is fairly mild, but sometimes completely blackening the pleura when exposure has been heavy. CWP is not usually associated with pleural thickening unless subpleural nodules or PMF is present. Intrapulmonary, hilar, and mediastinal lymph nodes are typically enlarged, black, and firm; microscopically they contain large numbers of pigmented histiocytes. Collagenous nodules identical to silicotic nodules are common in the lymph nodes in coal workers, but should not be diagnosed as silicosis.

In simple CWP the cut sections of the lung show black pigmentation in the centers of the lobules, often associated with mild emphysema. These lesions constitute the coal macule with associated focal emphysema. In theory coal macules are nonfibrotic and not palpable, but in practice may be quite fibrotic. Microscopically, the macule is composed of macrophages laden with coal dust within the walls of the respiratory bronchioles and adjacent alveoli. Focal emphysema resembles a mild form of cigarette smoke-induced centrilobular emphysema. In the US National Coal Workers Autopsy Study, roughly 45% of the cases had only macules, and 35% had both macules and focal emphysema [45]. Further features of simple CWP are the coal nodules. These are rounded lesions with collagenous centers and a rim of dust and macrophages. They represent a form of mixed dust fibrosis (i.e. coal dust plus silica exposure). Nodules are usually found in association with macules, and in some instances may develop from preexisting macules.

PMF (complicated CWP) almost invariably occurs in workers who have simple CWP, more commonly nodules rather than just macules; there is some morphologic evidence that CWP develops by fusion of smaller coal nodules. PMF lesions appear as black fibrotic masses that may be round, oval, or irregular in shape and are usually bilateral. They are sharply separated from the surrounding lung. More than one nodule may be present in a lung (i.e. 'satellite nodules'). PMF lesions transgress normal anatomic boundaries and in doing so obliterate fissures, bronchi, and vessels, all of which end up trapped in a mass of dust and fibrous tissue. At the microscopic level PMF lesions show bundles of haphazardly arranged hyalinized collagen fibers and/or reticulin fibers and coal dust. Necrosis of PMF lesions is common, and may be manifested clinically by the sudden expectoration of thick black material. A giant cell reaction may be seen in association with the necrotic collagen. Caplan nodules differ morphologically from ordinary PMF lesions: they are typically rounded, may be multiple, and histologically show a necrotic center with a peripheral palisade of histiocytes and giant cells. They are not distinguishable pathologically from necrobiotic nodules of rheumatoid disease unassociated with coal-dust exposure, and may be difficult to separate morphologically from tuberculous granulomas.

Pathogenesis

The pathogenesis of pneumoconiosis is similar to that of all interstitial lung diseases. There is a chronic inflammatory state (alveolitis) in which inflammatory cells are activated and damage the pulmonary architecture. This produces fibrotic scarring. Inorganic particles are phagocytosed by alveolar macrophages, causing activation and the release inflammatory mediators such as cytokines [47] and arachidonic acid metabolites [48]. The mediators in turn induce the recruitment of other inflammatory cells within the alveolar wall and on the alveolar epithelial surface. The alveolitis is dominated by alveolar macrophages [49]. Toxic oxygen derivatives and proteolytic enzymes are released by the inflammatory cells, which cause cellular damage and disruption of the extracellular matrix [50]. Prominent among these proteolyic enzymes are matrix metalloproteinases, elastase, and proteolytic enzymes directed against extracellular matrix components. They are secreted by inflammatory cells, such as activated alveolar macrophages and neutrophils [51].

The inflammatory phase is followed by a reparative phase in which growth factors stimulate the recruitment and proliferation of mesenchymal cells and regulate neovascularization and reepithelialization of injured tissues. During this phase abnormal, or uncontrolled, reparative mechanisms may result in the development of fibrosis [52].

Fibrogenic particles activate proinflammatory cytokine production within the respiratory tract. *In vivo* studies show that alveolar macrophages from animals exposed to silica overproduce tumor necrosis factor-α (TNFα) and interleukin-1 (IL1) early after exposure [53]. Proinflammatory cytokines such as chemokines are also expressed after exposure to fibrogenic dusts. For example, expression of macrophage inflammatory protein 1α (MIP1α) and MIP2 mRNA protein are increased in rats exposed to silica, and the upregulation of these chemokines precedes the influx of inflammatory cells into the respiratory airways [54–56]. TNFα seems to play a key role in the recruitment of inflammatory cells induced by toxic dusts [57].

In addition, neutrophils recruited in the area of inflammation may contribute to the alveolitis by secreting TNFα or IL1 [58], and respiratory and endothelial cells may play a further role by releasing inflammatory mediators like MIP2, IL-8, and intracellular adhesion molecule-1 (ICAM1) [54,55].

Several studies demonstrate a key role of transforming growth factor-β (TGFβ) in the pathogenesis of lung fibrosis, and in humans elevated TGFβ expression has been observed in CWP [59]. Thus, increased levels of TNFα and IL1 have been observed in both human and animal lungs under conditions of developing fibrosis such as CWP [60]. Several human studies have shown that alveolar macrophages of individuals with silicosis and CWP spontaneously release significant amounts of growth factors such as platelet-derived growth factor (PDGF) [59], insulin-like growth factor (IGF) [59], and fibroblast growth factor (FGF) [61]. These mediators are involved in the proliferative response of type II epithelial cells that occurs in progressive massive fibrosis.

MANAGEMENT

Of the worker

No specific treatment affects the course of CWP, though treatment options are available for complications such as tuberculosis and chronic hypoxemia.

Early pneumoconiosis is easily detected by regular chest radiographic examination. When a miner is found to have CWP, further dust exposure should be excluded and ongoing underground work prohibited. This may, however, cause financial hardship despite compensation and, since simple pneumoconiosis is not generally associated with any disabling impairment of lung function, few countries have statutory regulations preventing further work underground when simple CWP is detected. In practice early retirement with pension (and compensation) is often offered but, if the affected miner chooses to continue working, ongoing exposure is minimized by a change in underground job. This is particularly so for older miners, who are less likely to obtain alternative work above ground in other industries and are less likely anyway to develop disabling complicated pneumonconiosis. This is partly because simple CWP has taken longer to arise, implying less susceptibility, and partly because continued exposure is more limited by advancing age. When PMF is detected, however, all further dusty works should be prevented.

Since an obstructive loss of ventilatory function may develop in the absence of CWP, there is a need for regular spirometric tests in addition to regular radiographic surveillance. Progressive impairment provides an independent indication for cessation of dust exposure and underground work, irrespective of the presence or absence of CWP.

Miners who smoke should additionally by given appropriate advice and support for smoking cessation, and, if there is disablement from CWP, the affected miner should be directed towards whatever mechanism exists for compensation.

Of the workforce

Regular radiographic and spirometric surveillance should allow the early detection of CWP and chronic obstructive pulmonary disease (COPD) in other members of the workforce, and so enable activation of the above management options before there is respiratory disablement. More important is regular surveillance of dust exposure levels so that potentially hazardous exposures are avoided.

PREVENTION

In the workplace

The prevention of pneumoconiosis depends on controling exposure concentrations of ambient dust to levels known to be associated with minimal and acceptable risk. Dust control is effected primarily by ventilation, though water sprayed at points of dust generation is a useful measure of dust suppression. When each process is limited by practical constraints in unusual situations (e.g. during development or in emergencies), the individual miner can be provided with respiratory protection equipment or his duration of exposure can be limited.

The effectiveness of such measures should be monitored by regular measurement of dust concentrations, and by regular clinical and radiological surveillance of the workforce. Static samplers are commonly used at the coal face and other potential sites of exposure to monitor exposure levels, relevant respirable particles of 1–7 mm diameter being collected by size-selective gravimetric elutriators. In other mining situations, personal samplers worn by individual miners can be used. Surveillance allows early recognition of workers with simple pneumoconiosis, who are likely to be those with greatest susceptibility, so that ongoing exposure can be restricted (perhaps by transfer to jobs with lower exposure) and the risk of future disablement from PMF reduced [2,18,62].

Variability of individual susceptibility is likely to be an important determinant for CWP, as it is for most occupational disorders, and a number of predictive factors may be useful in identifying miners with higher than average risk. In a longitudinal study, Bourgkard and colleagues [63] followed three groups of 80 coal miners for 4 years. Group 1 had minimal chest radiographic abnormalities initially; group 2 had similar levels of exposure, but no radiographic abnormalities; group 3 had lower levels of exposure and normal chest radiographs. Four years latter, there was radiographic progression for 24/80 miners in group 1, 6/80 in group 2, and only 1/80 in group 3. Of the 31 miners with progression, 79% had expiratory wheezes initially and 100% had an obstructive pattern of lung function. They additionally had more micronodules on CT scans, suggesting a predictive value for the initial radiographic and CT abnormalities, for these early symptoms and lung function abnormalities, and for the higher level of exposure.

An alternative approach for the future might involve genetic screening. TNFα is known to be important in the development of fibrosis due to silica exposure, and is probably relevant to the development of PMF in coal miners. A recent study showed a polymorphism in the promoter of TNFα gene in coal miners with a predominance of the genotype A308 in miners with PMF, compared to simple pneumoconiosis [64], and a further study has shown an increased plasma level of soluble TNFα receptor in coal miners with pneumoconiosis [65].

These findings may provide markers of undue susceptibility.

National regulatory strategies

Permissible levels of respirable dust inevitably differ in different countries, though are often based on the same epidemiological studies. The following standards are active at present [11]:

USA	1 mg/m^3
UK	3.8 mg/m^3
Australia	3 mg/m^3
Germany	4 mg/m^3

Control of exposure levels alone is likely to prevent most cases of disabling PMF, and it has been predicted that an exposure concentration over 35 working years that does not exceed an average of 4.3 mg/m^3 is associated with a probability for the development of category 2 or more CWP of no more than 3.4% [66]. This represents a dramatic reduction in risk over the last 50 years.

DIFFICULT CASE

History

A 69-year-old retired man was referred because of increased dyspnea. He had been a coal miner for 30 years, and had a 30% disability pension for CWP. He had moderate hypertension treated with a diuretic, but there was no history of other cardiorespiratory diseases, nor medication of possible relevance. There were no animals at home.

His worsening breathlessness had been present for 3–4 months, and had been progressive. At presentation it forced him to rest after walking 100 m on the level. He had a nonproductive cough and had lost 3 kg in weight in 2 months. Examination revealed fine inspiratory crackles at the lung bases, and lower limb edema. There was no cyanosis, pyrexia, sweating, or finger clubbing.

Chest radiography revealed large oval opacities in the upper zones bilaterally (5 cm right, 9 cm left) and diffuse small nodular shadows, consistent with complicated CWP, together with reticular interstitial shadowing in the lower zones, mediastinal lymphadenopathy, and bilateral pleural effusions. Computed tomography confirmed the presence of large noncavitated masses with irregular margins in both upper lobes which were partly calcified, together with diffuse micronodules, peripheral calcification within mediastinal and hilar lymph nodes (eggshell calcification), and bilateral pleural effusions. There were additionally irregularly thickened interlobular septa in the lower lobes with microcysts.

Pulmonary function tests revealed a severe restrictive pattern (FEV$_1$ 39% predicted; FVC 34% predicted; TLC 44% predicted) and hypoxemia at rest (PaO$_2$ = 55 mmHg, 7.31 kPa).

Hematological studies showed features of inflammation with increased sedimentation rate (67 mm/h) and C-reactive protein level (132 mg/liter). Antinuclear antibodies (Scl 70) were noted. The pleural fluid was exudative (protein = 43 g/liter) without microorganisms on culture or malignant cells. The glucose level was 0.8 g/liter.

Fiberoptic bronchoscopy revealed diffuse inflammation of the bronchial mucosa. Bronchoalveolar lavage was not performed because of breathlessness. Capillaroscopy showed an abnormal appearance of capillary vessels in the nailfold, and oesophageal manometry revealed kinetic abnormalities of the lower three-quarters of the esophagus.

He was treated with oral corticosteroids (prednisolone 1 mg/kg per day) and supplemental oxygen. The radiographic and biological abnormalities were unchanged after 6 weeks and after 4 months of steroid treatment.

Issues

The primary issue is whether this coal miner has developed scleroderma of the lung. If so, the secondary issues are whether it is occupational in origin, and whether it is a consequence of exposure to coal dust, silica dust, or both.

Comment

A clear majority of the book's contributors did consider this to be a case of occupationally induced scleroderma of the lung, mostly with a high level of confidence. However, a modest minority did not. Of those who did, almost all considered silica to be the responsible agent, though a small minority attributed causality jointly to silica and coal. The occurrence of scleroderma with CWP and silica exposure has been discussed by Rodnan et al. [67].

SUMMARY POINTS

Recognition

- Simple CWP is symptomless without abnormalities of lung function, and so is recognized only from the identification on chest radiographs or CT scans of diffuse small rounded (nodular) opacities <10 mm in diameter.
- If complicated by progressive massive fibrosis (PMF), there may be a significant loss of lung function which has both obstructive and restrictive features, and this may be associated with clinical disablement together with productive cough and wheeze.
- PMF is also recognized from radiographic or CT imaging, and by the specific identification of one or more large opacities with a diameter exceeding 10 mm, on a background diffuse small opacities.
- The standard pneumoconiotic films of the International Labor Office provide a useful basis of radiographic classification.

Management

- No specific treatment modality is available for the management of the individual miner affected by CWP, but non-specific therapy for complications such as hypoxemia or cor pulmonale may be appropriate.

- Miners with simple CWP, particularly older miners, may reasonably be permitted to continue working underground if they choose, but on-going exposure should be minimized.
- Miners with complicated CWP should cease further exposure.
- The affected miner should be advised concerning compensation rights.

Prevention

- Prevention is centered on suppressing dust generation (water spraying) and in providing uncontaminated air in the working environment (ventilation) so that there is compliance with regulatory dust exposure standards.
- To be successful, preventative strategies require regular monitoring of respirable exposure levels and the regular medical surveillance of the population of workers at risk.
- With current exposure levels in most industrially developed countries, the risk for disabling CWP after a lifetime's work is very low (a few per cent) and, with careful surveillance and the early detection of the few individuals with undue susceptibility, no disablement should occur for newly employed miners.

REFERENCES

1. Rom WM, Crystal RG. Consequences of chronic inorganic dust exposure. In: Crystal RG, West JB *et al.*, eds. *The Lung: Scientific Foundations*. New York: Raven Press, 1991.
2. Seaton A, Coal workers' pneumoconiosis. In: *Occupational Lung Diseases*, Morgan WK, Seaton A, eds. 3rd edn, pp. 374–406. London: WB Saunders, 1995.
3. Hurley JF, Burns J, Copland L *et al.* Coal workers' simple pneumoconiosis and exposure to dust at 10 British coal mines. *Br J Ind Med* 1982; 39: 120–127.
4. Hurley JF, Alexander WP, Hazledine DJ *et al.* Exposure to respirable coalmine dust and incidence of progressive massive fibrosis. *Br J Ind Med* 1987; 44: 661–672.
5. Green FHY, Laqueur WA. Coal worker's pneumoconiosis. *Pathol Ann* 1980; 15: 333–341.
6. Borm PJ. Toxicity and occupational health hazards of coal fly ash (CFA). A review of data and comparison to coal mine dust. *Ann Occup Hyg* 1997; 41:659–676.
7. Gregory JC. Case of peculiar black infiltration of the whole lungs, resembling melanosis. *Edin Med Surg J* 1831; 36: 389.
8. Hart Pd'A, Aslett EA. *Medical Research Council, Special Report Series No. 243*. London: HMSO, 1942.
9. Fay JWJ. The National Coal Board's Pneumoconiosis Field Research. *Nature* 1957; 180: 309.
10. Lainhart WS, Doyle HM, Enterline PE *et al. Pneumoconiosis in Appalachian Bitumous Coal Miners*. US Department of Health, Education and Welfare. Washington, DC: US Government Printing Office, 1969.
11. National Institute for Occupational Safety and Health. *Criteria for a Recommended Standard: Occupational Exposure to Respirable Coal Mine Dust*. Publication 95–106, pp. 1–336. Cincinnati: National Institute for Occupational Safety and Health. 1995.
12. Carpenter GR, Cochrane AL, Clarke WG *et al.* Death rates of miners and ex-miners with and without CWP in South Wales. *Br J Ind Med* 1956; 13: 102–109.
13. Sadler RL. Attributability of death to pneumoconiosis in beneficiaries. *Thorax* 1974; 29: 699–702.
14. Cochrane AL, Haley TJL, Moore F, Hole D. The mortality of men in the Rhondda Fach 1950–1970. *Br J Ind Med* 1979; 36: 15–22.
15. Morgan WKC, Burgess DB, Jacobsen B *et al.* The prevalence of coal workers' pneumoconiosis in US coal miners. *Arch Environ Health* 1973; 27: 221–226.
16. Jacobsen M, Rae S, Walton W *et al.* The relation between pneumoconiosis and dust exposure in British coal mines. In: Walton WH, ed. *Inhaled Particles*. III, pp. 903–917. Woking: Unwin Brothers, 1971.
17. McLintock JS, Rae S, Jacobsen M. The attack rate of progressive massive fibrosis in British coal miners. In: Walton WH, ed. *Inhaled Particles*. III, pp. 933–950. Woking: Unwin Brothers, 1971.
18. LeRoy Lapp N, Parker JE. Coal workers' pneumoconiosis. In: Epler GR, ed. *Clinics in Chest Medicine: Occupational Lung Diseases*, pp. 243–252. London: WB Saunders, 1992.
19. Brichet A, Salez F, Lamblin C, Wallaert B. Coal workers' pneumoconiosis and silicosis. In: Mapp CE, ed. *Occupational Lung Disorders. European Respiratory Monograph* Vol. 4, monograph 11, Monograph from European Respiratory Journal Ltd, Sheffield, UK, pp. 136–157, 1999.
20. Brichet A, Wallaert B, Gosselin B *et al.* Fibrose interstitielle diffuse primitive du mineur de charbon: une entité nouvelle? *Rev F Mal Respir* 1997; 14: 277–285.

21. Caplan A, Payne RB, Withey JL. A broader concept of Caplan's syndrome related to rheumatoid factors. *Thorax* 1962; 17:205.

22. Mosquera JA, Rodrogo L, Gonzalvez F. The evolution of pulmonary tuberculosis in coal miners in Asturia, northern Spain. An attempt to reduce the rate over a 15-year period 1971–1985. *Eur J Epidemiol* 1994; 10: 291–297.

23. Une H, Esaki H. An epidemiological study of tuberculosis in the former coal-mining area of Chikuho. An analysis of newly registered tuberculosis patients in Iizuka Health Center District. *Nippon Eiseigaku Zasshi* 1993; 47: 994–1000.

24. James WRL. The relationship of tuberculosis to the development of massive pneumoconiosis in coal workers. *Br J Tuberc* 1954; 48: 89–101.

25. Gernez-Rieux C, Tacquet A, Devulder B *et al*. Experimental studies of interactions between pneumoconiosis and mycobacterial infection. *Ann NY Acad Sci* 1972; 200: 106–126.

26. Nomoto Y, Kuwano K, Hagimoto N *et al*. Aspergillus fumigatus Asp-f-1 DNA is prevalent in sputum from patients with coal workers pneumoconiosis. *Respiration* 1997; 64: 291–295.

27. International Agency for Research on Cancer. *Silica, some Silicates, Coal Dust and Para-aramid Fibers*. Lyon: IARC, 1996.

28. Honma K, Chiyotani K, Kimura K. Silicosis, mixed dust pneumoconiosis and lung cancer. *Am J Ind Med* 1997; 32: 595–599.

29. Cochrane AL, Higgins ITT. Pulmonary ventilatory function of coal miners in various areas in relation to the X-ray category of pneumoconiosis. *Br J Prev Soc Med* 1961; 15: 1–11.

30. Morgan WKC, Haudelsman L, Kibelstis J *et al*. Ventilatory capacity and lung volumes of U.S. coal miners. *Arch Environ Health* 1974; 28: 182–189.

31. Coggon D, Newman Taylor A. Coal mining and chronic obstructive pulmonary disease: a review of the evidence. *Thorax* 1998; 53: 398–407.

32. Frans A, Veriter C, Brasseur L. Pulmonary diffusing capacity for carbon monoxide in simple CWP. *Bull Physiopathol Respir* 1975; 11: 479–502.

33. International Labour Office. *Guidelines for the Use of ILO International Classification of Radiographs of Pneumoconiosis*. Revised edition. International Labour Office Occupational Safety and Health Series No. 22 (Rev. 80). Geneva: International Labour Office, 1980.

34. Remy-Jardin M, Degreef JM, Beuscart R *et al*. Coal worker's pneumoconiosis: CT assessment in exposed workers and correlation with radiographic findings. *Radiology* 1990; 177: 363–371.

35. Leigh J, Driscoll TR, Cole BD *et al*. Quantitative relation between emphysema and lung mineral content in coal workers. *Occup Environ Med* 1994; 51: 400–407.

36. Cockroft AE, Wagner JC, Seal EME *et al*. Irregular opacities in coal workers' pneumoconiosis – correlation with pulmonary function and pathology. *Ann Occup Hyg* 1982; 26: 767–787.

37. Remy-Jardin M, Remy J, Farre I, Marquette CH. Computed tomography evaluation of silicosis and coal worker's pneumoconiosis. *Radiol Clin N Am* 1992; 30: 1155–1176.

38. Lippmann M, Eckert HL, Hahon N, Morgan WKC. Circulating antinuclear and rheumatoïd factor in coal miners. *Ann Intern Med* 1973; 79: 807–811.

39. Soutar CA, Turner-Warwick M, Parkes WR. Circulating antinuclear antibody and rheumatoid factor in coal pneumoconiosis. *Br Med J* 1974; 3: 145–147.

40. Hahon N, Morgan WKC, Petersen M. Serum immunoglobulin levels in coal workers' pneumoconiosis. *Ann Occup Hyg* 1980; 23: 165–174.

41. Robertson MD, Boyd JE, Collins HPR, Davis JMG. Serum immunoglobulin levels and humoral immune competence in coal workers. *Am J Ind Med* 1984; 6: 387–393.

42. Wallaert B, Deflandre J, Ramon PH, Voisin C. Serum angiotensin-converting enzyme in coal worker's pneumoconiosis. *Chest* 1985; 87: 844–845.

43. Lapp NL, Lewis D, Schwegler-Berry D *et al*. Bronchoalveolar lavage in asymptomatic underground coal miners. *Chest* 1990; 98: 67S.

44. Wallaert B, Lasalle P, Fortin F *et al*. Superoxide anion generation by alveolar inflammatory cells in simple pneumoconiosis and in progressive massive fibrosis of non-smoking coal workers. *Am Rev Respir Dis* 1990; 141: 129–133.

45. Green FHY. Coal workers' pneumoconiosis and pneumoconiosis due to other carbonaceous dusts. In: Churg A, Green FHY (eds) *Pathology of Occupational Lung Disease*, 2nd edn, pp. 129–208. Baltimore, MD: Williams and Wilkins, 1998.

46. Kleinerman J, Green FHY, Harley R *et al*. Pathology standards for coal workers' pneumoconiosis: Report of the Pneumoconiosis Committee of the College of American Pathologists to the National Institute for Occupational Safety and Health. *Arch Pathol Lab Med* 1979; 103: 375–431.

47. Vanhee D, Gosset P, Boitelle A *et al*. Cytokines and cytokine network in silicosis and coal workers' pneumoconiosis. *Eur Respir J* 1995; 8: 1–9.

48. Demers LM, Kuhn DC. Influence of mineral dusts on metabolism of arachidonic acid by alveolar macrophage. *Environ Health Perspect* 1994; 102 (Suppl 10): 97–100.

49. Rom WN, Bitterman PB, Rennard SI *et al*. Characterization of the lower respiratory tract inflammation of nonsmoking individuals with interstitial lung disease associated with chronic inhalation of inorganic dust. *Am Rev Respir Dis* 1987; 136: 1429–1434.

50. Weiss SJ. Tissue destruction by neutrophils. *N Engl J Med* 1989; 320: 365–376.

51. Ferry G, Lonchampt M, Pennel L *et al*. Activation of MMP-9 by neutrophil elastase in an *in vivo* model of acute lung injury. *FEBS Lett* 1997; 402: 111–115.

52. Limper AH, Roman J. Fibronectin. A versatile matrix protein with roles in thoracic development, repair and infection. *Chest* 1992; 101: 1663–1673.

53. Oghiso Y, Kubota Y. Enhanced interleukin 1 production by alveolar macrophages and increase in Ia-positive lung cells in silica-exposed rats. *Microbiol Immunol* 1986; 30: 1189–1198.

54. Driscoll KE, Hassenbein DG, Carter J *et al*. Macrophage inflammatory proteins 1 and 2: expression by rat alveolar macrophages, fibroblasts, and epithelial cells and in rat lung after mineral dust exposure. *Am J Respir Cell Mol Biol* 1993; 8: 311–318.

55. Driscoll KE, Howard BW, Carter JM *et al*. Alpha-quartz-induced chemokine expression by rat lung epithelial cells: effects of *in vivo* and *in vitro* particle exposure. *Am J Pathol* 1996; 149: 1627–1637.

56. Yuen IS, Hartsky MA, Snajdr SI, Warheit DB. Time course of chemotactic factor generation and neutrophil recruitment in the lungs of dust-exposed rats. *Respir Cell Mol Biol* 1996; 15: 268–274.

57. Vanhee D, Molet S, Gosset P *et al*. Expression of leucocyte–endothelial adhesion molecules is limited to intercellular adhesion molecule-1 (ICAM-1) in the lung of pneumoconiotic patients: role of tumor necrosis factor-alpha (TNF-alpha). *Clin Exp Immunol* 1996; 106: 541–548.

58. Kusaka Y, Cullen RT, Donaldson K. Immunomodulation in mineral dust-exposed lungs: stimulatory effect and interleukin-1 release by neutrophils from quartz-elicited alveolitis. *Clin Exp Immunol* 1990; 80: 293–298.

59. Vanhee D, Gosset P, Wallaert B *et al*. Mechanisms of fibrosis in coal workers' pneumoconiosis. Increased production of platelet-derived growth factor, insulin-like growth factor type I, and transforming growth factor beta and relationship to disease severity. *Am J Respir Crit Care Med* 1994; 150: 1049–1055.

60. Lassalle P, Gosset P, Aerts C *et al*. Abnormal secretion of interleukin-1 and tumor necrosis factor alpha by alveolar macrophages in coal workers' pneumoconiosis: comparison between simple pneumoconiosis and progressive massive fibrosis. *Exp Lung Res* 1990; 16: 73–80.

61. Lesur O, Melloni B, Cantin AM, Begin R. Silica-exposed lung fluids have a proliferative activity for type II epithelial cells: a study on man and sheep alveolar fluids. *Exp Lung Res* 1992; 18: 633–654.

62. Beckett W, Abraham J, Becklake M *et al*. Adverse effects of crystalline silica exposure (Official Statement of ATS). *Am J Respir Crit Care Med* 1997; 155: 761–765.

63. Bourgkard E, Bernadac P, Chau N *et al*. Can the evolution to pneumoconiosis be suspected in coal miners? A longitudinal study. *Am J Respir Crit Care Med* 1998; 158: 504–509.

64. Zhai R, Jetten M, Schins RP, Franssen H, Borm J. Polymorphisms in the promoter of the tumor necrosis factor alpha in coal miners. *Ann J Ind Med* 1998; 34: 318–324.

65. Schins RPF, Borm JPA. Plasma level of soluble tumor necrosis factor receptors are increased in coal miners with pneumoconiosis. *Eur Respir J* 1995; 8: 1658–1663.

66. Jacobsen M. Progression of coal workers' pneumoconiosis in Britain in relation to environmental conditions underground. Proceeding of the Conference on Technical Measures of Dust Prevention and Suppression in Mines, pp. 77–93. Luxembourg: Commission of the European Communities, 1973.

67. Rodnan GP, Benedek TG, Medsger TA Jr, Cammarata RJ. The association of progressive systemic sclerosis (scleroderma) with coal miners' pneumoconiosis and other forms of silicosis. *Ann Intern Med* 1967; 66: 323–334.

9 | ASBESTOSIS

Paul De Vuyst and Pierre Alain Gevenois

BACKGROUND

Asbestosis is defined as diffuse interstitial fibrosis of the lung resulting from the inhalation and retention of considerable numbers of asbestos fibers, usually after prolonged exposure [1,2]. The degree of fibrosis increases with the fiber burden, which can approach 2×10^9 fibers/g of dry lung in severe asbestosis [3,4].

The term 'asbestos' refers to six naturally occurring fibrous silicate minerals, which can be usefully classified by their physical and chemical structures Figs 9.1 and 9.2.

Chrysotile (white) asbestos has been, and still is, mined commercially in many countries, principally Canada, China, Russia, and more recently Brazil. It is the only serpentine (curved) asbestos fiber of importance. The other asbestos fiber types are all amphibole (straight and needle-like) in nature. Crocidolite (blue) asbestos is no longer mined; it came predominantly from South Africa and Western Australia. Amosite (brown) asbestos was mined only

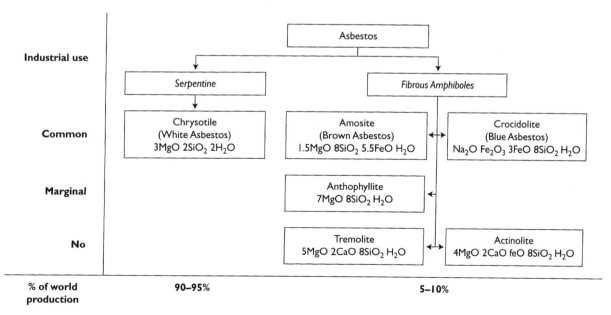

Figure 9.1 Classification of asbestos minerals.

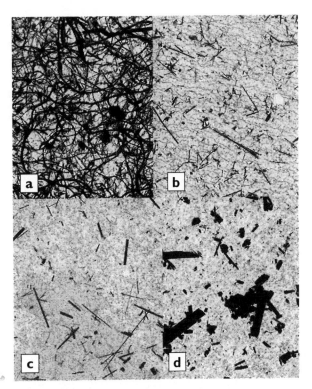

Fig. 9.2 Different types of asbestos fibers (a: chrysotile, b: crocidolite, c: amosite, d: anthophyllite) as seen by transmission electron microscopy (UICC reference material).

in South Africa. Anthophyllite has been locally exploited in Finland. Tremolite asbestos is of relatively little commercial importance, although it has been mined in Turkey, Italy, Pakistan, and South Korea [5]. Tremolite is, however, a frequent contaminant (geological component) of other mineral ores, including chrysotile and talc. Tremolite and anthophyllite are associated with environmental asbestos-related diseases in the Mediterranean area (Turkey, Greece, Corsica) and Finland, respectively.

Currently, annual global production is about 2 million tons, of which Canada and Russia produce more than 50%. The users are more difficult to identify; about 20% of consumption now takes place in developing countries, and 60% in Eastern and Central European countries, where regulations for exposure control and disease prevention are limited or have even declined [6,7]. In 1996, Canada produced 520 000 tons and consumed 6000 tons. In many industrially developed Western countries, the ongoing use of asbestos has been banned. The peak global incidence of asbestos-related diseases is now expected 30–40 years after the consumption peak of the 1960s and 1970s, and so incidence is not likely to decline much until 2020 [8].

Asbestos has been used in a wide variety of settings, largely because of its excellent thermal- and noise-insulating properties, its physical strength, and its marked durability against mechanical, thermal, and chemical stress. As a result occupa-

tional exposure has occurred extensively. Its physical properties and fibrous form endow it with considerable versatility in that it can be woven to produce fire-resistant cloth, added to cement to improve strength as well as provide fire resistance, and mixed with water to produce a slurry. The latter can then be applied as a fire retardant and insulation material by spraying, or it can be subjected to a number of industrial processes (mold setting, compression, rolling, drying, sawing) in order to make specific insulation and fire-retardant products. It has consequently been used very widely indeed in industry, until increasing awareness and acknowledgment of its dangers led to its ongoing use being discontinued in many countries. In the interim many of these manufacturing processes and many of its uses led to the release of substantial amounts of respirable dust in working environments, and to clinically meaningful exposure for many workers in many industries, well beyond those of mining, milling, and transport of the raw material.

Such exposures have led to a variety of respiratory disorders, and to considerable public awareness and concern. There is, nevertheless, a good deal of public misunderstanding, and misplaced alarm – much of it arising because of the common lay and news media (and occasional professional) tendency to use the term asbestosis to describe indiscriminately all of the associated adverse respiratory effects. Since they have profoundly different implications with regard to disability and survival, it is important that the one is clearly distinguished from the other:

- Asbestosis
- Lung cancer (Chapter 20)
- Benign pleural disease (Chapter 21)
  - Pleural plaques
  - Pleural effusion
  - Diffuse pleural thickening
  - Folded (entrapped) lung, known also as rounded atelectasis (Blesovsky's syndrome)
- Malignant mesothelioma (Chapter 22).

This chapter will review only asbestosis. It is inevitable, however, that in some individuals more than one effect will be manifested, demanding particular clarity when diagnoses are explained and information is passed to patients, their relatives, and healthcare personnel. In addition, some risk is likely to be evident for the future development of other asbestos-associated disorders.

Epidemiology

The majority of patients with asbestosis have been exposed directly in the asbestos-handling industry (i.e. mining, milling, and the production or installation of

Table 9.1 Main occupations consistent with a risk for asbestosis (historical)

Asbestos production:	Mining, milling
Asbestos transportation:	Packing, handling
Manufacture of insulation products	Friction products (brake linings) Asbestos cement products (pipes, tiles) Textile (fireproof clothes)
End-use of asbestos-containing material	Spraying Heating trades (boilermakers, heating mechanics) Glass factories Power stations Iron foundry industry (furnace builders) Pipe fitting Building construction (electricians, plumbers, carpenters, roofers) Railroads and shipyards
Occupations where a potential risk is still present	Removal of insulation, asbestos removal and asbestos waste handling Demolition of structures containing asbestos (ships, heating systems, buildings)

asbestos-containing material), or in the construction of buildings, automobiles, rail vehicles, or ships (Table 9.1). Some encounter exposure only during refurbishment or demolition work, when asbestos insulation is removed or disturbed. The greater the cumulative exposure, the greater is disease severity; and the shorter the period over which it is sustained, the shorter is the latency period between exposure onset and disease onset. There are, however, considerable differences in individual susceptibility.

The prevalence of asbestosis, usually defined by the presence of small irregular opacities on the chest radiograph and by a profusion score 1/0 using the classification devised by the International Labor Office (ILO) (see Chapter 31), is highly variable according to the type of fiber, type of industry, cumulative exposure, and age. Epidemiological studies involving 33 different cohorts between 1971 and 1994 show prevalence ranges of 2–16% in asbestos miners (chrysotile or crocidolite), 7.5–40% in workers manufacturing insulation products, and 0.8–60% in end-users [9]. The highest prevalence was found among a cohort of 2790 insulation workers [10].

Cumulative exposures estimated to exceed 200 [f/ml].yr (i.e. the product of the average airborne fiber concentration in fibers/ml to which the worker has been exposed and the number of years worked at this level) have not been uncommon, and some exposures have exceeded 1000 [f/ml].year [9]. The level of exposure has sometimes been so high that exceptionally a few months only of work has been sufficient to induce lung fibrosis. Mineral analyses performed decades later may still demonstrate the retention of large numbers of amphibole fibers in such cases [11]. Most asbestos-exposed workers have sustained substantially lesser cumulative levels of exposure, however, and most do not develop asbestosis.

Owing to better control of dust emissions and more strict regulations in industrialized countries, the fiber levels in the air of the workplace have substantially decreased over recent decades. As a consequence, the incidence of severe asbestosis has diminished over time, and most cases seen today are the result of exposures dating back several decades, or of exposures in unusual circumstances. However, the use of high-resolution computed tomography (HRCT) in the diagnosis of asbestos-related disease has led to an increased detection of subclinical cases. The vast majority of currently recognized asbestos-induced disorders are benign pleural lesions with little or no impact upon lung function. The incidence of symptomatic asbestosis has diminished so markedly that nowadays the development of interstitial lung fibrosis in an individual previously exposed to low asbestos fiber concentrations raises the meaningful possibility of coincidental idiopathic lung fibrosis [12]. It is surprising, therefore, that certified death rates from asbestos-related diseases appear to have remained stable. This probably reflects an increasing incidence of asbestos-related mesothelioma and lung cancer, balanced by a decreasing mortality from asbestosis, though inaccuracy of death certification may have played a contributory role [2].

Since the introduction of strict asbestos exposure regulations in most industrially developed countries, 'primary asbestos workers' (essentially asbestos removers) are now greatly outnumbered by workers encountering asbestos only inadvertently in other trades, for example, electricians, plumbers, carpenters, and demolition workers. Such tradesmen are more likely to work independently and, therefore, without the protection of industrial hygiene regulations prevailing in large factories. They currently face a variable chance of encountering asbestos in the course of daily work, and constitute the population at most risk for the development of asbestos-induced diseases for the future.

In subjects with environmental exposure to tremolite asbestos in Turkey, mineral analyses have shown in some cases very high fiber burdens in the lungs. These may reach the same magnitude as in industrial settings and may lead to similar diseases, including asbestosis. These may consequently be diagnosed in Turkish migrants to other countries [11–14].

Prognosis

The radiographic abnormalities of asbestosis may progress well beyond the time when exposure ceases, but the rate of progression is usually slow [15]. Overall, progression is observed in less than 50% of cases after exposure cessation, depending on the exposure conditions, the initial radiographic profusion score, and the interval between radiographs [15–19]. In Corsican chrysotile miners with a mean cumulative exposure of 30 [f/ml].yr, the progression rate was 46% after a mean of 14 years, reaching 63% for those with an initial ILO reading of 1/1 [17].

The probability of progression and its rate, as demonstrated by an observed increase in profusion of radiographic opacities over time, are influenced by a number of factors, some of which are interrelated. The principal determinants are cumulative dose, fiber type, and individual susceptibility, there being considerable variability among subjects with apparently similar exposure profiles. The probability of progression is correlated positively with the radiographic severity, and its rate is correlated negatively with the latency period.

Chrysotile is less hazardous than amphiboles [20]. This is likely to be a consequence of the greater durability (biopersistence) of amphiboles, which are much more resistant than chrysotile to the lung's clearance mechanisms. The respective half-lives are of the order of decades for amphiboles, and months for chrysotile. This progressive decline in the burden of retained fibers might be expected to slow the rate of progression of asbestosis over time. With the decrease in cumulative levels of exposure over the last 20 years, progression can be expected to become increasingly less common and less fast.

In a 1981 mortality study of 655 subjects with asbestosis, Berry reported that 20% died from respiratory failure attributable to asbestosis, 30% from lung cancer, and 10% from mesothelioma [21]. For subjects developing asbestosis now or in the future, cumulative levels of exposure are likely to be of lesser magnitude than was the case over the last 50 years, and disease severity is likely to be less. Prognosis will consequently differ from that observed over recent decades. In particular, death from respiratory failure

and cor pulmonale as a direct consequence of asbestosis will become rare, though asbestosis may still cause death indirectly by continuing to modify adversely any existing risk for lung cancer. The magnitude of this is difficult to quantify and poses a major outstanding issue of uncertainty associated with asbestosis since there is still a controversy as to whether asbestosis itself is the primary cause of the excess of lung cancer mortality or whether the associated level of exposure is independently responsible.

RECOGNITION

Clinical features

History

The symptoms of asbestosis are those common to other interstitial diseases of the lung. The most important, and the primary cause of disablement, is breathlessness without wheeze. It appears first only on exertion, but with progressive disease it increases in severity until it is present even at rest. A dry cough, often induced by deep breathing, is frequent in severe cases, and may occasionally provoke more distress than breathlessness. Thoracic pain is reported additionally by some severely dyspneic patients, and has been attributed to fatigue of the respiratory muscles consequent to the increased work of inflating stiff lung. Haemoptysis is not characteristic, and should be investigated as a possible symptom of complicating lung cancer.

Whether diffuse interstitial fibrosis might be asbestosis depends on the cumulative level of asbestos exposure sustained. Asbestosis results from exposure to high dust levels for extended periods of time – usually many years. It is commonly accepted that asbestosis will not develop to produce clinical manifestations below lifetime ex-posures of 25 [f/ml].yr [22,23]. This conclusion of the Royal Commission on Asbestos in 1984, supported by Doll and Peto, has faced few challenges over the following years, but it is probable that minimal or mild degrees of parenchymal fibrosis, detectable only by histology or HRCT scanning, will occur at lower exposure levels.

The relation between cumulative exposure and risk for asbestosis is considered to be approximately linear; the more intense and prolonged the exposure, the greater is the proportion of workers with evidence of asbestosis, and the greater is the severity of the disease. Nevertheless, a large proportion of similarly exposed workers will not develop asbestosis, implying important differences in indi-vidual susceptibility which are possibly genetic in origin [24]. At least 50% of heavily exposed workers demonstrate 'resistance' to the fibrogenic effects of asbestos.

Excess retention of fibers could be a major determinant in susceptibility to develop asbestosis, and several observations suggest that the efficacy of lung clearance mechanisms is linked to the risk of parenchymal disease. Experimental studies in a sheep model by Begin and colleagues documented a high level of fiber retention in those animals with interstitial lung disease than in those without, despite similar exposure [25,26]. Excess alveolar dust deposition, evaluated by bronchoalveolar lavage (BAL) samples, preceded the disease. Studies on mineral analyses of lung tissue or BAL fluid have generally demonstrated much higher asbestos fiber and asbestos body burdens in patients with asbestosis than in exposed subjects without apparent disease or with asbestos-related pleural disorders alone [3,27,28]. Asbestos bodies are fibers, almost exclusively amphibole, that have become coated within the lung by iron-containing proteinaceous material. This may produce a striking and readily detectable appearance under the light microscope, and so allow dust exposure to be quantified more easily (see Chapter 34).

Asbestosis is also more likely to be associated with regular or continuous exposure, whereas intermittent exposures are related more to pleural lesions [29]. Intermittent exposure could permit a more efficient lung clearance of fibers (aside from resulting in a lesser level of cumulative exposure), reducing the amount of retained fibers and hence the asbestosis risk. The amount of fibers retained in the pleura could be less influenced by the rate of dose delivery to the lung [30].

Cumulative exposure is related further, though negatively, to the latency period between exposure onset and the initial development of radiological or clinical manifestations of asbestosis. With the average levels of exposure measured over recent decades, there is typically a delay of at least 15 years before a radiological diagnosis can be made from chest radiographs. For the future, however, with occupational exposures controlled up to the limit currently permitted in most industrialized countries (<1 f/ml), asbestosis is not likely to be detected during a working career or even after retirement. With very low fiber levels (<0.01 f/ml), such as are detected most consistently in buildings, the development of asbestosis is virtually impossible [31].

It is, of course, exceptional for any estimate of cumulative exposure in [f/ml].yr to be available in an individual patient, and the consulted physician is usually obliged to assess exposure from the history alone. A lifetime job history should be obtained, with questions addressing fiber type (often not known), exposure concentration, and duration. The nature of the job tasks involved will usually provide a useful guide to the probable intensity of any airborne dust released into the working environment, and enquiry about work in confined environments, the presence of effective local exhaust ventilation, and the use of personal masks or respirators, should allow a rough quantitative assessment of cumulative exposure. By contrast, with mesothelioma and even pleural plaques, the issue is often not one of whether sufficient cumulative exposure has occurred, but whether any exposure can be identified, since these disorders frequently occur after much lower levels of exposure [32].

Environmental (or domestic) exposure outside recognized regions of asbestos geological outcropping is otherwise unlikely to be sufficiently high to pose any risk of asbestosis.

Physical signs

No physical signs are pathognomonic of asbestosis, the two most characteristic features being common to other interstitial diseases of the lung. Gravity-dependent inspiratory crackles may precede respiratory symptoms (and chest radiograph abnormalities) and thus be early indicators. Equally, they may remain unassociated with any other evidence of the disease, and so be non-specific. They are heard bilaterally, first laterally in the axillary segments, and then in the posterior parts of the lower lung fields. Finger clubbing is a much less constant sign in asbestosis than in idiopathic pulmonary fibrosis, though is common in severe disease. When clubbing is marked, or is present in mild asbestosis, a complicating lung cancer should be suspected.

Investigation

Lung function

Asbestosis is characterized by the pattern of lung function abnormalities typical of diffuse interstitial fibrosis in general: a restrictive ventilatory defect (reduction of total lung capacity, TLC, and forced vital capacity, FVC) and a reduction of carbon monoxide diffusion capacity (D_LCO) [33,34]. A reduction of FVC without reduction of TLC may be due to airway obstruction and air trapping, without implying the presence of ventilatory restriction, if the FEV_1/FVC ratio is additionally lowered and/or the residual volume (RV) is elevated.

A negative relationship between FVC and the profusion of small radiographic opacities has been clearly demonstrated [33]. In a large group of heavily exposed insulation workers, the mean FVC (as a percentage of predicted) was respectively 88% for cases with 0/0 profusion, 81.8% for category 1/1, 72.7% for category 2/2 and 65% for category 3/3. In 'never-smokers', the FVC and FEV_1 were both reduced by a similar extent, indicating a pure restrictive defect. These profusion scores are explained in the following section on imaging, and in Chapter 31. The mean results reflected a broad range of individual values, and included some workers with profusion categories of 0/0 whose FVC was significantly reduced, and others with 3/3 radiographs whose FVC was still normal.

This illustrates the low diagnostic sensitivity of lung volume measurements. It can be attributed, at least partly, to the wide range of normal values. Thus, an observed longitudinal loss of one liter of vital capacity in an individual with progressive asbestosis may still leave spirometric values within normal limits. Lung function measurements cannot provide definitive early markers of lung disease, unless longitudinal data are available. Normal longitudinal decline in FVC does not usually exceed 25–30 ml/year (and may be much less in young or middle-aged subjects) and so higher values observed over a minimum of 3–5 years may provide useful diagnostic information. This assumes that a minimum of three (preferably more) measurements at even intervals contribute to the slope estimation, and that the change cannot be attributed to worsening airway obstruction. The demonstration of decreased lung compliance may help to identify interstitial lung disease before a reduction of lung volume can be detected, but compliance measurements are not easy to perform or interpret in clinical practice.

A lowered $D_L co$ has been reported to be a more useful early indicator of asbestosis than reduction in total lung capacity and FVC, and it may be the only functional manifestation of asbestos-induced parenchymal disease [35]. Diminished $D_L co$ reflects loss of parenchymal function from cause, however, and is greatly influenced by emphysema in cigarette smokers. In such circumstances, which are common, the presence and degree of any airway obstruction will help differentiate the parenchymal loss attributable to emphysema from that due to asbestosis. Such differentiation is aided by the appearances on HRCT scans (see Chapter 31). Exercise tests can be done to detect desaturation of arterial blood on exertion.

When asbestosis and diffuse pleural thickening occur together, both will limit lung expansion. The restrictive effect of asbestosis on ventilation is consequently enhanced as is the associated decrease in compliance [36]. The effects of diffuse pleural thickening may be severe and respiratory failure has been described as a result, and so the degree of functional impairment attributable to asbestosis alone may be difficult to assess. The pleural disease will increase the decrement in FVC above that expected for asbestosis at any profusion score of the ILO classifi-

cation [33], and it will widen the discrepancy between $D_L co$ and the gas transfer coefficient, KCO, since $D_L co$ will decrease further because of increased restriction, but KCO will increase because the increased restriction is not associated with further loss of parenchymal function.

Although ventilatory restriction is the characteristic effect of asbestosis on lung function, it has been suggested that asbestos-induced inflammation and fibrosis of the terminal and respiratory bronchioles might cause airway obstruction [37]. Functional abnormalities considered to reflect peripheral obstruction in the small airways have been reported, such as decreased forced expiratory flow at midlung volumes (FEF_{25-75}), increased slope of the alveolar plateau in nitrogen washout curves, and increased RV/TLC ratios [38–41]. There is speculation that asbestos inhalation might promote small airway lesions induced by tobacco smoke, and in animal experiments a combined exposure to asbestos and tobacco smoke led to more severe fibrosis of small airways than was produced by each agent alone [42].

However, standard spirometric tests do not show an obstructive pattern (defined by a reduced FEV_1/FVC) in non-smoking workers with asbestosis. In a study by Miller *et al.* the mean FEV_1/FVC ratio was 100% of predicted among the group of asbestos insulators who were never-smokers, and a reduction in flow rates and mean FEV_1/FVC was seen only in smokers [33]. In fact the FEV_1/FVC increased in the never-smokers with increasing profusion of radiographic small opacities, overcoming a very small decrease observed at lesser profusion scores. This can be explained by increases in elastic lung recoil masking the effects of small airways disease.

In conclusion, asbestosis is not currently thought to contribute to chronic obstructive pulmonary disease (COPD) [43] and there is no evidence for a role of asbestos in producing emphysema. When COPD is detected with asbestosis, it is likely to be coincidental and a consequence of cigarette smoking. There is speculation that asbestos, like other dusts and mineral fibers, might augment the effect of tobacco smoke on airflow obstruction due to small airways disease, but airway disease attributable to asbestos should anyway be considered separately from asbestosis [44–46].

The use of lung function measurements is discussed more fully in Chapter 32.

Imaging

On a posteroanterior chest radiograph, asbestosis is characterized by irregular small opacities which predominate in the lower lung fields. A fine reticulation in mild disease progresses to a coarse linear pattern and honeycombing at the most severe stage. The different sized irregular opacities are designated by codes *s*, *t*, and *u* of the ILO classification and are described fully in Chapter 31 [47].

These findings are not specific for asbestosis and can be expected in other infiltrative and fibrotic diseases of the interstitium. The most common is idiopathic interstitial pulmonary fibrosis (cryptogenic fibrosing alveolitis). These small irregular opacities may additionally be related to age and smoking [48–50], and may be seen in patients with emphysema or bronchiectasis [51]. In asbestos-exposed subjects their association with pleural plaques tends to support a radiographic diagnosis of asbestosis, but pleural plaques are by no means invariably detectable. Furthermore, extensive pleural plaques or diffuse thickening may obscure interstitial abnormalities, and patients with histopathologically proven infiltrative lung disease may have a normal chest radiograph [52].

The posteroanterior chest radiograph remains the first-line imaging technique in asbestos-exposed subjects but suffers from weak sensitivity, weak specificity, and weak interreader reproducibility. The recently evolved technique of computed tomographic (CT) scanning with thin 1-mm sections, HRCT, has been proved to be considerably more accurate than both chest radiographs and conventional 1-cm thick CT scans in detecting and characterizing infiltrative lung disorders, including asbestosis, in asymptomatic subjects [53–57]. Consequently, thin-section CT has dramatically changed the imaging approach for asbestosis in clinical as well as medicolegal settings.

On thin-section CT, asbestosis is characterized by several signs that are seen best in the posterior subpleural area of the lung, at the lung bases, in the prone position [58]. These include septal lines, intralobular lines, subpleural curvilinear lines, and honeycombing [59]. The septal line is defined as a thin linear opacity that corresponds to an interlobular septum [60] (Fig. 9.3). The intralobular lines are present in the lobule when the intralobular interstitium is thickened. When numerous, they may appear as a fine reticular pattern [60] (Fig. 9.4). The subpleural curvilinear line is defined as a thin subpleural linear opacity, a few millimeters or less in thickness and usually less than 1 cm from the pleural surface, which runs parallel to the pleura [60] (Fig. 9.5). Honeycombing is defined as clustered cystic air spaces usually of comparable diameter, of the order of 0.3–1.0 cm but as much as 2.5 cm, usually subpleural and characterized by well-defined walls, which are often thick [60] (Fig. 9.6).

Septal lines, intralobular lines, and the curvilinear subpleural line are not definitive of pulmonary fibrosis and may be seen in a variety of other conditions. By themselves they are non-specific findings [61]. In

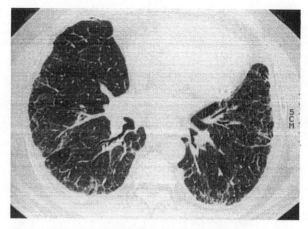

Fig. 9.3 CT scan showing interlobular septal lines: single or branching interlobular lines up to 1–2 cm in length are seen in the subpleural lung parenchyma.

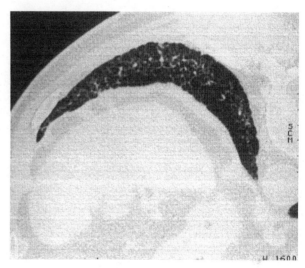

Fig. 9.4 CT scan showing intralobular non-septal lines: single or branching intralobular lines up to 1–2 cm in length are seen in the subpleural lung parenchyma.

comparison, honeycombing is a specific indicator of pulmonary fibrosis, though not specifically of asbestosis. It is a feature of all causes of pulmonary fibrosis [62]. HRCT may additionally show a 'ground-glass' opacification of the lung parenchyma which is common in idiopathic fibrosis, though is said to be less common in asbestosis [62]. The presence of pleural plaques reinforces the possible relationship between asbestos exposure and lung fibrosis but pleural plaques may be absent in patients with histopathologically proven asbestosis [62,63].

Thin-section CT is more specific than the chest radiograph since this technique is able to distinguish different types of lung disorder, such as pulmonary fibrosis, other infiltrative lung diseases, emphysema, and bronchiectasis, all being potentially responsible for irregular small opacities on chest radiographs [51]. It may also allow ventilatory restriction to be

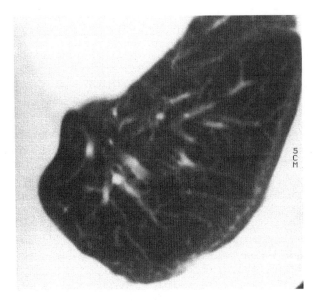

Fig. 9.5 CT scan showing a subpleural curvilinear line: a linear area of increased attenuation is seen within 1 cm of the pleura running parallel to the inner chest wall.

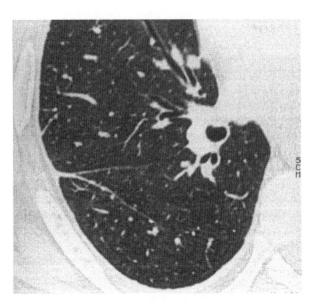

Fig. 9.7 CT scan showing a parenchymal band: a linear and branching line shadow 2–5 cm in length is seen extending through the lung to the thickened pleural surface.

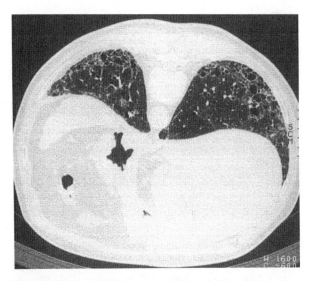

Fig. 9.6 CT scan showing honeycombing: cystic air spaces 0.3–1.0 cm in diameter are seen with well-defined and often thick walls.

attributed more accurately between asbestosis and pleural thickening. Thin-section CT is also more sensitive than chest radiographs, since it may reveal opacities that are too small or too few to be visible on the radiographs [64]. Nevertheless, thin-section CT is not the gold standard for diagnosis since patients with histopathologically proven asbestosis may have normal or near-normal thin-section CT scans. In practical terms, thin-section CT is currently the most accurate non-invasive technique, and is used widely in the investigation of asbestosis.

Two other CT signs may be seen in the parenchyma of asbestos-exposed subjects, the parenchymal band and rounded atelectasis (folded lung),

though neither is a defining characteristic of asbestosis. A parenchymal band is defined as an elongated opacity, usually several millimeters wide and up to about 5-cm long, often extending to the pleura, which may be thickened and retracted at the site of contact [60] (Fig. 9.7). Rounded atelectasis is defined as a mass shadow due to folded and collapsed lung which is closely related to an area of overlying pleural thickening. A characteristic 'comet tail' of vessels and bronchi may be seen sweeping into the lateral, or medial/lateral aspect of the mass thereby helping to distinguish it from a peripheral tumor [65] (Fig. 9.8). Both signs are intrapulmonary reflections of diffuse pleural thickening that is often the result of a previous benign asbestos-induced effusion [66,67]. They are not specific for asbestos exposure, since they can be seen in unexposed subjects with pleural disease attributable to trauma, infection, or drugs [68,69].

These thin-section CT findings are thus not specific for asbestosis but compared to standard chest radiographs, diagnostic confidence is increased and interreader variability is reduced. This is despite there being no standard set of CT films comparable to those of the ILO system. The American Thoracic Society established criteria for the clinical diagnosis of asbestosis which includes s, t, or u small irregular opacities on the chest radiograph at a profusion of 1/1 or greater according the ILO classification [70]. When absent, considerable diagnostic caution is warranted in an asbestos-exposed individual. Histopathological evidence of asbestosis (see Box 9.1 Histopathology) may, nevertheless, be evident, and when it is there is a reported 10–20% probability of

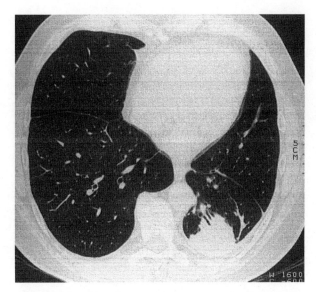

Fig. 9.8 CT scan showing rounded atelectasis: a mass is seen adjacent to overlying pleural thickening. Note the backward displacement of the fissure reflecting the volume loss in the left lower lobe, and the associated parenchymal band.

the chest radiograph being interpreted as normal [71]. The use of HRCT should consequently replace chest radiography for the diagnostic imaging criteria of asbestosis.

Bronchoscopy/bronchoalveolar lavage

Bronchoscopy reveals no obvious macroscopic abnormality in asbestosis, but BAL fluid may show a number of characteristic cellular, biochemical, and mineralogical features in asbestos-exposed workers and in patients with asbestosis. BAL is useful in the clinical diagnosis of asbestosis by documenting alveolitis and asbestos bodies or fibers, and by eliminating other causes of interstitial lung disease. The alveolitis of asbestosis is characterized by an increased total number of cells, mainly macrophages, and a mild but inconstant increase in neutrophil and eosinophil numbers [72–74]. The predominant presence of macrophages is consistent with the pivotal role of activated alveolar macrophages in the pathogenesis of the disease. The severity of BAL changes is better correlated with lung function abnormalities, such as lowered D_LCO, than with radiological alterations [35,75]. BAL profiles in asbestos workers may, however, be abnormal in the absence of clinical or radiological evidence of asbestosis.

The presence of a neutrophil and eosinophil alveolitis has been shown to be a prognostic factor, higher cell concentrations being associated with a greater progressive loss of D_LCO [34,75,76]. In a longitudinal study of 117 asbestos-exposed workers, increased macrophage and eosinophil numbers in BAL fluid together with an increased fibronectin concentration were associated additionally with the

persistence of lowered total lung capacity values throughout the period of observation, though the rate of decline of total lung capacity was not related significantly to these factors. These observations are consistent with studies in patients with idiopathic pulmonary fibrosis, which have shown that excess neutrophils and eosinophils in BAL fluid are associated with a higher probability of disease progression and a failure to respond to immunosuppressive therapy [34]. This cellular response is therefore not specific for asbestosis in a diagnostic sense.

A lymphocytic alveolitis, generally with an increase in CD4/CD8 ratio, may also be seen in asbestosis. It is, however, the most commonly reported abnormality in asbestos-exposed workers without clinical or radiological evidence of asbestosis, though some may have pleural fibrosis [72,77,78]. Smoking may also increase the number of macrophages and eosinophils, perhaps more than asbestosis itself [79].

A significant correlation has been found between the severity of asbestosis or asbestos alveolitis and the BAL levels of fibronectin and procollagen III [24]. Studies on mediators in BAL fluid are interesting for understanding the basic mechanisms of the disease, but are not relevant in clinical practice [80].

Mineralogy

Mineral analyses performed on BAL or lung tissue may be invaluable when exposure histories are ill-defined, and they provide an alternative tool in research for assessing the risks associated with asbestos exposure. Very high burdens, two to three orders of magnitude greater than the fiber burdens detected in unexposed controls, are consistently reported in asbestosis and increase with the severity of fibrosis [46,81,82].

A number of factors are crucial for the interpretation of the results from BAL and lung tissue of mineralogic analyses. These include standardized methodologies, adequate reference populations, a comprehensive understanding of the factors affecting the retention, deposition, and clearance of fibers in the lungs, and awareness of the different dose–response relationships of the various asbestos-induced diseases. It is particularly important to realize that most airborne dust is not inhaled into the intrathoracic airways (it is deposited in the upper airway), that few fibers entering the trachea reach the alveoli to be retained within the lung interstitium, and that, following interstitial retention, there is a slow dissolution and removal of fibers which varies considerably between chrysotile (serpentine) asbestos and the various amphiboles. Thus the half-lives of chrysotile and amphiboles are of the order months and decades, respectively.

Once deposition and retention have occurred, a proportion of fibers becomes coated in an iron-containing proteinaceous material to produce the widely recognized ferruginous body (an asbestos body if the fiber is asbestos). This occurs largely with amphiboles, and only rarely with chrysotile. Bodies are readily observed by light microscopy and so can serve usefully as markers of amphibole fiber numbers. The body-to-fiber ratio is highly variable, depending on fiber type, fiber lengths, and even on the amount of iron present in the lung [28]. Asbestosis is associated with high fiber and body burdens in both lung tissue and BAL, and so a fiber or body count within the normal range of an unexposed reference population provides strong evidence against asbestosis if there is no obvious history of asbestos exposure which could have involved only chrysotile.

Quantitative lung tissue analysis is the 'gold standard' by which to quantify the concentration of bodies, but results may differ markedly from one laboratory to another despite being satisfactorily repeatable in the laboratory of their source. They must consequently be compared to the reference (background) values from the particular source laboratory, the absolute concentration being largely meaningless otherwise. Nevertheless, results from all experienced laboratories indicate that asbestosis is invariably associated with high fiber burdens, whether counted as bodies or uncoated fibers [82–84]. The subject is discussed in more detail in Chapter 34. To give the reader some idea of the order of magnitude of the concentrations observed in some analytical laboratories, uncoated fiber counts >1000/g dry lung have been considered as indicative of occupational exposure [83,84], while in asbestosis concentrations are usually higher than 50 000/g. Indeed several millions, even hundreds of millions, may be found [82].

Asbestos bodies are rarely found in BAL of control subjects without occupational or specific environmental/domestic exposure, and if present are usually in concentrations below 1.0/ml. By contrast, asbestos bodies were found in BAL in 98% of 59 patients with asbestosis, with a median value of 121/ml. Corresponding mean values associated with benign pleural disease and exposure without evidence of any asbestos-induced disorder were 4 and 5/ml, respectively [81]. Asbestos bodies in sputum provide a highly specific marker of past asbestos exposure, but are a very inaccurate measure of asbestos fiber burden within the lung [85].

A mineralogic analysis may contribute to the assessment of past cumulative exposure, especially when data from other sources are unavailable, unreliable, or difficult to interpret quantitatively. It can reveal an indirect exposure which can not be recalled or comprehended by the patient, for example, an environmental or domestic exposure during childhood. While positive results confirm past exposures, negative results do not satisfactorily overrule a clear exposure history, especially one involving chrysotile. In surgically treated lung cancer patients, systematic counting of asbestos bodies in the resected lung tissue can be used to detect cases that require evaluation for a possible occupational cause. In particular an excess of feruginous bodies should stimulate a careful assessment of the histological appearances for interstitial fibrosis and the possible need for fiber-counting analysis. This can easily be performed routinely by optical microscopic analysis of digested lung samples, though an electron microscopic assessment may be preferred [28].

Atmospheric characterization

Asbestos levels in air samples from the workplace are usually evaluated by a membrane filter method [86]. The collected fibers are identified by phase-contrast optical microscopy (PCOM) with the following criteria: length >5 mm, aspect ratio (length/width) >3/1, and diameter <3 mm (broader fibers are considered non-respirable). The detection limit for fiber diameter by PCOM is 0.25–0.4 mm, and so fibers thinner than 0.25 mm and shorter than 5 mm are not counted. Examples of historic exposure levels that were clearly associated with an asbestosis risk are as follows [87]:

Crocidolite mine (South Africa)	650–1500 f/ml
Shipyard (removal of insulation, crocidolite)	200–400 f/ml
Chrysotile mines (Corsica)	20–282 f/ml
Asbestos processing (various)	0.1–2000 f/ml.

Current exposure standards, if respected throughout a working life, are associated with a very low probability for the development of asbestosis.

Differential diagnosis

Many interstitial lung diseases may be confused with asbestosis because of similar clinical and radiographic features. Most are, at least potentially, treatable by exposure cessation (e.g. hypersensitivity pneumonitis, drug-induced lung disease) and/or by immunosuppressive therapy (e.g. connective tissue disorders, idiopathic pulmonary fibrosis), and so need to be distinguished from asbestosis. A study by Gaensler showed that approximately 5% of cases of diffuse interstitial fibrosis in asbestos-exposed workers were found to be a consequence of idiopathic pulmonary fibrosis [12]. This percentage can

Box 9.1 Histopathology (Andrew Churg)

The gross appearance of asbestosis is similar to that of usual interstitial pneumonia (UIP; also called 'idiopathic interstitial pulmonary fibrosis', IPF; or 'cryptogenic fibrosing alveolitis', CFA) with lower zone fibrosis and honeycombing in advanced cases. Disease is always more severe in the lower lung zones; disease that is more severe in the upper zones is almost certainly not asbestosis.

The microscopic appearance of well-established asbestosis is similar to that of idiopathic interstitial pulmonary fibrosis except for the presence of asbestos bodies in tissue. The fibrotic component consists of a variable pattern of interstitial collagen and inflammatory cells. Both diffuse fibrosis and asbestos bodies (at least one) must be found to make the diagnosis microscopically (Fig. 9.9). The patho-logist should be sure that the process he or she is calling asbestosis is diffuse, preferably by finding that there is functional or radiographic evidence of diffuse disease, and not just a local reaction to tumor or radiation or some other process, since this type of fibrosis can mimic asbestosis in a small area of tissue. More detailed descriptions and illustrations of the pathological findings in asbestosis are provided in more specialized text [46].

Asbestos as well as other mineral dusts produce abnormalities in the region of the respiratory bronchioles and alveolar ducts: the walls of these airways become fibrotic and asbestos bodies may be present when the inciting dust is asbestos. This lesion should be interpreted with great caution. Although some authors regard it as a form of early asbestosis, it more likely represents a non-specific airway reaction to a variety of inorganic dusts [46], and it is not associated with the radiographic, clinical, or physiologic changes of classical asbestosis.

Rarely one sees cases of diffuse interstitial fibrosis without histologic evidence of asbestos bodies in patients with histories of asbestos exposure. In such instances mineralogic analysis may show that substantial amounts of asbestos are actually present and that the disease is really ('occult') asbestosis. Much more often, however, analysis fails to reveal increased amounts of asbestos and the process must be considered to have some other basis, e.g. UIP [12].

Most cases of asbestosis can be diagnosed on clinical grounds if an appropriate history is combined with

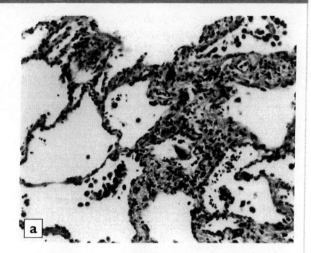

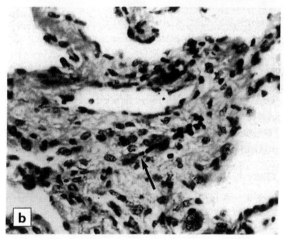

Fig. 9.9 Histologic appearances of asbestosis from open biopsy: (a) low power; (b) high power. The arrow identifies an asbestos body

characteristic roentgenographic and functional changes, and biopsy should be reserved for clinically atypical cases. Open biopsy is the procedure of choice when tissue is needed. As is true of UIP and any other type of diffuse interstitial fibrosis, transbronchial biopsy may be inadequate and lead to an incorrect or incomplete diagnosis.

---

be expected to increase in the future, since the prevalence of asbestosis is now decreasing, whereas that of idiopathic pulmonary fibrosis appears to be increasing [88]. The main differences distinguishing these two disorders are listed in Table 9.2.

Smoking may exert a confounding influence in the interpretation of several of the diagnostic procedures for asbestosis. Occupational exposure to dust is associated with an increased probability of smoking, and smoking is associated with small irregular opacities on

chest radiographs simulating asbestosis. It may also lead to a reduction in D_{LCO} when lung function is measured, and to the demonstration of macrophage and neutrophil alveolitis in BAL. Not surprisingly, asbestosis, as defined from its radiological appearances, seems to be more prevalent among the smokers than non-smokers of workers with asbestos exposure [33,89]. This may simply reflect the tendency among individuals who are most able to tolerate cigarette smoking being those who are most likely to tolerate work in a

Table 9.2 Clinical differential diagnosis of asbestosis and idiopathic lung fibrosis

	Asbestosis	Idiopathic lung fibrosis
Physical signs		
Clubbing	±	++
Lung function		
D_LCO decrease	+	++
Imaging (chest radiographs and HRCT)		
Location	Subpleural, lower zones	More widespread (mid, even upper zones) posterior and anterior
Honeycombing	+	++
Ground-glass opacities	±	+
Associated lesions		
Pleural lesions (plaques, thickening)	++	—
Parenchymal bands	+	—
Progression of disease	Slow or absent	Variable, might be rapid
BAL	Asbestos bodies ++	Rare or absent

dusty environment. Alternatively, smoking might increase fiber retention because excess mucus or airway narrowing enhances deposition, or because smoking interferes with clearance [42].

The recognition that asbestosis itself is the diagnosis relies upon three major criteria [2,90,91]:

- There is diffuse interstitial pulmonary fibrosis.
- There has been sufficient cumulative exposure to asbestos, as shown by:
  - an appropriate history with respect to intensity, duration, and latency; or
  - mineralogic analysis of BAL or lung tissue.
- The absence of more plausible causes.

Direct histopathological examination of lung tissue is the most reliable method of diagnosis, since it may provide definitive information concerning all three criteria, and may show evidence of asbestosis even when chest radiographs and lung function appear normal. It provides the 'gold standard', and is critical to ongoing research with material made available from lung resections or autopsy examinations. Biopsy is rarely necessary, however, in investigating the individual patient and, in practice, chest radiographs, HRCT scans, and lung function tests provide adequate data for the confirmation of interstitial pulmonary fibrosis and the assessment of its severity. This can be attributed to asbestosis if the exposure history is consistent and alternative causes appear improbable [70]. Nevertheless, doubt sometimes remains between asbestosis and other types of interstitial lung disease, and so biopsy may be indicated. Transbronchial biopsy may occasionally be useful, though larger and more satisfactory samples

can be obtained almost as readily from video-assisted thoracoscopy and are generally required for a confident pathologic diagnosis of asbestosis. The matter is the source of some controversy, since some pathologists take the view that transbronchial biopsies are too prone to sampling error to be reliable. A clear benefit following steroid therapy, confirmed by physiological improvement, implies that some other disorder is present rather than asbestosis, though occasionally asbestosis is present additionally.

Table 9.3 summarizes the diagnostic criteria for asbestosis of the American Thoracic Society, among which chest radiography showing grade 1/1 or more opacities is considered the most important [70]. There has been some evolution in their application subsequently and, when Harber reviewed the diagnostic criteria as used in published literature, he found that most investigators used a profusion of small opacities equal to or greater than 1/0 as the main (only) defining criterion of asbestosis, irrespec-

Table 9.3 American Thoracic Society criteria for asbestosis [70]

- A reliable history of asbestos exposure

- An appropriate time interval between exposure and detection

- Clinical criteria
  Chest roentgenographic evidence of type s, t, u, small irregular opacities of a profusion of 1/1 or greater.
  A restrictive pattern of lung impairment with an FVC below the lower limit of normal.
  A diffusing capacity below the lower limit of normal.

- Bilateral inspiratory crackles at the posterior lung bases not cleared by cough.

tive of functional abnormalities [90]. The increasing use of HRCT has, of course, led to the recognition of asbestosis much earlier and at much less serious degrees of severity than has been possible using traditional chest radiographs, and it has been suggested that its definition has changed over the years in consequence. A diagnostic approach which includes increasingly sensitive techniques of investigation implies that the severity and the prevalence of the disease will respectively decrease (so-called 'diagnostic dilution') and increase, and so it is important to understand the diagnostic base before considering the natural history of the disease – particularly the probability of progression [90].

Reliance upon chest radiographs and the ILO classification is no longer appropriate to confirm or refute a diagnosis of asbestosis. The vast majority of recent studies have shown HRCT to be more sensitive (it detects abnormalities not shown on chest radiographs) and more specific (it distinguishes opacities due to emphysema or pleural disease from those due to interstitial fibrosis) than chest radiographs, and is particularly useful in evaluating lung fibrosis. Gallium scanning has also proved to be more sensitive than chest radiography in detecting early interstitial disease, but the abnormalities have poor specificity and the technique has no practical value in the investigation of asbestosis at present.

MANAGEMENT

Of the individual

There is no effective specific therapy for asbestosis. Some symptoms (e.g. cough) may be amenable to palliation with medication, and if hypoxemia and cor pulmonale develop long-term oxygen therapy should be considered. Although oxygen supplementation from concentrators for 16 hours or more daily for cor pulmonale from COPD has been shown to improve survival (in the absence of continued smoking), a survival benefit has not been investigated in asbestosis.

Once asbestosis is diagnosed, there should be no further exposure. In practice occupational exposure will usually have ceased anyway, since most cases now present after retirement. Even when this is not so, current exposure regulations in most countries should prevent ongoing exposure to any meaningful degree. There may consequently be a dilemma if asbestosis is recognized in an individual who remains sufficiently fit to work and whose livelihood depends on continued work with asbestos, though in circumstances which should pose negligible risk. An evaluation of the true risk is crucial. For an insulation worker engaged daily in the removal of asbestos

material, the risk depends primarily on the effectiveness of the respiratory protection equipment with which he is supplied. Any accident or equipment failure could increase the lung fiber burden by a clinically important degree, particularly in a subject shown already to be susceptible, and so the risk may not be acceptable. By contrast, an electrician with frequent previous work in contaminated occupational environments may be able to adjust future engagements to sites in which asbestos is likely to be encountered only rarely and briefly. If insulation material is encountered in unexpected situations, a respirator can be used with little risk of failure. Alternatively, the task can be postponed pending an analytical inspection.

Asbestosis indicates a high cumulative exposure to asbestos and is associated with an increased risk for the development of lung cancer, and by a multiplicative not additive degree with respect to the existing risk. If the subject is a smoker, the combined multiplicative risk may be substantial and he should be informed of this and advised most strongly to avoid smoking. The concomitant presence in current smokers of COPD provides a further pressing indication for smoking cessation, though smoking has not been shown to increase the risk of progression of asbestosis once asbestos exposure has ceased.

The high risk for lung cancer in smokers (and former smokers) with asbestosis suggests a possible benefit from emerging surveillance programs based on low-dose CT scanning [92]. Earlier surveillance programs for lung cancer using chest radiographs and sputum cytology proved to be disappointing, and no survival benefit was observed, but there is optimism that the greater sensitivity of these new imaging procedures may identify some resectable lung cancers before they become incurable. If such programs are to succeed, regular surveillance will be necessary, which poses a major problem with regard to resources and compliance. The relative risk for lung cancer increases proportionally with the severity of lung fibrosis, whether demonstrated radiologically or pathologically, and by the cumulative exposure to tobacco smoke, and so surveillance programs should be focused accordingly [93,94]. A possible increased risk for lung cancer has also been reported in asbestos-exposed workers in the absence of small radiographic opacities, but the issue is controversial and the increase in risk in such circumstances is not likely to exceed two-fold [95].

Last but not least, the physician diagnosing asbestosis should provide advice concerning the administrative procedures which may help the afflicted worker obtain appropriate recognition and compensation (see Chapters 35–37). Ongoing surveillance with regular pulmonary function tests and, when indicated, chest radiographs or HRCT should be provided to detect progression, if this is not provided by compensation authorities. Intervals of 2–5 years are generally justified for a revised assessment of respiratory disablement and an appropriate adjustment in financial benefit.

Of the workforce

If one member of a workforce is found to have asbestosis, it is important to ensure that there is no unsuspected asbestos hazard for other workers. In most cases, the disease will have resulted from earlier work elsewhere in an environment well known to be associated with asbestos exposure, and so no further action will be required. If the probable source of dust exposure is not recognized to be an asbestos hazard, appropriate enquiries should be made about the work process and the work environment, and the physician should make contact with the employer, or the relevant occupational physician.

PREVENTION

In the workplace

Regulations concerning the protection of workers against the risk of asbestosis necessarily differ from country to country. In most there have been marked changes over recent decades. In some industrialized countries the use of asbestos is now forbidden, and in most of the remainder permitted exposure levels have reached very low levels. If there is compliance with these legislative controls, asbestosis will be prevented. Such levels represent very substantial reductions indeed from the several thousands of fibers per milliliter measured historically in asbestos mines and shipyards [87]. Within public buildings and schools, the ambient levels are usually below 0.01 f/ml (mean values < 0.0005 f/ml) and so there is no risk of asbestosis from such environments [31].

In many countries the greatest persisting risk for asbestosis is associated with asbestos removal. This has the potential to produce high fiber concentrations, and efficient measures of personal protection (airfed respirators, clothing) are essential, together with the use of effective extraction and filtering equipment so that any environmental contamination is minimized.

An essential additional element in prevention is the evaluation of risk associated with different levels of ambient exposure. This is enhanced by the use of the most sensitive method for detecting early disease. A recent study compared HRCT with chest radiographs to detect probable asbestosis in 585 asbestos-exposed workers in Normandy, France [96]. From serial exposure measurements and standardized job questionnaires, four cumulative exposure groups were identified: <25, 25–99, 100–199, and 200 [f/ml].yr. The HRCT scans demonstrated a significant trend of increasing prevalence of diffuse interstitial fibrosis with increasing level of exposure (0.0, 5.8, 5.1, 12.9%; $P < 0.01$), but the chest radiographs proved to be much less specific and no significant trend was observed when an ILO profusion of small irregular opacities category 1/0 was taken as evidence of interstitial fibrosis (18.0, 18.7, 14.6, 16.1%). The study consequently produced reassuring evidence that even HRCT could not detect asbestosis after a cumulative exposure <25 [f/ml].yr.

In a subsequent longitudinal study using the same cumulative exposure groups, 113 of the workers underwent a second HRCT after 2–5 years. New 'incident' cases of diffuse interstitial fibrosis were observed in 0.0, 5.3, 3.3, and 11.6%, respectively, of the exposure groups, but the trend was not statistically significant. Interestingly, out of 20 cases who had shown discrete interstitial abnormalities at the first HRCT examination (mainly ground-glass opacities and nonseptal lines), four (20%) developed fibrosis against three in the subgroup with an initially normal scan (3.4%). These observations are again reassuring that cumulative exposure <25 [f/ml].yr carries little or no risk for asbestosis. Moreover, they confirm that only a small proportion of workers will develop the disease, even in the more heavily exposed groups. It should be noted that the studied population comprised retired workers without previously recognized occupational disease. There is thus a selection bias (healthy worker effect) in the sense that they are likely to represent a population without high susceptibility to asbestos.

Table 9.4 shows the statistical trends for incident cases of non-malignant asbestos-related disorders in Belgium over four periods, 1953–1997. The number of cases recognized each year is increasing, but this

Table 9.4 Incident cases of non-malignant asbestos-related diseases (including pleural lesions only) and breakdown of the prevalent cases according to the rate of permanent invalidity. *Source: Occupational Diseases Fund, Brussels, Belgium* [97]

	Incident cases recognized/year	Percentage of disability in prevalent cases	
		< 25%	> 75%
1953–1972	6.7	8%	50.6%
1972–1979	35.6	40.8%	21%
1984–1985	140	65%	14.9%
1996–1997	238.5	75%	9.4%

is chiefly a consequence of benign pleural disease with low or no functional impairment. This is illustrated by the continuous decline in corresponding disability.

Another illustration of effective prevention of asbestosis has been reported by Gaensler and colleagues [98]. Of 1764 employees evaluated during industrial surveys, 254 (14.4%) were presumed to have asbestosis because of ILO radiograph profusion readings of ≥1/0. The prevalence decreased from 47.6% for those first exposed before 1950, to 18% for first exposure during 1950–1959, and to 2% for first exposure after 1960. The use of category 1/1 as the diagnostic threshold would reduced these figures, respectively, to 36.4%, 10.2%, and 0.6%.

National regulatory strategies

Table 9.5 provides a summary of the exposure controls for asbestos legislated within the European Union. In 1996 the European Commission postponed the adoption of any further restriction on asbestos use, but an increasing number of member

Table 9.5 Occupational exposure limits for asbestos (f/ml)

	Chrysotile	Other forms of asbestos
European Union	0.60	0.30
Austria	0.15	0.15
Belgium	0.50	0.15
Denmark	0.30	0.30
Finland	0.30	0.30
France	0.30	0.10
Germany	0.15	0.15
Greece	1.00	0.50
Italy	0.60	0.20
Netherlands	0.30	0.10
Spain	0.60	0.30
United Kingdom	0.50	0.20

states have implemented exposure limits that are more stringent than those specified by current legislation of the European Union as a whole (see table). For instance, Denmark, France, Germany, Italy, the Netherlands, and Sweden have passed regulations which, with some exceptions, practically phase out the future use of all varieties of asbestos.

DIFFICULT CASE

History

An electrician aged 63 years developed breathlessness and cough in 1994. His work from 1956 until 1987 had led to regular, almost daily, close contact with asbestos in the large buildings in which he installed electric cables. Asbestos insulation (chrysotile and amosite) had been used particularly extensively in such buildings to provide fire insulation and false ceilings, because a major fire of 1967 in a department store in his town had caused over 300 deaths. He had smoked to 1984, consuming a total of 30 pack-years.

Rheumatoid arthritis was diagnosed in 1980, which caused his premature retirement in 1987. He was treated from 1989 with prednisolone (5–10 mg daily) and methotrexate (7.5–15 mg weekly). Rheumatoid serology was strongly positive. Between 1994 and 1999, the erythrocyte sedimentation rate ranged from 42 to 100 mm/h and the C-reactive protein from 0.5 to 22 mg/dl.

By 2000 there was moderate respiratory disablement, largely masked by his rheumatoid disease. Auscultation then revealed bilateral crackles, and there were typical bone and joint deformities of rheumatoid arthritis. A plain chest radiograph was considered to show small irregular opacities (s/t, 1/1 by the ILO classification) and pleural plaques.

HRCT scans were carried out in 1994 (Fig. 9.10) and 2000 without apparent change, pleural plaques being evident in some sections. Lung function tests had been carried out at 2-yearly intervals since 1990. The results are illustrated in Fig. 9.11.

BAL was performed twice. In 1994: total cells; 200/mm³ (macrophages 93%, neutrophils 5%, lymphocytes 1%,

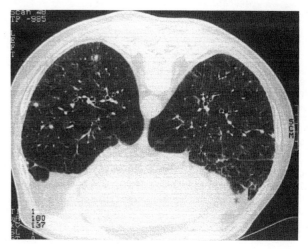

Fig. 9.10 Difficult case: HRCT, 1994.

eosinophils 1%), mineral analysis, 5.4 asbestos bodies/ml. In 2000: total cells; 430/mm³ (macrophages 81%, neutrophils 14%, lymphocytes 3%, eosinophils 2%).

Issues

The chief issues here are the nature of this man's respiratory disease (bronchiolitis, emphysema, fibrosing alveolitis, or a combination of these), the nature of any alveolitis if this is present (rheumatoid lung, asbestosis, or methotrexate lung), and the contribution if any of asbestosis to his disablement.

Comment

The book's contributors considered fibrosing alveolitis to be the major cause of respiratory disablement, though some concluded there was additionally smoking-induced COPD. A majority thought the fibrosing interstitial disease was a consequence of both asbestosis and rheumatoid lung.

Electricians are often exposed occupationally to asbestos, and mesothelioma or benign pleural disorders are not uncommonly seen among them. Asbestosis is much less common, since cumulative levels of exposure are usually insufficient. In his case, however, exposures are likely to have been unusually heavy (the evidence of the history and the BAL lavage findings), and they are known to have involved the amphibole, amosite. The possibility of rheumatoid-associated fibrosing alveolitis (rheumatoid lung) is not readily dismissed either, particularly as his rheumatoid disease was clearly active and progressive over the relevant years, and the physicians managing him concluded that both asbestosis and rheumatoid lung are contributing. The lung function tests suggest a possible reduction of FEV_1/FVC over the course of the last 10 years together with an increase rather than decrease of TLC, and so there is additionally physiological evidence of COPD, but the HRCT scan (including cuts not illustrated here) indicates that emphysema is not playing a major role in his lung disease.

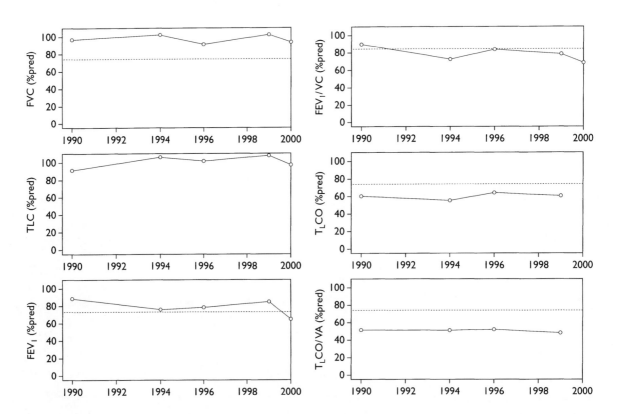

Fig. 9.11 Serial lung function tests. Dashed line denotes lower limit of normal range.

SUMMARY POINTS

Recognition

- The gold standard for diagnosis is histologic examination of lung tissue, and the demonstration of diffuse interstitial fibrosis with asbestos bodies in the tissue sections; in practice, biopsy is rarely needed.
- A clinical diagnosis relies on:
  - the demonstration of diffuse interstitial disease on chest radiographs or HRCT scans;
  - the identification of probable heavy asbestos exposure by history, or mineralogic analysis of sputum or bronchoalveolar lavage fluid;
  - the improbability of other causes.
- Although mesothelioma and pleural plaques may develop after low levels of cumulative exposure, asbestosis is not likely to arise after exposures < 25[f/ml].year.
- Imaging by HRCT is preferable to that by chest radiography because of its superior sensitivity and specificity.
- Lung function abnormalities (restricted ventilation with diminished D_LCO and KCO) provide supporting evidence of diffuse interstitial fibrosis, and characterize its severity, but are otherwise non-specific.

Management

- Once established, the disease process cannot be modified by any currently available treatment.
- Some symptoms may be palliated, e.g. cough.
- Long-term oxygen therapy should be considered if there is persistent hypoxemia.

- There should be no further exposure, but small risks of unexpected exposure may be acceptable in regions of legally enforced exposure controls, if continued employment is otherwise not feasible.
- The high risk of lung cancer attributable to the interactive effect between asbestosis, asbestos exposure, and tobacco smoke should be explained, and smoking cessation strongly encouraged.
- Regular surveillance with HRCT may be justified in smokers and former smokers in the hope of identifying lung cancer at a resectable and curable stage.
- Advice should be provided concerning the right to compensation.
- Consideration should be given to the possible risks faced by fellow workers, and hence the possible need for exposure-level monitoring and exposure control.

Prevention

- Exposure should be avoided by using alternative materials wherever economically possible.
- Where exposure may exceed statutory limits, there should be a program of regular monitoring to evaluate compliance, coupled with a possible need for exposure controls and/or personal protection devices.
- Where asbestos has to be used (or has to be removed) and exposure levels are likely to exceed statutory limits, dust emission should be minimized by the use of local exhaust ventilation fitted with appropriate filters, and workers should be protected with appropriate respirators and clothing.

REFERENCES

1. Consensus report: Asbestos, asbestosis, and cancer: the Helsinki criteria for diagnosis and attribution. *Scand J Work Environ Health* 1997; 23: 311–316.
2. Rosenberg DM. Asbestos-related disorders. A realistic perspective. *Chest* 1997; 111: 1424–1426.
3. Gibbs AR, Gardner MJ, Pooley FD *et al*. Fibre levels and disease in workers from a factory using predominantly amosite. *Environ Health Perspect* 1994; 102 (Suppl 5): 261–263.
4. Ashcroft T, Heppleston AG. The optical and electron microscope determination of pulmonary asbestos fibre concentrations and its relation to the human pathological reaction. *J Clin Pathol* 1973; 26: 224–234.
5. Hammar SP, Dodson RF. Asbestos. In: Dail DH, Hammar SP, eds. *Pulmonary Pathology*, pp. 901–983. New York: Springer-Verlag 1989.
6. Kendall T. Asbestos production: survivors counting Asian cost. *Ind Minerals* 1998; 384: 80–87.
7. Virta R. *Asbestos*. US Geological Survey: Mineral Commodity Summaries 1999: 1–29.
8. Peto J, Hodgson JT, Matthews FE, Jones JR. Continuing increase in mesothelioma mortality in Britain. *Lancet* 1995; 345: 535–539.
9. Expertise Collective INSERM. *Effects sur la Santé des Principaux Types d'Exposition à l'Amiante*. Paris: Editions INSERM, 1997.
10. Lilis R, Miller A, Godbold J *et al*. Radiographic abnormalities in asbestos insulators: effects of duration from onset of exposure and smoking. Relationships of dyspnea with parenchymal and pleural fibrosis. *Am J Ind Med* 1991; 20: 1–15.
11. De Vuyst P, Dumortier P, Gevenois PA. Analysis of asbestos bodies in BAL from subjects with particular exposures. *Am J Indust Med* 1997; 31: 699–704.
12. Gaensler EA, Jederlinic PJ, Churg A. Idiopathic pulmonary fibrosis in asbestos-exposed workers. *Am Rev Respir Dis* 1991; 144: 689–696.
13. De Vuyst P, Dumortier P, Jacobovitz D *et al*. Environmental asbestosis complicated by lung cancer. *Chest* 1994; 105: 1593–1595.
14. Dumortier P, Coplü L, De Maertelaer V *et al*. Assessment of environmental exposure in Turkey by bronchoalveolar lavage. *Am J Respir Crit Care Med* 1998; 158: 1815–1824.
15. Cookson W, De Klerk N, Musk AW *et al*. The natural history of asbestosis in former crocidolite workers of Wittenoom Gorge. *Am Rev Respir Dis* 1986; 133: 994–998.

16. Jakobsson K, Strömberg U, Albin M et al. Radiological changes in asbestos cement workers. *Occup Environ Med* 1995; 52: 20–27.

17. Viallat JR, Boutin C, Pietri JF, Fondarai J. Late progression of radiographic changes in Canari crysotile mine and mill exworkers. *Arch Environ Health* 1983; 38: 54–58.

18. Becklake M, Liddell FDK, Manfreda J, McDonald JC. Radiological changes after withdrawal from asbestos exposure. *Br J Ind Med* 1979; 36: 23–28.

19. Jones RN, Diem JE, Hughes JM et al. Progression of asbestos effects: a prospective longitudinal study of chest radiographs and lung function. *Br J Ind Med* 1989; 46: 97–105.

20. Browne K. Asbestos-related disorders. In: Parkes WR, ed. *Occupational Lung Disorders*, 3rd edn., pp. 411–504. Oxford, Butterworth Heinemann, 1994.

21. Berry G. The mortality of workers certified by pneumoconiosis medical panels as having asbestos disease. *Br J Ind Med* 1981; 38: 130–137.

22. Ontario Royal Commission on Matters of Health and Safety Arising from the Use of Asbestos in Ontario. Toronto: 1984. Ontario Ministry of the Attorney General.

23. Peto J, Doll R, Hermon C et al. Relationship of mortality to measures of environmental asbestos pollution in an asbestos textile factory. *Ann Occup Hyg* 1985; 29:304.

24. Cowden JD, Will JG, Schwartz DA. Genetics of environmental lung disease. *Sem Respir Crit Care Med* 1999; 20: 531–540.

25. Begin R, Martel M, Desmarais Y et al. Fibronectin and procollagen 3 levels in bronchoalveolar lavage of asbestos-exposed human subjects and sheep. *Chest* 1986; 89: 237–243.

26. Begin R, Sebastien P. Excessive accumulation of asbestos fibre in the bronchoalveolar space may be a marker of individual susceptibility to developing asbestosis: experimental evidence. *Br J Ind Med* 1989; 46: 853–855.

27. De Vuyst P, Karjalainen A, Dumortier P et al. Guidelines for mineral fibre analyses in biological samples: report of the ERS working group. *Eur Respir J* 1998; 11: 1416–1426.

28. Becklake M, Case B. Fiber burden and asbestos-related lung disease: determinants of dose response relationship. *Am J Respir Crit Care Med* 1994; 150: 1488–1492.

29. Becklake M. The epidemiology of asbestosis. In: Liddell D, Miller K, eds. *Mineral Fibers and Health*. pp. 103–119. Boca Raton, FL: CRC Press 1991.

30. Boutin C, Dumortier P, Rey F et al. Black spots concentrate oncogenic asbestos fibers in the parietal pleura. *Am J Respir Crit Care Med* 1996; 153: 444–449.

31. Health Effects Institute–Asbestos Research. *Asbestos in Public and Commercial Buildings*. A literature review and synthesis of current knowledge. HEI-AR publication available from HEI-AR, 141 Portland Street, Suite 7100, Cambridge, MA USA 02139, 1991.

32. Iwatsubo Y, Pairon JC, Boutin C et al. Pleural mesothelioma: dose-response relation at low levels of asbestos exposure in a French population-based case–control study. *Am J Epidemiol* 1998; 148: 133–142.

33. Miller A, Lilis R, Godbold J et al. Relationship of pulmonary function to radiographic interstitial fibrosis in 2611 long-term asbestos insulators. *Am Rev Respir Dis* 1992; 145: 263–270.

34. Schwartz DA, Davis CS, Merchant JA et al. Longitudinal changes in lung function among asbestos-exposed workers. *Am J Respir Crit Care Med* 1994; 150: 1243–1249.

35. Garcia JG, Griffith DE, Williams JS et al. Reduced diffusing capacity as an isolated finding in asbestos-and silica-exposed workers. *Chest* 1990; 98: 105–111.

36. Schwartz DA, Galvin JR, Dayton CS et al. Determinants of restrictive lung function in asbestos-induced pleural fibrosis. *J Appl Physiol* 1990; 68: 1932–1937.

37. Wright JL, Cagle P, Churg A et al. Diseases of the small airways. *Am Rev Respir Dis* 1992; 146: 240–262.

38. Fournier-Massey G, Becklake M. Pulmonary function profiles in Quebec asbestos workers. *Bull Physiopathol Respir* 1975; 11: 429–445.

39. Begin R, Cantin A, Berthiaume T, et al. Airway function in lifetime-nonsmoking older asbestos workers. *Am J Med* 1983; 75: 631–638.

40. Begin R, Boileau R, Peloquin S. Asbestos exposure, cigarette smoking, and airflow limitation in long-term Canadian chrysotile miners and millers. *Am J Ind Med* 1987; 11: 55–66.

41. Churg A, Wright JL, Wiggs B et al. Small airways disease and mineral dust exposure. *Am Rev Respir Dis* 1985; 131: 139–143.

42. Tron V, Wright J, Harrison N et al. Cigarette smoke makes airway and early parenchymal asbestos-induced lung disease worse in the guinea pig. *Am Rev Respir Dis* 1987; 136: 271–275.

43. Jones RN, Glindmeyer HW, Weill H. Review of the Kilburn and Warshaw Chest article. Airways obstruction from asbestos exposure. *Chest* 1995; 107: 1727–1729.

44. Trethowan WN, Burge PS, Rossiter CE et al. Study of the respiratory health of employees in seven European plants that manufacture ceramic fibres. *Occup Environ Med* 1995; 52: 97–104.

45. Hansen EF, Rasmussen FV, Hardt F, Kamstrup O. Lung function and respiratory health of long-term fiber-exposed stonewool factory workers. *Am J Respir Crit Care Med* 1999; 160: 466–472.

46. Churg A. Nonneoplastic diseases caused by asbestos. In: Churg A, Green FHY, eds. *Pathology of Occupational Lung Disease*, Vol 8, pp. 279–285. New York: Igaaku-Shoin Publications, 1988.

47. International Labour Office. Guidelines for the Use of ILO International Classification of Radiographs of Pneumoconioses. Revised Edition International Labour Office Safety and Health series No. 22 (Rev. 80). Geneva: International Labour Office, 1980.

48. Dick JA, Morgan WKC, Muir DFC et al. The significance of irregular opacities on the chest roentgenogram. *Chest* 1992; 102: 251–260.

49. Barnhart S, Thornquist M, Omenn GS et al. The degree of roentgenographic parenchymal opacities attributable to smoking among asbestos-exposed subjects. *Am Rev Respir Dis* 1990; 141: 1102–1106.

50. Hnizdo E, Sluis-Cremer GK. Effect of tobacco smoking on the presence of asbestosis at postmortem and on the reading of irregular opacities on roentgenograms in asbestos-exposed workers. *Am Rev Respir Dis* 1988; 138: 1207–1212.

51. Friedman AC, Fiel SB, Fisher MS et al. Asbestos-related pleural disease and asbestosis: a comparison of CT and chest radiography. *AJR* 1988; 150: 269–275.

52. Epler GR, McLoud TC, Gaensler EA et al. Normal roentgenograms in chronic diffuse infiltrative lung disease. *N Engl J Med* 1978; 298: 934–939.

53. Grenier P, Valeyre D, Cluzel P et al. Chronic diffuse interstitial lung disease: diagnostic value of chest radiography and high-resolution CT. *Radiology* 1991; 179: 123–132.

54. Remy-Jardin M, Remy J, Deffontaines C, Duhamel A. Assessment of diffuse infiltrative lung disease: comparison of conventional CT and high-resolution CT. *Radiology* 1991; 181: 157–162.

55. Gevenois PA, De Vuyst P, Dedeire S *et al.* Conventional and high-resolution CT in asymptomatic asbestos-exposed workers. *Acta Radiol* 1994; 35: 226–229.

56. Neri S, Antonelli A, Falaschi F *et al.* Findings from high resolution computed tomography of the lung and pleura of symptom free workers exposed to amosite who had normal chest radiographs and pulmonary function tests. *Occup Environ Med* 1994; 51: 239–243.

57. Aberle DR, Gamsu G, Ray CS, Feuerstein IM. Asbestos-related pleural and parenchymal fibrosis: detection with high-resolution CT. *Radiology* 1988; 166: 729–734.

58. Lynch DA. CT for asbestosis: value and limitations. *AJR* 1995; 164: 69–71.

59. Aberle DR, Gamsu G, Ray CS. High-resolution CT of benign asbestos-related diseases: clinical and radiographic correlation. *AJR* 1988; 151: 883–891.

60. Austin JHM, Müller NL, Friedman PJ *et al.* Glossary of terms for CT of the lungs: recommendations of the nomenclature committee of the Fleischner Society. *Radiology* 1996; 200: 327–331.

61. Bergin CJ, Castellino RA, Blank N, Moses L. Specificity of high-resolution CT findings in pulmonary asbestosis: do patients scanned for other indications have similar findings? *AJR* 1994; 163: 551–555.

62. Al-Jarad N, Strickland B, Pearson MC *et al.* High resolution computed tomographic assessment of asbestosis and cryptogenic fibrosing alveolitis: a comparative study. *Thorax* 1992; 47: 645–650.

63. Gamsu G, Salmon CJ, Warnock ML, Blanc PD. CT quantification of interstitial fibrosis in patients with asbestosis: a comparison of two methods. *AJR* 1995; 164: 63–68.

64. Staples CA, Gamsu G, Ray CS, Webb RW. High resolution computed tomography and lung function in asbestos-exposed workers with normal chest radiographs. *Am Rev Respir Dis* 1989; 139: 1502–1508.

65. Doyle TC, Lawler GA. CT features of rounded atelectasis on the lung. *AJR* 1984; 143: 225–228.

66. Gevenois PA, de Maertelaer V, Madani A *et al.* Asbestosis, pleural plaques and diffuse pleural thickening: three distinct benign responses to asbestos exposure. *Eur Respir J* 1998; 11: 1021–1027.

67. McLoud T, Woods BO, Carrington CB *et al.* Diffuse pleural thickening in an asbestos-exposed population: prevalence and causes. *AJR* 1985; 144: 9–18.

68. De Vuyst P, Pfitzenmeyer P, Camus Ph. Asbestos, ergot drugs and the pleura. *Eur Respir J* 1997; 10: 2695–2698.

69. McLoud T. The use of CT in the examination of asbestos-exposed persons. *Radiology* 1988; 169: 862–863.

70. Murphy RL, Becklake MR, Brooks SM *et al.* The diagnosis of nonmalignant diseases related to asbestos. *Am Rev Respir Dis* 1986; 134: 363–368.

71. Rockoff SD, Schwartz A. Roentgenographic underestimation of early asbestosis by International Labor Organization classification. *Chest* 1988; 93: 1088–1091.

72. Harkin TJ, McGuinness G, Goldring G *et al.* Differentiation in the ILO boundary chest roentgenograph (0/1 to 1/0) in asbestosis by high-resolution computed tomography scan, alveolitis, and respiratory impairment. *J Occup Environ Med* 1996; 38: 46–52.

73. Costabel U, Bross KJ, Huck E *et al.* Lung and blood lymphocyte subsets in asbestosis and in mixed dust pneumoconiosis. *Chest* 1987; 91: 110–112.

74. Robinson BW, Rose AH, James A *et al.* Alveolitis of pulmonary asbestosis. Bronchoalveolar lavage studies in crocidolite- and chrysotile-exposed individuals. *Chest* 1986; 90: 396–402.

75. Al-Jarad N, Gellert AR, Rudd RM. Bronchoalveolar lavage and ^{99m}Tc-DTPA clearance as prognostic factors in asbestos workers with and without asbestosis. *Respir Med* 1993; 87: 365–374.

76. Cullen MR, Merrill WW. Association between neutrophil concentration in bronchoalveolar lavage fluid and recent losses in diffusing capacity in men formerly exposed to asbestos. *Chest* 1992; 102: 682–687.

77. Rom WN, Travis WD. Lymphocyte–macrophage alveolitis in nonsmoking individuals occupationally exposed to asbestos. *Chest* 1992; 101: 779–786.

78. Sprince NL, Olivier LC, McLoud TC *et al.* Asbestos exposure and asbestos-related pleural and parenchymal disease. Associations with immune imbalance. *Am Rev Respir Dis* 1991; 143(4 Pt 1): 822–828.

79. Schwartz DA, Galvin JR, Merchant RK *et al.* Influence of cigarette smoking on bronchoalveolar lavage cellularity in asbestos-induced lung disease. *Am Rev Respir Dis* 1992; 145: 400–405.

80. Schwartz DA, Galvin JR, Frees KL *et al.* Clinical relevance of cellular mediators of inflammation in workers exposed to asbestos. *Am Rev Respir Dis* 1993; 148: 68–74.

81. De Vuyst P, Dumortier P, Moulin E *et al.* Diagnostic value of asbestos in bronchoalveolar lavage fluid. *Am Rev Respir Dis* 1987; 136: 1219–1224.

82. Gibbs A. In: WK Morgan A Seaton, eds. *Occupational Lung Diseases*, London: WB Saunders p. 149. 1995

83. Roggli VL, Greenberg SD, Pratt PhC. *Pathology of Asbestos-associated Diseases*, pp. 299–345. Boston: Little, Brown, 1992.

84. Craighead JE, Abraham JL, Churg A *et al.* The pathology of asbestos-associated diseases of the lungs and pleural cavities: diagnostic criteria and proposed grading schema. *Arch Pathol Lab Med* 1982; 106: 544–596.

85. Teschler H, Thompson AB, Dollenkamp R *et al.* Relevance of asbestos bodies in sputum. *Eur Respir J* 1996; 9: 680–686.

86. Walton WH. Airborne dusts. In: Liddell D, Miller K, eds. *Mineral Fibers and Health*, pp. 56–77. Boca Raton: CRC Press, 1991.

87. Esmen NA, Erdal S. Human occupational and nonoccupational exposure to fibers. *Environ Health Perspect* 1990; 88: 277–286.

88. Johnston I, Britton J, Kinnear W, Logan R. Rising mortality from cryptogenic fibrosing alveolitis. *Br Med J* 1990; 301: 1015–1017.

89. Weiss W. Cigarette smoking and small irregular opacities. *Br J Ind Med* 1991; 48: 841–844.

90. Harber P, Smitherman J. Asbestosis: diagnostic dilution. *J Occup Med* 1991; 33: 786–793.

91. Parkes WR. An approach to the differential diagnosis of asbestosis and non-occupational diffuse interstitial pulmonary fibrosis. In: Parkes WR, ed. *Occupational Lung Disorders*, pp. 505–535. Oxford: Butterworth Heinemann, 1994.

92. Henschke CI, McCauley DI, Yankelevitz DF *et al.* Early lung cancer action project: overall design and findings from baseline screening. *Lancet* 1999; 354: 99–105.

93. Hughes JM, Weill H. Asbestosis as a precursor of asbestos related lung cancer: results of a prospective mortality study. *Br J Ind Med* 1991; 48: 229–233.

94. Sluis Cremer GK, Bezuidenhout BN. Relation between asbestosis and bronchial cancer in amphibole asbestos miners. *Br J Ind Med* 1989; 46: 537–540.

95. Wilkinson P, Hansell DM, Janssens J *et al.* Is lung cancer associated with asbestos exposure when then are no small opacities on the chest radiograph? *Lancet* 1995; 345: 1074–1078.

96. Paris C, Letourneux M, Catilina P *et al.* Programmes de prévention chez les personnes exposées à l'amiante: bilan des expériences en cours. *Rev Mal Respir* 1999; 16: 1332–1349.

97. Thimpont J, De Vuyst P. Occupational asbestos-related diseases in Belgium. In: Peters GA, Peters BJ, eds. *Pathology, Immunology and Gene Therapy*, Vol. 13, p. 311. Charlottesville: Lexis Law Publishing, 1998.

98. Gaensler EA, Jederlinic PJ, McLoud C. Progression of asbestosis. *Proceedings of the Seventh International Pneumoconioses Conference, Pittsburgh.* DHSS (NIOSH) Publication no. 90–108, pp. 386–392.

10 DISORDERS DUE TO MINERALS OTHER THAN SILICA, COAL, AND ASBESTOS, AND TO METALS

Douglas Mapel and David Coultas

BACKGROUND

This chapter discusses the clinical evaluation and management of lung diseases caused by minerals and metals. The discussion includes a review of the factors that must be considered in establishing a causal relationship between a dust exposure and lung disease, and examines the relationships between the exposure–disease pathway and the histopathologic features. A large section also reviews the unique clinical features of the more commonly used minerals and metals, and discusses current epidemiologic, toxologic, and occupational health data. The three most commonly encountered minerals (silica, coal, and asbestos) and their related diseases are reviewed in detail in previous chapters; they are therefore discussed here only as they exist as important confounding exposures commonly found mixed with other minerals and metals. Some occupations that routinely expose workers to mineral and metal dust and fume (mining, welding, automotive industries) are also discussed in other chapters to which readers should refer for an expanded review.

The basic terminology used in this chapter is defined as follows:

- Minerals are defined as any of the over 3500 naturally occurring crystalline inorganic substances that are usually obtained by mining.

- Metals are defined as the 77 chemical elements of the periodic table that are opaque, fusible, ductile, and usually lustrous.
- Alloys are mixtures of metals brought together to enhance special characteristics such as strength and malleability.
- Compounds are the oxides, sulfides, and other products formed when metals are combined with non-metals in stoichiometric fashion.
- 'Pneumoconiosis' is a term used for any non-neoplastic disease of the lungs caused by the habitual inhalation of mineral or metallic particles or dusts excluding asthma, bronchitis, or emphysema. It should be noted that the diffuse diseases of the lungs caused by dusts are not limited to the classic pneumoconioses; in fact, bronchitis is the most common consequence of occupational exposure to dust, and many regard it as an integral step in the pathogenesis of many dust-related diseases.

The threat of mining to health and respiration was noted in ancient times, but only since the 1970s have there been comprehensive national and international occupational health and safety programs and policies designed to eliminate disease from dust exposure. These are still in relatively early phases of their scientific and political development. Although working conditions in most industries have undoubtedly improved, our understanding of the toxicology and pathophysiology of many common dusts is still limited, particularly in the area of individual susceptibility and genetically determined inflammatory responses. Many modern cases of mineral- and metal-caused diseases occur in workers who mistakenly assume that the materials they work with are safe, and a growing literature suggests that idiopathic pulmonary fibrosis, the largest group of diffuse parenchymal lung diseases, is often associated with occupational exposure to dusts that include minerals and metals [1–3]. The reader should keep in mind that, as in most areas of medicine, the study of occupational pulmonary disease is an evolving science, and the discussions presented in this chapter represent a limited review of the current state of the art of that science.

RECOGNITION

The diagnosis of diffuse parenchymal lung diseases caused by the minerals and metals considered in this chapter is based on classic clinical manifestations, which include symptoms, physical signs, radiology, physiology, and in selected cases histopathology and tissue mineralogical analysis combined with an appropriate history of exposure. In practice, making a specific diagnosis of an occupationally related lung disease is often very difficult, owing to the non-specific nature of most of the clinical syndromes, and because few patients can provide detailed and comprehensive information about their lifetime work exposures. This section reviews the major clinical features that must be considered to establish the diagnosis of a mineral- or metal-related lung disease.

Clinical features

Occupational history

Establishing the type and severity of mineral or metal exposure is usually the most problematic component of making a diagnosis of an occupation-related lung disease. The development of pneumoconiosis typically requires 5 or more years of exposure to the causative agent(s) with a latency between exposure and diagnosis of 10 or more years. By this time a patient may have forgotten important details about his or her work activities and exposures. Although current standards of workplace safety may be high, and workers are now generally entitled to all health information related to their working environments, there are often few data about the specific exposures of previous and more relevant years.

It must be remembered that exposure to mineral and metal dust is not confined to workers engaged in mining and metallurgy. Many pneumoconioses have been associated with what may be considered relatively clean occupations, such as jewelry-making, the production of dental appliances, movie projection, and printing. Families may also be exposed to significant quantities of hazardous dust if the worker brings dusty clothes home for cleaning. Although simple questionnaires and checklists may be useful for obtaining a chronology of the patient's work history and for prompting memory of specific exposures, it is essential that the clinician spends time reviewing each patient's occupational and environmental history. Consultation with an industrial hygienist may be needed if the nature of exposures encountered in a particular industry or job description is unclear. In the USA, workers or their representatives may request a health hazard evaluation from the National Institute for Occupational Safety and Health if the health risks of a particular exposure are unknown.

A comprehensive listing of all of the potential sources of exposure to minerals and metals is beyond the scope of this chapter. Several extensive occupational health databases are now available on the Internet and World Wide Web that include reviews of specific occupational situations and exposures (see Chapters 33 and 38–40).

Symptoms

Symptoms of chronic respiratory diseases caused by minerals and metals are highly variable and may range from no respiratory complaints in the case of a mild simple pneumoconiosis to debilitating dyspnea in the case of advanced complicated pneumoconiosis (progressive massive fibrosis). The most commonly noted symptoms in most chronic mineral and metal lung diseases include progressive dyspnea on exertion and chronic cough that may or may not be productive. Systemic symptoms such as weight loss or fever are uncommon except in certain conditions such as berylliosis or cobalt/hard metal disease, and should prompt consideration of other major illnesses commonly associated with chronic lung disease such as tuberculosis or cancer. Acute disorders associated with high concentration mineral or metal exposures, such as acute silicosis and metal fume fever, are described in detail in Chapters 7 and 23, and 12 and 30; respectively.

It is not unusual for the severity of respiratory symptoms to correlate poorly with the degree of impairment found on objective tests, such as spirometry or chest radiographs. With chronic disease and slow progression, respiratory impairment is often attributed to advancing age. Symptoms may also be minimized due to a fear of losing employment or medical insurance; conversely, they may be exaggerated in the hope of attracting sympathy or compensation. When symptoms appear inconsistent with the outcome of simple spirometric or radiographic testing, it may be necessary to obtain more definitive evidence from, for example, exercise tests, computed tomography (CT) scans, or lung biopsies.

Physical examination

The physical findings in most diffuse parenchymal lung diseases reflect the stage of disease progression, with most mild or early cases having normal examinations. Among patients with moderately advanced pulmonary fibrosis, who are enrolled in the New Mexico Interstitial Lung Disease Registry, 85% had crackles on chest examination, but only 17% had finger clubbing [4,5]. Evidence of chronic hypoxemia and cor pulmonale from end-stage occupational lung diseases is now seen much less commonly than just a generation ago [6,7], but unfortunately can still be found in some patients at the time of initial presentation.

Investigation

Imaging

Chest radiographic abnormalities provide the essential features for diagnosing pneumoconiosis from mineral and metal dusts. The subject is reviewed in Chapter 31. The International Labour Office (ILO) classification offers a useful method for standardizing the description of the radiographic abnormalities [8,9]. It was originally intended for epidemiologic surveys, but has become the most common method for radiological characterization, and is often used as a standard for compensation purposes [10,11]. It is largely concerned with describing the density (profusion), shape (rounded or irregular), size, and extent of small radiographic opacities. Additional features include film quality, large opacities (i.e. complicated pneumoconiosis), and pleural abnormalities. When combined with a clinical history and a working knowledge of the various radiographic features of different occupational diseases, the ILO system is an efficient and reproducible method for describing the radiographic changes associated with dust exposure. It has a number of well-described limitations, however, and its ongoing usefulness may be limited by the advent of CT scanning.

Although demonstrating radiographic changes is an essential part of establishing the diagnosis of pneumoconiosis, the correlation between radiographic changes, physiologic tests, and functional impairment is often weak in interstitial lung diseases [12,13]. Thus pneumoconiosis caused by metals with very high radiodensity such as barium or tin often have a very impressive radiographic appearance but usually cause few symptoms or pulmonary function abnormalities.

Lung function

While radiographs are helpful in demonstrating that a dust exposure has resulted in parenchymal lung changes, only physiologic testing can prove that the exposure has resulted in impairment. Standard spirometry is an indispensable tool in confirming the presence of ventilatory limitation caused by mineral- or metal-related lung disease and describing its severity. Compensation criteria for many occupational lung diseases, including coal workers' pneumoconiosis and uranium mining-related lung disease, are based on characterization of the airflow abnormality and on percent of predicted spirometry values.

Classically, most diffuse lung diseases caused by minerals and metals are associated with restrictive ventilatory defects because they cause parenchymal fibrosis and loss of alveolar airspace, and hence reduction in vital capacity. It has not been until recently that the uptake of dusts by tracheobronchial and alveolar epithelial cells was appreciated as an integral and important part of the mechanism of pneumoconiosis [14]. Inflammation, fibrosis, and distortion of the airways with subsequent airway obstruction can be found in many of the dust-related lung diseases [15]. Large reviews of coal miners from the USA and Britain have demonstrated significant loss in airflow associated with dust exposure even in the absence of smoking or radiographic evidence of pneumoconiosis [16,17]. Obstructive or mixed ventilatory defects are often seen in certain metal-related lung diseases that cause pathologic lesions similar to sarcoidosis or hypersensitivity pneumonitis, where the majority of the injury is localized at or near the airways. Reversible obstructive defects can be demonstrated in some pneumoconioses that cause an asthma-like picture, and specific bronchoprovocation testing has been performed as a research tool for some metals. Because of the high prevalence of smoking in most industrial populations, it is often difficult to distinguish the effects of dusts from the effects of tobacco smoke as a cause of obstructive lung disease, and in most occupational populations the effect of tobacco smoke on lung function is much stronger than that of any dust exposure.

Exercise testing should be considered whenever the results of spirometry and other pulmonary function tests are inconclusive. In addition to providing objective evidence for the existence and severity of a physiologic limitation, exercise tests can provide data that help to differentiate cardiac from pulmonary exercise limitation. A variety of exercise tests and protocols are available, and some compensation programs dictate their own specific protocols, so the clinician must be careful to choose the protocol that uses the best methodology to address the specific clinical questions [18–20].

Dust burden

'Dust burden' is a term that usefully addresses the quantity of inhaled dust that is retained in the body. Most of the metals that cause pneumoconiosis can be absorbed into blood and distributed systemically, and the demonstration of abnormally high concentrations in blood or urine may provide important objective support for a diagnosis of a specific metal-related disease. However, the absence of a metal in body fluids does not necessarily rule it out as a cause of lung disease.

Magnetopneumography is a technique that has been been used indirectly to support the diagnosis of a ferrous (iron-containing) metal-related lung disease. The normal constituents of the body have little potential for being magnetized, so any magnetic field that can be induced in a miner, welder, or other person exposed to ferrous metal can be assumed to be a consequence of inhaled dust that has been retained in the lungs. This technique has been particularly valuable in epidemiologic surveys of welders [21,22].

Lung biopsy

Transbronchial biopsy through the flexible fiberoptic bronchoscope is most often insufficient to make a specific diagnosis because of the limited tissue available for evaluation of lung architecture and mineral analysis. Open lung biopsy, usually from video-assisted thoracoscopic procedures or minithoracotomy, is most often needed to obtain adequate tissue. Specialized pathologic examination may be necessary if any mineralogic assay is to be undertaken (see Chapter 34).

Exposure–response relationships and pathologic findings

The toxicology of inhaled dusts, fumes, and other aerosols is quite complex and that of several minerals and metals has unique features. For relatively few dusts are there detailed toxicological data, but there are steps in the exposure–disease pathway that are shared by all, and several modifying factors at each step are important in any pneumoconiosis (Fig. 10.1).

The first step in the causal pathway is the relationship between environmental exposure to a dust and the actual dose of the dust that is delivered to the lungs. The major factors affecting this relationship are the natural airway clearance and defense mechanisms. Upper airway filter mechanisms are usually highly efficient at preventing any particle larger than 10 µm in diameter from reaching the tracheobronchial tree, and particles smaller than 0.1 µm tend not to settle on or impact the airway due to loss of gravitational and inertial effects [23]. However, these filtering mechanisms can be overwhelmed in any individual, and have variable efficacy from person to person because of differences in breathing mode (e.g. mouth breathing versus nasal breathing), airflow rates, and confounding exposures such as smoking and solvents [24]. Because of these individual differences in exposure–dose relationships, it cannot be assumed that exposure to any constant level of dust will result in a similar degree of disease in all. It is usually not practical to characterize all relevant factors in each individual in an occupational cohort, so most epidemiologic surveys are forced to assume constant levels of exposure and dose over time and to accept the bias and variability introduced by these assumptions.

The next step in assessing the exposure–disease relationship is the uptake of dust particles by tracheobronchial and alveolar epithelial cells. This is again a highly complex step with multiple factors that affect particle phagocytosis, oxidation, movement, and ultimately the quantity of particles

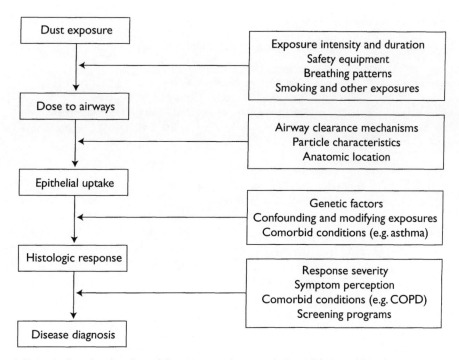

Fig. 10.1 Fundamental steps in the mineral- and metal-dust exposure disease pathway and their modifying factors.

retained in the lungs [14]. Whether particles that reach the airway are taken up at all is a complicated issue that is affected by the integrity of the normal mucociliary and macrophage clearance mechanisms. The great majority of particles that land on the airway surface stay in the dense superficial gel phase of the mucous blanket that covers all airways, and are swept by ciliary motion to the trachea or pharynx, where they are eventually coughed out or swallowed to pass through the digestive tract. Dust particles that manage to penetrate the mucous layer to contact epithelial cells will inevitably trigger an inflammatory response, most commonly an influx of polymorphonuclear leukocytes and macrophages. Most of these particles are phagocytized by macrophages and transported proximally along the airways for eventual expulsion, or carried through the lymphatic system to lymph nodes. It is suspected that this lung airway defense system can be overcome by several different mechanisms: by the physical characteristics of the particle that prevent phagocytosis or cell movement, as seen in asbestosis; by direct cytotoxicity, as in the case of silica dust or cytotoxic metals and compounds; or by simply overloading the clearance capacity of the system, which is most likely the mechanism of injury from normally non-fibrogenic 'nuisance' dusts [25]. Dusts that defeat the epithelial protective mechanisms can then become permanently fixed in airway submucosa, alveolar airspaces, and interstitial and lymphatic structures, where they can provoke a variety of secondary inflammatory reactions.

The retained dust particles may cause one or more of a spectrum of possible histopathologic reactions that characterize the dust-related lung diseases (Table 10.1). At one end of this spectrum are the fibrogenic reactions: those that cause a proliferative inflammatory response that results in collagen formation and loss of the normal lung architecture. Chronic silicosis (nodular silicosis) from inhalation of crystalline silicon dioxide is the classic example of this type of response. Most of the other histologic forms of fibrosis represent variants of this response caused by mixtures of silica with other materials (mixed dust fibrosis), unique forms of crystalline silicates (asbestosis), or coalescence of hyaline nodules (progressive massive fibrosis). At the other end of the pneumoconiosis spectrum are the inert dust or macular reactions: accumulations of dust and dust-filled macrophages with little or no collagen deposition. Coal workers' pneumoconiosis from carbon dust and welders' pneumoconiosis from iron oxide dust are classic examples of this type of lesion. In between these two extremes are the foreign-body granuloma reactions, which have focal accumulations of dust like the macular reactions, but less collagen formation and parenchymal damage than the classic fibrogenic reactions.

In addition to the typical histologic reactions to dust, many metals also cause chronic airway and interstitial inflammation (Table 10.1). Several metals, especially arsenic, chromium VI and nickel, are also known for their ability to cause lung cancer (see Chapter 20). The mechanisms for these various

Table 10.1 Pulmonary reactions to mineral and metal exposure

Histologic reaction	Etiological dusts and clinical disorder
Pneumoconioses	
Concentric hyaline nodules	Silica (*nodular silicosis*)
Stellate interstitial nodules	Silica plus other dust (*mixed dust pneumoconiosis*)
Diffuse interstitial fibrosis	Asbestos (*advanced asbestosis*), silica (*accelerated silicosis*)
Progressive massive fibrosis	Silica (*complicated silicosis*), coal dust (*complicated coal workers' pneumoconiosis*)
Peribronchiolar fibrosis	Asbestos (*early asbestosis*)
Granulomas	
Sarcoid-like	Beryllium (*berylliosis*)
Foreign-body	Talc (*talc pneumoconiosis*)
Dust macules	Coal dust (*uncomplicated coal workers' pneumoconiosis*), iron oxides (*siderosis*), other non-fibrogenic dusts (*simple pneumoconiosis*)
Airways diseases	
Acute tracheobronchitis	Welding fumes
Chronic bronchitis	Aluminum oxide (*industrial bronchitis*), non-asbestos mineral dust
Asthma	Cobalt (*occupational asthma*)
Interstitial diseases	
Giant cell interstitial pneumonia	Cobalt (*hard metal pneumoconiosis*)
Non-specific interstitial pneumonia	Asbestos (*asbestosis*)
Usual interstitial pneumonia	Metal dusts (*idiopathic pulmonary fibrosis*)
Acute interstitial pneumonia	Cadmium fume (*adult respiratory distress syndrome*)
Alveolar proteinosis	Silica dust (*acute silicosis*)
Emphysema	Cadmium fume (*chronic obstructive pulmonary disease*)

inflammatory and neoplastic reactions are still largely unknown, but they clearly depend upon interactions between the dust and the host's inflammatory system at the molecular and genetic level. Epidemiologic studies indicate that some people, such as those with familial idiopathic pulmonary fibrosis, appear to have inheritable inflammatory defects that predispose them to abnormal proliferative responses when stimulated with an environmental exposure [26]. The genetic susceptibility factor is one important explanation why only a few people in a large group with a common dust exposure will develop a pneumoconiosis or other lung disease.

The final step of the exposure–disease pathway, clinical diagnosis, may also be affected by multiple factors that obscure or confound the exposure–disease relationship. The insidious nature of most of the pneumoconioses raises a difficult but common clinical question: if a patient has a history of mineral or metal dust exposure and radiographic changes consistent with a pneumoconiosis, but does not perceive any impact on his physical function or general health, do these findings represent 'disease'? Affected individuals are often unaware of any problem unless they participate in a screening program or a chest radiograph is taken for other purposes, so a large number of cases may never be diagnosed. Coexisting diseases that cause similar respiratory symptoms, such as heart disease or smoking-related pulmonary illnesses, may increase

the chance that a pneumoconiosis is detected, but may also make it impossible to determine reliably the degree of physical disability attributable to dust exposure.

Because of the complexity of the exposure–disease pathway, and because any individual can have multiple exposures and diseases, establishing a causal association between one exposure and one disease is a difficult task. Hill described nine separate aspects that should be considered when examining causal associations [27]:

- Strength
- Consistency (repeated observations of association under different circumstances)
- Specificity
- Temporality (the cause precedes the effect with appropriate latency)
- Biologic gradient (presence of a dose–response relationship)
- Biologic plausibility
- Coherence
- Experimental evidence
- Analogy.

These were not intended to be absolute criteria for inductive inference, and the relevance of some of these criteria is debated. Nevertheless, Hill's criteria are useful in identifying the limitations in our current understanding of the many different mineral- and metal-related lung diseases.

Our current concepts in pneumoconiosis are largely based on our knowledge of the pathogenesis of crystalline silica, which is a potent cause of disease and historically has been one of the most common exposures sustained occupationally. By comparison, most other occupational dusts are not as effective in causing a fibrotic histologic reaction, and thus the terms 'inert dust', 'non-fibrogenic dust', and 'nuisance dust' have come into common use. Unfortunately, these terms are misleading; no dust that is deposited in the human airway is truly inert in the chemical sense – it will inevitably result in some form of inflammatory reaction and thus has the potential to cause tissue damage and clinical disease [14]. However, it can be difficult to recognize the importance of a particular dust because exposure may be rare, because it may cause more than one type of pathologic response, and because of the myriad factors affecting the exposure–disease mechanisms within and among individuals. Absence of information does not mean absence of association; it took more than 40 years to firmly establish the relationship between cigarette smoking and lung cancer. It will take several more decades before we fully appreciate the importance of many of the minerals and metals discussed in this chapter.

MINERALS

Compared with asbestos, silica, and coal there is only limited toxicologic or epidemiological evidence linking the other minerals considered here with diffuse parenchymal lung diseases. Further, investigation of the adverse effects of these other minerals on the lungs is complicated by their highly variable composition, and by frequent contamination by silica, asbestos, and other fibrogenic minerals. Because minerals are often mixed in this way, it is not surprising that the clinical manifestations may be variable with features of silicosis, asbestosis, or both. Nevertheless, careful questioning about exposure to minerals is essential in a patient with diffuse parenchymal lung disease, despite scientific uncertainty and controversy about causation for many of them (Table 10.2).

Talc

Surveys of talc miners and millers provide evidence that exposures associated with these jobs may cause pneumoconiosis [7,28,29]. Among 100 workers from Vermont who were exposed to talc free of both asbestos and silica [29], 12 had small round opacities (1/0 or greater), nine had small irregular opacities (1/0 or greater), and four had pleural plaques and diffuse pleural thickening. In contrast, no evidence of pneumoconiosis was found among another group of miners of talc free of asbestos and silica [30]. Radiographic patterns of mixed, small, rounded and irregular opacities together with pleural abnormalities were, however, described among 121 miners and millers of talc contaminated with asbestiform fibers from New York [28]. Small rounded and irregular opacities were found only with a history of 15 or more years of work, and 31% had diffuse pleural thickening. These results suggest that talc mining and milling may be associated with at least two types of pneumoconioses that are consistent with silicosis (i.e. nodular opacities) and asbestosis (i.e. irregular opacities with pleural plaques and diffuse thickening).

Talc mining and milling have been associated with decrements in spirometric indices in active

Table 10.2 Minerals associated with diffuse parenchymal lung diseases

Mineral	Clinical disorder	Uses and exposures
Fuller's earth	Pneumoconiosis Mixed-dust fibrosis	Wool processing Filler for paints and cosmetics Cat litter
Kaolin (china clay)	Pneumoconiosis Mixed-dust fibrosis (?) Interstitial fibrosis	Ceramics manufacture Pharmaceutical adsorbents Firebrick manufacture
Mica	Pneumoconiosis Mixed-dust fibrosis	Electrical and thermal insulation Dry lubricant
Talc	Nodular silicosis Mixed-dust fibrosis Interstitial fibrosis Foreign body granuloma	Filler for paint, ceramics, cosmetics, textiles Fire extinguishing powders Dry lubricant Thermal insulation

workers [28,29], but the results obtained have limited relevance for describing the severity and pattern of impairment among retired workers, who may develop diffuse parenchymal lung diseases years after exposure ceases.

Small case series of talc-exposed workers provide limited, but the best available, evidence on the complex pathological and mineralogical features associated with talc [31]. The most consistent feature is peribronchiolar dust-laden macrophages. Other more variable characteristics include rounded and irregular nodules, foreign body granulomas, ferruginous bodies, and variable degrees of fibrosis including progressive massive fibrosis [31]. Analysis of lung mineral dust content of talc-exposed workers has also shown a wide variety of minerals including talc, mica, kaolin, chlorite, quartz, and asbestos. These variable pathologic and mineralogic findings provide further evidence of the mixed-dust exposure that often occurs in talc workers.

Mica

Mica is largely obtained as a byproduct from the mining of other minerals (e.g. kaolin, feldspar) and metals (e.g. lithium), and is used in a wide variety of industrial applications (Table 10.2). The role of mica as a cause of diffuse parenchymal lung disease has been controversial because of contamination by other fibrogenic agents. Moreover, the evidence linking mica exposure to diffuse parenchymal lung diseases is limited to case reports and case series [31–34]. An example of the potential role of mixed mineral dust exposures, and the difficulty in diagnosing the various mineral dust pneumoconioses, is provided in a case series of talc pneumoconiosis reported by Gibbs and coworkers [31]. In the 17 talc-exposed patients they described, mineralogic analysis of lung tissue in one patient showed that mica was the predominant mineral and thus more likely than talc to be the cause of diffuse pulmonary fibrosis.

The radiographic, spirometric, and pathologic findings in mica pneumoconiosis are based on only a few case reports [32,34]. After more than 5 years of exposure small nodular opacities, predominately in the bases, have been reported, and with continued exposure small irregular densities have been found also. In one case larger nodules, consistent with progressive massive fibrosis, developed [32]. On spirometric testing, a restrictive pattern has been the main finding, and worsening impairment despite discontinued exposure has been reported. The pathologic findings have included small fibrous nodules, mainly in the lower lobes, and interstitial fibrosis in all lobes, but predominately in the lower lobes, together with abundant, polarizable, intracellular, crystalline material. Mica can be identified in lung tissue with mineralogic analysis.

Kaolin

Most of the available evidence on pneumoconiosis associated with kaolin exposure comes from china clay workers in the UK [35,36] and from kaolin processing plants in the USA [37–39]. Among 3689 china clay workers surveyed in 1985, 8.5% had radiologic evidence of pneumoconiosis with both nodular and irregular opacities that were predominately in the lower and middle lung zones, and 0.4% had large opacities consistent with progressive massive fibrosis (i.e. complicated pneumoconiosis). In the USA, radiologic evidence of pneumoconiosis was found in 9.2% of 459 workers at two kaolin-processing plants, and 1.7% had complicated pneumoconiosis [37]. Although both irregular and nodular opacities were seen in the US workers, irregular opacities predominated, and the opacities were equally distributed between lower, middle, and upper lung zones. Factors independently associated with an increased risk of pneumoconiosis in these workers were age over 55 years, increased years of working in production, and working in a plant with a high percentage of calcined kaolin (heated to remove moisture) [38].

Decrements in spirometric parameters have been found among workers exposed to kaolin [36,38,40]. The levels of forced vital capacity (FVC) and forced expired volume in 1 s (FEV$_1$) are inversely related to severity of profusion of radiographic opacities [36]. Moreover, greater decrements in FVC have been associated with exposure to calcined kaolin than with exposure to hydrous (natural moisture-containing) clay [38]. While these spirometric changes found in working populations suggest a restrictive pattern, the generalizability of these results to the clinical setting is uncertain.

Wagner *et al.* have described the pathological findings associated with kaolin exposure among cases referred to the Medical Research Council Pneumoconiosis Unit in the UK [35]. The findings showed two major patterns of parenchymal abnormalities: nodular fibrosis and interstitial fibrosis. These two pathologic patterns are consistent with the radiologic findings of nodular and irregular opacities [36,37]. Mineralogic analysis demonstrated a high quartz content with the nodular pattern and high kaolinite dust with the interstitial fibrosis. Kaolin has also been found in lung tissue of talc-exposed workers and may have a pathogenic role in talc pneumoconiosis [31].

Fuller's earth

This term refers to a group of absorbent clays comprised of fibrous silicates (e.g. attapulgite, sepiolite, montmorillonite). In a survey of 218 Spanish sepiolite workers, 20% had small opacities and clay dust exposure was associated with decrements in both FVC and FEV_1 [41]. A single case report suggests that attapulgite may be associated with pulmonary fibrosis [42]; however, a mortality study of attapulgite miners and millers found no increase in mortality from non-malignant respiratory diseases [43].

Perlite

Perlite is a non-crystalline silica that occurs naturally as small beads of volcanic glass [44]. Perlite's most useful characteristic is that it can be 'popped' or expanded when cooked at high temperatures to form lightweight particles similar to styrofoam pellets. Expanded perlite is commonly used as a soil conditioner and as a filler in construction materials. Most commercial-grade perlite is fairly pure, but perlite ores may be contaminated by a number of the other minerals found in volcanic ash, including free crystalline silica and fibrous silicates.

Three cross-sectional studies of perlite workers found no increased risk of pneumoconiosis, but each of the studies was subject to a number of methodologic problems, including inadequate exposure measurements and inappropriate reference standards [45,46]. Early unpublished animal studies reportedly found no evidence of fibrogenicity [45], but two published animal studies found evidence of an acute lymphocytic inflammatory reaction to expanded perlite with aggregation of lymphocytes, giant cells, and fibroblasts [47,48]. Cases of pulmonary fibrosis consistent with a complicated mixed-dust pneumoconiosis have been identified among perlite workers in New Mexico (Fig. 10.2).

Perlite is an excellent example of how the concept of 'nuisance dust' is potentially misleading. Most 'inert' or 'nuisance' minerals are contaminated with silica, asbestos, and other fibrogenic mineral particles, and must be treated as a potential health hazard [44].

METALS

Although this section of the text focuses primarily on lung parenchymal and interstitial diseases, it is important to note that metals have highly variable adverse effects on health both within and among individuals (Table 10.3). With some metals, such as arsenic, nickel, and uranium, the most clearly recognized and important pulmonary disease is cancer,

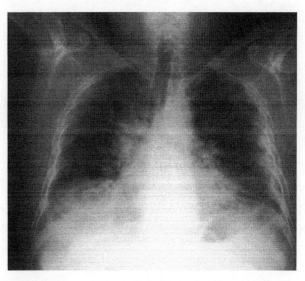

Fig. 10.2 Chest radiograph of a perlite worker. Note the diffuse peripheral reticular and nodular densities suggestive of a mixed-dust fibrosis.

which is discussed in more detail in Chapter 20. Because metals may have substantially different health effects from those of their compounds, we have included the major compounds that are known to cause lung disease when appropriate. It should also be noted that, for some highly toxic metals such as lead and mercury, inhalation of fume is an important mechanism of entry into the body, although the pulmonary system is rarely affected. More comprehensive listings of the systemic health effects and toxicology of metals are available on the Internet (see Chapters 38–40).

Aluminum

The respiratory pathogenicity of aluminum varies with the type of compound and by the type of exposure. Some forms of aluminum, such as aluminum metal powder, are quite clearly potent causes of pulmonary fibrosis, while aluminum oxides and silicates appear to be less fibrogenic [49]. Aluminum compounds have also been associated with industrial bronchitis and asthma, but these disorders are beyond the scope of this (see Chapter 4). Numerous epidemiologic surveys have been carried out in a variety of aluminum industries, but most have limited methodology and have not been able to establish clear relationships between aluminum exposure and lung disease [50]. Nevertheless, approximately 22 billion pounds of aluminum are produced in the USA each year, and the aluminum industry employs over 143 000 workers, so its importance as an occupational exposure cannot be overlooked.

Pure aluminum powder is a potent cause of lung disease (aluminum lung), which is characterized by

Table 10.3 Uses, exposures, and respiratory disorders associated with metals and metal compounds

Metal and related compounds	Clinical disorder	Uses and exposures
Aluminum (Al)		
Aluminum powder	Aluminum lung (interstitial fibrosis)	Fireworks manufacture
Bauxite (aluminum ore)	Industrial bronchitis	Aluminum ore processing
Aluminum smelting	Potroom asthma (occupational asthma)	Aluminum smelting and refining
Aluminum oxide (AlO_2)	Shaver's disease (acute silicosis)	Corundum manufacture and processing
	(?) Interstitial fibrosis	Metal grinding and polishing
	(?) Granulomatosis	Abrasives
Aluminum silicates (Al_2O_3–$2SiO_2$)	Pneumoconiosis	Kaolin (china clay) mining
	Mixed-dust fibrosis	Ceramics manufacture
	(?) interstitial fibrosis	Refractory material
Antimony (Sb)		
Stibnite (antimony ore)	Pneumoconiosis	Ore processing
Antimony oxides	Pneumoconiosis	Ceramic and glass pigments and glazes
Metal fume	Acute pneumonitis	Ore smelting and welding
		Lead products manufacture and munitions
Barium (Ba)		
Barium sulfate ($BaSO_4$)	Baritosis (pneumoconiosis)	Glass and paper manufacture
Barite (barium ore)	Mixed-dust fibrosis	Oil- and gas-well drilling
Beryllium (Be)		
Metal and alloys	Berylliosis (granulomatosis)	Metals for dental alloys and electronic parts
	Lung cancer	
Cadmium (Cd)		
Metal and fume	Acute pneumonitis	High-friction metal alloys
	Adult respiratory distress syndrome	Welding and metal cutting
	(?) Interstitial fibrosis	
CdO and various cadmium	Emphysema	Battery manufacture
compounds	Chronic bronchitis	Zinc, lead, and copper smelting
	(?) Interstitial fibrosis	Silver solder
	(?) Lung cancer	Paint, ceramic, and plastic pigments and glazes
Chromium (Cr)		
Chromite (chrome-iron ore)	Pneumoconiosis	Mining ore processing
Chromium metal, alloy, and fume,	Industrial bronchitis	Steel and chromium-alloy production
and various chromium compounds	Respiratory mucosal toxicity	Electroplating and welding
	Asthma	Chromate pigments
	(?) Interstitial fibrosis	Leather tanning
	Lung cancer	
Cobalt (Co)		
Cobalt fume, metal, or compounds	Occupational asthma	Cobalt metal smelting and refining
	Mucosal irritation and acute alveolitis	Paint, ceramic, and glass pigments
	(?) Pulmonary fibrosis	Chemical catalysts
Cobalt sintered metals (e.g.,	Hard metal pneumoconiosis (giant cell	Hard metal manufacture and use
titanium oxide and diamond	pneumonia)	Saw-blade and tool sharpening and polishing
polishing tools)	Pulmonary fibrosis	Diamond polishing
Dental metal (CoCrMo)	(?) Hypersensitivity pneumonitis	
	Dental technician's pneumoconiosis	Polishing of partial dentures and bridges
Copper		
Copper ore and copper fume	Respiratory mucosal irritation	Copper mining, smelting, and refining
Copper sulfate ($CuSO_4$)	Vineyard sprayers' lung (interstitial	Bordeaux mixture – antifungal solution for
	fibrosis and granulomatosis)	grapevines and agricultural applications
Iron		
Iron fume and oxide dust	Siderosis (pneumoconiosis)	Arc welding and metal cutting

continued

Table 10.3 (continued)

Metal and related compounds	Clinical disorder	Uses and exposures
Lanthanides		
Metal, fume, and alloys	Rare earth pneumoconiosis	Carbon arc-lamp fume: photoengraving, lithography, movie projectionists
Cerium oxide (CeO_2)	Interstitial fibrosis and granulomatosis	Manufacture and use of CeO_2 as a polish for glass lenses
Manganese		
Metal, fume, and alloys	Acute pneumonitis (?) Pneumoconiosis	Steel and specialty metal production
Nickel		
Metal, fume, and alloys	Acute and chronic pneumonitis Lung cancer Asthma and eosinophilic pneumonia	Steel and specialty metal production Welding, metal cutting, and electroplating
Tin		
Metal and fume	Stannosis (pneumoconiosis)	Tin mining, smelting, and refining Tin electroplating and soldering
Titanium		
Metal, fume, and oxide (TiO_2)	Mixed-dust fibrosis, asbestosis	TiO_2 mining and refining Titanium metal machining Paint and ceramics manufacture
Vanadium		
Metal, fume, and alloys	Acute bronchitis Occupational asthma	Cleaning of oil-fired turbines, boilers, and flumes Vanadium smelting and refining
Vanadium pentoxide (V_2O_5)	Acute bronchitis and pneumonitis Occupational asthma	Vanadium milling, smelting, and refining
Zirconium		
Metal, fume, and alloys	Industrial bronchitis (?) Interstitial fibrosis (?) Granulomatosis	Zirconium milling and refining Refining of other metals associated with zirconium (lanthanides, hafnium, thorium, antimony)
Zircon ($ZrSiO_4$)	Industrial bronchitis	Zirconium milling and refining Sand for sand-blasting and foundry work
Zirconia (ZrO_2)	(?) Interstitial fibrosis	Glass lens polish

pulmonary fibrosis involving dominantly the lung apices. It may result in severe respiratory impairment and death [51]. Aluminum powder is highly chemically active and is used in the manufacture of explosives and fireworks. It is likely that inhaled aluminum particles lead to exothermic reactions in the lungs with subsequent inflammation and fibrosis [52]. Commercially available aluminum powder is usually coated with sodium or potassium stearate, a fatty acid derivative from tallow, which helps to protect the powder against oxidation and hydrolysis. Animal studies have demonstrated that stearate-coated aluminum powder causes a much milder inflammatory response in the lungs than that seen with pure aluminum or with aluminum coated with other agents [53,54].

Aluminum oxide is often used in abrasives, particularly in the form of corundum, which is a very hard crystalline aluminum oxide. Corundum is the primary component of emery, a commonly used natural occurring abrasive. Aluminum oxide is not particularly fibrogenic by itself [49]; however, many aluminum abrasives also contain silicon dioxide, so the dust generated by grinding materials may be considered a mixed-dust exposure. Shaver's disease, described in workers engaged in the manufacture of corundum, is probably acute silicosis [55,56]. More recent reports suggest that aluminum oxide dust may cause diffuse fibrosis independent of silica exposure. Histologic and mineralogic analysis of fibrotic lung tissue from one aluminum polisher [57] and from three workers from an aluminum abrasives factory [58] found high concentrations of aluminum but minimal evidence of changes suggestive of silicosis or asbestosis. Case reports have also described granulomatous reactions in people exposed to high concentration of aluminum oxide dusts [59,60], but the incidence appears to be very low among the large number of exposed subjects and so might represent the chance occurrence of sarcoidosis.

Aluminum silicates are found in hydrated form (Al_2O_3 $2SiO_2$ $2H_2O$) as kaolin, which is also known as china clay (see above). They are also found in unhydrated form ($3Al_2O_3$ $2SiO_2$) in a crystalline product known as mullite. Mullite has been proposed as a possible cause of pneumoconiosis [61], although animal studies suggest that it is not particularly fibrogenic [62]. Both of these aluminosilicates are usually found with variable quantities of free silica or asbestos, so lung disease occurring in people exposed to these products may represent a mixed-dust fibrosis.

Antimony

Antimony is a white–silvery metal that is rarely used alone, but is commonly mixed with lead as a hardening alloy for use in battery plates and in ammunition. It is also combined with other metals in antifriction products such as machine bearings. Antimony oxides are often used as pigments for ceramic glazes, glass, and paints.

Antimony ore, known as stibnite (Sb_2S_3), may include high concentrations of silica and is implicated as a cause of a mixed-dust pneumoconiosis [63], although silica-free antimony oxide has also been described as causing a pneumoconiosis [64]. Two surveys of workers in antimony industries from the 1960s reported a prevalence of pneumoconiosis on chest radiographs as high as 16%, although spirometric abnormalities were rare [65,66]. A more recent survey found evidence of obstructive or mixed ventilatory defects in approximately 25% of a cohort with long-term exposure [63]. Animal and autopsy studies suggest that antimony oxides do not provoke a strong fibrotic reaction in the lung [65,66].

Exposure to high concentrations of antimony fume is described as causing a reversible mucositis and pneumonitis among workers in an antimony smelter [67]. A mortality study of workers at an antimony smelter in Texas found a slightly increased rate of death from lung cancer, but not from other lung diseases [68].

Barium

Barium is most commonly extracted and used in its sulfated form ($BaSO_4$), known as barite or barytes, and was once mined as witherite ($BaCO_3$). Barite has a wide variety of uses, and it is often employed as a weighting agent in papers, paints, textiles, vinyl, rubber, plastics, and glass. Barite ore is also used in drilling muds for oil and gas wells [69].

Like other metals of high radiodensity, such as tin and iron, barium dusts may cause a pneumoconiosis that produces a profound appearance on chest radio-graphs but only minimal clinical or physiologic impairment. The radiographic appearance of this pneumoconiosis, known as 'baritosis', is usually described as an even and diffuse distribution of discrete opacities ranging from 1 to 5 mm in diameter that are usually very densely radiopaque [69]. In a prospective follow-up of five workers with baritosis, Doig observed substantial radiographic clearance in all five several years after they were removed from the exposure [69]. Although most processed barite is relatively pure, quartz deposits may be found in barite formations, so silicosis or mixed-dust fibrosis must also be considered in barium miners [70].

Barium sulfate is commonly used as a contrast agent for radiographic procedures, particularly for studies of the esophagus. Barium contrast is usually considered inert, although a few case reports describe diffuse interstitial and granulomatous inflammatory reactions to aspirated or instilled contrast material in the lungs [71].

Beryllium

Beryllium is one of the best described causes of occupational or environmental lung disease from metal exposure, partly because of its unusual but striking effects [72–74]. These are described in Box 10.1.

Cadmium

Cadmium is a metal with excellent resistance to corrosion and is used as an alloy for steel and copper, for electroplating, and in a variety of low-temperature solders including silver solder. Its compounds are found in a wide variety of products including pigments in glazes and enamels, dyeing and printing textiles, and television phosphors, and its metal is commonly used in rechargeable nickel–cadmium batteries. Cadmium is found in significant quantities in cigarettes, and increased serum levels of cadmium may be found in smokers and people exposed to second-hand smoke [75]. While cadmium exposure has been linked to a number of adverse health effects, including nephrotoxicity, emphysema, acute lung injury, pulmonary fibrosis, and lung cancer, only the diffuse effects on the lung parenchyma are considered here.

Cadmium fumes are highly toxic, which is compounded by the fact that it has a very low melting point (320°C) and can be generated in high concentrations quite quickly when heated [76]. Cadmium fume is easily released when cadmium-containing metals are cut with an oxyacetylene torch or welded, and may lead to acute toxicity and death among unsuspecting individuals working in inadequately ventilated areas [77–80]. Inhalation of as little as

5 mg/m^3 over an 8-hour period can result in an acute fatal pneumonitis that initially is difficult to distinguish from typical metal fume fever. Symptoms usually do not start until several hours after exposure and begin with throat irritation, cough, dyspnea, and occasionally fever and gastrointestinal complaints. During the following few days, the patient may develop a diffuse pneumonitis with pulmonary edema and respiratory failure. The pathologic appearance is that of diffuse alveolar damage, which can be seen in a wide variety of toxic insults. The only diagnostic features of the acute disease are a history of metal fume exposure and the demonstration of high levels of cadmium in tissue, blood, or urine. Survivors of the acute disorder may go on to develop a permanent pulmonary fibrosis with a restrictive ventilatory defect [80,81], although most appear to recover within a few days and return to their normal activity [78].

Workers chronically exposed to cadmium have an increased risk of chronic obstructive pulmonary disease, although they are more likely to develop cadmium-induced renal tubular damage and proteinuria first [82,83]. Several surveys in the 1950s suggested that chronic exposure to cadmium could cause emphysema, but these studies did not take into account the effects of cigarette smoking [84], and other early surveys did not find an association. Several more recent case-control studies, that have controlled for cigarette smoking, have confirmed an increased risk of emphysema and obstructive ventilatory defects in workers from a variety of cadmium industries [82,85–87]. Mortality studies have also found that cadmium workers have approximately twice the risk of death from chronic bronchitis and emphysema compared with local and population-based controls [88–90]. Prolonged exposure to cadmium oxide has been shown to induce emphysematous changes in rabbit lung and rat lung, but the mechanisms by which cadmium causes emphysema in humans are unclear [91]. Although the association of emphysema with cadmium is not as strong as that with cigarettes, the weight of epidemiologic and laboratory evidence suggests a causal association with cadmium that may be modified by smoking.

Cadmium is listed by the International Agency for Research on Cancer (IARC) as a cancer-causing agent [92]; however, the epidemiologic studies examining the risk of lung cancer among cadmium workers are inconsistent. The few studies that have found a significant relationship between cadmium and lung cancer were confounded by concurrent exposures to nickel, arsenic, beryllium, chromium, or other suspected carcinogens, so the importance of cadmium as a carcinogen is suspect [93].

An association between chronic cadmium fume exposure and pulmonary fibrosis was suggested in one small study of workers at a cadmium production plant [94]. In this report, 29% had evidence of mild-to-moderate fibrosis on chest radiographs, and there was a significant association between decreased FVC and urine cadmium levels, suggesting a dose–response relationship. Acute cadmium chloride inhalation has been shown to provoke a fibrotic response in the lungs in several animal studies; however, because most human exposure is to cadmium oxide, the significance of these studies is uncertain. Few other epidemiologic studies have included analyses of chest radiographs, so the importance of cadmium as a cause of pulmonary fibrosis is still unknown.

Chromium

Chromium metal is commonly used as an alloy in ferrous metals, such as stainless steel, to confer oxidation and corrosion resistance, and in non-ferrous metals including aluminum, copper, and titanium to control microstructure [95]. It is also combined with other metals, especially cobalt and nickel, as alloys for special metals, such as those involving surgical implants. Chromium metal for decorative use is usually electroplated, using baths of chromium trioxide mixed with sulfuric acid and various organic acids. Chromium may also be found in high concentration in welding fumes. Chromium is found in many compounds with a wide range of uses, and over 80 occupations have been identified as having potential exposure to chromium. The hexavalent chromium compounds (chromium VI), including sodium and potassium dichromate, chromium trioxide, and calcium chromate, are the most commonly used and are most strongly associated with toxicity and carcinogenesis. Numerous surveys of workers in a variety of chromium industries have established a firm association between chromium VI and lung cancer [96], and case-series reports suggest that chromium workers also have increased risk for cancer of the head and neck [97]. In addition, chromium metals, alloys, and compounds are potent causes of an allergic dermatitis known as 'chromate dermatitis', and inhalation of these products may also produce severe respiratory mucosal irritation and ulceration [98]. Several case and case-series reports have described occupational asthma in workers exposed to chromium salts or to chromium electroplating [99–101].

Chromium is isolated from chromite ore, a mineral that also contains varying amounts of iron, aluminum, magnesium oxides and silica. Chromite has been associated with pneumoconiosis in a cohort of South African miners [102], and chronic bronchitis in a cohort of mostly non-smoking miners in Sudan [103]. Chromite miners also had a higher prevalence of spirometric and radiographic abnormalities than ferrochromium and stainless-steel production workers or non-chromium exposed controls in a study in Finland [104].

Rare case reports have described interstitial lung disease and fibrosis in welders exposed to chromium fume [105–107]. One animal study found only a mild fibrotic reaction to chromium dioxide dust, and rat-lung studies using fume from stainless-steel welding have found a mild fibrotic and nodular histologic response to chronic exposure that may be due in part to chromium VI [107–109]. However, welding fumes may contain a variety of substances, including silica and different metals, and the available epidemiologic data do not suggest that chromium is an important cause of pulmonary fibrosis [110].

Cobalt

Cobalt oxide and other cobalt compounds have been used for thousands of years as blue pigments for ceramics, glass, and paints, but it was not until 1907 that cobalt was used for industrial purposes [111]. Currently over 25 000 tons of cobalt metal are produced worldwide, mostly for use in alloys. Cobalt is commonly used in superalloys in high-temperature applications such as gas turbine and jet engines, in magnetic alloys for magnetic devices in electronic equipment, and in steels and other high-strength alloys for mechanical parts. One of cobalt's unique and important uses is as the binding or cementing metal for sintered products such as hard metal (tungsten carbide) and diamond tools [112]. A variety of cobalt compounds are used as catalysts, pigments, and adhesives in petrochemical, rubber, and paint industries.

Cobalt was recognized as a cause of pulmonary disease soon after its first industrial use, but historically there has been much confusion about the clinical characteristics and histopathology. This confusion stems from the many different types of cobalt exposure, the confounding influence of associated dusts, the variety of pathologic responses, and the possibility that an affected worker may have more than one type of exposure or disease. It is important to distinguish these features when examining the pulmonary toxicity of cobalt [113]. While it has been well established that inhalation of pure cobalt metal dust, cobalt compounds, or cobalt in combination with other dusts may cause asthma [113], only the association with diffuse parenchymal lung diseases is considered further here.

Cobalt, in combination with tungsten carbide or diamond dust, is well known for causing an intersti-

tial lung disease known as 'hard metal disease' or 'hard metal pneumoconiosis' [114–116]. The clinical features are variable and may be complicated by concurrent asthma or features of hypersensitivity pneumonitis. The length of exposure prior to development of symptoms may range from a few months to several years [114,115]. A variety of histopathologic findings have been described in hard metal disease, but the pattern that has come to be considered pathognomonic is giant cell interstitial pneumonia (GIP) [112,117]. It is described as a patchy interstitial inflammation, that is accentuated around bronchioles, plus the accumulation of large numbers of intra-alveolar macrophages. The appearances are similar to those seen in desquamative interstital pneumonia. The most unique feature of GIP is the presence of intra-alveolar multinucleated macrophages, also known as 'giant cells', which have been described as 'cannibalistic' because they often contain phagocytosed macrophages or neutrophils (Fig. 10.3). These giant cells can often be found in the bronchoalveolar lavage (BAL) fluid of affected patients, although BAL alone is probably not sufficient for diagnosis or exclusion of GIP [118]. The natural history of this disease is variable: if the patient presents relatively early and is removed from the dust exposure, there is an excellent chance for complete recovery; if the disease has been indolent or there has been a delay in presentation or diagnosis, permanent fibrosis or death may occur [115,117].

A few studies have suggested that hard metal lung disease is a form of hypersensitivity pneumonitis also known as 'extrinsic allergic alveolitis', based on the similarities in their clinical presentations, improvement with removal from exposure, and predominance of lymphocytes with reduced helper/suppressor ratio on BAL [114,115]. However, the radiographic and spirometric abnormalities in hard metal disease are

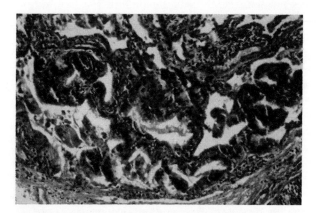

Fig. 10.3 Giant-cell pneumonia in a metal worker exposed to 'hard-metal' (tungsten carbide with cobalt). Note the intraalveolar giant cells, interstitial inflammation, and bronchiolar proliferation. (Courtesy of Dr Richard E. Sobonya, Tucson, AZ, USA.)

usually not as extensive as those seen in hypersensitivity pneumonitis, and few histologic studies of hard metal lung disease have found a hypersensitivity pneumonitis histologic pattern [113,115]. Patients with hard metal disease may have enlarged hilar lymph nodes and interstitial changes on chest radiographs making it difficult to distinguish from sarcoidosis [119].

Pure cobalt metal may cause respiratory mucosal irritation and an acute alveolitis, but studies of workers in cobalt refineries have found only rare cases of interstitial fibrosis, and cobalt alone does not appear to be a serious pathogen [113]. Animal studies have found that pure ultrafine cobalt dust causes an acute inflammatory reaction in lung airways and parenchyma comparable to that of silica dust, but in contrast to silica, these lesions heal relatively quickly [120,121]. However, in these models, when cobalt dust is combined with tungsten carbide, the inflammatory reaction is much greater than that seen with either of the dusts alone [121]. The mechanism of this synergistic reaction is unclear, but heightened free-radical generation by cobalt has been suggested [120].

Cobalt-chromium-molybdenum (CoCrMo) alloys are commonly used to make metal frames for partial dentures and bridges. Technicians in dental laboratories have recently been found to have a high prevalence of a lung disease known as 'dental technicians' pneumoconiosis', which is thought to be the result of exposure to CoCrMo alloy dust in addition to other fine dusts generated by metal polishing [122,123].

Copper

Copper is rarely cited as a cause of lung disease, which is notable considering that it is one of the most commonly produced metals. Copper fume released during smelting or welding is known to cause metal fume fever, and chronic exposure to high concentrations of copper dust are described as causing upper respiratory mucosal irritation, ulceration, and a mild, flu-like syndrome [124]. An animal model using intratracheally instilled cupric oxide (CuO), the primary component of copper metal fume, found that it causes a mild acute inflammatory response, but that most of the copper is solublized and relatively quickly cleared as compared with other metals [125].

A cross-sectional survey of the respiratory health of workers in a copper refinery in Canada did not find any increased risk of chronic obstructive pulmonary disease compared to the general population [126]. However, the survey did find that 11% of the 494 workers studied had pleural plaques that were most likely due to the widespread use of asbestos

for insulating pipes and furnaces in this refinery. Sulfur dioxide (SO_2) is produced during copper ore smelting, and an early study found an association between chronic exposure to SO_2 and reduced ventilatory function [127]. However, subsequent studies in this and another smelter did not confirm this association [128,129].

Copper sulfate ($CuSO_4$) is commonly used as a fungicide and is associated with a diffuse granulomatous and interstitial lung disease known as 'vineyard sprayers' lung'. The disorder was initially described in Portugal where an aqueous solution known as 'Bordeaux Mixture', containing 1–2.5% of copper sulfate neutralized with hydrated lime ($CaCO_3$), was liberally sprayed over grape vines several times a year to prevent mildew [130,131]. Most affected persons were vineyard workers who had used the solution for several years and who presented with symptoms of gradually progressive dyspnea or who were found to have abnormal findings on chest radiographs during mass screenings for tuberculosis. Patients with advanced disease often have diffuse reticulonodular opacities that are most pronounced in the upper third of the lungs in a pattern that is similar to that of tuberculosis or progressive massive fibrosis from other pneumoconioses [132]. On open biopsy or autopsy the lung has an unusual appearance with large blue–green patches over the visceral pleura with nodules and fibrous bands palpable below these areas. Microscopic examination of the affected lung reveals sheets of alveoli filled with macrophages with stainable copper particles in their cytoplasm, and septal granulomas that are macroscopically indistinguishable from those seen in silicosis but do not have birefringent particles under polarized light. Similar lesions were produced in the lungs of guinea-pigs exposed to Bordeaux Mixture [130]. Many affected subjects have clinical and radiographic improvement after discontinuing exposure, but if presentation is delayed for several years after exposure ceased, progressive fibrosis may be seen ultimately leading to death.

Iron

Iron and iron oxides are not thought to be a major cause of lung disease, which is fortunate given that over 1.3 million people are engaged in the production of more than 800 million tons of iron and steel worldwide each year (1999 figures, International Iron and Steel Institute). However, iron and steel workers may be exposed to a wide variety of known respiratory hazards that are commonly involved in iron mining and the production of iron products, including silica dust, polynuclear aromatic compounds, and numerous alloying metals. Many studies have found an increased risk for lung cancer among iron miners and among iron, steel, and ferroalloy foundry workers, but most of the excess risk is attributable to exposure to known carcinogens including radon, nickel, and cigarette smoking [133–135]. In general, disabling lung disease in a worker exposed to iron, steel, or iron fume should prompt a search for other respiratory hazards in the workplace.

Chronic exposure to iron dust, iron oxide dust, or iron fume may result in a lung disease known as 'siderosis', although the terms 'arc-welders' lung', 'welders' pneumoconiosis', and 'hematite lung' are also used. This condition was discovered in welders not long after the technique of arc-welding was invented. Welding is by far the most common cause of siderosis, although it has also been described in metal polishers and others exposed to high concentrations of iron oxide [110]. Iron ore and welding fume commonly contain silica, and so any resulting interstitial disease should be considered a type of mixed-dust pneumoconiosis or siderosilicosis.

Pathologically, siderosis is characterized by the formation of dust macules similar to those seen in coal workers pneumoconiosis, with irregular dense accumulations of iron oxide particles surrounded by numerous hemosiderin-laden macrophages (Fig. 10.4). In advanced stages, the accumulation of iron oxide and hemosiderin gives the entire lung an impressive rusty brown appearance.

The usual radiographic appearance in siderosis is similar to that of simple silicosis, with numerous, diffuse, small, rounded opacities of variable but often very high density [110]. In advanced disease, the radiograph may include fine dense linear opacities in the lung parenchyma, and as iron accumulates in

the lymphatics, the radiograph may also reveal Kerley's B-lines and radiodense but not enlarged lymph nodes. In contrast to silicosis or coal workers' pneumoconiosis, siderosis is not thought to be a cause of complicated pneumoconiotic lesions (progressive massive fibrosis). The radiographic appearance in siderosis does not correlate well with symptoms or physiologic changes, and radiographic abnormalities may improve over time after removal from exposure [136–138].

The clinical importance of siderosis has become a controversial issue [139]. Classic descriptions of siderosis found little evidence of fibrosis associated with iron macules except in cases where silica was also present, and animal studies also concluded that iron oxide was non-fibrogenic. These findings, coupled with early clinical studies of welders that found only minimal evidence of physiologic impairment, led most to conclude that siderosis is a benign condition [136,138]. However, recent animal studies of welding fume have found fibrogenic activity [106,109], and a few case reports and two case-series reports have described extensive interstitial fibrosis associated with iron deposits without evidence of an increased burden of silica. This suggests that welding fume may lead to fibrosis in some individuals [106,140]. Furthermore, in contrast to earlier clinical studies, several recent studies in welders using modern techniques of spirometric testing and exposure assessment have clearly demonstrated an increased risk of chronic bronchitis and airflow obstruction associated with welding exposure [21,22,141–143]. Although modern studies in welding cohorts have adjusted for cigarette use, the possibility of interactive effects and inadequate statistical adjustment is always a concern, as is any failure to control for change in weight.

Welding produces a very complex exposure, and further animal and clinical studies are needed to better understand the relationships between iron fume, the other components of welding fume, and lung disease. Until further information is available, siderosis should be regarded a marker, at least, of exposure to potentially hazardous vapors, and welders and others exposed to iron fume should observe standard preventive interventions against excessive exposure [110,139]. The respiratory effects of welding fume are considered further in Chapter 30.

Lanthanides

The lanthanides are the 14 metals ranging in atomic number from 58 to 71 that are characterized by the gradual filling of the 4f electron orbital. The Group IIIB elements of the periodic table [lanthanum (La), scandium (Sc), yttrium (Y), and

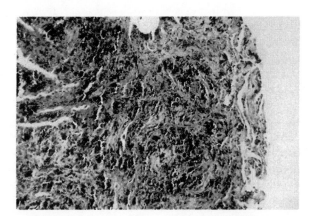

Fig. 10.4 A fibrous nodule in an arc-welder. The granular dark pigmented material is iron and hemosiderin. Note the mild fibrosis surrounding the granular deposits. (Courtesy of Dr Richard E. Sobonya, Tucson, AZ, USA.)

actinium (Ac)], and the actinide series (atomic numbers 90 through 103) are occasionally included in discussions of the lanthanides owing to their similarities in chemistry and because they are often associated with exposures to lanthanides. The lanthanides are also known as the 'rare earths', although they are not rare (all but one are more abundant in the earth than gold or silver) and they are not earths (i.e. metal oxides) [144].

Lanthanides are most commonly used as alloys for special metals. For example, the efficiency of control rods for nuclear reactors is improved by using a combination of dysprosium, erbium, europium, and gadolinium [145]. Samarium is an important component of the strongest known permanent magnets, and iron–lanthanide combinations are used for flints for cigarette lighters. Lanthanides are used in laser crystals and in glass coatings, and cerium oxide dust is commonly used as a soft polish for glass lenses. Lanthanides have unique electrochemical properties that make them essential components of superconducting ceramics and metals, and for microscopically small magnetic memory devices for computers [144].

Lanthanides are associated with a lung disease known as 'cerium or rare earth pneumoconiosis'. This condition has been most commonly reported in workers exposed to the fume from carbon arc lamps, but it has also been identified among lens polishers and others engaged in the manufacture and use of cerium oxide polishing powder [146,147]. Carbon arc lamps are used to generate an intense white light and are found in movie projectors, lithography and photoengraving equipment, and floodlights. The carbon rods in these lamps use lanthanide blends as an arc-stabilizing metal core. As the electrical arc gradually burns the carbon rods away in these lamps, the metal core is vaporized, and the fume may be inhaled or deposited on surrounding surfaces as a fine white dust. Soon after movie projectors came into widespread use in the 1930s, it was recognized that exposure to carbon arc lamp fume could result in acute and chronic respiratory symptoms, but these were attributed mostly to the oxides of nitrogen generated by the electrical spark [148]. Only after several decades have sufficient data accumulated to firmly implicate the lanthanides as a cause of granulomatous and fibrotic lung changes [145–147]. Clinical descriptions of rare earth pneumoconiosis have ranged from asymptomatic nodular chest radiograph infiltrates to a progressive fibrotic lung disease resulting in a severe restrictive ventilitory defect. A few reports have found very high levels of lanthanides in BAL fluid or lung tissues more than a decade after cessation of exposure [146,147,149,150].

The pulmonary toxicity of stable lanthanides has been the subject of debate [145]. Radioactive lanthanides (e.g. [44]Ce) quite clearly are both fibrogenic and carcinogenic, and lanthanide ores may also contain thorium ([228]Th) and other radioactive metals, which has caused some researchers to speculate that most lanthanide-related lung disease may be attributable to radioactive contaminants. Furthermore, early animal studies did not consistently find evidence of chronic lung injury associated with lanthanide exposure. However, most processed lanthanide metals and alloys are free of significant radioactivity, and [228]Th has a very long half-life (1.4×10^{10} years), so it is very unlikely that the trivial amounts of radiation found in some occupationally encountered lanthanide dusts would have had any appreciable pathologic effects [151]. Also, more recent animal studies using longer durations of exposure to purer lanthanide dusts have found granulomatous and fibrotic lesions similar to those found in occupational cases [145].

Manganese

Manganese is a brittle white–gray or silvery metal that is most often used as an alloy to improve the rolling quality and strength of steel. In nature it occurs as an oxide and it may be found in the form of nodules on many ocean floors. Manganese dioxide is used in a wide variety of products including dry-cell batteries, paint, ink, matches, fireworks, and fertilizers. Permanganate compounds are potent oxidizing agents and are commonly used in the glass and chemical industries.

Industrial and environmental inhalation exposure to manganese has long been cited as a risk factor for the development of respiratory tract infections. Animal studies have suggested that manganese oxide dust and fume exposure reduces both the number and the viability of alveolar macrophages and the phagocytic activity of these cells [152,153]. Bacterial, viral, and fungal infections of the lungs are all potentiated by preceding exposure to manganese dioxide in experimental models [154]. Acute inhalation of manganese dusts and fume may also cause a chemical pneumonitis and metal fume fever [155,156].

Although the respiratory toxicity of manganese appears to be limited, manganese is known to cause serious effects on the central nervous system, including a Parkinsonian-like syndrome. In two cross-sectional studies of workers exposed to manganese dusts, only mild effects on respiratory health were noted, but there were significant neurobehavioral impairments [157,158].

Nickel

Exposure to a variety of nickel compounds is mainly found among nickel refinery workers, and workers involved in the fabrication and production of products from nickel alloys. The main health effects associated with the various nickel compounds include acute poisoning [159] and respiratory tract malignancies [160]. Asthma and pulmonary eosinophilia have been described only in case reports [161]. Exposure to the volatile liquid, nickel carbonyl, causes acute poisoning manifested by upper airway irritation, dizziness, and headache, and in severe cases, chemical pneumonitis [159]. An increased risk of sinonasal and lung cancer has been found among nickel refinery workers; while the causal agent is not known, the risk is most strongly associated with soluble nickel compounds [160]. Muir and coworkers reviewed chest radiographs from 745 former nickel sinter plant workers and used five independent interpretations using the International Labour Office classification to describe the prevalence of small opacities [162]. The prevalence of small rounded opacities with a profusion of 1/0 or greater among workers with 5 or more years of exposure was extremely low, ranging from 0% to 1.3%. While the prevalence of irregular opacities using the same criteria was higher, ranging from 2.7% to 15.4%, the occurrence was similar to that in published studies of smokers and other workers exposed to dusts of low fibrogenic potential.

Tin

Although tin miners have been the subject of a large number of investigations, tin and its ores were not the primary exposures of concern. The respiratory effects associated with tin mining include lung cancer from radon exposure [163,164] and silicosis [164]. Exposure to metallic tin may occur during the smelting process that produces tin fumes or during bagging of the metal. In these jobs, exposure to tin oxide (SnO_2) may cause a pneumoconiosis known as 'stannosis', which is characterized by small rounded radiodense nodules on chest radiography. They may have an impressive appearance, but affected subjects are usually asymptomatic and there is no parenchymal fibrosis [165]. In the USA, tin is mainly used for plating steel and in solder, and there is little information on lung disease in these industries.

Titanium

Titanium is well known for its use in aircraft, spacecraft, joint prostheses, and other applications where a metal with high strength, light weight, and excellent corrosion resistance is needed. Titanium dioxide (TiO_2) is used extensively as a white pigment in paint, paper, plastics, cosmetics, and many other household products. The vast majority of studies examining the epidemiology and pathogenesis of titanium-associated lung disease are based on TiO_2 exposure, although exposure to titanium metal dust may occur during machining operations.

Epidemiologic surveys for lung disease in workers exposed to TiO_2 have given conflicting results. A case–control study including 1576 workers occupationally exposed to TiO_2 for at least 1 year did not find any increased risk of chronic respiratory disease, radiographic abnormalities, or lung cancer [166]. On the other hand, a study of workers in a Nigerian paint factory found that over 50% had chronic respiratory symptoms and evidence of restrictive lung disease [167]. Evidence of pulmonary fibrosis has also been reported in other small studies [168]. A survey of 207 workers in a titanium dioxide processing plant did not find evidence of excess radiographic abnormalities including fibrosis, but did find a higher risk of airflow obstruction [169]. Another survey found evidence of pleural disease in 17% of 209 titanium metal production workers [170]. Almost all titanium and TiO_2 refining and manufacturing processes also involve exposure to asbestos, silica dust, talc, or other fibrogenic minerals, thus obscuring titanium's possible role in these surveys.

TiO_2 used commercially is found in one of two crystalline forms – rutile and anastase. It also occurs naturally in a third form, ilmenite. There is some suggestion that the biological activity of TiO_2 varies with its morphology, with synthetically produced rutiles having substantially higher toxicity [171].

Histopathologic findings from case series reports suggest that retention of large amounts of TiO_2 dust particles in the lungs may cause chronic inflammation and fibrosis in humans. Lung biopsies from three workers occupationally exposed to TiO_2 found diffuse pulmonary fibrosis with accumulations of TiO_2 dust-filled macrophages in alveolar spaces and around bronchioles and blood vessels, plus large deposits of TiO_2 surrounded by fibrotic interstitium [172]. X-ray crystallography also revealed evidence of silica in each of the three cases and talc in two, but the amount of mineral dust was reportedly slight in comparison with the TiO_2, and the histopathology was not characteristic of silicosis or talcosis. Fibrosis associated with TiO_2 dust was also found in another study of three workers from a titanium-processing factory [168,173], although silica dust was also found in these cases. Because of the presence of silica dust in each of these cases, it is unclear whether the fibrosis is primarily due to TiO_2 dust or due to a synergistic reaction between TiO_2 and silica.

In addition to fibrosis, there are limited data suggesting that TiO_2 may also cause granulomatous and hypersensitivity reactions. Lung biopsies have revealed non-caseating granulomas in two case reports of persons exposed to TiO_2 [173,174], but coincidental sarcoidosis cannot be excluded as the explanation. Lymphocyte transformation tests from one of these cases showed a positive stimulation to titanium chloride, but not to other metals, suggesting a hypersensitivity to titanium [174]. Case reports also describe reactions to titanium in other tissues suggestive of an allergic response [172].

Titanium tetrachloride ($TiCl_4$) is a highly caustic liquid that may cause chemical burns after contact with skin or mucous membranes. Inhalation of $TiCl_4$ fumes may result in bronchitis, pneumonitis, or endobronchial polyposis [175].

Uranium

Uranium is a well-known radioactive element that is found naturally in minute quantities throughout the environment. The pathogenicity of uranium is primarily in its breakdown products, particularly radium, radon, and the radon progeny, which release highly destructive alpha particles as they decay. Radon is a gas with a half-life of approximately 4 days, which allows sufficient time for it to seep through rock formations and accumulate in trapped spaces such as unventilated mine tunnels. Modern houses with tight insulation may also accumulate high concentrations of radon if built on rock formations that channel its dispersion.

In addition to the well-established causal association between radon and lung cancer, uranium dust and radon are also thought to cause non-malignant respiratory disease. Animal studies have found evidence of pulmonary fibrosis and emphysema in rodents and dogs exposed to uranium dust, uranium ore, and very high concentrations of radon, and epidemiologic surveys of uranium miners in the USA, Newfoundland, and the Czech Republic have found an increased risk of death from non-malignant respiratory diseases. The risk is most pronounced in cigarette smokers, but also may be demonstrated in non-smokers. A cross-sectional survey of 1359 miners from the southwestern USA found a significant association between uranium mining, pneumoconiosis, and obstructive lung disease among native American miners, most of whom had never smoked, but most non-malignant lung disease in non-Native American miners was attributable to smoking [176].

Because uranium is usually found in rock formations with high silica content, it is likely that most non-malignant respiratory disease is due to silica dust and not uranium. However, Archer *et al.* have described a series of uranium miners with advanced pulmonary fibrosis who had little or no evidence of silicosis from lung biopsies [177]. The diffuse interstitial fibrosis found in these miners was reportedly very similar to that seen in animal studies of radon and uranium dust exposure.

Vanadium

Vanadium is most commonly used as an alloy in steels and brass. Because vanadium occurs naturally in some oil deposits, it can be found in high concentration in the soot and residue from oil-fired furnaces [178,179]. Vanadium pentoxide and ammonium vanadate ($NH_4 VO_3$) are used as catalysts in petroleum refining and chemical manufacturing processes. Vanadium pentoxide is also used as a dye in ceramics, paints, varnishes, glass, and inks.

Vanadium may be extracted from carnotite ($K_2O.2UO_3.V_2O_5.3H_2O$), a mineral found in southern Australia and the Colorado plateau region of the USA. Carnotite deposits that were originally mined in the early part of this century for their vanadium content were later reprocessed for their uranium [180]. Although cases of interstitial fibrosis have been identified among carnotite miners and others exposed to vanadium [181], most of these exposures are confounded by exposure to other fibrogenic materials including silica dust.

Zirconium

Zirconium is used as an alloy in steel and for specialty metals for the nuclear industry. Zirconium occurs naturally as zircon ($ZrSiO_4$), a very heavy sand with excellent refractory properties that make it valuable for foundry work. Zirconium dioxide, known commercially as 'zirconia', is used in powder form for polishing lenses, and in crystalline form in thermal and electric insulation, in abrasives, and in enamels and glazes.

Limited studies of workers in zirconium smelting and refining facilities have found an increased prevalence of chronic respiratory symptoms, but no evidence of spirometric or radiographic abnormalities [182,183]. A few cases of radiographic pneumoconiosis have been identified in workers exposed to zirconium who were also exposed to other dusts, including titanium ore [184], and antimony [65,66].

Although lung disease caused by zirconium appears to be rare, zirconium compounds are known to cause granulomatous skin reactions with chronic exposure, and recent case reports suggest that zirconium dusts may cause fibrotic and granulomatous reactions in the lungs as well. Bartter and colleagues reported on a lens grinder who used zirconia polish and was found to have extensive deposits of zirconium compounds in densely fibrotic lung tissue more than 15 years after his last exposure [185].

Another case report of a worker in a refractory brick factory found interstitial granulomas containing zirconium particles by transbronchial biopsy [186]. Both of these workers were also exposed to other dusts that could have caused a tissue reaction.

Box 10.1 Beryllium (William S. Beckett)

- Beryllium is unusually light for its strength, and is used in special applications in the aerospace industry, the manufacture of nuclear weapons, and the production of copper–beryllium alloy.
- Inhaled beryllium causes systemic disease with a prominent respiratory component in a minority of those occupationally exposed. Manifestations are similar to those of sarcoidosis, and include non-necrotizing (non-caseating) granulomatous disease of lungs, hilar lymph nodes, liver, and skin (but not uveitis, as is seen in sarcoidosis). Diagnosis is usually based on a history of inhalation exposure to beryllium, a consistent clinical picture, exclusion of other causes of non-necrotizing granulomatous lung disease (such as hypersensitivity pneumonitis) and confirmation of beryllium sensitization by immunologic testing (beryllium lymphocyte transformation tests of BAL cells or peripheral blood lymphocytes). Reference laboratories where this testing is available in North America are listed in the chapter on information sources and investigation centers (Chapter 38). Alternatively, the diagnosis of beryllium lung disease can be made by quantitative analysis of beryllium in ashed lung tissue from open biopsy or autopsy material (Chapter 34).
- Beryllium disease can be fatal, and complete cessation of exposure is essential to minimize morbidity. It may have its onset many years or even decades after a relatively brief period of exposure. As with sarcoidosis, systemic glucocorticosteroids may be helpful in the short-term treatment of respiratory symptoms, but their effectiveness as chronic medication in reducing long-term effects of the disease is uncertain.

MANAGEMENT

Unfortunately, with rare exceptions, there are few specific treatment options available for any of the mineral or metal lung diseases. Corticosteroids may be considered for some dust diseases associated with acute or semiacute inflammatory features such as hard-metal disease, but avoidance of continued dust exposure should be the key to management of these conditions. Because the effectiveness of corticosteroids for diffuse parenchymal lung diseases is highly variable for different pathologic types, and because the risk of serious complications from corticosteroids is high, the decision to treat these patients is best guided by a lung biopsy if the diagnosis is uncertain [187]. Many new therapies for interstitial lung disease are in clinical trials at present, and some may be found to be effective for mineral and metal-induced disease in the future.

Although nothing can be done to reverse the lung damage caused by most of the pneumoconioses, the clinician may still play an important role in helping to reduce the risk of complications and further health deterioration, activities often described as 'tertiary prevention'. Patients with chronic lung disease of any kind, including the pneumoconioses, have an increased risk of death from respiratory infections and need to be vaccinated annually with the current influenza vaccine, in addition to the multivalent pneumococcal vaccination every 7–10 years. Several mortality studies in occupational lung disease cohorts have found an increased risk of lung cancer that is mostly attributable to cigarette smoking. Many patients with pneumoconioses continue to smoke cigarettes and need assistance with smoking cessation, and clinicians need to be aware of the high risk of lung cancer found with some combined dust and cigarette smoking exposures. An increased risk for protein malnutrition has been reported in some chronic lung disease populations, and nutritional status may have a significant effect on outcome [188]. Nutrition is usually addressed as a part of most pulmonary rehabilitation and exercise programs, which have been proven to improve the physical functioning and quality-of-life of patients affected with chronic lung disease [189].

PREVENTION

In the workplace

Diffuse parenchymal lung diseases associated with minerals and metals are preventable, but the risks presented by the various dusts are often not recognized. Interventions designed to reduce health risks are classified as 'primary prevention' (usually to minimize or eliminate exposures), or 'secondary prevention' (essentially early detection of disease in at-risk populations). While these interventions are largely the responsibility of occupational medicine physicians or other health professionals at the work site and of regulatory agencies, a clinician who makes a diagnosis of a lung disease from a mineral or metal has the opportunity to prevent new cases by alerting the industry and regulatory agencies.

National regulatory strategies

In 1970 the United States Congress passed the Occupational Safety and Health Act, with the intention 'to assure, as far as possible, every working man and woman in the country safe and healthful working conditions'. This simple and noble goal, clearly based in the concept of primary prevention, contains a difficult problem – what is safe? Because completely eliminating occupational exposure to dusts is in many cases impossible or impractical, it is necessary to develop safety standards for each dust of interest. The process of developing these standards, known as *risk assessment*, involves bringing together epidemiologic and experimental data, knowledge of the basic mechanisms of toxicology, and exposure measurements from the workplace to form reasoned opinions [190]. Risk assessment is a dynamic process

because all of the disciplines involved are continually discovering new information and developing new techniques. Exposure standards for many mineral and metal dusts have been established by the American Conference of Governmental Industrial Hygienists (ACGIH), the United States Occupational Safety and Health Administration (OSHA), and other international professional and regulatory agencies. However, it should be recognized that for many dusts standards are based on remarkably little clinical information and that old standards need to be revised or new standards created as our knowledge of dust-related diseases evolves.

Unfortunately, the availability of safety standards and safety equipment does not guarantee that workers will use them, and surveillance of populations exposed to hazardous dusts is necessary to detect early evidence of lung disease before the damage becomes symptomatic or incurable. Secondary prevention of mineral- and metal-related lung diseases involves the development of screening programs that typically use spirometry, respiratory symptom questionnaires, and in some cases chest radiographs, to look for evidence of early disease on a periodic basis. Recommended health screening programs for workers in several different mineral and metal industries are available from ACGIH, OSHA, and industrial and professional societies, and sources of relevant information can be found in Chapters 38–40.

DIFFICULT CASE

History

A 65-year-old man, who had never smoked, presented with dry cough for about 6 months and dyspnea from climbing one flight of stairs [34]. On further questioning he recognized that mild undue breathlessness on exertion had started about 20 years earlier while he was still working, but this had never interfered with his ability to work and he had not previously sought medical attention. He had retired aged 62 years, when the breathlessness had gradually worsened. He had no symptoms or signs of sinus, skin, joint, renal, or systemic disease.

He had worked in a rubber manufacturing plant for about 40 years. During this time had spent 5 years in the 'core' department, where he was exposed to mica, process oils, carbon black, and blowing agents, but not talc. He had shoveled mica into mixing chambers and so was exposed to visible clouds of mica dust. During the following 17 years he worked in the maintenance department where he encountered additional exposure to agents used in urethane foam manufacture, including toluene diisocyanate. Mild dyspnea with wheezing had begun by the end of this period, at which

time he was transferred to the engineering department. He worked there until his retirement.

Physical examination revealed a respiratory rate of 20, with no accessory muscle use, and bibasilar late inspiratory crackles. There was no clubbing. Spirometry showed no airway obstruction, but the FVC was 73% of predicted, the total lung capacity (TLC) 77% of predicted, and the gas transfer factor for carbon monoxide (D_LCO) 65% of predicted. A chest radiograph suggested diffuse interstitial lung disease (Fig. 10.5), and high-resolution CT demonstrated an interstitial fibrotic process with peripheral honeycombing (Fig. 10.6). An open-lung biopsy confirmed extensive interstitial fibrosis with architectural remodeling, and showed abundant polarizable crystalline material (Fig. 10.7).

Over the following 2 years, his exercise capacity worsened and the diffusing capacity progressively declined, but his lung volumes remained stable. A 3-month trial of prednisone 60 mg per day had no effect on his dyspnea or diffusing capacity. Progressive disease led to hypoxemia, initially only when walking, eventually at rest, and he was given supplemental oxygen.

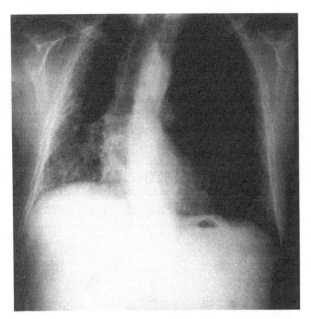

Fig. 10.5 Chest radiograph of Difficult Case. Note the volume loss in the right lung with diffuse peripheral reticular markings, especially on the right. (Courtesy of Dr David A. Schwartz, Duke University, Durham, NC, USA.)

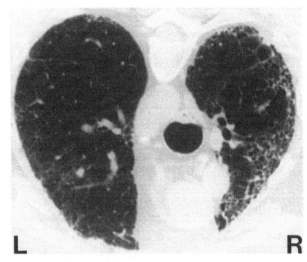

Fig. 10.6 Chest CT scan of Difficult Case. Note the bronchial dilatation and 'honeycomb' change, especially in the right lung. (Courtesy of Dr David A. Schwartz, Duke University, Durham, NC, USA.)

Issues

The chief issue for this case is whether this man's interstitial lung disease can be attributed to his occupation and, more specifically, to mica. An additional issue is whether further investigation is appropriate.

Comment

A clear majority of the book's contributors did consider that mica was responsible, mostly with a high degree of confidence. Some recommended a mineralogic analysis of lung tissue, but most considered this unnecessary. A small minority (20%) considered the mica exposure to be irrelevant and preferred a diagnosis of idiopathic pulmonary fibrosis (cryptogenic fibrosing alveolitis). The distinction is of limited significance, however, in view of the growing evidence linking idiopathic pulmonary fibrosis to dust exposure in the workplace [1–3].

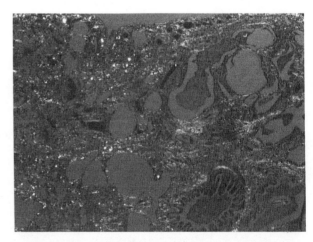

Fig. 10.7 Polarized light micrograph of the open-lung wedge biopsy of Difficult Case. Note the polarizable crystalline mica fragments (bright white granules and fragments) deposited within regions of fibrous scarring. The architectural remodeling and airspace dilatation has resulted in a honeycombed appearance. (Courtesy of Dr David A. Schwartz, Duke University, Durham, NC, USA.)

SUMMARY POINTS

Recognition

- The symptoms and clinical characteristics of most of the lung disease caused by mineral and metal dusts are non-specific, and many affected patients are unaware of the significance of their occupational dust exposures.
- Consultation with a physician who specializes in occupational lung diseases and an industrial hygienist should be considered whenever a dust-related lung disease is suspected.
- The clinical and pathological characteristics of lung diseases caused by minerals and metals are variable and are often confounded or modified by exposures to silica, asbestos, or cigarette smoke.
- Open-lung biopsy may be necessary in symptomatic patients with interstitial lung disease to demonstrate the histopathology, estimate the benefit of corticosteriod therapy, and better define prognosis.

- Biopsy confirmation of a dust-related disease provides the highest standard to establish a causal association, but may not be practical or necessary in many situations.

Management

Specific treatment is not available for most of the mineral- and metal-related lung diseases, but much can be done to help relieve symptoms, improve the quality of life, and prevent further lung damage in affected patients.

Prevention

- A diagnosis of diffuse parenchymal lung disease from mineral or metal dust exposure is a 'sentinel' event that should alert the clinician to the need for primary and secondary preventive interventions in the workplace in order to prevent new cases.
- Legislative regulations and sources of relevant information can be found from Chapters 35–40.

REFERENCES

1. Hubbard R, Lewis S, Richards K et al. Occupational exposure to metal and wood dust and aetiology of cryptogenic fibrosing alveolitis. Lancet 1996; 347: 284–289.
2. Baumgartner KB, Samet JM, Coultas DB et al. Occupational and environmental risk factors for idiopathic pulmonary fibrosis: A multicenter case–control study. Am J Epidemiol 2000; 152: 307–15.
3. Mapel DW, Coultas DB. The environmental epidemiology of idiopathic interstitial lung disease including sarcoidosis. Semin Respir Crit Care Med 1999; 20: 521–529.
4. Coultas DB, Zumwalt RE, Black WC, Sobonya RE. The epidemiology of interstitial lung diseases. Am J Respir Crit Care Med 1994; 150: 967–972.
5. Mapel DW, Hunt WC, Utton R et al. Idiopathic pulmonary fibrosis: survival in population based and hospital based cohorts. Thorax 1998; 53: 469–476.
6. Naeye RL, Laqueur WA. Chronic cor pulmonale. Its pathogenesis in Appalachian bituminous coal workers. Arch Pathol 1970; 90: 487–493.
7. Kleinfield M, Messite J, Kooyman O, Zaki MH. Mortality among talc miners and millers in New York State. Arch Environ Health 1967; 14: 663–667.
8. International Labour Office. Guidelines for the Use of ILO International Classification of Radiographs of Pneumoconioses. Occupational Safety and Health Series No. 22 (revised, 1980). Geneva: International Labour Office, 1980.
9. Milne ENC. Inorganic dust diseases: issues and controversies. J Thorac Imaging 1988; 3: 1–85.
10. Mulloy KB, Coultas DB, Samet JM. Use of chest radiographs in epidemiological investigations of pneumoconioses. Br J Ind Med 1993; 50: 273–275.
11. Wagner GR, Attfield MD, Parker JE. Chest radiography in dust-exposed miners: promise and problems, potential and imperfections. Occup Med 1993; 8: 127–141.

12. Watters LC, King TE, Schwarz MI et al. A clinical, radiographic, and physiologic scoring system for the longitudinal assessment of patients with idiopathic pulmonary fibrosis. Am Rev Respir Dis 1986; 133: 97–103.
13. Wells AU, Rubens MB, du Bois RM, Hansell DM. Functional impairment in fibrosing alveolitis: relationship to reversible disease on thin section computed tomography. Eur Respir J 1997; 10: 280–285.
14. Churg A. The uptake of mineral particles by pulmonary epithelial cells. Am J Respir Crit Care Med 1996; 154: 1124–1140.
15. Churg A, Colby TV. Diseases caused by metals and related compounds. In: Churg A, Green FHY, eds. Pathology of Occupational Lung Disease, 2nd edn., pp. 77–128. Baltimore: Williams & Wilkins, 1998.
16. Attfield MD, Hodous TK. Pulmonary function of US miners related to dust exposure estimates. Am Rev Respir Dis 1992; 145: 605–9.
17. Stenton SC, Hendrick DJ. Airflow obstruction and mining. Occup Med 1993; 8: 155–170.
18. European Respiratory Society. Clinical exercise testing with reference to lung diseases: indications, standardization and interpretation strategies. Eur Respir J 1997; 10: 2662–2689.
19. Sood A, Beckett WS. Determination of disability for patients with advanced lung disease. Clin Chest Med 1997; 18: 471–482.
20. Wasserman K. Diagnosing cardiovascular and lung pathophysiology from exercise gas exchange. Chest 1997; 112: 1091–1101.
21. Freedman AP, Robinson SE, O'Leary K et al. Non-invasive magnetopneumographic determination of lung dust loads in steel arc welders. Br J Ind Med 1981; 38: 384–388.
22. Nakadate T, Yoshiharu A, Yagami T et al. Change in obstructive pulmonary function as a result of cumulative exposure to welding fumes as determined by magnetopneumography in Japanese arc welders. Occup Environ Med 1998; 55: 673–677.

23. Chan TL, Lippmann M. Experimental measurements and empirical modeling of the regional deposition of inhaled particles in humans. *Am Ind Hyg Assoc J* 1980; 41: 399–409.

24. Miller FJ, Martonen TB, Menache MG *et al*. Influence of breathing mode and activity level on the regional deposition of inhaled particles and implications for regulatory standards. *Ann Occup Hyg* 1988; 32(Suppl 1): 3–10.

25. Morrow PE. Dust overloading of the lungs: update and appraisal. *Toxicol Appl Pharmacol* 1992; 113: 1–12.

26. Bitterman PB, Rennard SI, Keogh BA *et al*. Familial idiopathic pulmonary fibrosis: evidence of lung inflammation in unaffected family members. *N Engl J Med* 1986; 314: 1343–1347.

27. Hill AB. The environment and disease: association or causation? *Proc R Soc Med* 1965; 58: 295–300.

28. Gamble JF, Fellner W, Dimeo MJ. An epidemiologic study of a group of talc workers. *Am Rev Respir Dis* 1979; 119: 741–753.

29. Wegman DH, Peters JM, Boundy MG *et al*. Evaluation of respiratory effects in miners and millers exposed to talc free asbestos and silica. *Br J Ind Med* 1982; 39: 233–238.

30. Hildick-Smith GY. Talc-recent epidemiologic studies. In: Walton WH and McGovern B, eds. *Inhaled Particles*, 4th edn, pp. 655–664. Oxford: Pergamon Press. 1977.

31. Gibbs AE, Pooley FD, Griffiths DM, *et al*. Talc pneumoconiosis: a pathological and mineralogic study. *Hum Pathol* 1992; 23: 1344–1354.

32. Davies D, Cotton R. Mica pneumoconiosis. *Br J Ind Med* 1983; 40: 22–27.

33. Skulberg KR, Glyseth B, Skaug V *et al*. Mica pneumoconiosis-a literature review. *Scand J Work Environ Health* 1985; 11: 65–74.

34. Landas SK, Schwartz DA. Mica-associated pulmonary interstitial fibrosis. *Chest* 1991; 144: 718–721.

35. Wagner JC, Pooley FD, Gibbs A *et al*. Inhalation of china stone and china clay dusts: relationship between the mineralogy of dust retained in the lungs and pathological changes. *Thorax* 1986; 41: 190–196.

36. Ogle CJ, Rundle EM, Sugar ET. China clay workers in the southwest of England: analysis of chest radiography readings, ventilatory capacity, and respiratory symptoms in relation to type and duration of occupation. *Br J Ind Med* 1989; 46: 261–270.

37. Kennedy T, Rawlings W, Baser M *et al*. Pneumoconiosis in Georgia kaolin workers. *Am Rev Respir Dis* 1983; 127: 215–220.

38. Baser ME, Kennedy TP, Dodson R *et al*. Differences in lung function and prevalence of pneumoconiosis between two kaolin plants. *Br J Ind Med* 1989; 46: 773–776.

39. Morgan WK, Donner A, Higgins IT *et al*. The effects of kaolin on the lung. *Am Rev Respir Dis* 1988; 138: 813–820.

40. Sheers G. The china clay industry – lessons for the future of occupational health. *Respir Med* 1989; 83: 173–175.

41. McConnochie K, Bevan C, Newcombe RG *et al*. A study of Spanish sepiolite workers. *Thorax* 1993; 48: 370–374.

42. Sors H, Gaudichet A, Sebastien P *et al*. Lung fibrosis after inhalation of fibrous attapulgite. *Thorax* 1979; 34: 695–696.

43. Waxweiler RJ, Zumwalde RD, Ness GO *et al*. A retrospective cohort mortality study of males mining and milling attapulgite clay. *Am J Ind Med* 1988; 13: 305–315.

44. Elmes PC. Perlite and other nuisance dusts. *J R Soc Med* 1987; 80: 403–440.

45. Cooper WC, Sargent EN. Study of chest radiographs and pulmonary ventilatory function in perlite workers. *J Occup Med* 1986; 28: 199–206.

46. Cooper WC. Pulmonary function in perlite workers. *J Occup Med* 1976; 18: 723–729.

47. McMichael RF, DiPalma JR, Blumenstein R *et al*. A small animal study of perlite and fir bark dust on guinea pig lungs. *J Pharmacol Meth* 1983; 9: 209–217.

48. Ueda A, Ueda T, Nomura S. An experimental study on fibrogenesity of the oil absorbant particles made of perlite expanded. *Jap J Ind Health* 1978; 20: 367–373.

49. Lindenschmidt RC, Driscoll KE, Perkins MA *et al*. The comparison of a fibrogenic and two nonfibrogenic dusts by bronchoalveolar lavage. *Toxicol Appl Pharmacol* 1990; 102: 268–281.

50. Abramson MJ, Wlodarczyk JH, Saunders NA, Hensley MJ. Does aluminum smelting cause lung disease? *Am Rev Respir Dis* 1989; 139: 1042–1057.

51. Mitchell J, Manning GB, Molyneux M, Lane RE. Pulmonary fibrosis in workers exposed to finely powdered aluminum. *Br J Ind Med* 1961; 18: 10–20.

52. Dinman BD. Aluminum in the lung: the pyropowder conundrum. *J Occup Med* 1987; 29: 869–876.

53. Corrin B. Aluminum pneumoconiosis. I. In vitro comparison of stamped aluminium powders containing different lubricating agents and granular aluminium powder. *Br J Ind Med* 1963; 20: 264–267.

54. Corrin B. Aluminum pneumoconiosis. II. Effect on the rat lung of intratracheal injections of stamped aluminium powders containing different lubricating agents and of a granular aluminium powder. *Br J Ind Med* 1963; 20: 268–276.

55. Shaver CG, Riddell AR. Lung changes associated with the manufacture of alumina abrasives. *J Ind Hyg Toxicol* 1947; 29: 145–157.

56. Shaver CG. Further observations of lung changes associated with the manufacture of alumina abrasives. *Radiology* 1948; 50: 760–769.

57. De Vuyst P, Dumortier P, Rickaert F *et al*. Occupational lung fibrosis in an aluminium polisher. *Eur J Respir Dis* 1986; 68: 131–140.

58. Jederlinic PJ, Abraham JL, Churg A *et al*. Pulmonary fibrosis in aluminum oxide workers. Investigation of nine workers, with pathologic examination and microanalysis in three of them. *Am Rev Respir Dis* 1983; 127: 465–469.

59. De Vuyst P, Dumortier P, Schandene L *et al*. Sarcoid-like lung granulomatosis induced by aluminum dusts. *Am Rev Respir Dis* 1987; 135: 493–497.

60. Chen WJ, Monnat R, Chen M *et al*. Aluminum induced pulmonary granulomatosis. *Hum Pathol* 1978; 9: 705–711.

61. Golden EB, Warnock ML, Hulett LD, Churg AM. Fly ash lung: a new pneumoconiosis. *Am Rev Respir Dis* 1982; 125: 108–112.

62. Musk AW, Beck BD, Greville HW *et al*. Pulmonary disease from exposure to an artificial aluminium silicate: further observations. *Br J Ind Med* 1988; 45: 246–250.

63. Pontkonjak V, Pavlovich M. Antimoniosis: a particular form of pneumoconiosis. Etiology, clinical, and X-ray findings. *Int Arch Occup Environ Health* 1983; 51: 199–207.

64. Klucik I, Juck A, Gruberova J. Lesions of the respiratory tract and the lungs caused by antimony trioxide dust. *Prac Lek* 1962; 14: 363–368.

65. Cooper D, Pendergrass EP, Vorwald JA *et al.* Pneumoconiosis among workers in an antimony industry. *Am J Roentgenol* 1968; 103: 495–508.

66. McCallum RI. Detection of antimony in process workers' lungs by X-radiation. *Trans Soc Occup Med* 1967; 17: 134–138.

67. Renes LE. Antimony poisoning in industry. *Arch Ind Hyg* 1953; 7: 99–108.

68. Schnorr TM, Steenland K, Thun MJ, Rinsky RA. Mortality in a cohort of antimony smelter workers. *Am J Ind Med* 1995; 27: 759–770.

69. Doig AT. Baritosis: a benign pneumoconiosis. *Thorax* 1976; 31: 30–39.

70. Seaton A, Ruckley VA, Addison J, Rhind Brown W. Silicosis in barium miners. *Thorax* 1986; 41: 591–595.

71. Erickson LM, Shaw D, MacDonald FR. Prolonged barium retention in the lung following bronchography. *Radiology* 1979; 130: 635–636.

72. Saltini C, Amicosante M, Franchi A *et al.* Immunogenetic basis of environmental lung disease: lessons from the berylliosis model. *Eur Respir J* 1998; 12: 1463–1475.

73. Newman LS, Lloyd J, Daniloff E. The natural history of beryllium sensitization and chronic beryllium disease. *Environ Health Perspect* 1996; 104 (Suppl 5): 937–943.

74. Meyer KC. Beryllium and lung disease. *Chest* 1994; 106: 942–946.

75. Shaham J, Meltzer A, Ashkenazi R, Ribak J. Biological monitoring of exposure to cadmium, a human carcinogen, as a result of active and passive smoking. *J Occup Environ Med* 1996; 38: 1220–1228.

76. Anthony JS, Zamel N, Aberman A. Abnormalities in pulmonary function after brief exposure to toxic metal fumes. *Can Med Ass J* 1978; 119: 586–588.

77. Nicholson G, Fynn J, Coroneos N. Cadmium poisoning in a crematorium worker. *Anaesthesia Intensive Care* 1997; 25: 163–165.

78. Lucas PA, Jariwalla AG, Jones JH *et al.* Fatal cadmium fume inhalation. *Lancet* 1980; ii(205): 26.

79. Patwardhan JR, Finckh ES. Fatal cadmium-fume pneumonitis. *Med J Aust* 1976; i: 962–966.

80. Beton DC, Andrews GS, Davies HJ *et al.* Acute cadmium fume poisoning. Five cases with one death from renal necrosis. *Br J Ind Med* 1966; 23: 292–301.

81. Townshend RH. Acute cadmium pneumonitis: a 17-year follow-up. *Br J Ind Med* 1982; 39: 411–412.

82. Lauwerys RR, Roels HA, Buchet JP *et al.* Investigations on the lung and kidney function in workers exposed to cadmium. *Environ Health Perspect* 1979; 28: 137–145.

83. Edling C, Elinder CG, Randma E. Lung function in workers using cadmium containing solders. *Br J Ind Med* 1986; 43: 657–662.

84. Editorial. Cadmium and the lung. *Lancet* 1973; 2: 1134–1135.

85. Sakurai H, Omae K, Toyama T *et al.* Cross-sectional study of pulmonary function in cadmium alloy workers. *Scand J Work Environ Health* 1982; 8, suppl 1: 122–130.

86. Cortona G, Apostoli P, Toffoletto F *et al.* Occupational exposure to cadmium and lung function. In: Nordberg GF, Herber RFM, Alessio L, eds. *Cadmium in the Human Environment: Toxicity and Carcinogenicity.* Lyon: IARC Scientific Publications 1992; 118: 205–210.

87. Davidson AG, Fayers PM, Taylor AJ *et al.* Cadmium fume inhalation and emphysema. *Lancet* 1988; 1; 663–667.

88. Armstrong BG, Kazantzis G. Prostatic cancer and renal disease in British cadmium workers: a case control study. *Br J Ind Med* 1985; 42: 540–545.

89. Kazantzis G, Lam TH, Sullivan KR. Mortality of cadmium-exposed workers. A five-year update. *Scand J Work Environ Health* 1988; 14: 220–223.

90. Sorahan T, Lister A, Gilthorpe MS, Harrington JM. Mortality of copper cadmium alloy workers with special reference to lung cancer and non-malignant diseases of the respiratory system, 1946–92. *Occup Environ Med* 1995; 52: 804–812.

91. Oberdorster G. Pulmonary depostion, clearance and effects of inhaled soluble and insoluble cadmium compounds. In: Nordberg GF, Herber RFM, Alessio L, eds. *Cadmium in the Human Environment: Toxicity and Carcinogenicity.* Lyon: IARC Scientific Publications 1992; 118: 189–204.

92. IARC working group on the evaluation of carcinogenic risks to humans: beryllium, cadmium, mercury, and exposures in the glass manufacturing industry. In: *IARC Monographs on the Evaluation of Carcinogenic Risks to Humans.* Lyon: IARC Scientific Publications 1993; 58: 119–237.

93. Kazantizis G, Blanks RG, Sullivan KR. Is cadmium a human carcinogen? In: Nordberg GF, Herber RFM, Alessio L, eds. *Cadmium in the Human Environment: Toxicity and Carcinogenicity.* Lyon: IARC Scientific Publications 1992; 118: 435–446.

94. Smith TJ, Petty TL, Reading JC, Lakshminarayan S. Pulmonary effects of chronic exposure to airborne cadmium. *Am Rev Respir Dis* 1976; 114: 161–169.

95. IARC Working Group on the Evaluation of Carcinogenic Risks to Humans: chromium, nickel and welding. In: *IARC Monographs on the Evaluation of Carcinogenic Risks to Humans,* Vol. 49, pp 42–256. Lyon: IARC Scientific Publications, 1990.

96. Hayes RB. The carcinogenicity of metals in humans. *Cancer Causes Control* 1997; 8: 371–385.

97. Satoh N, Fukuda S, Takizawa M *et al.* Chromium-induced carcinoma in the nasal region. A report of four cases. *Rhinology* 1994; 32: 47–50.

98. Lindberg E, Hedenstierna G. Chrome plating: symptoms, findings in the upper airways and effects on lung function. *Arch Environ Health* 1983; 38: 367–374.

99. Bright P, Burge PS, O'Hickey SP *et al.* Occupational asthma due to chrome and nickel electroplating. *Thorax* 1997; 52: 28–32.

100. Olaguibel JM, Basomba A. Occupational asthma induced by chromium salts. *Allergol Immunopathol* 1989; 17: 133–136.

101. Park HS, Yu HJ, Jung KS. Occupational asthma caused by chromium. *Clin Exp Allergy* 1994; 24: 676–681.

102. Sluis-Cremer GK, Du Toit RS. Pneumonconiosis in chromite miners in South Africa. *Br J Ind Med* 1968; 25: 63–67.

103. Ballal SG. Respiratory symptoms and occupational bronchitis in chromite ore miners, Sudan. *J Trop Med Hyg* 1986; 89: 223–228.

104. Huvinen M, Utti J, Zitting A *et al.* Respiratory health of workers exposed to low levels of chromium in stainless steel production. *Occup Environ Med* 1996; 53: 741–747.

105. Glass WI, Taylor DR, Donoghue AM. Chronic interstitial lung disease in a welder of galvanized steel. *Occup Med* 1994; 53: 158–160.

106. Stern RM, Pigott GH, Abraham JL. Fibrogenic potential of welding fumes. *J Appl Toxicol* 1983; 3: 18–30.

107. Siegesmund KA, Funahashi A, Pintal K. Identification of metals in lung from a patient with interstitial pneumonia. *Arch Environ Health* 1974; 28: 345–349.

108. Lee KP, Ulrich CE, Geil RG, Trochimowicz HJ. Effects of inhaled chromium dioxide dust on rats exposed for two years. *Fundam Appl Toxicol* 1988; 10: 125–145.

109. Hicks R, Lam HF, Al-Shamma KJ, Hewitt PJ. Pneumoconiotic effects of welding-fume particles from mild and stainless steel deposited in the lung of the rat. *Arch Toxicol* 1984; 55: 1–10.

110. Sferlazza SJ, Beckett WS. The respiratory health of welders. *Am Rev Respir Dis* 1991; 143: 1134–1148.

111. IARC Working Group on the Evaluation of Carcinogenic Risks to Humans: chlorinated drinking water; chlorination by-products; some other halogenated compounds; cobalt and cobalt compounds. In: *IARC Monographs on the Evaluation of Carcinogenic Risks to Humans*, Vol. 52, pp. 363–472. Lyon: IARC Scientific Publications, 1991.

112. Newman LS, Maier LA, Nemery B. Interstitial lung disorders due to beryllium and cobalt. In: Schwarz MI, King TE Jr, eds. *Interstitial Lung Disease*, pp. 377–392. Hamilton: BC: Marcel Decker, 1998.

113. Lison D. Human toxicity of cobalt-containing dust and experimental studies on the mechanism of interstitial lung disease (hard metal disease). *Crit Rev Toxicol* 1996; 26: 585–616.

114. Cugell DW. The hard metal diseases. *Clin Chest Med* 1992; 13: 269–279.

115. Cugell DW, Morgan WKC, Perkins DG, Rubin A. The respiratory effects of cobalt. *Arch Intern Med* 1990; 150: 177–183.

116. Van den Oever R, Roosels D, Douwen M, *et al.* Exposure of diamond polishers to cobalt. *Ann Occup Hyg* 1990; 34: 609–614.

117. Ohori NP, Sciurba FC, Owens GR *et al.* Giant-cell interstitial pneumonia and hard-metal pneumoconiosis. *Am J Surg Pathol* 1989; 13: 581–587.

118. Michetti G, Mosconi G, Zanelli R *et al.* Bronchoalveolar lavage and its role in diagnosing cobalt ung disease. *Sci Total Environ* 1994; 150: 173–178.

119. Rizzato G, Fraioli P, Sabbioni E *et al.* The differential diagnosis of hard metal lung disease. *Sci Total Environ* 1994; 150: 77–83.

120. Zhang Q, Kusaka Y, Kazuhiro S. Differences in the extent of inflammation caused by intratracheal exposure to three ultrafine metals: role of free radicals. *J Toxicol Environ Health* 1998; 53: 423–438.

121. Lison D, Lauwerys R, Demedts M, Nemery B. Experimental research into the pathogenesis of cobalt/hard metal disease. *Eur Respir J* 1996; 9: 1024–1028.

122. Selden A, Sahle W, Johansson L *et al.* Three cases of dental technician's pneumoconiosis related to cobalt–chromium–molybdenum dust exposure. *Chest* 1996; 109; 837–842.

123. Selden A, Persson B, Bornberger-Dankvardt SI *et al.* Exposure to cobalt chromium dust and lung disorders in dental technicians. *Thorax* 1995; 50: 769–572.

124. Cohen SR. A review of the health hazards from copper exposure. *J Occup Med* 1974; 16: 621–624.

125. Hirano S, Ebihara H, Sakai S *et al.* Pulmonary clearance and toxicity of intratracheally instilled cupric oxide in rats. *Arch Toxicol* 1993; 67: 312–317.

126. Ostiguy G, Vaillancourt C, Begin R. Respiratory health of workers exposed to metal dusts and foundry fumes in a copper refinery. *Occup Environ Med* 1995; 52: 204–210.

127. Smith TJ, Peters JM, Reading JC, Castle CH. Pulmonary impairment from chronic exposure to sulfur dioxide in a smelter. *Am Rev Respir Dis* 1977; 116: 31–39.

128. Rom WN, Stephen DW, White GL *et al.* Longitudinal evaluation of pulmonary function in copper smelter workers exposed to sulfur dioxide. *Am Rev Respir Dis* 1986; 133: 830–833.

129. Federspiel CF, Layne JT, Auer C, Bruce J. Lung function among employees of a copper mine smelter: lack of effect of chronic sulfur dioxide exposure. *J Occup Med* 1980; 22: 438–844.

130. Pimental JC, Marques F. Vineyard sprayers lung: a new occupational disease. *Thorax* 1969; 24: 678–688.

131. Villar TG. Vineyard sprayers lung. Clinical aspects. *Am Rev Respir Dis* 1974; 110: 545–555.

132. Stark P. Vineyard sprayers lung – a rare occupational disease. *J Can Ass Radiol* 1981; 32: 183–184.

133. Icso J, Szollosova M, Sorahan T. Lung cancer among iron ore miners in east Slovakia: a case–control study. *Occup Environ Med* 1994; 51: 642–643.

134. Xu Z, Pan GW, Liu LM *et al.* Cancer risks among iron and steel workers in Anshan, China, part I: proportional mortality ratio analysis. *Am J Ind Med* 1996; 30: 1–6.

135. Starzynski Z, Marek K, Kujawska A, Szymczak W. Mortality among different occupational groups of workers with pneumoconiosis: results form a register-based cohort study. *Am J Ind Med* 1996; 30: 718–725.

136. Kleinfeld M, Messite J, Keoyman O *et al.* Welder's siderosis: a clinical, roentgenographic, and physiological study. *Arch Environ Health* 1969; 19: 70–73.

137. Morgan WKC, Kerr HD. Pathologic and physiologic studies of welder's siderosis. *Ann Intern Med* 1963; 55: 293–305.

138. Hunnicutt TN Jr, Cracovaner DJ, Myles JT. Spirometric measurements in welders. *Arch Environ Health* 1964; 8: 661–669.

139. Billings CG, Howard P. Occupational siderosis and welder's lung: a review. *Monaldi Arch Chest Dis* 1993; 48: 304–314.

140. Funahashi A, Schlueter DP, Pintar K *et al.* Welder's pneumoconiosis: tissue elemental microanalysis by energy dispersive X-ray analysis. *Br J Ind Med* 1988; 45: 14–18.

141. Kilburn KH, Warshaw RH. Pulmonary functional impairment from years of arc welding. *Am J Med* 1989; 87: 62–69.

142. Ozdemir O, Numanoglu N, Gonullu U *et al.* Chronic effects of welding exposure on pulmonary function tests and respiratory symptoms. *Occup Environ Med* 1995; 52: 800–803.

143. Bradshaw LM, Fishwick D, Slater T *et al.* Chronic bronchitis, work related respiratory symptoms, and pulmonary function in welders in New Zealand. *Occup Environ Med* 1998; 55: 150–154.

144. Muecke GK, Moller P. The not-so-rare earths. *Sci Am* 1988; 258(1): 72–77.

145. Haley PJ. Pulmonary toxicity of stable and radioactive lanthanides. *Health Physics* 1991; 61: 809–820.

146. Waring PM, Watling RJ. Rare earth deposits in a deceased movie projectionist. A new case of rare earth pneumonconiosis? *Med J Aust* 1990; 153: 726–730.

147. McDonald JW, Ghio AJ, Sheehan CE et al. Rare earth (cerium oxide) pneumoconiosis: analytical scanning electron microscopy and literature review. *Mod Pathol* 1995; 8: 859–865.

148. La Towsky LW. Effects on health of gases produced by the electric arc. *Am J Public Health* 1939; 21: 912–916.

149. Pairon JC, Roos F, Sebastien P et al. Biopersistence of cerium in the human respiratory tract and ultrastructural findings. *Am J Indust Med* 1995; 27: 349–358.

150. Dufresne A, Krier G, Muller JF et al. Lanthanide particles in the lung of a printer. *Sci Total Environ* 1994; 151: 249–252.

151. Vocaturo G, Colombo F, Zanoni M et al. Human exposure to heavy metals. Rare earth pneumoconiosis in occupational workers. *Chest* 1983; 83: 780–783.

152. Graham JA, Gardner DE, Waters MD et al. Effect of trace metals on phagocytosis by alveolar macrophages. *Infect Immun* 1975; 11: 1278–1283.

153. Waters MD, Gardner DE, Aranyi C, Coffin DL. Metal toxicity for rabbit alveolar macrophages in vitro. *Environ Res* 1975; 9: 32–47.

154. Maigetter RZ, Ehrlich R, Fenters JD, Gardner DE. Potentiating effects of manganese dioxide on expermental respiratory infections. *Environ Res* 1976; 11: 386–391.

155. Nemery B. Metal toxicity and the respiratory tract. *Eur Respir J* 1990; 3: 202–219.

156. Lison D, Lardot C, Huaux F et al. Influence of particle surface area on the toxicity of insoluble manganese dioxide dusts. *Arch Toxicol* 1997; 71: 725–729.

157. Kilburn KH. Neurobehavioral and respiratory findings in jet engine repair workers: a comparison of exposed and unexposed volunteers. *Environ Res* 1999; 80: 244–252.

158. Roels H, Lauwerys R, Buchet JP et al. Epidemiological survey among workers exposed to manganese: effects on lung, central nervous system, and some biological indices. *Am J Ind Med* 1987; 11: 307–327.

159. Zhicheng S. Acute nickel carbonyl poisoning: A report of 179 cases. *Br J Ind Med* 1986; 43: 422–424.

160. IARC Working Group on the Evaluation of Carcinogenic Risks to Humans: nickel. In: *IARC Monographs on the Evaluation of Carcinogenic Risks to Humans*, Lyon: IARC Scientific Publications, 1990; Vol. 49, pp. 119–237.

161. Block G, Chan-Yeung M. Asthma induced by nickel. *JAMA* 1982; 247: 1600–1602.

162. Muir DCF, Julian J, Jadon N et al. Prevalence of small opacites in chest radiographs of nickel sinter plant workers. *Br J Ind Med* 1993; 50: 428–431.

163. Xiang-Zhen Xuag, Lubin JH, Jun-Yao et al. A cohort study in southern china of tin miners exposed to radon and radon decay products. *Health Phys* 1993; 64: 120–131.

164. Hodgson JT, Jones RD. Mortality of a cohort of tin miners 1941–86. *Br J Ind Med* 1990; 47: 665–676.

165. Sluis-Cremer GK, Thomas RG, Goldstein B et al. Stannosis. A report of 2 cases. *S Afr Med J* 1989; 75: 124–126.

166. Chen JL, Fayerweather WE. Epidemiologic study of workers exposed to titanium dioxide. *J Occup Med* 1988; 30: 937–942.

167. Oleru UG. Respiratory and non-respiratory morbidity in a titanium oxide paint factory in Nigeria. *Am J Ind Med* 1987; 12: 173–180.

168. Elo R, Maata K, Uksila E et al. Pulmonary deposits of titanium dioxide in man. *Arch Pathol* 1972; 94: 417–424.

169. Daum S, Anderson HA, Lilis R et al. Pulmonary changes among titanium workers. *Proc R Soc Med* 1977; 70: 31–32.

170. Garabrant DH, Fine LJ, Oliver C et al. Abnormalities of pulmonary function and pleural disease among titanium metal production workers. *Scand J Work Environ Health* 1987; 13: 47–51.

171. Nolan RR, Langer AM, Weisman I, Herson GB. Surface character and membranolytic activity of rutile and anastase: two titanium ore polymorphs. *Br J Ind Med* 1987; 44: 687–698.

172. Moran CA, Mullick FG, Ishak KG, et al. Identification of titanium in human tissues: probable role in pathologic processes. *Hum Pathol* 1991; 22: 450–44.

173. Maata K, Arstila AV. Pulmonary deposits of titanium dioxide in cytologic and lung biopsy specimens: light and electron microscopic X-ray analysis. *Lab Invest* 1975; 33: 342–346.

174. Redline S, Barna BP, Tomashefski JF Jr, Abraham JL. Granulomatous disease associated with pulmonary deposition of titanium. *Br J Ind Med* 1986; 43: 652–656.

175. Park T, DiBenedetto R, Morgan K et al. Diffuse endobronchial polyposis following a titanium tetrachloride inhalation injury. *Am Rev Respir Dis* 1984; 130: 315–317.

176. Mapel DW, Coultas DB, James DS et al. Ethnic differences in the prevalence of nonmalignant respiratory disease among uranium miners. *Am J Public Health* 1997; 87: 833–838.

177. Archer VE, Renzetti AD, Doggett RS et al. Chronic diffuse interstitial firbosis of the lung in uranium miners. *J Occup Environ Med* 1998; 40: 460–874.

178. Levy BS, Hoffman L, Gottsegen S. Boilermakers' Bronchitis: Respiratory tract irritation associated with vanadium pentoxide exposure during oil-to-coal conversion of a power plant. *J Occup Med* 1984; 26: 567–570.

179. Sjoberg SG. Vanadium bronchitis from cleaning oil-fired boilers. *Arch Ind Health* 1955; 12: 505–512.

180. Samet JM, Mapel DW. Diseases of uranium miners and other underground miners exposed to radon. In: Rom WN, ed. *Environmental and Occupational Medicine*, 3rd edn, Philadelphia: Lippincott-Raven, 1998; pp. 1307–1315.

181. Lees REM. Changes in lung function after exposure to vanadium compounds in fuel ash. *Br J Ind Med* 1980; 37: 253–256.

182. Reed CE. Effects of the lungs of industrial exposure to zirconium dust. *Arch Ind Health* 1956; 13: 578–581.

183. Hadjimichael OC, Brubaker RE. Evaluation of an occupational exposure to a zirconium-containing dust. *J Occup Med* 1981; 23: 543–547.

184. Uragoda CG, Pinto MRN. An investigation into the health of workers in an ilmenite extraction plant. *Med J Aust* 1972; i: 167–169.

185. Bartter T, Irwin RS, Abraham JL et al. Zirconium compound-induced pulmonary fibrosis. *Arch Intern Med* 1991; 151: 1197–1201.

186. Romeo L, Cazzadori A, Bontempini L, Martini S. Interstitial lung granulomas as a possible consequence of exposure to zirconium dust. *Medicina Lavoro* 1994; 85: 219–222.

187. Bjoraker JA, Ryu JH, Edwin MK et al. Prognostic significance of histopathologic subsets in idiopathic pulmonary fibrosis. *Am J Respir Crit Care Med* 1998; 157: 199–203.

188. Mannix ET, Manfredi F, Farber MO. Elevated O_2 cost of ventilation contributes to tissue wasting in COPD. *Chest* 1999; 115: 708–713.

189. Mahler DA. Pulmonary rehabilitation. *Chest* 1998; 115(4 Suppl): 263–268.

190. McClellan RO. Risk assessment. In: Rom WN, ed. *Environmental and Occupational Medicine*, 3rd edn, pp. 1691–1708. Philadelphia: Lippincott-Raven, 1998.

11 DISORDERS DUE TO MANMADE VITREOUS FIBERS

Mark J. Utell and James E. Lockey

BACKGROUND

Classification

Manmade vitreous fibers (MMVF) have historically been classified into three main groups: (1) glass fiber (with subcategories of glass wool, continuous glass filament, and special purpose glass fiber); (2) mineral wool (with subcategories rock and slag wool); and (3) refractory ceramic fiber (Table 11.1). Mineral wool was first in production late in the 19th century with peak production in the 1950s [1]. In the USA slag wool is the predominant mineral wool and is manufactured primarily by the melting and fiberizing of iron ore slag. In Europe rock wool manufactured from igneous rock is the predominant mineral wool. Glass fiber was initially manufactured successfully in the 1930s and subsequently overtook mineral wool as the primary MMVF in thermal insu-

Table 11.1 Industrial categorization of manmade vitreous fibers*

Major groups	Subcategories
Glass fiber	Glass wool
	Continuous glass filament
	Special purpose glass fiber
Mineral wool	Rock wool
	Slag wool
Refractory ceramic fiber	

* Synonyms for manmade vitreous fibers: synthetic vitreous fibers, manmade mineral fibers, manufactured vitreous fibers.

lation products. Refractory ceramic fiber (RCF) has been a more recent addition to the MMVF range with initial production in the 1950s. RCF is produced from melted kaolin clay or alumina and silica, and is used in high-temperature insulation applications [2]. Other names for manmade vitreous fibers include manmade mineral fibers, synthetic vitreous fiber, and manufactured vitreous fibers.

There is increasing overlap within the above classification with the introduction of new types of fiber and new production processes over the last decade. Changes in chemical composition of fibers have occurred with the addition of stabilizers, such as oxides of aluminum, titanium, and zinc, and modifiers such as oxides of barium, calcium, lithium, manganese, potassium, and sodium. These can markedly influence the physical properties of fibers such as thermal non-transference (insulating quality), resistance to moisture and corrosion, elasticity and tensile strength [2]. For example, fibers in the glass category can differ significantly in the biologic responses they cause, depending on their chemical composition, size distribution, and durability in physiologic fluids [3]. The chemical constituents of glass fiber that is produced for fibrous glass (fiberglass) home insulation can differ markedly from glass fiber used in specialty applications.

Manufacturing processes

All the manufacturing processes for MMVF allow for variation in average fiber diameter, and include fibers well within the respirable range [2]. The majority of MMVF are manufactured through a melting and fiber-forming (fiberization) process. Glass wool is used for residential and commercial thermal and acoustic insulation as batts, blankets, and blowing wool, and in such products as ceiling panels, and air-handling ducts. It consists of discontinuous fibers that average 3–15 μm in diameter. The fibers are held together predominantly through the use of phenol-formaldehyde resins that are subsequently heat cured to insoluble polymers. Continuous glass filaments, which are predominantly used in textiles and in plastic re-enforcement, are produced by a process that allows for variation in average fiber diameters that range from 3 to 25 μm. Special purpose glass fibers, which average less than 3 μm in diameter, are manufactured through a flame attenuation process that produces discontinuous fibers. They are used for high temper-

ature and acoustic applications such as in the aerospace industry. Mineral wool is manufactured through wheel centrifuge and 'Downey' processes, resulting in discontinuous fibers that average 3.5–7 μm in diameter. Binders can be added depending on the end-uses. Mineral wool products are similar to glass wool but are generally used in higher temperature commercial processes [2].

Refractory ceramic fibers have been manufactured for approximately 35 years and constitute 1–2% of all MMVF production. The vast majority are produced through a steam blowing or spinning process utilizing molten kaolin clay or an alumina–silica mixture to produce fibers that average 1–5 μm in diameter. Fibers less than 1 μm in diameter can also be produced [4]. Owing to their capacity to withstand temperatures up to 2300°F, the primary application for RCF is in lining furnaces and kilns. Final products include bulk fibers, blanket and felts, boards, various types of paper, and

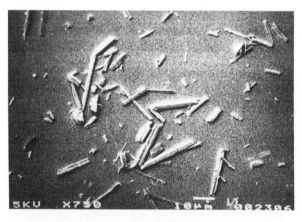

Fig. 11.1 Electron photomicrograph of Wollastonite fibers (note 10 μm scale bar in margin). Wollastonite is a naturally occurring fibrous silicate mineral (cf. longer, narrower morphology of crocidolite asbestos fibers in Fig. 11.3). All figures courtesy of Teresa Liberati Ph.D. and Jacob Finkelstein Ph.D., University of Rochester School of Medicine and Dentistry.

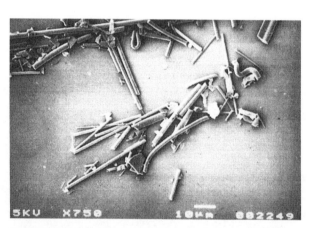

Fig. 11.2 Electron photomicrograph of refractory ceramic fibers. Wollastonite and refractory ceramic fibers are more similar to each other in morphology than to the longer, narrower fibers of crocidolite asbestos.

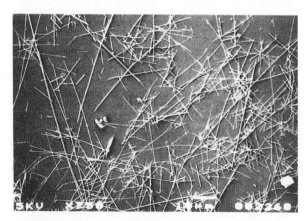

Fig. 11.3 Electron photomicrograph of naturally occurring crocidolite asbestos (mineral) fibers.

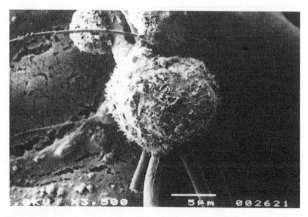

Fig. 11.4 Refractory ceramic fiber in cell culture with primary rat alveolar macrophage. Note that the fiber is partially phagocytosed by macrophages.

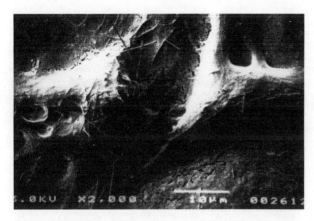

Fig. 11.5 Naturally occurring asbestos (crocidolite) fiber in culture with rat Type II epithelial cells. Note the contrast in size and shape with the refractory ceramic fiber in Fig. 11.4.

textile products, as well as vacuum-formed or cast shapes. Temperatures above 1800°F will cause RCF to undergo partial conversion to cristobalite, a form of crystalline silica highly fibrogenic to lungs. This represents a potential hazard for workers involved with relining furnaces and kilns [2]. A morphological comparison of naturally occuring Wollastonite fibers to RCF is provided in Figures 11.1 through 11.5.

Determinants of pathogenicity

Fiber diameter is a critical factor determining the likelihood of MMVF penetration into mucous membranes (and skin) when their surfaces are exposed to fiber-contaminated air. Fibers of 4–5 μm diameters can cause intense skin itching and associated excoriations. Factors related to pulmonary toxicity are fiber length, dose delivered to the target organ, and fiber durability within biological fluids. The most recent understanding of toxicologic mechanisms has identified biopersistence as the primary determinant of fiber toxicity [5]. Pulmonary biopersistence for MMVF refers to the time that an intact fiber remains in the lung or pleura, including its movement and residence in target cells and tissues. For example, asbestos fibers are highly biopersistent or durable. Of the MMVF, special purpose glass fibers and refractory ceramic fibers have the greatest durability, followed by rock and slag wool, and then fibrous glass. Characteristics such as chemical composition, surface charge, and site of deposition appear to be additional determinants of fiber toxicity within the lungs [6].

RECOGNITION

Investigation of the possible adverse respiratory effects of MMVF has been limited by both the relatively short periods during which some fibers have been available and by the relatively few workers with meaningful cumulative levels of exposure. In this chapter, the focus is directed to the evidence currently available for specific lung disorders that may possibly arise from occupational exposure to MMVF, rather than on how such disorders may be recognized, managed, or prevented. The emphasis is on whether any adverse respiratory effects have been recognized in association with the various MMVF and, when appropriate, on their nature. Methods of clinical recognition of particular disorders, principles of management for individual cases, and strategies of prevention are as described in Chapters 7, 9, 11, 12, 22, and 23.

Non-malignant respiratory effects

Glass fiber and mineral wool

Skin irritation is a common health complaint from exposure to MMVF. Skin areas that come in frequent contact with MMVF, such as forearms and areas in close contact with clothing openings like the neck, are the major sites of irritation particularly in hot and humid weather. It is estimated that approximately 5% of new workers involved in MMVF production leave employment because of problems with skin irritation. Work practices that help control the exposures, use of long-sleeved shirts and pants that are loose fitting, changing clothes at work, and washing clothes daily (and separately from other clothes) all help prevent these problems [7].

Irritation of the eyes, upper, and lower airways can also occur depending on the nature of exposure. Residential contamination with MMVF from improperly installed air-handling ducts resulted in irritation of the upper and lower expiratory tract in a family necessitating extensive cleaning of the residence including replacement of upholstered furniture and carpet [8].

A study of US workers from five fibrous glass and two mineral wool manufacturing plants did not, however, demonstrate any increase in upper or lower respiratory tract symptoms in comparison to a non-exposed group. Furthermore, chest radiographic evaluation did not demonstrate an overall increase in small opacities when compared to a non-MMVF exposed comparison group. Small opacities [International Labour Office (ILO) profusion level 1/0 or 1/1] were, nevertheless, observed in 23 subjects (1.6%) who worked in production facilities with exposure to fibers of respirable size. They were predominantly irregular in shape and there was an association with various exposure indices at profusion level 1/0 (but not 1/1), thereby providing a hint of fiber-induced diffuse interstitial pulmonary fibrosis. The plant was identified as manufacturing ordinary diameter fibers (over 3 μm) and fine diameter fibers (average 1–3 μm). No relationship was identified between spirometric measurements and exposure indices or radiographic changes [9].

No such hint of pulmonary fibrosis was found in a study of rock wool and glass wool factory workers in eight plants in Australia, nor was there evidence of asthma, lung cancer, or occupational pleural disease [10]. A Danish study of rock wool workers similarly showed no increased prevalence of respiratory symptoms in comparison to a non-exposed control group, and there were no abnormalities of transfer factor ($D_L$co) or transfer coefficient ($D_L$co/Va). The forced expired volume in 1 s /forced vital capacity (FEV_1/FVC) ratio was, however, moderately lower in the exposed group, with smoking accounting for some of the difference. There was no correlation with duration of exposure, but an elevated risk of airway obstruction associated with fiber exposure was identified in a subgroup of heavy cigarette smokers (>40 pack year). This suggested an additive or synergetic interaction between heavy smoking and fiber exposure on the risk of airway obstruction. Historical fiber exposure levels were estimated to range from 0.1 to 0.2 fibers/ml extending back to 1955 [11].

The most recent analysis of non-neoplastic mortality in the European cohort of MMVF workers followed by the International Agency for Research on Cancer (IARC) did not demonstrate increased mortality from bronchitis, emphysema, or asthma, or any type of trend, related to time since the first employment, duration of employment, or technological phase. There were only a small number of deaths from non-malignant renal disease, but the investigators noted some suggestion of an increase in mortality risk among rock and slag wool workers with duration of employment or employment in an early technological phase. Within this analysis only the underlying cause of death as reported on death certificates was used, which may have underestimated the importance of renal disease as a potential adverse effect of MMVF exposure. Mortality from ischemic heart disease was increased in rock and slag wool workers and continuous fiber workers after 30 years since first employment, which may be explained in part from exposure to heat, carbon monoxide, and physical strain in this particular cohort in the earlier phase of MMVF production [12].

A study was conducted to determine if nephritis or nephrosis was either the primary cause of death or a contributing factor in glass wool manufacturing facilities in the USA. No association was found between respirable fibers or silica levels and these outcomes

[13]. A study of US mineral wool plants did, however, demonstrate increased mortality from nephritis and nephrosis (observed 12; standardized mortality ratio, SMR 204) when compared against both national and local rates [14]. This subject is a focus of particular attention because of a previous association described between crystalline silica exposure and renal disease [15]. Whether this applies to non-crystalline silica remains to be further delineated.

There is limited information on adverse health effects in those who use these materials after manufacture. A case report of a carpenter who used fiberglass for insulation in construction projects did raise the possibility of an association between mild interstitial fibrosis and deposition of small glass fibers less than 2.5 microns in length and 0.3 microns in diameter, as detected by analytical electron microscopy [16]. A study of workers using rotary spun fiberglass for insulating appliances demonstrated a 3.5% prevalence of irregular opacities >1/0 to 2/1, and 7.7% prevalence when including profusion category 0/1 and greater, after exposure of 15 years or longer. Airborne asbestos fiber may, however, have contaminated the plant site [17,18]. Clausen *et al.* found lower values of FEV_1 in insulation workers compared to a non-exposed control group independent of smoking habits and self-assessed former asbestos exposure [19].

Refractory ceramic fiber

In a group of RCF workers followed in the USA since 1987, cross-sectional spirometric data demonstrated that 10 years of employment in production tasks were associated with a significant reduction in the FVC for current (165 ml) and past (156 ml) male smokers, respectively, but not 'never-smokers'. For FEV_1 the decrement, 135 ml, was significant only for current smokers. For women, the decrement was significant for FVC among non-smokers at 350 ml per 10 years of employment in production job tasks [20]. The longitudinal analysis of workers who had provided five or more pulmonary function tests between 1987 and 1994 demonstrated no further decline in either the FVC or FEV_1 between the initial and last tests in male workers [21].

Chest radiographs demonstrated pleural plaques in 8 of 70 (11.4%) employees with more than 20 years since first RCF production job. Of the 29 workers with more than 20 years duration in RCF production, 20.7% had pleural plaques [22]. There was an overall prevalence of pleural plaques of 3.1%. A case-control study confirmed that asbestos exposure did not account for the observed association between RCF exposure and the occurrence of pleural plaques. No significant interstitial radiographic changes were noted; the prevalence of small opacities of 1/0 or greater (ILO classification) was 0.5%, similar to the background rate in a non-exposed population [23].

An initial study of workers at seven European manufacturing facilities of refractory ceramic fiber concluded that irritant symptom prevalences were similar to those seen in other types of manmade mineral-fiber manufacturing facilities, and that there was an interactive effect between cumulative RCF exposure and cigarette smoking in producing airway obstruction. Small opacities were noted on 13% of chest radiographs but these did not correlate with estimated cumulative exposure to refractory ceramic fiber [24]. A subsequent study found a negative association between estimated cumulative exposure to RCF and FEV_1 and FVC in current smokers, with an estimated effect of 100 ml for average lifetime RCF exposure. No association was demonstrated with diffusing capacity measurements. There was no consistent relationship between the presence of small opacities and cumulative exposure to respirable fibers or dust. In addition, the prevalence of small opacities was similar in the study population and a non-exposed group. In contrast to the US study, the occurrence of pleural plaques in the study population was felt to be secondary to historical asbestos exposure and not refractory ceramic fiber [25].

Respiratory malignancy

Lung cancer

A working group of the IARC determined that 'there is inadequate evidence of the carcinogenicity of glass wool in humans' [26]. Again, there is evidence in support of such an effect from glass wool and other MMVF, but it is not consistent and not convincing.

In a study of US workers producing MMVF (fibrous glass and mineral wool) [27–29], there was a statistically significant increase of respiratory cancer (SMR 112) but no association with various indices of exposure. Differences in the prevalences of cigarette smoking in the local community compared with national rates may have been a contributing factor in the excess lung cancer seen in one glass manufacturing facility [30]. A case-control study of nine US slag wool plants demonstrated an association between lung cancer mortality and smoking, but not MMVF exposure [31].

A study of Canadian insulating glass wool manufacturing employees also demonstrated a statistically elevated SMR of 176 for lung cancer, but it was not associated with the length of exposure or time since the first exposure (the inclusion of short-term workers may have exerted an influence), and smoking data were not available [32].

Analysis of the cohort of US workers from five rock and slag wool plants demonstrated an overall increase of lung cancer mortality (SMR 129) based on US (but not local) expected rates. The excess was concentrated in short-term workers (duration of employment less than 5 years) and was not associated with measures of respirable fiber exposure [14].

Since 1976, IARC has conducted a cohort study of mortality and cancer incidence among workers at 13 MMVF factories throughout Europe. An initial analysis in 1982 demonstrated an overall increase in lung cancer incidence related to time from first employment but not duration of employment, with higher mortalities occurring among rock and slag wool workers than glass wool workers [33,34]. The most recent analysis among workers with 1 year or more of employment demonstrated a significant increase in lung cancer mortality in rock and slag wool workers [SMR 134; confidence interval (CI) 1.08–1.63] and glass wool workers (SMR 127; CI 1.07–1.50) compared with national mortality rates, and a non-significant increase in the subcohort manufacturing continuous glass filament (SMR 111; CI 0.61–1.86). When compared against local adjustment factors to national mortality rates, the SMR for glass wool workers was substantially reduced to 112 (95% CI 0.95 to 1.31) with no association with duration of employment or time since initial employment. With removal of glass wool workers who were employed for less than one year, no excess lung cancer was noted and no trend was noted with duration of employment in a sub-group of workers with 20 years or more since first employment [35].

In the rock and slag wool cohort, which represented seven of the 13 MMVF factories in the study, there was an overall increase in lung cancer mortality in five of the seven factories. The possible relevance of exposure during the early technologic phase of production was less clear in the most recent analysis, and overall the investigators felt that the results were not sufficient to conclude that the increased lung cancer risk was specifically related to rock and/or slag wool exposure. Fiber exposure may, nevertheless, have contributed non-specifically to the increased risk [35].

Similar findings were noted from a cancer incidence study of six rock and slag wool facilities located in countries covered by cancer registries [36].

A study of a glass-filament textile factory in Canada demonstrated a slight but non-significant increase in lung cancer (SMR 136) that was not related to duration of employment or cumulative exposure [37]. A similar US study did not demonstrate any significant association between exposure and respiratory cancer or non-malignant respiratory disease. The overall risk of lung cancer for white males was mildly elevated [odds ratio (OR) 126; 95% CI 92.5–167.5] compared with US mortality rates as well as local mortality rates (OR 116.6; 95% CI 85.7–155.1). Within this facility, respirable size glass fibers with an average diameter of approximately 3.5 microns were manufactured from 1963 through 1968 [38,39].

A mortality study of end-users of glass and rock wool in the prefabricated house industry did not demonstrate an increased risk of lung cancer. This study was limited by the small number of workers and relative short time frame from initial exposure [40].

Ceramic fibers and glass wool fibers of respirable size are listed by the US National Toxicology Program as follows: There is sufficient evidence for carcinogenicity in experimental animals. No data were available on the carcinogenicity of ceramic fibers for humans [41].

Mesothelioma

There have been five cases of mesothelioma reported within the IARC study of European MMVF manufacturing plants, but two occurred in workers with less than 1 year of employment and two occurred in workers with a high probability of prior asbestos exposure [35]. Historical exposure levels were felt to be less than 0.5 fibers/ml (f/ml) [33].

Inhalation toxicology studies

Inhalation studies constitute the best available laboratory model for assessing human health risks posed by respiratory exposure to fibers [6,42], since it is the route by which occupational lung exposures occur and the inhaled fibers are then subjected to the variety of natural pathophysiological processes. Investigations in humans are justified only for fully reversible reactions, such as those which occur in subjects with asthma or hypersensitivity pneumonitis, neither of which appear to be probable consequences of occupational exposure to MMVF. Inhalation studies with MMVF are in practice confined to laboratory animals, and provide invaluable insight to the possible long-term adverse effects of MMVF exposure in man. Major limitations of this method of investigation include high cost, a need for sophisticated equipment, and rigorously defined experimental conditions.

The outcomes of inhalation toxicity studies in rodents must be extrapolated to man cautiously. In general, rats or other rodent species are exposed experimentally to high concentrations of aerosol enriched by long fibers. Such exposures may not, however, simulate adequately occupational or environmental exposures to lower fiber concentrations or to mixtures of fibers of varied lengths; the experi-

mental exposure studies are designed to represent a worst-case scenario.

Numerous inhalation studies of various types of glass fibers have been conducted in multiple species of laboratory animals, such as guinea pigs [43], hamsters [44–46], and rats [43,44,46–52]. While none of these studies demonstrated a significant increase in pulmonary or pleural fibrosis, or pulmonary neoplasms, even in the presence of hundreds of thousands of retained fibers per milligram dry lung, only one of these studies (in rats) was conducted using size-selected fiber with nose-only exposure [53]. In a more recent study of a more durable and biopersistent specialty type of fiberglass (MMVF 33) in hamsters, inhalation caused irreversible fibrosis and one mesothelioma.

There have been several reports of chronic inhalation studies with mineral wool. As with those for fibrous glass, none have shown that slag or rock wool cause significant numbers of tumors by this route of exposure [46,49,52,54]. In contrast to slag wool, rock wool exposure began to show evidence of interstitial pulmonary fibrosis after 6 months exposure to 30 mg/m³ and after 18 months exposure to 16 mg/m³. The fibrosis was not progressive with time [54].

Recent reports have used rats and hamsters as the primary species for assessing the chronic effects of inhaled RCF [45,47,48]. In all cases the RCF was specially sized to provide a rat-respirable material approximately 1 µm in diameter and 20 µm long. Despite efforts to remove non-fiberized material, a substantial amount of respirable particulate remained (particulate: fiber ratio 9:1, a ratio significantly greater than that found in the workplace) [42]. Groups of rats were exposed 6 hours/day, 5 days/week for 24 months to 30 mg/m³ (maximum tolerated dose, approximately 200–250 f/ml) of four different types of RCF, and hamsters were exposed to RCF-1 only. In hamsters, RCF-1 induced pulmonary and pleural fibrosis and led to the development of malignant mesotheliomas in 42% of animals. No pulmonary tumors occurred. In the rats, the RCF also induced pulmonary and pleural fibrosis. It additionally induced a low incidence of mesotheliomas (in 1–2% over 2 years) and a significantly increased prevalence of lung tumors (7–19%). This dramatic difference in responses between rats and hamsters suggests a unique sensitivity to the induction of mesothelioma and a resistance to the development of lung tumors in the hamster as compared to the rat with this particular MMVF material.

Following estimation of the maximum tolerated fiber level, a multiple-dose exposure study was performed in rats with RCF-1 at concentrations of 3, 9, and 16 mg/m³ (approximately 25, 75 and 150 f/ml) [48]. Time-and dose-dependent pulmonary and pleural changes were seen. Interstitial fibrosis and minimal pleural fibrosis occurred after 12 months of exposure to 16 mg/m^3, while only minimal interstitial fibrosis was seen after 18 months exposure to 9 mg/m^3. In the lowest exposure group (3 mg/m^3) no pleural or parenchymal fibrosis was seen. There was no significant increase in lung tumor numbers at any dose compared to controls. Further studies in hamsters suggest unusual pleural sensitivity to this species to nearly all MMVF examined to date [48].

Under appropriate conditions and with sufficient exposure to large quantities of rodent-respirable RCF fibers with particles, rats developed lung fibrosis and an excess of benign and malignant lung tumors in a time- and concentration-dependent manner [42]. In hamsters, RCF-1 induced lung fibrosis, no pulmonary tumors of any kind, and a high incidence of pleural tumors.

MANAGEMENT

Since there is currently no conclusive evidence of any adverse respiratory disorder attributable to MMVF in man, the issue of management in individual cases is obviously an irrelevancy. Respiratory disorders arising in MMVF must, at present, be considered a consequence of other etiologic factors, and management is provided accordingly.

PREVENTION

In the workplace

The prevention of skin irritation and any potential adverse effects on the lungs requires minimizing exposure. Workplace exposures can be controlled with worker training, proper work practices, and environmental controls. Where skin contact or inhalation cannot be prevented, personal protection is essential: protective equipment can be as simple as long-sleeved shirts to minimize skin effects or safety glasses to prevent eye irritation, or more sophisticated to include respirators to avoid inhalation of airborne fibers. Regular sampling of fiber levels in

the workplace should be a standard component of worker protection. Finally, product stewardship programs (in which the manufacturer provides instruction for safe use to the production worker and purchaser) are an important prerequisite to protecting both the production worker and the end-user.

National regulatory strategies

No specific regulations govern exposure to manmade vitreous fibers. The US Occupational Safety and Health Administration regulates MMVF as 'particulate not otherwise regulated' with a workplace permissible exposure limit of 5.0 mg/m^3 for respirable dust, and 15.0 mg/m^3 for total dust. In 1998, the American Conference of Governmental Industrial Hygienists (ACGIH) adopted a threshold limit value (TLV) of 1 f/ml (one fiber per milliliter of air) for conventional glass fibers, and rock and slag wool. It has recommended a lower exposure level for RCF but has provided little scientific rationale for the proposed level; to date, no specific standard has been adopted by ACGIH. However, regulatory agencies in other countries have examined the issue and adopted standards for RCF that generally range from 0.5 to 1.0 f/ml [55].

In 1997, the Refractory Ceramic Fiber Coalition, a trade organization of US manufacturers of RCF, adopted a recommended exposure guideline of 0.5 f/ml. This was based in part on the results of a quantitative risk assessment [56] that estimated the excess working lifetime risk of lung cancer to workers exposed to 0.5 f/ml RCF at approximately 7.3×10^{-5} or even lower.

It is encouraging that new MMVF are being developed for high-temperature insulation applications with high solubility and, thus, low *in vivo* biodurability. Two new synthetic fibers have *in vitro* and *in vivo* dissolution rate kinetics such that they would not be expected to produce either pulmonary fibrosis or lung tumors in well-designed animal inhalation bioassays, or result in excess cancer incidence in human cohorts [6]. Clearly, ongoing human and animal research studies will continue to redefine the database for determining the health risks of MMVF inhalation.

DIFFICULT CASE

Since an adverse clinical effect of MMVF on the lung has not been confirmed in man, a Difficult Case cannot be included in this chapter.

SUMMARY POINTS

Recognition

- The most common effects in man of MMVF are skin, eye, and upper and lower respiratory tract irritation.
- Pleural plaques have been found in workers exposed during the manufacturing process of refractory ceramic fiber.
- To date there is no convincing evidence of any other adverse occupational effect in man, but studies of laboratory animals indicate some risk from some fibers of interstitial pulmonary fibrosis, pleural fibrosis, lung cancer, and mesothelioma, with considerable differences between different rodent species.

Management

- The effects described in studies to date have no specific treatment, and are most amenable to prevention.

Prevention

- Attention to appropriate skin protection by clothing and personal protective equipment is needed.
- In addition, respiratory protective devices can protect against airway irritation, since most fibers are relatively large and are easily filtered out by protective devices.

REFERENCES

1. *Occupational Exposure to Fibrous Glass. Proceedings of a Symposium.* HEW Publication (NIOSH), April 1976. No. 76–151.
2. Nomenclature Committee of TIMA, Inc. In: Eastes W, ed. *Manmade Vitreous Fibers: Nomenclature, Chemical and Physical Properties*, 2nd edn. Stamford, CT: Time Inc., 1993.
3. McConnell EE, Axten C, Hesterberg TW *et al.* Studies on the inhalation toxicology of two fiberglasses and amosite asbestos in the Syrian golden hamster. Part II. Results of chronic exposure. *Inhal Toxicol* 1999; 11: 785–835.
4. Lentz TJ, Rice CH, Lockey JE *et al.* Potential significance of airborne fiber dimensions measured in the U.S. refractory ceramic fiber manufacturing industry. *Am J Ind Med* 1999; 36: 286–298.
5. Cherrie JW, Bodsworth PL, Cowie HA *et al.* A report on the environmental conditions at seven European ceramic fibre plants. IOM Report TM/89/97. Edinburgh: Institute of Occupational Medicine, 1989.
6. World Health Organization European Program for Occupational Health. *Validity of Methods for Assessing the Carcinogenicity of Man-made Fibres. Executive Summary of a WHO Consultation, 19–20 May 1992.* Copenhagen: WHO Regional Office for Europe.
7. Björnberg A. Glass fiber dermatitis. *Am J Ind Med* 1985; 8: 395–400.
8. Newhall HH, Brahim SA. Respiratory response to domestic fibrous glass exposure. *Environ Res* 1976; 12: 201–207.
9. Hughes JM, Jones RN, Glindmeyer HW *et al.* Follow up study of workers exposed to man made mineral fibres. *Br J Ind Med* 1993; 50: 658–666.
10. Woodcock AJ, Mellis CM. *Respiratory Health of Workers in the Australian Glasswool and Rockwool Manufacturing Industry.* Final report prepared for Insulation Wools Research Advisory Board by Institute of Respiratory Medicine, Royal Prince Alfred Hospital, Sydney, Australia, 1994.
11. Hansen EF, Rasmussen FV, Hardt F, Kamstrup O. Lung function and respiratory health of long-term fiber-exposed stonewool factory workers. *Am J Respir Crit Care Med* 1999; 160: 466–472.
12. Sali D, Boffetta P, Anderson A *et al.* Non–neoplastic mortality of European Workers who produce man made vitreous fibres. *Occrup Environ Med* 1999; 56: 612–617.

13. Chiazze L, Watkins DK, Fryar C, Fayerweather W, Bender JR, Chiazze M. Mortality from nephritis and nephrosis in the fibreglass manufacturing industry. *Occup Environ Med* 1999; 56: 164–166.
14. Marsh G, Stone R, Youk A *et al.* Mortality among United States rock wool and slag wool workers: 1989 update. *J Occup Health Safety–Anst NZ* 1996; 12: 297–312.
15. Calvert GM, Steenland K, Palu S. End–stage renal disease among silica-exposed gold miners: a new method for assessing incidence among epidemiologic cohorts. *JAMA* 1997; 277: 1219–1223.
16. Takahashi T, Munakata M, Takekawa H *et al.* Pulmonary fibrosis in a carpenter with long-lasting exposure to fiberglass. *Am J Ind Med* 1996; 30: 596–600.
17. Kilburn KH, Powers D, Warshaw RH. Pulmonary effects of exposure to fine fibreglass: Irregular opacities and small airways obstruction. *Br J Ind Med* 1992; 49: 714–720.
18. Bender JR. Pulmonary effects of exposure to fine fibreglass: irregular opacities and small airways obstruction. *Br J Ind Med* 1993; 50: 381–382.
19. Clausen J, Netterstrom B, Wolff C. Lung function in insulation workers. *Br J Ind Med* 1993; 50: 252–256.
20. Lemasters GK, Lockey JE, Levin LS *et al.* An industry-wide pulmonary study of men and women manufacturing refractory ceramic fibers. *Am J Epidemiol* 1998; 148: 910–919.
21. Lockey JE, Levin LS, Lemasters GK *et al.* Longitudinal estimates of pulmonary function in refractory ceramic fiber manufacturing workers. *Am J Respir Crit Care Med* 1998; 157: 1226–1233.
22. Lemasters G, Lockey J, Rice C *et al.* Radiographic changes among workers manufacturing refractory ceramic fibre and products. *Ann Occup Hyg* 1994; 38(1): 745–751.
23. Lockey J, Lemaster G, Rice C *et al.* Refractory ceramic fiber exposure and pleural plaques. *Am J Respir Crit Care Med* 1996; 154: 1405–1410.
24. Trethowan MN, Burge PS, Rossiter CE *et al.* Study of the respiratory health of workers in seven European plants that manufacture ceramic fibres. *Occup Environ Med* 1995; 52: 97–104.
25. Cowie HA, Beck J, Wild P *et al. Institute of Occupational Medicine. Epidemiological research in European Ceramic Fibre Industry 1994–1998.* IOM Report TM/99/01, June 1999.
26. IARC Monographs. *Evaluation of Carcinogenic Risks to Humans*, Vol. 43, 39–46. IARC: Lyon, France 1988.
27. Enterline PE, Marsh GM, Esmen NA. Respiratory disease among workers exposed to man-made mineral fibers. *Am Rev Respir Dis* 1983; 128: 1–7.

28. Enterline PE, Marsh GM, Henderson VL, Callahan C. Mortality update of a cohort of US man-made mineral fiber workers. *Ann Occup Hyg* 1987; 31: 625–656.

29. Marsh GM, Enterline PE, Stone RA *et al*. Mortality among a cohort of US man-made mineral fiber workers: 1985 follow-up. *J Occup Med* 1990; 32: 594–604.

30. Chiazze L, Watkins DK, Fryar C. A case-control study of malignant and non-malignant respiratory disease among employees of a fibreglass manufacturing facility. *Br J Ind Med* 1992; 49: 326–331.

31. Wong O, Foliart D, Trent LS. A case-control study of lung cancer in a cohort of workers potentially exposed to slag wool fibres. *Br J Ind Med* 1991; 48: 818–824.

32. Shannon HS, Jamieson E, Julian JA *et al*. Mortality experience of Ontario glass fibre workers-extended follow-up. *Ann Occup Hyg* 1987; 31(4B): 657–662.

33. Simonato L, Fletcher AC, Cherrie JW *et al*. The International Agency for Research on cancer historical cohort study of MMMF production workers in seven European countries: extension of the follow-up. *Ann Occup Hyg* 1987; 31: 603–623.

34. Simonato L, Fletcher AC, Cherrie J *et al*. The man-made mineral fiber European historical cohort study. *Scand J Work Environ Health* 1986; 12: 34–47.

35. Boffetta P, Saracci R, Andersen A *et al*. Cancer mortality among man–made vitreous fiber production workers. *Epidemiology* 1997; 8: 259–268.

36. Boffetta P, Anderson A, Hansen J *et al*. Cancer incidence among European man–made vitreous fiber production workers. *Scan J Work Environ Health* 1999; 25: 222–226.

37. Shannon HS, Jamieson E, Julian JA, Muir DC. Mortality of glass filament (textile) workers. *Br J Ind Med* 1990; 47: 533–536.

38. Watkins DK, Chiazze L, Fryar C. Historical cohort mortality study of a continuous filament fiberglass manufacturing plant. *J Occup Environ Med* 1997; 39: 548–555.

39. Chiazze L, Watkins DK, Fryar C. Historical cohort mortality study of a continuous filament fiberglass manufacturing plant. *J Occup Environ Med* 1997; 39: 432–441.

40. Gustavsson P, Plato N, Axelson O *et al*. Lung cancer risk among workers exposed to man–made mineral fibers (MMMF) in the Swedish prefabricated house industry. *Am J Ind Med* 1992; 21: 825–834.

41. USDHHS. *9th Report on Carcinogens, 1999. Summary*. National Toxicology Program Washington DC 1998.

42. Maxim LD, Mast RW, Utell MJ *et al*. Hazard assessment and risk analysis of two new synthetic vitreous fibers. *Reg Toxicol Pharmacol* 1999; 30: 54–74.

43. Hesterberg TW, Müller WC, McConnell EE *et al*. Chronic inhalation toxicity of size-separated glass fibers in Fischer 344 rats. *Fund Appl Toxicol* 1993; 20: 464–476.

44. Wagner JC, Berry GB, Hill RJ *et al*. Animal experiments with MMM(V) F – effects of inhalation and intrapleural inoculation in rats. In: *Biological Effects of Man-made Mineral Fibres*. Proceedings of a WHO/IARC Conference, Copenhagen, 20–22 April, Vol. 2. Geneva: World Health Organization, 1982.

45. Mitchell RI, Donogrio DJ, Moorman WJ. Chronic inhalation toxicity of fibrous glass in rats and Monkeys. *J Am Coll Toxicol* 1986; 5: 545–575.

46. Le Bouffant L, Daniel H, Henin JP *et al.*, Experimental study on long-term effects of inhaled MMMF on the lung of rats. *Ann Occup Hyg* 1987; 31: 765–790.

47. Mast RW, McConnell EE, Hesterberg TW *et al*. Multiple dose chronic inhalation study of size-separated kaolin refractory fiber in male Fischer 344 rats. *Inhal Toxicol* 1995; 7: 469–502.

48. Everitt JI, Gelzleichter TR, Bermudez E *et al*. Comparison of pleural responses of rats and hamsters to subchronic inhalation of refractory ceramic fibers. *Environ Health Perspect* 1997; 105: 1209–1213.

49. McConnell EE, Mast RW, Hesterberg TW *et al*. Chronic Inhalation Toxicity of a Kaolin Based Refractory Ceramic Fiber (RCF) in Hamsters. pp. 1–69. Littleton, CO: Mountain Technology Center, 1991. MTC Report 092518.

50. Muhle H, Pott F, Bellmann B *et al*. Inhalation and injection experiments in rats to test the carcinogenicity of MMMF. *Ann Occup Hyg* 1987; 31: 755–764.

51. Smith DM, Ortiz LW, Archuleta RF and Johnson NF. Long-term health effects in hamsters and rats exposed chronically to man-made vitreous fibres. *Ann Occup Hyg* 1987; 31: 731–754.

52. Lee KP, Barras E, Griffith FD, Waritz RS and Lapin CA. Comparative pulmonary responses to inhaled inorganic fibers with asbestos and fiber glass. *Environ Res* 1981; 24: 167–191.

53. Hesterberg TW, Chase G, Axten C *et al*. Biopersistence of synthetic vitreous fibers and amosite asbestos in the rat lung following inhalation, a joint study of NAIMA and EURIMA. *Toxicol Appl Pharmacol* 1998; 151: 262–275.

54. Mast RW, Maxim LD, Utell MJ *et al*. Refractory ceramic fiber: toxicology, epidemiology, and risk analysis – a review. *Inhal Toxicol* 2000; 12: 359–399.

55. Bunn WB III, Bender JR, Hesterberg TW *et al*. Recent studies of man-made vitreous fibers: chronic animal inhalation studies. *J Occup Med* 1993; 35: 101–113.

56. Mast RW, Utell MJ. Man-made vitreous fibers. In: Zenz C, Dickerson OB, Horvath EP, eds. *Occupational Medicine*, pp. 185–193. St Louis, MO: Mosby, 1994.

TOXIC PNEUMONITIS: CHEMICAL AGENTS

Benoit Nemery

BACKGROUND

The notion of 'toxic pneumonitis' is not strictly defined; in this chapter the definition is essentially operational. The terms toxic pneumonitis and chemical-induced lung injury, and the underlying concepts, are often used interchangeably, usually with the implicit notion that disease presentation is acute (or subacute). In a broad sense, even the traditional pneumoconioses might be considered examples of toxic pneumonitis, because minerals such as crystalline silica or fibrous asbestos are obviously toxic for the lung in which they induce some degree of 'pneumonitis', but the term is not usually applied in the context of slowly evolving processes. In this chapter, toxic pneumonitis refers to acute or subacute disorders of chemically induced injury in the lung parenchyma. In this sense, alveolar lipoproteinosis caused by brief heavy exposure to crystalline silica is included more appropriately within the category of toxic pneumonitis, than in that of pneumoconiosis.

Another somewhat confusing aspect of 'toxic pneumonitis' is that it is sometimes difficult to dissociate toxic injury to the lung parenchyma from injury to the airways, particularly when the bronchioles are involved. Although the site of damage depends essentially on the nature of the inhaled agent, the circumstances of the exposure (such as

the concentration of the chemical, the duration of the exposure, and the depth of inhalation) also determine whether the lung parenchyma is affected in inhalation injury. Consequently, many agents that can cause toxic tracheo-bronchitis (Chapter 6) may also cause toxic pneumonitis, and some overlap is inevitable among disease descriptions. However, some agents, most notably the poorly water-soluble gases, may reach deeply into the lung without giving rise to much injury to the conducting airways.

In the occupational setting, toxic pneumonitis generally results from exposure by inhalation, but toxic lung injury may also be caused by chemicals (most often therapeutic drugs) that reach the lung via the circulation. Paraquat provides a further notable example (Chapter 23). The inhaled agents capable of causing toxic pneumonitis are very diverse. They include gases, vapors, and aerosols (particles and liquid droplets) and they range from single and well-defined chemicals to complex and poorly characterized mixtures, such as the combustion products from fires or explosions. Moreover, toxic lung damage may not only be caused by man-made compounds, it may also result from exposure to 'biologic' agents, such as bacterial or fungal toxins (Chapter 13). For most compounds, pneumonitis results from direct toxic injury, but for some chemical agents, such as methylene diphenyl diisocyanate (MDI) or trimellitic anhydride (TMA), the damage results from immunologic mechanisms (Chapters 14, 23).

Epidemiologic data about the occurrence of toxic pneumonitis are virtually non-existent. The literature on toxic pneumonitis is based, to a large extent, on anecdotal reports of accidental inhalation injuries in one or more individuals and by more or less defined chemicals. Poison control center data from the San Francisco Bay area indicate that symptomatic inhalational exposures are common, but severe acute and persistent morbidity is uncommon [1]. In this series, 62% of subjects had sustained the exposure outside work. In the subjects with work-related inhalations, approximately one-fifth reported closed-space exposure [2]. In the SWORD (Surveillance of Work-related and Occupational Respiratory Disease) voluntary surveillance scheme in Britain, less than 10% of the 24 108 reported cases of occupational lung disease between 1990 and 1997 concerned inhalation accidents [3]. Such accidents may take catastrophic proportions [4] and involve hundreds of victims, as occurred after the explosion of a tank containing methyl isocyanate in Bhopal in 1984, or as a result of chemical warfare during the First World War or the more recent Iran–Iraq War. However, the epidemiologic information that could have been gained from these catastrophes has been rather limited [5].

Rarely, outbreaks of toxic pneumonitis have occurred without accident or warfare, as in the case of the 'Ardystil' syndrome that was caused by exposure to sprayed polymeric paints. Some epidemiologic data suggest that individuals exposed occupationally to metals, wood smoke, etc. have higher risks of 'idiopathic' pulmonary fibrosis [6]. The latter may be partly a reflection of inadequate occupational and environmental histories in unaffected 'control' populations, but there is speculation that 'low-grade' toxic pneumonitis occurs in some individuals within exposed occupational groups who then develop fibrotic lung disease.

Although the focus of this chapter is on occupational disorders, it is clear that chemical-induced lung injury is not restricted to the traditional workplace: it may occur in other environments such as the home (e.g. during cleaning or leisure activities), or the urban and general environment (e.g. after industrial or transport accidents) [7–9]. It is also important to realize that toxic pneumonitis may result from inhaling or injecting illegal drugs [10], as well as from an adverse effect of prescribed drugs [11].

Toxic pneumonitis may have various clinical presentations which, for convenience, are divided here in three main categories. A first category concerns relatively mild, febrile reactions, collectively known as inhalation fevers; the second category is that of the acute and often life-threatening chemical pneumonitis with non-cardiogenic pulmonary edema, that follows a single brief exposure to a toxic agent; the third category covers subacute pulmonary inflammation resulting from more prolonged exposure to pneumotoxic agents.

INHALATION FEVERS

Inhalation fever is the name given to cover a group of 'flu-like clinical syndromes, such as metal fume fever, polymer fume fever, and the organic dust toxic syndrome (ODTS) [12]. The term 'inhalation fever' is of relatively recent adoption [12] and for a while it competed with the term 'toxic alveolitis' [13]. There are arguments in favor of both terms, because the former emphasizes the clinical and relatively benign nature of the condition, whereas the latter indicates the (presumed) main site of the toxic (i.e. non-immunological) inflammatory reaction. Inhalation fever is currently the term preferred by most authors, largely because clinical evidence of alveolar involvement is often lacking. Inhalation fever occurs in many settings, and so is addressed additionally in several other chapters within the book.

Recognition

Causes

Metal fume fever is a long-recognized syndrome, known best by those who are especially at risk of suffering from it, such as welders or other workers in metal trades, than by most doctors [14,15]. The most frequent and best documented cause is heating zinc. Zinc fumes, which oxidize to fine particles of zinc oxide (ZnO), are produced, for instance, when zinc is smelted to make alloys, when zinc-containing scrap metal is melted, when metal surfaces are sprayed with zinc, and when galvanized (zinc-covered) steel is welded or cut. Metal fume fever occurs when the fumes are not properly exhausted, which is often the case when these jobs are carried out in enclosed spaces. Not only freshly formed zinc fumes, but also fine zinc oxide dust, has the ability to cause metal 'fume' fever [15]. The fumes of many other metals are also said to cause metal fume fever, but this is much less satisfactorily documented, except for copper [15].

Polymer fume fever is a less common cause of inhalation fever [16]. It occurs principally after exposure to the fumes that are produced when fluorine-containing polymers, such as polytetrafluoroethylene (PTFE, also known as Teflon), are heated above 300°C. This may occur when such polymers are extruded (e.g. as a consequence of malfunction with overheating) or machined, or when metals coated with PTFE are welded. PTFE may also be sprayed, for example as a mold-releasing agent [17], and pyrolysis of airborne PTFE aerosols may occur within burning cigarettes. This explains why polymer fume fever occurs mainly in those who smoke at work. Although polymer fume fever has been well described only after exposure to the fumes of fluorine-containing polymers, it may possibly occur after exposure to fumes evolved from heating other plastics, such as polyvinylchloride (PVC) or other polymers containing chlorine [18,19], polyurethane, or polymers containing bromine-based flame retardants [20] (Fig. 12.1).

It has been argued that polymer fume fever is not an appropriate descriptive term for inclusion within the category of the inhalation fevers, because severe incidents with pulmonary edema and long-term sequelae have been described after the inhalation of pyrolysis products of such polymers, probably when the heating temperatures are higher (see later).

Organic dust toxic syndrome is caused by the inhalation of large quantities of agricultural and other dusts of biologic origin (Chapter 13). It has clinical and pathogenetic features that are essentially similar to those of metal fume fever and polymer fume fever.

Clinical features

The clinical features of the inhalation fevers are best described as influenza-like. The actual exposure may or may not have been experienced as irritant or troublesome for the eyes and respiratory tract. Four to eight hours after the exposure (i.e. often in the evening after work), the affected subject begins to feel unwell with fever, chills, headaches, malaise, nausea, and muscle aches. In the case of metal fume fever, there may be a metallic taste in the mouth. Respiratory symptoms are usually mild and consist mainly of cough and/or sore throat, but occasionally subjects may have more severe responses with dyspnea. The body temperature may rise as high as 39–40°C, but there are also less full-blown inhalation 'fevers' with malaise, headache, or systemic symptoms, but without detectable fever.

In general, chest auscultation and chest radiographs are normal, but in more severe cases, which are more likely to attract medical attention, crackles may be heard, and there may be transient radiographic infiltrates [21,22]. In the latter circumstances, a diagnosis of inhalation fever could reasonably be challenged, and one of chemical pneumonitis substituted. The difference is essentially quantitative rather than qualitative, the two diagnostic terms representing opposite ends of a disease spectrum. Although pulmonary function is often within normal limits, reductions in vital capacity and forced expired volume in 1 s (FEV_1) are perhaps more frequent than commonly accepted; in severe cases there may be a decrease in transfer factor and arterial

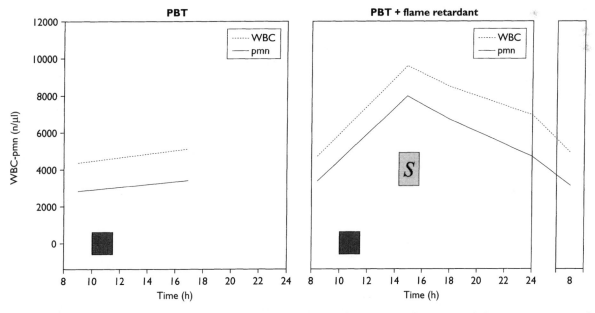

Fig. 12.1 Results of a provocation test in a production worker from a polyester extrusion plant who complained of symptoms suggestive of inhalation fever only after exposure to fumes of heated polyester containing polybrominated flame retardants. The subject was a 30-year-old male non-smoker with a history of atopic rhinitis. He was exposed, in a cabin, to the fumes produced by heating (to 300°C) approximately ~ 500 g of polybutyleneterephthalate (PBT) without (left panel) or with (right panel) the flame retardant. Exposures are indicated by black squares (90 min and 80 min, respectively). There were no symptoms after exposure to PBT fumes, but after exposure to the fumes containing the flame retardant, the subject complained of malaise and myalgia, and had noticeable chills (S), without fever or changes in pulmonary function. WBC and pmn are peripheral blood leukocytes and polymorphonuclear neutrophils, respectively. The horizontal axis represents time of day.

hypoxemia, thereby pointing to more obvious alveolar involvement. Peripheral blood leukocytosis, with a rise in neutrophils, is a consistent finding for 24 hours after the exposure (see Fig. 12.1); other blood tests should give normal results except, probably, for indices of an inflammatory response, but few published data are available about this. Bronchoalveolar lavage studies have shown very pronounced increases in polymorphonuclear leukocyte proportions (between 19% and 63% of cells) on the day after exposure to zinc fumes [23,24].

Metal fume fever and ODTS are considered to be mediated non-specifically (i.e. non-immunologically) through activation of macrophages and/or pulmonary epithelial cells and the local and systemic release of pyrogenic and chemotactic mediators, such as tumor necrosis factor-alpha (TNF-α), interleukin - (IL) 6 and IL8 [25,26]. The mechanism of polymer fume fever is unknown and the causal components within the fume are also unknown. It has been shown that the heating rate of PTFE influences the type and quantity of thermal decomposition products, some of which appear to be extremely toxic [16].

Inhalation fever is generally a self-limiting syndrome, with recovery after a night's rest. Tolerance usually develops to exposures recurring shortly after a bout of metal fume fever or ODTS, but it seems that this feature is less typical of polymer fume fever [16].

Differential diagnosis

Arguably, the most important issue concerning diagnosis is that physicians know of the existence of occupational febrile influenza-like reactions and the circumstances in which they occur. The diagnosis rests essentially on the exposure history and the clinical condition, and when these clearly point to inhalation fever, no sophisticated investigations are required. In practice, those workers who are most familiar with the condition rarely seek medical attention for it. If they do, there is greater need to consider an alternative diagnosis.

Because many doctors are unfamiliar with occupationally induced disease, inhalation fever is often not recognized and, instead, the condition is attributed simply to a viral infection or, more trivially, 'indigestion'. Migraine and even prostatitis may be suspected initially. With more severe or recurrent episodes, patients may undergo invasive procedures (e.g. emergency lumbar puncture to exclude meningitis) or extensive investigations for 'fever of unknown origin' until the possibility of an occupational cause is considered.

Sometimes, hypersensitivity pneumonitis or occupational asthma is suspected. As a rule, the typical respiratory symptoms and functional characteristics of hypersensitivity pneumonitis or asthma are absent, although subjects with these disorders may, of course, suffer also from inhalation fever. It is conceivable, though not established, that subjects with preexisting high levels of non-specific airway responsiveness are more susceptible to zinc or polymer fumes. Thus, fume fever and asthma occasionally occur together [27,28], and it may be difficult to ascertain which is primarily responsible for the symptoms. Systematic studies of sequential measurements of peak expiratory flow (PEF) from patients with recurrent bouts of metal fume fever have not been published, but experience with a few patients suggests that they may show small, but consistent, work-related decreases in peak expiratory flow. It is worth asking patients to measure their temperature daily when inhalation fever is suspected. Increases in blood leukocyte numbers may be useful to document changes in individuals or groups.

It is also important not to confuse inhalation fever with more serious conditions. In particular, it is critical to ensure that the exposure fumes did not include highly toxic gases (such as nitrogen dioxide and phosgene) or the vapors or condensation products from metals such as cadmium, mercury, or osmium. Such exposures may lead to fatal pulmonary edema (i.e. chemical pneumonitis, see below), which in its early phases could be mistaken for inhalation fever. The physician should also be aware that some fumes from heated polymers, including fluorinated polymers, may be extremely hazardous and lead to severe pulmonary injury.

Management

No specific treatment (other than palliative analgesics or antiinflammatory agents) is required for inhalation fever, and the patient may be reassured about the generally benign nature and course of the disease. It is important to recognize that 'allergy' is not involved in the pathogenesis of inhalation fevers. Consequently, there is no rationale for advising complete and definitive avoidance of further exposure in subjects who have suffered from inhalation fever – in contrast to occupational asthma caused by sensitization.

Prevention

It is unacceptable from an occupational hygiene point of view that metal fume fever occurs in the workplace, and working conditions should be improved to prevent any recurrence of symptoms. Although metal fume fever is generally considered not to lead to long-term sequelae, this has not been investigated fully satisfactorily, and there are indications that a history of metal fume fever may be associated with an excess of ongoing respiratory symptoms and poorer lung function [29]. Such associations may, however, reflect the higher exposure levels likely to be encountered in such circumstances.

It should be noted that, at least in the case of zinc, compliance with the occupational exposure limit (threshold limit value; TLV) of 5 mg/m^3 does not necessarily prevent the occurrence of fume fever [26]. For as yet unknown reasons, some subjects appear to be more susceptible than others to non-specific stimuli of inflammation. Metal fume fever may also occur in some individuals because of 'ergonomic errors', such as holding the head between the source of the fume and the exhaust hood or port for local exhaust ventilation, or a leak in respiratory protective equipment. Since smokers are at particular risk of polymer fume fever, because PTFE particles burn in the cigarette, a further useful preventive measure is the prohibition of smoking within the working environment.

ACUTE CHEMICAL PNEUMONITIS

A great variety of substances can cause inhalation injury. The toxic compounds may be in a gaseous state, or they may consist of aerosols of liquid or solid particles; often both gases and particles are present, as is the case with burning plastics, wood, and other materials. The site and severity of the respiratory damage caused by inhaled compounds depend mainly on the nature of the agent and the amount inhaled. The subject has been amply covered in a number of textbooks and review articles [7–9].

Recognition

As a general rule, gaseous irritants that have a high solubility in water mainly affect the upper respiratory tract, causing laryngitis, tracheitis, or bronchitis (Chapter 6). Such water-soluble irritants are easily trapped in the aqueous surfaces of the upper respiratory tract and the eyes, where they rapidly cause irritation, thus leading the subject to avoid further exposure whenever this is possible. In contrast, poorly water-soluble gases are not so well scrubbed by the upper respiratory tract and reach the deep lung more easily, where they may cause pulmonary edema, usually after a latency of several hours. Moreover, as they cause much less sensory irritation, significant exposure to such gases may be tolerated with little or no difficulty. These insoluble gases are consequently more hazardous. Gases of intermediate solubilities mainly affect the upper respiratory tract and large bronchi, but high or prolonged exposures to these agents may also injure the lung parenchyma and cause chemical pneumonitis. This may also occur when massive quantities of highly water-soluble gases are inhaled.

With aerosols, the degree of penetration into the respiratory tract depends mainly on the size of the particles, with the smallest particles (<5 μm aerodynamic diameter) having the greatest probability of reaching the distal airways and alveoli. Such small particles are often produced by combustion processes or by the condensation of vapors. The particles may be toxic by themselves (e.g. cadmium oxide) or they may carry adsorbed irritants, such as sulfates or aldehydes.

Chemical pneumonitis may also result from the ingestion and subsequent aspiration of liquids, such as solvents or hydrocarbon fuels. Some chemicals, most notably agrichemicals such as paraquat and cholinesterase inhibitors, may cause chemical lung injury by routes other than inhalation.

Clinical features

The response to acute chemical injury in the respiratory tract is rarely compound-specific. Following exposure to water-soluble irritants, there may be pronounced signs of upper airway irritation, with severe cough, hoarseness, stridor or wheezing, retrosternal pain, and discharge of bronchial mucus – possibly with blood, mucosal tissue, and soot. Death may occur as a result of laryngeal edema. If the lung parenchyma is also involved, non-cardiogenic pulmonary edema may develop over the course of several hours. It is important to realize that victims of serious inhalation accidents may feel perfectly well and walk into the hospital or emergency room, or even go home following the inhalation, and then experience progressive dyspnea, shallow breathing, cyanosis, frothy pink sputum, and eventually respiratory failure. The clinical picture of adult respiratory distress syndrome (ARDS) may thus develop gradually over 4–72 hours, even after a period of clinical improvement. In the days that follow severe acute inhalation injury, pulmonary infectious complications are common because of the impairment of the normal protective mechanisms of the airways (epithelial disruption, impaired ciliary clearance, plugging by debris and inflammation). The possible late effects and sequelae of inhalation injury are discussed below.

Depending on the circumstances of the accident, there may be thermal or chemical facial burns, as well as signs of mucosal irritation and edema, and even hemorrhage and ulcerations in the air passages. Auscultation of the chest may or may not be abnormal, with wheezing, rhonchi, or crepitations. Pulmonary function can be used to monitor ambulatory subjects; spirometry is expected to show an obstructive or mixed obstructive and restrictive impairment, depending on the site of the injury. Arterial blood gases show varying degrees of hypoxemia and respiratory acidosis, depending on the severity of the injury. The chest radiograph is usually normal if only the conducting airways are involved, but there may be signs of peribronchial cuffing. Following the deep penetration of toxic chemicals, the chest radiograph is unremarkable in the first hours after presentation, but signs of interstitial and alveolar edema then become visible and, with time, patchy infiltrates, areas of atelectasis and even 'white lungs' may develop (Fig. 12.2). These changes may be due to tissue damage and organization, or they may reflect superimposed infectious bronchopneumonia.

Depending on the causal agent, the circumstances of the accident, and subsequent complications, other organ systems may also be affected.

Causes

Table 12.1 lists the more important agents that can cause chemical inhalation injuries. They are grouped for convenience, rather than on the basis of their pathophysiological effects, into four general categories: (1) irritant gases; (2) organic chemicals; (3) metallic agents; and (4) complex mixtures.

Irritant gases

Irritant gases with high water solubility, such as ammonia (NH_3), sulfur dioxide (SO_2), hydrogen chlor-

Table 12.1 Posible causes of acute chemical pneumonitis

- Irritant gases
    High water-solubility: NH_3, SO_2, HCl, ...
    Moderate water-solubility: Cl_2, H_2S, ...
    Low water-solubility: O_3, NO_2, $COCl_2$
- Organic chemicals
    Organic acids: acetic acid, ...
    Aldehydes: formaldehyde, acrolein, ...
    Isocyanates: methyl isocyanate (MIC), toluene
        diisocyanate (TDI)
    Amines: hydrazine, chloramines, ...
    Tear gas (CS) and mustard gas
    Organic solvents, including some leather
        treatment sprays
    Some agrichemicals (paraquat, cholinesterase
        inhibitors)
- Metallic compounds
    Mercury vapours
    Metallic oxides: CdO, V_2O_5, MnO, Os_3O_4, ...
    Halides: $ZnCl_2$, $TiCl_4$, $SbCl_5$, UF_6, ...
    $Ni(CO)_4$
    Hydrides: B_2H_5, LiH, AsH_3, SbH_3
- Complex mixtures
    Fire smoke
    Pyrolysis products from plastics
    Solvent mixtures
    Spores and toxins from microorganisms

ide (HCl), formaldehyde (HCHO), and acetic acid (CH_3COOH), have good warning properties and so, in general, exposure to them is rapidly curtailed and only mild upper airway irritation ensues. When ongoing exposure cannot be curtailed, there is the potential for serious toxicity to the upper respiratory tract, the intrathoracic airways, and the lung parenchyma sequentially, especially if the exposure concentration (or duration) has been considerable. Notable recent examples of such massive inhalation accidents followed explosions or accidents in mines or chemical installations causing the release of SO_2 [30–32] or NH_3 [33,34].

Similar considerations apply to chlorine (Cl_2), hydrogen sulfide (H_2S), and methyl isocyanate (CH_3CNO), which have intermediate water solubilities. Accidental release of chlorine is probably one of the most frequent causes of inhalation injury, not only in industry, but also in the community, as a result of transportation accidents or the use of chlorine for the disinfection of swimming pools [35]. An important cause in the domestic setting is that which results from the mixing of bleach (NaClO) with acids, releasing gaseous chlorine, or with ammonia, releasing volatile chloramines (monochloramine, NH_2Cl, dichloramine, $NHCl_2$, and trichloramine, NCl_3) [36]. The mixing of household cleaners and their over-enthusiastic use has been reported to cause severe

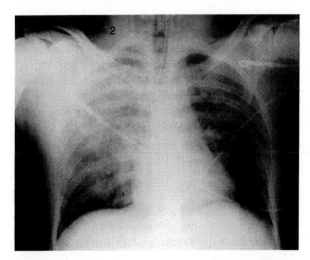

Fig. 12.2 Chest radiograph 1 day after the accidental inhalation of hydrogen sulfide (H_2S). The subject was a 31-year-old male non-smoker with a history of asthma in his youth. When attempting to sample oil on a tanker, a massive quantity of H_2S escaped because the normal venting procedures had not been followed. The man became comatose within an hour of exposure and needed artificial ventilation for 10 days. One day after the accident he had bilateral infiltrates on a chest radiograph. During the following 2 years he suffered from severe bronchorhea and asthma symptoms. (Courtesy of Dr P. Bomans, Stuivenberg Hospital, Antwerp.)

pneumonia that was not immediately recognized as being of toxic origin [37]. Chloramines are also implicated in the irritant effects of swimming pool atmospheres [38,39].

Hydrogen sulfide (H_2S), which is formed by the putrefaction of organic material in sewage drains, manure pits, and ship holds, and is also a frequent contaminant in the petrochemical industry, has special properties as an irritant gas because it does not only cause mucosal irritation but also leads to chemical asphyxia by mechanisms similar to those of cyanide. Victims who survive massive inhalation of H_2S may exhibit (hemorrhagic) pulmonary edema, as well as pneumonia in the days following the event [40,41] (see Fig. 12.2). Methyl isocyanate (CH_3CNO) has gained notoriety as the chemical that caused the highest number of casualties in a single accident, when it was released from a tank in a pesticide factory in Bhopal, India, in December 1984 [5,42–44]. Methyl isocyanate causes intense eye and upper airway irritation, and may also lead to pulmonary edema.

Poorly water-soluble gases are potentially the most hazardous, because the absence of immediate irritant effects allows them to penetrate to the distal airways and gas-exchanging tissues in increasing cumulative dose. This leads to delayed non-cardiogenic pulmonary edema. The best known examples are nitrogen dioxide (NO_2), ozone (O_3) and phosgene ($COCl_2$). NO_2 (which is generally in equilibrium with other oxides of nitrogen, NO and N_2O_4) is a reddish brown gas, heavier than air. It is often incorrectly referred to as 'nitrous fumes'. It may be encountered in a wide variety of occupational settings. A well-known example in agriculture is 'silo-filler's disease' [45]. This occurs because NO_2 is produced within a few days of fermentation of silage, thus posing a risk of fatal inhalation injury for anyone entering the silo soon after it is filled. Silo-filler's disease must not be confused with 'silo-unloader's syndrome', an inhalation fever which may occur later (after microbial toxins have formed) when the silo is decapped.

Fatally high concentrations of NO_2 may also be produced when special jet fuels explode [46], when tanks of nitric acid (HNO_3) explode [47], and when materials containing large quantities of nitrogen are burned or when nitric acid reacts with metals, wood, or other cellulose materials. Further sources of NO_2 exposure include the production and use of fertilizers, explosives, and other nitrogen-containing synthetic chemicals; the detonation of explosives in mining or tunneling; the normal combustion of fuels, particularly diesel; and the welding or torch cutting of metals. However, air concentrations of NO_2 produced in the latter instances are only rarely, if ever, a cause of acute pulmonary edema.

Nevertheless, outbreaks of acute respiratory illness in players and spectators attending ice-hockey matches have been attributed to NO_2 as a result of malfunctioning ice-resurfacing machines [48,49].

Although ozone is a very potent oxidant and although, as an outdoor air pollutant, it is a well-established cause of respiratory irritation, functional impairment, and airway inflammation, there are no documented instances of serious acute lung damage caused by exposure to ozone during occupational operations such as welding, office photocopying, or laser printing. By contrast, phosgene (carbonyl chloride) is a well-known cause of pulmonary edema, since it was used in chemical warfare during the First World War [50]. At present, it is used most in chemical syntheses, notably in the manufacture of isocyanates, and it may be released as a byproduct by the thermal or ultraviolet decomposition of chlorine-containing compounds such as methylene chloride or trichloroethylene [51,52].

Organic chemicals

Some organic chemicals are made intentionally to cause respiratory irritation. The most common lachrymating agents, known as tear gases (they are in fact aerosol-dispersed chemicals) are *ortho*-chlorobenzylidene malononitrile (CS) and ω-chloroacetophenone (CN). They are used in riot-control operations or as personal antiharassment weapons. Their action is usually short-lived and limited to the mucous membranes of the eyes and upper respiratory tract, but their use in confined spaces (e.g. prison cells) may lead to more serious lung damage [53–55]. Lung-damaging chemical warfare agents include the choking agents (chlorine, phosgene, diphosgene, and chloropicrin) and the vesicant (or blister agent), mustard gas (sulphur mustard). The latter caused severe bronchopulmonary damage in soldiers during the Iran–Iraq war [56,57].

Exposure to organic solvents is only rarely a cause of toxic pneumonitis. However, acute exposure to very high concentrations of solvent vapors in confined spaces (e.g. in chemical tanks) may be a cause of chemical pneumonitis and pulmonary edema, often in victims who have been unconscious [58]. Pneumonitis and ARDS caused by loss of alveolar surfactant may also result from the aspiration of ingested solvents or fuels, whether this was intentional ('fire eating' [59]) or unintentional (petrol siphoning). When pulmonary edema occurs after exposure to chlorinated aliphatic solvents (methylene chloride, trichloroethylene, tetrachloroethylene), the actual toxic agent may be phosgene generated from their (thermal) degradation.

A special mention should also be given to cases of severe acute respiratory illness caused, in the domestic environment, by acute exposure in confined spaces to water-proofing sprays [60], leather conditioners [61], or similar agents [62]. The exact causative agent(s) and mechanisms of injury in these cases are not always clear, but the solvents or fluorinated polymers are likely to play a role.

Some agrichemicals may cause toxic pneumonitis after non-inhalatory exposure. The best known of these agents is the herbicide paraquat which gains access to the lung via the circulation after gastrointestinal or (rarely) dermal absorption, and exerts a selective toxicity for the pulmonary epithelium. It may cause death, either through acute multiorgan failure or delayed pulmonary fibrosis [63,64]. Paraquat poisoning is discussed more fully in Chapter 23. Poisoning by cholinesterase inhibitors, such as the organophosphate or carbamate insecticides, is also associated with significant respiratory effects such as bronchospasm, bronchorrhea, respiratory depression, and sometimes (delayed) pulmonary edema [65].

Metallic agents

In general, the principles governing the site and type of damage caused by inhaled irritant gases and organic chemicals apply also to metallic compounds, many of which may cause lung injury [66]. Metallic compounds may be inhaled as fumes (generally as oxides), very fine particles, or salts. It is important to realize that many metals also exert toxic effects in non-pulmonary organs.

Cadmium-pneumonitis is perhaps the best-documented example of metal-induced acute pneumonitis, and accidental cases still occur [67–71]. Cadmium is a byproduct in the zinc and lead industry. It is used in metal plating and in special alloys, as well as in the production of batteries, pigments, and plastic stabilizers. From a practical point of view, it is important to be aware that cadmium may be liberated, often unknowingly to the worker, from the welding or burning of cadmium-containing alloys and cadmium-plated metal, from the use of hard solders, or from the smelting of zinc or lead (or scrap metal), which often contain significant levels of contaminating cadmium. As with other pneumotoxic agents, exposure to toxic levels of cadmium fume does not necessarily lead to immediate respiratory symptoms, but symptoms of pneumonitis may start many hours after the exposure. Although cadmium accumulates in various organs with chronic exposure, there are no reports of even detectable concentrations in the pulmonary tissue of victims of acute and fatal cadmium pneumonitis. Chronic exposure to cadmium oxide is one of the few well-documented causes of pulmonary emphysema of occupational origin [72].

Severe chemical pneumonitis may also result from exposure to high concentrations of mercury vapor. Several fatalities (and cases of severe pulmonary involvement) have been reported as a result of the refining of gold or silver (using amalgams) in confined spaces [73–76]. In a recent interesting report, 'smelter disease' was attributed to mercury poisoning via skin absorption among workers replacing pipes in plants producing sulfuric acid [77]. It included respiratory, gastrointestinal, dermal, and general symptoms. Exposure to low levels of mercury, for example, that resulting from breaking a thermometer or other types of spillage, does not appear to be associated with significant respiratory damage. It may, however, be a serious, but elusive cause of neurological disease [78–80]. The embolization of droplets of metallic mercury in the pulmonary circulation following deliberate injection or accidental inoculation leads to a peculiar pattern of small very radiodense dots on the chest radiograph. This condition does not appear to be associated with either pulmonary or systemic disease [81,82].

Vanadium pentoxide (V_2O_5) may be present in significant quantities in slags from the steel industry (ferrovanadium) and, because some fuel oils contain high quantities of vanadium, in furnace residues from oil refineries or in soot from oil-fired boilers. Dust containing V_2O_5 may cause upper and lower airway irritation: rhinitis with sneezing and nose bleeds, pharyngitis and acute tracheobronchitis with cough, wheeze, and (possibly) airway hyperreactivity ('boilermakers' bronchitis'), as well as possibly bronchopneumonia [83–87].

The older literature also indicates that exposure to high levels of oxides of beryllium, cobalt, manganese, and osmium may cause airway irritation and even bronchopneumonia. Newer technologies, such as those involving the thermal spraying of metals, may also prove to be hazardous, as is shown by a recently described fatal case caused by spraying nickel [88].

Cases of ARDS, some with a protracted course, have been reported in military and civilian personnel accidentally exposed to smoke bombs which liberate zinc chloride ($ZnCl_2$) [89–91]. Accidental exposure (e.g. as a result of explosions, burst pipes, or leaks in chemical plants) to antimony trichloride ($SbCl_3$) and pentachloride ($SbCl_5$) [92], zirconium tetrachloride ($ZrCl_4$), titanium tetrachloride ($TiCl_4$) [93], and uranium hexafluoride (UF_6) [94] may also lead to inhalation injury.

Nickel carbonyl [$Ni(CO)_4$] is a volatile liquid of very high toxicity for the lungs and brain. Acute inhalation may cause hemorrhagic pulmonary edema [95]. Lithium hydride (LiH), phosphine (hydrogen phosphide, PH_3, used as a doping agent for the manufacture of silicon crystals, or released from aluminum phosphide grain fumigants or zinc phosphide rodenticides), hydrogen selenide (SeH_3), and diborane (B_2H_5, used as high-energy fuel) have also been reported to cause acute inhalation injury with, possibly, pulmonary edema [92].

The inhalation of the hydrogenated forms of arsenic (arsine, AsH_3) or antimony (stibine, SbH_3) can also be lethal as a result of fulminant hemolysis, which may sometimes manifest itself initially as dyspnea, besides abdominal and lumbar pain with hemoglobinuria.

Complex mixtures

Of the various complex mixtures that pose a risk of acute chemical pneumonitis following inhalation, the most common is smoke from domestic, industrial, or other fires. Respiratory morbidity is often the major complication in burn victims [96]. It may be caused by direct thermal injury (particularly if hot vapors have been inhaled), but more generally the lesions are caused by chemical injury. The composition of smoke is highly complex and variable depending on the materials that are involved and the stages of the fire [97–99]. The toxic components of smoke are numerous and involve gaseous asphyxiants (CO, HCN) and irritants, as well as particulates. Of particular concern are conditions which involve the burning or pyrolysis (e.g. overheating) of plastics, such as polyurethanes, polyacrylates, and other polymers that are known to give off numerous, generally poorly characterized but potentially highly toxic chemicals. The topic of smoke inhalation and ensuing lung injury is well covered in a number of texts [96–100].

Pathology and bronchiolitis obliterans organizing pneumonia

The pathology of acute toxic pneumonitis is that of diffuse alveolar damage with epithelial disruption, interstitial and alveolar edema, hemorrhage, and formation of hyaline membranes. Depending on the stage of the lesions, there are additionally varying degrees of infiltration by polymorphonuclear leukocytes, hyperplasia of the alveolar and bronchiolar epithelium, and interstitial or intraalveolar fibrosis. Understandably, only few human pathology reports of acute toxic pneumonitis are available, except from autopsies of the most fulminant cases.

A feature of chemically induced lung injury of particular interest is that of organizing pneumonia, or bronchiolitis obliterans organizing pneumonia (BOOP), as it is often called. It is an entity with fairly distinct clinical, functional, and radiological features [101], which is characterized pathologically by the presence of (polyps of) granulation tissue in the bronchiolar and alveolar lumina. Most cases are related to a recent infection or the cause

remains unclear; hence the term cryptogenic organizing pneumonia (COP), which is often used interchangeably with BOOP. However, it is also stated that BOOP may result as a late or delayed consequence of the inhalation of toxic substances, although the body of evidence linking toxic exposures to the development of BOOP is not large. The matter has been reviewed in remarkable detail by Douglas and Colby [102].

Almost all published instances of (alleged) irritant-induced BOOP have been attributed to single acute inhalation exposures. In Epler and coworkers' seminal publication on BOOP [103] only two subjects out of the reported 57 patients had suffered an acute inhalation, but the agent and time course were not mentioned. Similarly, Gosink et al. [104], who reported eight cases of toxic inhalation (including three with aspiration) among their 52 cases of bronchiolitis obliterans (most of which would have satisfied the diagnostic criteria for BOOP), did not clearly specify the causal agents. The exception was one case of nitrous fume inhalation, which is arguably the best-single documented toxic cause of BOOP. In a paper from 1955, it is stated that the inhalation of NO_2 is the 'single most common cause of bronchiolitis obliterans', which the author considered was nearly always accompanied by alveolar involvement [105]. It has been known for many years that, following resolution of the acute pulmonary edema caused by massive exposure to NO_2, a clinical relapse may occur after 2–6 weeks with dyspnea, cough, fine crackles, a radiographic picture of miliary nodular infiltrates, arterial hypoxemia, and a restrictive or mixed impairment, with low diffusion capacity [7,102]. The site of cellular damage caused by NO_2 is the centriacinar region [106], and the relapse phase has been attributed to bronchiolar scarring with peribronchiolar and obliterating fibrosis of the bronchioles. It is not clear whether these instances of BOOP result from the 'normal' repair of a particularly severe form of epithelial injury (i.e. with disruption of the basement membrane [107]), or whether they result from an abnormal pattern of cellular proliferation in this critical region of the lung.

In the past 20 years, other agents besides NO_2 [46,108] have been reported to cause bronchiolitis obliterans in humans, including SO_2 [30,109], poorly defined fumes from fires involving plastics [110], cleansing agents [111], trichloroethylene degradation products (perhaps phosgene) [51], cocaine smoking [112,113], and a mycotoxin [114]. In several of the cited studies, the diagnosis of bronchiolitis obliterans has been inferred mainly from clinical and functional criteria, without the distinct radiological appearance of BOOP or its definitive pathological features, and so could be challenged. Thus, in some instances, most notably in case reports describing the inhalation of water-soluble agents (SO_2 and NH_3), the inflammatory lesions in the small airways may have caused a 'constrictive' bronchiolitis obliterans (i.e. inflammation and constrictive fibrosis of the bronchiolar walls), rather than true BOOP (i.e. intraluminal granulation tissue accompanied with interstitial inflammation). These distinctions are, however, of doubtful importance for the management of the patient.

The literature on BOOP of toxic origin remains limited and some issues remain unresolved; it could be argued, nevertheless, that any severe chemical injury to the epithelium of the bronchioloalveolar region has the potential to be followed by organizing pneumonia with obliterating bronchiolitis. Myers and Katzenstein [115] have demonstrated epithelial cell damage well in cases of idiopathic BOOP, and it has been said in an authoritative review [101] that the pathological pattern of organizing pneumonia 'reflects one type of inflammatory process resulting from lung injury [and] it may also be a feature of the organizing stage of adult respiratory distress syndrome'. This is supported by studies of phosgene poisoning in dogs [116]: 'if animals which have apparently recovered from the acute symptoms following gassing and which give no signs of pneumonia are killed 3 to 10 days later, they show a widespread, organizing bronchiolitis, which clearly represents the sequel of the acute bronchial and peribronchial inflammatory reaction, so prominent in the acute period'. The authors described miliary peribronchial nodules after 33 days as 'a perfect example of obliterative bronchiolitis', which clearly represented a more advanced stage of the organizing bronchiolitis and pneumonia found in dogs killed 3–10 days after gassing.

If any chemical pneumonitis may give rise to organizing pneumonia, then it may be surmised that many inhaled irritant agents could cause BOOP. Inhaled cadmium in particular is widely accepted as a cause of (delayed) chemical pneumonitis, and scrutiny of the available experimental data [117] and some published observations in human cases [69,71] suggest that BOOP also occurs following exposure to cadmium. It follows that in clinical cases of 'cryptogenic' organizing pneumonia, the possibility of an underlying toxic cause should always be seriously considered. This is particularly true in view of the occurrence of outbreaks of organizing pneumonia, as in the case of the 'Ardystil syndrome' (see below).

Sequelae

Following acute inhalation injury, there is often complete recovery, but this is not always the case. The experience with ARDS caused by etiologies other than acute inhalation injury suggests that a substantial proportion of surviving patients are left with some degree of dyspnea and functional impairment, often a reduced diffusing capacity [118]. However, it is not yet clear whether, and how frequently, pulmonary fibrosis occurs after diffuse lung injury of toxic origin. The possible occurrence of residual abnormalities within the airways is better documented, though the evidence is often based on single instances only. Thus, various chronic sequelae, such as constrictive bronchiolitis, bronchiectasis, bronchial strictures, and bronchial polyps, have been reported to result from acute inhalation injury, depending on the severity of the initial damage and, perhaps, the treatment modalities. As yet there have been no controlled studies regarding the latter issue [5].

Even in the absence of structural sequelae (which may be identified by imaging studies or through bronchoscopy) or significant defects in basal spirometry, a state of permanent non-specific airway hyperresponsiveness may be observed, often associated with asthmatic symptoms. This condition of adult-onset, non-allergic asthma has been named 'reactive airways dysfunction syndrome' (RADS) [119] and occurs in a number of survivors of (severe) airway injury. Its incidence and the mechanisms giving rise to it remain to be elucidated [5].

An important, but in practice often neglected, issue is the documentation of sequelae and their severity in victims of inhalation injury. This may cause difficult medicolegal problems when victims seek compensation, sometimes many months or years after the event. It is, therefore, important that physicians treating victims in the early days after the incident document accurately the clinical condition and all relevant data. Documentation of the degree of any injury using bronchoscopy and high resolution computed tomography (CT) may be particularly useful, and repeated measurements of lung function and arterial blood gas tensions are essential. Victims of acute inhalation injury should never be discharged without a comprehensive assessment of their pulmonary function. The latter should include diffusing capacity and an assessment of non-specific airway responsiveness, either by a bronchodilatation test, or by a histamine or methacholine bronchoconstrictor test. Neurological evaluation may be indicated, if there has been loss of consciousness or severe anoxia.

A common difficult medicolegal issue is the condition of the patient before the accident. Most often, there are few or no objective data concerning the subject's ventilatory function (let alone diffusing capacity, airway responsiveness, or exercise capacity), and it becomes a matter of judgment to disentangle the possible contributions of previous smoking, personal traits (such as atopy), or preexisting disease, from that of the accident. All workers at risk of acute inhalation injury should undergo routine measurements of at least spirometry.

Management

When inhalation injury occurs, appropriate medical intervention includes removal from exposure, resuscitation, and supportive treatment. This may require intensive care treatment with intubation and artificial ventilation. Antibiotics are only to be given if there are signs of infection.

In some instances, emergency (rescue) personnel must also be protected from chemicals that remain present on victims or their clothes, and decontamination procedures must be available.

When there has been exposure to water-insoluble gases (such as phosgene or NO_2), or when there is doubt about the nature and severity of the exposure, even asymptomatic persons must remain under observation for 24 hours. There is anecdotal evidence, as well as physiological grounds, that persons at risk of developing pulmonary edema should not exercise, nor should they be overinfused with intravenous fluids.

It is common practice to administer oxygen to any victim of an inhalation accident. However, oxygen treatment should probably be given sparingly and only as required by the level of arterial oxygen saturation, because oxygen potentially has a considerable pulmonary toxicity of its own. It is conceivable that adding further oxidant stress to an already damaged and inflamed lung may hamper the resolution of any damage. Few studies have addressed the matter, however, except in the case of paraquat intoxication, where adverse synergy between paraquat and oxygen is well known [120].

The administration of (systemic) corticosteroids probably is justified in the hope of preventing complications arising from (excessive) inflammation, such as bronchiolitis obliterans [9]. Although there are no controlled studies on this issue, the available data concerning NO_2-induced bronchiolitis obliterans suggest that this complication does not occur when steroids have been administered. Moreover, BOOP is known to resolve rapidly with corticosteroids treatment [101]. Consequently, in the present state of knowledge, it seems advisable to administer corticosteroids to victims of severe inhalation injury. It is not known whether inhaled steroids should be given prophylactically in victims of less severe inhalation injuries to prevent the occurrence of irritant-induced asthma (RADS). The usefulness of other therapeutic agents, such as antioxidants, metal chelators, and other drugs, in particular forms of toxic lung injury is beyond the scope of this text.

When a worker has had an inhalation accident, questions often arise over his/her subsequent return to work. In principle, there should be no other reason to consider than the subject's physical ability to perform the job. Thus, if there is no or only minimal residual respiratory impairment, he/she may resume normal working activities, provided that the necessary preventive measures have been taken to avoid a new accident (this applies to any other person working in that job). If the subject has developed non-specific airway hyperresponsiveness (i.e. RADS), the return to work should be guided by the same considerations as those that apply for any other asthmatic subjects, except in the rather exceptional circumstance where the offending toxic exposure involved a sensitizer (e.g. toluene diisocyanate) and the subject has become sensitized by the accident.

Prevention

The first consideration with regard to the prevention of chemical pneumonitis is obviously prevention of accidents that result in the release of toxic chemical agents. Much can be learned from earlier incidents and, when they occur, a thorough enquiry should be conducted of the cause or causes (both direct and indirect factors). This principle underlies improvements in safety after any major accident or catastrophe. Technical, organizational, and human errors should be identified clearly in an accident report, and appropriate preventive measures should be proposed, implemented, and verified.

Regardless of any earlier incident, an inventory should be made of all chemical agents and processes that could give rise to inhalation injury on the premises, both in large plants and small workshops. Material safety data sheets must be within easy reach and available to all concerned employees; they are generally adequate with regard to major acute hazards (although they may be deficient with regard to sensitization hazards or chronic health risks). Appropriate warning labels and signs should be displayed according to national legislation, and specific regulations regarding the shipping and transportation of dangerous chemicals should be carefully followed.

All necessary technical and administrative measures must be taken to prevent explosions, leaks, and spills; monitoring devices and alarm systems should be installed when appropriate, and the possible need for emergency evacuation should be anticipated with clearly planned and understood procedures. Often such measures will be part of an existing disaster plan involving the local or regional emergency services.

Particular attention should be paid to mixing incompatibilities, operations in confined spaces (e.g. cleaning tanks), start-up phases of new work processes, special maintenance jobs performed by subcontractors, and unusual working conditions. Workers (including trainees, temporary workers, and subcontractors) should be informed about existing dangers, and should receive adequate protective equipment and be trained in the use of respirators. A particular issue for the non-occupational environment is that of domestic accidents caused by mixing bleach with acids or ammonia; it appears that the labels on cleaning products are often insufficiently explicit about the risks of inhalation injury.

SUBACUTE TOXIC PNEUMONITIS

The concept of 'subacute toxic pneumonitis' is not widely recognized. The term 'subacute' is used here to indicate both the clinical presentation of the disease and the pattern of exposure, as is the practice in toxicology. Thus, subacute toxic pneumonitis refers to conditions of toxic lung injury in which the onset of the disease is not so sudden as that caused by an accidental exposure, and where the exposure itself consists of repeated peaks (or more uniform concentrations) over weeks to months. There are not many published examples of lung disease occurring in such situations, but pulmonary alveolar proteinosis caused by heavy exposure to silica ('acute silicosis') and possibly by other agents [121] can readily be classified in this category. So too can some instances of exogenous lipoid pneumonitis, the somewhat obscure 'hairspray lung', and the pulmonary hemorrhagic syndrome associated with exposure to trimellitic anhydride and possibly methylene diphenyl diisocyanate. The latter, however, is likely to be primarily immunologic in mechanistic origin rather than toxic [121–123]. Such miscellaneous disorders of the lung are discussed more fully in Chapter 23.

The focus within the present chapter for 'subacute toxic pneumonitis' is the recent occurrence of a newly recognized disorder, the so-called 'Ardystil' syndrome. This occurred in workers exposed to air-sprayed paints in the textile industry, and it represents the most convincing example, hitherto, of occupationally induced BOOP.

The Ardystil syndrome

In the spring of 1992, an outbreak of severe respiratory disease occurred in the area of Alcoy, Community of Valencia, Spain. Several workers,

often young women, from factories where textiles were air-sprayed with dyes were affected by what appeared to be organizing pneumonia. Six subjects died from the disease over the course of a few months. Most of the affected workers had worked in a factory named Ardystil – hence Ardystil syndrome. An epidemiological study, conducted among 257 workers from eight factories, identified 22 subjects meeting the radiological and histological criteria for organizing pneumonia [124]. Shortly thereafter, a similar, though smaller, outbreak was reported from Algeria in workers from a factory near Tlemcen, where the same paints had been used as in Spain [125]. The clinical features of the pulmonary disease have been described by Romero et al. [126]. The most common clinical findings were cough, epistaxis (an unusual feature in other forms of BOOP), dyspnea, and chest pain, together with crackles on auscultation. Chest radiographs showed patchy infiltrates in two-thirds of patients and a micronodular pattern in one-third (Fig. 12.3). There was a restrictive impairment of ventilatory function, and rapid progression to irreversible respiratory failure, despite corticosteroid treatment, in several patients.

On the basis of the strong temporal and geographical relationships found in the epidemiological study [124], it was suggested that the outbreak was linked to the substitution of Acramin FWR (a polyurea) by Acramin FWN (a polyamideamine) in the paint system used (Acramin F). Acramin F is a three-component water-based printing system, which had been widely used since the early 1950s. It had generally been used with brush or sponge application or in screen printing, and it had never been associated with respiratory or any other significant health problems. However, in the factories where the disease occurred, the paste was sprayed by air guns, with a solvent (petroleum naphtha) to facilitate the spraying. In addition, hygiene conditions were reportedly very poor. The chemical structures of Acramin FWR and Acramin FWN did not indicate particular 'structural alerts' and conventional toxicity testing of these polymeric compounds in experimental animals had not revealed any significant adverse effects, nor any potential for dermal or ocular irritation. However, no inhalation studies had been performed.

Subsequent in vivo [127] and in vitro [128] experimental studies could not establish any significant difference in the intrinsic toxicities of Acramin FWR and Acramin FWN, but it did emerge that both agents were unexpectedly toxic for the lungs. The current hypothesis to explain the pathogenesis of the Ardystil syndrome is that the aerosol characteristics of the sprayed paint were altered in such a way, probably by the inclusion of organic solvents in the mixture, that the polymer could be inhaled into the

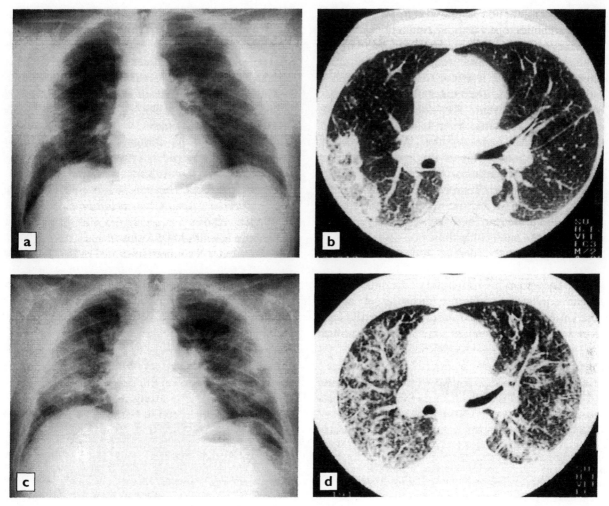

Fig. 12.3 The Ardystil syndrome. Patchy infiltrates on (a) the chest radiograph with (b) predominantly subpleural distribution on high-resolution computed tomography (HRCT). Progression of diffuse alveolar and interstitial infiltrates on (c) the chest radiograph and (d) HRCT of the same patient. Reproduced from Romero *et al.* [126].

deeper regions of the lung where it exerted a marked toxicity as a result of its polycationic character.

The Ardystil syndrome seems to differ from the common forms of BOOP with respect to its severity, with a rapidly fatal outcome in several patients and an evolution towards chronic pulmonary fibrosis in others [129,130].

Other causes

The Ardystil syndrome is reminiscent of another recent outbreak of 'subacute' interstitial lung disease caused by occupational exposure to a synthetic polymer, namely the 'nylon flock worker's lung' [131,132]. Although the clinical presentation and pathology of this disease caused by synthetic organic microfibers appear to be different from those of the Ardystil syndrome [133], this further recently discovered subacute disorder warns against complacency about occupational exposures to reputedly innocuous or 'chemically inert' compounds. The explanation

appears to lie primarily with the way the microfibers are cut, thus allowing small respirable fragments to be produced [134,135]. Nylon flock worker's lung is characterized by interstitial lung disease of low to high severity and has a distinct pathologic pattern of bronchiolar and peribronchiolar lymphocytic inflammation and lymphoid hyperplasia [133].

Solvent exposure provides a further possible cause of (subacute) toxic pneumonitis but the issue is controversial and insufficiently resolved. Solvent vapors are often incriminated by patients as causing respiratory symptoms, but clinicians should know that organic solvents are rarely primary causes of pulmonary disease. It must be admitted, however, that the respiratory effects of solvent exposure have not been widely investigated [58]. Organic solvents consist of a broad spectrum of chemicals, which, by virtue of their intended use, generally have little chemical reactivity. The central nervous system is the main target for the acute and chronic toxicity of solvents as a group, with some solvents having particular selective toxicity for certain other organs, e.g. the peripheral nervous system, the liver, and bone marrow.

When a patient reports pronounced effects upon exposure to a solvent, it is wise to pay attention first to the chemicals (e.g. isocyanates) that are being dissolved by that solvent. For example, the solute formaldehyde, off-gassing from its solution in water (formalin), causes more irritation than the solvent acetone. Some solvent vapors do, however, produce mucus membrane irritation, the intensity of which depends on the type of solvent. The effects on the airways also depend on the degree of non-specific airway responsiveness, and asthmatic subjects are generally more susceptible than non-asthmatic subjects. However, with odorous and centrally active compounds such as organic solvents, individual subjective perception of respiratory discomfort may appear unrelated to objective measures of airway function (e.g. spirometric measurements or the level of airway responsiveness). In some patients, exposure to solvents may trigger manifest attacks of hyperventilation, while in others this is not so evident and a diagnosis may be made of 'multiple chemical sensitivity' (or 'idiopathic environmental intolerance'), after a careful consideration of other conditions that may result from excessive solvent exposure, such as sleep apnea and solvent-induced encephalopathy (or 'organic psychosyndrome').

In conclusion, the existence of subacute toxic disease of the lung parenchyma has only been well documented for the Ardystil syndrome and nylon flock workers' lung. However, it is likely that chemicals known to cause acute pneumonitis when the inhalation exposure is accidental and massive, will also cause less dramatic forms of lung injury when lesser exposure levels are sustained over a period of days to months. The Ardystil syndrome and the development of organizing pneumonia with obliterating bronchiolitis suggest that in some cases the repair process rather than the initial injury may be the major cause of the disabling disorder.

DIFFICULT CASE

History

A man, aged 34 years, was referred in June 1999 by his occupational physician for advice regarding a possible return to work after a serious respiratory illness of July 1998.

He had never been ill previously and had smoked about 10 cigarettes a day. He denied taking illicit drugs. He lived alone, his house was without apparent mold, and he kept no animals. His hobbies had been cycling and walking. After completing his military service, he had been employed from December 1987 as a technician in a large chemical plant that produced titanium dioxide (TiO_2). During the first 10 years he had worked (usually with adequate respiratory protection) in various areas of the plant, with potential exposure to dusts, oxides of sulfur and nitrogen, ammonia, and hydrazine. He had never had any accidental excess exposure and had never experienced any respiratory problem.

In September 1997 he started working as a maintenance technician in a new division where slags resulting from the production of TiO_2 were treated with 'additives' and diluted sulphuric acid to produce ammonium sulphate. One job required him to replace the 'mats' that filtered the effluent of this production process. Replacement should have been required every 3 months, but the process had unforeseen difficulties and the frequency was steadily increased. The job was physically demanding and very dusty, and despite wearing a dust mask he often had black–brown discolored nasal secretions. In the period immediately preceding his illness only he and one workmate were available to carry out this task, and they had done it almost daily – sometimes for 10 hours per day. From May to July 1998 he had had the impression that he was less able to carry out hard physical work, but he had not sought medical attention for this because he had considered it a consequence of back trouble. His mother later reported that he used to produce a lot of foamy sputum for 1–2 hours after returning from work. Two days after the start of annual leave in July 1998, he developed a 'flu-like illness, leading to a hospital admission in severe respiratory distress 19 days later. He had received Augmentin over the preceding week. His workmate was apparently unaffected.

He had extreme respiratory distress (respiratory rate >50/min) and was cyanotic (SaO_2 <85%); his pulse was 146/min, and the blood pressure was 165/100. The chest radiograph showed diffuse bilateral interstitial infiltrates. He was intubated and ventilated (IPPV). A thoracic CT on day 3 showed multiple areas of airspace consolidation in all lung lobes, a right pneumothorax, and a pneumomediastinum. Bronchoalveolar lavage revealed Candida albicans, but there was no evidence of any other infection. No significant abnormalities were found in the blood, except for an initial transient neutrophilia. There was no cardiac insufficiency or pulmonary hypertension (Swann–Ganz catheter). He was treated intravenously with corticosteroids (from day 5) and broad-spectrum antibiotics (from day 6). On day 8, he was transferred to a university hospital and underwent a surgical lung biopsy on day 9. This gave a pathological diagnosis of 'bronchiolitis obliterans with organizing pneumonia' (BOOP) of unknown origin (Fig. 12.4).

He was ventilated for a further 8 days. No evidence of connective tissue disease or specific bacterial, viral, or fungal infection was found. He was discharged in a clinically good condition, and was treated with oral prednisolone for a further 6 months. He remained well. In December 1998, his chest radiograph was almost normal and his pulmonary function showed slight ventilatory restriction with a low diffusing capacity. By June 1999 he was asymptomatic.

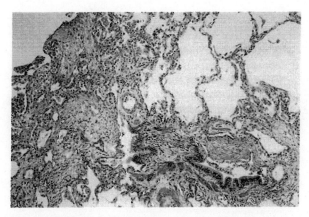

Fig. 12.4 Histopathology of the lung in Difficult Case showing typical features of bronchiolitis obliterans organizing pneumonia. There is an interstitial inflammatory infiltrate of variable density with some interstitial and mainly alveolar fibrosis (left part of figure). There is also partial obliteration of the membraneous bronchioles (two bronchioles are seen in the lower half of the figure). The lesions have a mainly centrilobular distribution. Hematoxylin and eosin staining; original magnification × 50. (Courtesy of Professor E.K. Verbeken, Department of Pathology, Katholieke Universiteit Leuven.)

Only limited information was received regarding the potential occupational exposures in the plant. They included titanium dioxide, salts of aluminum, alkylaluminum, antimony pentoxide, ammonia, sodium hydroxide, sulfuric acid and other inorganic acids, hexamethylene tetramine, and other organic agents in small amounts. The composition of the dusts in the filter remains unknown.

Issues

The chief issue in this case is whether this man's respiratory illness was a consequence of exposure to a toxic agent(s) encountered at work. Secondary issues, if the illness was occupational in origin, center on the action that should be taken within the workplace and the advice he should be given regarding a return to work.

Comment

The book's authors were evenly divided as to whether the workplace was relevant; those who favored an occupational cause reporting a wide range of confidence. They suggested a thorough industrial hygiene assessment (and a mineralogic evaluation of the biopsy material) to evaluate the causal agent, and did not advise any return to the same work tasks unless the cause could be identified and any ongoing risk eliminated. There was more general agreement that close medical surveillance should follow any return to work and should involve other exposed workers.

At the time of the first consultation, the main points in favor of an occupational etiology were: the patient's young age (BOOP generally affects older people [101]); the homogeneous distribution of the lesions throughout the lungs; the reasonable exclusion of infectious causes; the notion that BOOP may be caused by inhaled agents; the nature of the work (exposure to presumably high levels of dust originating from acid-treated metal slags); and the chapter author's personal experience of a case of similarly severe (but equally controversial) BOOP in a young man who had removed slags from a gutter in a metal recycling plant. The main points against were the delay between the last day of exposure and disease onset, the lack of qualitative and quantitative exposure data, and the absence of supporting evidence from the literature for the occurrence of BOOP in this particular occupational setting.

Paraffin-embedded lung tissue was examined by transmission electron microscopy with electron dispersive X-ray analysis (David Dinsdale, MRC Toxicology Unit, Leicester, UK). This did not reveal any specific metallic element with pneumotoxic potential (such as cadmium, antimony, or vanadium), but this does not exclude the possibility that these elements had been present (e.g. as soluble salts) only to be cleared from the lungs by the time of the biopsy. An industrial hygiene evaluation was carried out in September 2000. Personal air sampling (2 liters/min) was carried out for 75 min in two workers while they replaced the filters. Total inhalable dust amounted to 9.15 mg/m^3 and respirable dust amounted to 0.68 mg/m^3. The largest metal fraction of the dust consisted of iron. The concentrations of vanadium were 0.12 mg/m^3 and 0.009 mg/m^3, in inhalable and respirable dust, respectively, the TLV for vanadium being 0.014 mg/m^3 for respirable dust. No cadmium or other known pneumotoxic metals were detected in significant amounts. These measurements, which were made in much better working conditions than those experienced by the patient, confirmed that this was a dusty job and they indicated that vanadium, a known pulmonary irritant, was a plausible culprit (as was, perhaps, the residues of sulfuric acid with which the slags had been treated). They do not provide definitive proof for an occupational etiology, however, and in this case the true cause will probably remain elusive. At the time of writing, no decision had been made by the national funding body responsible for compensating occupational diseases.

Following recovery, the patient (who was then completely asymptomatic with normal pulmonary function and a normal chest CT) was advised to return to work in the same plant, but without further exposure to high concentrations of dusts or irritants. Absolute cessation of contact with his previous work environment was not felt to be necessary. Close medical surveillance of relevant symptoms and pulmonary function (including $D_{L}CO$) was arranged, but no suitable job could be found in the same company and he was eventually made redundant. He then had difficulty finding a job in the chemical industry and elsewhere, because of his history of severe pulmonary disease.

SUMMARY POINTS

Recognition

- The presentation of pneumonitis caused by the inhalation of toxic chemicals ranges from relatively benign febrile illnesses to life-threatening non-cardiogenic pulmonary edema with ARDS.
- Recognition of the nature of the injury depends primarily on an evaluation of the causal exposure.
- The inhalation fevers are caused by exposure to certain metal fumes (mainly zinc) and heated plastics (mainly fluorine-containing polymers), as well as by organic dusts contaminated by microbial agents.
- Toxic pneumonitis results chiefly from exposure to poorly water-soluble agents (various gases, organic chemicals, metals, and complex aerosol mixtures), which often cause little irritation during the period of exposure allowing dangerous cumulations.
- High concentrations of water-soluble irritants may also cause damage to the bronchioloalveolar region.
- Repeated or prolonged exposure to pneumotoxic agents may lead to 'subacute toxic pneumonitis', best exemplified by the Ardystil syndrome, a form of BOOP caused by some spray paints.

Management

- Inhalation fevers do not require specific treatment, nor any change of employment, but they do indicate a need for reduced exposure level.
- Because pulmonary edema may take several hours to become clinically manifest after toxic injury, asymptomatic workers exposed accidentally to respirable pneumotoxic agents should be kept under close medical supervision for 24 hours.
- Although there are no controlled studies in this area, it seems prudent to administer systemic corticosteroids to victims of severe inhalation injuries

to reduce the chances of inflammatory and/or fibrotic sequelae.

- The management of the possible medicolegal consequences of inhalation accidents is often complex, and so patients injured by inhaled toxic chemicals should never be discharged without a complete evaluation of pulmonary function.

Prevention

- The risk of inhalation injury is best reduced by appropriate administrative and technical measures to prevent accidents.
- Strategies include:
  - avoidance of the most hazardous agents and work processes
  - preparation of a complete inventory of the agents used on the premises
  - adequate product labelling
  - use of well-functioning monitoring devices and alarm systems
  - use of personal protective equipment
  - worker education and training
  - emergency planning.
- Workers at risk of inhalation injuries should undergo regular measurements of spirometry so that any sequelae following an inhalation accident can be readily recognized.
- The occurrence of outbreaks of subacute toxic pneumonitis, such as the Ardystil syndrome, shows that chemicals should never be sprayed without prior adequate evidence that it is safe to do so.
- This implies a determination of the size of the aerosol particles and appropriate inhalation experiments in animals.

REFERENCES

1. Blanc PD, Galbo M, Hiatt P, Olson KR. Morbidity following acute irritant inhalation in a population-based study. *JAMA* 1991; 266: 664–669.
2. Blanc PD, Galbo M, Balmes JR *et al.* Occupational factors in work-related inhalations: inferences for prevention strategy. *Am J Ind Med* 1994; 25: 783–791.
3. Ross DJ. Ten years of the SWORD project. *Clin Exp Allergy* 1999; 29: 750–753.
4. Ferner RE. Chemical disasters. *Pharmacol Ther* 1993; 58: 157–171.
5. Nemery B. Late consequences of accidental exposure to inhaled irritants: RADS and the Bhopal disaster. *Eur Respir J* 1996; 9: 1973–1976.
6. Hubbard R, Lewis S, Richards K *et al.* Occupational exposure to metal or wood dust and aetiology of cryptogenic fibrosing alveolitis. *Lancet* 1996; 347: 284–289.
7. Schwartz DA. Acute inhalation injury. *Occup Med* 1987; 2/2: 297–318.
8. Schwartz DA, Blaski CA. Toxic inhalations. In: Fishman AP, ed. *Pulmonary Diseases and Disorders*, Vol. 1, pp. 925–940. New York: McGraw-Hill, 2000.

9. do Pico GA. Toxic gas inhalation. *Clin Pulm Med* 1994; 1: 84–92.
10. Wesselius LJ. Pulmonary disorders associated with use of illicit drugs. *Clin Pulm Med* 1997; 4: 71–75.
11. Foucher P, Biour M, Blayac JP *et al.* Drugs that may injure the respiratory system. *Eur Respir J* 1997; 10: 265–279.
12. Rask-Andersen A, Pratt DS. Inhalation fever: a proposed unifying term for febrile reactions to inhalation of noxious substances. *Br J Ind Med* 1992; 49: 40.
13. Rylander R, Malmberg P. Non-infectious fever: inhalation fever or toxic alveolitis? *Br J Ind Med* 1992; 49: 296.
14. Gordon T, Fine JM. Metal fume fever. *Occup Med* 1993; 8: 505–517.
15. Blanc P, Boushey HA. The lung in metal fume fever. *Semin Respir Med* 1993; 14: 212–225.
16. Shusterman DJ. Polymer fume fever and other fluorocarbon pyrolysis-related syndromes. *Occup Med* 1993; 8: 519–531.
17. Albrecht WN, Bryant CJ. Polymer-fume fever associated with smoking and use of a mold-release spray containing polytetrafluoroethylene. *J Occup Med* 1987; 29: 817–819.

18. Goldstein M, Weiss H, Wade K *et al.* An outbreak of fume fever in an electronics instrument testing laboratory. *J Occup Med* 1987; 29: 749.

19. Sjögren B, Bäckström I, Fryk G *et al.* Fever and respiratory symptoms after welding on painted steel. *Scand J Work Environ Health* 1991; 17: 441–443.

20. Nemery B, Willems H, Laureyssens R *et al.* Polymer fume fever and brominated flame retardants in plastics – preliminary observations. In: Chiyotani K, Hosoda Y, Aizawa Y, eds. *Advances in the Prevention of Occupational Respiratory Diseases*, pp. 756–758. Amsterdam: Elsevier, 1998.

21. Langham Brown JJ. Zinc fume fever. *Br J Radiol* 1988; 61: 327–329.

22. Castet D, Bouillard J. Pneumopathie aiguë au cours d'une exposition à l'oxyde de zinc. *Rev Mal Respir* 1992; 9: 632–633.

23. Vogelmeier C, Konig G, Beneze K *et al.* Pulmonary involvement in zinc fume fever. *Chest* 1987; 92: 946–948.

24. Blanc P, Wong H, Bernstein MS *et al.* An experimental human model of metal fume fever. *Ann Intern Med* 1991; 114: 930–936.

25. Blanc PD, Boushey HA, Wong H *et al.* Cytokines in metal fume fever. *Am Rev Respir Dis* 1993; 147: 134–138.

26. Fine JM, Gordon T, Chen LC *et al.* Metal fume fever: characterization of clinical and plasma IL-6 responses in controlled human exposures to zinc oxide fume at and below the threshold limit value. *J Occup Environ Med* 1997; 39: 722–726.

27. Malo JL, Cartier A. Occupational asthma due to fumes of galvanized metal. *Chest* 1987; 92: 375–377.

28. Malo JL, Malo J, Cartier A *et al.* Acute lung reaction due to zinc inhalation. *Eur Respir J* 1990; 3: 111–114.

29. Cotes JE, Feinmann EL, Male VJ *et al.* Respiratory symptoms and impairment in shipyard welders and caulker/burners. *Br J Ind Med* 1989; 46: 292–301.

30. Charan NB, Myers CG, Laksminarayan S *et al.* Pulmonary injuries associated with acute sulfur dioxide inhalation. *Am Rev Respir Dis* 1979; 119: 555–560.

31. Rabinovitch S, Greyson ND, Weiser W *et al.* Clinical and laboratory features of acute sulphur dioxide inhalation poisoning: two year follow-up. *Am Rev Respir Dis* 1989; 139: 556–558.

32. Harkonen H, Nordman H, Korhonen O, Winblad I. Long-term effects of exposure to sulfur dioxide. Lung function four years after a pyrite dust explosion. *Am Rev Respir Dis* 1983; 128: 890–893.

33. Leduc D, Gris P, Lheureux P *et al.* Acute and long term respiratory damage following inhalation of ammonia. *Thorax* 1992; 47: 755–757.

34. de la Hoz RE, Schlueter DP, Rom WN. Chronic lung disease secondary to ammonia inhalation injury: a report on three cases. *Am J Ind Med* 1996; 29: 209–214.

35. Das R, Blanc PD. Chlorine gas exposure and the lung: a review. *Toxicol Indust Health* 1993; 9: 439–455.

36. Olson KR, Shusterman DJ. Mixing incompatibilities and toxic exposures. *Occup Med* 1993; 8: 549–560.

37. Reisz GR, Gammon RS. Toxic pneumonitis from mixing household cleaners. *Chest* 1986; 89: 49–52.

38. Hery M, Hecht G, Gerber JM *et al.* Exposure to chloramines in the atmosphere of indoor swimming pools. *Ann Occup Hyg* 1995; 39: 427–439.

39. Massin N, Bohadana AB, Wild P *et al.* Respiratory symptoms and bronchial responsiveness in lifeguards exposed to nitrogen trichloride in indoor swimming pools. *Occup Environ Med* 1998; 55: 258–263.

40. Reiffenstein RJ, Hulbert WC, Roth SH. Toxicology of hydrogen sulfide. *Annu Rev Pharmacol Toxicol* 1992; 32: 109–134.

41. Guidotti TL. Occupational exposure to hydrogen sulfide in the sour gas industry: some inresolved issues. *Int Arch Occup Environ Health* 1994; 66: 153–160.

42. Anonymous. Calamity at Bhopal. *Lancet* 1984; ii: 1378–1379.

43. Dhara R, Dhara VR. Bhopal – a case study of international disaster. *Int J Occup Environ Health* 1995; 1: 58–69.

44. Cullinan P, Acquilla S, Dhara VR. Respiratory morbidity 10 years after the Union Carbide gas leak at Bhopal: a cross sectional survey. *Br Med J* 1997; 314: 338–343.

45. Douglas WW, Hepper NGG, Colby TV. Silo filler's disease. *Mayo Clin Proc* 1989; 64: 291–304.

46. Yockey CC, Eden BM, Byrd RB. The McConnell missile accident. Clinical spectrum of nitrogen dioxide exposure. *JAMA* 1980; 244: 1221–1223.

47. Hajela R, Janigan DT, Landrigan PL *et al.* Fatal pulmonary edema due to nitric acid fume inhalation in three pulp-mill workers. *Chest* 1990; 97: 487–489.

48. Hedberg K, Hedberg CW, Iber C *et al.* An outbreak of nitrogen dioxide-induced respiratory illness among ice hockey players. *JAMA* 1989; 262: 3014–3017.

49. Brauer M, Spengler JD. Nitrogen dioxide exposures inside ice skating rinks. *Am J Publ Health* 1994; 84: 429–433.

50. Diller WF, Schnellbächer F, Wüstefeld E. Pulmonale Spätfolgen nach Phosgenvergiftung bzw. inhalationstoxischem Lungenödem. *Zbl Arbeitsmed* 1979; 29: 6–16.

51. Sjögren B, Plato N, Alexandersson R *et al.* Pulmonary reactions caused by welding-induced decomposed trichloroethylene. *Chest* 1991; 99: 237–238.

52. Snyder RW, Mishel HS, Christensen GC. Pulmonary toxicity following exposure to methylene chloride and its combustion product, phosgene. *Chest* 1992; 102: 1921.

53. Hu H, Fine J, Epstein P *et al.* Tear gas – harassing agent or toxic chemical weapon? *JAMA* 1989; 262: 660–663.

54. Breakell A, Bodiwala GG. CS gas exposure in a crowded night club: the consequences for an accident and emergency department. *J Accid Emerg Med* 1998; 15: 56–64.

55. Fraunfelder FT. Is CS gas dangerous? Current evidence suggests not but unanswered questions remain. *Br Med J* 2000; 320: 458–459.

56. Willems JL. Clinical management of mustard gas casualties. *Ann Med Milit Belg* 1989; 3(Suppl): 1–61.

57. Freitag L, Firusian N, Stamatis G *et al.* The role of bronchoscopy in pulmonary complications due to mustard gas inhalation. *Chest* 1991; 100: 1436–1441.

58. De Raeve H, Nemery B. Lung diseases induced by metals and organic solvents. In: Mapp CE, ed. *European Respiratory Monograph II*, pp. 178–213 Genève: 1999.

59. Birolleau S, Belleguic C, Lena H *et al.* Le poumon du cracheur de feu: à propos de six cas. *Rev Pneumol Clin* 1999; 55: 29.

60. Jinn Y, Akizuki N, Ohkouchi M *et al.* Acute lung injury after inhalation of water-proofing spray while smoking a cigarette. *Respiration* 1998; 65: 486–488.

61. Burkhart KK, Britt A, Petrini G *et al.* Pulmonary toxicity following exposure to an aerosolized leather protector. *Clin Toxicol* 1996; 34: 21–24.

62. Bracco D, Favre J-B. Pulmonary injury after ski wax inhalation exposure. *Ann Emerg Med* 1998; 32: 616–619.

63. Bismuth Ch, Hall AH. *Paraquat Poisoning. Mechanisms, Prevention, Treatment.* New York: Marcel Dekker, 1995.

64. Wesseling C, Hogstedt C, Micado A *et al.* Unintentional fatal paraquat poisonings among agricultural workers in Costa Rica: report of 15 cases. *Am J Ind Med* 1997; 32: 433–441.

65. Tsao TCY, Juang YC, Lan RS *et al.* Respiratory failure of acute organophosphate and carbamate poisoning. *Chest* 1990; 98: 631–636.

66. Nemery B. Metal toxicity in the respiratory tract. *Eur Respir J* 1990; 3: 202–219.

67. Barnhart S, Rosenstock L. Cadmium chemical pneumonitis. *Chest* 1984; 86: 789–791.

68. Taylor A, Jackson MA, Burston J, Lee HA. Poisoning with cadmium fumes after smelting lead. *Br Med J* 1984; 288: 1270–1271.

69. Yates DH, Goldman KP. Acute cadmium poisoning in a foreman plater welder. *Br J Ind Med* 1990; 47: 429–431.

70. Seidal K, Jörgensen N, Elinder CG *et al.* Fatal cadmium-induced pneumonitis. *Scand J Work Environ Health* 1993; 19: 429–431.

71. Fernandez MA, Sanz P, Palomar M *et al.* Fatal chemical pneumonitis due to cadmium fumes. *Occup Med* 1996; 46: 372–374.

72. Davison AG, Newman Taylor AJ, Darbyshire J *et al.* Cadmium fume inhalation and emphysema. *Lancet* 1988; i: 663–667.

73. Liles R, Miller A, Lerman Y. Acute mercury poisoning with severe chronic pulmonary manifestations. *Chest* 1985; 88: 306–309.

74. Levin M, Jacob J, Polos PG. Acute mercury poisoning and mercurial pneumonitis from gold ore purification. *Chest* 1988; 94: 554–556.

75. Rowens B, Guerrero-Betancourt D, Gottlieb CA *et al.* Respiratory failure and death following acute inhalation of mercury vapor. A clinical and histologic perspective. *Chest* 1991; 99: 185–190.

76. Moromisato DY, Anas NG, Goodman G. Mercury inhalation poisoning and acute lung injury in a child. Use of high-frequency oscillatory ventilation. *Chest* 1994; 105: 613–615.

77. Koizumi A, Aoki T, Tsukada M *et al.* Mercury, not sulphur dioxide, poisoning as cause of smelter disease in industrial plants producing sulphuric acid. *Lancet* 1994; 343: 1411–1412.

78. Bonhomme C, Gladyszaczak-Kholer J, Cadou A *et al.* Mercury poisoning by vacuum-cleaner aerosol. *Lancet* 1996; 347: 1044–1045.

79. Rennie AC, McGregor-Schuerman M, Dale IM *et al.* Mercury poisoning after spillage from a sphygmomanometer on loan from hospital. *Br Med J* 1999; 319: 366–367.

80. Forman J, Moline J, Cernichiari E *et al.* A cluster of pediatric metallic mercury exposure cases treated with meso-2,3-dimercaptosuccinic acid (DMSA). *Environ Health Perspect* 2000; 108: 575–577.

81. Shaffer BA, Schmidt-Nowara WW. Multiple small opacities of metallic density in the lung. *Chest* 1989; 96: 1179–1181.

82. dell'Omo M, Muzi G, Bernard A *et al.* Long-term toxicity of intravenous mercury injection. *Lancet* 1996; 348: 64.

83. Lees REM. Changes in lung function after exposure to vanadium compounds in fuel oil ash. *Br J Ind Med* 1980; 37: 253–256.

84. Musk AW, Tees JG. Asthma caused by occupational exposure to vanadium compounds. *Med J Aust* 1982; 1: 183–184.

85. Levy BS, Hoffman L, Gottsegen S. Boilermakers bronchitis. Respiratory tract irritation associated with vanadium pentoxide exposure during oil-to-coal conversion of a power plant. *J Occup Med* 1984; 26: 567–570.

86. Hauser R, Elreedy S, Hoppin JA *et al.* Airway obstruction in boilermakers exposed to fuel oil ash. *Am J Respir Crit Care Med* 1995; 152: 1478–1484.

87. Hauser R, Elreedy S, Hoppin JA *et al.* Upper airway response in workers exposed to fuel oil ash: nasal lavage analysis. *Occup Environ Med* 1995; 52: 353–358.

88. Rendall REG, Phillips JI, Renton KA. Death following exposure to fine particulate nickel from a metal arc process. *Ann Occup Hyg* 1994; 38: 921–930.

89. Hjortso E, Qvist J, Bud MI *et al.* ARDS after accidental inhalation of zinc chloride smoke. *Intensive Care Med* 1988; 14: 17–24.

90. Matarese SL, Matthews JI. Zinc chloride (smoke bomb) inhalational lung injury. *Chest* 1988; 89: 308–309.

91. Allen MB, Crisp A, Snook N, Page RL. 'Smoke-bomb' pneumonitis. *Respir Med* 1992; 86: 165–166.

92. Cordasco EM, Stone FD. Pulmonary edema of environmental origin. *Chest* 1973; 64: 182–185.

93. Park T, Di Benedetto R, Morgan K *et al.* Diffuse endobronchial polyposis following a titanium tetrachloride inhalation injury. *Am Rev Respir Dis* 1984; 130: 315–317.

94. Brooks SM, Weiss MA, Bernstein IL. Reactive airways dysfunction syndrome (RADS). Persistent asthma syndrome after high level irritant exposures. *Chest* 1985; 88: 376–384.

95. Zhicheng S. Acute nickel carbonyl poisoning: a report of 179 cases. *Br J Ind Med* 1986; 43: 422–424.

96. Ryan CM, Schoenfeld DA, Thorpe WP *et al.* Objective estimates of the probability of death from burn injuries. *N Engl J Med* 1998; 338: 362–366.

97. Beritic T. The challenge of fire effluents. Poisonous gases are potential killers. *Br Med J* 1990; 300: 696–698.

98. Orzel RA. Toxicological aspects of firesmoke: polymer pyrolysis and combustion. *Occup Med* 1993; 8: 415–429.

99. Peterson JE. Toxic pyrolysis products of solvents, paints, and polymer films. *Occup Med* 1993; 8: 533–547.

100. Loke JS. Thermal lung injury and acute smoke inhalation. In: Fishman AP, ed. *Pulmonary Diseases and Disorders*, Vol. 1, pp. 989–1000. New York: McGraw-Hill, 2000.

101. Cordier J-F. Organising pneumonia. *Thorax* 2000; 55: 318–328.

102. Douglas WW, Colby TV. Fume-related bronchiolitis obliterans. In: Epler GR, ed. *Diseases of the Bronchioles*, pp. 187–213. New York: Raven Press, 1994.

103. Epler GR, Colby TV, McLoud TC *et al.* Bronchiolitis obliterans organizing pneumonia. *N Engl J Med* 1985; 312: 152–158.

104. Gosink BB, Friedman PJ, Liebow AA. Bronchiolitis obliterans. Roentgenologic–pathologic correlation. *Am J Radiol* 1973; 117: 816–832.

105. McAdams J Jr. Bronchiolitis obliterans. *Am J Med* 1955; 19: 314–322.

106. Crapo JD, Marsh-Salin J, Ingram P *et al*. Tolerance and cross-tolerance using NO_2 and O_2. II. Pulmonary morphology and morphometry. *J Appl Physiol Respir Environ Exercise Physiol* 1978; 44: 370–379.

107. Corrin B. Pathology of interstitial lung disease. *Semin Respir Med* 1994; 15: 61–76.

108. Fleming GM, Chester EH, Montenegro HD. Dysfunction of small pulmonary airways following pulmonary injury due to nitrogen dioxide. *Chest* 1979; 75: 720–721.

109. Woodford DM, Coutu RE, Gaensler EA. Obstructive lung disease from acute sulfur dioxide exposure. *Respiration* 1979; 38: 238–245.

110. Seggev JS, Mason UG, Worthen S *et al*. Bronchiolitis obliterans. Report of three cases with detailed physiologic studies. *Chest* 1983; 83: 169–174.

111. Murphy DMF, Fairman RP, Lapp NL *et al*. Severe airway disease due to inhalation of fumes from cleansing agents. *Chest* 1976; 69: 372–376.

112. Patel RC, Dutta D, Schonfeld SA. Free-base cocaine use associated with bronchiolitis obliterans organizing pneumonia. *Ann Intern Med* 1987; 107: 186–187.

113. Haim DY, Lippmann ML, Goldberg SK, Walkenstein MD. The pulmonary complications of crack cocaine. A comprehensive review. *Chest* 1995; 107: 233–240.

114. Bates C, Read RC, Morice AH. A malicious mould. *Lancet* 1997; 349: 1598.

115. Myers JL, Katzenstein AL. Ultrastructural evidence of alveolar epithelial injury in idiopathic bronchiolitis obliterans-organizing pneumonia. *Am J Pathol* 1988; 132: 102–109.

116. Winternitz MC. *Collected Studies on the Pathology of War Gas Poisoning*. New Haven: Yale University Press, 1920.

117. Damiano VV, Cherian PV, Frankel FR *et al*. Intraluminal fibrosis induced unilaterally by lobar instillation of CdCl2 into the rat lung. *Am J Pathol* 1990; 137: 883–894.

118. Ghio AJ, Elliott CG, Crapo RO *et al*. Impairment after adult respiratory distress syndrome. An evaluation based on American Thoracic Society recommendations. *Am Rev Respir Dis* 1989; 139: 1158–1162.

119. Brooks SM, Bernstein IL. Reactive airways dysfunction syndrome or irritant-induced asthma. In: Bernstein IL, Chan-Yeung M, Malo JL *et al*. eds. *Asthma in the Workplace*, pp. 533–549. New York: Marcel Dekker, 1993.

120. Fisher HK, Clements JA, Wright RR. Enhancement of oxygen toxicity by the herbicide Paraquat. *Am Rev Respir Dis* 1973; 107: 246–252.

121. Blanc PD, Golden JA. Unusual occupationally related disorders of the lung: case reports and a literature review. *Occup Med* 1992; 7: 403–422.

122. Glynn KP, Gale NA. Exogenous lipoid pneumonia due to inhalation of spray lubricant (WD-40 lung). *Chest* 1990; 97: 1265–1266.

123. Carby M, Smith SR. A hazard of paint spraying. *Lancet* 2000; 355: 896.

124. Moya C, Antó JM, Newman Taylor AJ, the Collaborative Group for the Study of Toxicity in Textile Aerographic Factories. Outbreak of organising pneumonia in textile printing sprayers. *Lancet* 1994; 343: 498–502.

125. Ould Kadi F, Mohammed-Brahim B, Fyad A *et al*. Outbreak of pulmonary disease in textile dye sprayers in Algeria. *Lancet* 1994; 344: 962–963.

126. Romero S, Hernández L, Gil J *et al*. Organizing pneumonia in textile printing workers: a clinical description. *Eur Respir J* 1998; 11: 265–271.

127. Clottens FL, Verbeken EK, Nemery B. Pulmonary toxicity of components of textile paint linked to the Ardystil syndrome: intratracheal administration in hamsters. *Occup Environ Health* 1997; 54: 376–387.

128. Hoet PHM, Gilissen LPL, Leyva M *et al*. In vitro cytotoxicity of textile paint components linked to the 'Ardystil syndrome'. *Toxicol Sci* 1999; 52: 209–216.

129. Solé A, Cordero PJ, Morales P *et al*. Epidemic outbreak of interstitial lung disease in aerographics textile workers – the 'Ardystil syndrome': a first year follow up. *Thorax* 1996; 51: 94–95.

130. Ould Kadi F, Abdesslam T, Nemery B. Five-year follow-up of Algerian victims of the 'Ardystil syndrome'. *Eur Respir J* 1999; 13: 940–941.

131. Kern DG, Crausman RS, Durand KTH *et al*. Flock worker's lung: chronic interstitial lung disease in the nylon flocking industry. *Ann Intern Med* 1998; 129: 261–272.

132. Lougheed MD, Roos JO, Waddell WR *et al*. Desquamative interstitial pneumonitis and diffuse alveolar damage in textile workers. Potential role of mycotoxins. *Chest* 1995; 108: 1196–1200.

133. Eschenbacher WL, Kreiss K, Lougheed MD *et al*. Nylon flock-associated interstitial lung disease. *Am J Respir Crit Care Med* 1999; 159: 2003–2008.

134. Burkhart J, Piacitelli C, Schwegler-Berry D *et al*. Environmental study of nylon flocking process. *J Toxicol Environ Health* 1999; 57: 1–23.

135. Kern DG, Kuhn C III, Ely EW *et al*. Flock worker's lung: broadening the spectrum of clinicopathology, narrowing the spectrum of suspected etiologies. Chest 2000; 117: 251–259.

13 TOXIC PNEUMONITIS: 'ORGANIC' AGENTS

Martin Iversen

BACKGROUND

Febrile reactions caused by exposure to organic dust or aerosols have been known for decades and have been given various names according, generally, to the specific workplace or causal agent: mill fever or Monday morning fever in cotton mills [1], grain fever [2], swine confinement fever [3], farmers fever [4], mycotoxicosis from work with moldy material [5,6], and humidifier fever in environments with malfunctioning air-conditioning equipment [7–9]. Metal fume fever and polymer fever are comparable responses in occupational environments contaminated by fumes of non-'organic' origin. In 1986 during an international congress the term organic dust toxic syndrome (ODTS) was formulated as a general term to encompass this type of reaction caused by any organic dust, and ODTS is used widely today as the standard term [10]. 'Inhalation fever' is a popular alternative term in some circles, and accommodates additionally fever arising from the inhalation of metal fume and the pyrolysis products from plastics. It is possibly more appropriate for communications with the public [11]. Toxin fever and toxic pneumonitis are other terms used interchangeably with ODTS.

Causes

Organic dust exposure takes place in a variety of occupations and repeated environmental surveys in various environments have shown that dust exposure is always associated with a very high exposure to bacteria, fungi, and toxins (especially endotoxins) [12,13]. In some occupations ODTS is reported to occur in 2–5% of exposed workers [14].

Typical occupations at risk are in the textile and grain industries, livestock farming, and horticulture, but every occupation associated with the handling of organic material poses some risk, especially if it can give rise to substantial exposures to dust or other aerosols. Exposure to microbially contaminated aerosols may occur particularly with air conditioning in both industrial and office environments (even automobiles), and in the most recent decade there has been concern about similar exposures in private homes. Occasionally, new and unexpected occupations are associated with ODTS, such as refuse cycling (or recycling) work, the distribution of various composts or gardening mulch, and the use of cooling and lubricating fluids in metal working [15].

Prognosis

ODTS is a benign self-limiting disorder and the available evidence shows that there are no long-term consequences even with recurring episodes [16,17].

RECOGNITION

Clinical features

History

For some occupations, for example those within the cotton or grain industries, the clinical picture of ODTS has been known for a long time, yet affected workers rarely seek medical attention. The same probably applies to most cases in farming. In occupations where there is a substantial exposure most symptoms occur on the first work day after weekends, holidays, or other days off work because an adaptative tolerance seems to take place with prolonged exposure, hence 'Monday morning fever'.

ODTS does not depend on immunologic sensitization, so can occur during or immediately after the first exposure. Typical examples of this occur when silos are cleaned, when compost or garbage is handled, or when there is faulty air conditioning. On occasions there are sudden 'epidemics' of ODTS, an illustrative example being an outbreak during a college fraternity gathering where moldy straw was used to cover the floor [18]. Out of 67 participants, 55 (82%) fell ill within 1.3–13 hours of arriving. In a further similar example, 16 of 28 (57%) workers in a print shop fell ill owing to bacterial contamination of a humidifier [19].

When organic material gives rise to ODTS on being handled, it is nearly always described as extremely moldy with visible airborne dust, often to the degree of reducing visibility. Airborne bacterial and fungal spore counts are mostly higher than in environments associated with allergic alveolitis [5,6,12].

The clinical picture is an influenza-like reaction with 70–95% of affected individuals experiencing shivering with fever and myalgias. Approximately half will experience chest tightness and cough, whereas constitutional symptoms like headache and nausea will occur in approximately one-third. Irritation of the eyes, nose, and throat is seen in a small minority of patients, and gastrointestinal upset occurs rarely. Symptoms will usually appear 4–12 hours after the start of exposure, but rarely persist beyond 1 or 2 days [19–24].

Physical signs

The patient will usually appear unwell with an elevated temperature (38.5–40.0°C). Respiratory frequency is increased and there is evident respiratory discomfort during exercise. Bibasilar lung crackles are often, but not always, present, but wheezing is typically absent unless there is preexisting airways obstruction [20,22].

Investigation

Lung function

Spirometry usually shows a mild restrictive pattern, with a normal forced expired volume in 1s/forced vital capacity (FEV_1/FVC) ratio and a FVC below 80% predicted, but some patients will have normal spirometry [20,22,24–27]. Most patients have a mildly reduced total lung capacity and a mildly reduced diffusion capacity. Those who are most severely afflicted have a reduced oxygen tension in arterial blood (levels to 7.7 kPa have been reported), but most patients have a normal oxygen saturation and tension.

Imaging

The chest radiograph usually gives normal appearances [24,26], but in some patients there are small patchy infiltrates that persist for a few days. Progression of ODTS to acute pulmonary edema has been reported [28] but is very unusual. The appearances of ODTS on high-resolution computed tomography (CT) scanning have yet to be described.

Blood tests

A mild leukocytosis ($10–15 \times 10^9$/liter) is usually present for a few days [20,22,24] together with a mildly elevated erythrocyte sedimentation rate, but the C-reactive protein is normal or only slightly elevated. The leukocytosis is due to an increased number of granulocytes.

By definition ODTS does not require sensitization to inhalant allergens, though where there is chronic exposure to allergenic organic agents, antibody responses may be detected coincidentally. In workers chronically exposed to farm allergens, more than 10% may have low titers of precipitating antibodies. In most cases of humidifier disease there will not be antibodies against the agents most commonly responsible for allergic alveolitis, such as *Aspergillus*, *Streptomyces*, *Penicillium*, and *Thermopolyspora*, but 10–40% will have serum precipitins against microbial antigens in extracts from the humidifier reservoir containing contaminated water [23–26]. Although there is an association between these antibodies to antigens in humidifier water and symptoms of ODTS [26,29], many exposed individuals have precipitating antibodies without symptoms. As in farming and other environments, the presence of precipitating immunoglobulin G (IgG) antibodies reflects exposure but not necessarily disease, and is more common in non-smokers than in smokers [26]. Over time the titer of precipitating antibodies will fall [30]. The use of intradermal testing with organisms occurring in the workplace has generally not been useful [31].

Bronchoscopy/bronchoalveolar lavage

Bronchoscopy and studies of bronchoalveolar lavage (BAL) fluid have demonstrated increased cell numbers, a polymorphonuclear leukocytosis (40–60%) and a low percentage of lymphocytes (<10%) in the first days after exposure [5,6,22,32]. Later this pattern gradually changes to one of lower cell numbers with a dominant lymphocytosis (20–30%) and few granulocytes (<5%). The CD4/CD8 ratio has been reported as low (<1.5).

Histopathology

Very limited knowledge is available on the pathological changes in ODTS, and biopsy will usually not be necessary for its diagnosis and management. A case study with transbronchial biopsies reported a moderate cellular infiltrate with peribronchiolar distribution. There was no granuloma formation or fibrosis [4].

Atmospheric characterization

With nearly all case studies of ODTS occurring during the handling of organic material (straw, grain, hay), very high levels of endotoxin have been reported along with very high bacterial and fungal spore counts – of the order $10 \times 10^9/m^3$ [12,33]. In most cases, mold contamination is obvious, and airborne spores produce a smoke-like appearance when the material is disturbed. It should be recognized, however, that work with apparently uncontaminated organic material is often associated with the release of airborne dust and substantial exposure to fungi, bacteria, and endotoxin [34].

Poultry and swine farming is associated with the greatest levels of exposure, with 5–10 mg/m³ of total dust, 10^5–10^6 colony-forming units (cfu)/m³ of bacteria and fungi, and 20–200 ng/m³ of endotoxin encountered during normal work procedures. Dairy and grain farming, mushroom cultivation, work in cotton and wool mills, work with animal feed, and the handling of garbage and waste generally yield considerably lower levels of exposure (approximately one-tenth), but exposures may still be substantial [34]. Air sampling in heavily contaminated environments is difficult to perform and to interpret, and the measurement of endotoxin content in air is particularly difficult to standardize [35,36]. Nevertheless, a relatively close correlation has been demonstrated in a number of studies between the number of airborne Gram-negative bacteria (but not the total number of bacteria) and airborne endotoxin [36,37].

In cases arising from contamination of air-conditioning and humidification equipment, the cause is much less obvious and dust levels are comparatively low. The causal exposure usually arises from droplet aerosols released from reservoirs of microbially contaminated water. Inspection of the ventilation and air-conditioning equipment or the equipment for water handling (e.g. for recycling or cleaning) will usually show signs of contamination, but further investigation with cultures for bacteria and moulds may be necessary [24]. Similarly, inspection and culture of metal-working fluids usually reveals evidence of microbial contamination if ODTS symptoms arise in this setting [38]. In contrast to dust-related ODTS, the organisms responsible for humidifier fever are usually not thermophilic fungi like *Thermoactinomyces*, but various strains of Gram-negative bacteria. In many cases *Pseudomonas* or other Gram-negative species will be found (Table 13.1), but a wide range of organisms may be encountered, including amoebae [24,39,40]. The levels of airborne microorganisms and endotoxin will usually be much higher when air-conditioning and water treatment facilities are turned on than when closed down. The spraying or vaporization of stored or recycled water is often involved.

Table 13.1 shows the analytical results from several studies of ODTS associated with air conditioners and humidifiers. High levels of endotoxin were found in both air (up to 3600 ng/m³) and reservoir water (up to 580 000 ng/m³) during operation. In a case with *Pseudomonas* contamination of a water tank, the airborne concentration of colony-forming units rose from a background level of 8/m³ to 10 000/m³ with the spraying of water [24]. Although endotoxin measurement from Gram-negative bacteria is widely available, the measurement of fungal toxins (mycotoxins) is not.

Differential diagnosis

The differential diagnoses are mainly viral illness, pneumonia, and allergic alveolitis. Occasionally chemical toxicity has to be considered, especially if silos are decapped and exposure to nitrogen dioxide is possible, or pesticide sprays have been in use.

Exposure to organic dust causing ODTS is usually heavy, with onset within a few hours only. As a consequence, the diagnosis is usually obvious, unless the circumstances of exposure are unusual and the disorder is unexpected. If infection results from the exposure, a longer period of incubation is generally necessary before symptoms arise, but symptoms from allergy or chemical toxicity share similar timing characteristics to those of ODTS. If a single subject becomes ill among many with a shared similar level of exposure, the possibility of an unrelated infection

Table 13.1 Microbiological samples from various environments with humidifier fever

Facility	Bacteria species	cfu/m³ air	Endotoxin ng/m³ air	cfu/ml water	Endotoxin ng/ml water
Office [41] (humidifier)	Flavobacteriae	3×10^3		8×10^4	
Laboratory [24] (water for cleaning)	Pseudomonas	1×10^4			2900–5700
Ten sites [37] (waste water)	84% various Gram-negative	10^2–10^5 (mean 10^4)	0.6–320		
Fiberglass factory [36] (washwater)	Gram-negative	10–7.5×10^3 (mean 1200)	20–3600 (mean 580)	1.2×10^6–4.9×10^8 (mean 1.8×10^8)	25–580×10^3 (mean 170×10^3)
Printing factory [39] (humidifier)	Pseudomonas		130–390		
Fiber plant [42] (humidifier)	Gram-negative	292	0.06		

cfu, colony-forming units.

is strengthened. However, ODTS often affects only single individuals among a lightly exposed population, illustrating the importance of individual susceptibility. With heavy exposure, attack rates of 50–80% are common, but episodes are short lasting. High fever after 48 hours and persistent symptoms after 3 days make a diagnosis of ODTS unlikely. When the exposure is not typical and the diagnosis of ODTS is tentative, the health of other exposed workers should be sought, and a site visit may be advisable.

In cases not caused by dust exposure but by aerosol generation from air-conditioning equipment or humidifiers, the causal exposure may not obvious. In the index case, in particular, a diagnosis of ODTS may not be readily made. Most cases appear in clusters, however, and this together with repeated episodes in the affected individual should lead speedily to the correct diagnosis.

MANAGEMENT

Of the individual

The management of the affected individual person should be flexible; it depends considerably on the circumstances and the timing of any medical consultation. During acute symptoms, medical management is supportive with paracetamol or non-steroidal antiinflammatory agents as needed. Corticosteroids are not recommended; in circumstances of marked exposure to fungi, they may encourage infection and pulmonary invasion. The patient should be instructed to seek further medical attention if symptoms have not disappeared by the third day, since in these circumstances there is a need to consider an alternative diagnosis. For the

longer term, the causal environment should be identified and improved to prevent further symptoms. Alternatively, and less satisfactorily, the individual's job tasks may be modified or respiratory protection equipment provided.

The benign nature of the disorder and the lack of long-term sequelae should be made clear to the patient. There is very rarely any need for a change in employment.

Of the workforce

The most typical cases of ODTS are caused by point exposures to organic dust, such as the unloading of moldy grain or feedstuffs, or the handling of moldy straw, wood chips, or fruit. Environmental measurements are unnecessary in most cases, though documentation by photography may be advisable. Work by unprotected workers should cease until the source of exposure is contained. This may require a thorough cleaning of the occupational environment by workers wearing high-efficient respiratory protection, or confinement of the moldy product. When the latter is impractical, respiratory protection equipment will be needed when the product is handled.

When ODTS results from air conditioners or humidifiers, there is usually a need to sample water reservoirs and air for bacterial and fungal counts together with endotoxin content in order to locate the source of contamination. Clustering of ODTS cases in a manufacturing facility using air conditioners or humidifiers is often a dramatic event, and it usually leads to closing the facility for a short period. Once the equipment is turned off, the airborne levels of bacteria and endotoxin generally fall, and inspection, sampling, and cleaning can be done with only a small risk of symptoms. If production cannot be closed down for technical reasons, the use of high-efficiency respiratory filtering equipment [corresponding to the HEPA (High Efficiency Particulate Air filter) standard from National Institute for Occupational Safety and Health, USA (NIOSH)] or respirators with an independent air supply, is recommended for the workers involved during the period of sampling, location of the source of contamination, and cleaning. In typical cases both microbial sampling and endotoxin measurements will give high values, though this is not always so [41–43].

PREVENTION

In the workplace

ODTS usually reflects deviation from good working practice with regard to the regular maintenance of air conditioners and humidifiers, and the storage and handling of organic material. The measures discussed above concerning the management of workforces and workplaces found to be affected by cases of ODTS, are relevant also to its prevention in any working environment at risk.

National regulatory strategies

Because many different etiologic agents may be relevant to the ODTS in different situations, it is difficult to regulate occupational exposure levels through defined standards. As a result, few countries have specific legislation governing exposure to organic dust. In many, however, there is a more general requirement of employers to provide safe working conditions for their employees, and such legislation provides the regulatory strategy in most countries.

DIFFICULT CASE

History

A 42-year-old male 'never-smoking' farmer had been engaged in pig fattening for 15 years. He had every third weekend off duty, but otherwise worked 7 days a week inside a swine confinement building, usually for 6 hours daily. Straw had been used as a bedding material for the animals, which may at times have been moldy.

He complained that for 2 years he had noted shortness of breath, cough, or 'flu-like symptoms for the first 1 or 2 days at work after periods off duty. On days with long working hours he often experienced wheezing in addition. His temperature on symptomatic days was mostly in the range 37.8–38.5°C, but on some days it rose as high as 39.5°C and on some days he was without fever. Symptoms occasionally occurred at other times. He was otherwise well and was not using any medications. He had one employee for 6 years, who was without symptoms.

A chest radiograph was normal. Spirometry showed the FEV_1 and FVC to be respectively 87% and 95% of predicted, and the diffusing capacity (T_LCO) was 91% of predicted. Peak expiratory flow (PEF) measurements showed a variability of 5–13% over work shifts, but there was no meaningful circadian change during periods away from work. A methacholine challenge test was interpreted to show moderate bronchial hyperreactivity. Skin-prick tests with extracts of common allergens, and grain and pig allergens gave negative results, but there was a small though probably insignificant reaction to storage mites (*Lepidoglyphus destructor*). Serum precipitin tests showed positive reactions to *Aspergillus fumigatus* (titer 1:8) and *Thermoactinomyces* (titer 1:4).

The technical service of a national association of pork producers was consulted and dust levels in the working environment were measured. In the farmer's breathing zone during work in the pig confinement building, the mean total dust level was 7.3 mg/m^3 and the mean endotoxin content was 89 ng/m^3.

Issues

The chief issue here is one of diagnosis. Were this man's symptoms primarily due to asthma (and if so occupational asthma), bronchitis, ODTS, or hypersensitivity pneumonitis, or could they have represented a non-specific response to endotoxin? Additional issues are the choice of management, and the probable long-term outcome.

Comment

The environmental measurements showed that the exposure was significant at a level that is well associated with ODTS. The development of recurrent fever, which was self-limiting within 1 or 2 days, is best explained by an ODTS type of reaction; allergic alveolitis with repeated episodes would generally lead to a more severe illness. The wheezing and asthma-like symptoms cannot be explained satisfactorily by an ODTS type of reaction. Since there was a moderately high level of airway responsiveness, it is likely that he additionally had asthma, though this gave rise to symptoms and variability in peak flow measurements only during work days. This raises the possibility that he had occupational asthma as well as ODTS, but the asthmatic symptoms may simply have been a consequence of non-specific bronchial irritation.

The low antibody titers against molds probably resulted independently from his occupational exposures as a farmer. Such levels have been reported in several studies in about 10% of farmers. The positive prick-test to storage mites probably reflects occupational exposure and is found in approximately 5% of farmers in temperate climates.

SUMMARY POINTS

Recognition

- ODTS is an acute-onset, febrile, influenza-like illness, that is self-limiting within 2–3 days.
- It is the result of substantial exposures to airborne bacterial endotoxin and a variety of microorganisms, principally fungi.
- Physical signs are absent or subtle.
- A causal exposure is often obvious, usually involving dust from moldy vegetable produce or aerosols from microbially contaminated air conditioners, humidifiers, or metal-working fluids.
- A clustering of cases is nearly always found when many individuals are exposed.
- ODTS does not require a latent period of sensitization; it can occur on first exposure.
- Serum IgG antibodies to microbial antigens are not diagnostic; ODTS often occurs in their absence, and they are often found in exposed individuals without evidence of ODTS.
- Many working environments are associated with substantial levels of exposure.

Management

- Acute episodes of ODTS require no specific treatment.

- If symptomatic therapy is needed, paracetamol or non-steroidal antiinflammatory agents are recommended, not corticosteroids.
- There should be follow-up to exclude alternative diagnoses if symptoms persist beyond 3 days.
- The workplace should be investigated to identify the causal exposure source, and there should be documentation (preferably by photography) where the occupational environment can be improved.
- Biologic sampling of air and contaminated water (measurement of endotoxin levels and fungal colony forming units) is complex and expensive, and may not be necessary in typical cases, but it may be required if the presumed source is a contaminated air conditioner or humidifier.
- A change of occupation is not normally indicated.

Prevention

- ODTS is usually prevented by good maintenance standards and working practices.
- When a contaminated working environment is to be inspected, sampled, or cleaned, there may be a need for respiratory protection equipment.

REFERENCES

1. Holness DL, Taraschuk IG, Goldstein RS. Acute exposure of cotton dust. A case of mill fever. *JAMA* 1982; 247: 1602–1603.
2. doPico GA, Flaherty D, Bhansali P *et al*. Grain fever syndrome induced by inhalation of airborne grain dust. *J Allergy Clin Immunol* 1982; 69: 435–443.
3. Vogelzang PFJ, van der Gulden JWJ, Folgering H *et al*. Organic dust toxic syndrome in swine confinement farming. *Am J Ind Med* 1999; 35: 332–334.
4. Cormier Y, Fournier M, Laviolette M. Farmer's fever. *Chest* 1993; 103: 632–634.
5. Lecours R, Laviolette M, Cormier Y. Bronchoalveolar lavage in pulmonary mycotoxicosis (organic dust toxic syndrome). *Thorax* 1986; 41: 924–926.
6. May JJ, Stallones L, Darrow D, Pratt DS. Organic dust toxicity (pulmonary mycotoxicosis) associated with silo unloading. *Thorax* 1986; 41: 919–923.
7. Pickering CAC, Moore WKS, Lacey J *et al*. Investigation of a respiratory disease associated with an air-conditioning system. *Clin Allergy* 1976; 6: 109–118.
8. Ganier M, Lieberman P, Fink J *et al*. Humidifier lung. An outbreak in office workers. *Chest* 1980; 77: 183–187.
9. Pestalozzi C. Febrile Gruppenerkrankungen in einer Modelschreinerei durch Inhalation von mit Schimmelpilzen kontaminiertem Befeuchterwasser ('Befeuchterfieber'). *Schweiz Med Wochenschr* 1959; 89: 710–713.
10. doPico GA. Health effects of organic dust in the farm environment. Report on diseases. *Am J Ind Med* 1986; 10: 261–265.
11. Rask-Andersen A. Inhalation fever. In: Harber P, Schenker MB, Balmes JR, eds. *Occupational and Environmental Respiratory Disease*, pp. 243–258. St Louis: Mosby.

12. Malmberg P, Rask-Andersen A, Palmgren U *et al*. Exposure to microorganisms, febrile and airway-obstructive symptoms, immune status and lung function of Swedish farmers. *Scand J Work Environ Health* 1985; 11: 287–293.
13. Dutkiewicz J, Olenchock SA, Sorensen WG *et al*. Levels of bacteria, fungi, and endotoxin in bulk and aerosolized corn silage. *Appl Environ Microbiol* 1989; 55: 1093–1099.
14. Simpson JCG, Niven RM, Pickering CAC *et al*. Prevalence and predictors of work related respiratory symptoms in workers exposed to organic dust. *Occup Environ Med* 1998; 55: 668–672.
15. Poulsen OM, Breum NO, Ebbehøj N Sorting and recycling of domestic waste. Review of occupational health problems and their possible causes. *Sci Total Environ* 1995; 168: 33–56.
16. May JJ, Marvel LH, Pratt DS, Coppolo P. Organic dust toxic syndrome: A follow-up study. *Am J Ind Med* 1990; 17: 111–113.
17. Pal TM, de Monchy JGR, Groothoff JW *et al*. Follow up investigation of workers in synthetic fibre plants with humidifier disease and work related asthma. *Occup Environ Med* 1999; 56: 403–410.
18. Brinton WT, Vastbinder EE, Greene JW *et al*. An outbreak of organic dust toxic syndrome in a college fraternity. *JAMA* 1987; 258: 1210–1212.
19. Mamolen M, Lewis DM, Blanchet MA *et al*. Investigation of an outbreak of 'Humidifier Fever' in a print shop. *Am J Ind Med* 1993; 23: 483–490.
20. Rask-Andersen A. Organic dust toxic syndrome among farmers. *Br J Ind Med* 1989; 46: 233–238.
21. Malmberg P, Rask-Andersen A, Höglund S *et al*. Incidence of organic dust toxic syndrome and allergic alveolitis in Swedish farmers. *Int Arch Allergy Appl Immunol* 1988; 87: 47–53.

22. Wintermeyer SF, Kuschner WG, Wong H *et al.* Pulmonary responses after wood chip mulch exposure. *J Occup Environ Med* 1997; 39: 308–314.

23. Anderson K, Watt AD, Sinclair D *et al.* Climate, intermittent humidification, and humidifier fever. *Br J Ind Med* 1989; 46: 671–674.

24. Anderson K, McSharry CP, Clark C *et al.* Sump Bay Fever: inhalational fever associated with a biologically contaminated water aerosol. *Occup Environ Med* 1996; 53: 106–111.

25. Pal TM, Kaufmann HF, de Monchy JGR, de Vries K. Lung function of workers exposed to antigens from a contaminated air-conditioning system. *Int Arch Occup Environ Health* 1985; 55: 253–266.

26. Cockroft A, Edwards J, Bevan C *et al.* An investigation of operating theatre staff exposed to humidifier antigens. *Br J Ind Med* 1981; 38: 144–151.

27. Ashton I, Axford AT, Bevan C *et al.* Lung function of office workers exposed to humidifier fever antigen. *Br J Ind Med* 1981; 38: 34–37.

28. Yoshida K, Ando M, Araki S. Acute pulmonary edema in a storehouse of moldy oranges: a severe case of the organic dust toxic syndrome. *Arch Environ Health* 1989; 44: 382–384.

29. McSharry C, Anderson K, Speekenbrink A *et al.* Discriminant analysis of symptom pattern and serum antibody titres in humidifier disease. *Thorax* 1993; 48: 496–500.

30. Lewis C, McSharry C, Anderson K *et al.* Quantifying antibody class and subclass responses by enzyme immunoassay in humidifier-related disease. *Clin Exp Allergy* 1991; 21: 601–607.

31. Kremer AM, Pal TM, de Monchy JG *et al.* Precipitating antibodies and positive skin tests in workers exposed to airborne antigens from a contaminated humidification system. *Int Arch Occup Environ Health* 1989; 61: 547–553.

32. Raymenants E, Demedts M, Nemery B. Bronchoalveolar lavage findings in a patient with the organic dust toxic syndrome. *Thorax* 1990; 45: 713–714.

33. Weber S, Kullman G, Petsonk E *et al.* Organic dust exposures from compost handling: case presentation and respiratory exposure assessment. *Am J Ind Med* 1993; 24: 365–374.

34. Simpson JCG, Niven RM, Pickering CA *et al.* Comparative personal exposures to organic dust and endotoxin. *Ann Occup Hyg* 1999; 43: 107–115.

35. Eduard W, Heederich D. Methods for quantative assessment of airborne levels of noninfectious microorganisms in highly contaminated work environments. *Am Ind Hyg Assoc J* 1998; 59: 113–127.

36. Walters M, Milton D, Larsson L *et al.* Airborne environmental endotoxin: a cross-validation of sampling and analysis techniques. *Appl Environ Microbiol* 1994; 60: 996–1005.

37. Laitinen S, Nevalainen A, Kotima M *et al.* Relationship between bacterial counts and endotoxin concentrations in the air of wastewater treatment plants. *Appl Environ Microbiol* 1992; 58: 3774–3776.

38. Woskie SR, Virji MA, Kriebel D *et al.* Exposure assessment for a field investigation of the acute respiratory effects of metalworking fluids. Summary of findings. *Am Ind Hyg Assoc J* 1996; 57: 1154–1162.

39. Rylander R, Haglind P. Airborne endotoxins and humidifier disease. *Clin Allergy* 1984; 14: 109–112.

40. Finnegan MJ, Pickering CA, Davies PS *et al.* Amoebae and humidifier fever. *Clin Allergy* 1987; 17: 235–242.

41. Rylander R, Haglind P, Lundholm M *et al.* Humidifier fever and endotoxin exposure. *Clin Allergy* 1978; 8: 511–516.

42. Kateman E, Heederick D, Pal TM *et al.* Relationship of airborne microorganisms with the lung function and leucocyte levels of workers with a history of humidifier fever. *Scand J Work Environ Health* 1990; 16: 428–433.

43. Pal TM, de Monchy JG, Groothoff JW *et al.* The clinical spectrum of humidifier disease in synthetic fiber plants. *Am J Ind Med* 1997; 31: 682–692.

14 HYPERSENSITIVITY PNEUMONITIS

Yvon Cormier

BACKGROUND

Hypersensitivity pneumonitis (HP), also known as extrinsic allergic alveolitis, is a parenchymal disease of the lung caused by a hyperimmune response to inhaled antigens in sensitized individuals. The primary site of the allergic response is alveolar/bronchiolar tissue and the lung's interstitium. The duration of exposure required to induce sensitization is unknown, but HP does not develop after a first contact with the antigenic source. This is a useful distinguishing characteristic from the organic dust toxic syndrome, which may show similar clinical features and arise in similar circumstances, though after a single unduly heavy exposure (see Chapter 13). The causal antigens are varied in nature and can be present in a wide range of environments including the home as well as the workplace. The antigens most commonly involved occupationally are proteins derived from bacteria, fungi, and a number of animal species; less commonly inhaled reactive chemicals act as haptens and become antigenic when bound to the host's proteins.

The first cases of HP were described by Campbell in 1932 in farm workers, and the cause of that form of the disease (farmers' lung) was identified by Pepys 30 years later [1,2]. If forage is stored damp or in humid conditions it becomes moldy, and with the exothermic process there is a sequential contamin-ating growth of antigenic spore-forming thermo-philic bacteria or fungi. Farmer's lung remains an important form of HP in many countries, but many additional causes are now recognized.

Causes

There are exhaustive and ever-expanding listings of individual causes and the relevant environments in which they may be encountered [3–5]. The most prominent types of HP, besides farmers' lung, are bird breeders' (fanciers') disease, Japanese summer-type HP, and humidifier lung, but in regions cultiv-ating sugar cane and mushrooms, bagassosis and mushroom workers' lung may be more prevalent. Most of the reported causal agents are encountered occupationally, and most result from microbial con-tamination when vegetable produce is stored without being adequately dried or is stored under damp conditions. Table 14.1 provides a summary.

Epidemiology

The prevalence and incidence of HP are difficult if not impossible to quantify, and the reported estimates are difficult to compare, since different definitions and diagnostic methods have been used [6–11]. Furthermore, few studies have been carried out and published. The disease is seen worldwide, different

Table 14.1 Agents reported to cause extrinsic allergic alveolitis. Modified from Hendrick DJ. Extrinsic allergic alveolitis. In: Weatherall DJ, Ledingham JGG, Warrell DA, eds. *Oxford Textbook of Medicine*, 3rd edn. Oxford: Oxford University Press, 1990.

Agent	Source	Appellation
Microorganisms		
Alternaria	Paper mill wood pulp	Wood pulp workers' lung
Aspergillus clavatus	Whisky maltings	Malt workers' lung
Aspergillus fumigatus	Vegetable compost	Farmers' lung
Aspergillus versicolor	Dog bedding (straw)	Dog house disease
Aureobasidium pullulans	Redwood	Sequoiosis
Bacillus subtilis	Domestic wood	
Cephalosporium	Sewage	Sewage workers' lung
Cryptostroma corticale	Maple	Maple bark stripper's lung
Graphium	Redwood	Sequoiosis
Lycoperdon	Puffballs	Lycoperdonosis
Merulius lacrymans	Domestic wood	
Mucor stolonifer	Paprika	Paprika splitters' lung
Penicillium casei	Cheese	Cheese washers' lung
Penicillium chrysogenum/Penicillium cyclopium	Domestic wood/peat moss	
Penicillium frequentens	Cork	Suberosis
Saccharomonspora viridis	Logging plant	
Sporobolomyces	Horse barn straw	
Streptomyces albus	Soil/peat	
Thermophilic actinomycetes (Saccharopolyspora rectivirgula)	Hay/straw/grain/mushroom compost/bagasse	Farmers' lung Mushroom worker's lung Bagassosis
Trichosporon cutaneum Saccharo polyspora rectivirgula, T. vulgaris	Japonese summer air	Summer-type hypersensitivity pneumonitis
Miscellaneous ?bacteria/?fungi/?amoebae/ ?nematode debris	Air conditioners/humidifiers/ tap water	Humidifier lung, ventilation pneumonitis, sauner takers' lung
Unknown	Roof thatch	New Guinea lung
Animals		
Arthropods (S. granarius)	Grain dust	Wheat weevil disease
Birds	?Bloom/?excreta	Bird breeder's/fanciers' lung
Fish	Fish meal	Fish meal workers' lung
Mammals		
Pituitary (cattle, pig)	Pituitary extracts	Pituitary snuff takers' lung
Hair	Fur	Furriers' lung
Mollusc shell	Nacre-button manufacture	
Urine (rodents)	Urinary protein	Rodent handlers' lung
Vegetation		
Coffee	Coffee bean dust	Coffee workers' lung
Wood (Gonystylus bacanus)	Wood dust	Wood workers' lung
Chemicals		
Bordeaux mixture (fungicide)	Vineyards	Vineyard sprayers' lung
Cobalt dissolved in solvents	Tungsten carbide grinding	
Diphenyl methane diisocyanate	Plastics industry	
Formaldehyde*	Laboratory	
Hexamethylene diisocyanate	Plastics industry	
Pauli's reagent	Laboratory	
Pyrethrum	Insecticide spray	
Toluene diisocyanate	Plastics industry	
Trimellitic anhydride	Plastics industry	

*One subject, possibly toxic not allergic response.

regions associating it with different occupational environments and different causal antigens. For example, farmers' lung is frequent in cold humid climates like those of eastern North America or northern Europe, pigeon breeders' disease is the most important type in Central and South America, summer-type HP predominates in Japan, and humidifier lung may occur with dramatic prevalence (15–70%) without regard to geographic region in small populations working in contaminated offices [7,12–14].

Most cases of pigeon breeders' disease and summer-type HP occur in domestic or social environments, not in the workplace, and the epidemiology of occupational HP is particularly difficult to ascertain. This is largely a consequence of HP being an uncommon cause of occupational lung disease. Recent experience over 3 years from a British surveillance project suggested that HP of occupational origin accounts for only 2% of occupational lung diseases [15]. Contaminating microorganisms were thought to underlie over 50% of the reported cases, followed in order of importance by animal antigens in 6% and chemicals in 5%. In 27% a causal agent was not specified. Almost 50% of the British cases affected farmers or farm workers, among whom the average incidence was 41 per million per year. This approached 100/million per year in some regions, but the true incidence must have been underestimated since in areas of high rainfall where 'traditional' farming methods are used, the prevalence of farmers' lung may reach 10%. A more realistic incidence of 3000/million per year has been estimated in Quebec, Canada, but all estimates are necessarily crude, since the number of cases vary from year to year depending on climatic conditions during the hay-making season, and most cases are not reported or even diagnosed [16].

It is reasonable to assume that the incidence of HP in general is underestimated: transient acute forms are often misclassified as infectious diseases, cases are often not reported, and patients (especially farmers) may minimize their symptoms or not consult a physician. Few farmers are willing to give up farming, even after a confirmed diagnosis, though in one study an unreasonable fear of the prognosis was the most important reason why affected farmers quit their profession [17].

Prognosis

The prognosis of HP is quite varied. If the diagnosis is made early and the causative agent or agents removed from the patient's environment, HP will heal and usually leave no permanent damage. Acute cases can be severe in terms of dyspnea, hypoxia, fever, and general weakness but are very rarely fatal. Continued exposure will often lead to recurrent acute episodes or a low-grade progression of the disease causing irreversible lung damage in the form of fibrosis, emphysema or a combination of both [13,18,19]. Respiratory failure and death from these forms of HP can be as high as 25% of the affected individuals over

a 5-year period [13]. Treatment of HP with corticosteroids will not alter the long-term course of the disease, only accelerate the initial improvement [20].

RECOGNITION

Clinical features

HP can manifest itself in very different ways. Classically the clinical presentations have been described as acute, subacute, and chronic [21]. The symptoms of acute HP comprise febrile influenza-like reactions with chills, dyspnea, cough, chest tightness and malaise occurring 3–8 hours after the beginning of exposure to the causal antigen. These symptoms wane spontaneously over a few hours, only to recur on subsequent exposure. The associated physical signs, if the subject is seen during the time course of the acute reaction, are fever and bilateral inspiratory crackles on chest auscultation. More obviously the subject appears ill, as if he/she has influenza. Severity depends on exposure dose and individual susceptibility, and only exceptionally is there any threat to survival. After multiple episodes, the more indolent forms may supervene (though these may occur independently of the acute form) and undue breathlessness becomes persistent. Weight loss may then occur as well. In many cases, however, the affected individual recovers fully after each acute episode, and there is no persisting pulmonary damage.

The subacute form is characterized by progressive increasing shortness of breath, cough which is generally dry, and weight loss, but there are no prominent recurrent episodes of influenza-like illness. Inspiratory crackles can again be heard but fever is not prominent. Digital clubbing has been described in this form of HP, though is not common [22].

The chronic form is the least well defined, largely because its features of irreversible scarring or parenchymal destruction are indistinguishable from those of other chronic fibrotic diseases of the lung. Two research groups have reported that, while interstitial fibrosis is the most likely long-term outcome in most forms of HP, farmers' lung more frequently evolves to produce emphysema [18,19]. The explanation for such a difference is unknown, but CT scanning showed clear evidence of emphysema in non-smoking subjects with farmers' lung, without there being any emphysema excess in farmers without farmers' lung. Thus emphysema appears not to be a coincidental and independent phenomenon of farm dust exposure. It is possibly related to differences in the intensity or duration of exposure, or in the nature of the inducing agent. The latter, in farmers' lung, often involves a mixture of microbes and endotoxin, whereas in many types of HP a single antigen is responsible, for example, pigeon breeders' disease and summer-type HP [13,23]. There may consequently be an interactive effect between the agents within farm dust and farmers' lung which changes the usual outcome of HP.

The symptoms of chronic HP, when present, are shortness of breath and chronic cough, often with sputum production [23]. It therefore simulates chronic bronchitis, though chronic bronchitis may occur independently as a consequence of chronic antigen inhalation as may airway obstruction attributable to asthma [24,25]. Physical signs are non-specific and include crackles, rhonchi, and 'squawks' on auscultation, the rare presence of clubbing and, in very advanced cases, signs of cor pulmonale [22,23]. If the patient is no longer in contact with the causal environment, a diagnosis of chronic HP may be very difficult. These chronic abnormalities are non-specific, a specific serum antibody response may no longer be detectable, and the characteristic numbers of lymphocytes and granulomas from bronchoalveolar lavage or biopsy material will not be evident. Often only a clear and thorough clinical history orients the physician to the diagnosis, and this may not be sufficient for most compensation or insurance agencies.

Why an individual patient presents with one or another form of HP is not clearly understood. The nature of the antigen, its airborne concentration, the duration of contact, and the patient's genetic susceptibility are all factors of hypothetical importance. In general, however, episodic high-level exposures tend to precipitate acute events, while continuous low-level exposures are more likely to cause subacute or chronic HP.

The importance of a detailed clinical history in the diagnosis of HP cannot be overstated. Thorough questioning about environmental exposure in the home, at work, or socially is essential for all patients presenting with either recurrent febrile episodes with dyspnea or progressive dyspnea without fever. This is especially true if inspiratory crackles are heard bilaterally. Sometimes the source of relevant allergen is obvious (e.g. dairy farm), but sometimes it is extremely difficult to find (e.g. a patient's girlfriend who keeps a dove in her apartment). Once HP is suspected by a primary-care physician, further investigation should be undertaken in a referral center with appropriate facilities and expertise.

Investigation

The investigation of suspected HP generally requires the following four clinical procedures in order to confirm the diagnosis and document the extent of involvement. For cases which prove to be unusually challenging, the additional listed procedures may be required.

Lung function

Physiological tests should include flow rates (spirometry), volumes, diffusion capacity, and blood gas analysis. They are possibly more useful in assessing disease severity than diagnosis, but serial tests may show fluctuation as exposure waxes and wanes, and so provide some diagnostic clues. When impaired function is demonstrable, there is typically a restrictive loss of ventilatory function [similar or greater impairment of forced vital capacity (FVC) than forced expired volume in 1 s (FEV_1), and a reduction of total lung capacity] coupled with impaired parenchymal function (a reduction of T_LCO and KCO). With mild involvement the arterial blood gases often show no abnormality at rest, but hypoxemia occurs with exercise together with lowered carbon dioxide tension because hyperventilation is stimulated. All these features are characteristic of diffuse parenchymal/interstitial disease of the lungs, and so are not specific to HP, but they usefully distinguish such diseases from those characterized by airway obstruction. If the physiological assessment takes place days or weeks after the most recent exposure, disease activity may have subsided and these physiological tests may show no abnormality. Conversely, if there is active disease and extensive involvement, the degree of impairment provides a useful measure of disease severity.

Some of the environmental agents that cause HP are, however, recognized to cause asthma [and possibly chronic obstructive pulmonary disease (COPD)], and so a mixed restrictive/obstructive physiological picture is sometimes observed. Furthermore, in the acute and subacute forms of HP the characteristic involvement of distal bronchioles may cause widespread obstruction at the level of the small airways and so the residual volume is often increased not decreased, despite the dominant restrictive effect on ventilation; in the chronic form, an obstructive, restrictive, or mixed pattern may dominate [13,18,19,23,24,26]. It should also be recognized that measurements obtained within the normal (i.e. predicted) range, may nevertheless represent significant reductions from the values existing before HP developed. Serial measurements may consequently be particularly useful in monitoring the effect of treatment and the natural history of the disease in each affected individual. Further details concerning physiological measurements are presented in Chapter 32 (lung function).

Chest radiology

Standard chest radiographs are abnormal in 80% of cases of HP [27]; a normal film does not therefore rule out HP. In acute and subacute cases the characteristic abnormalities are fine interstitial infiltrates which predominate in the lower lung fields. A typical example is presented in Fig. 14.1, a case of subacute HP attributable to *Saccharopolyspora rectivirgula*, the thermophilic bacteria most commonly responsible for farmers' lung. In advanced stages of the chronic form of the disease, the radiological appearances are of irregular scarring typical of diffuse pulmonary fibrosis (Fig. 14.2) or diffuse emphysema (Fig. 14.3). Both are cases of farmers' lung.

High-resolution computed tomography (HRCT) is a very sensitive and important tool in establishing the diagnosis of HP [6,28–30]. It is abnormal in most, if not all, cases of active disease [31,32]. In

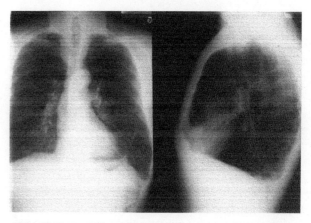

Fig. 14.3 Posteroanterior and lateral chest films showing typical emphysematous changes. The patient was a non-smoker with longstanding farmer's lung.

the acute and subacute cases, HRCT shows ground-glass patchy infiltrates and a mosaic pattern (particularly in expiration), which predominate in the lower zones [33]. A HRCT cut from the case whose chest radiograph is shown in Fig. 14.1 is presented in Fig. 14.4. Further details concerning the radiological appearances are presented in Chapter 31.

Bronchoscopy

Bronchoscopy with bronchoalveolar lavage, and in some cases transbronchial biopsy, is now a standard procedure in the evaluation of suspected HP. The visual aspect of the airways is not altered in most cases but mild inflammation can sometimes be seen. Infection is the major alternative consideration in differential diagnosis of the acute and subacute forms of HP, and the presence of purulent secretions would favor this. Bronchial secretions, lavage fluid, and brushing samples should be sent for bacterial, mycobacterial, and fungal analyses. Infectious processes

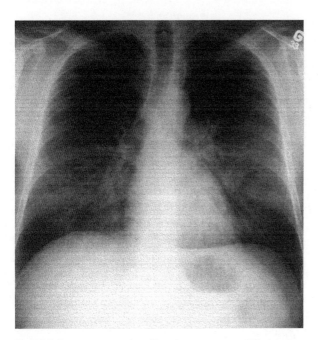

Fig. 14.1 Posteroanterior chest film of an acute case of HP showing fine interstitial infiltrates which predominate in the lower lung fields.

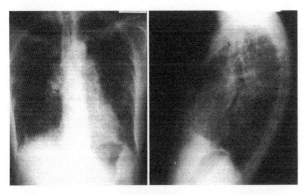

Fig. 14.2 Posteroanterior and lateral films of another case of longstanding and poorly controlled farmer's lung where the outcome was that of end-stage fibrosis. This patient died of this disease and necropsy confirmed the fibrotic nature of the chest film's findings.

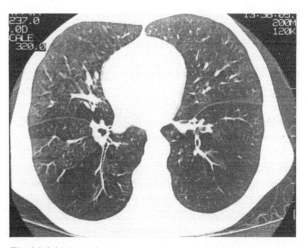

Fig. 14.4 High-resolution computed tomography image of the same case of acute HP as shown in Fig. 14.1. Note the patchy ground-glass alveolar infiltrates and mosaic pattern.

most likely to simulate HP include atypical pneumonias attributable to mycoplasma, legionnella, chlamydia (e.g. psittacosis in bird keepers), *Pneumocystis carinii* pneumonia, invasive fungal infection (e.g. aspergillosis) and mycobacteriosis (tuberculous or non-tuberculous). For the more chronic forms of HP, the differential diagnosis includes all types of chronic diffuse pulmonary fibrosis.

The bronchoalveolar lavage (BAL) yield is usefully separated into cell pellet and supernatant. Although the supernatant contains increased levels of various cytokines and growth factors, surfactant protein A, specific antibodies to the causal antigens, and several other substances, these are seldom measured in clinical practice and are not relevant in the diagnosis and staging of the disease [34–36]. Cell counts and differentials are, however, very useful. The total number of cells is increased, the lymphocytes accounting for most of the increase. Alveolar macrophages are also increased in number but their percentage decreases because of the greater increase in lymphocyte numbers. Neutrophils are transiently increased in the hours that follow exposure [37].

The major pitfall from counting lymphocytes in the lavage yield is that an increase in their number is not specific for HP. Other diseases that are also associated with alveolar lymphocytosis include: sarcoidosis, miliary tuberculosis, *Pneumocystis carinii* pneumonia, lymphocytic leukemia, bronchiolitis obliterans with organizing pneumonitis (BOOP), drug reactions (e.g. amiodarone, methotrexate), and berylliosis. Furthermore, many asymptomatic individuals exposed in an environment associated with HP (e.g. dairy barns) also have increased numbers of lymphocytes in BAL [38]. HP is, however, the disease in which the largest numbers and percentages of lymphocytes are recovered by BAL, and analysis of their subsets can be useful. The lymphocytes in HP are predominantly of the T-suppressor subtype (CD8+) and the ratio CD4+/CD8+ is generally less than 1 [14,39]. By contrast, in sarcoidosis the T-helper (CD4+) cells usually dominate, giving a high CD4+/CD8+ ratio (40).

Transbronchial biopsies are often obtained during the bronchoscopic procedure. HP produces interstitial inflammation characterized by monocytic infiltrates and poorly formed granulomas [41]. Biopsy specimens are necessarily small, and the samples may not be adequately representative of the underlying disease process. Their usefulness is consequently limited, though in individual cases an unequivocal diagnosis may still be possible [42].

Specific antibodies

Antigen-specific immunoglobulin G (IgG) antibodies (precipitins) are present in the serum and lavage fluid of most cases of HP, though active smoking may impair, even inhibit, this antibody response without necessarily 'protecting' the individual from the disease. There is, however, some evidence of protection [43]. When antibodies are not found, as in one-third of patients with presumed farmers' lung, it is possible that inappropriate antigens were used in the tests. Specific IgA antibodies are also commonly found in BAL fluid, but generally reflect exposure rather than disease. They do not aid diagnosis, except for confirming that sufficient exposure has occurred to stimulate a local immune response. Much the same might be said for specific IgG responses, since these are not infrequently found among exposed though apparently unaffected subjects, but IgG antibodies imply a more systemic and potentially more relevant immune response, and in practice negative serology makes the diagnosis of HP unlikely.

The traditional double diffusion method of Ouchterlony is less sensitive than the more recent enzyme-linked immunosorbent assay (ELISA) technique, and the latter is often preferred [44–45]. The increase in sensitivity is associated with diminished specificity, however. Between 10% and 30% of individuals exposed to moldy hay or pigeons have been found to have preciptins against, respectively, *Saccharopolyspora rectivirgula* or avian antigens without presenting a clinical picture of HP, even with the double-diffusion technique of precipitin assay [46,47]. The falsely seropositive proportion can be expected to be much higher with the ELISA technique and, when it was used in a recent survey within a peat moss-processing plant, IgG antibodies to *Penicillium* sp. (the cause of HP in that environment) were found in all but one of the non-smokers [4]. Half the exposed, but asymptomatic, precipitin-positive workers nevertheless showed evidence of lymphocytic alveolitis from BAL [38].

Atmospheric characterization

The use of air sampling in the hope of identifying sources of potentially relevant antigens is difficult, and it requires equipment and expertise that are often not readily available. The procedure may nevertheless be invaluable, particularly when a potentially novel environmental setting for HP is suspected, but the precise causal antigen is unclear and specific antibody tests have proved unrewarding.

Surgical lung biopsy

Surgical biopsy is rarely required for the diagnosis of HP, but when suspected HP is not confirmed from the investigations described already, and the cause of progressive diffuse parenchymal/interstitial lung disease remains unclear, surgical biopsy is not readily avoided. The presence of loosely formed

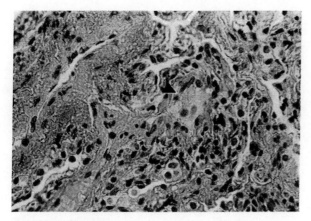

Fig. 14.5 Histopathology of a lung biopsy in HP showing mononuclear cellular infiltrate with early granuloma formation (arrow head).

granulomas with interstitial mononuclear cell infiltrates, typically centered around respiratory bronchioles, is characteristic of the majority of biopsies from cases of HP. Interstitial fibrosis is usually only seen in the chronic form of the disease, along with evidence of old granulomas (Schaumann bodies). These features allow a specific diagnosis of HP in most instances. It is important to note the presence of true interstitial fibrosis, since this finding signifies irreversible changes. The inducing antigens will not, however, be found in the biopsy specimen, even if they are microbial. Figure 14.5 shows the histological appearances of HP diagnosed in this way in a case of farmers' lung.

Inhalation challenge tests

Inhalation provocation tests with the relevant specific antigen possibly provides the most convincing method of confirming that the underlying disease is HP and that the challenge agent is the causal antigen. Such tests are rarely needed, which is fortunate since there is limited experience of them, they are time consuming, not readily standardized, and available in only a few referral centers. Furthermore, positive results are associated with

uncomfortable influenza-like symptoms, which often persist for 24 hours or more, and significant changes in lung function may be difficult to demonstrate [48,49]. An acute neutrophil response in BAL fluid usefully confirms a positive outcome, but bronchoscopy is also likely to be uncomfortable in the circumstances [37]. The febrile reaction together with characteristic hematological responses in circulating blood (neutrophilia and lymphopenia) and changes in breathing pattern offer an alternative method of confirming a positive result with confidence. The diagnostic features are summarized in Table 14.2.

MANAGEMENT

Of the individual

HP in an individual patient is best managed by removing him/her from the responsible working environment (e.g. dairy barn). If this is achievable then the immediate medical problem is solved. Unfortunately, it is not usually that simple; for many occupations the causal environment cannot readily be avoided, and for many affected workers alternative employment is not readily available. Farmers and farm workers in particular are often very reluctant to change their profession, and so management may involve the compromise of reducing the individual's level of exposure to a practical minimum rather than eliminating it altogether.

First, the affected individual (or his employer) may be able to rearrange the particular tasks of his/her job so that others with less susceptibility carry out those associated most heavily with exposure.

Secondly, he/she should use respiratory protection equipment for the tasks that cannot readily be passed to others [50–52]. A simple surgical-type face mask is usually inadequate. Most countries regulate the standards required for the use of respirators in particular circumstances, and appropriate advice is essential before any individual device is

Table 14.2 Diagnostic features of positive inhalation challenge tests. Adapted from Hendrick DJ. Extrinsic allergic alveolitis. In: Weatherall DJ, Ledingham JGG, Warrell DA, eds. *Oxford Textbook of Medicine*, 3rd edn. Oxford: Oxford University Press, 1990.

Diagnostic changes within 36 hours of challenge exposure	Sensitivity (%)
1 Increase in body temperature to >37.2°C	78
2 Increase in circulating neutrophils by ≥2.5 × 10⁹/liter	68
3 Decrease in circulating lymphocytes by ≥0.5 × 10⁹/liter with lymphopenia (<1.5 × 10⁹/liter)	52
4 Decrease in forced vital capacity by ≥15%	48
5 Increase in exercise minute volume by ≥15%	85
6 Increase in exercise respiratory frequency by ≥25%	64

The data were taken from a series of 144 antigen and control challenge tests in 31 subjects. Diagnostic end-points were chosen to produce specificities of approximately 95%, after mean changes associated with positive challenges tests were shown to be highly significant. When each monitoring parameter was given a score of 1 for a significant result, a total score of 2/6 or more was associated with a specificity of 100% and a sensitivity of 78% for the 144 challenge tests.

selected. One with charcoal filters may be needed if the working environment is contaminated with reactive chemicals. A helmet directing the flow of air from a battery-powered filtering device is the most effective for dusty environments, but these are cumbersome, expensive, and uncomfortable; they may be used only reluctantly. Furthermore, the circulation of air over the head may make them unsuitable in cold environments. In very dusty environments, the filters may become obstructed, thereby increasing the work of breathing through them if there is not an additional source of power for filtration.

Thirdly, treatment may be offered with systemic corticosteroids. These drugs shorten the time required for recovery following acute episodes, and they reduce the probability and severity of recurrence when there is ongoing exposure [53]. They do not, however, alter the long-term outcome of HP [20].

Of the workforce

HP is usually a sporadic disease, and only a few members of an exposed workforce are characteristically affected. Whether their undue susceptibility is a consequence of genetic predisposition or a need for triggering cofactors is currently unknown. Once the disease has been detected in one worker, however, there is some risk for its development in others, and the employer has a responsibility to provide reasonable protection. Thus exposure levels should be reduced whenever practical, whether by altering storage or processing procedures to reduce microbial contamination, or by improving ventilation. When neither is possible, workers should wear appropriate respiratory protection devices, and a surveillance program should be instituted to ensure that the working environment remains adequately controlled. If it does not and new cases arise, they will be detected promptly. This in turn reduces the chance of chronic, and hence irreversible, disease, and it should stimulate further improvement of the causal environment.

PREVENTION

In the workplace

Decreasing the levels of relevant airborne antigens is the only practical way of preventing HP. The feasibility of this and how it can be done depend on the environment involved. Improving hay drying so that the water content falls below 30% and avoiding the barns at peak antigen levels (when the animals are eating hay) will help prevent farmers'

lung. In wet countries it is often difficult to dry hay adequately before baling it, and drying machines are sometimes used. Hay preservatives, like lactobacteria, do not decrease airborne levels of *Saccharopolyspora rectivirgula* [54] and are probably not useful. The value of propionic acid has not been determined. The modern practice of storing wet hay in hermetically sealed plastic bags decreases the subsequent levels of aerosolized antigens, both by trapping initial decomposition products such as aldehydes (which 'pickle' the remaining intact hay) and by preventing drying.

The surveillance of antigenic exposure by monitoring dust levels may not be appropriate, since different antigens may be relevant to different cases, and their levels are not necessarily correlated with measured total dust. In swine confinement buildings, the levels of airborne bacteria are actually negatively related to the dust levels [55], suggesting that dust can actually help sediment these microbes. A regulatory standard for organic dust level (commonly a threshold limit value of 10 mg/ml) is probably not applicable to HP, and there are no current regulatory data that specifically address the risks for HP.

The levels of specific serum IgG levels against the more likely antigens in that workplace probably reflect the risk of workers in developing HP. There are more cases of HP in a workforce where a large number of workers are precipitin positive [4]. However, the presence of precipitating antibodies does not predict the eventual development of HP in a given worker [56]. The turnover of these antibodies being slow, persisting up to over 2 years after contact cessation [57], antibody surveillance may be useful only in the initial evaluation of a workforce and of little value to evaluate the effectiveness of an intervention program.

National regulatory strategies

The regulation of exposure levels for the very wide range of agents responsible for HP poses considerable practical difficulties, and in many countries there are no provisions for regulating dust exposure on farms or other relevant working environments. In the UK, farm dusts are covered by the regulations for controlling dusts generally in the workplace. The Occupational Exposure Standard is 10 mg/m^3 as an 8-hour time weighted average, but the respirable component should not exceed 4 mg/m^3. For identified dusts considered to pose special risks, there are specific maximum exposure limits, but these are not generally relevant to farms, nor to most situations in which HP arises.

DIFFICULT CASE

History

A lifelong dairy farmer sold his farm to his son when he was aged 50 years, and took ongoing employment as a janitor in a wood furniture workshop. He swept the floor of wood shavings and sawdust, and fed them into a wood-burning furnace. During the evenings and at weekends he helped his son on the farm. He noted the onset of undue dyspnea on exertion 8 years later, which proved to be progressive, and after 3 months was referred to a respiratory physician. There were no other symptoms, in particular no wheeze, cough, weight loss, or febrile episodes. His breathlessness was not obviously exacerbated by work on the farm or in the workshop. He had never smoked regularly, gave no history of other respiratory disease, and was taking no medication. There was no relevant family history, and physical examination revealed nothing remarkable apart from the presence of bilateral inspiratory crackles.

A chest radiograph showed diffuse interstitial infiltrates predominantly in the lower zones and HRCT showed patchy ground-glass images (Fig. 14.6). Spirometry gave 2.20/2.88, respectively 72% and 68% of the predicted levels, and the total lung capacity and residual volume were respectively 71% and 75% of predicted. The gas transfer factor for carbon monoxide was 65% of predicted. Arterial blood gases breathing room air at sea level gave: PaO_2, 77 mmHg (10.2 kPa); $PaCO_2$, 33 mmHg (4.4 kPa); pH 7.44. A sample of the wood dust grew *Penicillium* sp. on culture, and serological tests (ELISA) for antibodies to *Penicillium* and *Saccharopolyspora rectivirgulis* (the microorganism most commonly responsible for farmers' lung in the region) gave negative results. BAL yielded 139 ml of fluid which contained 57×10^6 cells, 73% lymphocytes. Transbronchial biopsy was interpreted to show 'granulomatous interstitial pneumonitis' (Fig. 14.7).

Issues

The key issue here is whether a diagnosis can be made of HP, or whether additional investigation is required. If HP is dia-

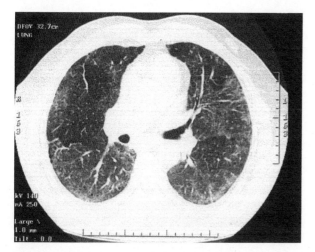

Fig. 14.6 High-resolution tomography image of Difficult Case. Ground-glass infiltrates are separated by more translucent areas giving a mosaic pattern.

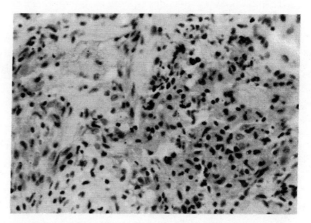

Fig. 14.7 Transbronchial lung biopsy of the Difficult Case showing a mononuclear infiltrate with early granulomatous organization.

gnosed, additional issues are whether the farm or the furniture shop is responsible, whether he should cease work in one or other occupational environment, and whether he should have corticosteroid treatment.

Comment

A clear majority of the book's contributors did consider this to be a case of HP, and most thought the farm was the source of the causal antigen. Some thought the furniture workshop was responsible, either alone or (mostly) together with the farm. Almost all recommended corticosteroid treatment. A number of additional investigations were suggested, particularly IgG antibody tests to a wider range of potential causes (e.g. avian protein and other molds) and an inspection of both working environments. Periods of monitoring progress while discontinuing work in one environment but continuing in the other were also recommended.

In a non-smoker the apparent absence of a relevant IgG antibody response (at least initially) is a pointer against HP, particularly as the history did not include characteristic systemic symptoms nor any obvious relation to periods of exposure in either workplace. This may have been a consequence of exposure being unremitting at similar levels on most days (perhaps unlikely) or of there being an inherently low level of responsiveness in this particular individual so that only the subacute form of HP was manifested. He did not, however, have evidence of farmers' lung during his earlier long years of farming, and so some scepticism over a diagnosis of HP was expressed among a small minority of contributors. They offered the suggestions that serial HRCT scans should be used to monitor progress and that a thoracoscopic lung biopsy might be indicated in order to obtain a larger (and possibly more representative) sample of lung tissue.

The patient was initially considered to have HP by the physicians managing him. He was given prednisolone 20 mg daily for 5 weeks and advised to avoid both working environments for 2 months. Symptoms and lung function improved, during both the initial period of steroid treatment and the ongoing period of antigen avoidance. After 2 months all symptoms had resolved, lung volumes had returned to normal, and the gas transfer factor for carbon monoxide had increased to 80% of predicted. Subsequent tests revealed a positive precipitating antibody response to *Aspergillus fumiga-* *tus.* The patient returned to work in the furniture workshop but not the farm, and remained asymptomatic. The final diagnosis was considered to be farmers' lung.

SUMMARY POINTS

Recognition
- A detailed history of environmental exposures is essential.
- Occupational HP should be considered in all patients presenting with recurrent febrile episodes and dyspnea, who work with organic dusts.
- Suspect HP when there is interstitial infiltration on chest radiographs and a mosaic pattern on computed tomography scans (especially on expiration).
- Active HP is always associated with a lymphocytic alveolitis.
- The absence of serum precipitins to the relevant antigen generally excludes the diagnosis, but there are often false-positive tests.

Management
- Removal from contact is the best treatment of HP and the only one needed when total avoidance is possible.

- Compromise, by reducing not eliminating exposure, is often necessary since many affected individuals cannot or will not change employment.
- Reduced exposure for the affected individual may be achieved by a redistribution of work tasks and the use of respirators.
- Systemic corticosteroids, the only effective drug treatment, will not change long-term outcome.

Prevention
- The causal antigen should be identified.
- Strategies for reducing exposure levels to a minimum (e.g. adequate drying of forage before storage) should be carried out.
- Surveillance programs are needed to ensure the working environment is adequately safe, and to identify new cases before permanent lung damage is likely.

REFERENCES

1. Campbell JM. Acute symptoms following work with hay. *Br Med J* 1932; ii: 1143–1144.
2. Pepys J, Jenkins PA, Festenstein GN *et al.* Farmer's lung: thermophilic actinomycetes as a source of 'farmer's lung hay' antigen. *Lancet* 1963; 2: 607–611.
3. Cormier Y, Schuyler M. Hypersensitivity pneumonitis. In: Bone RC, ed. *Textbook of Pulmonary Medicine*, Vol. 2, Part M: *Interstitial Lung Disease*, pp. 1–9. St Louis: Mosby-Year Book, 1992.
4. Y. Cormier, E. Israël-Assayag, G. Bédard, C. Duchaine. Hypersensitivity pneumointis (HP) in peat moss processing plant workers. *Am J Respir Crit Care Med* 1998; 158: 412–417.
5. Fox J, Anderson H, Moen T *et al.* Metal working fluid-associated hypersensitivity pneumonitis: an outbreak investigation and case-control study. *Am J Ind Med* 1999; 35: 58–67.
6. Boyd DHA. The incidence of farmer's lung in Caithness. *Scott Med J* 1971; 16: 261–262.
7. Depierre A, Dalphin JC, Pernet D *et al.* Epidemiological study of farmer's lung in five districts of the French Doubs province. *Thorax* 1988; 43: 429–435.
8. Fink JN. Epidemiologic aspects of hypersensitivity pneumonitis. *Monogr Allergy* 1987; 21: 59–69.
9. Grant IWB, Blyth W, Wardrop VE *et al.* Prevalence of farmer's lung in Scotland: a pilot survey. *Br Med J* 1972; 1: 530–534.
10. Terho EO, Heinonen OP, Lammi S. Incidence of clinically confirmed farmer's lung disease in Finland. *Am J Ind Med* 1986; 10: 330.
11. Hendrick DJ, Faux JA, Marshall R. Budgerigar fancier's lung: the commonest variety of allergic alveolitis in Britain. *Br Med J* 1978; 2: 81–84.

12. Gump DW, Babbott FL, Holly C *et al.* Farmer's lung disease in Vermont. *Respiration* 1979; 37: 52–60.
13. Pérez-Padilla R, Salas J, Chapela R *et al.* Mortality in Mexican patients with chronic pigeon breeder's lung compared to those with usual interstitial pneumonitis. *Am Rev Respir Dis* 1993; 148: 49–53.
14. Ando M, Knoishi K, Yoneda R *et al.* Differences in the phenotypes of bronchoalveolar lavage lymphocytes in patients with summer-type hypersensitivity pneumonitis, farmer's lung, ventilation pneumonitis, and bird fancier's lung: report of a nationwide epidemiologic study in Japan. *J Allergy Clin Immunol* 1991; 87: 1002–1009.
15. Meredith SK, Taylor VM, McDonald JC. Occupational respiratory disease in the United Kingdom 1989: a report to the British Thoracic Society and the Society of Occupational Medicine by the SWORD project group. *Br J Indust Med* 1991; 48: 292–298.
16. Cormier Y, Belanger J. The fluctuant nature of precipitating antibodies in dairy farmers. *Clin Digest* 1990; 3: 26–27.
17. Bouchard S, Morin F, Bédard G *et al.* Farmer's lung and variables related to the decision to quit farming. *Am J Respir Crit Care Med* 1995; 152: 997–1002.
18. Erkinjuntti-Pekkanen R, Rythönen H, Kokkarinen JI *et al.* Long-term outcome of farmer's lung evaluated by high resolution computed tomography: a case control study. *Am J Respir Crit Care Med* 1998; 158: 662–665.
19. Lalancette M, Carrier G, Ferland S *et al.* Long term outcome and predictive value of bronchoalveolar lavage fibrosing factors in farmer's lung. *Am Rev Respir Dis* 1993; 148: 216–221.
20. Kokkarinen JI, Tukiainen HO, Terho EO. Effect of corticosteroid treatment on the recovery of pulmonary

function in farmer's lung. *Am Rev Respir Dis* 1992; 145: 3–5.

21. Richerson HB, Bernstein IL, Fink JN, *et al.* Guidelines for the clinical evaluation of hypersensitivity pneumonitis. *J Allergy Clin Immunol* 1989; 84: 839–844.

22. Sansores R, Salas J, Chapela R *et al.* Clubbing in hypersensitivity pneumonitis: its prevalence and possible prognostic role. *Arch Int Med* 1990; 150: 1849–1851.

23. Yoshizawa Y, Ohtani Y, Hayakawa H *et al.* Chronic hypersensitivity pneumonitis in Japan: a nationwide epidemiologic survey. *J Allergy Clin Immunol* 1999; 103: 315–320.

24. Freedman PM, Ault B. Bronchial hyperreactivity to methacholine in farmer's lung disease. *J Allergy Clin Immunol* 1981; 67: 59–63.

25. Bourke S, Anderson K, Lynch P *et al.* Chronic simple bronchitis in pigeon fanciers. Relationship of cough with expectoration to avian exposure and pigeon breeders' disease. *Chest* 1989; 95: 598–601.

26. Braun SR, doPico GA, Tsiatis A *et al.* Famers's lung disease: a long-term clinical and physiological outcome. *Am Rev Respir Dis* 1979; 119: 185–191.

27. Hodgson MJ, Parkinson DK, Karpf M. Chest X-rays in hypersensitivity pneumonitis: a meta-analysis of secular trend. *Am J Indust Med* 1989; 16: 45–53.

28. Buschman DL, Gamsu G, Waldron JA Jr *et al.* Chronic hypersensitivity pneumonitis: use of CT in diagnosis. *Am J Roentgenol* 1992; 159: 957–960.

29. Lynch DA, Newell JD, Logan PM *et al.* Can CT distinguish hypersensitivity pneumonitis from idiopathic pulmonary fibrosis? *Am J Roentgenol* 1995; 165: 807–811.

30. Silver SF, Müller NL, Miller RR *et al.* Hypersensitivity pneumonitis: evaluation with CT. *Radiology* 1989; 173: 441–445.

31. Akira M, Kita N, Higashihara T *et al.* Summer-type hypersensitivity pneumonitis: comparison of high-resolution CT and plain radiographic findings. *Am J Roentgenol* 1992; 158: 1223–1228.

32. Lynch DA, Rose CS, Way D *et al.* Hypersensitivity pneumonitis: sensitivity of high-resolution CT in a population-based study. *Am J Roentgenol* 1992; 159: 469–472.

33. Cormier Y, Racine G, Brown M *et al.* Tomodensitometric characterization of different phases of hypersensitivity pneumonitis (HP). *Am J Respir Crit Care Med* 1999; 159: A742.

34. Denis M, Bédard M, Laviolette M *et al.* A study of monokine release and natural killer activity in the bronchoalveolar lavage of subjects with Farmer's lung. *Am Rev Respir Dis* 1993; 147: 934–939.

35. Cormier Y, Israël-Assayag E, Desmeules M *et al.* Effect of contact avoidance or treatment with oral prednisolone on bronchoalveolar lavage surfactant protein A levels in subjects with farmer's lung. *Thorax* 1996; 51: 1210–1215.

36. Calvanico NJ, Ambegaonkar SP, Schlueter DP *et al.* Immunoglobuline levels in bronchoalveolar lavage fluid from pigeon breeders. *J Lab Clin Med* 1980; 96: 129–140.

37. Fournier E, Tonnel AB, Gosset Ph *et al.* Early neutrophil alveolitis after antigen inhalation in hypersensitivity pneumonitis. *Chest* 1985; 88: 563–566.

38. Cormier Y, Bélanger J, Beaudoin J *et al.* Abnormal bronchoalveolar lavage in asymptomatic dairy farmers:

Study of lymphocyutes. *Am Rev Respir Dis* 1984; 130: 1046–1049.

39. Costabel U, Bross KJ, Marxen J *et al.* T-lymphocytes in bronchoalveolar lavage fluid of hypersensitivity pneumonitis. *Chest* 1984; 84: 514–518.

40. Godard P, Clot J, Jonquet O *et al.* Lymphocyte subpopulations in bronchoalveolar lavage of patients with sarcoidosis and hypersensitivity pneumonitis. *Chest* 1981; 80: 447–452.

41. Richerson HB. hypersensitivity pneumonitis: pathology and pathogenesis. *Clin Rev Allergy* 1983; 1: 469–486.

42. Lacasse Y, Fraser RS, Fournier M *et al.* Diagnostic accuracy of transbronchial biopsy in acute farmer's lung. *Chest* 1997; 112: 1459–1465.

43. Warren CPW. Extrinsic allergic alveolitis: a disease commoner in non-smokers. *Thorax* 1977; 32: 567–569.

44. Ouchterlony O. Antigen–antibody reactions in gels. *Acta Pathol Microbiol Scand* 1953; 32: 231.

45. Sandoval J, Banales JL, Cortés JJ *et al.* Detection of antibodies against avian antigens in bronchoalveolar lavage from patients with pigeon's breeders disease: usefulness of enzyme-linked immunosorbent assay and enzyme immunotransfer blotting. *J Clin Lab Anal* 1990; 4: 81–85.

46. Cormier Y, Bélanger J. Precipitating antibody in Québec dairy farmers: a follow-up study. *Thorax* 1989; 44: 469–473.

47. Fink JN, Schlueter DP, Sosman AJ *et al.* Clinical survey of pigeon breeders. *Chest* 1972; 62: 277–281.

48. Hargreaves FE, Pepys J. Allergic respiratory reactions in bird fanciers provoked by allergen inhalation provocation tests. *J Allergy Clin Immunol* 1972; 50: 157–173.

49. Hendrick DJ, Marshall R, Faux JA *et al.* Positive 'alveolar' responses to antigen inhalation provocation tests: their validity and recognition. *Thorax* 1980; 35: 415–427.

50. Dalphin JC, Pernet D, Roux C *et al.* Investigation of the protective value of breathing masks on thermophilic actinomycetes. *Am Rev Respir Dis* 1993; 147: A903.

51. Hendrick DJ, Marshall R, Faux JA *et al.* Protective value of dust respirators in extrinsic allergic alveolitis: clinical assessment using inhalation provocation tests. *Thorax* 1981; 36: 917–921.

52. Müller-Wening D, Repp H. Investigation of the protective value of breathing masks in farmer's lung using an inhalation provocation test. *Chest* 1989; 95: 100–105.

53. Cormier Y, Desmeules M. Treatment of hypersensitivity pneumonitis (HP): comparison between contact avoidance and corticosteroids. *Can Respir J* 1994; 1: 223–228.

54. Duchaine C, Mériaux A, Brochu G *et al.* Airborne microflora in Quebec dairy farms: lack of effect of bacterial hay preservatives. *Am Indust Hyg Assoc J* 1999; 60: 89–95.

55. Duchaine C, Grimard Y, Cormier Y. Influence of building maintenance, environmental factors and seasons on airborne contaminants of swine confinement buildings. *AIHAJ* 2000; 61: 56–63.

56. Gariépy L, Cormier Y, Leblanc P *et al.* Longterm outcome of asymptomatic dairy farmers with BAL lymphocytosis. *Am Rev Respir Dis* 1989; 140: 1386–1389.

57. Leblanc P, Bélanger J, Laviolette M *et al.* Farmer's lung disease: between continued exposure, alveolitis, and clinical status. *Arch Int Med* 1986; 146: 153–157.

15 SICK BUILDING SYNDROME

Jouni J.K. Jaakkola and Maritta S. Jaakkola

BACKGROUND

The concept 'sick building syndrome' (SBS) was introduced to occupational medicine in the 1980s as a health problem related to indoor air quality and ventilation in office buildings. A World Health Organization (WHO) working group on indoor air and health characterized the 'sick' building syndrome in its report [1]. A UK epidemiological study [2] compared symptoms of workers in nine buildings with different ventilation systems. The investigators empirically postulated the main components of the sick building syndrome: nasal, eye and mucous membrane symptoms, dry skin, lethargy, and headaches. The WHO working group indicated the association between the symptoms and forced (mechanical) ventilation systems, and the British study reported an excess of symptoms related to air handling, more specifically air conditioning. The concept SBS has also been used to characterize health problems in non-industrial occupational environments such as day-care centers and hospitals. In this chapter, the focus will center on the office environment although the data presented can be applied to other environments.

Expanding research has revealed a complex set of modern occupational health problems underlying the SBS. It has become clear that there is no single disease entity that could be diagnosed within individual subjects, and so the chapter is focused on buildings rather than individuals working within them [3]. The symptoms described as SBS are symptoms and signs of a number of different health outcomes with different manifestations and etiologic factors. One, or a set of, environmental determinants of different ontological nature, i.e. physical or social, can cause the symptoms and signs. Consequently, the phenomenon SBS consists of several types of relations between environmental determinants and health outcomes, and, as a result, a singular exposure can cause different health outcomes, and a given symptom can be caused by one, several, or a combination of different exposures and exposure patterns. The SBS should be considered as a figurative concept of everyday language rather than as a single disease entity in clinical medicine. Therefore, the approach of presenting the SBS differs slightly from the approaches to specified occupational diseases.

First a model is presented that will help to explain the complex multidimensional relations between the office environment and health [3]. Second, an environmentally oriented approach is used to characterize the physical factors in the office environment that may influence human health and well-being. Third, a disease-oriented approach is followed that addressed the social and psychological influences of the office environment and the symptoms, signs, and illnesses typically related to SBS. Finally, the chapter discusses the recognition, management, and prevention of these health problems.

The office environment model

Figure 15.1 presents schematically the worker (inner circle) and the office environment (outer circle – inner

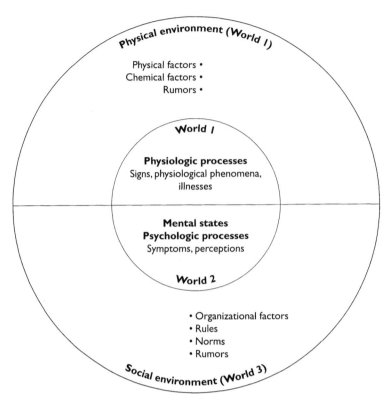

Fig. 15.1 The office environment model: the worker (inner circle), the office environment (outer circle – inner circle), and phenomena of different ontological nature involved in the sick building syndrome. Adapted from Jaakkola [3].

circle) and illustrates the phenomena that are relevant in the SBS [3]. First, the office environment is divided conceptually into physical and social environments, which both include determinants of human health and well-being. Second, the human being is divided into two different domains, the one belonging to the physical phenomena and the other to the psychological phenomena, and the outcomes related to the environmental determinants are thus either physical or psychological. This is a simplified theoretical model for describing the different types of phenomena. The relations between these phenomena theoretically describe how the environmental determinants can affect human health and well-being and can cause both physical (objective) and mental outcomes (subjective).

A disease or a state can have physiologic and/or psychologic underlying mechanisms and manifestations. As the first step in identifying the relations between possible health problems and their environmental and constitutional determinants, the components of the SBS have to be considered. In Table 15.1 the symptoms and signs are categorized into two dimensions: anatomic site and hypothesized underlying mechanism. The main anatomic sites are the eyes; the respiratory tract, including nose, airways,

Table 15.1 Dimensions of the outcomes related to the sick building syndrome. Adapted from Jaakkola [3].

Dimension	Symptoms and signs
Anatomic site	Eyes
	Respiratory tract, including nose, airways and parenchyma
	Skin
	Central nervous system
Possible underlying mechanisms	Mechanical irritation and inflammation
	Allergic reactions
	Toxicity
	Infectious
	Environmental psychologic stress

and lung parenchyma; the skin; and the central nervous system. Possible underlying mechanisms include mechanical irritation and inflammation, immunological/allergic reactions, toxicity, infection, and environmental psychologic stress.

The symptoms arising at the different anatomic sites are non-specific as to their causes. However, inferences about their causes and underlying mechanisms can be made by characterizing the type and intensity of the symptoms and the time and place of their occurrence. This means, for example, that a number of environmental factors, such as artificial mineral fibers, formaldehyde, and pollen can cause similar eye symptoms via mechanical irritation and/or chemical toxicity and/or allergic reactions. Biochemical or immunologic investigation of tear fluid or conjunctiva may help to identify the underlying mechanisms and environmental causes of the symptoms. Exposure to a given environmental factor can cause different symptoms and signs; these may depend on constitutional characteristics of the individual, duration of exposure, or other exposure patterns. For example, the effect of a complex mixture of office air could cause different types of symptom and different health outcomes in different individuals depending on personal susceptibility. These effects could also be mediated via more than one mechanism.

The physical environment comprises physical determinants, such as thermal climate, electromagnetic fields, lighting, and chemical and biological indoor air pollutants. The social environment includes the rules, norms, and organizational factors that have been created by human beings but can be considered to be autonomous by any one individual. Psychologic processes mediate the effects of social determinants, and psychologic factors can be considered as constitutional determinants of health outcomes. Psychologic factors may also modify the relationship between the physical environment and health. For example, experience of stress may intensify the effects of high temperature on headache.

The occurrence of symptoms and signs in individuals varies according to personal characteristics such as age, gender, and past and present health status. Personal characteristics may also imply susceptibility to environmental factors. For example, individuals with allergic diseases are often more sensitive to the effects of both chemical and microbiologic pollutants. Individual mental states and psychological processes, which may or may not be affected by the environment, are also considered as acquired constitutional determinants of the outcomes.

According to the theoretical model presented above, the following types of causal relation are possible: (i) the physical environment causes physical effects via physiologic and/or psychologic processes; (ii) the physical environment causes psychologic effects via physiologic and/or psychologic processes; (iii) the social environment causes physical effects via psychologic processes; (iv) the social environment causes psychologic effects. Psychologic, social, and physiologic factors can modify all of these relations.

Determinants of indoor air quality

The main route of exposure to the physical environment in the office is probably inhalation, though skin contact with air and physical surfaces may contribute. Indoor air quality is an important characteristic of the office environment and is determined by: outdoor sources, the building envelope, occupants and their activities, physical indoor sources, and heating, ventilation, and air-conditioning (HVAC) systems. Table 15.2 gives examples of different determinants of indoor air quality in buildings, with special reference to office buildings.

Outdoor sources

All of the environmental elements surrounding the building, including air, water, and soil, have a potential impact on indoor air quality. The role of air pollutants from industry, traffic, heating, and natural sources have received most interest, but only a few studies of outdoor–indoor penetration have been conducted. Geographic location of the office building is an important factor that determines the exposure to many environmental factors indoors. Vicinity of industrial plants or busy traffic routes may contribute substantially to total exposure to various environmental pollutants in the office environment, although the type of building envelope and ventilation system plays an important role in controlling these exposures.

Building envelope

The type of building, the structures, openings, and the type of ventilation system influence the penetration of outdoor pollutants into buildings as well as the elimination of air pollutants from indoor sources. In a sealed building, penetration and elimination depend mainly on the function of the ventilation system. The location of the air inlet in a building may influence the penetration of outdoor pollutants from local point sources or background air into indoors.

Occupants

Office workers constitute an important sources of indoor air pollution. The human body produces carbon dioxide, carbon monoxide, ammonia, acetone,

Table 15.2 Determinants of indoor air quality in the office environment

Determinant	Pollutants or type of influence
Outdoor sources	
Traffic	NO_x, CO, SO_2, particulate matter
Industry	NO_x, CO, SO_2, particulate matter
Heating	
Natural sources	Pollen, particulate matter
Building envelope	Influences outdoor–indoor penetration and dilution of indoor concentrations
Occupants	
Metabolic products	CO_2, CO, ammonia, acetone, alcohol, and various other odorous organic gases
Infectious agents	Viruses and bacteria
Skin	Particles
Activities	Smoking, office work
Physical indoor sources	
Surface materials, (floors, walls, ceilings, furniture)	VOCs, physical and biological particles
Damp materials	Enhance growth of fungi
HVAC systems	
Ventilation	Influences dilution and distribution of pollutants
Heating	Direct and indirect effects of temperature
Humidification	Direct and indirect effects of relative humidity; potential source of microbial pollutants

CO, carbon monoxide; CO_2, carbon dioxide; HVAC, heating/ventilation/air conditioning; NO_x, oxides of nitrogen; SO_2, sulfur dioxide; VOCs, volatile organic compounds.

alcohol, and various other odorous organic gases, which may be released into indoor air through breathing and perspiration. Occupants are also sources of bacteria and viruses, which may cause infectious diseases. Clothing materials may release various types of particles, and clothes may carry particles and absorbed gas from one microenvironment to another. For example, individuals can bring animal dander on their clothes from homes to office space. Typically office activities, such as paper handling, photocopying, and printing, may generate important exposures to gases and particles. Tobacco smoking produces a large number of chemicals and particles into indoor air and is an important source of irritant chemicals as well as carcinogens in office buildings where smoking is allowed. In some countries and some occupational environments, smoking restrictions have decreased or eliminated such exposure in the workplace.

Physical sources

Building materials used in floors, walls, and ceiling are potential sources of indoor air pollution. In the 1970s, exposure to formaldehyde from building materials emerged as a large-scale health problem [4]. Materials used in furniture, curtains, and carpets are potential sources of volatile organic compounds (VOCs) or particles and may serve as a reservoir for allergens. Structural deficiencies in buildings may cause dampness, a problem that varies with climate. Dampness promotes microbial growth and creates suitable conditions for house dust mites and cockroaches to flourish. Cleaning chemicals may also contribute substantially to the exposure of occupants [5].

Heating, ventilation, and air-conditioning

Heating, ventilation, and air-conditioning may influence indoor air quality in several ways. Air change dilutes the concentrations of pollutants from indoor sources, given that outdoor concentrations are substantially lower than indoor concentrations. Ventilation systems may also increase indoor air pollution by introducing pollutants to indoor air. Air humidification may alleviate health problems related to dry air, but the equipment may serve as a source of microbial growth and lead to adverse health effects.

Physical environment

Indoor air temperature

The percentage of dissatisfied subjects in a given indoor environment can be predicted relatively well using information on the air temperature, radiant heat, relative humidity, velocity of air, metabolic rate, clothing, and thermal insulation as independent variables [6]. The thermal environment affects directly the neural sensors of mucous membranes and skin, and, may provoke neurosensoral responses indirectly by changes in blood circulation [7]. According to epidemiological studies in the office environment, temperatures above 23°C seem to increase the occurrence of skin, respiratory, and general symptoms, such as headache and lethargy [8,9]. Relative humidity probably modifies the effects of temperature in that the adverse effects are stronger in dry air.

Relative humidity

Relative humidity may influence the symptoms of the SBS independently of, as well as in synergy with, temperature. There are two biologically plausible mechanisms. First, drying of mucosae and skin may give rise to symptoms of the eyes, upper respiratory tract, and skin. Second, disturbance of thermal balance may induce general symptoms, such as headache and lethargy, and disturbances in neuro-behavioral functions. Relative humidity has been shown to influence thermal comfort in controlled laboratory studies [6]. Air movement can be an independent determinant of some general symptoms through effects on the thermal balance.

Office workers commonly complain of dryness of air during the heating season in cold climates [9–12]. In experimental studies carried out in office buildings [13] and hospitals [14], humidification was found to alleviate the sensation of dryness and the associated symptoms of the eyes and respiratory tract. The relation between dry air, air humidification, and mucosal symptoms is complicated. First, chemical and particulate air pollution, as well as low relative humidity, may cause dryness and irritation of the eyes and respiratory tract [15]. Second, level and change in relative humidity and temperature may influence emission and adsorption of VOCs and influence air particle concentrations to the extent that it may be difficult to separate the direct and indirect effects of relative humidity. Third, non-hygienic air humidification equipment may serve as a source of microbial air pollution.

Air change

Air change affects the concentrations of indoor air pollutants, which can be expressed simply as follows [16]:

$$C = \frac{G}{Q_v \varepsilon_v}$$

where C is the concentration of the contaminant, G is the generation of contaminant (volume flow), Q_v is the clean air flow to the room, and ε_v is pollutant removal efficiency.

Insufficient air change or ventilation may lead to accumulation of contaminants and to moisture problems, which in turn may lead to adverse health effects. Conversely, excessive ventilation may increase emission rates in two ways. Increased air velocities above interior surfaces increase the emission rate for some materials [17,18]. High levels of ventilation may also increase the resuspension of sedimented particulate matter into indoor air [19]. Ventilation rates below 5 liters/s per person are likely to result in indoor air pollution problems in facilities with high emissions. The minimum ventilation rate for office buildings is recommended to be 10–15 liters/s per person, given the current average emissions and activities [20,21].

The occurrence of SBS symptoms has been associated with the type of ventilation system in an office building. Generally, air-conditioning has consistently been related to an increased prevalence of lethargy and upper respiratory/mucous membrane symptoms compared with mechanical or natural ventilation [11,22,23]. Humidification as well as air recirculation has also been found to determine SBS symptoms. However, the role of humidification illustrates the complexity of the relations between ventilation systems and symptoms. On the one hand, several population-based studies have indicated a higher risk of typical SBS symptoms in buildings with air humidification [11,22,24]. On the other hand, results of a Finnish crossover trial indicate that SBS symptoms can be alleviated by hygienic steam humidification under cold climatic conditions when indoor air relative humidity in non-humidified conditions falls below 20% [13]. These findings are not contradictory: hygienic humidification alleviates the irritation of the mucosa caused by very low humidity, and poorly maintained, especially evaporative, humidification equipment creates a risk of symptoms through microbiological contamination [11].

Ventilation type should be thought as a risk indicator of certain environmental problems in a given building stock [11]. Thus, the ventilation system affects the probability of the occurrence of causal exposures in the indoor environment. It is likely that there exist a number of causal pathways, some of which are directly and some indirectly related to the function of the ventilation system.

Volatile organic compounds

Outdoor air contains low concentrations of VOCs. Some office buildings have contained several times higher concentrations, which suggests the existence of important indoor sources [25,26]. The main sources have proved to be building materials and furnishings, maintenance products (for cleaning, disinfecting, and polishing), insecticides, consumer products, combustion processes, occupants, and outdoor air. Typical office work activities, such as photocopying and the handling of self-copying paper, may also contribute to indoor air VOC concentrations. Low concentrations of many different VOCs from several sources may create a chemical 'cocktail'. In a Danish exposure chamber study, a 2-hour exposure to a mixture of 22 common hydrocarbons with a total VOC concentration of 5 mg/m^3 caused irritation of the eyes, nose, and throat and led to decreased scores in the digit span test, which measures short-term memory impairment [15]. The concentration of each individual compound was well below occupational standards. A 4-hour exposure to 25 mg/m^3 of a similar mixture caused an inflammatory response of the upper respiratory tract, expressed as the number of polymorphonuclear cells in the nasal lavage [27].

Mølhave [28] suggested three mechanisms for the effects of exposure to low-level VOCs: sensory perception of the environment, weak inflammatory reactions, and environmental stress reactions. Humans use several senses to identify VOCs, including the sense of smell in the nasal cavity, the sense of taste in the tongue, and/or the stimulation of sensory nerves in skin areas. The perceived indoor air quality is formed from an integration of these sensations. The stimulation of sensory nerves in the skin is felt as irritation, smarting, or stinging (i.e. symptoms). Protective physiologic reflexes such as tear formation, cough, or sneezing (i.e. signs) may also occur. Chemical mediators usually cause acute reversible inflammatory reactions leading to dilatation of vessels and changes in color and temperature of the tissue. Environmental stress may lead to increases of stress hormone levels and blood pressure, and consequently to fatigue, irritability, reduced tolerance, as well as psychologic processes and symptoms.

A commonly used general measure of chemical burden is total VOC (TVOC) concentration. Use of TVOC has several limitations; it is an ambiguous concept, individual VOCs making up the total can be expected to have different adverse effects, and different definitions and interpretations for TVOC have been used [29]. Some empirical studies have provided evidence of a relation between the total VOC concentration in the indoor environment and reported symptoms in occupants [30–33], but the results are inconsistent [34]. There have been major difficulties in assessing long-term exposure to the complex mixtures present in office environments and the effects of different compounds are likely to be very variable. This may explain the inconsistent results.

Microbial pollution

Moisture may accumulate in building constructions resulting in dampness and microbial growth. The usual signs are color changes in and loosening of the surface materials, wet spots on the surfaces, visible mold, and mold odor. Air humidity influences the materials in areas where the climate is moist and warm throughout the year but has little influence in cold climates where outdoor air humidity is relatively low throughout the year. Rainwater, melted water, surface water, ground water, damp materials from construction, domestic water, and occupants are other sources of moisture. Common causes of water damage include water leaks through the building envelope from water or drainage pipes, and condensation.

Dampness supports the growth of fungi, some bacteria, and house dust mites. Fungi produce spores and metabolic products that may cause adverse health effects through both allergic and non-allergic (toxic or irritative mechanisms) reactions. *Dermatophagoides pteronyssinus* and *D. farinae* are the most common house dust mites in damp buildings. Exposure to their faeces and desquamated skin can cause allergic sensitization. Several studies have reported an association between dampness and mold-associated respiratory illnesses, including respiratory infections, asthma, and allergic alveolitis [35]. Harrison and colleagues [36] reported that the prevalence of SBS symptoms was associated with the mean levels of airborne viable bacteria and fungi in British office buildings. Among office workers in 19 buildings in Taipei, the prevalence of eye symptoms, cough, and lethargy was related to indicators of dampness and mold problems [2]. In Canadian office workers, occurrences of respiratory symptoms were related to levels of *Altenaria* spp. in the indoor air, as well as total dust mite concentration and relative humidity [37]. In addition, workers with respiratory symptoms had a positive skin prick test reaction to molds, in particular *Alternaria altenata*, more commonly than those without symptoms.

Dampness and mold problems in office buildings are common globally, despite the wide range of climatic conditions in different countries, although the causes of dampness vary substantially from one climatic region to another. Current knowledge suggests there are substantial health effects related to dampness.

Environmental tobacco smoke

Exposure to environmental tobacco smoke (ETS) increases any irritation of the eyes and the respiratory tract, and may also cause headache. It is therefore, one of the potential determinants of SBS. Several epidemiological studies have reported an association between exposure to tobacco smoke and SBS [10,38] but there has been debate about its relative importance. It is argued that ETS has provided a convenient focus of attention allowing other occupational hazards to be ignored. It is clear that its relative role depends on both smoking behavior and the influence of other environmental factors in the office environment. Some countries have forbidden smoking in the workplace outside isolated and ventilated smoking rooms, and implementation of tobacco law in Finland has reportedly reduced ETS exposure [Heloma *et al.* unpublished]. ETS should therefore play a much smaller role in SBS in the future.

Office equipment and supplies

Modern office work requires an increasing use of equipment and supplies that may have adverse effects. Self-copying paper is a potential source of various particle and volatile substances, including solvents and color-forming chemicals [39]. Exposure of the eyes, nasal mucosa, and skin may be direct, through contaminated air, or indirect because of later contact with fingers that have handled the chemical-containing paper. Studies from Denmark [40], Sweden [12], the USA [41], and Finland [42] have consistently shown an increased risk of SBS symptoms in relation to handling self-copying paper. A recently published study from Finland showed a strong link also to the risk of chronic respiratory symptoms and the occurrence of some respiratory infections [42].

Photocopiers may also emit chemicals, such as VOCs, ozone, particles, and resin [43], but studies on the health effects of photocopying have provided inconsistent evidence for an association with SBS [40–44]. This inconsistency of results may reflect large variations in emission level depending on the type of equipment, and large differences in volume and ventilation rate of the spaces where photocopying takes place. There is little information on emissions from modern photocopiers.

Work with video display terminals has been linked with exposure to electromagnetic fields [43]. Some studies have reported associations with headache, lethargy, skin and eye problems, and musculoskeletal and ocular symptoms [40,42,45]. However, musculoskeletal symptoms and headache could be related to ergonomic factors rather than to exposure to electromagnetic fields [45,46]. Furthermore, glare, poor contrast of the monitor, and ocular distress could be explanations for the eye symptoms [47].

Social environment

Stress research in occupational medicine provides two theoretical models of interest, which can be used to elaborate the SBS. According to the occupational stress model, stress arises when there is perceived imbalance between external demand and response capabilities, especially under conditions where failure to meet demand has important consequences [48,49]. In addition to exceeding demand, too little environmental stimulus may also lead to stress.

The job strain model was used to elaborate the role of work stress as a determinant of the symptoms and signs of cardiovascular disease in a population-based cohort study of Swedish men [50]. According to this model, stress results from the joint effects of demands of the work situation and environmental moderators of stress, particularly the range of decision-making freedom available to the workers facing those demands. Job demands or stressors place the individual in a motivated state of 'stress'. If no action can be taken, or if the individual has in general low decision latitude (control), the unreleased stress may have adverse psychologic and physiologic consequences. This model could be generalized to include both stressors of the physical environment, such as poor indoor air quality or thermal discomfort, and stressors of the social environment, such as job demand, conflicts, etc. [49]. Low decision latitude of the work could be generalized to lack of control of both the physical environment (considered uncomfortable or unhealthy) and the social environment, including work characteristics [3].

The distinction between the social environment and psychologic phenomena is important. Overemphasis of individual psychology may disregard the role of the social determinants of health. The common use of the term 'psychosocial factors' is likely to blur this distinction. The social universe has been defined as a human product, though autonomous from the point of view of any single person. Therefore, social phenomena can and should be studied as primary objects (in the domain of social sciences), separately from psychologic phenomena (in the domain of psychology and psychiatry). The social environment affects individual psychologic processes, and the stress theory provides a model for both physiologic and psychologic outcomes. It is conceivable that a combination of the individuals' psychological processes affects the development of social environment.

Earlier epidemiological studies are consistent with the hypothesis that both psychologic and social factors are of importance in the etiology of the SBS symptoms [12,24,31,40,51,52]. These investigations usually analyzed a construct that includes different aspects of both psychologic and social determinants. Moreover, some studies have tried to evaluate psychologic and social factors separately. In the Danish Town Hall Study, an affirmative answer to the question of whether the quantity of work inhibited job satisfaction was a determinant of both mucosal irritation and general symptoms [40]. This could be taken as an indirect indicator of the role of work stress. In agreement with the job strain model, little influence on work demand combined with a high work pace was a determinant of general symptoms.

In the Helsinki Office Environment Study the occurrence of symptoms was related to reported experience of work stress. In the Pasila Office Center Study, a reported negative social atmosphere at work was a strong determinant of the SBS index [10,51]. To our knowledge, no study has simultaneously evaluated the characteristics of social environment independently of workers' perceptions and assessed the effect of social factors on the symptom occurrence. However, a substantial amount of work has been carried out on organizational factors that belong to the domain of social environment in office work [49].

In summary, there is consistent evidence of a relation between workers' perceptions of both psychologic stresses from work and social environment at work, and their experienced health. More research is needed for a better understanding of the separate roles of these factors. Psychologic stress can have direct physiologic effects as well as psychologic effects that become manifest as symptoms. Stress can also modify the relations between physical environment and health, although so far there exists no empirical evidence of this type of modification.

RECOGNITION

A practical approach is necessary for the identification and evaluation of problem buildings. The methods of outcome and exposure assessment are similar, or the same, in occupational health practice and scientific research. Occupational health practice is aimed at identification, treatment, and prevention of SBS, and the measurements serve practical problem solving. The purpose of scientific research is to provide knowledge about etiology, identification, and treatment of health problems related to SBS. In research, the hypotheses and aims of the study should guide the study design and choice of methods.

Assessment of occupants

SBS is not a single disease entity that can be diagnosed readily in an individual. The typical symptoms and signs may indicate a particular disorder and may fulfill established diagnostic criteria, and sometimes the disorder will be occupational in origin. There are several allergic diseases, for example, for which the typical symptoms and signs are encompassed by those associated with SBS. These include asthma, allergic rhinitis, allergic conjunctivitis, and hypersensitivity pneumonitis; the etiology and diagnostic criteria of these are described in other chapters. Headache and lethargy are non-specific symptoms that occur in a large number of diseases and conditions and may or may not be related to occupational exposures.

Clinical examination of an office worker with one or several SBS symptoms has three aims. First, it is important to identify and make a diagnosis in individuals who have a disease fulfilling diagnostic criteria. Part of the purpose is to consider the role of occupational exposure in causation and prognosis. Second, in individuals with a chronic disease, it is necessary to consider whether occupational exposures influence symptoms and the natural history of the disease. Third, identification and characterization of non-specific symptoms and signs in otherwise healthy workers (i.e. those without an evident specific illness) may provide an important lead to the detection of relevant occupational exposures.

Symptoms and signs of SBS in an individual may indicate adverse effects related to the office environment. Recognition of these symptoms and signs in one or several individuals from the same work environment may be the first step in identification and management of environmental problems. Often a history of symptoms and signs and clinical examination is sufficient for identification and treatment of health problems. Information about the presence and intensity of symptoms in relation to workplace and other environments may give information concerning the potential causes. However, this may not differentiate the relative impacts of physical and social environment. There are a number of relevant questions. Are the symptoms most intense at work? Are there changes over the day, week, and season? Do symptoms alleviate after the workday, during the weekends (or other days off duty), and on vacation? Symptoms appearing mainly at work identify the work environment as a potential cause and imply a short induction period for the exposure–response relation and reversibility of the effects. However, the lack of apparent work-related symptoms does not exclude the possibility that the work environment is relevant, since long induction periods and slow recoveries may mask the causal association.

In some situations and in certain patient groups, particular methods may be useful in assessing the observed outcome (Table 15.3). Clinical tests may be useful to elaborate immunologic sensitivity or airway reactivity in relation to the occupational

Table 15.3 Assessment of outcomes in investigations of problem buildings

Outcome	Methods
Symptoms	Standardized questionnaires, interviews
Nasal irritation, redness	Nasal lavage
Eye irritation, redness	Tear-film stability
Bronchial reactivity	Methacholine challenge, peak expiratory flow, spirometry
Type I skin allergy	Skin prick tests
Immunologic responses	Specific IgE measurement

environment. A brief description follows of the most common responses detected in relation to SBS and the available methods of investigation.

History

Perceptions of undesirable odors and annoyance reactions often coincide with symptoms. The type of odor (e.g. molds or certain chemicals) may indicate a source of a relevant exposure. There is a large variation in individual sensitivity to odors. Odor sensitivity is often related to susceptibility to other reactions.

Self-administered questionnaires have been used to assess the prevalence of symptoms in populations and occupants of large buildings. That developed at the Department of Occupational and Environmental Medicine, Örebro Medical Center Hospital, is perhaps the most widely used standardized instrument for evaluation of indoor air and health problems and provides a reference for workplaces including offices and other indoor environments [53]. The basic health questionnaire includes questions regarding 12 symptoms, 12 items of work environment, four items of work conditions and four questions of past and present allergic diseases. The characteristics of the study group, such as age and gender distribution and proportion of atopic subjects, determine strongly the prevalence of a given symptom. This limits the use of cross-sectional surveys as a diagnostic tool in SBS. However, repeated surveys in a stable population may be useful for evaluating the effects of changes in the environment. Use of a reference ('control') group is crucial, because there is substantial variation over time in the occurrence of symptoms and signs of interest.

Irritation of eyes, nose, respiratory tract

Irritation of the conjunctivae and the mucous membrane of the nose is a typical effect of exposure to reactive chemicals, whether gaseous or particulate. They can also cause skin irritation and itching,

and irritation may additionally be caused directly or indirectly by high temperature and dry air. The tear-film stability test has been used to measure ocular reactions in office workers [54,55]. Subjects with ocular symptoms had reduced tear-film stability and the mean tear-film stability was lower in workers of a problem building than in those of a comparison building [56]. Lower tear-film stability was found also in workers in a damp hospital building, where there were emissions from polyvinyl chloride (PVC) flooring induced by dampness. As a consequence, increased levels of 2-ethyl-l-hexanol was measured in the air [57]. In the same study, an increased concentration of lysozyme was found in nasal lavage among exposed workers. Another study reported increased concentrations of lysozyme and eosinophilic cationic protein in nasal lavage as a response to emissions from newly painted walls [58]. These methods are currently used in research, but there are no guidelines for clinical applications.

A methacholine test is a standardised method for studying bronchial reactivity. Measuring reactivity at and out of work can be used to study an individual's response to office air. Peak expiratory flow or other measures of lung function such as FEV_1 (forced expired volume in 1 s) measured with a pocket size spirometer can be used to assess an individual's airways reactivity to the office environment in a similar way. Bronchial reactivity and variation in lung function are important differential diagnostic tools for asthma. Further, challenge tests with specific compounds and lung function measurements over time can be used to detect occupational asthma.

Type I hypersensitivity

Measurement of serum immunoglobulin E (IgE) can be used to assess the probability of specific type I allergic reactions to allergens within the office environment. Identification of specific sources of emissions, such as fungal growth, together with specific IgE responsiveness provide evidence of a possible causal pathway for occupational health problems. However, many allergens occur commonly in other microenvironments encountered by individual workers. Therefore, increased specific IgE in serum is not by itself sufficiently diagnostic. Information on population distributions of immunoglobulins is needed before immunoglobulin distributions in an occupational setting can be used to make inferences about SBS. Recently, Malkin and colleagues [59] studied IgE and IgG antibody levels in office workers but did not find differences between workers from areas with high and low airborne fungal concentrations. High IgE antibody levels to one or more fungi were detected in 40% of the workers, and high IgG levels in 67%.

Skin prick tests may be used as an alternative to serologic assays for specific IgE. Reactions to fungi and dust mites are perhaps the most informative.

Intervention studies

Controlled intervention studies have been used to study the effects on symptoms and other outcomes of a number of physical environmental factors, such as humidification, [13], ventilation rate [9,10], air recirculation [60], and enhanced particle filtration [61]. A similar, but perhaps simplified, approach can be used to evaluate the clinical effects on office occupants of changes in physical or social environment.

Assessment of environment

A four-step approach can be used to assess the office environment: assessment of potential emission sources, measurement of basic physical parameters and air change, measurement of chemical and microbiological pollutants (selected by the type of SBS problem), and evaluation of social environment (Table 15.4).

Source inventory

Evaluation of potential sources of indoor pollutants, such as new surface materials, damp constructions, and the location of office equipment, should be conducted before any indoor air quality measurements. Occupants' perceived indoor air quality might provide complementary information on relevant sources of indoor air pollutants.

Basic physical parameters

Measurements of room temperature, relative humidity, and air change rate will provide important information on the office environment and should be conducted as the second step of office environment investigation. Carbon dioxide concentrations (which can be measured with a direct-reading infrared detector) combined with information on the volume of the space and the number of occupants can be indirectly used to assess air change rate.

Specific pollutants

Meaningful assessment of exposure to specific pollutants can be conducted by planning a measurement protocol on the basis of emission sources and/or health outcomes. Table 15.4 shows a list of relevant agents that can be measured with current techniques. The principles and methods of assessment are described in more detail in a recent document [62]. The measurement of TVOCs in locations with suspected sources of emission gives a reasonable view of the general levels, given that the limitations described above are understood [29]. The samples are collected in charcoal tubes with volumetric air pumps and are analysed by flame ionization and gas chromatography/mass spectrometry. Measurement of formaldehyde, a known airway irritant, may provide additional information. Formaldehyde can be col-

Table 15.4 Assessment of exposure in investigations of problem buildings

Step	Factors assessed
1 Source inventory	Surface materials in floors, walls and ceilings Dampness and microbial growth in building materials Type of ventilation Heating system Cleaning routines and materials
2 Basic physical parameters	Temperature Relative humidity Air change rate
3 Specific air, dust, and material measurements selected according to the study problem	VOCs + total VOC Nicotine Carbon dioxide Carbon monoxide Particulate matter: PM_{10} and $PM_{2.5}$ Aeroallergens: airborne fungal spores Floor dust allergens: house dust mite antigens (immunoassays Der p 1, Der f 1), culturable fungi Damp building material: fungi
4 Social environment	Organizational evaluation Experience of social environment (interview, questionnaire)

PM, particles of mean diameter (≤ 10 µm and 2.5 µm); VOCs, volatile organic compounds.

lected using passive samplers during an 8-hour period and analyzed as described elsewhere [63].

Exposure to particulate matter with aerodynamic diameter less than 10 μm or fine particles of less than 2.5 μm can cause various effects in the eyes and respiratory tract. The sources of such particles vary from traffic exhaust from outside and other combustion products to resuspension of floor dust.

The qualitative and quantitative assessment of viable fungal spores suspended in the air is commonly conducted using a two-stage Andersen sampler, which divides particles into respirable and non-respirable fractions and deposits particles onto separate agar plates. Exposed plates with respirable fungal spores are incubated in darkness at 25°C for 4 days. The resulting fungal colonies are identified on the basis of colony and spore morphology. Counts are usually expressed as colony-forming units per cubic meter of air. The total fungal biomass in floor dust can be evaluated using fungal membrane lipid ergosterol as an indicator [64]. The most common fungi found within the office environment include *Cladosporium, Alternaria, Penicillium,* and *Aspergillus* spp.

Floor dust samples may be collected by vacuuming according to standardized protocols, which specify area and time. Samples are sieved through a mesh to extract the fine dust. Two-site monoclonal antibody immunoassays are used for measurement of most common house dust mites (Der p 1, Der f 1) as well as for pet dander. Allergen concentrations are reported in micrograms per gram of dust.

Social environment

Simple questions in self-administered questionnaires can be used for a crude assessment of the social environment. Differences in reported indicators of social atmosphere and psychologic problems between organizational units may reveal the importance of social factors. Furthermore, a relation of reported symptoms and perceptions to assessed social atmosphere may elaborate the role of the social environment in a given building. Further evaluation of organizational problems by qualitative methods requires expertise in social sciences.

MANAGEMENT

The management of affected individuals should be based on avoidance or reduction of the environmental exposures causing the symptoms, and on modifying any relevant social and psychologic factors. Symptomatic treatment should also be available, according to the specific nature of the symptoms and the clinical disorder. Subjects with a history of atopic diseases are more sensitive to the environmental ex-

posures and may, therefore, need a more strict control of environmental exposures.

PREVENTION

Strategies for improving the office building environment can be made on the basis of the information presented above. These will help to prevent SBS.

The location of the office building is an important determinant of indoor exposures. Therefore environmental conditions in the location should be taken into account when designing buildings.

Environmental and health issues should be considered explicitly in architecture and building engineering. Use of building materials with low emissions of chemicals is an important part of source control to diminish indoor air pollution. Producers of building materials should be encouraged to develop materials with lower emissions, using international accreditation and certification. An important part of prevention is testing of new materials introduced to the market. The emission from a given material may vary substantially in different microenvironments and depends on a number of factors such as the level and variation of temperature and relative humidity. The choice of materials used to cover large surfaces, such as floors and walls, is critical for indoor air quality [65]. The component materials and their emission rates should be readily available. Appropriate models should be developed in the design phase of new buildings for predicting the overall emission rates and likely concentrations in a given space. The need for cleaning is another important factor in choosing an appropriate surface material. This may be in conflict with the requirement for low emission rates. The cleaning materials too are potential sources of emission [5].

Sufficient air change is the most important characteristic of a good office environment and must take account of emissions from both occupants and other sources. The minimum acceptable ventilation rate for office buildings according to epidemiological studies is 10–15 l/s per person, given current average emissions and activities [20,21,66]. Ventilation rates below 5 l/s per occupant are likely to result in indoor air pollution problems in facilities with high emissions. Air change can be easily measured directly or indirectly and so can be regulated and monitored. An increase of air change is often the first aid for apparent indoor air-quality problems. This should be a secondary solution to removing strong indoor sources of emission. There is strong evidence that emphasizes a need for close control over air temperature in offices (23 ± 2°C provides an acceptable range). At present, no recommendations can be made about the usefulness of air humidification, although some findings in office environments suggest a preventive benefit from hygienic steam humidification when heating is required and the indoor air is very dry.

Restriction of smoking to spaces with a separate ventilation system will reduce exposure to a large number of particulate and gaseous air pollutants, which has both short-term and long-term health effects. Although limited by national regulations in some countries, exposure to ETS is globally a large problem and an important determinant of SBS in many countries.

A general program for providing training about indoor environmental issues should be developed for building maintenance personnel as well as for occupational health personnel. Understanding the principles of hygiene and indoor air quality, in combination with practical tools and advice, is needed.

DIFFICULT CASE

History

A 39-year-old teacher contacted her local occupational health center in early 1999 because of eye irritation, respiratory symptoms of both upper and lower respiratory tract, tiredness, and headache. She had experienced these symptoms over several years and considered they had initially been clearly related to the work environment. Over the years, they had become persistent and were alleviated only during the 2-month summer vacation. In addition, she complained of 'stuffiness' of the indoor air in the classroom. She had no previous history of asthma or allergies, was a never-smoker, and had no pets at home. Her father had experienced symptoms of asthma, but no clinical diagnosis was ever made.

She worked in 1987–9 in a temporary building, which was later closed because of mold problems. She worked thereafter in the main school building. It was constructed in the 1960s, but the roof was renovated a few years before her presentation, apparently because of water leakage problems. An initial examination of the building had not revealed any obvious mold problems, but a new examination was taking place when the patient first contacted the occupational physician.

She was referred to the Finnish Institute of Occupational Health for evaluation. Clinical examinations were undertaken in the fall of 1999, when the results from the new and detailed school building examination became available.

The clinical examination revealed no signs of oronasopharyngeal inflammation. Skin prick tests with a set of typical water-damage microbes, including *Acremonium kiliense*, *Aspergillus fumigatus*, *Cladosporium cladosporioides*, *Geotrichum candidum*, *Penicillium brevicompactum*, *Rhodotorula* spp., and *Trichoderma viride* were negative; so too were placebo-controlled nasal challenge tests with *A. fumigatus* and *P. brevicompactum*. Spirometric parameters were normal, a methacholine challenge test did not indicate a level of airways responsiveness within the asthmatic range, and serial peak expiratory flow monitoring was not indicative of occupational asthma.

Examination of the indoor environment of the school was conducted by a commercial firm. It included a careful evaluation of the HVAC system and building structures as well as indoor air and material measurements. A standard Örebro Questionnaire Survey (MM-40) was carried out among the occupants. The ventilation system was deemed to function relatively well. Investigators observed signs of previous roof and pipe leakages, but no damp structures. Air change rate varied from 2.3 to 4 h^{-1}, providing sufficient ventilation per person as indicated by carbon dioxide levels of 929–1220 mg/m^3. The levels of total VOC, formaldehyde, and carbon monoxide were acceptable and were within the standard values (3.8–4.7 mg/m^3). The concentrations of ammonium ions were unusually high (0.3–4.5 mg/m^3), but no apparent sources were detected. The levels of spores and bacteria were unremarkable. Species typical for damp buildings were present, but the low levels did not indicate building-related growth.

It was concluded from the specialist clinical evaluation that there was no evidence of immediate reactivity to specific molds. The history suggested a work-related worsening of symptoms and this was considered consistent with non-specific mucosal reactions to various indoor environmental factors. Verification of ammonium ion concentrations and a search for a source in the case of high concentrations was recommended. Improvement of the workplace environment was recommended since the indoor air was perceived to be poor.

Issues

The primary issue here is whether this is a case of the sick building syndrome. Secondary issues are whether the clinical examination of the patient and the environmental study of the school were sufficient to confirm or exclude this diagnostic possibility; in particular how should the acquired information be interpreted?

Comment

It is important to consider separately a possible occupational etiology and a work-related exacerbation of symptoms of a disease from non-occupational cause. Here the work environment history indicated the possibility of both past and current exposure to molds. The clinical examination provided no diagnostic criteria for asthma or specific allergic sensitivity, which excluded the possibility of specific occupational diseases, and there was little evidence of a specific cause–effect relation. The environmental studies gave equivocal results, the levels of most measured contaminants falling within acceptable standards, though an unexplained high concentration of ammonia was noted.

The history, nevertheless, pointed clearly towards work-relatedness of these symptoms, and the specialist clinician suspected that poor indoor air quality at work may have caused irritative and central nervous symptoms, or at least it may have aggravated such symptoms. The overall picture is typical of SBS.

Certain recommendations concerning the work environment were made to the employer, but there were no clear requirements for which fulfilment could be verified. If measures to improve the workplace indoor quality were implemented, a follow-up of the patient's symptom experience would be useful to confirm the work-relatedness of her illness.

 ## SUMMARY POINTS

Recognition

- SBS is not a single disease entity that can be diagnosed readily in an individual.
- The typical symptoms and signs may indicate a particular disorder and may fulfill established diagnostic criteria, and sometimes the disorder will be occupational in origin.
- Clinical examination of an office worker with one or several SBS symptoms has three aims:
  - to make a diagnosis in individuals who have disease-fulfilling diagnostic criteria and to consider the role of occupational exposure in causation and prognosis
  - to consider whether occupational exposures influence symptoms and the natural history of a preexisting chronic disease
  - to identify and characterize non-specific symptoms and signs in otherwise healthy workers (i.e. those without an evident specific illness) and so detect relevant noxious occupational exposures.
- Self-administered questionnaires can be used to assess the prevalence of symptoms in occupants of large buildings.
- Environmental assessment involves four steps:
  - assessment of potential emission sources
  - measurement of basic physical parameters and air change
  - measurement of chemical and microbiological pollutants (selected by the type of SBS problem)
  - evaluation of social environment.

Management

- Provide specific or symptomatic treatment according to the nature of the symptoms and the clinical disorder.
- Reduce the environmental exposures causing the symptoms, or provide specific facilities for the affected individual so that these exposures are avoided.
- Improve social factors that may cause SBS symptoms or contribute to them.

Prevention

- Environmental and health issues should be considered explicitly in architecture and building engineering.
- The use of building materials with low emissions of chemicals is an important part of source control to diminish indoor air pollution.
- Sufficient air change is the most important characteristic of a good office environment and must take account of emissions from both occupants and other sources: the minimum acceptable ventilation rate for office buildings is 10–15 liter/s per person.
- Close control over air temperature in offices ($23 \pm 2°C$) will help to prevent SBS symptoms.
- Restriction of smoking to spaces with a separate ventilation system will reduce exposure to a large number of particulate and gaseous air pollutants which have both short-term and long-term health effects.

REFERENCES

1. WHO. *Indoor Air Pollutants: Exposure and Health Effects. EURO Reports and Studies No 78: Report on a WHO meeting*, Copenhagen, Denmark, Geneva: World Health Organization Regional Office for Europe, 1983.
2. Finnegan MJ, Pickering CAC, Burge PS. The sick building syndrome: prevalence studies. *Br Med J* 1984; 289: 1573–1575.
3. Jaakkola JJK. The office environment model: a conceptual analysis of sick building syndrome. *Indoor Air* 1998; 8: 7–16.
4. Marbury MC, Krieger RA. Formaldehyde. In: Samet JM, Spengler JD, eds. *Indoor Air Pollution. A Health Perspective*. Baltimore, MD: The Johns Hopkins University Press, 1991.
5. Wolkoff P, Schneider T, Kildeso J *et al*. Risk in cleaning: chemical and physical exposure. *Sci Total Environ* 1998; 215: 135–156.
6. Fanger PO. Calculations of thermal comfort, introduction of a basic comfort equation. *ASHRAE Trans* 73(II):III.4.1–20. 1967; 73(Suppl II): 4.1–4.20.
7. Berglund B, Gustafsson L, Lindvall T. Thermal climate. *Environ Int* 1991; 17: 185–204.
8. Jaakkola JJK, Heinonen OP, Seppänen O. Sick building syndrome, sensation of dryness and thermal comfort in relation to room temperature in an office building: need for individual control of temperature. *Environ Int* 1989; 15: 163–168.
9. Menzies R, Tamblyn R, Farant JP *et al*. The effect of varying levels of outdoor-air supply on the symptoms of sick building syndrome. *N Engl J Med* 1993; 328: 821–827.
10. Jaakkola JJK, Heinonen OP, Seppänen O. Mechanical ventilation in office buildings and the sick building syndrome. An experimental and epidemiological study. *Indoor Air* 1991; 1: 111–121.

11. Jaakkola JJK, Miettinen P. Type of ventilation system in office buildings and sick building syndrome. *Am J Epidemiol* 1995; 141: 755–765.

12. Stenberg B, Mild KH, Sandström M *et al.* A prevalence study of the sick building syndrome and facial skin symptoms in office workers. *Indoor Air* 1993; 3: 71–81.

13. Reinikainen LM, Jaakkola JJK, Seppänen O. The effect of air humidification on symptoms and the perception of air quality in office workers. A six period cross-over trial. *Arch Environ Health* 1992; 47: 8–15.

14. Nordström K, Norbäck D, Akselsson R. Effect of air humidification on the sick building syndrome and perceived indoor air quality in hospitals: a four month longitudinal study. *Occup Environ Med* 1994; 51: 683–688.

15. Mølhave L, Bach B, Pedersen OF. Human reactions to low concentrations of volatile organic compounds. *Environ Int* 1986; 12: 167–175.

16. ASHRAE. *ASHRAE Handbook, Fundamentals*. Atlanta, GA: American Society of Heating, Refrigeration and Air-Conditioning Engineers Inc., 1993.

17. Tichenor BA, Guo Z. The effect of ventilation on emission rates of wood finishing materials. *Environ Int* 1991; 17: 317–323.

18. Wolkoff P, Clausen PA, Nielsen JB *et al.* The influence of specific ventilation rate on the emissions from construction products. In: Saarcla K, Kalliokoski P, Seppänen O eds. *Indoor Air '93*, Vol. 2, *Chemicals in Indoor Air, Material Emissions*, pp. 9–14. Jyväskylä, 1993.

19. Thatcher TL, Layton DW. Deposition, resuspension, and penetration of particles within a residence. *Atmos Environ* 1995; 29: 1487–1497.

20. Jaakkola JJK, Miettinen, P. Ventilation rate in office buildings and sick building syndrome. *Occup Environ Med* 1995; 52: 709–714.

21. Godish T, Spengler JD. Relationships between ventilation and indoor air quality: a review. *Indoor Air* 1996; 6: 135–145.

22. Mendell MJ, Smith AH. Consistent pattern of elevated symptoms in air-conditioned office buildings: a reanalysis of epidemiologic studies. *Am J Public Health* 1990; 80: 1193–1199.

23. Wan GH, Li CS. Dampness and airway inflammation and systemic symptoms in office building workers. *Arch Environ Health* 1999; 54: 58–63.

24. Zweers T, Preller L, Brunekreef B, Boleij JSM. Health and indoor climate complaints of 7043 office workers in 61 buildings in the Netherlands. *Indoor Air* 1992; 2: 127–136.

25. Daisey JM, Hodgson AT, Fisk WJ *et al.* Volatile organic compounds in twelve Californian office buildings: classes, concentrations and sources. In: Saarela K, Kalliokoski P, Seppänen O, eds. *Indoor Air '93* Vol. 2. *Chemicals in Indoor Air, Material Emissions*, pp. 9–14. Jyväskylä, 1993.

26. Shields HC, Fleischer DM. VOC survey: sixty-eight telecommunication facilities. In: Saarela K, Kalliokoski P, Seppänen O eds. *Indoor Air '93*, Vol. 2. *Chemicals in Indoor Air, Material Emissions*, pp. 93–98. Jyväskylä, 1993.

27. Koren HS, Devlin RB, House D *et al.* The inflammatory response of human upper airways to volatile organic compounds (VOC). In: *Proceedings of the 5th International Conference on Indoor Quality and Climate*, Vol. 1, *Indoor Air '90*, Toronto, pp. 325–330, 1990.

28. Mølhave L. Volatile organic compounds, indoor air quality and health. In: *Proceedings of the 5th International Conference on Indoor Quality and Climate*, Vol. 5, *Indoor Air '90*, Toronto, pp. 15–34, 1990.

29. Andersson K, Bakke JV, Bjørseth O *et al.* TVOC and health in non-industrial indoor environments. *Indoor Air* 1997; 7: 78–91.

30. Bergland B, Bergland U, Lindvall T, Nicander-Brefberg H. Olfactory and chemical characterization of indoor air - towards a psycho-social model of air quality. *Environ International* 1982; 8: 327–332

31. Norbäck D, Michel I, Widström J. Indoor air quality and personal factors related to the sick building syndrome. *Scand J Work Environ Health* 1990; 16: 121–128.

32. Norbäck D, Torgen M, Edling C. Volatile organic compounds, respirable dust, and personal factors related to prevalence and incidence of sick building syndrome in primary schools. *Br J Ind Med* 1990; 47: 733–741.

33. Hodgson MJ, Frohliger J, Permar E *et al.* Symptoms and microenvironmental measures in non-problem buildings. *J Occup Med* 1991; 33: 527–533.

34. Sundell J, Andersson B, Andersson K, Lindvall T. Volatile organic compounds in ventilating air at different sampling points in the building and their relationships with the prevalence of occupant symptoms. *Indoor Air* 1993; 3: 82–93.

35. Husman T. Health effects of indoor-air microorganisms. *Scand J Work Environ Health* 1996; 22: 5–13.

36. Harrison J, Pickering CA, Faragher EB *et al.* An investigation of the relationship between microbial and particulate indoor air pollution and the sick building syndrome. *Respir Med* 1992; 86: 225–235.

37. Menzies D, Comtois P, Pasztor J *et al.* Aeroallergens and work-related respiratory symptoms among office workers. *J Allergy Clin Immunol* 1998; 101: 38–44.

38. Robertson AS, Burge PS, Hedge A *et al.* Relation between passive smoke exposure and 'building sickness'. *Thorax* 1988; 43: 263P.

39. Buring JE, Hennekens CH. Carbonless copy paper: a review of published epidemiologic studies. *J Occup Med* 1991; 33: 486–495.

40. Skov P, Valbjørn O, Pedersen BV. Influence of personal characteristics, job-related factors and psychosocial factors on the sick building syndrome. *Scand J Work Environ Health* 1989; 15: 286–292.

41. Fisk WJ, Mendell MJ, Daisey JM *et al.* Phase 1 of the California Healthy Building Study: a summary. *Indoor Air* 1993; 3: 246–254.

42. Jaakkola MS, Jaakkola JJK. Office equipment and supplies – a modern occupational health concern? *Am J Epidemiol* 1999; 150: 1223–1228.

43. Stenberg B. *Office Illness. The Worker, the Work and the Workplace*: Umeå University Medical Dissertations, New Series No 399. Umeå, Sweden: Umeå University Press, 1994.

44. Wallace LA, Nelson CJ, Highsmith R *et al.* Association of personal and workplace characteristics with health, comfort and odor: a survey of 3948 office workers in three buildings. *Indoor Air* 1993; 3: 193–205.

45. Rossignol AM, Morse EP, Summers VM, *et al.* Video display terminal use and reported health symptoms among Massachusetts clerical workers. *J Occup Med* 1987; 29: 112–118.

46. Ong CN, Chia SE, Jeyratnam J *et al.* Musculoskeletal disorders among operators of visual display terminals. *Scand J Work Environ Health* 1995; 21: 60–64.

47. Murata K, Araki S, Kawakami N *et al.* Central nervous system effects and visual fatigue in VDT workers. *Int Arch Occup Environ Health* 1991; 63: 109–113.

48. Baker DB. Occupational stress. In: Levy BS, Wegman DH, eds. *Occupational Health,* 2nd edn, pp. 297–318. Boston, MA: Little, Brown, 1988.

49. Baker DB. Social and organizational factors in office building-associated illness. *Occup Med* 1989; 4: 607–624.

50. Karasek R, Baker D, Marxer F *et al.* Job decision latitude, job demands, and cardiovascular disease: a prospective study of Swedish men. *Am J Public Health* 1981; 71: 694–705.

51. Jaakkola JJK. Indoor air in office building and human health. Experimental and epidemiologic study of the effects of mechanical ventilation. [In Finnish with an English summary] Doctoral Thesis. University of Helsinki, Department of Public Health. Helsinki: Health Services Research by the National Board of Health in Finland, Nr 41, 1986.

52. Hedge A, Burge PS, Robertson AS *et al.* Work-related illness in offices: a proposed model of the 'sick building syndrome'. *Environ Int* 1989; 15: 143–158.

53. Andersson K. 1998 Epidemiologic approach to indoor air problems. *Indoor Air* 1998; 8: 32–39.

54. Franck C. Eye symptoms and signs in buildings with indoor climate problems ('office eye syndrome'). *Acta Ophthalmol* 1986; 64: 306–311.

55. Franck C, Palmvang IB, Palmvang IB. Break-up time and lissamine green epithelial damage in 'office eye syndrome'. Six-month and one-year follow-up investigations. *Acta Ophthalmol* 1993; 71: 62–64.

56. Muzi G, dell'Omo M, Abbritti G *et al.* Objective assessment of ocular and respiratory alterations in employees in a sick building. *Am J Ind Med* 1998; 34: 79–88.

57. Wieslander G, Norbäck D, Nordström K *et al.* Nasal and ocular symptoms, tear film stability and biomarkers in nasal lavage, in relation to building-dampness and building design in hospitals. *Int Arch Occup Environ Health* 1999; 72: 451–461.

58. Wieslander G, Norbäck D, Walinder R *et al.* Inflammation markers in nasal lavage, and nasal symptoms in relation to relocation to a newly painted building: a longitudinal study. *Int Arch Occup Environ Health* 1999; 72: 507–515.

59. Malkin R, Martinez K, Marinkovich V *et al.* The relationship between symptoms and IgG and IgE antibodies in an office environment. *Environ Res* 1998; 76: 85–93.

60. Jaakkola JJK, Tuomaala P, Seppänen O. Air recirculation and sick building syndrome. A blinded crossover trial. *Am J Public Health* 1994; 84: 422–428.

61. Mendell MJ, Fisk WJ, Dong MX *et al.* Enhanced particle filtration in a non-problem office environment: preliminary results from a double-blind crossover intervention study. *Am J Ind Med* 1999; Suppl 1: 55–57.

62. Jantunen MJ, Jaakkola JJK, Krzyzanowski M (eds.). *Assessment of Exposure to Indoor Air Pollutants: WHO Regional Publications, European Series,* No. 78. Geneva: World Health Organization 1997.

63. ASTM (ed.) ASTM standard test method for measurement of formaldehyde in indoor air (passive sampler method). In: *Occupational Health and Safety,* American Society of Testing Materials. Philadelphia, PA: pp. 425–430. 1990.

64. Martin F, Delaruelle C, Hilbert JL. An improved ergosterol assay to estimate fungal biomass in ectomycorrhizas. *Mycol Res* 1990; 94: 1059–1064.

65. Jaakkola JJK, Tuomaala P, Seppänen O. Textile wall materials and sick building syndrome. *Arch Environ Health* 1994; 49: 175–181.

66. Seppänen OA, Fisk WJ, Mendell MJ. Association of ventilation rates and CO_2 concentrations with health and other responses in commercial and institutional buildings. *Indoor Air* 1999; 9: 226–252.

16 TUBERCULOSIS

P. Sherwood Burge

BACKGROUND

Tuberculosis acquired at work is the same disease as the more usual non-occupational tuberculosis. The main occupational issue is the prevention of infection in those exposed at work. Whilst occupationally acquired tuberculosis remained relative infrequent and treatable, there was little interest in occupational medicine in the subject. With the emergence of multidrug-resistant tuberculosis, and spread from infected individuals to carers, the situation has become more serious. There is a clear increase in incidence in clinical tuberculosis in some worker groups, particularly those exposed to silica, and those in contact with infected humans or animals (or infected biological material).

There remain some who believe that healthcare workers are no longer at increased risk of developing tuberculosis compared with others not occupationally exposed [1]. This chapter will review in particular the evidence for risks in healthcare workers over time, identify others at increased risk, review methods of linking infected workers with potential source cases, and review the different approaches to prevention. Before starting it is important to understand the different definitions of what constitutes a 'case'.

Case definition

Tuberculosis starts with a primary infection, with an 'illness' that is usually subclinical and self-limiting, and conversion of tuberculin skin sensitivity from negative to positive. In some countries, particularly in the USA, this constitutes a case. In most of Europe this is regarded as tuberculin conversion, but not a disease. Tuberculin conversion also occurs as a result of bacille Calmette–Guérin (BCG) vaccination, which is recommended in many countries for the prevention of tuberculosis, both in the general population, and (in particular) in healthcare workers. BCG vaccination therefore prevents tuberculin conversion being used as a marker of primary infection. Skin positivity may result from infection acquired at work, and in some countries this constitutes an occupational 'case', even if there is no clinical disease.

Epidemiology

Primary tuberculin conversion may progress to clinical disease; the lifetime risk is in the order of 10%. It is this clinical disease which constitutes the occupation disease in many countries.

Some workers are at particular risk of developing disease after infection. In the past, silica exposure was the principal risk factor. It has been difficult to separate the effects of silica from the crowded living conditions of many, mainly miners, who have been exposed. Recent work suggests that dust exposure (as a rock driller) increases the risk 2.3 times compared with that of a surface worker in South African gold mines [2]. Human immunodeficiency virus (HIV) infection is now the most widespread risk factor; drugs which suppress the immune system, such as cyclosporin, are also implicated. Such factors are not normally a consequence of occupation, but their presence coincidentally will greatly increase the risk of occupational infection.

Tuberculosis is usually transmitted by droplet nuclei from an infected individual coughing. The source case must have disease in the lungs (or larynx). Those with non-respiratory tuberculosis are generally not infectious. The exceptions are in the autopsy room, where aerosols from bone saws, etc. can generate infected droplet nuclei from otherwise non-infectious sources, and in laboratories handling infected specimens. Laennec, the inventor of the stethoscope, died of tuberculosis, which he thought he had caught from performing autopsies. Valsalva and Morgani in Italy avoided doing autopsies for this reason.

Most occupational risk relates to healthcare workers, for whom infected patients and their biological specimens are a potential source of infection. Others at risk include farm workers [3], veterinarians, and slaughterhouse workers, where infected livestock are the principal source of infection. Tuberculosis has become common in some prisons and hostels; those working in such institutions may be at increased risk. In one study, one-third of tuberculin conversions in New York state prison staff were thought to be occupational [4]. The primary route of infection is nearly always via the respiratory tract; tuberculosis used to be transmitted through infected milk, but this is not a current occupation risk factor. There are occasional cases of tuberculosis transmitted via direct skin penetration, for instance, during surgery through a hand wound (prosectors wart), where the primary infection would be on the finger. Primary infection in the conjunctiva has been recorded in a bronchoscopist when infected material came back along the suction channel of a direct viewing bronchoscope.

The risks of occupational tuberculosis have changed over time. They depend principally on the likelihood of primary infection in childhood, and on the period of infectivity of a source case. In the late 19th century, it was generally thought that sanatorium workers were not at increased risk of tuberculosis. At this time the great majority of teenagers starting healthcare work would have had a primary infection in childhood. A study at the Brompton Hospital, London, considered the cause of death in resident medical officers, physicians, clinical assistants, matrons, dispensers, and chaplains; the study was rather vague about nurses and gallery maids. There were 12 cases of tuberculosis with nine deaths amongst 215 workers followed for many (at least 15) years [5,6]; at this time the annual death rate from tuberculosis in England and Wales was 4/1000, giving an expected 13 expected deaths over 15 years in the Brompton workers [7]. The results were not corrected for social class or affluence.

In the first half of the 20th century the likelihood of primary tuberculous infection in childhood declined, whilst the sanatorium movement concentrated infectious patients together. Without anti-tuberculous therapy they generally remained infectious for their time in the sanatorium, which was often several years in the survivors. Norwegian nurses were studied between 1924 and 1935 [8]. All 280 who started nursing with negative tuberculin tests became positive during the training period of 3 years, 96 developed clinical tuberculosis and 10 died. The actual incidence of clinical disease was 171/1000/year. Of the 625 who started student training with positive tuberculin tests, 27 developed clinical tuberculosis and none died (incidence 10/1000 per year). BCG vaccination was offered to tuberculin-negative student nurses from 1927 onwards and, following BCG vaccination, the annual rate of clinical tuberculosis fell to 26/1000 in those starting nurse training with a negative tuberculin test.

By the mid-20th century tuberculosis was a recognized and serious risk for those working in sanatoriums. Between 1930 and 1950 their rates of tuberculosis were 5–9 times the rate of healthcare workers in other hospitals in the USA [9,10]. A study of medical students from 62 medical schools between 1940 and 1950 found 557 cases of tuberculosis (rate 3.34/1000 per year) with an age-corrected population risk of 1/1000 per year [11]. A prospective study in the UK between 1935 and 1944 studied 5016 nurses, 1547 medical students, and 1592 office workers as controls. A total of 80% were already tuberculin positive at the start of their training (representing childhood infection). In those who were initially tuberculin negative, conversion rates within the first year of training were 80% for nurses in hospitals with a tuberculosis ward, 54% for nurses in other hospitals, 36% for medical students, and 26% for office workers [12]. The rates for clinical tuberculosis for female nurses were twice that of their office worker controls (10.7 vs 5.5/1000 per year); for male medical students the risk was three times that of the controls (5.1 vs 1.4/1000 per year).

Triple therapy for tuberculosis became widespread in the early 1950s. It is believed that infectivity is reduced to a negligible degree about 2 weeks after the start of therapy, even when mycobacteria can still be cultured from the sputum [13]. Occupational tuberculosis in healthcare workers then became less apparent [14]. However, a study of healthcare workers in British Columbia, Canada, between 1969 and 1979 still showed the risk to be 1.9 times that of controls matched by age and place of birth, although there was no increased risk compared with the whole Canadian population [15]. Three studies in the UK in the 1980s showed no increased risk in healthcare workers compared with the general population, with the possible exception of autopsy and microbiology laboratory workers [16–18]. Laboratory workers have been shown to have high risks of tuberculosis in a number of studies from the UK (five times the general population [19]), and Japan (6–11 times the general population [20–22]), and morticians in the USA have also shown an increased risk (3.9-fold) [3]. Exposure need not be frequent; there is a report of one case of tuberculosis and six tuberculin conversions among medical students attending a single postmortem examination, that of an immunosuppressed patient with tuberculosis [23]. There is also a rather sad case report of a trainee pathologist doing an autopsy as part of her specialist examinations. She was failed for diagnosing urogenital tuberculosis, and soon after developed tuberculosis herself without any other recognizable tuberculous contact over recent years. A review of the specimens that she took from the bladder at the original autopsy showed a positive culture for *Mycobacterium tuberculosis*. She passed next time [24].

Tuberculosis in the West is a disease with a marked social-class gradient, making the general population a poor control group. In the UK Meredith took data from national surveys of tuberculosis in 1988 and 1993, and compared these with 1991 census data [25]. Doctors were compared with other professions, and nurses with similar (associate) professional groups. Both comparisons were corrected for ethnicity. The study identified 119 healthcare workers with clinical tuberculosis (61 nurses and 42 doctors). The overall risk ratio was 2.4 (confidence intervals 2–3), slightly higher for doctors (2.7) than nurses (2.0). There were no gender differences, but the risks for Indian subcontinent ethnicity compared with white UK ethnicity was elevated 26.8 times for nurses, and 43.7 times for doctors. The crude rate for clinical tuberculosis for all healthcare workers was 0.12/1000 per year. It is possible that countries with low immigration rates from places with a high tuberculosis incidence, such as Finland, do not have an increased incidence of tuberculosis in healthcare workers. The studies, however, compare healthcare workers with the general population [1]; it is unclear whether the social gradients promoting tuberculosis in many countries are also present in Finland.

In some African countries, such as Malawi, tuberculosis remains a substantial threat to healthcare workers, whose risk depends on the number of tuberculous patients admitted annually to their hospital. In one study there was no increased risk to workers in hospitals admitting less than 100 tuberculous patients per year. The overall risk for notified and treated tuberculosis for all hospital workers was 11.9 times that for the adult general population, with a mortality of 24% [26].

Attempts have generally failed to identify higher risk employees for whom heightened surveillance could be implemented. In a prospective study of tuberculosis clinics and wards, in healthcare workers in the West Midlands, UK, only 2 of 26 cases came from identified high-risk areas (laboratories, autopsy rooms, tuberculosis clinics and wards, thoracic surgery) [27]. Similar results were found in New York where the highest risk for tuberculin conversion was in a group including housekeepers, and personnel in security, portering, engineering, and transport services, who had an adjusted relative risk of 6.7. Increased risks were also found in finance staff, physicians, and nurses having a combined relative risk of 3 [28]. It appears that infection often comes from unexpected sources, such as the elderly, where the diagnosis may not be suspected (and appropriate precautions taken) before death.

RECOGNITION

Investigation

The diagnosis of active pulmonary tuberculosis requires the same tools whether it is occupational in origin or not (chest radiography, sputum smear and culture, bronchoscopy and bronchoalveolar lavage, tuberculin skin tests, tissue biopsy, etc.). The details are widely familiar and can be obtained from any general respiratory text. In the occupational setting associated with notably high risk, there is additional benefit from regular screening with tuberculin skin tests (if BCG is not used). Workers at high risk should also recognize a need for prompt chest radiographs if suspicious symptoms arise, such as cough in non-smokers, worsening cough in smokers, hemoptysis, fever, and weight loss.

Identification of an occupational source

DNA fingerprinting has revolutionized the monitoring of person-to-person spread of tuberculosis, and has identified clusters of cases in the general population, which evidently shared the same infective source, whether directly or indirectly [29,30]. In one study a patient was shown to have developed tuberculosis from the same organism as an earlier patient who had been in the same room 2 years previously [31]. For DNA fingerprinting to be possible, there must be positive cultures for *Mycobacterium tuberculosis* from both source and case, which can be run side by side on the same plate. Less definitive assessments of mycobacterial identity can be made without culture from techniques using the polymerized chain reaction (PCR) and genetic probes. Tuberculosis is often diagnosed in the absence of positive cultures, particularly from pleural fluid, lymph nodes or other tissue. Positive cultures were obtained in only 11/26 cases in one study of tuberculosis in healthcare workers [27].

MANAGEMENT

Of the individual

The individual worker infected with tuberculosis is treated along conventional lines, details again being available in standard respiratory texts. It is particularly important in areas where drug resistance is endemic, that sensitivities are obtained to ensure that appropriate chemotherapy regimens are used, and genetic probes may be very helpful in identifying drug resistance without the need to wait for culture results. When the organism is fully sensitive to standard drugs, and when there is full compliance, a cure is to be expected. Adverse side-effects occasionally require modifications to the standard regimen, and close surveillance is advisable at regular intervals (usually monthly) with serological tests of liver function.

In general, the treated individual does not remain infectious beyond a couple of weeks, though completion of the full-treatment protocol is essential to effect a long-term cure and to prevent the emergence of drug resistance. If the individual works with others who are unduly susceptible (e.g. nurses or doctors working with immunocompromised patients, or miners working with exposure to silica), it is wise to delay any return to work until the sputum is negative on culture for *M. tuberculosis*.

Of the workforce

If any fellow worker has had regular close contact with the index case, he/she should be identified for 'contact testing'. The procedure may vary from country to country, and may be an irrelevance in those in which tuberculosis is endemic with high prevalence. Where low prevalences are found, there is benefit in screening close contacts (generally defined as individuals living in the same household or having a similar level of repeated close contact) with tuberculin skin tests and/or chest radiographs so that other infected individuals are promptly identified and treated before there is illness and further disease dissemination. If the index case has a negative sputum smear, the chances of close contacts becoming infected are remote, and the screening procedure serves more to identify the probable source of infection in the index case. A single evaluation is then sufficient. If the index case is smear positive, the chance of disease dissemination is much greater (of the order 3–10%) and repeated screening evaluations over the following 12 months are indicated, if the initial evaluation produces a negative outcome. There are no studies showing benefit from prolonged surveillance following occupational contact in healthcare workers.

PREVENTION

In the workplace

Tuberculosis is no longer distributed uniformly in economically developed countries, being more common in the poor and unemployed. These individuals often have different access to healthcare than the more affluent population, and may be cared for in different hospitals. There are many hospitals where tuberculosis amongst patients is infrequent, making control measures less of a priority, and there are major differences in the approach to control between countries who use and do not use BCG vaccination.

Tuberculin skin test conversion, assessed annually amongst staff, can be used to assess the risks for the institution as a whole, and determine the priority for tuberculosis control measures amongst the staff [14,32,33]. Healthcare workers with identified tuberculin conversions can be treated with isoniazid chemoprophylaxis, which reduces the risks for clinical disease developing following primary infection. The problems with this strategy are several. Tuberculin sensitivity, at least as measured with the Mantoux test, is not very reproducible, as it necessitates accurate intradermal injection. Once chemoprophylaxis is indicated, completion rates in healthcare workers are often low (e.g. 25% at 6 months [34–38]), and isoniazid alone is probably ineffective for multidrug-resistant tuberculosis. Some healthcare workers are themselves HIV positive [39,40]; in more advanced HIV disease, the capacity to mount a positive tuberculin test is very limited, and cases of clinical tuberculosis may be present despite negative tuberculin tests.

BCG vaccination

The risks of developing clinical tuberculosis after contact with an infected patient are significantly higher in those with a negative tuberculin test than those who are already positive [8,35,41,42]. BCG vaccination has been shown to reduce the risks of clinical tuberculosis in many, but not all, parts of the world [35,41]. It must be given before primary infection has occurred, necessitating vaccination at birth when the risks of tuberculosis are high, but can be delayed when the risks of primary infection in childhood are low. It can be given safely to tuberculin-negative entrants to healthcare work. There is evidence of reduced (or absent) efficacy in countries nearer to the Equator, for reasons that are not fully understood [41,43]. Successful BCG vaccination protects against multidrug resistant and fully drug-sensitive tuberculosis, and facilitates healthcare workers moving between low and higher risk employment. BCG vaccination results in tuberculin conversion, so that this cannot be used to monitor hospital-acquired infection. This policy is recommended in most of Europe, Australia, and New Zealand.

Isolation

The emergence of multidrug-resistant tuberculosis, which has causes death in healthcare workers [29,39,44], has increased the need for effective containment of infected patients (who may remain infectious for the rest of their lives) and infected aerosols. Tuberculosis may spread via return air ducts, particularly when recirculation of return air occurs. In the UK, recirculation of return air in not recommended in any hospital, but in regions of extreme temperature the use of recirculated conditioned air may be common. Patient areas should be under negative pressure compared to surrounding rooms, but a problem remains when patients need moving around a hospital. The patient's use of respiratory protection equipment is then recommended for the benefit of other patients and healthcare personnel [45]. Portable HEPA filters in the room of an infectious patient have reduced mycobacterial loads more efficiently than negative air pressure ventilation [46]. Labeling and safe packaging of patient specimens is also important for the control of tuberculosis in laboratory workers.

National regulatory strategies

National strategies relate to the incidence of tuberculosis and to the organization (or lack of organization) of the tuberculosis services. When the organization is limited, the statistics tend to be less reliable; but the tuberculosis risk is then often at its highest. The World Health Organization (WHO) identifies high-risk countries or areas as those with an annual incidence of over 40/100 000. High-risk areas include South-East Asia (mean 165/100 000 – range 180/100 000 for India to 35/100 000 for Sri Lanka); Africa (mean 78/100 000); Eastern Europe and countries of the former USSR except the Czech and Slovak republics; some South and Central American countries (Belize, Bolivia, Brazil, Chile, Dominican Republic, Ecuador, El Salvador, French Guiana, Haiti, Honduras, Nicaragua, Panama, Paraguay, and Peru); and a few others (Portugal, Djibouti, and Yemen).

DIFFICULT CASE

History

A male 44-year-old theater attendant in a hospital thoracic surgery unit developed a left-sided pleural effusion. Pleural fluid from thoracoscopy grew M. tuberculosis, fully sensitive to standard drugs, and pleural biopsy showed granulomatous inflamation without evidence of other pathology. There were two possible occupational sources for his infection. First he had assisted a surgeon with a pleurectomy for diffuse pleural thickening 6 months earlier, following which the surgeon had developed a primary tuberculous lesion on a finger. The mycobacterium that was isolated from the surgeon had an identical pattern of restriction fragment length polymorphism (RFLP) to that cultured from pleurectomy tissue. Secondly, the attendant had assisted at a cardiopulmonary resuscitation following the cardiac arrest in the operating theatre of another patient with probable active tuberculosis.

He had been born in India, however, and had migrated to Britain as a child. His brother, who also lived in Britain, developed tuberculosis when the patient was aged 8 years, and so he was examined as a close contact. The outcome was presumably satisfactory since no specific treatment nor advice was given, and he was not followed further. At the time of employment, prior to working in the surgical theater, a tuberculin (Heaf) test proved to be positive, Grade 2.

Issues

The chief issue here is whether this man developed active tuberculosis as consequence of his work, or from other sources (most obviously his childhood contact). Secondary issues are the precautions, if any, which should have been taken to protect him from such an occurrence.

Comment

He was tuberculin positive at preemployment (apparently without receiving BCG vaccination), suggesting a primary infection in childhood. This should provide a degree of protection against occupational tuberculosis. As organisms were cultured from him, and from a possible occupational source (the pleurectomy tissue), RFLP analysis was used to compare the two organisms. They proved to be indistinguishable, implying that his current disease was indeed occupationally acquired.

Epidemiological estimates in the UK, where the incidence of tuberculosis is fairly low, suggest that about 50% of tuberculosis in healthcare workers is likely to be occupational. The source case was not identified as having possible tuberculosis at the time, and so special precautions were not taken to protect him or the surgeon. This unfortunately is often the case.

SUMMARY POINTS

Recognition

- The incidence of tuberculosis varies widely between and within countries and geographic areas, and this exerts an overwhelming influence on the risk for developing the disease occupationally.
- In countries with high incidences, there may be a place for routine surveillance.
- Surveillance of 'at-risk' workers has not been found helpful in countries with low incidences.
- Apart from autopsy and microbiology workers, it is rarely possible to identify groups of healthcare workers at increased risk as many of the source cases are not identified.
- Healthcare workers and others 'at risk' should receive written information of the risks of tuberculosis, and the symptoms and signs of early disease.
- Prompt investigation of those with early symptoms is probably the best approach to aid early recognition and limit the chances of dissemination.
- Active tuberculosis of occupational origin is otherwise recognized no differently from active tuberculosis in the community at large.
- When tuberculosis is occupational in origin, this is best demonstrated from studies of mycobacterial identity between organisms recovered from the affected worker and the index case.

Management

- The individual affected by tuberculosis of occupational origin is treated along standard lines using protocols

that take account of drug sensitivities and adverse effects.
- Infected workers should be isolated from work while infectious (generally for the first 2 weeks of chemotherapy).
- The identification of a worker with tuberculosis of suspected occupational origin should additionally lead to a search for a source case, for which DNA fingerprinting may link cases to a common source with reasonable certainty.
- Close contacts, both occupational and non-occupational, should be evaluated for the presence of active infection.

Prevention

- Healthcare workers who are tuberculin negative at employment onset have an increased risk of disease following contact with an infected patient.
- A metaanalysis has shown protection from BCG vaccination, which should be effective against multidrug-resistant organisms as well as fully sensitive organisms.
- Workers who are HIV positive, or who are immunosuppressed through some other cause, should not work in areas with recognized increased risks of tuberculosis.
- Patients with active and potentially infectious disease should be nursed in negative-pressure rooms whenever possible, and be supplied with filtering respirators/masks for journeys to other environments.

REFERENCES

1. Raitio M, Tala E. Tuberculosis among health care workers during three recent decades. *Eur Respir J* 2000; 15: 304–307.
2. Kleinschmidt I, Churchyard G. Variation in incidences of tuberculosis in subgroups of South African gold miners. *Occup Environ Med* 1997; 54: 636–641.
3. McKenna MT, Hutton M, Cauthen G *et al.* The association between occupation and tuberculosis. a population-based survey. *Am J Respir Crit Care Med* 1996; 154: 587–593.
4. Steenland K, Levine AJ, Sieber K *et al.* Incidence of tuberculosis infection among New York State Prison employees. *Am J Public Health* 1997; 87: 2012–2014.
5. Williams CT. The contagion of phthisis. *Br Med J* 1882; i: 618–621.
6. Williams CT. A lecture on the infection of consumption. *Br Med J* 1909; i: 433–437.
7. Springett VH. An interpretation of statistical trends in tuberculosis. *Lancet* 1952; i: 521–524.
8. Heimbeck J. Tuberculosis in hospital nurses. *Tubercle* 1936; 18: 97–99.
9. Childress WG. Occupational tuberculosis in hospital and sanatorium personnel. *JAMA* 1951; 146: 1188–1190.
10. Mikol EX, Horton R, Lincoln NS *et al.* Incidence of pulmonary tuberculosis among employees of tuberculosis hospitals. *Am Rev Tuberc* 1952; 66: 16–27.
11. Abruzzi WA, Hummel RJ. Tuberculosis: incidence among American medical students, prevention and control and the use of BCG. *N Engl J Med* 1953; 248: 722–729.
12. Daniels M, Ridehalgh F, Springett VH. *Tuberculosis in Young Adults – Report of the Prophit Tuberculosis Survey 1935–1948.* London: H.K. Lewis, 1948.
13. Jindani A, Aber VR, Edwards EA *et al.* The early bactericidal activity of drugs in patients with

pulmonary tuberculosis. *Am Rev Respir Dis* 1980; 121: 939–949.

14. Menzies D, Fanning A, Yuan L *et al.* Tuberculosis among health care workers. *N Engl J Med* 1995; 332: 92–98.

15. Burrill D, Enarson DA, Allen EA *et al.* Tuberculosis in female nurses in British Columbia: implications for control programs. *Can Med Assoc J* 1985; 132: 137–140.

16. Capewell S, Leaker AR, Leitch AG. Pulmonary tuberculosis in health service staff – is it still a problem? *Tubercle* 1988; 69: 113–118.

17. Loughrey C, Riley M, Varghese G. Tuberculosis among National Health Service employees. *Am Rev Respir Dis* 1992; 145: A103.

18. Lunn JA, Mayho V. Incidence of pulmonary tuberculosis by occupation of hospital employees in the National Health service in England and Wales 1980–1984. *J Soc Occup Med* 1989; 39: 30–32.

19. Harrington JM, Shannon HS. Incidence of tuberculosis, hepatitis, brucellosis and shigellosis in British medical laboratory workers. *Br Med J* 1976; i: 759–762.

20. Shishido S, Mori T, Tokudome O *et al.* Investigation of tuberculosis among the necropsy staff and environment in necropsy rooms. *Kekkaku* 1994; 69: 549–553.

21. Sugita M, Tsutsumi Y, Suchi M *et al.* Pulmonary tuberculosis. An occupational hazard for pathologists and pathology technicians in Japan. *Acta Pathol Jap* 1990; 40: 116–127.

22. Sugita M, Tsutsumi Y, Suchi M *et al.* High incidence of pulmonary tuberculosis in pathologists at Tokai University Hospital: an epidemiological study. *Tokai J Exp Clin Med* 1989; 14: 55–59.

23. Wilkins D, Woolcock AJ, Cossart YE. Tuberculosis: medical students at risk. *Med J Aust* 1994; 160: 395–397.

24. Stenton SC, Hendrick DJ. Occupational tuberculosis and failed postgraduate medical examination. *Occup Med* 1986; 46: 87–88.

25. Meredith SK, Watson JM, Citron KM *et al.* Are healthcare workers in England and Wales at increased risk of tuberculosis? *Br Med J* 1996; 313: 522–525.

26. Harries AD, Nyirenda TE, Banerjee A *et al.* Tuberculosis in health care workers in malawi. *Trans Roy Soc Trop Med Hyg* 1999; 93: 32–35.

27. Hill A, Burge A, Skinner C. Tuberculosis in National Health Service hospital staff in the west Midlands region of England, 1992–5. *Thorax* 1997; 52: 994–997.

28. Louther J, Rivera P, Feldman J *et al.* Risk of tuberculin conversion according to occupation among health care workers at a New York City hospital. *Am J Respir Crit Care Med* 1997; 156: 201–205.

29. Jereb JA, Klevens RM, Privett TD *et al.* Tuberculosis in health care workers at a hospital with an outbreak of multidrug-resistant Mycobacterium tuberculosis. *Arch Internal Med* 1995; 155: 854–859.

30. Bifani PJ, Plikaytis BB, Kapur V *et al.* Origin and interstate spread of a New York City multidrug-resistant mycobacterium tuberculosis clone family. *JAMA* 1996; 275: 452–457.

31. Lambregts-van Weezenbeek CS, Keizer ST, Sebek MM *et al.* Transmission of multiresistant tuberculosis in a Dutch hospital. *Ned Tijdsch Geneeskunde* 1996; 140: 2293–2295.

32. Anonymous. Guidelines for preventing the transmission of Mycobacterium tuberculosis in health-care facilities, 1994. Centers for Disease Control and Prevention. *MMWR – Morbid Mortal Weekly Rep* 1994; 43(RR-13): 1–132.

33. Anonymous. The role of BCG vaccine in the prevention and control of tuberculosis in the United States. A joint statement by the Advisory Council for the Elimination of Tuberculosis and the Advisory Committee on Immunization Practices. *MMWR – Morbid Mortal Weekly Rep* 1996; 45(RR-4): 1–18.

34. Geiseler PJ, Nelson KE, Crispen RG. Tuberculosis in physicians. Compliance with preventive measures. *Am Rev Respir Dis* 1987; 135: 3–9.

35. Geiseler PJ, Nelson KE, Crispen RG, Moses VK. Tuberculosis in physicians: a continuing problem. *Am Rev Respir Dis* 1986; 133: 773–778.

36. Clague JE, Fields P, Graham DR *et al.* Screening for tuberculosis: current practices and attitudes of hospital workers. *Tubercle* 1991; 72: 265–267.

37. Raad I, Cusick J, Sheretz RJ *et al.* Annual tuberculin skin testing of employees at a university hospital: a cost-benefit analysis. *Infect Control Hosp Epidemiol* 1989; 10: 465–469.

38. Greenberg PD, Lax KG, Schechter CB. Tuberculosis in house staff. A decision analysis comparing the tuberculin screening strategy with the BCG vaccination. *Am Rev Respir Dis* 1991; 143: 490–495.

39. Valway S, Pearson ML, Ikeda R *et al.* HIV infected healthcare workers with multidrug-resistant tuberculosis, 1990–1992. *33rd Interscience Conference on Antimicrobial Agents and Chemotherapy.* American Society of Microbiology, Washington. 1993, 231 p.

40. Sepkowitz KA, Friedman CR, Hafner A *et al.* Tuberculosis among urban health care workers: a study using restriction fragment length polymorphism typing. *Clin Infect Dis* 1995; 21: 1098–1101.

41. Colditz GA, Brewer TF, Berkey CS *et al.* Efficacy of BCG vaccine in the prevention of tuberculosis. Meta-analysis of the published literature. *JAMA* 1994; 271: 698–702.

42. Fine PE, Ponnighaus JM, Maine N. The distribution and implications of BCG scars in northern Malawi. *Bull World Health Organization* 1989; 67: 35–42.

43. Colditz GA, Berkey CS, Mosteller F *et al.* The efficacy of bacillus Calmette–Guerin vaccination of newborns and infants in the prevention of tuberculosis: meta-analyses of the published literature. *Pediatrics* 1995; 96: 29–35.

44. Pearson ML, Jereb JA, Frieden TR *et al.* Nosocomial transmission of multidrug-resistant Mycobacterium tuberculosis. A risk to patients and health care workers. *Ann Internal Med* 1992; 117: 191–196.

45. Bozzi CJ, Burwen DR, Dooley SW *et al.* Guidelines for preventing the transmission of Mycobacterium tuberculosis in health-care facilities, 1994. *MMWR – Morbid Mortal Weekly Rep* 1994; 43: 1–33.

46. Rutala WA, Jones SM, Worthington JM *et al.* Efficacy of portable filtration units in reducing aerosolized particles in the size range of Mycobacterium tuberculosis. *Infect Control Hosp Epidemiol* 1995; 16: 391–398.

17 NON-TUBERCULOUS INFECTIONS

Edmund Ong

INTRODUCTION

The risk of respiratory infection from occupation depends largely on the nature of the pathogen and on the nature of the occupational environment. These are the major determinants of the transmissibility rate. The immunologic status of exposed individuals is also a crucial factor, as is susceptibility attributable to underlying chronic lung disease.

Infectious diseases may be classified by various methods. In the occupational setting the disorders associated with different microorganisms are conveniently considered according to the source from which they are acquired, and in this chapter (which does not address tuberculosis) transmissions from three particular sources are reviewed:

- from infected humans
- from infected animals (the zoonosis)
- from contaminated environmental vegetation, soil, dust, or air.

Inevitably a large range of pathogenic microorganisms may contribute to respiratory infections acquired occupationally, some being almost exclusively occupational in origin, some arising additionally from non-occupational settings; only those with the greatest clinical or epidemiological impact will be discussed in detail. Table 17.1 provides a quick reference for clinicians faced with animal handlers for whom the occupational environment is possibly relevant to suspected respiratory and systemic infection.

Clinical approach to diagnosis

There are multiple causes of respiratory infections acquired through occupational contact, and no single symptom complex is common to all. Constitutional symptoms are often present initially including fever, chills, and malaise. Progressive anorexia and weight loss usually indicate chronic illness. Pulmonary symptoms may be present early, though they are frequently delayed until late in the course of the illness. Any patient with a prolonged illness involving non-specific constitutional complaints and pulmonary symptoms such as a new or worsening cough, sputum production, hemoptysis, chest pain (especially pleuritic), or dyspnea deserves a medical evaluation and a chest radiograph.

The history should address the possibility of similar disease in fellow workers, family members, or recreational contacts, and both inquiry and examination should also be directed to the possibility of involvement of extrapulmonary organs. For example, skin lesions might suggest coccidioidomycosis, cryptococcosis, blastomycosis, nocardiosis, or even sporotrichosis,

Table 17.1 Acute febrile illness among animal handlers[a]

Clinical presentation	Possible infectious agent	Possible animal sources
Fever sweats, anorexia, headache, back pain	Brucella abortus	Cattle, buffalo, camels
	Brucella melitensis	Goats, sheep, camels
	Brucella suis biovars 1–3	Swine
	Brucella suis biovar 4	Reindeer, caribou
	Brucella canis	Dogs
Non-specific illness or atypical pneumonia	Coxiella burnettii (Q-fever)	Cattle, sheep, goats
	Chlamydia psittaci (psittacosis)	Birds (poultry, ducks, parrot family, finches, pigeons, pheasants, seagulls, puffins)
Abrupt onset fever, chills, headache, malaise, anorexia, fatigue, tender lymphadenopathy	Francisella tularensis (tularemia)	Voles, squirrels, rabbits, hares, muskrats, beavers, hamsters
	Yersinia pestis (plague)	Rats, squirrels, prairie dogs
Enlarging papule, which ulcerates and develops eschar	Bacillus anthracis (anthrax)	Herbivores, e.g. cattle, goats, donkeys, horses, and bone meal

[a] Animal handlers include animal farmers, fishermen, livestock handlers, veterinarians, zoo workers, animal laboratory workers, slaughter house workers, butchers, meat inspectors, and raw animal product processors.

whereas mucous membrane lesions would suggest histoplasmosis or paracoccidioidomycosis.

HUMAN SOURCES

Influenza

Background

Influenza is probably the commonest cause of occupationally acquired respiratory infection and indeed it is the commonest cause of absence from work. Influenza is an acute usually self-limited febrile illness caused by infection with influenza type A or B virus that occurs in outbreaks of varying severity almost every winter. The attack rates during such outbreaks may be as high as 10–40% over a 5- to 6-week period. Some of the other respiratory viruses (e.g. respiratory syncytial virus, adenovirus, rhinovirus) may produce infections with clinical manifestations indistinguishable from those of influenza, but such infections do not occur in epidemics and do not have the same mortality, which results in part from the pulmonary complications of influenza.

Influenza virus infection is acquired by the transfer of virus-containing respiratory secretions from an infected to a susceptible person [1]. Small particle aerosols (<10 μm median diameter) are the predominant factor in such person-to-person transmission. First, large amounts of virus are present in respiratory secretions of infected persons at the time of illness and are thus available for aerosol dispersion by sneezing, coughing, and talking. Second, the explosive nature and simultaneous onset in many persons suggest that a single infected person can transmit virus to a large number of susceptible individuals.

Recognition

Most infected individuals develop a classical abrupt onset of symptoms after an incubation period of 1–2 days. Initially systemic symptoms predominate including fever, chills, headaches, myalgias, malaise, and anorexia. Respiratory symptoms, particularly a dry cough and nasal discharge, are usually present at the onset of the illness but are overshadowed by the systemic symptoms. Fever is the most important physical finding and early in the course of illness the patient appears toxic, the face is flushed, and the skin is hot and moist. The eyes are watery and reddened and small tender cervical lymph nodes are often present. As the systemic signs and symptoms diminish, respiratory complaints and findings become more apparent. Cough is the most frequent and troublesome of these symptoms and may be accompanied by substernal discomfort or burning. Nasal obstruction and discharge occur but not to the degree seen in rhinovirus common colds. Such symptoms and signs usually persist for 3–4 days after the fever subsides. A convalescent period of 2 or more weeks to full recovery then ensues. Cough, lassitude, and malaise are the most frequent symptoms during this period [2].

Influenza is associated with the following complications:

- primary influenzal viral pneumonia
- secondary bacterial pneumonia
- croup

- exacerbation of chronic obstructive pulmonary disease
- myositis
- myocarditis and pericarditis
- toxic shock syndrome
- Guillain–Barré syndrome, transverse myelitis, and encephalitis
- Reye syndrome.

Virus isolation, or detection of viral antigen in respiratory secretions, is the best diagnostic technique in the setting of acute illness. Serological tests comparing acute and convalescent sera, although sensitive and specific, do not yield data in time to effect clinical decisions. Virus can be isolated readily from nasal swab specimens, throat swab specimens, nasal washes, or sputum by various cell culture techniques or by inoculation of embryonated hens' eggs. If the patient is expectorating sputum, this is perhaps the best specimen. Complement fixation or hemagglutination antibody tests are commonly used for serologic diagnosis with paired specimens, and fourfold or greater rises or falls in titer are diagnostic of infection [3].

Management

Amantadine, rimantidine, and zanamivir may be used in the treatment of influenza, but they should be considered early in the course of the infection. These antiviral agents have minimal side-effects, but nausea and vomiting occasionally occur. They have been shown to reduce the duration of signs and symptoms of clinical influenza and they may accelerate the rate of recovery of small airways dysfunction to normal [4]. Acutely ill febrile patients should stay in bed and their fluid intake should be adequate.

Prevention

Since the late 1940s, the mainstay for the prevention of influenza has been inactivated virus vaccines. A number of trials in military and civilian populations have demonstrated the efficacy of inactivated, parenterally administered influenza vaccines in the prevention of naturally occurring outbreaks of H1N1, H2N2, and H3N2 viruses [5,6]. Efficacy rates have generally ranged between 67 and 92%, particularly when vaccine and circulating strains were closely related. Studies in young adults and the elderly show that vaccination also reduces the frequency of severe illness among those who become infected.

Individuals with chronic diseases such as cystic fibrosis, asthma, chronic obstructive pulmonary disease (COPD), interstitial pulmonary fibrosis, diabetes, human immunodeficiency virus (HIV) infection, renal disorders, and endocrine disorders should be routinely offered vaccination [7–9]. A Medicare project in the USA indicated that the vaccine usage had a beneficial effect on reducing hospital admissions associated with laboratory documented influenza A or B infection [10]. Amantadine and rimantadine are used as prophylactic agents in close contacts and when there are outbreaks or epidemics of influenza A [11]. Nosocomial influenza has produced major problems in several epidemics in the past and, therefore, special attention to the prevention of nosocomial spread of influenza should be undertaken when an epidemic is identified in the community. Vaccination supplemented with amantidine or rimantadine for the hospital staff is one good option, and if staff members develop illness they should be required to stay away from work. Visitors with any illness should be restricted and patients with acute illness should be isolated in single rooms or grouped together, and staff should be grouped to care either for patients with suspected influenza or for patients felt not to have influenza. Gowns, masks, and handwashing are a logical part of the isolation procedure for influenza [12], but there is no general consensus in control of infection guidelines for dealing with such nosocomial outbreaks.

Streptococcus pneumoniae

Pneumococci spread from one individual to another as a result of extensive close contact. Day care centers consequently provide very likely sources for spread of these organisms in toddlers and their carers. For adults more generally crowded living and working conditions (e.g. military barracks, camps, prisons, and shelters for the homeless) are associated with epidemics [13].

Chlamydia pneumoniae

Chlamydia pneumoniae is believed to be transmitted from person to person by respiratory tract secretions but direct evidence is lacking. Spread of the infection is slow, and the case to case interval has averaged 30 days. Epidemics, even in closed populations, have spread only slowly. It appears that many infected persons are ineffective transmitters of the organism and that some persons with asymptomatic infections play a role in spread of the disease [14].

ANIMAL SOURCES

Zoonosis are a complex group of diseases caused by a remarkable diversity of pathogenic microorganisms that ordinarily reside in and cause disease in the non-human animal world. The possibility of a zoonotic infection may quickly surface from an occupational history (e.g. slaughterhouse worker, veterinarian, farmer) or an account of outdoor interests (e.g. hunting, trapping, other activities with animals or in forests).

Anthrax

Background

Anthrax is usually a disease of herbivores and only incidently infects humans who come into contact with infected animals or their products. Human cases may occur in an industrial or in an agricultural environment. Industrial cases result from contact with anthrax spores that contaminate raw materials used in manufacturing processes. In the USA, occasional epidemics occurred in industrial settings that were probably related to the processing of batches of highly contaminated imported animal bones and bone meal, and fibers, particularly goat hair. These epidemics were primarily of cutaneous (direct contact) rather than respiratory (inhalant) infection although sporadic respiratory cases occurred, and a recent outbreak in Swiss textile factory included one respiratory infection among a total of 25 affected workers [15,16].

In developed countries, approximately 95% of anthrax infections are cutaneous and 5% are respiratory; in developing countries there have additionally been confirmed epidemic cases of gastrointestinal anthrax.

Recognition

Respiratory anthrax shows a biphasic clinical pattern with a benign initial phase followed by an acute, severe second phase that is almost always fatal. The initial phase begins as a non-specific illness consisting of malaise, fatigue, myalgia, mild fever, and non-productive cough. Findings on physical examination are unremarkable, except that rhonchi may be present. The illness may resemble a mild respiratory tract infection such as a cold or viral influenza, and so it is difficult to diagnose early. After 2–4 days, the patient may show signs of improvement only to develop acute severe respiratory distress subsequently that is characterized by severe hypoxemia and dyspnea. The pulse, respiratory rate, and temperature become elevated and there may be evidence of rales over the lungs and possibly pleural effusion. Patients may become hypotensive. Septicemia and meningitis may develop. Death occurs in most persons with respiratory anthrax within 24 hours after the onset of the acute phase.

Cutaneous anthrax, which should alert the physician to the possibility of concomitant respiratory anthrax, occurs in exposed skin: mainly over the arms and hands followed by the face and neck. The infection begins as a pruritic papule that resembles an insect bite. It ulcerates within 1–2 days and it is then surrounded by vesicles. A characteristic black necrotic central eschar develops later with associated edema. The lesion is most often painless. After 1–2 weeks it dries and the eschar begins to loosen, revealing a scar. Regional lymphangitis and lymphadenopathy and systemic symptoms of fever, malaise, and headache may be present. Antibiotic treatment does not appear to change the natural progression of the lesion itself but it will help to resolve the systemic symptoms. The differential diagnosis includes other conditions caused by contact with infected animals, such as plague and tularemia.

An enzyme-linked immunosorbent assay (ELISA) has been developed that measures antibodies to the lethal and edema toxins. The diagnosis may be confirmed serologically by demonstrating a fourfold change in titer in acute and convalescent phase serum specimens collected 4 weeks apart or by a single titer of greater than 1:32. For both cutaneous and pulmonary forms of the disease, vesicular fluid and sputum should reveal *B. anthracis* organisms microscopically on Gram stain smears and on culture.

Management

It is estimated that approximately 20% of untreated cases of cutaneous anthrax will result in death from sepsis, whereas inhalation anthrax is almost always fatal. Death is, however, rare after antimicrobial treatment in the cutaneous form. Intravenous benzylpenicillin (penicillin G) is the drug of choice. Although the skin lesions become culture negative in a few hours [17] therapy should continue for 7–10 days. For the penicillin-allergic patient, erythromycin, a tetracycline, or chloramphenicol are good alternatives. Excision of the lesion is contraindicated. Systemic corticosteroids have been used for patients with extensive or cervical edema, and with meningitis.

Dressings with drainage from the lesions should be incinerated, autoclaved, or otherwise disposed of as biohazardous waste. Person-to-person transmission has not been documented, including experience with patients with inhalation anthrax.

Prevention

The resistance of the spore form of *B. anthracis* to physical and chemical agents is reflected in the survival of the organism in the inanimate environment. Organisms can persist for years in factories in which the environment was contaminated. Paraformaldehyde vapor has been shown to kill *B. anthracis* spores; working surfaces may be decontaminated with either 5% hypochlorite or 5% phenol.

Employees should be educated about the disease and the recommendations for reducing risk in working environment with potential contamination. Both an attenuated live vaccine and a killed vaccine have been developed, but only the killed vaccine derived from a component of the exotoxin is in current human use. It was field tested in employees of four textile mills in the USA, and an effectiveness of 92.5% was demonstrated. Currently the vaccine is given parenterally over three doses at 2-week intervals, followed by three booster inoculations at 6-month intervals and annual booster inoculations. Veterinarians and other persons with potential occupational contact with anthrax should be immunized with this vaccine [18].

Coxiella burnettii (Q-fever)

Background

Q-fever is an acute (on occasion chronic) febrile illness that occurs worldwide. The most common animal reservoirs of the causative organism, *Coxiella burnettii*, are cattle, sheep, and goats. These domestic ungulates, when infected, shed the desiccation-resistant organisms in urine, feces, milk, and (especially) birth products. Humans are infected by inhalation of contaminated aerosols; after an incubation period of 20 days (range 14–39 days) they become ill with severe headache, fever, chills, fatigue, and myalgia. Other symptoms depend on the organs involved.

Recognition

Humans are the only animals known to develop illness regularly as a result of *C. burnettii* infection [19]. In one large series of 207 patients, the mortality rate was 2.4% [20]. There are several clinical syndromes:

- a self-limited febrile illness (2–14 days)
- pneumonia
- endocarditis
- hepatitis
- osteomyelitis
- Q-fever in the immunocompromized host
- Q fever in infancy
- neurologic manifestations: encephalitis, aseptic meningitis, toxic confusional states, dementia, extrapyramidal disease, manic psychosis.

Self-limited febrile illness is probably the most common form of Q-fever. In many farming areas 11–12% of individuals have antibodies to *C. burnettii*; most do not recall pneumonia or other severe illness [21]. It is likely that the age at which infec-

tion occurs and the dose of the agent determine whether or not Q-fever remains a mild self-limited febrile illness [22,23].

There are three presentations of the pneumonic form of Q-fever: atypical pneumonia, rapidly progressive pneumonia, and pneumonia presenting as fever with no pulmonary symptoms. The last is probably the most common presentation. Physical examination of the chest is often unremarkable. The most common physical finding is the presence of inspiratory crackles [24]. Patients with rapidly progressive pneumonia usually have pulmonary consolidation. About 5% of patients have splenomegaly. The rapidly progressive form of Q-fever mimics legionnaires' disease and the pneumonic form of tularemia; indeed all the causes of rapidly progressive pneumonia enter the differential diagnosis.

The radiological appearances of Q-fever pneumonia is variable. Non-segmental and segmental pleural-based opacities are common [24–26]. Pleural effusion is found in 35% of patients. Atelectasis, an increase in reticular markings, and hilar adenopathy may occur. In one series, the resolution time ranged from 10 to 70 days with a mean of 30 days [25].

The diagnosis of Q-fever pneumonia is confirmed serologically but, with the recent development of primers derived from the *C. burnetti* superoxide dismutase gene, amplification of the DNA by polymerase chain reaction is now possible in some laboratories [27]. Microagglutination [28], complement fixation [29], and microimmunofluorescence tests [30] have all been used in the serologic diagnosis of this illness. A fourfold rise in titer between acute and convalescent samples is diagnostic.

It is now recognized that Q-fever has a variety of chronic manifestations: endocarditis, infection of a vascular prosthesis, infection of aneurysms, osteomyelitis, hepatitis, interstitial pulmonary fibrosis, prolonged fever, and purpuric eruptions [31].

Management

The treatment of choice of *C. burnettii* pneumonia is tetracycline [32]. Useful alternatives include chloramphenicol [33], and a macrolide with rifampicin (rifampin) [34,35].

Prevention

Because of the lack of person-to-person spread there is no need to isolate affected patients [36,37]. The pasteurization of milk serves to eliminate most cases. In Cyprus, the incidence of infection among sheep and goats was reduced by destroying aborted material, isolating affected dams, and disinfecting their shelters [38,39]. Control of ectoparasites in the transmission of the disease amongst cattle, sheep, and goats is also important in preventing Q-fever.

Brucellosis

Background

Brucellosis is a disease of domestic and wild animals that is transmittable to humans [40]. The disease exists worldwide especially in the Mediterranean basin, the Arabian peninsula, the Indian subcontinent, and in parts of Central and South America. *Brucella abortus* is found principally in cattle but other species such as buffalo, camels, and yaks can be of local importance. *Brucella melitensis* occurs primarily in goats and sheep, although camels appear to be an important source in some countries. *Brucella suis* biovars 1–3 occur in domestic and feral swine and can cause abattoir-associated infections [41]. *Brucella suis* biovar 4 is confined to reindeer and caribou, or their predators, in the tundra regions of the subarctic. Occupations associated with an increased risk of brucellosis include animal husbandry, veterinary medicine, slaughterhouse work, meat inspection, and laboratory science [42]. Human-to-human transmission of brucellosis is extremely rare [43].

Recognition

The onset of symptoms of brucellosis is acute in about 50% of patients and insidious in the remainder. Symptoms usually begin from 2 to 8 weeks after exposure [44]. They are non-specific (fever, sweats, malaise, anorexia, headache, and back pains) and patients are sometimes misdiagnosed as suffering from influenza [45]. An undulant fever pattern is observed if patients are untreated for long periods. Depression is common. Mild lymphadenopathy occurs in 10–20% and splenomegaly in 20–30% [46,47]. It is a systemic infection that can involve many organs, leading to potential complications in the gastrointestinal tract, skeletal system, central nervous system, cardiovascular, and genitourinary system. Cutaneous manifestations have also been described.

Respiratory symptoms are reported in up to 25% of patients with brucellosis [48] after inhalation of contaminated aerosols or via bacteremic spread to the lungs [49]. The spectrum of respiratory features ranges from influenza-like symptoms with a normal radiograph, to bronchitis, bronchopneumonia, solitary or multiple lung nodules, lung abscesses, miliary lesions, hilar lymphadenopathy, and pleural effusions [50–52]. Rarely are brucellae identified in stains or cultures of expectorated sputum.

The serum agglutination test is the simplest and most widely used serological method of diagnosis [53,54]. Some laboratories use ELISA, which is reported to be more sensitive [55]. The diagnosis of brucellosis is made with certainty when the organisms are recovered from blood, bone marrow, or other tissues.

Management

The use of a 6-week course of doxycycline (200 mg/day) plus rifampicin (600–900 mg/day) administered orally for at least 6 weeks is the combination of choice for uncomplicated brucellosis adopted by most clinicians. It is recommended by the World Health Organization [56]. The treatment of complications such as meningitis and endocarditis pose special problems.

Prevention

Prevention of brucellosis in humans is dependent on the control or eradication of the disease in domestic animals. In the USA, the federal bovine brucellosis program is based on certification of disease-free herds by serologic testing and elimination of reactor cattle [57]. Immunization of cattle with *B. abortus* strain 19 vaccine and *B. melitensis* strain Rev-1 vaccine has resulted in a decrease of human infection [58]. No vaccine is currently available for human use.

Psittacosis

Background

Chlamydia psittaci is common in birds and domestic animals. Infection is, therefore, a hazard for pet owners, pet shop employees, poultry and duck farmers (turkey-associated psittacosis has the highest attack rate in psittacosis epidemics), workers in slaughterhouses and processing plants, and veterinarians. However anyone in contact with an infected bird or animal is at risk. Human cases can occur sporadically and as outbreaks [59,60]. The infection is spread by the respiratory route, by direct contact, or aerosolization of infective discharges or dust. Rarely, the bird may spread the infection by bite. If untreated, 10% of infected birds become asymptomatic carriers [61,62].

Recognition

The disease begins after an incubation period of 5–15 days. Onset may be insidious or abrupt and the clinical manifestations tend to be non-specific. Several syndromes have been described resembling a non-specific viral illness with fever and malaise; a mononucleosis-like syndrome with fever, pharyngitis, hepatosplenomegaly, and adeonopathy; or a typhoidal form presenting with fever, bradycardia, malaise and splenomegaly. Non-productive cough, fever, headache, and an abnormal chest radiograph suggesting atypical pneumonia are frequently encountered in clinical practice [63–65].

Specific end-organ involvement reflects the systemic nature of the disease. The organ most commonly affected in humans is the lung. Clinically this is manifested by cough, breathlessness, and a variety of non-specific auscultatory findings on physical examination. Cardiac complications include pericarditis, myocarditis, and culture-negative endocarditis. *C. Psittaci* is associated with preexisting heart disease and may cause valvular destruction [66,67,68]. Hepatitis, anemia (from hemolysis), disseminated intravascular coagulation, and reactive arthritis are well recognized complications [69]. Neurological manifestations include nerve palsy, cerebellar involvement, transverse myelitis, confusion, meningitis, encephalitis, transcient focal signs, and seizures [70]. Dermatologic phenomena include Horder's spots: pink blanching maculopapular eruptions resembling the rose spots of typhoid fever.

The chest radiograph is abnormal in approximately 75% of patients and it is usually more abnormal than auscultation would predict. The most frequent finding is consolidation in a single lower lobe (in 90% of the abnormal radiographs). However, a variety of patterns has been reported including a homogeneous ground glass appearance, a patchy reticular pattern radiating from the hila, segmental or lobar consolidation with or without atelectasis, a miliary pattern, and unilateral or bilateral hilar enlargement. Pleural effusions are seen in up to 50% [71,72].

Demonstrating the presence of complement-fixing antibodies in paired sera remains the most common serologic test for confirmation of the diagnosis. Techniques such as DNA hybridization, polymerase chain reaction, antigen detection utilizing direct fluorescent antibody, and ELIZA remain experimental [73].

Management

The treatment of choice is tetracycline or doxycycline for 10–21 days. Newer macrolides such as azithromycin and clarithromycin are alternatives. Most patients respond within 24 hours; the untreated fatality rate is about 20% [74].

Prevention

Infected birds should be treated with a tetracycline for at least 45 consecutive days [73]. Human-to-human transmission is rare but tends to be more severe than avian-acquired disease. Environmental sanitation is important since the organism is resistant to drying and can remain viable for a week at room temperature [75].

Tularemia

Background

Tularemia is widely distributed but it is primarily a disease of the northern hemisphere. *Francisella tularensis* is capable of infecting hundreds of differ-

ent vertebrates and invertebrates but no more than a dozen mammalian species (e.g. rodents). Transmission to humans occurs most often through the bite of an insect or contact with contaminated animal products. Other routes include aerosol droplets, contact with contaminated water or mud, and animal bites. Human-to-human spread does not occur [76]. Occupations that have been associated with an increased risk for tularemia are laboratory workers, farmers, veterinarians, sheep workers, hunters or trappers, cooks, and meat handlers [77].

Recognition

The clinical consequences of *F. tularensis* infection depend on the virulence of the particular organism, the portal of entry, the extent of systemic involvement, and the immune status of the host. The outcome can range from asymptomatic or inconsequential illness to acute sepsis and rapid death.

The incubation period averages from 3 to 5 days and the clinical illness usually starts abruptly with the onset of fever, chills, headache, malaise, anorexia, and fatigue [78]. The initial illness may be dominated by pulmonary infection. This is found in 7–20% of all cases [79]. It may result from direct inhalation of the organism or from hematogenous spread to the lungs. Common symptoms include fever, cough, substernal tightness, and pleuritic chest pain. Physical examination may be nonspecific or may reveal rales, consolidation, a friction rub, or signs of effusion. Adult respiratory distress syndrome may complicate any form of tularemia. Acute radiographic changes may include subsegmental or lobar infiltrates, hilar adenopathy, pleural effusion, and apical or miliary infiltrates [80].

The diagnosis is usually confirmed by serologic tests. Antibodies to *F. tularensis* may be demonstrated by tube agglutination, microagglutination, hemagglutination, and ELISA [81,82].

Management

The drug of choice for the treatment of tularemia (except the meningitic form) is streptomycin, although gentamicin is an acceptable substitute [83]. The usual treatment for meningeal infection has been chloramphenicol plus streptomycin, but third-generation cephalosporins may prove to be effective.

Prevention

Avoiding exposure to the organism is the best prevention of tularemia. Wild animals should not be skinned or dressed using bare hands; special care is needed when the animal appeared ill. Gloves, masks, and protective eyecovers should be worn when performing such tasks and when disposing of dead animals brought home by household pets. Wild game should be cooked thoroughly prior to ingestion. Well water or other water that might be contaminated by dead animals should not be used. The most important measure to avoid tick bites in infested areas is wearing clothing that is tight at the wrists and ankles and that covers most of the body. No effective vaccine is currently available [84].

Plague

Background

Plague is primarily a zoonotic infection. *Yesinia pestis* is transmitted among the natural animal reservoirs (predominantly rodents) by flea bites or by ingestion of contaminated animal tissues. The most common clinical form is an acute febrile lymphadenitis called bubonic plague. Less common forms include septicemic, pneumonic, and meningeal plague.

Recognition

One of the most serious complication of bubonic plague is secondary pneumonia. The infection reaches the lungs by hematogenous spread of bacteria from the bubo. In addition to high mortality, plague pneumonia is highly contagious by airborne transmission. It presents in the setting of fever and lymphadenopathy as cough, chest pain, and often hemoptysis. Radiologically there is patchy bronchopneumonia, cavities, or confluent consolidation [85]. The sputum is usually purulent and contains plague bacilli. Primary inhalation pneumonia is rare but is a potential threat following exposure to a patient with plague who has a cough. Recent cases in the USA resulted from exposure to sick domestic cats that had pneumonia or submandibular abcesses. Plague pneumonia is invariably fatal when antibiotic therapy is delayed more than 1 day after the onset of the illness.

A bacteriologic diagnosis is readily made in most patients by smear and culture of a bubo aspirate. A serologic test involving the passive hemagglutination test utilizing fraction I of *Y. pestis* can be performed on acute and convalescent phase serum.

Management

A 10-day course of intramuscular streptomycin is the treatment of choice. Tetracycline is a satisfactory alternative [86].

Prevention

Patients with plague must be placed in strict respiratory isolation for at least 48 hours after the initiation of therapy or until the sputum culture is negative. The bubo aspirate and blood must be handled with gloves and with care to avoid aerosolization of these infected fluids. A formalin-killed vaccine, Plague Vaccine USP (Cutter Laboratories, Berkeley, CA 94710, USA) is available.

ENVIRONMENTAL SOURCES

Sporotrichosis

Background

Sporotrichosis is an endemic fungal infection caused by *Sporothrix schenckii*. Infection begins when the fungus is inoculated into a site of skin injury and produces an ulcerated, verrucous, or erythematous nodule, sometimes associated with local lymphatic spread. On rare occasions the fungus is inhaled and it causes a granulomatous pneumonitis that often cavitates, producing a clinical pattern very similar to tuberculosis. The fungus may also disseminate hematogenously and cause isolated osteoarticular, central nervous system, or ocular lesions in the normal host, or widespread, multifocal disease in the immunocompromized host. *S. schenckii* is mostly isolated from soil, plants, or plant products such as straw and wood. A conspicuous host is sphagnum moss.

Most cases are related to occupational or avocational exposure to these materials, typically through gardening or farming.

Recognition

Patients with pulmonary sporotrichosis are occasionally asymptomatic but will usually have a productive cough. Low-grade fever or weight loss. The chest radiograph reveals unilateral or bilateral cavitary lesions usually with an associated parenchymal infiltrate. Pleural effusions and hilar enlargement are occasionally noted [87]. Gram stain of sputum or bronchial washings will sometimes reveal characteristic yeast appearances, and sputum culture will usually yield the organism [88]. Untreated, the cavities of pulmonary sporotrichosis will gradually enlarge.

Management

The pulmonary form of the disease must be treated with systemic amphotericin (amphotericin B); cure of more advanced disease may require surgical resection of the affected section of lung.

Prevention

There are no documented measures that have been shown to prevent sporotrichosis effectively although epidemics that are caused by mine timbers, thorned plants (especially roses), hay, straw, and armadillos have all been described.

Coccidioidomycosis

Background

Coccidioidomycosis is endemic in certain areas of North, Central, and South America. It resembles tuberculosis in its pathologic manifestations [89]. A notorious site is the San Joaquin valley of California.

Recognition

Of those infected, 10% are asymptomatic or have illness indistinguishable from ordinary upper respiratory infections [90] and 40% develop symptoms of a primary infection 1–3 weeks after exposure. Symptoms comprise cough, sputum production, chest pain, malaise, fever, chills, night sweats, anorexia, weakness and arthralgias. Chest radiographs show minimal changes, patchy infiltrates, frank pneumonia, or pleural effusion. Hilar nodes may be prominent. About 5% will develop nodules; some will develop progressive pneumonia with a fatal outcome, others chronic pulmonary disease [91]. About 0.5% develop disseminated (extrapulmonary) disease involving musculoskeletal and central nervous system [92]. The skin is a common target organ in disseminated coccidioidomycosis.

Coccidioides immitis organisms can be demonstrated by examination of tissues and culture with relative ease. The mycelial phase antigen coccidioidin is most useful in detecting humoral antibody [93]. Serum IgM precipitins can be demonstrated by tube precipitin, latex agglutination, ELISA, or immunodiffusion methods. These antibodies occur 1–3 weeks after the onset of symptoms of primary infection and disappear after 4 months. Positive skin tests (>5 mm induration) to coccidioidal antigens are detectable 2–21 days after the first symptoms appear, usually before the first serologic reactions are detectable [94].

Management

Pulmonary involvement of the infection requires systemic treatment with amphotericin. The new oral azoles, such as itraconazole, are reasonable alternatives [95].

Prevention

No control measures have been shown to be effective in this disease, and the incidence of infection will likely rise over time because of the rapidly growing population in endemic areas of the US sunbelt states and Latin America, and the on-going increases in mobility and travel. In addition, there are occasional marked periodic clusters of cases: after dust storms, or cycles of drought followed by heavy rains, which facilitate spore formation. The only instances of person-to-person transmission have been in special circumstances when the fungus reverts from its tissue mycelial phase to its airborne spore form in contaminated secretions. An example of such transmission is drainage of pus into the interior of a cast, a moist environment where aerial structures can develop. The spores are then released into the air when the cast is opened [96].

Non-tuberculous mycobacteriosis

Background

Most of the non-tuberculous mycobacteria species are ubiquitous. They have been found in soil, water, domestic and wild animals, milk, and other foodstuffs. Despite their widespread distribution in nature, many of the potentially pathogenic mycobacterial species appear to be relatively more common in certain geographic locations. Most infections appear to be acquired by aspiration or inoculation of the organisms from a natural reservoir. There is little evidence of person-to-person transmission of disease [97]. Although there are exceptions, serious infections that are caused by non-tuberculous mycobacteria tend to occur more commonly in males, in adults of middle age or older, and in persons with one or more predisposing conditions.

Recognition

Individual patients pose unique problems, and much time and effort may be required to produce a specific diagnosis. The patient's illness should be consistent with one or more of the syndromes associated with the non-tuberculous mycobacteria, and other causes of disease such as *Mycobacterium tuberculosis* or fungi should be excluded. The species of the mycobacterium isolated is crucial. Certain species are rarely, if ever, associated with human disease whereas other species are seldom environmental contaminants and, therefore, demand further attention. The site of origin of a positive culture is equally crucial, and the quantity of culture growth is important. For patients with a radiographic cavitary infiltrate, definite non-tuberculous mycobacteria disease is considered to be present when both of the following apply:

- two or more sputum samples (or sputum and a bronchial washing) are smear positive for acid-fast bacilli (AFB) and/or result in moderate to heavy growth on culture
- other plausible causes for the disease process have been excluded, e.g. fungal disease, malignancy, tuberculosis.

In the presence of a non-cavitary infiltrate not known to be caused by another disease, non-tuberculous mycobacterial lung disease is considered to be present when all of the following apply:

- two or more sputum samples (or sputum and a bronchial washing) are AFB smear positive and/or result in moderate to heavy growth on culture
- failure of the sputum cultures to convert to negative with either bronchial hygiene or 2 weeks of specific mycobacterial drug therapy
- other plausible causes for the disease have been excluded.

The important species in causing disease are *M. kansasii*, *M. simiae*, *M. scrofulaceum*, *M. sculgai*, *M. xenopi*, *M. malmoense*, *M. haemophilum*, *M. avian-intracellulare* complex and the rapidly growing mycobacteria such as *M. fortuitum*, *M. chelonae*.

Management and prevention

There are no controlled trials defining optimal treatment regimens for non-tuberculous disease and expert advice should be sought as *in vitro* susceptibility studies are usually unhelpful in this context. Various regimens for treatment and prophylaxis have been advocated [98,99].

Legionellosis

Background

In 1976, an outbreak of pneumonia occurred at a hotel at the site of the American Legion Convention in Philadelphia [100]. A total of 221 persons were affected and 43 died. The causative organism, *Legionella pneumophila*, was subsequently diagnosed in this outbreak and linked to the air-conditioning system of the hotel. The mode of transmission of legionellae to humans is likely to be multiple and there is evidence for aerosolization, aspiration, and even lung instillation during respiratory tract manipulation [101,102,103].

Recognition

Legionella infection presents in two very different forms: Pontiac fever and pneumonia (legionnaires' disease). It is not known why these two different forms occur, but inoculum of the organism, differing modes of transmission, and host factors are probably important.

Pontiac fever is an acute self-limiting influenza-like illness without pneumonia [104]. The incubation period is 24–48 hours and the attack rate of those exposed is quite high (>90%). The predominant symptoms are malaise, myalgias, fever, chills, and headache. Non-productive cough, dizziness, and nausea have also been noted. The chest radiograph

remains clear. Only symptomatic therapy is required and complete recovery within 1 week is the rule.

Pneumonia is the predominant clinical finding in legionnaires' disease. The disease encompasses a broad spectrum of illness ranging from a mild cough and slight fever to stupor with widespread pulmonary infiltrates and multisystem failure. The incubation period for legionnaires' disease ranges from 2 to 10 days. Early in the illness, patients experience non-specific symptoms including fever, malaise, myalgia, anorexia, and headache. The cough is initially mild and only slightly productive. Occasionally the sputum may be streaked with blood. Watery diarrhea is seen in about 25–50% and neurologic involvement ranges from headache to encephalopathy [105].

Physical examination typically reveals rales early in the course of the disease and the signs of consolidation. Hypotension is frequently seen and fever is virtually always present. Although the clinical presentation is non-specific, the following should raise the possibility of legionnaires' disease in patient with an undiagnosed pneumonia:

- Gram staining of respiratory secretions shows neutrophils in large numbers but few if any organisms
- hyponatremia (serum sodium less than 130 mmol/l)
- failure to respond to β-lactam and aminoglycoside antibiotics
- occurrence in a hospital or an environment in which the potable water supply is known to be contaminated with legionellae.

The vast majority of patients have abnormal chest radiographic findings on presentation. The initial involvement is usually unilateral and with lower lobe predominance, and the initial infiltrate is typically alveolar, and segmental-lobar or diffuse and patchy. It progresses to more widespread consolidation over the following several days. The extent of radiographic infiltration does not correlate well with the severity of the clinical manifestations or with the ultimate outcome [106]. The period required for complete clearing of the infiltrates ranges from 1 to 4 months.

The definitive method for diagnosis is isolation of the organism from respiratory secretions by buffered charcoal yeast extract agar [107]. Direct fluorescent antibody stain is a rapid diagnostic test but the sensitivity is less than that of culture. Serological detection of antibodies (e.g. by ELISA) is less useful. Although urinary antigen provides a good rapid test, it is only available for sero-group 1 species, which account for about 80% of *L. pneumophila* infection.

Management

Erythromycin has been the antibiotic of choice historically. However, the newer macrolides (azithromycin, clarithromycin) and quinolones (ciprofloxacin) have superior *in vitro* activity and improved pharmacokinetics when compared to erythromycin [108,109]. Although controlled studies are not available, combination therapy with a macrolide or a quinolone combined with rifampicin are recommended as initial treatment.

Prevention

Superheat and flush has emerged as the most widely used method for disinfection of water distribution systems in the control of legionella growth [110], and hyperchlorination is no longer recommended. Routine environmental culturing for legionella should be performed in hospitals in which organ and bone marrow transplants are performed, given the high risk for legionnaires' disease in these patients [111].

DIFFICULT CASE

The author and editors are indebted to Dr C. Ellis for the following case.

History

A previously fit 32-year-old maintenance engineer developed an influenza-like illness in early summer, and was admitted to hospital 5 days later following the onset of pleuritic pain. He was then pyrexial and confused. He responded to a macrolide antibiotic and was later shown to have been suffering from Q-fever. Two colleagues experienced a similar illness in the same month, and both were shown subsequently to have unequivocally raised titers in serum for Q-fever. They too responded to a macrolide antibiotic, but all three men were unwell for several months, and all experienced undue fatigue for up to 12 months after all objective abnormalities had resolved.

During the 3 weeks before the onset of symptoms, all three men had worked on a radio mast surrounded by pasture on which sheep had been grazing. Furthermore, on one occasion they recalled that waste from a nearby dairy (a mixture of milk, water, and excreta) had been spread on the pasture while they were working. They argued that their employer should have taken special measures to protect them against hazardous airborne pathogens, and that 'washings' from the dairy should not have been spread in their working environment. It transpired, however, that there was no evidence of relevant infection among the livestock in the pasture or in the dairy over the period in question, and so the employer contended that there had been no reason to take any special precaution.

Issues

The chief issues here are whether this man's infection was truly occupational in origin, and whether there was a recognisable risk of Q-fever from the nature of this work? If so, should the employer have taken preventive measures?

Comment

The contributors to this volume were of the unanimous opinion that the infection was primarily occupational in origin, mostly with a high degree of confidence. The majority, however, did not consider such an outcome to be predictable from work of this nature. Individuals commented that a period of lambing might increase the risk of exposure by inhalation, that ingestion of contaminated food (perhaps unpasteurized milk) was a more plausible cause than inhaled material, and that 'organic' fertilizer of this type should not be spread in the presence of other workers.

The most likely sequence of events in the cycle of transmission of *C. burnettii* to humans is that the organism is maintained in ticks and other arthropods. These ectoparasites infest domestic and other animals including a variety of small mammals. Infected domestic ungulates are usually asymptomatic although abortion may result. The heavily infected placenta contaminates the environment at the time of parturition. Air samples may remain positive for up to 2 weeks after parturition and viable organisms may be present in the soil for periods up to 150 days; consequently, the sheep could have been the source of these infections. Humans are infected by the inhalation of contaminated aerosols, and because of the close proximity of these workers to the waste spread over the pastures, their infections are more likely to have come from this source. They are likely to have been occupational in origin but could not have been predicted by the nature of the work that the men were doing.

SUMMARY POINTS

Recognition
- Characteristic symptoms and signs of each disease should alert clinicians to the possibility of an occupational cause.
- Special emphasis on the occupational and environmental history is of utmost importance in suspecting such disease entities.

Management
- The natural history of the diseases described should form the basis for the management principles, specific antimicrobial therapy, and supportive treatment.

- It is important to bear in mind that some diseases may have systemic involvement in addition to their pulmonary manifestations.

Prevention
- Where there are safe vaccines available for occupationally acquired infections, a risk-assessment exercise should be carried out to evaluate whether they should be made available and recommended.
- The potential for transmission of any pathogens to humans in the workplace should be carefully assessed, controlled, and regulated.

REFERENCES

1. Douglas RG Jr. Influenza in man. In: Kilbourne ED, ed. *Influenza Viruses and Influenza*, p. 395. London: Academic Press, 1975.
2. Stuart-Harris CH. Twenty years of influenza epidemics. *Am Rev Respir Dis* 1961; 83: 54.
3. Schild GC, Dowdle WR. Influenza virus characterization and diagnostic serology. In: Kilbourne ED, ed. *Influenza Viruses and Influenza* p. 315. London: Academic Press, 1975.
4. Little JW, Hall WJ, Douglas RG et al. Amantadine effect on peripheral airways abnormalities in influenza. *Ann Intern Med* 1976; 85: 177.
5. Hoskins TW, Davies JR, Allchin A et al. Controlled trial of inactivated influenza vaccine containing the A/Hong Kong strain during an outbreak of influenza due to the A/England/42/72 strain. *Lancet* 1973; 2: ii; 116.
6. Stiver HG, Graves P, Eickhoff TC et al. Efficacy of Hong Kong vaccine in preventing England variant influenza A in 1972. *N Engl J Med* 1973; 289: 1267.
7. Ong ELC, Bilton D, Abbot J, Webb AK et al. Influenza vaccination in adults with cystic fibrosis. *Br Med J* 1991; 28: 309.
8. Ong ELC, Ellis ME, Webb AK et al. Infection exacerbations of young adults with cystic fibrosis: role of viruses and atypical micro-organisms. *Thorax* 1989; 44: 739–742.
9. Dorell L, Hassan ISA, Marshall S et al. Clinical and serological responses to an inactivated influenza vaccine in adults with HIV infection, diabetes, obstructive airways disease, elderly adults and healthy volunteers. *Int J AIDS STD* 1997; 8: 776–779.
10. Barker W, Raubertas R, Menegus M et al. Case control study of influenza vaccine effectiveness in preventing pneumonia hospitalisation among older persons, Monroe county, New York 1989–1992. In: Hannoun C, Kendal AP, Klenk HD et al. eds. *Options for the Control of Influenza* II, pp. 143–151. North Holland Elsevier, 1998.
11. Dolin R, Reichman RC, Madore HP et al. A controlled trial of amantadine and rimantadine in the prophylaxis of influenza A infection. *N Engl J Med* 1982; 307: 580.
12. Dolin R. Antiviral chemotherapy and chemoprophylaxis. *Science* 1985; 227: 1296–1303.

13. Mercat A, Nguyen J, Dautzenberg B. An outbreak of pneumococcal pneumonia in two men's shelters. *Chest* 1991; 99: 147–151.
14. Berdal BP, Scheel O, Ogaard AR et al. Spread of subclinical *Chlamydia pneumoniae* infection in a closed community. *Scand J Infect Dis* 1992; 24: 431–436.
15. Winter H, Pfisterer RM. Inhalation anthrax in a textile worker: Non-fatal course. *Schweiz Med Wochenschr* 1991; 121: 832–835.
16. Pfisterer RM. An anthrax epidemic in Switzerland. Clinical, diagnositic and epidemiological aspects of a mostly forgotten disease. *Schweiz Med Wochenschr* 1991; 813–825.
17. Ronaghy HA, Azadeh B, Kohout E. Penicillin therapy of human cutaneous anthrax. *Curr Ther Res* 1972; 14: 721–725.
18. Turnball PC. Anthrax vaccines: past, present and future. *Vaccine* 1991; 9: 533–539.
19. Stoker MGP, Marmion BP. The spread of Q fever from animals to man. The natural history of a rickettsial disease. *Bull WHO* 1955; 13: 781–806.
20. Dupont HT, Raoult D, Brouqui P et al. Epidemiologic features and clinical presentation of acute Q fever in hospitalised patients: 323 French cases. *Am J Med* 1992; 93: 427–434.
21. Clark WH, Romker MS, Holmes MA et al. Q fever in California VIII. An epidemic of Q fever in a small rural community in Northern California. *Am J Hyg* 1951; 54: 25–34.
22. Gonder JC, Kishimoto RA, Kastello MR et al. Cynomologus monkey model for experimental Q fever infection. *J Infect Dis* 1979; 139: 191–196.
23. Tigertt WD, Benenson AS, Goscheneur WS. Airborone Q fever. *Bacteriol Rev* 1961; 25: 285–293.
24. Feinstein M, Yesner R, Marks JL. Epidemic of Q fever among troops returning from Italy in the spring of 1945. I. Clinical aspects of the epidemic at Fort Patrick Henry, Virginia. *Am J Hyg* 1946; 44: 72–87.
25. Gordon JD, MacKeen AD, Marrie TJ et al. The radiographic features of epidemic and sporadic Q fever pneumonia. *J Can Assoc Radiol* 1984; 35: 293–296.
26. Millar JK. The chest film findings in 'Q' fever- a series of 35 cases. *Clin Radiol* 1978; 329: 371–375.
27. Stein A, Raoult D. Detection of *Coxiella burnetii* by DNA amplification using polymerase chain reaction. *J Clin Microbiol* 1992; 30: 2462–2466.

28. Fiset P, Ormsbee RA, Siberman R et al. A microagglutination technique for detection and measurement of rickettsial antibodies. *Acta Virol* 1969; 13: 60–66.

29. Murphy AM, Field PR. The persistence of complement fixing antibodies to Q fever (*Coxiella burneti*) after infection. *Med J Aust* 1970; 1: 1148–1150.

30. Field PR, Hunt JG, Murphy AM. Detection and persistence of specific IgM antibody to *Coxiella burnetii* by enzyme-linked immunosorbent assay: a comparison with immunofluorescence and complement fixation tests. *J Infect Dis* 1983; 148: 477–487.

31. Brouqui P, Dupont HT, Drancourt M et al. Chronic Q fever: ninety-two cases from France including 27 cases without endocarditis. *Arch Intern Med* 1993; 153: 642–649.

32. Turck WPG. Q fever. In: Braude AL, Davis CE, Fierer, eds. *Medical Microbiology and Infectious Diseases*, Philadelphia, pp 932–937. Saunders 1981–1998.

33. Pierce TH, Yucht SC, Gorin AB et al. Q fever Pneumonitis: Diagnosis by transbronchoscopic lung biopsy. *West J Med* 1979; 130: 453–455.

34. D'Angelo LJ, Hetherington R. Q fever treated with erythromycin. *Br Med J* 1979; ii: 305–306.

35. Ellis ME, Dunbar EM. In vivo response of acute Q fever to erythromycin. *Thorax* 1982; 37: 867–868.

36. Worswick D, Marmion BP. Antibody response in acute and chronic Q fever and in subjects vaccinated against Q fever. *J Med Microbiol* 1985; 119: 281–296.

37. Levy PY, Drancourt M, Etienne J et al. Comparision of different antibiotic regimens for therapy of 32 cases of Q fever endocarditis. *Antimicrob Agents Chemother* 1991; 35: 533–537.

38. Grant CG, Ascher MS, Bernard KW et al. Q fever and experimental sheep. *Infect Control* 1985; 6: 122–123.

39. Polydourou K. Q fever in Cyprus-recent progress. *Br Vet J* 1985; 141: 427–430.

40. Corbell MJ. Brucellosis: Epidemiology and prevalence worldwide. In: Young EJ, Corbell MJ, eds. Boca Raton, *Brucellosis: Clinical and Laboratory Aspects*, pp. 25–40. FL: CRC Press 1989.

41. Buchanan TM, Hendricks SL, Patton CM et al. Brucellosis in the United States 1960–1972. An abattoir-associated disease. Part III. Epidemiology and evidence for acquired immunity. *Medicine* 1974; 53: 427–439.

42. Young EJ. Human brucellosis. *Rev Infect Dis*, 1983; 5: 321–342.

43. Naparstek E, Block C, Slavin S. Transmission of brucellosis in bone marrow transplantation. *Lancet* 1982; i: 574–575.

44. Trevor RW, Cluff LE, Peeler RN et al. Brucellosis. 1. Laboratory acquired acute infection. *Arch Intern Med* 1959; 103: 381–397.

45. Staszkiewicz J, Lewis CM, Colville J et al. Outbreak of *Brucella melitensis* among microbiology laboratory workers in a community hospital. *J Clin Microbiol* 1991; 29: 287–290.

46. Mousa ARM, Elhag KM, Khogali M et al. The nature of human brucellosis in Kuwait: Study of 379 cases. *Rev Infect Dis* 1988; 10: 211–217.

47. Lulu AR, Araj GF, Khateeb MI et al. Human brucellosis in Kuwait: a prospective study of 400 cases. *Q J Med* 1988; 66: 39–54.

48. Mili N, Auckenthaler R, Nicod LP. Chronic brucella empyema. Chest 1993; 103: 620–621.

49. Kaufmann AF, Fox MD, Boyce JM et al. Airborne spread of brucellosis. *Ann NY Acad Sci* 1980; 353: 105–114.

50. Al-Jam'a AH, Elbashier AM, Al-Faris SS. Brucella pneumonia. a case report. *Ann Saudi Med* 1993; 13: 74–77.

51. Patel PJ, Al-Suhaibami H, Al-Aska AK et al. The chest radiograph in brucellosis. *Clin Radiol* 1988; 39: 39–41.

52. Lubani MM, Lulu AR, Araj GF et al. Pulmonary brucellosis. *Q J Med* 1989; 71: 319–324.

53. Buchanan TM, Faber LC. 2-Mercaptoethanol brucella agglutination tests: usefulness for predicting recovery from brucellosis. *J Clin Microbiol* 1980; 11: 691–698.

54. Anderson RK, Jenness R, Brumfield HP et al. Brucella-agglutinating antibodies: relation of mercaptoethanol stability to complement fixation. *Science* 1964; 143: 1334–1335.

55. Araj GF, Kaufmann AF. Determination by enzyme-linked immunosorbent assay of immunoglobulin G (IgG), IgM and IgA to *Brucella melitensis* major outer membrane proteins and whole-cell heat killed antigens in sera of patients with brucellosis. *J Clin Microbiol* 1989; 27: 1909–1912.

56. World Health Organization *Sixth Report of the Joint FAO/WHO Expert Committee on Brucellosis*. Geneva: WHO, 1986.

57. Brown GM. The history of the brucellosis eradication programme in the United States. *Ann Sclavo* 1977; 19: 18–34.

58. Escalante JA, Held JR. Brucellosis in Peru. *J Am Vet Med Assoc* 1969; 155: 2146–2152.

59. Esposito AL. Pulmonary infections acquired in the workplace. *Clin Chest Med* 1992; 13: 355–365.

60. Schachter J. *Chlamydia psittaci* – 'reemergence' of a forgotten pathogen. *N Engl J Med* 1986; 315: 189–191.

61. Editorial. Psittacosis. *Br Med J* 1972; i: 1–2.

62. Centers for Disease Control. *Psittacosis Surveillance 19775–1984*. MMWR June 1987.

63. Yung AP. Grayson ML. Psittacosis – a review of 135 cases. *Med J Aust* 1988; 148: 228–233.

64. Schaffner W, Drutz DJ, Duncan GW et al. The clinical spectrum of endemic psittacosis. *Arch Intern Med* 1967; 119: 433–443.

65. Crosse B. Psittacosis. A clinical review. *J Infect* 1990; 21: 251–259.

66. Shapiro DS, Kenney SC, Johnson M et al. Brief report: *Chlyamydia psittaci* endocarditis disgnosed by blood culture. *N Engl J Med* 1992; 326: 1192–1195.

67. Page SR, Stewart JT, Bernstein JJ. A progressive pericardial effusion caused by psittacosis. *Br Heart J* 1988; 66: 87–89.

68. Coll R, Horner I. Cardiac involvement in psittacosis. *Br Med J* 1967; 4: 35–36.

69. Geddes DM, Skeates SJ. Ornitosis pneumonia associated with haemolysis *Br J Dis Chest* 1977; 71: 135–137.

70. Shee CD. Cerebellar disturbance in psittacosis. *Postgard Med J* 1988; 64: 382–383.

71. Sahn SA. Pleural effusions in the atypical pneumonias. *Semin Respir Infect* 1988; 3: 322–334.

72. Fraser RG, Pare JAP, Pare PD et al. *Diagnosis of the Chest*. Philadelphia, PA: Saunders, 1991.

73. Schacter J. Chlamydia. In: Rose NR, de Macario EL, Fahey JL et al. eds. *Manual of Clinical Laboratory Immunology*. Washington, DC: American Society for Microbiology, 1992.

74. Grimes JE. Zoonoses acquired from pet birds. *Vet Clin* 1987; 17: 209–218.

75. Centers for Disease Control and Prevention. Human psittacosis linked to a bird distributor in Mississippi,

Massachusetts and Tennesse, USA. *MMWR* 1992; 41: 793–797.

76. Boyce JM. Recent trends in the epidemiology of tularaemia in the United States. *J Infect Dis* 1975; 131: 197–199.

77. Sanders CV, Hahn R. Analysis of 106 cases of tularaemia. *J Louisians State Med Soc* 1968; 120: 391–393.

78. Cox SK, Everett ED. Tulaemia. An analysis of 25 cases. *Missouri Med* 1981; 78: 70–74.

79. Syrjala H, Kujala P, Myllyla V *et al*. Airborne transmission of tularaemia in farmers. *Scand J Infect Dis* 1985; 17: 371–375.

80. Evans ME, Gregory DW, Schaffner W *et al*. Tularemia: a 30 year experience with 88 cases. *Medicine* 1985; 64: 251–269.

81. Snyder MJ. Immune response to *Francisella tularensis*. In: Rose NR, Friedman H, Fahey JL, eds. *Manual of Clinical Laboratory Immunology*, pp. 377–378. Washington, DC: Americian Society for Microbiology 1986.

82. Sato T, Fujita H, Ohara Y *et al*. Microagglutination test for early and specific serodiagnosis of tularaemia. *J Clin Microbiol* 1990; 28: 2372–2374.

83. Mason WL, Eigelsbach HT, Little SF *et al*. Treatment of tularaemia, including pulmonary tularaemia and gentamicin. *Am Rev Respir Dis* 1980; 121; 39–45.

84. Burke DS. Immunization against tularaemia: Analysis of the effectiveness of live *Francisella tularensis* vaccine in prevention of laboratory acquired tularaemia. *J Infect Dis* 1977; 135: 55–60.

85. Centers for Disease Control and Prevention. Pneumonic plague – Arizona. *JAMA* 1992; 268: 2146–2147.

86. Welty TK, Grabman J, Kompare E *et al*. Nineteen cases of plague in Arizona. A spectrum including ecthyma gangrenosum due to plague and plague in pregnancy. *West J Med* 1985; 142: 641–646.

87. Pluss JL, Opal SM. Pulmonary sporotrichosis: review of treatment and outcome. *Medicine* 1986: 65: 143–153.

88. Kosinki RM, Axelrod P, Rex JH *et al*. *Sprothrix schenckii* fungaemia without disseminated sporotrichosis. *J Clin Microbiol* 1992; 30: 501–503.

89. Puckett TF. Hyphae of *Coccidioides immitis* in tissues of the human host. *Am Rev Tuberc* 1954; 70: 320.

90. Smith CE, Beard RR, Whiting EG *et al*. Varieties of coccidioidal infection in relation to the epidemiology and control of the disease. *Am J Public Health* 1946; 36: 1394.

91. Casellino RA, Blank N. Pulmonary coccidioidomycosis: The wide spectrum of roentgenographic manifestations. *Calif Med* 1968; 109: 41.

92. Bouza E, Dreyer JS, Hewitt WL *et al*. Coccidiodal meningitis: An analysis of thirty-one cases and review of the literature. *Medicine* 1981; 60: 139.

93. Pappagianis D, Zimmer BL. Serology of coccidioidomycosis. *Clin Microbiol Rev* 1990; 3: 247.

94. Galgiani JN and the Valley Fever Vaccine Group. Development of dermal hypersensitivity to coccidioidal antigens associated with repeated skin testing. *Am Rev Respir Dis* 1986; 134: 1035.

95. Drutz D. Amphotericin B in the treatment of coccidioidomycosis. *Drugs* 1983; 26: 337.

96. Eckmann BH, Schaefer GL, Huppert M. Bedside interhuman transmission of coccidioidomycosis via growth on fomites: an epidemic involving sick persons. *Am Rev Respir Dis* 1964; 89: 175.

97. Wolinsky E. Nontuberculous mycobacteria and associated diseases. *Am Rev Respir Dis* 1979; 119: 107–159.

98. Wallace RJ Jr, O'Brien R, Glassroth J *et al*. Diagnosis and treatment of disease caused by nontuberculosis mycobacteria. *Am Rev Respir Dis* 1990; 142: 940–953.

99. Ong ELC. Prophylaxis against disseminated *Mycobacterium avium* complex in AIDS. *J Infect* 1999; 38: 6–8.

100. Fraser DW, Tsai T, Orenstein W *et al*. Legionnaires' disease: description of an epidemic of pneumonia. *N Engl J Med* 1977; 297: 1189–1197.

101. Dondero TJ Jr, Rendtorff RC, Mallison GF *et al*. An outbreak of legionnaires' disease associated with a contaminated air-conditioning cooling tower. *N Engl J Med* 1980; 302: 365–370.

102. Woo AH, Goetz A, Yu VL. Transmission of Legionella by respiratory equipment aerosol generating devices. *Chest* 1992; 102: 1586–1590.

103. Blatt SP, Parkinson MD, Pace E *et al*. Nosocomial legionnaires' disease: Aspiration as a primary mode of transmission. *Am J Med* 1993; 95: 16–22.

104. Mangione EJ, Remus RS, Tait KA *et al*. An outbreak of Pontiac fever related to whirlpool use, Michigan 1982. *JAMA* 1985; 535–539.

105. Yu VL, Kroboth FJ, Shonnard J. *et al*. Legionnaires' disease: new clinical perspective from a prospective study. *Am J Med* 1982; 73: 357–361.

106. Kroboth FJ, Yu VL, Reddy S *et al*. Clinicoradiographic correlations with the extent of legionnaries' disease, *AJR* 1983; 141: 263–268.

107. Zuravleff JJ, Yu VL, Shonnard J *et al*. Diagnosis of Legionnaires' disease: an update of laboratory methods with new emphasis on isolation by culture. *JAMA* 1983; 250: 1981–1985.

108. Millar MF, Martin J, Johnson P *et al*. Erythromycin uptake and accumulation by human polymorphonuclear leukocytes and efficacy of erythromycin in killing of ingested legionella pneumophila. *J Infect Dis* 1984; 149: 714–718.

109. Dorrel L, Fulton B, Ong ELC. Legionnaires' pneumonia–salvage therapy with azithromycin. *Thorax* 1994; 49: 620–621.

110. Muraca PW, Yu VL, Goetz A. Disinfection of water distribution systems for Legionella: a review of application procedures and methodologies. *Infect Control Hosp Epidemiol* 1990; 11: 79–88.

111. Korvick J, Yu VL. Legionnaires' disease: an emerging surgical problem. *Ann Thorac Surg* 1987; 43: 341–347.

18 | ASPHYXIATION

Dennis Shusterman

INTRODUCTION

Definitions

Asphyxia, defined as 'impaired or absent exchange of oxygen' [1], is a toxicologic hazard in a variety of occupational and environmental settings. Asphyxiants (agents capable of producing asphyxia) are principally gases, the majority of which lack any warning properties (color, odor, or respiratory tract irritancy). Because of the ability of asphyxiants to produce, on the one hand, non-specific symptoms mimicking influenza (flu) or other common disorders and, on the other, incapacitation, anoxic brain injury, and even death, successful recognition, treatment, and prevention of asphyxia is a major industrial and environmental health concern.

Asphyxia, or more generally tissue hypoxia, can be divided physiologically into several types depending upon supplied oxygen (O_2) tension, the O_2-carrying capacity of the blood, local perfusion, and tissue O_2 extraction (Fig. 18.1). In the hypoxic state, the volume of O_2 extracted per volume of blood circulated may be less than normal (histotoxic hypoxia), greater than normal (stagnant hypoxia), or maintained at near-normal levels at the cost of reduced tissue O_2 tension (anemic hypoxia and hypoxic hypoxia). In histotoxic, anemic, and hypoxic hypoxia, compensatory cardiovascular reflexes (increased heart rate and stroke volume) typically act, at least initially, toward normalizing O_2 delivery. In stagnant hypoxia, it is the failure of the cardiovascular system to maintain adequate circulation that produces the hypoxic state. These distinctions are based upon the physiologist's classification of the form of disruption of O_2 delivery or utilization [2].

The toxicologist, by comparison, normally classifies asphyxiant agents according to their mode of action:

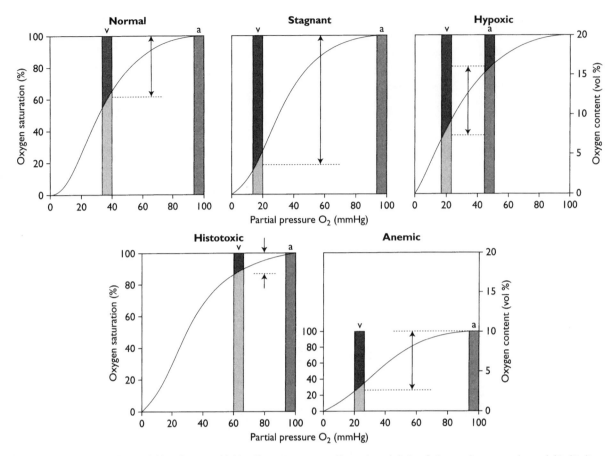

Fig. 18.1 Composition of arterial (a) and venous (v) blood in various types of hypoxia and their relation to the oxygen–hemoglobin binding curve. These relationships, although potentially demonstrable via simultaneous arterial and venous blood gas determination, are presented here for conceptual purposes. Adapted from Lenfant [2].

Table 18.1 Classification of asphyxiants. Adapted from Shusterman [4]

Type of hypoxia produced	Type of asphyxiant	
	Simple	Chemical
Hypoxic	Carbon dioxide, nitrogen, methane	
Anemic		Carbon monoxide, methemogobin-formers
Histotoxic		Hydrogen cyanide, hydrogen sulfide

simple asphyxiants produce tissue hypoxia by displacing O_2 from the inspired atmosphere, whereas chemical asphyxiants produce tissue hypoxia by interacting with biological molecules and there by interfering with normal O_2 transport or utilization [3].

Table 18.1 shows the relationship between agent and type of hypoxia for the most common asphyxiants.

Simple asphyxiants

Carbon dioxide (CO_2), nitrogen (N_2), methane (CH_4) and other simple asphyxiants produce hypoxia by the physical displacement of O_2 from an inspired atmosphere rather than by any direct biochemical effect. The resulting decreased inspired O_2 concentration produces a state of hypoxic hypoxia.

Chemical asphyxiants

Carbon monoxide (CO), hydrogen cyanide (HCN), hydrogen sulfide (H_2S), and methemoglobin (MetHb)-forming agents (particularly nitrogen oxides, NO_x) are all classified as chemical asphyxiants, since they disrupt either O_2 transport or utilization at a molecular level. Despite their similarities, these agents differ in the type of hypoxia they produce.

- Both carboxy- and met-hemoglobinemia reduce the O_2-carrying capacity of the blood; hence, the conditions resemble anemic hypoxia (the comparison is explored in greater detail below).

- HCN and H_2S act at the tissue level by poisoning cytochrome c oxidase, the terminal enzyme of the electron transport chain involved in cellular respiration. In HCN or H_2S poisoning, even adequate inspired O_2 concentration, respiratory gas exchange, hemoglobin O_2 binding/release, and blood flow cannot ensure proper tissue O_2 utilization; HCN and H_2S therefore produce histotoxic hypoxia.

In clinical practice, a severely asphyxiated patient may also suffer secondary stagnant hypoxia because of cardiopulmonary compromise. The type (or types) of hypoxia produced by an asphyxiant is important because it critically influences what mode of treatment is likely to be effective. Fortunately this may be deduced by the laboratory findings, as will be established below.

Clinical features

Asphyxiants produce a spectrum of clinical effects that are essentially similar irrespective of the causal pathway but are largely non-specific. They range from minor common symptoms such as headache, dizziness, fatigue and nausea at one extreme, to obtundation, coma, and cardiovascular collapse at the other. For example, wintertime headaches and nausea, easily misdiagnosed as influenza, have been traced in patients seen in inner-city emergency rooms to asphyxia from CO produced by malfunctioning combustion appliances and the inappropriate use of kitchen stoves and ovens for space heating [5].

Central nervous system (CNS) symptoms are particularly prominent, with headache, lightheadedness, cognitive impairment and then confusion preceding syncope and coma. Nausea and fatigue are common but similarly non-specific. Cardiovascular effects, including precipitation of angina and enhanced ventricular ectopy, have been demonstrated among subjects with preexisting coronary artery disease with experimentally produced carboxyhemoglobin (COHb) levels as low as 2% (angina) and 6% (ectopy) [6,7].

The ranges of susceptibility and tolerance can be wide, at least with mild asphyxia, with some subjects remaining apparently unaffected while others are quite distressed despite sharing the same polluted and/or O_2-deficient environment. In smokers with asphyxia from CO poisoning, this may be partly attributable to preexisting high levels of COHb.

Investigation

Laboratory tests

Tissue hypoxia cannot be quantified in the clinical setting, while arterial blood gas analysis (or percu-

taneous oximetry) will give different outcomes according to whether the mechanism of the hypoxic state is histotoxic, stagnant, anemic, or hypoxic. Useful tests in the investigation of asphyxia are consequently discussed within the sections addressing each particular type of asphyxiant.

Imaging

Chest radiographs have limited benefit in the investigation of asphyxia, their chief value being to exclude other causes of arterial O_2 desaturation. The brain is of more specific interest, once the acute asphyxiating episode is passed. Severe asphyxiation (i.e. exposures producing loss of consciousness) may produce lesions in the basal ganglia (specifically the globus pallidus), as well as in cerebral white matter. They have been demonstrated on both computed tomography (CT) and magnetic resonance imaging (MRI) scans, although the latter may be more sensitive [8]. They have been described most consistently after CO intoxication, and less commonly with cyanide poisoning, but may be seen after any prolonged insult producing cerebral hypoxia/hypoperfusion, including cardiogenic or septic shock.

General principles of management

The shared therapeutic approach to all asphyxiants includes removal from exposure, decontamination (e.g. if gastrointestinal or cutaneous exposure to cyanide salts is suspected), basic cardiopulmonary support, and oxygenation. Standard practice during prehospital care is to provide any patient suspected of suffering asphyxiation who has a patent airway and spontaneous adequate respirations with high-flow O_2, normally in the form of a 'non-rebreather' mask. For others, intubation may be necessary, particularly among smoke inhalation victims and those with severe obtundation. Beyond normobaric oxygenation, modes of therapy have included hyperbaric O_2 and, more recently, isocapneic hyperventilation. The controversy surrounding hyperbaric oxygen (HBO) is reviewed below in discussing therapy for CO intoxication.

SIMPLE ASPHYXIANTS

Carbon dioxide

Carbon dioxide (CAS 124–38–9), an odorless and colorless gas, is a byproduct of aerobic metabolism, the fermentation of carbohydrates, and the complete combustion of carbonaceous materials. Industrial processes in which high concentrations of CO_2 are encountered include food processing (particularly breweries and wineries), and metallurgical or biomedical settings in which liquid or solid CO_2 is allowed to off-gas without adequate ventilation [9]. It is also produced, along with the more toxic CO, by combustion of carbonaceous materials, and it is generated environmentally by the slow oxidation of underground coal and by volcanic emissions into stagnant lakes (see Box 18.1). It is normally present in the ambient atmosphere at approximately 350 ppm (i.e. 0.035%).

In indoor settings, somewhat higher than ambient concentrations are usual; the actual concentration is used as a surrogate marker of the adequacy of building ventilation relative to human occupancy. Whereas indoor CO_2 levels exceeding 800–1000 ppm may signal an unhealthy accumulation of other indoor air pollutants, asphyxia caused by CO_2 itself occurs at much higher levels of exposure. At very high levels (>20% or 200 000 ppm), CO_2 can act as a mucous membrane irritant by dissolving in mucous membrane water to give carbonic acid, thus exhibiting mild warning qualities [10]. However, such irritation is highly non-specific and should not be relied upon to guarantee the safety of CO_2-exposed workers. At somewhat lower concentrations (>2% or 20 000 ppm), CO_2 stimulates ventilation by its lowering of blood pH and its subsequent effect on the carotid chemoreceptor apparatus [11].

Nitrogen

Nitrogen (CAS 7727–37–0) is a primary constituent of the earth's atmosphere, constituting approximately 78% of sea level air, by volume. Except in situations of altered barometric pressure, N_2 lacks intrinsic toxicity. Among underseas divers, N_2 is responsible for nitrogen narcosis ('rapture of the deep') and decompression sickness (the 'bends') [12]. These effects are reviewed in Chapter 20. Nitrogen is used to control ripening and spoilage of fruits and vegetables and may be deliberately injected into closed spaces (e.g., railroad cars, food storage compartments, segments of low-grade combustion in coal mines) to exclude O_2. It is therefore

a potential health and safety concern in agriculture, food processing, transportation and (rarely) coal mines [13]. In addition, N_2 is used in metallurgy, oil-field production, and chemical synthesis [9].

Methane

Methane (CAS 74–82–8) is an organic molecule produced by the anaerobic fermentation of organic material. As such, it is frequently encountered in petroleum refineries, wastewater treatment plants, and in underground service work near sewer lines (often in the presence of H_2S); it is the principal component of 'natural gas' [4]. Methane (as well as the related short-chain hydrocarbon gases ethane, propane, butane, etc.) has minimal intrinsic toxicity, but like other simple asphyxiants it has the potential for displacing O_2 from the inspired atmosphere. Of at least equal concern is the flammability of aliphatic hydrocarbon gases, leading to utility companies' practice of odorizing natural gas, using either a mercaptan or thiophene additive, to warn consumers of gas leaks [14].

Pathophysiology

Asphyxia by simple asphyxiants (i.e. significant O_2 displacement) occurs at exposure concentrations in the percent range (i.e. tens of thousands of parts per million). Assuming normal cardiopulmonary function, the initial response to the inhalation of a hypoxic atmosphere will include tachycardia and tachypnea, with increased cardiac output and consequent partial normalization of O_2 delivery. The effects of O_2 deprivation from simple asphyxiants are similar to the effects of altitude, and are reviewed in Table 18.2. In general, symptoms begin with the CNS, followed by exercise intolerance, and then cardiovascular impairment. Despite the similarities of sea level exposure to O_2-deficient atmospheres and that of altitude, there are important differences: 'altitude sickness' includes such specific syndromes as high-altitude pulmonary edema (HAPE) and high-altitude cerebral edema (HACE). Further, aero-

Table 18.2 Effects of acute oxygen deprivation in healthy adults. Adapted from Lipsett *et al.* [15] and Peterson [16].

Inspired oxygen (vol % (torr))[a]	Equivalent altitude (m)	Symptoms
19–16 (145–123)	900–2100	Usually none
16–13 (122–100)	2100–3700	Tachycardia, tachypnea, ± headache
13–10 (99–76)	3700–6000	Dyspnea, fatigue, confusion
10–6 (75–46)	6000–9700	Nausea, vomiting, syncope
<6 (<45)	>9700	Coma, convulsions, death

[a]Normal oxygen partial pressure at sea level: 760 torr × 0.21 = 160 torr

space environments carry with them the hazard of rapid decompression. Altitude-related disorders, which are beyond the scope of this chapter, are reviewed in Chapter 20 and elsewhere [17].

Regardless of the specific identity of any simple asphyxiant(s) present, there is a consistent fractional inspired concentration of O_2 that defines an O_2-deficient atmosphere in regulatory terms. The US Occupational Safety and Health Administration (OSHA), considers any atmosphere containing less that 19.5% O_2, by volume, as being 'oxygen deficient', and any atmosphere containing less that 16% O_2, by volume, as 'oxygen deficient, immediately dangerous to life and health' [18]. Both situations require special respiratory precautions (see Prevention below). Actual physiologic alterations among healthy workers at sea level can be observed with fractional oxygen concentrations less than approximately 16% [15].

Recognition

There are no clinical features of asphyxia attributable to simple asphyxiants other than those attributable to asphyxia in general. The diagnosis consequently relies on prompt recognition that simple asphyxiants have contaminated the environmental atmosphere.

Laboratory tests

Both blood gas measurement and transcutaneous oximetry can be expected to show decreased oxygen saturation with simple asphyxia, regardless of the sample source (i.e. arterial or venous).

Management

Removal from exposure, administration of high-flow O_2, and general supportive therapy provide the basis of appropriate therapy for simple asphyxiant exposure.

CARBON MONOXIDE

Sources and epidemiology

Carbon monoxide (CAS 630–08–0) is a byproduct of the incomplete combustion of carbonaceous materials, including gasoline, coal, natural gas, wood, and plastics, among others. Improperly vented cooking and heating appliances, internal combustion engines, structural fires, tobacco products, and a variety of industrial operations produce CO at potentially toxic levels. Not surprisingly then, CO is one of the most common agents of inadvertent human intoxication, both in the workplace and general environment [19,20].

The discovery of CO is credited to Priestly in America (1772), although observations of the toxicity of 'coal fumes' dates back to Aristotle in the third century BC. The introduction of coal gas as an illuminating fuel in Prussia in the 1790s occasioned laws to protect citizens against its hazards. In 1842 in France, LeBlanc identified CO as the toxic constituent of coal gas, and some 15 years later Claude Bernard first demonstrated that CO reversibly combines with hemoglobin [21]. Over the last 150 years, technology has changed considerably, but CO remains an insidious and persistent threat to health.

In industry, CO is used as a feedstock for the synthesis of methanol, ethylene, aldehydes, isocyanates, acrylates, and phosgene; it is also used in metallurgy and as an industrial fuel [9]. Use of various CO-containing industrial gases derived from the partial combustion of coal and other carbonaceous materials (including synthesis, producer, and blast-furnace gases) continues to pose hazards to workers [22,23]. Occupational exposures to CO also occur among workers in mines (particularly after blasting or fires), petroleum refineries (near catalytic cracking units), pulp mills (near lime kilns and kraft recovery furnaces), and boiler rooms, as well as among those using or repairing internal combustion engines [24]. Of primarily historic significance, coal gas and water gas (also coal-derived) had CO contents approximating 8 and 30%, respectively, and at one time posed hazards in both occupational and home settings [25,26].

Carbon monoxide exposures are of particular concern for structural firefighters, who often enter enclosed spaces in which CO may be present at toxic levels. Although higher CO concentrations are encountered during the 'knockdown' phase of firefighting (when materials are actively burning) than during 'overhaul' (searching for 'hot spots' among smoldering materials), potentially hazardous levels may still be encountered during the latter period [27,28]. Use of respiratory protective gear, however, is often limited to the early phases of firefighting. Industrial hygiene evaluations of exposures to wildlands (outdoor) firefighters have demonstrated, in contrast to their urban counterparts, relatively low levels of CO exposure [29,30]. Among smoke inhalation victims (both fatalities and survivors), evidence of CO intoxication is the rule rather than the exception [31].

Vehicular sources of CO affect both working and non-working populations. Occupationally, virtually any work involving internal combustion engines (including automobile, bus, and truck drivers, mechanics, toll takers, garage attendants, and police officers) entails some exposure to CO [26,32,33]. The placement of exhaust pipes near the front bumpers of aircraft refueling trucks has been linked with at least one CO-related death in an airport employee [34]. The indoor use of propane-powered forklifts is another common source of CO exposure in industry, giving rise to the expression 'warehouse-worker's headache' [35,36].

Among the general public, vehicular emissions are a significant cause of CO poisoning. Malfunctioning exhaust systems, rusted or damaged auto bodies, and the use of pickup truck campers and camper shells as passenger compartments have all been linked with serious CO intoxications, particularly among children [37–40]. The indoor use of gasoline or propane-powered ice resurfacing ('Zamboni') machines has caused CO-related symptoms among both athletes and spectators [41,42]. It has also been documented that the passenger compartments of some ambulances expose both patients and emergency medical personnel to excessive CO levels [43].

Although automotive emissions controls have reduced per-mile CO emissions substantially since 1968, vehicular exhaust continues to be the principal contributor to atmospheric CO pollution in most developed countries [44]. Conditions favoring incomplete combustion of gasoline (with consequent raised CO emissions) include lack of engine repair or tuning, high-altitude and cold weather operation, and excessive idling or stop-and-go driving. Recent controversies have surrounded the use of oxygenated compounds in automotive gasoline (e.g. methyl tertiary butyl ether; MTBE), balancing potential reductions of CO emissions against a well-documented problem with ground water contamination [45,46].

Within residential and commercial buildings, combustion appliances are the principal source of CO exposure. Both fatal and non-fatal human CO poisonings have been documented because of improperly functioning (or inadequately vented) water heaters, furnaces, and kerosene space heaters [47–52]. Influenza-like symptoms (headaches, nausea, and lightheadedness) have been linked to the use of gas stoves and ovens as unvented space heaters during the wintertime [5,53,54]. Other sources of indoor CO exposure include reentrainment of vehicular exhaust through improperly placed building air intakes, indoor use of propane-powered floor buffers, gasoline-powered pressure washers, and concrete saws, and the use of electrical generators employed during storm-related power failures [55–59].

Formerly of considerable concern, the use of CO-containing domestic gas fuels has been phased out in both the USA and western Europe, leading to a dramatic decline in both accidental and suicidal poisonings [60]. In many parts of Asia, by contrast, the use of charcoal as an indoor heating and cooking fuel has led to an endemic problem with CO intoxication [61]. Similar problems have been reported domestically among individuals using charcoal 'hibachis' indoors [62–64].

On a population-weighted basis, the most significant source of CO exposure in the USA is tobacco smoke. So-called 'mainstream' smoke can contain up to 5% CO by volume [65]. 'Sidestream' smoke (the predominant source of environmental exposures) typically carries 70 to 90% of the total per-cigarette CO yield (2 to 11 times that in mainstream smoke) [66]. Indoor CO levels in smoking-allowed areas may exceed 11 ppm, compared with less than 2 ppm in most non-smoking areas [67]. Cigarette smokers normally exhibit significant elevations in the percentage of their hemoglobin combined with CO compared with non-smokers. In a large population-based study, 95% of non-smokers had COHb levels below 2%, while the 95th percentile for COHb among smokers was nearly 9% [68].

An unexpected source of both occupational and avocational CO exposure occurs among individuals using methylene chloride-containing products, particularly paint strippers [69]. Methylene chloride, along with other dihalomethanes, is metabolized to CO in the mammalian liver, leading to potential additive CNS impairment from both solvent narcosis and chemical asphyxia [70,71].

An unavoidable source of CO exposure is that produced within the body. The normal turnover of erythrocytes, specifically the breakdown of the porphyrin rings that make up the heme unit, releases from 0.5 to 1.0 ml CO per hour in normal adults. This endogenously produced CO gives rise to a baseline COHb level of 0.3–0.7%, even in the absence of any external source of exposure. Conditions that increase red blood cell turnover, including hemolytic anemias, polycythemia, blood transfusions (and, to a lesser degree, menstruation), may increase baseline COHb levels substantially [72–74].

Pathophysiology

CO exerts its toxic action via its competitive and allosteric effect on oxygen binding with hemoglobin. Hemoglobin binds CO with over 200 times the avidity with which it binds oxygen, as summarized in the following equilibrium equation:

$$\frac{[\text{COHb}]}{[\text{O}_2\text{Hb}]} = \frac{M \times P_{A\text{CO}}}{P_{A\text{O}_2}}$$

where [COHb] is the CO content of blood (ml/ml), [O_2Hb] is the O_2 content of blood (ml/ml), P_{ACO} is the alveolar partial pressure of CO (torr), P_{AO_2} is the alveolar partial pressure of oxygen (torr) and M is the relative affinity of hemoglobin for CO compared with O_2.

Experimentally, observed values for M (the Haldane constant) vary between approximately 210 and 240 [15]. Therefore, small concentrations of inspired CO can displace a much larger fraction of O_2 molecules from hemoglobin. Of at least equal importance toxicologically is the fact that when CO is bound to the hemoglobin complex, the remaining O_2 molecules are bound more tightly (i.e. they are less readily released to tissues). This 'left shift' in the HbO_2 dissociation curve is illustrated in Figure 18.2, in which 50% carboxyhemoglobinemia is compared with a comparable (50%) reduction of O_2 carrying capacity because of anemia. A CO-induced left shift requires that, for a given degree of O_2 delivery, capillary (and tissue) O_2 tensions fall to lower levels in the CO-intoxicated patient than in a patient with a comparably lowered O_2-carrying capacity caused by anemia alone.

The formula defining the Haldane constant describes the static situation in which CO and O_2 compete for binding sites on hemoglobin molecules

under equilibrium conditions. This situation might be approximated by an animal breathing a fixed-composition atmosphere for an extended period of time or, more appropriately, by hemoglobin in a test tube. The dynamic situation in a living organism must take into account endogenous CO production, ventilation rate, variations in alveolar O_2 pressure related to altitude, and individual differences in hemoglobin concentration and total blood volume. The best-known equation taking all of these variables into account is considerably more complicated than the Haldane formula and has come to be known as the 'Coburn–Forster–Kane' (or CFK) equation [76]. While the mathematical intricacies of modeling CO uptake (and elimination) are beyond the scope of this chapter, it is important to understand the influence of major exposure variables on CO uptake; the effects of exposure concentration and time are illustrated in Figure 18.3 [77].

Recognition

Clinical features

CO intoxication should be suspected among symptomatic individuals with a history of exposure to automobile (or other engine) exhaust, smoke from fires, or use of paint strippers (methylene chloride) without appropriate protective equipment. Even when there is no obvious etiology among patients presenting with headache and nausea or with altered sensorium, the potential for occult CO intoxication should be considered since exposures to malfunctioning (or inappropriately used) combustion appliances is an important source of CO exposure. Many appliance-related CO intoxications occur at the onset of cold weather (i.e. with first use of malfunctioning space heaters), and directed questioning and/or environmental investigation may be necessary.

Most CO-intoxicated individuals with either nonspecific findings or mild obtundation recover without permanent sequelae. However, once loss of consciousness has occurred, the potential for persistent neurologic effects is a major concern. Residual CNS impairment after significant CO intoxication, including the appearance of 'delayed' neuropsychiatric deterioration, was first documented more than 60 years ago [78]. In Korea (where indoor use of charcoal is an important cause of CO poisoning), Choi estimated that 5% of all patients evaluated for CO intoxication (or 24% of those hospitalized) experienced either prolonged coma or neuropsychiatric sequelae of immediate or delayed onset [61]. In the UK, Smith and Brandon found that approximately 11% of hospitalized patients with CO poisoning suffered gross neuropsychiatric sequelae, with

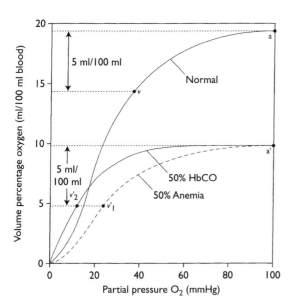

Fig. 18.2 Blood oxygen content as a function of oxygen tension in the normal state (hemoglobin (Hb) 14.4 g/dl (144 g/l)), 50% anemia (Hb 7.2 g/dl (72 g/l)) with an oxygen-binding capacity of 10 ml/dl (100 ml/l) blood, and normal Hb concentration but 50% bound to carbon monoxide (50% HbCO). Symbols a and v refer to the arterial and venous points in normal state; a' is the arterial point for both anemia and carboxyhemoglobinemia; v'₁ is the venous point for anemia and v'₂ the venous point for carboxyhemoglobinemia. Assuming constant tissue oxygen extraction of 5 ml/dl (50 ml/l) blood, note progressively lower venous oxygen tension from normal state to anemia to carboxyhemoglobinemia. Adapted from Bartlett [75].

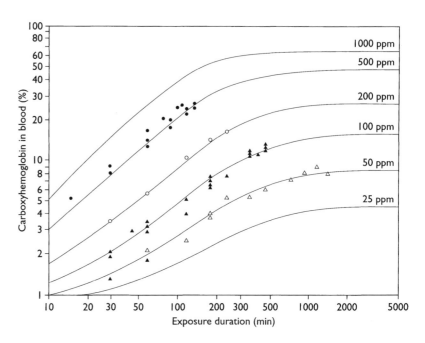

Fig. 18.3 Predicted versus observed carbon monoxide (CO) uptake (carboxyhemoglobin (COHb) formation) under varying exposure conditions. Observed COHb levels under four experimental conditions of inhaled partial pressure of CO: 50 ppm (△), 100 ppm (▲——▲), 200 ppm (○), 500 ppm (●——●). The solid lines are the values predicted by the Coburn–Forster–Kane equation, which closely approximate the experimental points. Barometric pressure 750 mmHg; partial pressure of oxygen 100 mmHg; alveolar ventilation 6000 ml/min; diffusing capacity of the lung for CO 30 ml/min per mmHg; baseline carboxyhemoglobin 0.8%; $\dot{V}$co, ventilation of CO, 0.007 ml/min. Adapted from Stewart [77].

about two to three times that fraction reporting less profound personality changes or memory loss; all of those who were severely affected had been in coma [79].

The range of neurologic and neuropsychiatric findings after significant CO intoxication includes not only personality and memory disturbances but also a Parkinson-like syndrome (including tremor, rigidity, and abnormal postural reflexes) [80,81], peripheral neuropathy of a sensory or mixed sensorimotor type [82,83], and severe psychiatric disturbances (including obsessive–compulsive disorder, 'psychic akinesia', and Tourette's syndrome) [84–86]. Of particular concern is the fact that some patients exhibit a lucid, asymptomatic period of days to weeks between clearing of their acute CO-related symptoms and manifestation of delayed neurologic or neuropsychiatric deficits [87–89]. Pathologic examination in fatalities may show necrosis within the basal ganglia and lesions of the periventricular white matter; less commonly, diffuse white and gray matter destruction may be found. Lesions in the basal ganglia on CT or MRI scanning frequently herald a poor clinical outcome [90–92].

CO intoxication of sufficient severity to impair consciousness has also been associated with various neuroophthalmologic sequelae, including retrobulbar neuritis and cortical blindness [93–95]. Retinal flame hemorrhages have been reported after symptomatic acute and subacute CO exposures [96,97]. Deafness has also been reported after severe CO intoxications. Baker and Lilly documented a symmetrical 'U-shaped' audiogram with sensorineural defect in a patient with severe CO poisoning with otherwise complete neurologic recovery;

they noted similar audiometric findings in their review of the literature on CO intoxication and hearing loss [98].

Another area of concern regarding persistent CO-related health effects is toxicity to the offspring of pregnant smoke-inhalation victims. Toxicokinetic studies in animals predict higher equilibrium COHb levels and delayed clearance of CO in the fetal compared with the maternal circulation [99,100]. The fetus' apparent heightened susceptibility to CO may derive from its limited cardiovascular reserve and the fact that both venous and arterial fetal oxygen tensions are shifted by CO loading [101]. Among clinically CO-poisoned patients, stillbirths have been reported, at times with fetal COHb levels as low as 23 to 24% [102–104]. Perinatal asphyxia and congenital malformations have also been reported [105,106]. While normal birth outcomes are most common, long-term neurobehavioral follow-up of the offspring of CO-poisoned mothers is the exception rather than the rule [107,108].

The three major targets of CO intoxication are the CNS, heart, and, in the pregnant female, the fetus. An oft-cited physical finding of cherry-red discoloration of the skin and mucous membranes is not seen with sufficient regularity to prove clinically useful [21]. Other physical signs seen infrequently include retinal venous engorgement and cutaneous bullae, the latter particularly in unconscious victims. Most often, the earliest symptoms of CO intoxication are referable to the CNS and include headache, fatigue, and lightheadedness. At higher COHb levels, vasodilatation (a compensatory response to decreased O_2 carrying capacity) produces flushing, tachycardia, and lowered systemic blood pressure. Dilated vessels are probably also responsible for the throbbing quality of CO-induced headaches. With progressively increasing COHb levels, headache, lightheadedness, and decreased vigilance are followed by nausea, vomiting, decreased coordination, syncope, coma, convulsions, and finally death.

Laboratory tests

Clinical laboratory diagnosis of CO intoxication most commonly involves analysis of venous or arterial blood COHb by differential spectrophotometry, also known as CO oximetry. In this method, the absorbance of a hemolyzed blood specimen is simultaneously determined at two or more wavelengths (wavelengths at which the known absorbance of various hemoglobin species differ). Through the algebraic solution of a set of simultaneous equations, the relative concentration of each Hb species is calculated. Modern instruments are programmed to perform these calculations automatically and typically utilize at least four test wavelengths in order to permit the simultaneous measurement of Hb, oxyhemoglobin (O_2Hb), COHb, and MetHb [109]. Extreme hyperlipidemia (as observed during diabetic ketoacidosis) may produce a falsely elevated COHb level using this method [110]. Of importance, conventional arterial blood gases, while showing decreased O_2 saturation and possible metabolic acidosis in CO poisoning, do not necessarily show decreased O_2 tension. Pulse oximetry likewise does not distinguish between COHb and O_2Hb and, therefore, cannot be used to make the diagnosis of CO poisoning [111].

An alternative to direct measurement of COHb in blood is the measurement of CO in breath air at the end of exhalation. This technique has found use in both field studies of firefighters and in emergency departments. Detectors of CO may utilize electrochemical, gas chromatographic, or infrared absorption methods. The empirical relationship of exhaled breath CO and whole blood COHb is given by the equation:

$$CO_{breath} = 0.132COHb^2 + 3.125COHb + 4.24$$

where CO_{breath} is expressed in ppm and COHb in percent [16].

Some instruments in use for breath CO analysis register falsely elevated CO levels when the sample contains hydrogen (H_2) gas. Clinical conditions known to increase H_2 in exhaled breath include lactose intolerance and various other types of intestinal malabsorption [112].

Whichever method is used to document CO exposure, the clinician should be aware of two critical variables in interpreting laboratory values:

- time (from exposure to sampling)
- inspired oxygen concentration (fraction of inspired O_2; FIO_2).

Back-extrapolation of observed COHb to estimated peak values can be attempted using kinetic toxicokinetic modeling.

The acute effects of CO exposure, by approximate COHb level, are listed in Table 18.3.

Table 18.3 Acute health effects of carbon monoxide exposure. Modified from Stewart [77]

Carboxyhemoglobin (%)	Response of healthy adults	Patients with severe coronary artery disease
0.3–0.7	Normal range from endogenous carbon monoxide production	No symptomatic effect
2–5	No symptomatic effect	Lower threshold for exercise-induced angina
5–10	Compensatory increase in CNS and coronary bloodflow	Lower threshold for exercise-induced ventricular arrhythmias
10–20	Slight headache, fatigue, lightheadedness	Lower threshold for exercise-induced myocardial infarction
20–30	Moderate headache, nausea, fine manual dexterity impaired, visual evoked response abnormal, flushing and tachycardia	
30–40	Severe headache, nausea and vomiting, hypotension, ataxia	
40–50	Syncope	
50–65	Coma and convulsions	
65–70 (or over)	Fatal if not treated	

Management

Forces similar to those governing CO uptake are involved in CO elimination, a process likewise dominated by concentration gradients between the pulmonary circulation and alveolar air. Since O_2 acts as a competitor to CO at hemoglobin-binding sites, increased inspired O_2 tensions displace CO from hemoglobin and speed its elimination via exhaled breath. The effect of three different inspired O_2 concentrations (including HBO) on CO elimination is illustrated in Figure 18.4 [113].

Although clinicians are unanimous in supporting the use of supplemental O_2 in confirmed or suspected CO intoxication, the subject of HBO constitutes an unusually contentious subject in the medical literature. Along with conflicting claims of clinical efficacy (or lack thereof), references to potential non-hemoglobin-mediated mechanisms of CO intoxication are frequently used as justification for one or another position in this debate. The criteria usually applied in the evaluation of therapeutic interventions include efficacy, safety, and underlying biological rationale. Evaluation of the efficacy of HBO has been hampered, at least until recently, by the lack of any randomized trials. Patients selected for HBO treatment generally include those with altered consciousness and/or with documented COHb levels in excess of 25–40%. Since obtunded patients are considered to be at risk for persistent neurologic impairment, medicolegal concerns are frequently cited as justification for not carrying out randomized trials of hyperbaric versus normobaric O_2 (NBO) therapy.

Despite this charged atmosphere, a small number of intrepid investigators have attempted to approach this question with randomized trials; only those including comatose patients are reviewed here. Raphael and colleagues randomized a total of 629 adults with non-occupational CO poisoning to one of four groups. Patients without initial impairment of consciousness received either 6 hours of NBO or 2 hours of HBO at 2 atmospheres plus 4 hours of NBO. Patients with initial obtundation or coma received either one or two 2-hour sessions of HBO along with 4 hours of NBO. Based upon the endpoint of full symptomatic neurologic recovery, they found no benefit from HBO among patients who had not lost consciousness, regardless of their presenting COHb level. Among patients with only brief initial loss of consciousness, there was no difference in outcome between those receiving one or two HBO sessions. Among patients with initial coma, there was a small (but not statistically significant) difference in outcome favoring two over one treatments [114]. Significantly, this study did not compare HBO with NBO in patients who had initial loss of consciousness, thus leaving open the ultimate question of the efficacy of HBO in that important group.

More recently, Scheinkestel's group in Australia randomized patients with CO intoxication presenting to a regional hyperbaric center over a period of over 2 years to either daily HBO (n = 104) or daily NBO (n = 87) treatments. Treatments were conducted on a blinded basis, with both HBO and NBO being carried out in an HBO chamber. The treatment protocol lasted 3–6 days, depending upon the clinical course, and subgroups received high-flow O_2 between HBO/NBO sessions. Pregnant women, children, and burn victims were excluded. Mini-mental status examinations were performed at the time of admission, and a battery of neuropsychological tests was administered after 3 days of treatment and again (if possible) a month later. The groups were well matched with respect to age and circumstances of intoxication (suicidal versus accidental). Roughly one half of subjects were comatose at the time of admission, again similar in the HBO and NBO groups. A high proportion of total subjects (71%) had persistent neurologic sequelae at time of discharge. However, the observed differences in neuropsychologic testing actually favored the NBO group, with subjects who underwent HBO treatment having a 20% greater rate of neuropsychologic abnormalities on testing ($p = 0.02$) and a greater rate of delayed-onset neuropsychologic abnormalities (5.8% versus 0%; $p = 0.03$) [115].

The safety of HBO treatment is another point of contention. Some HBO chambers are single-place cylinders that do not permit continuous hands-on care. If, in a fit of delirium or seizure, a patient removes an intravenous line or endotracheal tube in

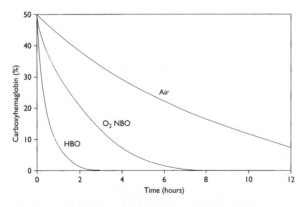

Fig. 18.4 Carbon monoxide elimination (carboxyhemoglobin (COHb) clearance) under varying conditions of oxygenation. In this example, an initial COHb concentration of 50% is halved in approximately 5 hours when breathing room air, in 1.5 hours when breathing 100% oxygen under normobaric conditions (NBO, 1 atm), and in 0.5 hours under conditions of hyperbaric oxygenation (HBO, 2.5 atm). Adapted from Winter and Miller [113].

a monoplace chamber, the consequences can be serious. Cardiac arrest and cardiopulmonary resuscitation also pose a challenge, since several minutes are normally allowed to depressurize a chamber from 2.5 atmospheres back to sea level. Most of the above concerns are addressed by the use of multiplace chambers, which can accommodate nursing or medical staff along with the patient (although this approach puts health professionals at risk of barotrauma). Finally, HBO treatment has been associated with tension pneumothorax (particularly among patients who have received cardiopulmonary resuscitation prior to HBO), tympanic membrane rupture, and, in conscious patients, ear and sinus pain [116–118].

A recent proposed method that holds some promise is the use of mechanical hyperventilation with NBO (100% O_2) with the addition of inspired CO_2 to the ventilator circuit to prevent the development of respiratory alkalosis. This approach has been tested so far only in a dog model, but in this setting it appears to be equivalent to HBO in the rate of removal of CO from hemoglobin.

HYDROGEN CYANIDE

Sources and epidemiology

Cyanide salts are employed in metal plating, chemical synthesis, extraction of gold and silver from ores, silver reclamation from spent photographic film, and metallurgy (heat treatment of metals, or 'case-hardening'). Liberation of highly toxic HCN gas from its solution in water (hydrocyanic acid) is normally avoided in these situations by maintaining any aqueous cyanide salt solutions at an alkaline pH. Nevertheless, accidental mixing of alkaline cyanide solutions with acids has occurred in industry with tragic consequences, particularly when workers entered enclosed spaces in which cyanide containing solutions are present [119].

HCN gas is also liberated when N_2-containing polymers are burned. In general, the yield of HCN is proportional to the fractional content of N_2 in the source material, as well as the temperature and O_2 concentrations at which combustion occurs (higher temperatures and limited O_2 concentrations favoring HCN production) [120]. The potential contribution of HCN to the lethality of smoke from structural fires was first appreciated by authorities in Detroit, Michigan, who included blood cyanide analysis on all coroner's cases, not suspecting an association with smoke inhalation [121]. This observation has subsequently been replicated in a number of different locales [122,123].

Pathophysiology

HCN is readily absorbed across the alveolar membrane, distributes itself with total body water, and tends to bind with serum proteins and concentrate in erythrocytes [124]. Its volume of distribution (V_d) has been variously estimated at 0.4 and 1.5 l/kg body weight [125,126].

At the cellular level, HCN combines with (and reversibly inhibits) cytochrome oxidase (cytochromes a–a_3), the terminal enzyme in the electron transport chain (Fig. 18.5) [127]; various other enzymes are also inhibited by cyanide, but with less dramatic physiologic consequences [124,126]. The immediate result of cytochrome inhibition is interference with normal aerobic glycolysis, accumulation of metabolic acids (particularly lactic acid), and a decrease in the adenosine trisphosphate to adenosine bisphosphate (ATP: ADP) ratio; there is a consequent slowing of all energy-utilizing physiologic processes, including membrane transport. Because of their lack of alternative anaerobic pathways, the brain and myocardium are the most sensitive organs to acute cyanide toxicity [124]. A more specific effect of cyanide is its direct stimulation of carotid and aortic chemoreceptors, resulting in hyperpnea and a subsequently increased internal dose of the airborne toxicant [126,128]. Since it appears to be the undissociated form of cyanide (HCN) that actively binds to cytochrome oxidase, the metabolic acidosis that occurs with severe cyanide poisoning may aggravate

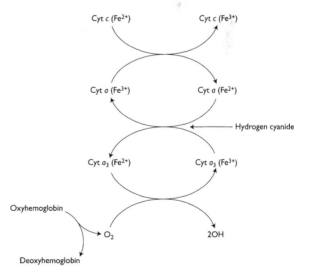

Fig. 18.5 Cyanide-related interruption of oxidative phosphorylation in mitochondria. The prosthetic heme iron of the cytochromes (cyt.) involved in oxidative phosphorylation is in the ferrous (Fe^{2+}) or ferric (Fe^{3+}) state. The step most affected by cyanide intoxication is coupling of the redox reactions between cyt. a and cyt. a_3. Interruption of oxidative phosphorylation results in impaired aerobic metabolism, with decreased tissue oxygen utilization (and abnormal tissue oxygen accumulation) and decreased energy (ATP) generation [127].

the underlying biochemical lesion [128]. Based upon animal data, Ballantyne extrapolated a human LC_{50} (lethal inhalation concentration for 50% of exposed individuals) of 1500 ppm for a 3 min exposure and 140 ppm for a 60 min exposure [124].

Cigarette smoking and dietary cyanogens (cassava, stone fruits, almonds) are common sources of low-level cyanide exposure in everyday life [129]. In nonlethal exposures, approximately 80% of absorbed cyanide is metabolized via the hepatic enzyme rhodanese (thiosulfate cyanide sulfur transferase), which detoxifies cyanide by conjugating it with various sulfur-containing substrates [124,130].

Thiocyanate (SCN), the principal product of cyanide detoxification, has on occasion been used as a surrogate measure of cyanide exposure in case series involving smoke inhalation. However, since SCN is eliminated via slow renal excretion (with a half life of approximately 14 days), an elevated SCN level may reflect:

- acute high-level cyanide exposure
- chronic low-level exposures either to cyanide (from cigarette smoking or dietary cyanogens) or to SCN (from cruciferous vegetables) [131].

As a consequence of these limitations, SCN has lost favor as a biomarker of cyanide exposure. Under conditions of overdose, the rate-limiting step in cyanide detoxification becomes the availability of sufficient sulfur donors for SCN production; this fact provides the rationale for the administration of thiosulfate in cyanide intoxication.

Recognition

Clinical features

HCN and cyanide salts are the fastest-acting lethal agents encountered in clinical toxicology practice; for many smoke-inhalation victims, the diagnosis of cyanide intoxication is made on an autopsy basis. Short of cardiopulmonary arrest, cyanide exposed patients may present with the symptoms of headache, nausea, postural dizziness, and confusion. Neurologic sequelae of severe cyanide intoxication have resembled those seen after other causes of postanoxic encephalopathy and include personality changes, intellectual impairment, and Parkinson-like findings.

With the possible exception of the extraordinarily rapid onset of action, intoxication caused by cyanide is generally indistinguishable from that caused by CO and other asphyxiants. Physical findings may include hypotension, tachycardia, flushing, and disorientation; seizures and cardiac arrhythmias may also be present. Nevertheless, a few specific diagnostic clues

may be present. First, cyanide salts, when ingested, may emit an almond-like odor, evident (cautiously!) on either exhaled breath or from evacuated stomach contents. Second, because of impaired peripheral utilization of O_2, 'arteriolarization of venous blood' (increased venous O_2 tension) may be present in significant cyanide intoxication. This finding can be documented by obtaining simultaneous arterial and venous blood gas determinations or, at the bedside, by documenting an abnormally reddish color to retinal venules (i.e. with a loss of distinction from retinal arterioles) [132].

Laboratory tests

Various laboratory methods have been devised for the detection and quantification of cyanide in blood [4,133]. The most widely used methods involve extraction of cyanide by gaseous diffusion, aeration, or microdistillation, with spectrophotometry after a subsequent colorimetric reaction. Less commonly used methods include specific ion electrodes, gas chromatography, and fluorometry. Finally, a rapid, semiquantitative method for whole-blood cyanide detection using a colorimetric reaction on a paper test strip has also been developed. Table 18.4 gives the approximate range of blood cyanide levels associated with specific clinical outcomes [134,135].

Because of its interference with normal aerobic metabolism, significant cyanide intoxication produces several indirect metabolic derangements, some of which may provide rapid diagnostic clues when whole-blood cyanide levels are not immediately available. One metabolic alteration relates to its interference with O_2 extraction/utilization from circulating blood. Under normal circumstances, arterial blood contains approximately 20 ml/dl (200 ml/l) dissolved O_2; after 5 ml/dl (50 ml/l) is extracted in the capillary bed, about 15 ml/dl (150 ml/l) remains in venous blood. Translated into terms of O_2 saturation, normal arterial blood is nearly 100% saturated with O_2 and mixed venous blood about 75%. In at least two published cyanide intoxication cases, blood gas determinations performed simultaneously on arterial and venous blood have shown decreased O_2

Table 18.4 Acute health effects of cyanide exposure. Adapted from Hall *et al.* [134] and Gonzales and Sabatini [135]

Cyanide concentration (µg/ml (µmol/l))	Symptoms/outcome
0.0–0.5 (<20)	Usually none
0.5–1.0 (20–38)	Tachycardia, hyperpnea, flushing
1.0–2.5 (38–95)	Obtundation
2.5–3.0 (95–114)	Coma, convulsions
>3.0 (>114)	Fatal if untreated

extraction, with venous O_2 saturation approximating 85% (rather than the normal 75%). This alteration may be taken as indirect evidence of the action of cyanide [136,137].

Impaired tissue O_2 utilization in cyanide intoxication also results in the accumulation of the metabolic byproducts of anaerobic metabolism, most notably lactic acid [138]. The serum lactic acid concentration is therefore an indirect indicator of cyanide poisoning; assays for lactic acid are widely available in clinical laboratories, with a typical normal range quoted as 0.5–2.0 mmol/l. Even more readily available is the serum anion gap (AG), which can be computed from routine serum electrolytes. This is raised by the presence of various metabolic and exogenous acids (including lactic acid) and is defined by the formula:

$$AG = (Na^+ + K^+) - (Cl^- + HCO^-_3)$$

The normal range is 12–20 mmol/l. The alternative formula for anion gap, omitting K^+, has a normal range of 8–16 mmol/l. Several conditions other than cyanide poisoning can produce an elevated anion-gap acidosis, as summarized by the mnemonic MUD-PILES. These include **m**ethanol intoxication, **u**remia, **d**iabetic ketoacidosis, **p**ropylene glycol/phenformin/paraldehyde, **i**ron/isoniazid/inhalants (CO, HCN, H_2S), **l**actic acidosis, **e**thanol (alcoholic ketoacidosis)/ethylene glycol poisoning, and **s**alicylates [139].

Management

A number of different therapeutic strategies have been devised to treat cyanide toxicity [140], as shown in Fig. 18.6 and Table 18.5. Cyanide antagonists act either to enhance normal cyanide elimination as SCN (via administration of sulfur donors) or to bind (complex) cyanide competitively. In this latter category are MetHb-forming agents (nitrites and dimethylaminophenol; DMAP), exogenous MetHb, dicobalt edetate (Kelocyanor), and hydroxocobalamin (vitamin B_{12} precursor). Experimental cyanide antagonists not further reviewed here include hydroxylamine (a MetHb former), primaquine (another MetHb-former), α-ketoglutaric acid (a cyanide-complexing agent), chlorpromazine (an enhancer of SCN formation), and HBO.

Administration of nitrites and sodium thiosulfate has been a documented mode of treatment for cyanide intoxication since the 1930s [141]. The kinetics and efficacy of this Food and Drug Administration (FDA) approved drug regimen have been reviewed in several publications [134,135,142].

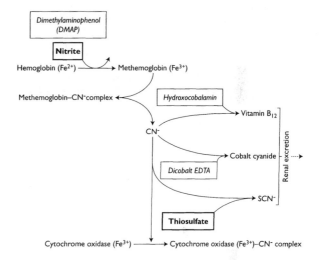

Fig. 18.6 Treatment approaches to cyanide (CN⁻) intoxication. Nitrite and thiosulfate are US Food and Drug Administration-approved antidotes (bold boxes); investigational antidotes are given in italics. EDTA, ethylenediaminetetraacetic acid. Adapted from Shusterman. [44].)

Table 18.5 Comparison of cyanide antagonists. Modified from Bright [140]

Antagonist	Advantages	Disadvantages
Substances that increase intrinsic cyanide detoxification		
Sodium thiosulfate	Low toxicity	Requires i.v. administration
Rhondanese		Requires i.v. administration, may cause sensitization
Substances that bind cyanide		
Methemoglobin-inducers	Some inducers can be given by inhalation	Causes decrement in oxygen carrying capacity
Methemoglobin (stroma-free)	No decrement in oxygen-carrying capacity	Requires i.v. administration, may cause sensitization
Dicobalt edetate (Kelocyanor)	Acts rapidly	Potential idiosyncratic reactions
Hydroxocobalamin (vitamin B_{12})	Low toxicity	Requires i.v. administration (high volume in current form)

i.v., intravenous.

This approach involves the induction of a state of methemoglobinemia (via administration of nitrites) and enhanced elimination of cyanide via administration of an exogenous sulfur donor (thiosulfate). The rationale for generating MetHb is its high affinity for cyanide, which allows it to act as a 'sink' thereby diverting cyanide from the mitochondrial enzymes of the electron transport train [143]. The cyanomethemoglobin formed by the interaction of cyanide with MetHb slowly dissociates in the presence of hepatic rhodanese and, along with sulfur donors (including intravenously administered thiosulfate), forms SCN, an acutely non-toxic ion that is excreted slowly in the urine [144]. One objection to the use of MetHb generators in smoke-inhalation victims (who are coexposed to CO) is the fact that neither COHb nor MetHb are capable of transporting O_2 thereby yielding an additive anemic hypoxia.

In likely or confirmed intoxication in an adult, the current (FDA approved) therapeutic recommendation includes:

- crushing 1 to 2 perles of amyl nitrite (0.3 ml each) in the breathing zone of the patient
- administering 300 mg sodium nitrite (10 ml of 3% solution) intravenously over 3 to 5 min
- administering sodium thiosulfate, 12.5 g (50 ml of 25% solution) intravenously at 2.5–5 ml/min (a half-dose may be repeated in 30–60 min, if indicated).

Although corresponding pediatric dosages are not relevant to occupationally induced toxicity, the Bhopal incident illustrated the potential for industrial accidents to affect neighboring communities. Pediatric dosage is:

- sodium nitrite, 6–10 mg/kg (0.2–0.33 ml/kg 3% solution, to a maximum of 300 mg or 10 ml)
- sodium thiosulfate, 400 mg/kg (1.6 ml/kg 25% solution, up to 50 ml).

Of importance, the pediatric dose of sodium nitrite is adjusted if the child's hemoglobin differs significantly from a 'normal' of 12 g (see Kim [145] and Keller [146] for further details of adult and pediatric dosage regimens). All of the above pharmaceuticals are packaged in a kit, available from Taylor Pharmaceuticals. General supportive measures include supplemental O_2, airway support (with possible assisted ventilation), cardiac monitoring, and treatment of seizures and arrhythmias [132].

Two other agents that increase the MetHb 'cyanide sink' deserve comment. Dimethylaminophenol (DMAP) is a MetHb-inducing agent; it is available in Europe but not the USA. Compared with nitrites, it produces a more rapid onset and reversal of methemoglobinemia, the latter probably related to the fact that DMAP does not appear to inhibit MetHb reductase enzymes (as do nitrites) [147]. Another approach is to administer exogenous MetHb, which does not detract from the O_2-carrying capacity of the blood. So-called stroma-free MetHb has been shown to be moderately protective against cyanide in animal experiments [148]. However, stroma-free MetHb poses several theoretical risks (including obstruction of renal tubules and allergic reactions), and its use in humans has been viewed with caution. Similar (sensitization) issues have been raised over the potential administration of exogenous rhodanese in an effort to speed cyanide detoxification [149].

A newer antidote, hydroxocobalamin, complexes cyanide to form cyanocobalamin (vitamin B_{12}), which is subsequently eliminated in the urine [125,150,151]. Hydroxocobalamin was designated an orphan drug by the FDA in 1985. In an investigational study of 2-pack-per-day smokers, 5 g hydroxocobalamin administered intravenously was efficacious and safe in acutely lowering subtoxic blood cyanide levels [152]. Hydroxocobalamin has been available in France since 1970 in an antidote kit with sodium thiosulfate for intravenous administration (Trousse Anticyanure, Anphar-Rolland Laboratories, Chilly-Mazarin, France). Hall and Rumack have reviewed the published case reports documenting the use of this antidotal combination [125]. Side-effects of hydroxocobalamin may include transient discoloration of the skin, mucous membranes, and urine, along with a slight increase in blood pressure and reflex decrease in heart rate. Adverse reactions appear to be limited to occasional urticaria, although chronic administration has been associated with anaphylaxis in a few patients. In order to achieve an optimal therapeutic effect, hydroxocobalamin must be administered in a 1 : 1 molar ratio to absorbed cyanide. However, given the drug's high molecular weight and the current formulation's dilute nature (0.1%), therapeutic doses may require the administration of several liters of intravenous fluid, a fact that must be weighed against the risk of fluid overload and subsequent development of acute respiratory distress syndrome in smoke-inhalation patients [125]. Fortunately, more concentrated preparations (5%) have been made available to clinical investigators and may be available in the future if the drug is approved in the USA [152].

The final cyanide-complexing agent to be discussed here is dicobalt edetate (Kelocyanor). In addition to the problem of questionable clinical efficacy, this drug may induce severe allergic, cardiovascular, or neurologic reactions, particularly if administered in the absence of an elevated cyanide level [135]. Dicobalt edetate is neither currently licensed for use in the USA nor are clinical trials currently in progress in this country.

Because acute cyanide intoxication can be rapidly fatal, some investigators have advocated early treatment of hypotensive or unconscious smoke-inhalation victims, particularly in the presence of refractory metabolic acidosis [153–155]. While the long-approved combination of nitrites and thiosulfate is efficacious in isolated cyanide intoxication, concern exists regarding its safety in patients simultaneously intoxicated with cyanide and CO, since neither COHb nor therapeutically produced MetHb are capable of carrying O_2 [156,157]. Of the various newer cyanide antagonists, the agent with the best combination of therapeutic efficacy and safety may be hydroxocobalamin, which, like nitrites, may be administered in combination with sodium thiosulfate [125].

HYDROGEN SULFIDE

Sources and epidemiology

Hydrogen sulfide (CAS 7783–06–4) is frequently encountered, along with aliphatic hydrocarbon gases, in sewage systems, oilfields, and petroleum refineries. In addition, H_2S is liberated from geothermal energy-production facilities, as well as from the digestion process in 'kraft' pulp mills. Hydrogen sulfide has a prominent role in 'environmental odor pollution', in large part because of its characteristic 'rotten egg' odor, and its extraordinary odorant versus irritant potency (an odor threshold of 8 parts per billion compared with an irritant threshold >10 ppm; i.e. more than an thousandfold difference in concentration). Although most community episodes of air pollution involve H_2S at subirritant concentrations, at least one incident (near a sulfur extraction facility of a Mexican oil refinery in 1950) involved both irritant and asphyxiant effects among community residents [158].

Irritant effects, ranging from conjunctivitis to pulmonary edema, have been reported in the 10–500 ppm range; however, it is the capacity of H_2S to act as a chemical asphyxiant that concerns us here. 'Olfactory paralysis' (profound and rapid olfactory fatigue) has been reported at exposure levels at or above 100 ppm, potentially depriving the exposed worker of a valuable warning sign. An equally rapid loss of consciousness caused by H_2S exposure ('knock-down') has been reported at exposure levels in the 500–1000 ppm range [159,160].

Pathophysiology

Asphyxia (and impairment of consciousness) by H_2S results from at least two mechanisms. Sulfide ions (which are liberated by H_2S in biological fluids) have been shown to inhibit cytochrome oxidase, much in the same manner as HCN [161]. Coupled with this mechanism, there may be selective uptake of sulfide ions in the brainstem [162]. Additionally, H_2S apparently inhibits monoamine oxidase in the CNS, resulting in elevated levels of serotonin and catecholamines, which in turn may interfere with proper regulation of respiratory drive. Respiratory arrest may occur suddenly (with respect to the dose–response curve) because of saturation of the intramitochondrial detoxification mechanism for sulfide ions [163].

Recognition

Clinical features

Hydrogen sulfide intoxication should be suspected when there is a history of impairment of consciousness after exposure to decaying organic material (e.g. sewage), geothermal energy sources, or underground utility work. A history of rapid loss of consciousness or olfactory paralysis may be present. Recovery of consciousness may be as rapid and dramatic as its onset; alternatively coma and even death can ensue.

Besides the non-specific CNS findings outlined above, there are no characteristic physical findings in H_2S poisoning.

Laboratory tests

Much has been written about 'sulfhemoglobin' a pigment that can be formed by bubbling concentrated H_2S through blood. The best information available is that this pigment does not play a role in the asphyxia produced by high-level H_2S exposure [127]. As a consequence, there is no specific laboratory diagnosis to be made in H_2S poisoning. However, determination of lactate levels and/or the anion gap can provide indirect evidence of chemical asphyxia (including that caused by H_2S) in the obtunded/acidotic patient.

Management

Therapy of symptomatic H_2S poisoning is primarily supportive. The rationale for administering MetHb-inducing agents, such as sodium nitrite, to divert H_2S away from cytochrome oxidase is not well-established, and it may even be harmful [164].

METHEMOGLOBIN FORMERS

Sources and epidemiology

Accumulation of MetHb (methemoglobinemia) is a molecular response to oxidative stress, and, depending upon the specific chemical stressor, host susceptibility factors may play an important role in this process. Classes of chemical capable of producing MetHb include organic and inorganic nitrites, some N-hydroxylamines, chlorites, chlorates, and various aromatic amino and nitro compounds [165,166]. MetHb elevations have been associated with administration of selected medications (dapsone, phenacetin, benzocaine, primaquine), incorporating nitrate-contaminated well water into infant formula, accidental ingestion of artificial fingernail removers containing nitroethane and cleaning solutions containing nitrites, and finally smoke inhalation from fires in which nitrogen oxides are prominent [167–173].

Pathophysiology

Normal hemoglobin metabolism involves an equilibrium between ferrous (Fe^{2+}) and ferric (Fe^{3+}) ions in the heme prosthetic group, with at least two metabolic pathways maintaining a large majority of heme iron in the Fe^{2+} state. Agents inducing MetHb formation push this reaction in the direction of Fe^{3+}, resulting in impairment of the O_2-carrying capacity of hemoglobin (anemic hypoxia). For some individuals with predisposing conditions (e.g. glucose 6-phosphate dehydrogenase deficiency), exposure to oxidizing agents can not only alter the functional status of hemoglobin but also overwhelm the enzymatic systems responsible for maintaining erythrocyte membrane integrity, resulting in a hemolytic anemia [127].

Recognition

Clinical features

Methemoglobin intoxication typically occurs in the context of an industrial exposure to, or accidental ingestion of, a MetHb-forming chemical, exposure to nitrogen oxide(s) in the context of smoke inhalation, or medical administration of selected MetHb-forming drugs in susceptible individuals.

The clinical presentation in severe cases is one of confusion, headache, and nausea, with obtundation, tachycardia, and tachypnea. In addition, myocardial ischemia may be produced in susceptible individuals. Notwithstanding these serious possibilities, cyanosis may occur out of proportion to the severity of symptoms, with some individuals showing cyanosis but being otherwise asymptomatic [174].

Laboratory tests

Methemoglobin has a characteristic absorption spectrum, and can be identified, along with COHb, by differential spectrophotometry (CO oximetry). Pulse oximetry does not reliably distinguish between MetHb and O_2Hb and hence underestimates the degree of Hb desaturation in methemoglobinemia [172]. A bedside diagnostic finding is that of 'chocolate brown' coloration of a drop of blood on filter paper [175].

Management

The therapy for symptomatic methemoglobinemia consists of supplemental O_2 and intravenous methylene blue, a reducing agent; MetHb levels below 15 to 20%, however, rarely require specific therapy. In the treatment of smoke inhalation victims (some of whom are coexposed to HCN), clinicians should exercise caution before correcting mild elevations of MetHb, since this maneuver could theoretically liberate cyanide ions complexed to MetHb molecules. Both hereditary MetHb reductase deficiency and glucose 6-phosphate dehydrogenase deficiency are contraindications to the administration of methylene blue, since the drug may induce hemolysis in such individuals. The recommended dose of methylene blue is 1–2 mg/kg (0.1–0.2 ml/kg of a 1% solution) given intravenously slowly (over several minutes); the dose may be repeated in 30 to 60 min. More specific management recommendations can be found in standard reference texts in toxicology [176].

Box 18.1 Black damp (David J. Hendrick)

Coal mines

Whenever coal comes into contact with O_2 there is a low level of spontaneous combustion. The process is exothermic and the heat produced increases the rate of ongoing combustion. In working coal mines a high level of mechanical ventilation provides an important cooling factor in inhibiting this unwanted combustion, and if, conversely, there is very little ventilation (for example, in unworked waste areas) O_2 is quickly depleted, thus preventing any further oxidation. Open conflagration is

consequently a very rare event in either working mines or disused mines.

The volume of air in disused mines or unworked sections does, however, create the potential for the slow replacement of substantial volumes of O_2 with CO_2, though with most types of coal (compared with the wooden debris commonly left in older mines when they cease to operate) not every molecule of O_2 is replaced by one of CO_2. This, curiously, simulates the combustion of fat compared with carbohydrate in the human body.

Box 18.1 (contd.)

The resulting gas mixture may ultimately contain only nitrogen (N_2) and CO_2, though the proportions of N_2, CO_2, and any surviving O_2 will obviously vary during the time course of the process. When the O_2 content at normal barometric pressure falls below 17%, the miner's lamp of yesteryear would become extinguished, but a danger of asphyxiation for miners encountering such a gas mixture, which is known most widely as black damp (or choke damp, stythe, or stythe gas), would not generally arise until the concentrations fall below 16%. This hazard from black damp is fully recognized in working coal mines and is effectively countered by suitable rates of mechanical ventilation and by monitoring continuously the concentrations of all important gases throughout the mine.

Surface buildings

By contrast, the potential risk from disused coal mines to communities working or living on the surface is very poorly recognized. At times of high atmospheric pressure, fresh air in quantities of several million liters per km^2 of mined area is forced into these mines, either through unsealed shafts or through permeable strata of the surrounding ground. This allows oxidation and the production of black damp to continue. As the atmospheric pressure returns to normal after a few days, the mine expires a similar volume, which consists of the inspired air mixed with residual black damp already present in the mine. This movement of gas, therefore, provides a further curious human analogy: that of breathing. The expired gas mixture may pose little hazard, but when weeks or months later there is a storm and a more profound fall in atmospheric pressure, the mine may expire black damp with little or no O_2 content. This can pose a serious hazard depending on its path of escape.

Most of the black damp necessarily escapes harmlessly to the atmosphere through the mine shafts or from the whole surface of the overlying land, but over the intervening period of weeks or months a good deal may diffuse through the ground surrounding the mine to accumulate under impervious layers of rock or clay. The rapidly falling barometric pressure then triggers its release through fissures or faults in the strata, or some other breach of an impervious layer. The outcome can be dramatic if occupied buildings are sited over these narrow escape routes. For example, during one episode in a former coal mining area in northeast England, a neighborhood of some 150 households suddenly experienced a widespread failure of heating appliances that used natural gas from a central (mains) source [177]. A major mains leakage (and hence loss of pressure) was initially suspected and so the area was evacuated as an emergency. This led to the speedy discovery of an elderly couple who had lost consciousness in their cellar. They were fortunately revived. A leakage of mains gas was quickly excluded but low concentrations of O_2 with high concentrations of CO_2 confirmed there had been a major escape of black damp. Similar escapes had been clearly documented in the same area 2, 6, and 30 years previously.

In one particular home (where the owner and her visitors had experienced dizziness, nausea, unsteadiness, and headaches until being driven from the house into the heavily falling rain outdoors) regular measurements of CO_2 and O_2 concentration were made over the following year [177]. The maximum recorded concentration of CO_2 was 7.05%. Oxygen concentrations reached extraordinarily low troughs of 8–9% in a cupboard under her kitchen sink, under which a defect in the concrete floor allowed the entry and exit of piped water. A partial 'shell' over the external pipework, which protected it from soil and other buildings above, unfortunately captured black damp from a much wider area and channelled it in greater volume into the house. Elsewhere in the house, concentrations varied from normality (mostly) to transitory lows of about 12% in confined downstairs sites. Some living areas gave occasional values in the range 16–19%, and in other homes concentrations of 13–15% were sometimes recorded. Measured levels of natural gas, CO, and CH_4 were negligible throughout. The lowest O_2 readings were consistently associated with bad weather and periods when the house was closed because the owner was away.

The particular geological features relevant to these incidents are illustrated in Figure 18.7. The problem was eventually controlled by sinking new shafts into the mine so that it could be ventilated mechanically once more. Sufficient flow rates were used to dilute and dissipate the ongoing production of black damp.

Other sources

Coal mines are not the only source of underground collections of O_2-depleted, CO_2-enriched, air. An unprecedented and far more calamitous episode occurred in Cameroon in 1986 when a massive release from Lake Nyos was responsible for suffocating as many as 1800 inhabitants of an adjacent village. CO_2 in large amounts from volcanic sources had entered the deeper recesses of the lake, and readily dissolved because of the high ambient pressure. Poor mixing of different water levels allowed exceptional accumulations (more dissolved CO_2 per unit volume than in champagne), but when mixing did eventualy occur and the deeper waters rose to be decompressed, CO_2 outgassed in lethal amounts [178]. There is optimism that continous controlled mixing between layers will alow a steady but safe release of CO_2 and thereby prevent further dangerous accumulations.

Other low lying 'water holes' in Africa have become notorious for suffocating animals that gather to drink or to scavenge, because the heavy CO_2 is slow to dissipate after its release from the soil in volcanic areas. Of more relevance to human occupations, have been the recorded

Box 18.1 (contd.)

episodes of fatal asphyxiation when wells were entered during periods of falling barometric pressure. These were a consequence of the outflow of O₂-depleted gas from the surrounding porous strata. Any organic matter within such strata will undergo oxidation and decomposition, thereby producing black damp.

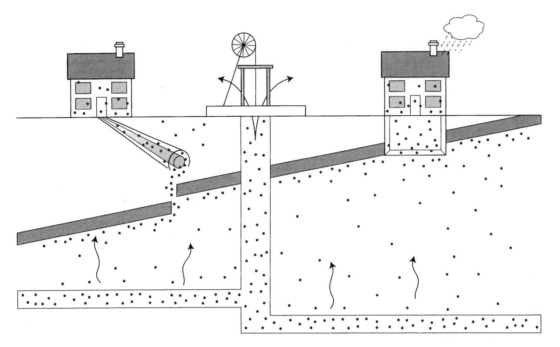

Fig. 18.7 With falling barometric pressure, signalled by poor weather, black damp escapes from the mineshaft and the soil. The house on the left is affected because black damp is collected over a fault in an impervious layer and is channelled through protective covering of servicing ducts. On the right black damp enters the cellar directly because it breached the impervious layer. (Courtesy of Sole Design.)

PREVENTION

In the workplace

Primary prevention (i.e. exposure control) should be the preferred approach to hazard abatement for asphyxiants in the workplace. In keeping with the 'hierarchy of industrial hygiene controls', substitution of a less hazardous product, ventilation and/or enclosure, and administrative controls (e.g. limitation of exposure time) can, in principle, all achieve the end of exposure reduction. An example of a successful primary prevention strategy for CO is the use of negative-pressure exhaust hoses connected to the tailpipes of motor vehicles being serviced in indoor shops (see the Difficult Case, below).

In some municipal and industrial settings, asphyxiants may be encountered on an unpredictable basis. In these situations, proper training, real-time air monitoring equipment, and personal protective gear (respiratory and dermal) are indicated. A particularly hazardous situation is posed by the cleaning of tanks and reaction vessels (confined spaces), in which chemical asphyxiants may be present with O₂-deficient and/or irritant-laden atmospheres. Use of air-supplied (particularly self-contained) breathing apparatus and work in teams (with harnesses and tether lines) can help to prevent the all too common (and tragic) scenario in which both worker and rescuer(s) are overcome by a toxic atmosphere.

In household settings, the likelihood of significant environmental exposures to CO may be reduced by the use of simple alarm-type monitors that alert household residents if a given exposure concentration is exceeded [179,180].

National regulatory strategies

An 'oxygen-deficient atmosphere' is defined by US OSHA as less than 19.5% O_2; such conditions require the use of air-supplied respirators. In addition, either a self-contained breathing apparatus (SCBA) or airline respirator with auxiliary self-contained air supply must be used when O_2 concentrations (at sea level) are less than 16%. At higher altitudes, stricter requirements for SCBA or auxiliary air sources may apply [18]. The US OSHA time-weighted-average permissible exposure limits (PELs) for various specific asphyxiant agents are summarized in Table 18.6 [181].

Of the asphyxiants reviewed in this chapter, only CO is subject to regulation in the US as a 'criteria air pollutant' The current standards of the US Environmental Protection Agency include time-weighted average levels of 35 ppm over a 1-hour period, and 9 ppm over an 8-hour period [182].

Table 18.6 US occupational exposure standards. Data taken from Occupational Safety and Health Administration [181]

Agent	Permissible exposure limit (PEL; ppm)^a	Other
Simple asphyxiants		
Carbon dioxide	5000	Oxygen deficient <19.5%
Nitrogen, methane		Oxygen deficient IDLH: <16% O_2
Chemical asphyxiants		
Carbon monoxide	50	
Hydrogen cyanide	10	
Hydrogen sulfide		20 ppm 'ceiling', 50 ppm (10 min) 'peak above ceiling'

IDLH, immediately dangerous to life and health
^{a}PEL is an 8-hour time-weighted average.

DIFFICULT CASE

History

A 32-year-old automobile mechanic consulted his family physician with the complaint of headaches that were global in location, daily in occurrence, and not associated with visual auras, nausea, localized weakness, or sensory disturbance. He was a non-smoker and denied any history of sinusitis or allergies. He reported that this problem was associated with the institution 1 month earlier of several heat-conserving measures in his workplace at the beginning of the cold weather season. He claimed that these included keeping the garage doors partially or completely closed (even when car engines were running), placing trash bags over the roof vents, and using an unvented catalytic kerosene heater indoors. He had been off work for several days at the time of the first consultation, and while there had been some improvement in his symptoms, occipital headache persisted.

The blood pressure was 140/90 mmHg, and there were normal findings on cardiopulmonary, neurologic, and fundoscopic examination. Musculoskeletal examination revealed moderate occipital and trapezius muscle group tenderness. Because of concern over possible CO intoxication caused by auto exhaust exposure, a baseline COHb level was obtained. This was reported as <2%. The patient was prescribed a muscle relaxant and a mild analgesic. He was instructed to return to work and to report for another COHb determination at the close of his second day back at work. At his next review he reported satisfactory improvement during the interval prior to returning to work, but his headache recurred within a few hours of his return to the workplace. A second COHb level, taken 1 hour after he completed an 8-hour shift, was reported to be 17%. A diagnosis of CO intoxication was made with secondary muscle tension persisting beyond the immediate period of exposure.

The patient was advised of his options under the California OSHA of filing an anonymous complaint, or of suggesting that his employer request a voluntary inspection without threat of penalty through the California OSHA Consulting Service. He chose the latter course. His employer, although initially cooperative, eventually contended that the workplace could not have been responsible for the intoxication and maintained that an inspection would prove that the workplace was not at fault. The industrial hygiene inspection duly found the workplace air to be within legal standards for CO, but the patient claimed that prior to the inspection the workplace environment had been modified. The obstructions were removed from the vents, and the garage doors were left wide open.

Issues

The primary issue here, assuming this man's CO intoxication was indeed occupational in origin, is how a consulted physician should deal with the inference that it was the result of non-occupational exposure. He/she should additionally be able to advise what measures could be available to provide a safe working atmosphere in garages in cold weather without sacrificing worker comfort unduly.

Comment

The book's contributors did not give serious thought to the employer's assertion that CO had been encountered from non-occupational sources. They agreed that, under ideal circumstances, COHb measurements should have been made before and after work shifts with the earlier heat-conserving practices in place and compared with measurements at similar times during days away from work. This sampling strategy was effectively precluded by the employer's actions, however. They advised a number of measures to provide a suitably warm working environment without risk of CO intoxication, principally direct exhaust extraction for automobiles (tailpipe hoses), adequate ventilation, and an approved source of heating (most obviously electric).

In this particular case the clinician interviewed the patient and his wife regarding potential household or other sources of CO exposure. There appeared to be none, and so the following calculation was performed. Assuming a 4-hour half life for CO elimination in an active individual, an 8-hour work day would represent two half lives, thereby allowing 75% decay in COHb from an initial level. Therefore, for the patient to have a 17% COHb level at the end of an 8-hour workday as the sole consequence of exposure sustained previously outside of the workplace the patient would have had to report to work with a COHb level four times that, or approximately 68%. With the range for coma being 40–60% COHb, this was unlikely to have been the sequence of events. The workers' compensation insurance carrier apparently agreed, and temporary disability was granted without adjudication.

The half life employed in this calculation, 4 hours, was approximate, and given the worker's level of activity may have underestimated the extent of elimination in 8 hours. More rigorous modeling of COHb levels is possible using the CFK equation, assuming ventilation rate, ambient CO levels, exposure times, blood volume, hemoglobin concentration, and endogenous COHb production rates.

The goal of maintaining a reasonably warm work environment while properly venting exhaust gases is best achieved by joining tailpipes to negative pressure hoses, which has become standard practice for larger garages. The work situation described was a particularly flagrant example of disregard for worker safety given the employer's failure to exhibit even commonsense protective measures. The worker in this case reported complete resolution of headaches when he was removed from the work situation and reported no recurrence in his subsequent place of employment (another garage with more adequate ventilation).

SUMMARY POINTS

Recognition

- Asphyxiants are viewed by toxicologists as belonging to two general classes: simple and chemical.
- Simple asphyxiants (including CO_2, N_2, CH_4, and the inert gases) are themselves relatively non-toxic, but impair tissue oxygenation by displacing-O_2 from the inspired atmosphere.
- Chemical asphyxiants (including CO, HCN, H_2S, and MetHb-forming agents) disrupt-O_2 transport or utilization at a molecular level.
- Sources of exposure for the simple asphyxiants include brewing and food processing (CO_2 and N_2) and underground utility work (CH_4).
- Sources of exposure for CO include internal combustion engines, combustion appliances, fires, endogenous production (from porphyrin metabolism), metabolism of dihalomethanes, and selected industrial processes.
- Sources of exposure for HCN include electroplating, gold and silver mining (leaching method), silver recovery from photographic film, incomplete combustion of nitrogen-containing polymers, and metabolism of cyanogenic glycosides (plant constituents).
- Sources of exposure for H_2S include wastewater treatment plants, refineries, pulp mills, and geothermal steam fields.

Management

- Therapy for asphyxia, in general, is supportive, emphasizing enhanced oxygenation (normobaric or hyperbaric).
- Specific antidotes are currently available for only one chemical asphyxiant: cyanide.

Prevention

- The primary method of prevention should be adequate control of any hazardous exposure using well-established standard methods: substitution of less hazardous agents, ventilation, enclosure, exhaust, administrative control.
- Risk is limited further by worker understanding of the major risks and the principles of prevention, and by training for the action required in emergency situations.
- Regular monitoring of hazardous agents may help to identify emerging failures of primary prevention, and compliance with regulatory controls (when enacted) will provide appropriate guidance.
- The use of personal protective equipment should be available when emergency situations arise or when adequate primary control is insufficient.
- There is particular need for understanding, training, and personal protective equipment when asphyxiation accidents can be anticipated so that rescuers do not become additional victims.

REFERENCES

1. Hensyl WR (ed.). *Stedman's Medical Dictionary*, Baltimore, MD: Williams & Wilkins, 1990.

2. Lenfant C. Gas transport and gas exchange. Ruch TC, Patton HD, Scher AM, eds. *Physiology and Biophysics*, 20th edn, Vol. 2, pp. 325–357. Philadelphia, PA: Saunders, 1974.

3. Peterson JE. *Industrial Health*, 2nd edn. Cincinnati: American Conference of Governmental Industrial Hygienists, 1991.

4. Shusterman DJ. Clinical smoke inhalation injury: systemic effects. *Occup Med* 1993; 8: 469–503.

5. Heckerling PS, Leikin JB, Maturen A, Perkins JT. Predictors of occult carbon monoxide poisoning in patients with headache and dizziness. *Ann Intern Med* 1987; 107: 174–176.

6. Allred EN, Bleecker ER, Chaitman BR *et al.* Short-term effects of carbon monoxide exposure on the exercise performance of subjects with coronary artery disease. *N Engl J Med* 1989; 321: 1426–1432.

7. Sheps DS, Herbst MC, Hinderliter AL *et al.* Production of arrhythmias by elevated carboxyhemoglobin in patients with coronary artery disease. *Ann Intern Med* 1990; 113: 343–351.

8. Silver DA, Cross M, Fox B, Paxton RM. Computed tomography of the brain in acute carbon monoxide poisoning. *Clin Radiol* 1996; 51: 480–483.

9. Sax NI, Lewis R. *Hawley's Condensed Chemical Dictionary* New York: Van Nostrand Reinhold, 1987.

10. Cometto-Muniz JE, Cain WS. Perception of nasal pungency in smokers and nonsmokers. *Physiol Behav* 1982; 29: 727–731.

11. Hornbein TF, Sorensen SC. The chemical regulation of ventilation. In: Ruch TC, Patton HD, Scher AM, eds. *Physiology and Biophysics*, pp. 378–392. Philadelphia, PA: Saunders, 1974.

12. US Naval Sea Systems Command. *US Navy Diving Manual*, Revision 3. Washington, DC: US Government Printing Office, 1991.

13. Anon. Cal/OSHA cites winery in worker death. *Cal-OSHA Reporter* 1999; 26(13): 1.

14. Cain WS, Turk A. Smell of danger: an analysis of LP-gas odorization. *Am Ind Hyg Assoc J* 1985; 46: 115–126.

15. Lipsett MJ, Shusterman DJ, Beard RR. Inorganic compounds of carbon, nitrogen, and oxygen. In: Clayton GD, Clayton FE, eds. *Patty's Industrial Hygiene and Toxicology*, 4th edn, pp. 4523–4643. New York: NY: John Wiley, 1994.

16. Peterson JE. Postexposure relationship of carbon monoxide in blood and expired air. *Arch Environ Health* 1970; 21: 172–173.

17. Ward MP, Milledge JS, West JB. *High Altitude Medicine and Physiology* Philadelphia, PA: University of Pennsylvania, 1989.

18. Occupational Safety and Health Administration. *OSHA Regulations – Standards*. 29 CFR 1910. 134; Section b, Subpart I – *Personal Protective Equipment*. Washington, DC: OSHA, 1998.

19. Cobb N, Etzel RA. Unintentional carbon monoxide-related deaths in the United States, 1979 through 1988. *JAMA* 1991; 266: 659–663.

20. Woolf A, Fish S, Azzara C, Dean D. Serious poisonings among older adults: a study of hospitalization and mortality rates in Massachusetts 1983–85. *Am J Public Health* 1990; 80: 867–869.

21. Jain K. *Carbon Monoxide Poisoning*, St Louis, MO: Warren Green, 1990.

22. Pruett RL. Synthesis gas: a raw material for industrial chemicals. *Science* 1981; 211: 11–16.

23. Hunter D. *The Diseases of Occupations*, 6th edn. London: Hodder and Stoughton, 1978.

24. National Institute for Occupational Safety and Health. *Occupational Diseases – A Guide to Their Recognition*, revised edn. Washington, DC: US Department of Health, Education, and Welfare, 1977.

25. Black NH, Conant JB. *Practical Chemistry*. New York: MacMillan, 1931.

26. Sayers RR, Davenport SI. US *Public Health Service. Review of Carbon Monoxide Poisoning: 1936*. Washington, DC: US Government Printing Office, 1937.

27. Brandt-Rauf PW, Fallon LF Jr, Tarantini T *et al.* Health hazards of fire fighters: exposure assessment. *Br J Ind Med* 1988; 45: 606–612.

28. Jankovic J, Jones W, Burkhart J, Noonan G. Environmental study of firefighters. *Ann Occup Hyg* 1991; 35: 581–602.

29. Brotherhood JR, Budd GM, Jeffery SE *et al.* Fire fighters' exposure to carbon monoxide during Australian bushfires. *Am Ind Hyg Assoc J* 1990; 51: 234–240.

30. Materna BL, Jones JR, Sutton PM *et al.* Occupational exposures in California wildland fire fighting. *Am Ind Hyg Assoc J* 1992; 53: 69–76.

31. Anderson RA, Watson AA, Harland WA. Fire deaths in the Glasgow area: II The role of carbon monoxide. *Med Sci Law* 1981; 21: 288–294.

32. Ayers SM, Evans R, Licht D *et al.* Health effects of exposure to high concentrations of automotive emissions: Studies in bridge and tunnel workers in New York City. *Arch Environ Health* 1973; 27: 168–178.

33. Stern FB, Lemen RA, Curtis RA. Exposure of motor vehicle examiners to carbon monoxide: a historical prospective mortality study. *Arch Environ Health* 1981; 36: 59–66.

34. Centers for Disease Control. Carbon monoxide exposure in aircraft fuelers – New York City. *MMWR* 1979; 28: 254–255.

35. Centers for Disease Control. Carbon monoxide poisoning in a garment-manufacturing plant – North Carolina. *MMWR* 1987; 36: 543–545.

36. Fawcett TA, Moon RE, Fracica PJ *et al.* Warehouse workers' headache: carbon monoxide poisoning from propane-fueled forklifts. *J Occup Med* 1992; 34: 12–15.

37. Centers for Disease Control. Fatal carbon monoxide poisoning in a camper-truck – Georgia. *MMWR* 1991; 40: 154–155.

38. Hampson NB, Norkool DM. Carbon monoxide poisoning in children riding in the back of pickup trucks. *JAMA* 1992; 267: 538–540.

39. Piatt JP, Kaplan AM, Bond GR, Berg RA. Occult carbon monoxide poisoning in an infant. *Pediatr Emerg Care* 1990; 6: 21–23.

40. Venning H, Roberton D, Milner AD. Carbon monoxide poisoning in an infant. *Br Med J* 1982; 284: 651.

41. Centers for Disease Control. Carbon monoxide intoxication associated with use of a gasoline-powered resurfacing machine in an ice-skating rink – Pennsylvania. *MMWR* 1984; 33: 49–50.

42. Paulozzi LJ, Satink F, Spengler RF. A carbon monoxide mass poisoning in an ice arena in Vermont. *Am J Public Health* 1991; 81: 222.

43. Iglewicz R, Rosenman KD, Iglewicz B *et al.* Elevated levels of carbon monoxide in the patient compartment of ambulances. *Am J Publ Health* 1984; 74: 511–512.

44. US Environmental Protection Agency. *National Air Pollutant Emission Estimates 1940–1989*. Washington, DC: US Environmental Protection Agency, 1991.

45. Stump FD, Knapp KT, Ray WD. Seasonal impact of blending oxygenated organics with gasoline on motor vehicle tailpipe and evaporative emissions. *J Air Waste Manage Assoc* 1990; 40: 872–880.

46. Office of Environmental Health Hazard Assessment. *Public Health Goals for Chemicals in Drinking Water: Methyl Tertiary-Butyl Ether (MTBE)*. Sacramento, CA: California Environmental Protection Agency, 1999.

47. Burney RE, Wu SC, Nemiroff MJ. Mass carbon monoxide poisoning: clinical effects and results of treatment in 184 victims. *Ann Emerg Med* 1982; 11: 394–399.

48. Caplan YH, Thompson BC, Levine B, Masemore W. Accidental poisonings involving carbon monoxide, heating systems, and confined spaces. *J Forensic Sci* 1986; 31: 117–121.

49. Centers for Disease Control. Carbon monoxide inhalation – Florida. *MMWR* 1980; 29: 574.

50. Sullivan BP. Carbon monoxide poisoning in an infant exposed to a kerosene heater. *J Pediatr* 1983; 103: 249–251.

51. Wharton M, Bistowish JM, Hutcheson RH, Schaffner W. Fatal carbon monoxide poisoning at a motel. *JAMA* 1989; 261: 1177–1178.

52. Centers for Disease Control. Use of unvented residential heating appliances – United States, 1988–1994. *MMWR* 1997; 46: 1221–1224.

53. Heckerling PS, Leikin JB, Maturen A. Occult carbon monoxide poisoning: validation of a prediction model. *Am J Med* 1988; 84: 251–256.

54. Heckerling PS, Leikin JB, Terzian CG, Maturen A. Occult carbon monoxide poisoning in patients with neurological illness. *Clin Toxicol* 1990; 28: 29–44.

55. Wallace LA. Carbon monoxide in air and breath of employees in an underground office. *J Air Pollut Control Assoc* 1983; 33: 678–682.

56. Centers for Disease Control. Carbon monoxide poisoning associated with a propane-powered floor burnisher – Vermont, 1992. *MMWR* 1993; 42: 726–728.

57. Centers for Disease Control. Unintentional carbon monoxide poisoning from indoor use of pressure washers – Iowa, January 1992–January 1993. *MMWR* 1993; 42: 777–9, 785.

58. Hawkes AP, McCammon JB, Hoffman RE. Indoor use of concrete saws and other gas-powered equipment. Analysis of reported carbon monoxide poisoning cases in Colorado. *J Occup Environ Med* 1998; 40: 49–54.

59. Centers for Disease Control. Unintentional carbon monoxide poisoning following a winter strom – Washington, January 1993. *MMWR* 1993; 42: 109–111.

60. Lester D. The effects of detoxification of domestic gas on suicide in the United States. *Am J Publ Health* 1990; 80: 80–81.

61. Choi IS. Delayed neurologic sequelae in carbon monoxide intoxication. *Arch Neurol* 1983; 40: 433–435.

62. Hampson NB, Kramer CC, Dunford RG, Norkool DM. Carbon monoxide poisoning from indoor burning of charcoal briquets. *JAMA* 1994; 271: 52–53.

63. Gasman JD, Varon J, Gardner JP. Revenge of the barbecue grill – Carbon monoxide poisoning. *West J Med* 1990; 153: 656–657.

64. Centers for Disease Control. Carbon monoxide poisoning deaths associated with camping – Georgia, March 1999. *MMWR* 1999; 48: 705–706.

65. Hawkins LH, Cole PV, Harris JRW. Smoking habits and blood carbon monoxide levels. *Environ Res* 1976; 11: 310–318.

66. Rickert WS, Robinson JC, Collishaw N. Yields of tar, nicotine, and carbon monoxide in the sidestream smoke from 15 brands of Canadian cigarettes. *Am J Publ Health* 1984; 74: 228–231.

67. Sterling TD, Collett CW, Ross JA. Levels of environmental tobacco smoking under different conditions of ventilation and smoking regulation. In: Harper JP, edn. *Combustion Processes and the Quality of the Indoor Environment* pp. 223–235. Pittsburgh, PA: Air & Waste Management Association, 1989.

68. Radford EP, Drizd TA. *Blood Carbon Monoxide Levels in Persons 3–74 Years of Age: United States, 1976–80.* Advance data, Vol. 76, pp. 1–24. Washington, DC: National Center for Health Statistics, US Dept. Health and Human Services, 1982.

69. Stewart RD, Hake CL. Paint-remover hazard. *JAMA* 1976; 235: 398–401.

70. Kubic VL, Anders MW. Metabolism of dihalomethanes to carbon monoxide: II. In vitro studies. *Drug Metab Dispos* 1975; 3: 104–112.

71. Winneke G. The neurotoxicity of dichloromethane. *Neurobehav Toxicol Teratol* 1981; 3: 391–395.

72. Sjostrand T. Endogenous formation of carbon monoxide in man under normal and pathological conditions. *Scand J Clin Lab Invest* 1949; 1: 201–214.

73. Delivoria-Papadapoulos M, Coburn RF, Forster RE. Cyclic variation of rate of carbon monoxide production in normal women. *J Appl Physiol* 1974; 36: 49–51.

74. Coburn RF. Endogenous carbon monoxide production. *N Engl J Med* 1980; 282: 207–209.

75. Bartlett D. Effect of carbon monoxide on human physiological processes. In: *Proceedings of the Conference on Health Effects of Pollutants*, Serial No. 93–15, pp. 103–126. Washington, DC: US Government Printing Office, 1973.

76. Coburn RF, Forster RE, Kane PB. Considerations of the physiological variables that determine the blood carboxyhemoglobin concentration in man. *J Clin Invest* 1965; 44: 1899–1910.

77. Stewart RD. The effect of carbon monoxide on humans. *Annu Rev Pharmacol* 1975; 15: 409–423.

78. Shillito FH, Drinker CK, Shaughnessy TJ. The problem of nervous and mental sequelae in carbon monoxide poisoning. *JAMA* 1936; 106: 669–674.

79. Smith JS, Brandon S. Morbidity from acute carbon monoxide poisoning at three-year follow-up. *Br Med J* 1973; 1: 318–321.

80. Jaeckle RS, Nasrallah HA. Major depression and carbon monoxide-induced parkinsonism: Diagnosis, computerized axial tomography, and response to L-dopa. *J Nerv Ment Dis* 1985; 173: 503–508.

81. Klawans HL, Stein RW, Tanner CM, Goetz CG. A pure parkinsonian syndrome following acute carbon monoxide intoxication. *Arch Neurol* 1982; 39: 302–304.

82. Choi IS. Peripheral neuropathy following acute carbon monoxide poisoning. *Muscle Nerve* 1986; 9: 265–266.

83. Wilson G, Winkleman NW. Multiple neuritis following carbon monoxid poisoning. *JAMA* 1924; 82: 1407–1410.

84. Laplane D, Levasseur M, Pillon B *et al.* Obsessive–compulsive and other behavioural changes with bilateral basal ganglia lesions. A neuropsychological, magnetic resonance imaging and positron tomography study. *Brain* 1989; 112: 699–725.

85. Lugaresi A, Montagna P, Morreale A, Gallassi R. 'Psychic akinesia' following carbon monoxide poisoning. *Eur Neurol* 1990; 30: 167–169.

86. Pulst SM, Walshe TM, Romero JA. Carbon monoxide poisoning with features of Gilles de la Tourette's syndrome. *Arch Neurol* 1983; 40: 443–444.

87. Norris CR, Trench JM, Hook R. Delayed carbon monoxide encephalopathy: clinical and research implications. *J Clin Psychiatry* 1982; 43: 294–295.

88. Sawa GM, Watson CP, Terbrugge K, Chiu M. Delayed encephalopathy following carbon monoxide intoxication. *Can J Neurol Sci* 1981; 8: 77–79.

89. Werner B, Back W, Akerblom H, Barr PO. Two cases of acute carbon monoxide poisoning with delayed neurological sequelae after a 'free' interval. *J Toxicol Clin Toxicol* 1985; 23: 249–265.

90. Kim KS, Weinberg PE, Suh JH, Ho SU. Acute carbon monoxide poisoning: computed tomography of the brain. *Am J Neuroradiol* 1980; 1: 399–402.

91. Nardizzi LR. Computerized tomographic correlate of carbon monoxide poisoning. *Arch Neurol* 1979; 36: 38–39.

92. Sawada Y, Takahashi M, Ohashi N *et al.* Computerised tomography, as an indication of long-term outcome after acute carbon monoxide poisoning. *Lancet* 1980; 1: 783–784.

93. Katafuchi Y, Nishimi T, Yamaguchi Y *et al.* Cortical blindness in acute carbon monoxide poisoning. *Brain Dev* 1985; 7: 516–519.

94. Quattrocolo G, Leotta D, Appendino L *et al.* A case of cortical blindness due to carbon monoxide poisoning. *Ital J Neurol Sci* 1987; 8: 57–58.

95. Reynolds NC, Shapiro I. Retrobulbar neuritis with neuroretinal edema as a delayed manifestation of carbon monoxide poisoning: case report. *Mil Med* 1979; 144: 472–473.

96. Dempsey LC, O'Donnell JJ, Hoff JT. Carbon monoxide retinopathy. *Am J Ophthalmol* 1976; 82: 692–693.

97. Kelley JS, Sophocleus GJ. Retinal hemorrhages in subacute carbon monoxide poisoning. *JAMA* 1978; 239: 1515–1517.

98. Baker SR, Lilly DJ. Hearing loss from acute carbon monoxide intoxication. *Ann Otol Rhinol Laryngol* 1977; 86: 323–328.

99. Hill EP, Hill JR, Power GG, Longo LD. Carbon monoxide exchanges between the human fetus and mother: A mathematical model. *Am J Physiol* 1977; 232(Suppl H3): 11–23.

100. Longo LD. Carbon monoxide: effects on oxygenation of the fetus in utero. *Science* 1976; 194: 523–525.

101. Longo LD. The biological effects of carbon monoxide on the pregnant woman, fetus, and newborn infant. *Am J Obstet Gynecol* 1977; 129: 69–103.

102. Cramer CR. Fetal death due to accidental maternal carbon monoxide poisoning. *J Toxicol Clin Toxicol* 1982; 19: 297–301.

103. Goldstein DP. Carbon monoxide poisoning in pregnancy. *Am J Obstet Gynecol* 1965; 92: 526–528.

104. Muller GL, Graham S. Intrauterine death of the fetus due to accidental carbon monoxide poisoning. *N Engl J Med* 1955; 252: 1075–1078.

105. Norman CA, Halton DM. Is carbon monoxide a workplace teratogen? A review and evaluation of the literature. *Ann Occup Hyg* 1990; 34: 335–347.

106. Woody RC, Brewster MA. Telencephalic dysgenesis associated with presumptive maternal carbon monoxide intoxication in the first trimester of pregnancy. *J Toxicol Clin Toxicol* 1990; 28: 467–475.

107. Koren G, Sharav T, Pastuszak A *et al.* A multicenter, prospective study of fetal outcome following accidental carbon monoxide poisoning in pregnancy. *Reprod Toxicol* 1991; 5: 397–403.

108. Margulies JL. Acute carbon monoxide poisoning during pregnancy. *Am J Emerg Med* 1986; 4: 516–519.

109. Small KA, Radford EP, Frazier JM *et al.* A rapid method for simultaneous measurement of carboxy- and methemoglobin in blood. *J Appl Physiol* 1971; 31: 154–160.

110. Hodgkin JE, Chan DM. Diabetic ketoacidosis appearing as carbon monoxide poisoning. *JAMA* 1975; 231: 1164–1165.

111. Hampson NB. Pulse oximetry in severe carbon monoxide poisoning. *Chest* 1998; 114: 1036–1041.

112. McNeill AD, Owen LA, Belcher M *et al.* Abstinence from smoking and expired-air carbon monoxide levels: lactose intolerance as a possible source of error. *Am J Public Health* 1990; 80: 1114–1115.

113. Winter PM, Miller JN. Carbon monoxide poisoning. *JAMA* 1976; 236: 1502–1504.

114. Raphael JC, Elkharrat D, Jars-Guincestre MC *et al.* Trial of normobaric and hyperbaric oxygen for acute carbon monoxide intoxication. *Lancet* 1989; ii: 414–419.

115. Scheinkestel CD, Bailey M, Myles PS *et al.* Hyperbaric or normobaric oxygen for acute carbon monoxide poisoning: a randomised controlled clinical trial. *Med J Aust* 1999; 170: 5: 203–210.

116. Murphy DG, Sloan EP, Hart RG *et al.* Tension pneumothorax associated with hyperbaric oxygen therapy. *Am J Emerg Med* 1991; 9: 176–179.

117. Sloan EP, Murphy DG, Hart R *et al.* Complications and protocol considerations in carbon monoxide-poisoned patients who require hyperbaric oxygen therapy: report from a ten-year experience. *Ann Emerg Med* 1989; 18: 629–634.

118. Youngberg JT, Myers RA. Complications from hyperbaric oxygen therapy? *Ann Emerg Med* 1990; 19: 1356–1357.

119. Anon. Idaho employer convicted of exposing employees to cyanide. *Cal-OSHA Reporter* 1999; 26: 7166.

120. Orzel R. Toxicological aspects of firesmoke: polymer pyrolysis and combustion. *Occup Med* 1993; 8: 415–430.

121. Wetherell HR. The occurrence of cyanide in the blood of fire victims. *J Forensic Sci* 1996; 11: 167–173.

122. Anderson RA, Harland WA. Fire deaths in the Glasgow area: III. The role of hydrogen cyanide. *Med Sci Law* 1982; 22: 35–40.

123. Jones J, McMullen MJ, Dougherty J. Toxic smoke inhalation: cyanide poisoning in fire victims. *Am J Emerg Med* 1987; 5: 317–321.

124. Ballantyne B. Toxicology of cyanides. In: Ballantyne B, Marrs TC, eds. *Clinical and Experimental Toxicology of the Cyanides*, pp. 41–126. Bristol, UK: Wright, 1987.

125. Hall AH, Rumack BH. Hydroxycobalamin/sodium thiosulfate as a cyanide antidote. *J Emerg Med* 1987; 5: 115–121.

126. Lovejoy FH. Cyanide. *Clin Toxicol Rev* 1980; 2: 1–2.

127. Smith RP. Toxic responses of the blood. In: Klaassen CD, ed. *Casarett and Doull's Toxicology* 5th edn, pp. 335–354. New York: McGraw-Hill, 1996.

128. Smith RP. Cyanate and thiocyanate: acute toxicity. *Proc Soc Exp Biol Med* 1973; 142: 1041–1044.

129. Homan ER. Reactions, processes and materials with potential for cyanide exposure. In: Ballantyne B, Marrs TC eds. *Clinical and Experimental Toxicology of the Cyanides*, pp. 1–21. Bristol, UK: Wright, 1987.

130. Westley J, Adler H, Westley L, Nishida C. The sulfur transferases. *Fundam Appl Toxicol* 1983; 3: 377–382.

131. Borgers D, Junge B. Thiocyanate as an indicator of tobacco smoking. *Prev Med* 1979; 8: 351–357.

132. Blanc PD. Cyanide. In: Olson KR ed. *Poisoning and Drug Overdose*, 3rd edn. pp. 150–152. Stamford, CT: Appleton and Lange, 1999.

133. Troup CM, Ballantyne B. Analysis of cyanide in biological fluids and tissues. In: Ballantyne B, Marrs TC, eds. *Clinical and Experimental Toxicology of Cyanides*, pp. 22–40. Bristol, UK: Wright, 1987.

134. Hall A, Rumack BH, Schaffer MI, Linden CH. Clinical toxicology of cyanide: North American experience. In: Ballantyne B, Marrs TC, eds. *Clinical and Experimental Toxicology of the Cyanides*, pp. 312–333. Bristol, UK: Wright, 1987.

135. Gonzales J, Sabatini S. Cyanide poisoning: pathophysiology and current approaches to therapy. *Int J Artif Organs* 1989; 12: 347–355.

136. Hall AH, Linden CH, Kulig KW, Rumack BH. Cyanide poisoning from laetrile ingestion: role of nitrite therapy. *Pediatrics* 1986; 78: 269–272.

137. Johnson RP, Mellors JW. Arteriolization of venous blood gases: a clue to the diagnosis of cyanide poisoning. *J Emerg Med* 1988; 6: 401–404.

138. Vogel SN. Lactic acidosis in acute cyanide poisoning. In: Ballantyne B, Marrs TC, eds. *Clinical and Experimental Toxicology of the Cyanides*, pp. 451–466. Bristol, UK: Wright, 1987.

139. Goldfrank LR, Starke CL. Metabolic acidosis in the alcoholic. In: Goldfrank LR *et al.* eds. *Goldfrank's Toxicological Emergencies*, 4th edn, pp. 465–472. Norwalk, CT: Appleton & Lange, 1990.

140. Bright JE. A prophylaxis for cyanide poisoning. In: Ballantyne B, Marrs TC, eds. *Clinical and Experimental Toxicology of the Cyanides*, pp. 359–382. Bristol, UK. Wright, 1987.

141. Chen KK, Rose CL, Clowes GHA. Comparative values of several antidotes in cyanide poisoning. *Am J Med Sci* 1934; 188: 767–781.

142. Vick JA, Froehlich H. Treatment of cyanide poisoning. *Mil Med* 1991; 156: 330–339.

143. Way JL, Leung P, Sylvester DM. Methaemoglobin formation in the treatment of acute cyanide intoxication. In: Ballantyne B, Marrs TC, eds. *Clinical and Experimental Toxicology of the Cyanides*, pp. 402–412. Bristol, UK: Wright, 1987.

144. Isom GE, Johnson JD. Sulphur donors in cyanide intoxication. In: Ballantyne B, Marrs TC, eds. *Clinical and Experimental Toxicology of the Cyanides*, pp. 413–426. Bristol, UK: Wright, 1987.

145. Kim S. Thiosulfate, sodium. In: Olson KR, ed. *Poisoning and Drug Overdose* 3rd edn, pp. 408–409. Stamford, CT: Appleton and Lange, 1999.

146. Keller KH. Nitrite, sodium and amyl. In: Olson KR, ed. *Poisoning and Drug Overdose* 3rd edn, pp. 390–392. Stamford, CT: Appleton and Lange, 1999.

147. Weger NP. Treatment of cyanide poisoning with 4-dimethylaminophenol (DMAP) – experimental and clinical overview. *Fundam Appl Toxicol* 1983; 3: 387–396.

148. Ten Eyck RP, Schaerdel AD, Ottinger WE. Stroma-free methemoglobin solution: an effective antidote for acute cyanide poisoning. *Am J Emerg Med* 1985; 3: 519–523.

149. Bhatt HR, Linnell JC. The role of rhodanese in cyanide detoxification: its possible use in acute cyanide poisoning in man. In: Ballantyne B, Marrs TC, eds. *Clinical and Experimental Toxicology of the Cyanides*, pp. 440–450. Bristol, UK: Wright, 1987.

150. Linnell JC. The role of cobalamins in cyanide detoxification. In: Ballantyne B, Marrs TC, eds. *Clinical and Experimental Toxicology of the Cyanides*, pp. 427–439. Bristol, UK: Wright, 1987.

151. Williams HL, Johnson DJ, McNeil JS, Wright DG. Studies of cobalamin as a vehicle for the renal excretion of cyanide anion. *J Lab Clin Med* 1990; 116: 37–44.

152. Forsyth JC, Mueller PD, Becker CE *et al.* Hydroxocobalamin as a cyanide antidote: safety, efficacy and pharmacokinetics in heavily smoking normal volunteers. *J Toxicol Clin Toxicol* 1993; 31: 277–294.

153. Ballantyne B. Hydrogen cyanide as a product of combustion and a factor in morbidity and mortality from fires. In: Ballantyne B, Marrs TC, eds. *Clinical and Experimental Toxicology of the Cyanides*, pp. 248–291. Bristol, UK: Wright, 1987.

154. Becker CE. The role of cyanide in fires. *Vet Hum Toxicol* 1985; 27: 487–490.

155. Kulig K. Cyanide antidotes and fire toxicology. [Editorial; comment] *N Engl J Med* 1991; 325: 1801–1802.

156. Moore SJ, Norris JC, Walsh DA, Hume AS. Antidotal use of methemoglobin forming cyanide antagonists in concurrent carbon monoxide/cyanide intoxication. *J Pharmacol Exp Ther* 1987; 242: 70–73.

157. Hall AH, Kulig KW, Rumack BH. Suspected cyanide poisoning in smoke inhalation: complications of sodium nitrite therapy. *J Toxicol Clin Exp* 1989; 9: 3–9.

158. Goldsmith JR. The 20-minute disaster: hydrogen sulfide spill at Poza Rica. In: Goldsmith JR, ed. *Environmental Epidemiology: Epidemiological Investigation of Community Environmental Health Problems* pp. 65–71. Boca Raton, FL: CRC Press, 1986.

159. Beauchamp RO Jr, Bus JS, Popp JA *et al.* A critical review of the literature on hydrogen sulfide toxicity. *Crit Rev Toxicol* 1984; 13: 25–97.

160. Guidotti TL. Hydrogen sulphide. *Occup Med (Oxf)* 1996; 46: 367–371.

161. Roth SH, Skrajny B, Bennington R, Brookes J. Neurotoxicity of hydrogen sulfide may result from inhibition of respiratory enzymes. *Proc West Pharmacol Soc* 1997; 40: 41–43.

162. Kombian SB, Warenycia MW, Mele FG, Reiffenstein RJ. Effects of acute intoxication with hydrogen sulfide on central amino acid transmitter systems. *Neurotoxicology* 1988; 9: 587–595.

163. Warenycia MW, Smith KA, Blashko CS *et al.* Monoamine oxidase inhibition as a sequel of hydrogen sulfide intoxication: increases in brain catecholamine and 5-hydroxytryptamine levels. *Arch Toxicol* 1989; 63: 131–136.

164. Roth B. Hydrogen sulfide. In: Olson KR, ed. *Poisoning and Drug Overdose*, 3rd edn, p. 188. Stamford, CT: Appleton and Lange, 1999.

165. Steffen C, Wetzel E. Chlorate poisoning: mechanism of toxicity. *Toxicology* 1993; 84: 217–231.

166. French CL, Yaun SS, Baldwin LA *et al.* Potency ranking of methemoglobin-forming agents. *J Appl Toxicol* 1995; 15: 167–174.

167. Reilly TP, Woster PM, Svensson CK. Methemoglobin formation by hydroxylamine metabolites of sulfamethoxazole and dapsone: implications for differences in adverse drug reactions. *J Pharmacol Exp Ther* 1999; 288: 951–959.

168. Severinghaus JW, Xu FD, Spellman MJ Jr. Benzocaine and methemoglobin: recommended actions. *Anesthesiology* 1991; 74: 385–387.

169. Fletcher KA, Barton PF, Kelly JA. Studies on the mechanisms of oxidation in the erythrocyte by metabolites of primaquine. *Biochem Pharmacol* 1988; 37: 2683–2690.

170. Gault MH, Shahidi NT. Methemoglobin formation in patients with renal disease associated with abuse of analgesics containing phenacetin. *J Lab Clin Med* 1971; 78: 810–811.

171. Shuval HI, Gruener N. Epidemiological and toxicological aspects of nitrates and nitrites in the environment. *Am J Public Health* 1972; 62: 1045–1052.

172. Hornfeldt CS, Rabe WH III. Nitroethane poisoning from an artificial fingernail remover. *J Toxicol Clin Toxicol* 1994; 32: 321–324.

173. Freeman L, Wolford RW. Methemoglobinemia secondary to cleaning solution ingestion. *J Emerg Med* 1996; 14: 599–601.

174. Blanc PD. Methemoglobinemia. In: Olson KR ed. *Poisoning and Drug Overdose*, 3rd edn, pp. 220–222. Stamford, CT: Appleton and Lange, 1999.

175. Rieder HU, Frei FJ, Zbinden AM, Thomson DA. Pulse oximetry in methaemoglobinaemia. Failure to detect low oxygen saturation. *Anaesthesia* 1989; 44: 326–327.

176. Keller KH. Methylene blue. In: Olson KR ed. *Poisoning and Drug Overdose*, 3rd edn, pp. 381–382. Stamford, CT: Appleton and Lange, 1999.

177. Hendrick DJ, Sizer KE. 'Breathing' coal mines and surface asphyxiation from stythe (black damp). *Br Med J* 1992; 305: 509–510.

178. Clarke T. Taming Africa's killer lake. *Nature* 2001; 409: 554–555.

179. Yoon SS, Macdonald SC, Partrish RG. Deaths from unintentional carbon monoxide poisoning and potential for prevention with carbon monoxide detectors. *JAMA* 1998; 279: 685–687.

180. Krenzelok EP, Roth R, Full R. Carbon monoxide – the silent killer with an audible solution. *Am J Emerg Med* 1996; 14: 484–486.

181. Occupational Safety and Health Administration. *OSHA Regulations – Standards. 29 CFR 1910.1000 – Air Contaminants.* Washington, DC: OSHA, 1997.

182. US Environmental Protection Agency. *National Primary and Secondary Ambient Air Quality Standards.* 40 CFR Part 50; Section 50.8 – *National Primary Ambient Air Quality Standards for Carbon Monoxide.* Washington, DC: US EPA.

19 LUNG CANCER

Michelle Ng Gong and David C. Christiani

BACKGROUND

Most of the exposures that have been judged to cause cancer in humans have occurred in the workplace [1]. A large proportion of these exposures involves lung carcinogens, although most lung cancer is known to be a consequence of tobacco smoke. The most important occupational lung carcinogen is asbestos. Tobacco and many workplace carcinogens are relatively strong causes of lung cancer, increasing the reported incidences 10–100-fold compared with unexposed groups. Workers may, however, be exposed to a wide range of carcinogens, and so epidemiological studies are more likely to identify a strong carcinogen than a weak one. Difficulty in identifying a weak carcinogen does not exclude its existence.

The designation of a substance as a human carcinogen requires judgment. The International Agency for Research on Cancer (IARC) has been reviewing the scientific literature on animal and human studies on potential carcinogens since 1971. Every year one or more working groups convene in Lyon, France, to review experimental and epidemiological studies in order to classify the carcinogenic potential of various substances in humans. The classification in use is given in Table 19.1. In 1979 the first comprehensive listing of agents judged to be definite (group 1) causes of human cancer was published by IARC [2]. A number of these agents are lung carcinogens (Table 19.2). One of these agents,

Table 19.1 IARC classification of the carcinogenicity of substances

Group	Characteristic
1	The agent is carcinogenic to humans
2A	The agent is probably carcinogenic to humans
2B	The agent is possibly carcinogenic to humans
3	The agent is not classifiable as to its carcinogenicity to humans
4	The agent is probably not carcinogenic to humans

arsenic, had been found to be a lung carcinogen before 1900, but the year an agent or process is first deemed to be carcinogenic is somewhat arbitrary and other dates are often suggested by researchers in the field [3]. A characteristic of many of the 'established' agents listed in Table 19.2 is their strong association with lung cancer (often a rate ratio of 10 or more) depending upon intensity and duration of exposure for the relevant working population.

Between 1980 and 1987, IARC expanded the list of occupational exposures considered to be carcinogenic for the lung (Table 19.3), and since 1987 the list has been expanded further (Table 19.4).

Table 19.5 lists occupational agents that, to date, have been classified by IARC as probable (group 2A) rather than definite human carcinogens. Some represent mixtures of chemical compounds or general manufacturing processes. More recently IARC has identified a further category of possible (group 2B)

Table 19.2 Agents and processes judged by IARC in 1979 to be carcinogenic for the human lung

Substance or process	Year of first report
Arsenic and certain arsenic compounds	(1822)[a]
Asbestos	1935
Chromium and certain chromium compounds	1948
Mustard gas	1955
Underground hematite mining	1956

[a] Refers to the work environment rather than to a specific compound.

Table 19.3 Agents and processes judged by IARC from 1980 to 1987 to be carcinogenic for the human lung

Substance or process	Year of first report
Coal gasification	1936
Coke production	1971
Iron and steel founding	1977
Talc containing asbestiform fibers	1979
Aluminum production	1981
Soot	1985

Table 19.4 Agents and processes judged by IARC from 1988 to 1996 to be carcinogenic for the human lung

Substance or process	Year of first report
Radon	(1879)[a]
Sulfuric acid mist	1952
Bis(chloromethyl) ether and chloromethyl methyl ether	1973
Cadmium and cadmium compounds	1976
Nickel	1960s
Spray painting	1976
2,3,7,8-Tetrachlorodibenzo-*para*-dioxin	1977
Beryllium and beryllium compounds	1979
Paint manufacturing and painting	1980
Crystalline silica	1986

[a] Refers to work environment rather than specific compound.

Table 19.5 Agents and processes judged by IARC from 1979 to 1995 as probable human lung carcinogens

Substance or process	Year of first report
Epichlorohydrin	1976
Non-arsenical pesticides (spraying)	1979
α-Chlorinated toluenes and benzoyl chlorides	1982
Diesel particulate	1983
Glass manufacture	1987

Table 19.6 Agents judged by IARC to be possible lung carcinogens

Acetaldehyde
Acrylonitrile
Very fine vitreous fibers
Welding fumes

lung carcinogens; they are identified in Table 19.6. For this group there is limited epidemiological information on which to provide an unambiguous judgment of causality. In parts of the industrializing world, however, there may be working populations of sufficient size and with a sufficient range of exposure to yield unambiguous information in the future.

Established carcinogens

There is a large body of information on IARC group 1 lung carcinogens. It comes chiefly from toxicologic and epidemiological studies of working populations in industrially developed countries since, with few exceptions, only sparse information is available from countries still undergoing industrial development.

Arsenic

Although arsenic has generally not been found to induce cancer in experimental animals, epidemiologic studies from around the world clearly show that inorganic arsenic is a human lung carcinogen. The evidence emanates mainly from observations among copper smelter workers who are exposed to arsenic trioxide. Inorganic arsenic is a constituent of most copper ores and, to a lesser extent, lead and zinc ores. It is removed during the smelting process and may be emitted within industrial effluent.

As early as 1948 Hill and Fanning reported a fivefold increase in lung cancer deaths among workers manufacturing arsenical pesticides for use as sheep dip [4]. Studies of larger populations in the 1960s [5] and 1970s showed increased standardized mortality ratios (SMR) for lung cancer among Montana copper smelter workers. Extended follow-up of the cohort confirmed an excess lung cancer risk among 8000 smelter workers and clarified the exposure–response relationship (Table 19.7) [6]. Similar observations have come from follow-up studies of workers in copper smelters elsewhere in the USA, as well as in Japan, Sweden, and China [7–10].

In some epidemiological studies, a potential interaction between cigarette smoking and arsenic has been evaluated. Only a minority of the participants in the US Montana smelter study were non-smokers, but the risk of lung cancer increased with rising arsenic exposure among both smokers and non-

Table 19.7 Standard mortality ratios (SMR) for lung cancer according to cumulative exposure to airborne arsenic among 8000 Montana copper smelter workers. Adapted from Lee-Feldstein [6]

Cumulative arsenic exposure: (mg/m³ × years)	No. lung cancer deaths	SMR
<0.9	20	168
0.9–1.9	33	256
2.0–8.3	43	167
8.4–41.6	115	315
41.7–208.3	54	429
208.4–416.6	20	571
>416.7	17	680

smokers [11]. The effects of exposure and smoking appeared more additive than multiplicative. Similar findings were reported in smelter workers in the southwest China province of Yunnan [12].

Another major source of occupational arsenical exposure around the world has been the production of pesticides, fungicides, and herbicides. Following the earliest report, above, of arsenic-related lung cancer in workers making arsenic trioxide pesticides, epidemiological studies of American workers revealed a ten-fold increase in lung cancer mortality with light exposures for 15 or more years [13].

Although systematic studies of cancer risk have not been performed on workers exposed to arsenic in other settings, it is important to note that airborne arsenic exposure can take place in a variety of industries, including pressure-treated wood and glass production.

Asbestos

Evidence for a lung carcinogenic effect of asbestos has been available since 1935, and in 1938 the German physician Nordmann suggested that lung cancer in subjects with asbestosis was an occupational disease [14]. Since then there have been multiple studies showing an elevated risk of lung cancer associated with asbestos exposure. A recent review by Steenland et al. [15] summarized the findings from six cohort studies of subjects with asbestosis and 20 cohort studies of asbestos workers without asbestosis. The combined relative risk for developing lung cancer compared with unexposed subjects was 5.91 (95% confidence interval (CI) 4.98–7.00) in the asbestosis group and 2.00 (95% CI 1.90–2.11) in the non-asbestosis group. In only four of the studies was the risk adjusted for smoking history, and in these the relative risk attributable to asbestos exposure alone ranged from 1.04 to 4.33 [16–19]. On the basis of such evidence IARC has, since 1979, classified asbestos as a lung carcinogen.

Although it is clear that asbestos exposure in general is associated with an increased risk of lung cancer, some studies have not shown an increased risk in asbestos-exposed individuals without pulmonary fibrosis. A number of investigators have argued that the increased risk is related primarily to asbestosis rather than exposure, and so it is an indirect rather than a direct effect of exposure [20,21]. The issue is complicated, and confounded, because the probability of asbestosis is itself related closely to exposure dose. This implies that a lower risk of lung cancer is to be expected in individuals without pulmonary fibrosis irrespective of whether exposure or asbestosis is of primary etiologic importance [15]. Further problems have been a lack of statistical power of many of the studies to detect a difference in lung cancer incidence at levels of exposure insufficient to cause asbestosis, and the use of different criteria to identify asbestosis (radiologic in some, histologic in others) [22,23]. The use of broader definitions may have resulted in over diagnosis of asbestosis in some of the studies of asbestos-related lung cancer [24].

Nevertheless, a number of studies have found an association between asbestos exposure and lung cancer in the absence of asbestosis. In a 1995 case-control study Wilkinson et al. compared 271 patients with lung cancer with 678 control patients (279 with other respiratory diseases, 399 with cardiac diseases) for a history of definite or probable occupational exposure to asbestos more than 15 years previously. They found an odds ratio for exposure (cases versus controls) of 2.03 (95% CI 1.00–4.13) in the subgroup of 211 patients who had a median pneumoconiosis profusion score of 1/0 or more on the International Labor Office (ILO) scale after adjusting for age, sex, and smoking [25]. The corresponding odds ratio for the remaining 738 patients with median ILO scores of 0/1 or less (i.e. those without evidence of pulmonary fibrosis on plain radiographs) was 1.56 (95% CI 1.02–2.39) after controlling for age, sex, and smoking. This suggests a modest increase in risk of lung cancer attributable to asbestos even in the absence of radiographic asbestosis, but the CI values for the odds ratio came very close to including 1. The CI did include 1 for the participants with radiographic evidence of pulmonary fibrosis. The outcome illustrates well some of the difficulties that investigation of the issue generates, and it explains why it readily generates controversy [20,21]. The matter has been reviewed again more recently [26], and in the authors' opinion the weight of evidence suggests that asbestos exposure is associated with an increased risk of lung cancer even in the absence of asbestosis.

Some studies have also indicated increased expected rates of lung cancer in patients with pleural plaques without evidence of asbestosis compared with age-matched males in Sweden. For example, in 1994 Hillerdal reported a relative risk of 1.4 (95% CI 1.04–1.97) for subjects with pleural plaques but no evidence of radiologic asbestosis [27]. This issue remains very controversial.

It is important, of course, to be clear which population is being compared with which. If subjects with and without pleural plaques are compared from within the general population, the former are likely to have sustained greater levels of exposure to asbestos, and so are more likely to develop asbestosis or any other type of asbestos-induced disorder. If, however, the starting point is a population of individuals with similar cumulative levels of asbestos exposure over similar time frames, then the presence or absence of pleural plaques is not thought to influence the probability for the development of any other type of asbestos-related disorder. In this sense pleural plaques are not predictors of the other disorders. Put another way, pleural plaques do not predispose to other asbestos-related disorders if adjustments are made for cumulative exposure dose, but they do serve as markers of asbestos exposure.

Although asbestos is a well-recognized carcinogen, our knowledge about how it causes cancer is incomplete. Asbestos has been demonstrated experimentally to induce the production of oxygen radicals by inflammatory cells, and it is possible that the oxidative effects may result in cellular and DNA damage and so contribute to the development of cancer [28]. In addition, asbestos has been shown in the laboratory to induce chromosomal deletions and rearrangements, and to be strongly mutagenic in mammalian cells [29,30]. More recently, mutations of the tumor suppressor gene p53 have been found to be associated with asbestos-related lung cancer [31].

As with mesothelioma, there have been suggestions that serpentine (chrysotile) fibers may be a less potent carcinogen for lung cancer than the amphibole fibers (crocidolite, amosite, tremolite, actinolite and anthophyllite) and that cancer secondary to suspected chrysotile exposure is actually caused by contamination with amphibole fibers [32]. This belief stems partly from the finding that the percentage of chrysotile fibers found in patients with lung cancer is low relative to other fiber types, even though chrysotile is the most common source of asbestos used [33]. This can be misleading as chrysotile is cleared from the lungs much faster than amphibole fibers (a half life of months rather than years). Given that lung cancer appears to have a latency of some 20 to 40 years after exposure onset [26,34], the lung burden of chrysotile or any other fibers at the time of disease presentation may not reflect accurately the carcinogenic potential at the time of initial tumorgenesis.

Several studies have found high risks of lung cancer in workers exposed to chrysotile fibers [34,35], and in 1996 Stayner et al. reviewed 12 retrospective cohort studies of workers exposed predominantly to chrysotile [33]. They calculated a pooled SMR of 150 compared with a reference population (95% CI 140–160), and found that the elevated risk persisted in the six studies that controlled for tobacco consumption. The current evidence seems to indicate, therefore, that chrysotile exposure is associated with an increased risk of lung cancer but it is not yet clear how potent a carcinogen it is relative to amphibole asbestos.

Asbestos confers an increased independent risk for lung cancer even in the absence of a tobacco history. In one study of 530 Chinese workers in an asbestos plant [34], the SMR for lung cancer for 370 non-smoking females was significantly elevated at 680 ($P<0.01$) compared with local Chinese women. It is clear that smoking in combination with asbestos exposure has a synergistic effect on the risk of lung cancer, and current evidence suggests a multiplicative association [36–38]. A study by Kjuus et al. [38] gave an odds ratio for lung cancer of 2.9 for light smokers (5–9 cigarettes) with no asbestos exposure and of 11.9 for light smokers with heavy asbestos exposure (defined as moderate asbestos exposure for 10 years or heavy exposure for 1 year) when compared with unexposed never-smokers. This increased to 370.2 in heavy smokers (>30 cigarettes a day) with heavy asbestos exposure compared with 90.3 for heavy smokers with no asbestos exposure. Among both the light smokers and the heavy smokers, heavy asbestos exposure was consequently associated with a 4.1-fold increase in risk; among both the subjects without asbestos exposure and those with asbestos exposure, the difference between heavy and light smoking was associated with a 31-fold increase in risk (Table 19.8).

Table 19.8 Multiplicative risk of smoking and asbestos exposure[a]

Smoking	No asbestos	Heavy asbestos	Increased risk
Light	2.9	11.9	×4.1
Heavy	90.3	370.2	×4.1
Increased risk	×31	×31	

[a] Given that the risk associated with no smoking and no asbestos exposure is 1.

Clinically, asbestos-induced lung cancer is indistinguishable from other lung cancers. Early reports had suggested an increased incidence of lower lobe tumors and of adenocarcinoma in association with asbestos exposure [39,40], but subsequent studies have not confirmed this and it is not possible to attribute causality to asbestos from location or histologic type [41,42].

Beryllium

Beryllium exposure occurs mainly in mining, refining, and in the manufacture of ceramics, electronic, and aerospace equipment. In 1980, IARC concluded that there was sufficient animal evidence for beryllium metal and several beryllium compounds to be considered carcinogenic [43]. Since that time two cohort mortality studies have been reported, and in both an excess of lung cancer was found. One was based on the US Beryllium Case Registry Mortality Study of 689 women and men in which an SMR for lung cancer of 200 (95% CI 133–289) was found [44]. Given the magnitude of the effect and after limited adjustment for smoking, the authors concluded that smoking was unlikely to be a major confounder. In the second study, Ward *et al.* [45] reported the results of a cohort mortality study of 9225 males from seven US beryllium plants. The overall lung cancer SMR was 124 (95% CI 110–139). Lung cancer SMR values increased with latency and with work in factories with higher SMR values for pneumoconiosis. In 1994, IARC concluded that the evidence was sufficient to conclude that beryllium is carcinogenic to humans [46].

Cadmium

Cadmium is principally used in electroplating, in compounds that serve as stabilizers for plastics and as pigments, in electrodes in batteries, and in alloys [47]. In experimental animals, cadmium induces tumors of the lung and other organs, including prostate and lymphoid tissue [48–50]. Cadmium exposure often takes place in settings with other carcinogens, such as nickel and arsenic, which results in confounding [51]. However, a US study of metal waste reclamation workers was able to assess the relative risk for lung cancer with increasing exposure to cadmium from the lowest negligible category (1.49; 95% CI 0.96–2.22) to the highest category (2.72; 95% CI 1.24–5.18) [52,53]. This provides important evidence that cadmium itself is carcinogenic, and hence its IARC classification [43].

Chloromethyl ethers

Bis(chloromethyl)ether (BCME) and chloromethyl methyl ether (CMME) have been recognized by IARC as definite lung carcinogens since 1987 [54].

Occupational exposure to BCME and CMME may occur in the production of ion-exchange resins. In animal studies, BCME is the more carcinogenic of the two compounds [55–57]. In addition, it is more volatile and therefore more readily inhaled. However, technical grade CMME used in industry is always contaminated with BCME so it impossible to separate the carcinogenic potential of the two compounds in occupational studies.

A series of epidemiological reports from the UK, France, and the USA has indicated an increased risk of lung cancer associated with occupational exposure to BCME and CMME in the manufacturing of ion-exchange resins [57–59]. In a group of 1203 male workers in a chemical plant in France, a statistically significant increase in the rate ratio of 5.0 (95% CI 2.0–12.3) was found for the development of lung cancer when exposed workers were compared with non-exposed workers [58]. When the exposed workers were compared with the male population of that part of France, the rate ratio increased to 7.6 (95% CI 4.3–13.5). An elevated risk was also found in a recent 30-year update of a cohort of 125 chemical workers in Philadelphia [59]. An elevated SMR of 1090 (95% CI 670–1680) was found only in the moderately to heavily exposed workers, the risk being highest in the first 10–19 years after first exposure (SMR 2860; 95% CI 1370–5260).

Several common features were found in these French and Philadelphia workers. There appeared to be a dose-dependent response with the elevated risk occurring mostly in moderately to heavily exposed workers. Compared with other occupational lung carcinogens, exposure to BCME and CMME appeared to be associated with a shorter latency for the development of lung cancer. Consequently, the disease occurred at a younger age than would be expected. While adjustment was not made for smoking in any of these studies, it is unlikely to have been an important confounder as the cancer occurred in both smokers and non-smokers. In the Philadelphia cohort, 25% of the lung cancers occurred in non-smokers. In addition, small cell lung cancer accounted for 80–90% of the cases unlike tobacco related lung cancer.

Chromium

Chromium is a metal that can exist in any oxidation state between −2 and +6. Most chromium compounds contain the metal in the +3 (trivalent) or +6 (hexavalent) state, and most naturally occurring chromium is found as oxides in chromite ore. Chromium (VI) causes cancer in animal studies and is the currently regulated form [60]. Most chromium consumed in the USA is used in the production of stainless (rust-resistant) steel. Exposure may occur during the production of stainless steel, other chrome alloys, and chrome-containing pigments, during chrome plating, and during stainless steel welding.

There have been over 50 epidemiological studies of chromium exposure and lung cancer [60]. The largest investigations have been performed on chromium production workers, chromate paint makers, and chrome platers. Steenland *et al.* estimated the overall relative risk of lung cancer in these studies at 2.78 (95% CI 2.47–3.52). In the studies that were able to address confounders (tobacco, asbestos, nickel), they rejected confounding as the major source of the observed elevated risk [15]. A retrospective cohort study of 2982 workers in Chinese chromate manufacturing plants revealed a very similar increased risk for lung cancer (relative risk (RR) 2.7; 90% CI 1.3–5.5) [61]. Risk was related to exposure latency, extent of exposure and smoking habits.

Nickel

The principal current uses of nickel and nickel salts are in the production of stainless steel, non-ferrous alloys, electroplating, and battery manufacture [62]. IARC considers the evidence for human carcinogenicity to be sufficient for nickel sulfate and for the 'combinations of nickel sulfides and oxides encountered in the nickel refining industry'. However, it considers the evidence for metallic nickel and nickel alloys to be inadequate.

The most current review of cancer among nickel-exposed workers is the 1990 report of The International Committee on Nickel Carcinogenesis in Man [62]. This review of nine cohort and one case-control study reports that lung cancer and nasal cancer were consistently and significantly increased among exposed workers at nickel refineries. Steenland *et al.* [15] used data from this report to estimate a combined RR of 1.56 (95% CI 1.41–1.73). Interestingly, studies of workers engaged in other nickel-related industries, such as nickel alloys and stainless-steel welding, have not shown consistently elevated lung cancer deaths.

Silica

IARC reviewed the evidence for carcinogenicity of crystalline silica in 1997 and concluded that there was sufficient evidence for carcinogenicity in humans to warrant designation of crystalline silica as a group 1 carcinogen [63].

In rats, inhaled silica causes both fibrosis and lung cancer at relatively low concentration (1 mg/m^3) [64]. In human studies, problems of confounding (smoking and radon exposure) and selection bias (participants with or without pneumoconiosis) have complicated the epidemiological assessment of silica exposure [65]. Its association with lung carcinoma has been examined in autopsy series, case-control series drawn from workers with silicosis or from patients with lung cancer, and population-based groups of silica-exposed workers. The balance of evidence indicates that silicotic patients have increased risk for lung cancer, but it is less clear whether silica exposure in the absence of silicosis carries an increased risk for lung cancer [66].

An elevated SMR, approximately 1.5-fold that expected, was detected for silica exposure in large population-based studies in Massachusetts and Canada [67,68]; in workers exposed to silica in Italy, the Netherlands and in some, but not all, Nordic countries there were three- to five-fold increases in lung cancer risk [69–71]. Reports from many countries have identified an increased frequency of lung cancer more specifically among workers compensated for silicosis [72–78]. The RR value compared with that of the general population ranged from 1.3 to 6.9. An excess lung cancer risk was found in never-smokers with an SMR of 222 [79].

Metal ore miners with silica exposure in the USA, UK, China, and South Africa experienced a significant raised mortality from lung cancer, with two to threefold increases in risk [80–86]. Several of these studies adjusted for the effects of smoking [80,83–86], though not for other potential confounders such as radon, arsenic, and diesel exhaust [87,88].

In addition, an increased lung cancer SMR of 150–200 has been demonstrated in workers exposed to silica in a variety of non-mining but dusty trades. These include granite workers in Vermont and China, foundry workers, German slate workers, workers in dusty trades in North Carolina, and California diatomaceous earth workers exposed to amorphous silica and cristobalite [89–94]. Ceramic or pottery workers demonstrated increased lung cancer risk in Sweden and Italy but not in China [95,96]. Workers in foundries, quarries, and manufacturing industries do not experience radon exposure, although some may be exposed to polycyclic aromatic hydrocarbons or other lung carcinogens.

The available data consequently support the conclusion that silicosis increases the risk for lung carcinoma, as may smoking and other carcinogens in the workplace. The epidemiological evidence is convincing among tobacco smokers with silicosis, but less information is available for never-smokers and for workers exposed to silica who do not have silicosis. For workers with silicosis who smoke, the risks demonstrated by investigators in various countries have been consistently high, though less than those associated with asbestosis.

2,3,7,8-Tetrachlorodibenzo-para-dioxin

Based on epidemiological and animal studies 2,3,7,8-tetrachlorodibenzo-*para*-dioxin (TCDD) was classified as a group 1 carcinogen by IARC in 1997. It is found as a contaminant in small concentrations in soil, sediments, and air. Higher exposures, as indicated by a several magnitude increase in tissue level, are encountered in a number of occupations [97]. It is produced during metal-processing, incineration, and in the chlorine bleaching of paper pulp. TCDD is also a byproduct of the production of chlorophenol and chlorophenoxy herbicides and is often found as a contaminant in these herbicides. The existing data on the occupational hazards of TCCD come mainly from studies of herbicide producers and applicators.

An elevated risk for several cancers including lung cancer, sarcoma, and lymphoma has been found in cohort studies from Germany and the USA [98–100]. An international cohort of herbicide producers and sprayers assembled by IARC [101] gave an SMR of 221 (95% CI 110–395) for lung cancer in probably exposed workers. However, in the same study the SMR for lung cancer was not elevated in the definitely exposed workers at 102 (95% CI 87–118). A German cohort of 1583 workers in a herbicide plant contaminated with TCDD revealed an elevated SMR of 167 (95% CI 109–244) for lung cancer compared with that of a cohort of German gas supply workers, but there was no adjustment for smoking [98]. In a US cohort of 5172 male workers from 12 different chemical plants engaged in the manufacture of products with TCDD contamination, a borderline significant elevation of lung cancer risk (SMR 139; 95% CI 99–189) was found in those workers with greater than 1 year of exposure, assuming a latency of 20 years [100]. The result is unlikely to be a result of smoking as the risks for other smoking-induced diseases were not elevated, and an adjustment in a subcohort for whom a smoking history was obtained did not change the SMR for lung cancer (SMR 137; 95% CI 98–187).

Established carcinogenic processes

While a specific carcinogenic agent has been demonstrated to be the cause of lung cancer in certain industries, in others there may be many different agents (often chemicals of the same or similar family) which inevitably occur together. Exposure to one is linked collinearly with exposure to another, and it becomes impossible to identify the actual causal agent (or agents) from epidemiological investigation in humans, even if there is no reasonable doubt that the industrial process itself is associated with an excess incidence of lung cancer. Nevertheless, the carcinogenicity of certain industrial processes is clear and is so recognized by the IARC as a known carcinogenic process.

Coke production and coal gasification

Coke production involves the controlled heating of coal in an oven until the gaseous content is removed. This leaves coke, a stronger burning fuel. Coal gasification refers to the retrieval by condensation of the gaseous content released by the complete distillation of coal. The heating of coal in both of these processes results in the production of polycyclic aromatic hydrocarbons (PAHs). They are formed from pyrolysis or incomplete combustion of organic matter generally, a large fraction being adsorbed to any particles that are produced by the combustion process. Other occupational settings where exposure may occur to PAHs include aluminum, iron, and steel founding, production or use of coal tar and coal tar pitches, refining of mineral oils, and combustion of diesel or other fuels.

Workplace exposures to PAHs are consequently common, though few data are available on exposures to specific individual compounds. In the mid-1980s, IARC estimated that worldwide over two million workers were exposed to PAHs in the basic processes of aluminum production, iron and steel founding, coke production, and coal gasification [102]. The strongest epidemiological evidence for a human lung cancer risk after exposure to PAHs comes from studies of coke oven workers. The highest risk occurs with work on the topside of coke ovens where the levels of PAHs are highest. The risk increases with increasing intensity and duration of exposure. In one study, the RR for lung cancer for topside workers compared with non-oven workers increased to 16 after 15 or more years of employment [103]. At a more extreme level of exposure, it has been estimated from another study that after 40 years work on a coke oven there is a 40% chance of developing lung cancer by age 85 [104].

There have been several cohort studies of workers exposed to PAHs in coking and coal-gas plants in China, all using as referents (controls) a cohort of workers at a primary steel rolling mill [61]. Reported standardized incidence ratios for lung cancer were of similar magnitude in two studies involving 21 coking plants (27 122 workers) and in one of six coal-gas plants (3107 workers): 2.55 (90% CI 2.13–3.03), 2.6 (90% CI 1.79–3.60), 3.66 (90% CI 2.36–5.43).

Similar studies from China have addressed the lung cancer risk in workers at shale refining and fuel oil producing plants, where PAH exposure is again to be expected. In a cohort of 6285 workers at a large shale-refining plant, increased SMRs for lung cancer (240; 90% CI 185–307) and esophageal cancer were observed [61]. By contrast a cohort of 12 422 workers at an oil-refining plant showed no elevated risk of lung cancer, though the SMR for liver cancer was raised. SMR values were raised also in a cohort of 3774 workers at a synthetic oil plant for both lung cancer (202; 90%; CI 134–293) and digestive tract cancer.

Coal tars or asphalts are byproducts from the distillation of coal for gasification and coke production. Coal tars are used in road-paving, roofing, and other industries. There have been a few epidemiological studies of workers exposed to PAHs in these settings. Mortality studies of roofers revealed a small excess in lung cancer mortality, but there were no adjustments for smoking [105]. A case-control study at an automobile metal stamping plant assessed cancer risk and its relationship to specific jobs. An elevated odds ratio (13.2; 95% CI 1.1–154.9) for lung cancer was found among maintenance welders and millwrights with known exposures to coal tar volatiles and welding fumes, compared with other workers in the plant [106]. Another case-cohort study of 1476 men from an aluminum plant demonstrated an increased relative risk of 2.25 (95% CI 1.50–3.38) for lung cancer deaths in those workers with a moderate cumulative exposure to coal tar pitch volatiles (expressed as 10–19 mg/m^3-years of benzene-soluble matter, compared with unexposed workers) [107].

Iron and steel founding

Approximately two million workers are employed in the iron- and steel-founding industry. They are exposed to a number of recognized lung carcinogens such as silica, PAHs, chromium, and nickel [102]. There have been a number of epidemiological studies involving iron- and steel-foundry workers from several countries indicating an increased risk of lung cancer [102,108–110]. A proportionate mortality study of 578 deceased South African iron workers was reported by Situs et al. [108]. Non-whites were excluded because of small sample size and lack of population comparison at that time. An increased proportionate mortality ratio (PMR) of 1.7 was found for lung cancer ($P < 0.05$). An elevated risk of lung cancer in groups of foundry workers compared with the general population has ranged from 1.5- to 2.5-fold, but not all were statistically significant [102]. In addition, a statistically increased SMR of 142 for lung cancer mortality was reported for male workers in nine English steel foundries compared with the general population [110]. Smoking was not controlled in most of these studies but in those that did have limited questionnaires on tobacco use, there was no difference in the smoking habits of the study cohort and the general population [102].

Although smoking was not controlled for in most of these studies and the specific carcinogens in iron

and steel founding were not identified, the IARC recognized iron and steel founding as a group 1 lung carcinogenic risk in 1987 based upon the consistent increase in risk reported [109].

Paint manufacture and painting

Worldwide there are approximately 200 000 workers employed in paint manufacturing and several million in painting [111]. They are exposed to a number of solvents including petroleum, toluene, xylene, ketones, alcohols, esters, and glycol ethers. Benzene (a common paint solvent before the 1950s) is no longer used. In addition, there is often exposure to titanium dioxides, chromium, iron, and lead in the paint pigments and to chlorinated hydrocarbons in paint strippers. For painters in the construction and shipyard industries, which constitute a large proportion of the painting industry, there are also potential exposures to asbestos and silica.

The IARC recognized paint spray as a group I carcinogen in 1989. The strongest data incriminating painting as a carcinogenic process comes from studies of lung cancer [112].

Steenland et al. reviewed the SMR for lung cancer of the largest existing cohort of painters (57 000 members of a US trade union) after 15 years surveillance [113]. It was significantly elevated compared with general US population at 123 (95% CI 117–129). Although there was no adjustment for smoking, the outcome is unlikely to have been confounded by tobacco consumption for several reasons. An indirect adjustment for smoking using previously reported smoking habits of painters did not account fully for the increased incidence of lung cancer; the risks for other smoking-related diseases were not elevated; an internal comparison within the trade union still showed an elevated risk for lung cancer in the painters compared with the non-painters; a nested case-control study had previously indicated a three-fold increased risk of lung cancer even after adjusting for smoking [114]. A further case-control study of women in Germany [111] demonstrated an elevated smoking adjusted odds ratio of 3.0 (95% CI 0.73–12.33) for lung cancer in female painters compared with population controls matched for sex, age, and region.

Underground mining

Following its early recognition in European hematite miners an elevated risk of lung cancer has been demonstrated worldwide in association with some hard rock mining industries. Although exposures to respirable silica and arsenic may play a role in some settings, radon (and its degradation products) is likely to be the principal causal agent in most.

Interactions among different exposures (particularly with cigarette smoking) may, however, play an important role. Radon is a naturally occurring radioactive noble gas emitted during the radioactive decay of uranium to stable lead. Radon decays and produces radioactive isotopes known as radon progeny (daughters), which can be inhaled and deposited in the respiratory tract where they irradiate surrounding tissue. As radon is emitted from the soil it is ubiquitous in the environment, entering homes and workplaces from the ground. Indoor radon has recently been postulated to contribute to 10–14% of lung cancer deaths in the USA, especially among smokers [115]. In underground mines, the level of radon is often several magnitudes higher than in most homes and surface workplaces, and so the impact on lung cancer is likely to be much greater in some mining industries.

Radon exposure is thought to be a causative agent in the increased risk of lung cancer in the underground mining of uranium, iron (hematite), tin, and niobium [81,116–120]. In a cohort of uranium miners in New Mexico, there was an elevated SMR for lung cancer of 400 (95% CI 310–510) that was unchanged after adjusting for smoking [116]. Among Chinese hematite miners an SMR of 370 compared with nationwide male population rates has been reported [84]. A case-control study among tin miners in the Yunnan province of China showed the estimated average cumulative exposure to radon and decay products was 2.1-fold greater in 107 prevalent cases of lung cancer than in 107 age-matched control miners without lung cancer [121]. In the 214 study participants as a whole, those in the highest quartile of cumulative exposure had an odds ratio of 9.5 (95% CI 2.7–33.1) compared with those unexposed for the development of lung cancer, after adjusting for arsenic exposure, age, year starting work, and tobacco use. A later study showed an even stronger association in these tin miners between lung cancer and cumulative exposure to arsenic. It is not clear, however, whether these relationships were influenced additionally by interactive effects between the various exposures and with smoking, and it appears that misclassification of exposure intensity has been common in such studies [12].

A possible interactive effect from occupational exposure and tobacco was addressed by two case-control studies from a further tin-mining area of China, where measured radon levels are low (Dachang in Guangxi Province). There were conflicting results. In the one (69 cases and 138 controls), the main risk factors for lung cancer were duration of exposure to smelting, duration of underground mining, and age at which last occupation began (all factors related to occupational exposures); and cig-

arette smoking was found to be synergistic with them [118]. In the other, the odds ratio for underground employment was 2.42 (95% CI 1.3, 4.4) for lung cancer compared with unaffected controls, after adjusting for smoking and silicosis and matching for age, but there was no interaction [122].

Much research has been carried out on men employed in southern African gold and other non-ferrous mines, but conflicting outcomes were noted when an association with lung cancer was sought [86,123]. Among several case-control studies, however, an elevated risk for lung cancer was noted among copper, gold, and nickel miners, though not among coal and chromium miners [124]. An important limitation may have been inadequate occupational information from some of the cases.

Probable carcinogens

Chlorinated toluenes and benzoyl chloride

A retrospective cohort mortality study of 953 workers in a UK organic chemical plant revealed five cases of lung cancer when 1.78 cases were expected (P < 0.05). An increased risk of gastrointestinal cancer was also found. The culprit was suspected to be benzotrichloride. A prospective cohort study of 610 Caucasian male workers of a chlorination plant in the USA demonstrated a statistically significant increase in the risk of lung and laryngeal cancer (SMR 265) but a non-significant increased risk of lung cancer alone (SMR 239) [126]. The workers in this plant were exposed to chlorinated toluene, benzoic acid, benzotrichloride, and benzyl chloride. When the data were analyzed further, significantly elevated risks were noted for lung cancer in workers with more than 15 years of employment (SMR 399; P < 0.05) and for latency of greater than 15 years after first exposure (SMR 329; P < 0.05).

Despite the limited information, IARC was sufficiently concerned to classify alpha-chlorinated toluenes and benzoyl chlorides as probable lung carcinogens in 1999.

Diesel exhaust

Diesel exhaust is a complex mixture of substances characterized by both aerosol (particle) and gas phases. Each particle comprises an elemental carbon core with adsorbed PAHs; the gas phase includes carbon monoxide and oxides of nitrogen.

Diesel exhaust has been shown to cause lung cancer in animals, and the particulate, rather than gaseous, phase appears to be responsible [127]. Two large epidemiological investigations have been conducted in North America in railroad workers exposed occupationally to diesel exhaust. Howe *et al.* studied the mortality of 43 826 retired workers at the Canadian National Railway Company and reported relative risks for lung cancer of 1.35 and 1.2, respectively, among workers probably or possibly exposed to diesel exhaust compared with unexposed workers [128]. A similar study of 55 407 US railroad workers by Garshick et al. showed a somewhat higher risk among workers with the longest duration of exposure (RR 1.45; 95% CI 1.11–1.89) [129]. An earlier case-control study of 1256 lung cancer deaths among the same cohort had found an odds ratio of 1.41 (95% CI 1.06–1.88) for subjects working in a job exposed to diesel exhaust for 20 or more years, after adjusting for smoking and asbestos exposure.

It should be noted that the RR observed in these studies was of modest degree only (<1.5-fold), and that the 95% CI came close to including 1. However, other investigations reached similar conclusions [130,132], and in 1989 IARC judged diesel exhaust in occupational settings to be a probable human lung carcinogen [131]. Since then several other epidemiologic studies of exposed workers have demonstrated an elevated risk of lung cancer, and a recent meta-analysis of 30 studies on diesel exhaust reported a pooled smoking adjusted relative risk of 1.47 (95% CI 1.29–1.67) [125,133–136].

There is currently no Occupational Safety and Health Administration (OSHA) standard specifically to limit exposure to diesel exhaust although there are OSHA standards for components of diesel exhaust such as carbon monoxide or nitrogen dioxide.

Epichlorohydrin

Occupational exposure to epichlorohydrin can occur during the production and use of resins, glycerine, and propylene-based rubbers. It is also sometimes used as a solvent, and it is considered by IARC to be a probable lung carcinogen [137].

A retrospective cohort study of 2642 men from a resin manufacturing plant in New Jersey included 32 men regularly involved in epichlorohydrin production and 12 other men who were intermittently involved [138]. Lung cancer developed in four compared with an expected 0.91 ($P = 0.03$). A subsequent nested case-control study from this cohort demonstrated an increased risk of lung cancer (smoking-adjusted odds ratio, 2.4; 95% CI 1.1–5.2) in those workers exposed to both anthraquinone dye and epichlorohydrin [139]. The smoking-adjusted odds ratio for those workers exposed to epichlorohydrin alone was 1.7, but the elevation was not significant (95% CI 0.7–4.1) and contrary to what one might expect from an occupational exposure, an odds ratio greater than 1.0 was found only in those workers with the shortest duration of exposure and the least cumulative exposure. More recently, a prospective cohort of 863

workers with potential epichlorohydrin exposure at two chemical plants in Texas and Louisiana showed a deficit, not excess, of lung cancer deaths in the exposed cohort (SMR 63.3), but there was no adjustment for smoking history [140].

Current evidence on the risk of lung cancer among epichlorohydrin-exposed workers is consequently equivocal.

Probable carcinogenic processes

Art glass manufacture

The manufacturing of glass and glassware has become increasing mechanized, but the production of art glass and other special varieties of glass still involves close handwork and mouth blowing. A number of lung carcinogens (or potential carcinogens) may be involved, including arsenic, asbestos, silica, other metal oxides, and polycyclic aromatic hydrocarbons, and IARC acknowledges that the manufacture of art glass is probably carcinogenic (group 2A) [46].

A recent case-control study of lung cancer in German women indicated an elevated odds ratio of 2.5 (95% CI 1.00–6.08) for female pottery and art glass workers compared with the general female population after adjusting for smoking [111]. A cohort of 625 male art glass workers in Sweden had an elevated but non-significant SMR of 236 for lung cancer ($p < 0.10$) and an SMR of 1589 ($p < 0.05$) for pharyngeal cancer [141]. The increased risk appeared to exist only for those workers who had over 15 years of exposure. Adjusting for tobacco consumption increased the SMR of lung cancer to 350 ($p < 0.05$). Increased risks of lung cancer (SMR 143; 90% CI 113–178) and laryngeal cancer (SMR 193; 95% CI 96–348) were also reported among an Italian cohort of glass workers whose jobs included glass blowing, casting, and pressing [142]. There was no change in the risk when smoking was taken into account.

Insecticide application

Many chemicals are used as insecticides and pesticides, the most common being organochlorines, organophosphates, carbamates, pyrethroid compounds, and various inorganic compounds (IARC 1991 [143]. Occupational exposure occurs in both manufacture and application (principally spraying).

A prospective cohort study of 1485 pest control officers in England and Wales showed deficits of lung cancer (SMR 63; 95% CI 38–98) and all cancers (SMR 79; 95% CI 61–100), though of borderline significance [144]. In the USA, however, a cohort of 3827 male pest-control workers demonstrated an increased risk of lung cancer with an SMR of 140 (95% CI 100–180) [145]. Again there was a borderline level of significance. Although there was no adjustment for smoking, a nested case-control study within this cohort showed a smoking adjusted odds ratio of 1.4 (95% CI 0.7–3.0) for lung cancer deaths in workers licensed for 10 to 19 years compared with those licensed for less than 10 years. This increased to 2.1 (95% CI 0.8–5.5) for those licensed for more than 20 years. Although a dose-dependent response is implied, the odds ratios did not achieve conventional levels of significance.

The data are not, consequently, definitive, and IARC classifies these agents as probable not definite carcinogens [143].

Epidemiology

Lung cancer is the leading cause of cancer mortality in the USA and its incidence is increasing in many industrializing countries. In the USA, lung cancer ranks second only to bladder cancer in the proportion of cases thought to be caused by occupational exposure. This epidemic pattern is likely to be reproduced in other industrialized countries and in many of the world's industrializing countries, as both tobacco and occupational exposures increase.

In the USA each year there are approximately 90 000 lung-cancer deaths among males, and approximately 100 000 newly diagnosed cases. In females, the comparable estimates are 45 000 and 60 000, respectively. Several attempts have been made to estimate the proportion caused by occupational exposure. From large case-control studies, Morabia et al. estimated 9% of male lung cancers were attributable to occupational exposures [146]. Using similar methodology, Vineis et al. estimated that between 3 and 17% were attributable to occupational exposures [147]. Doll and Peto estimated that 15% of male and 5% of female lung cancers in the USA were caused by occupational exposures but did not use any formal methodology [148].

Steenland et al. [15] based estimates on the proportion of the population exposed to specific occupational carcinogens and used estimated RR for these carcinogens, using a formula for calculating attributable risk (or etiologic fraction) from Kleinbaum et al. [149]. Excluding the contribution of radon at work, approximately 9000 annual lung cancers among US males were considered occupational (about 9%), and about 900 among females (2%). Of the yearly cases attributable to occupational exposure approximately 6000 in men (6%) and 600 in women (1%) were attributed to asbestos exposure. Radon exposure at work was estimated to cause an additional 1000 cases annually among both males and females.

These estimates apply to the USA only, and Steenland et al. [15] omitted from their analysis workplace carcinogens for which relatively few workers in the USA are exposed (<30 000). These carcinogens included BCME, coke production and coal gasification, and soot. In some parts of the world (e.g. east Asia), considerably larger numbers of workers may be exposed to these and other lung carcinogens. In Europe, where asbestos exposure is more common, 11.6% of all male lung cancers in the Netherlands [150] and 18.3% of all male lung cancers in the Italian asbestos cement manufacturing town of Casale Monferrato [151] were attributed to asbestos exposure.

Lung cancer is one of the most important human neoplasms, not only because of its incidence but also because of its dismal prognosis. Overall, only about 15% of patients survive 5 years or longer. However, the vast majority of cases are preventable. The critical preventive intervention is elimination or reduction in exposure to lung carcinogens. Although tobacco is the most obvious exposure for reduction, the impact of occupational exposure and its contributory role must also be addressed. This is particularly so for many parts of the industrializing world, where smoking and worker exposure to lung carcinogens are both increasing. Some countries, such as China, are undergoing societal transformations at an unprecedented rate [152,153]. In order to prevent epidemics of occupational lung cancer, preventive measures must be instituted now, not when the human and economic toll of disease beckons too loudly to be ignored.

Susceptibility

Individual susceptibility to lung cancer appears to vary widely among working populations exposed similarly to occupational carcinogens, as is the case with most diseases resulting from exposure to hazardous agents within the working environment and indeed the environment in general. Such variability adds considerably to the complexity of identifying the hazards since it implies there are likely to be different dose–response relations (and possibly different thresholds) among the various participants of epidemiologic investigations that aim fundamentally to detect only average effects. If individual susceptibility can not be quantified, thereby preventing adjustment for it, 'noise' is added to the dataset and adverse health effects are less readily revealed.

With lung cancer, for which causal effects of occupational agents are particularly difficult to demonstrate since smoking and ageing exert such powerful confounding influences, there have been important advances over recent years that are unraveling the pathogenic mechanisms at molecular level. These advances may soon make adjustments for individual susceptibility possible, and this in turn may allow occupational causes of (or contributors to) lung cancer to be identified with greater certainty. Individual variability in carcinogen metabolism may be a particularly important factor underlying differential susceptibility, and in recent years molecular techniques in the epidemiological study of cancer have been applied in three areas:

- determination of internal and biologically effective dose
- detection of early biologic effects (particularly mutations and cytogenic changes)
- assessment of variations in individual susceptibility to carcinogens, mainly via metabolic polymorphisms.

Among the 3800 chemicals that have been identified in tobacco smoke, a large number are biologically active compounds. The most important families of carcinogens are PAHs, which are of course encountered in some occupational environments irrespective of smoking (see above under coke production and coal gasification, and diesel exhaust), aromatic amines, nitroso compounds, volatile organic compounds (e.g. benzene, formaldehyde), and radioactive elements such as polonium-210. Chemical compounds derived from tobacco smoke have been measured in biological specimens of smokers and non-smokers. DNA adducts are formed when chemical carcinogens react with DNA. Several methods of detecting adducts in lung and other tissues, including the sensitive ^{32}P-postlabeling procedure for PAHs, have been described in detail. Among the class of pulmonary carcinogens known as PAHs, benzo[α]pyrene forms DNA adducts in the lung that are associated with smoking. Recent research indicates that adducts are found also in peripheral blood mononuclear cells in cancer patients [154].

Demonstrating the presence or absence of such adducts (or even assaying their quantity) may consequently provide a means of identifying (quantifying) susceptibility in individuals, and of assessing the effectiveness of hygiene interventions to control occupational exposures. The use of blood samples to investigate adducts may prove to be particularly valuable since they could be used readily in epidemiological studies, not only in occupational populations but in the population at large. The potential implications are obvious. They include screening to identify individuals with undue risk, and monitoring of populations to detect undue exposure (for example PAH–DNA adducts in peripheral blood mononuclear cells to assess the effectiveness of passive smoke elimination programs in public places).

Although the presence of PAH–DNA adducts has not been definitely associated with lung cancer, these adducts appear to be important in the pathway leading to cancer [155], and interventions aimed at reducing their presence in high-risk individuals are on the horizon. Focusing on this upstream marker of dose and early effect is particularly important in lung-cancer prevention, a condition for which there is no effective early detection marker and for which treatment is an ineffective means of disease control. The molecular epidemiology of lung cancer promises to lead to the development of exciting opportunities in environmental health research, and it will add greatly to our understanding of the human-health consequences of toxic exposures.

RECOGNITION

Clinical features

Exposure history

There is a tendency among clinicians to discard the possible diagnosis of lung cancer in lifelong non-smokers. This is a consequence of the well-accepted strong association between smoking and lung cancer, and a belief in consequence that lung cancer is improbable in the absence of smoking. It is a significant cause of misdiagnosis [156,157]. Full occupational and environmental histories should be considered in clinical practice, as well as the smoking history, and it should be remembered that there is a latency of some 12–40 years between onset of the relevant exposure and the development of lung cancer. Therefore, the occupational history should be obtained for the entire lifetime of the patient and not just the current or most recent work.

Determining the exact type of work and the duration of employment in each aspect of that work can help to determine the total estimated exposure to a particular agent. Under US federal law, patients or their physicians can request from current or former employers Material Safety Data Sheets (MSDS), which contain information about the potential toxicity of materials used in the workplace. If available, measured levels of exposure can be requested also. Inspection results of regulatory agencies such as OSHA serve as another potential source of information for the physician and patient.

If the history and supporting information confirms exposure to a known or suspected lung carcinogen and a latency interval of 12 years or more is present, the clinician may conclude that workplace exposure contributed to or, in the case of a non-smoker, was the sole cause of the disease.

Symptoms and signs

Occupational lung cancer displays no unique clinical features with which to inform the clinician regarding causation. Most patients who develop lung carcinoma do not consult a physician until symptoms of the disease become manifest, and in most cases the disease is already incurable. The initial symptoms may vary with the patient population and the cell type of the tumor. Common symptoms include cough, hemoptysis, hoarseness, bone pain, dyspnea, dysphagia, and weight loss, which may relate to the primary tumor itself, its local invasion, distant metastases, or even paraneoplastic effects. Signs depend primarily on site, size, and the presence of distant metastases. Most lung cancers arise in or around the large airways, and so they may cause local obstruction (and unilateral wheeze), distal infection, and atelectasis. Pleural effusion is common, and it usually implies pleural infiltration and inoperability. Fuller detail is the province of texts of respiratory medicine.

Investigation

The first call in the investigation of possible lung cancer lies with imaging: plain radiographs followed if necessary by computed tomography (CT scan). Confirmation comes from cytologic examination of sputum, the products of bronchoscopy (alveolar lavage fluid or brushings), or percutaneous aspiration; or from histologic examination of biopsy material (generally from bronchoscopy or video-assisted thoracoscopy). When there is evidence of metastatic spread, the distant metastases may provide a more convenient opportunity to obtain cytologic or biopsy material, especially lymph node or skin sites. Lung function has no meaningful role in diagnosis, but it becomes important if there is the possibility of curative surgery so the patient's suitability for lung resection is assessed. This becomes critical if lobectomy is likely to be tolerated but not pneumonectomy, and in such circumstances quantitative perfusion and ventilation scans are invaluable.

Imaging

There is nothing in the radiologic appearance of occupational lung cancer that might distinguish it from tobacco-related lung cancer. Briefly, the radiologic signs include isolated or multiple pulmonary nodules, hilar fullness or mass, persistent infiltrates, lobar or segmental collapse, pleural effusions, elevated hemi-diaphragm, and bony erosions. Occasionally, a chest radiograph appears normal and the cancer is only found on bronchoscopy or on CT scan.

In addition to the radiologic features of lung cancer, there may be radiologic evidence of an occupational exposure of relevance. In particular the presence of pleural plagues would suggest asbestos exposure, and if this is associated with evidence of interstitial lung disease (i.e. asbestosis) there may be a strong possibility that occupation has played a causal role. Diffuse pleural thickening is a less strong indicator of asbestos exposure since there are numerous other potential causes, but again it may point the way to identifying an occupational cause, as may interstitial disease suggesting pneumoconiosis. While small irregular opacities may suggest asbestos exposure, small rounded opacities may indicate exposure to silica or beryllium or some other industrial dust. Associated hilar adenopathy may be particularly suggestive of beryllium exposure while egg shell calcification of hilar nodes may help to identify silicosis. It is important, however, to combine the radiologic findings with an appropriate occupational history, as not all interstitial lung diseases are occupationally induced.

Mineralogic analysis

Except for the bronchoalveolar or peripheral blood lymphocyte transformation response to beryllium, there are no reliable cellular or serologic tests to evaluate the relevance of occupational exposures to the development of lung cancer. In the case of asbestos and other mineral dusts, however, it may be helpful to assay the fiber, body, or particle content from an uninvolved sample of resected lung if an exposure history remains uncertain (see Chapter 34). The number of asbestos bodies per milligram of dry lung can be determined in a number of laboratories to provide a quantitative estimate of cumulative exposure. Depending on the reference values of the examining laboratory, greater than 0.5 asbestos bodies/mg dry lung is generally indicative of greater than background exposure to asbestos [158,159]. Even the identification of a visible asbestos body in most high-power microscopic fields of examined resected tissue suggests qualitatively that excess exposure is likely to have occurred. However, given the long latency between exposure onset and the development of lung cancer, and the rapid clearance of chrysotile asbestos fibers, the finding of less than 0.5 bodies/mg dried lung may mask a meaningful period of occupational exposure. Likewise, the absence of asbestos bodies or any other occupational carcinogens in bronchoalveolar fluid, pleural fluid, sputum or lymph node is not helpful in evaluating a specific asbestos exposure history.

MANAGEMENT

Of the individual

Occupationally induced lung cancer is not managed any differently from lung cancer of other causes. Once a pulmonary mass is found there will be concern for malignancy, and a definitive diagnosis is usually necessary with tissue biopsy or cytologic examination. Staging with a CT scan, mediastinoscopy, pleural fluid examination, or (if clinically indicated) CT scans of head/abdomen or radioisotope scans of bone/liver/brain will help to determine the most appropriate treatment option and aid estimation of the prognosis. Pulmonary function tests and ventilation/perfusion scanning will help to assess whether segment, lobe, or lung can be safely removed.

Surgical resection, with or without adjuvant chemotherapy, provides the best chance of cure for tumors other than small cell tumors, but it is appropriate only in a minority of patients with limited disease. For advanced stages, chemotherapy and radiation therapy may provide valuable palliation. With small cell tumors, chemotherapy provides the best hope of immediate improvement, followed by radiotherapy to the primary site and mediastinum in responders. Combined sequential treatment is occasionally curative, but in most cases relapses occur within 1–2 years. Radiotherapy may also be valuable for palliating distant metastases. Specialized texts of respiratory medicine or clinical oncology will provide fuller detail.

In addition to therapies directed at the primary tumor, it is usually necessary to institute specific supportive remedies for its complications: thoracentesis, with or without pleurodesis, for symptomatic pleural effusions; medications for paraneoplastic syndromes such as hypercalcemia and inappropriate secretion of antidiuretic hormone; and radiation therapy, bronchial stenting, or antibiotics for obstructive lesions that result in hemoptysis, atelectasis, or pneumonia.

Compensation

Although compensation for occupationally induced mesothelioma is widely available, compensation for lung cancer of occupational origin often poses problems. The difficulty lies in establishing at the individual rather than population level that the evolution of lung cancer depended critically on an exposure (or exposures) in the workplace. There is a natural tendency, when lung cancer arises in a smoker exposed to an occupational carcinogen, to conclude that smoking is the more probable cause; conversely, in a never-smoker, lung cancer may be readily accepted to be the consequence of an occupational carcinogen. Both assumptions may be erroneous.

The key point is whether there is an interaction between smoking and the occupational carcinogen, as is well established in smokers working with asbestos. The data presented in Table 19.8 provide a useful illustration, to which may be added the more familiar data of Hammond and colleagues (Table 19.9) concerning mortality ratios for lung cancer among smoking and non-smoking workers with and without recognized occupational exposure to asbestos [160].

Table 19.9 Multiplicative risk of smoking and asbestos exposure[a]

	No asbestos	Asbestos	Actual average risk
Non smokers	1	5.17	× 5.17
Smokers	10.85	53.24	× 4.91
Actual average risk	× 10.85	×10.3	

[a] Given that the risk associated with no smoking and no asbestos exposure is 1.

Both smoking and asbestos are highly relevant to the risk of developing lung cancer, and in an interactive (multiplicative) fashion. For the average individual in this population, smoking increased the risk of lung cancer by about 10-fold, and asbestos increased the risk by about 5-fold; the two together increased the risk by about 50-fold not 15-fold, compared with that of the non smokers who were unexposed to asbestos. If the figure of 53 is used to quantify the actual average risk in a smoker with asbestos exposure, its components are 1 for the base risk, 10 (10.85-1) for the smoking risk, 4 (5.17-1) for the asbestos risk, and 38 (53-1-10-4) for the risk that depends on the interaction between smoking and asbestos. It is readily evident that the interaction is of major importance.

The real issue for compensation purposes is whether the individual would have developed lung cancer had he/she not sustained occupational exposure to asbestos. For the average worker so affected within this particular exposure group, the risk was increased about 5-fold, irrespective of smoking habit. Therefore the chances for its development would have been reduced to merely 20% had there been no asbestos exposure, and it can reasonably be concluded that it is unlikely to have occurred in such circumstances. Looked at another way, of five similarly exposed and affected individuals, whether they are smokers or not, only one is likely to have developed lung cancer had it not been for the asbestos exposure. At present, this one cannot be distinguished from the other four.

The critical value for the relative risk is obviously 2. If the increased lung cancer risk attributable to asbestos is estimated in the individual to be 2-fold or more, it can be concluded that asbestos probably did play a critical role, and that (on the balance of probabilities) the lung cancer would not have occurred in the absence of asbestos exposure. Conversely, an elevated risk less than 2, implies that the lung cancer would probably have occurred anyway. For 15 subjects with lung cancer and similar exposures to tobacco and asbestos, but a 1.5-fold increase in lung cancer risk attributable to asbestos, occupation would be irrelevant in 10 and critical in only a minority of 5. A parallel argument can be applied to smoking, but this is not relevant to the issue of whether the occupational environment played a critical role. Smoking does, however, play a very influential role, and in practice lung cancer is very rare in never smokers, irrespective of any occupational exposure to asbestos.

If there is known to be no interaction (a second exposure neither augmenting nor diminishing the effect of the first), the calculations are importantly different. Using the above example, but ignoring the observed true outcome from the interaction, the independent risks should be added to estimate the overall risk for a smoker with asbestos exposure $(1+10+4=15)$. Thus for 15 relevant cases of lung cancer, one is likely to have occurred anyway, 10 are likely to be a consequence of smoking, and 4 are likely to be a consequence of asbestos exposure. Again, the one category cannot be distinguished from any other, and for the affected individual the balance of probabilities lies clearly in favor of smoking, not asbestos (nor coincidence), being the cause. If the system of compensation depends absolutely on the balance of probabilities, no compensation would be payable to any of the 15 subjects. By contrast, the interactive model with 53 affected subjects (above) would lead to all 53 receiving compensation.

Since affected individuals do not, in fact, share precisely the same average exposure profiles, there is considerable difficulty in devising an equitable system of compensation, and it is not surprising that different countries have widely different procedures. In the USA, for example, some states require that the exposure in question be the major causal exposure, whereas others require only a substantial contribution. Moreover, the level of certainty required of a physician to make a judgment in any individual case varies by jurisdiction. In the USA and many other countries, the standard of proof is a 'more likely than not' level of certainty, not the 90% or 95% level of confidence used in the research studies reviewed in this chapter. For the clinician, judgment is best guided by a familiarity with the literature 'state-of-the-art' as well as the legal/administrative environment in which he/she works.

Of the workforce

Once it is established that lung cancer has arisen in one member of a workforce as a probable consequence of exposures in the workplace, there is a clear obligation to inform other members of relevant information, and to insure that any ongoing risk is minimized. The latter involves the principles of prevention, and these are discussed in the following section. Lung cancer is, however, a disease of long latency following the onset of the causal environmental exposure(s), and in many cases the relevant exposure will have occurred during a previous period of employment. There may consequently be no need for management action concerning the current workforce, and it may be that the matter has already been appropriately addressed within the earlier workforce of relevance. A check should, nevertheless, be made in case an unrecognized risk persists.

When there is a probable increase in risk of lung cancer for other members of the workforce, it is important that relevant information is clearly disseminated, in particular the circumstances associated with the most obvious risk, together with appropriate counselling and a clear description of the magnitude of the risk. The perceived risk is often exaggerated otherwise, causing unnecessary anxiety, and it is best explained with comparative analogies. For example, the estimated occupational risk may be similar to that from smoking 'x' cigarettes daily for 'y' years, or (when the risk is of minor degree) to that associated more generally with passive smoking. In active smokers, the potential for a multiplicative interaction should be explained, and hence the particular benefit from smoking cessation.

There is also an obligation to explain the need to recognize emerging disease at the earliest opportunity, while there remains some potential for cure, since the prognosis of bronchogenic lung cancer depends greatly on early detection and prompt resection. In practice most lung cancers are not curable once symptoms begin, and so the question arises whether there would be greater benefit from surveillance programs of subjects at high risk.

Surveillance

Three screening studies sponsored by the US National Cancer Institute proved disappointing in that no overall improvement in mortality occurred [161–165]. Chest radiographs and/or sputum cytology proved to be insufficiently sensitive in detecting early and curable tumors in male smokers 45 years of age or older. The matter has recently attracted renewed interest with the use of more sensitive screening procedures based on low-dose CT scanning [166]. If successful, the methodology should be particularly beneficial where the lung cancer risk attributable to smoking is enhanced by occupational factors. An obvious example would be the regular screening of smokers who have been exposed to occupational lung carcinogens and have pulmonary fibrosis (especially asbestosis). To be successful, the screening procedures will need to be repeated after short intervals (perhaps 3–6 months), and so there will be formidable problems with compliance and not an inconsequential risk from cumulative irradiation. It is obvious that the further development of molecular markers of susceptibility could greatly improve the potential benefits of surveillance programs.

PREVENTION

In the workplace

Worker selection

In most western countries the use of preemployment medical examinations to select workers deemed to have a low risk for lung cancer is considered either not feasible or discriminatory. Instead, all work environments should have an acceptable minimal risk for the development of lung cancer, irrespective of the inherent risks of the individual worker. One exception is the recommendation that non-smokers only are recruited for asbestos removal work. At present there are no generally recommended medical guidelines for worker selection regarding lung cancer, except for identifying smokers and encouraging cessation.

Exposure control

Limiting occupational exposure may not necessarily protect fully against an increased risk of lung cancer, since for the majority of occupational exposures no clear threshold has been demonstrated below which there is no increased risk. Therefore even at low exposure (exposure below OSHA standards, for example), there may still be some increased risk above background, especially if exposure is pro-

longed. Failure to demonstrate such a threshold (which is likely to vary anyway from individual to individual) does not, of course, prove that none exists, and a more important factor may be one of effect modification (i.e. multiplicative interaction) with other exposures, principally smoking. While there is no doubt that exposure levels should comply with national standards, the most prudent course of action is to limit exposures to known carcinogens further to the lowest possible levels.

Smoking cessation policy

For most of the agents discussed, a synergistic relationship between exposure and tobacco use has been demonstrated. Smoking cessation would, therefore, lower the overall risk of lung cancer, and this should be encouraged both within and without the work place. Advances in the treatment of nicotine dependence, neurochemical research, and addictive behavioral research have the potential to reduce tobacco-related morbidity and mortality from lung cancer. Employers need to provide positive incentives for smoking cessation, such as sponsoring smoking cessation treatment programs, work release to attend sessions, and discounts in insurance premiums for successful quitters.

National regulatory strategies

Regulatory strategies for the control of occupational cancer generally focus on the elimination (or minimization) of carcinogen exposure. In most western countries, IARC class I carcinogens are regulated such that permissible exposure limits are at or below the limit of detection, usually the lowest feasible concentration. These standards encourage exposure control procedures that either substitute the carcinogen with a less hazardous material or minimize exposure through engineering modifications. The use of personal protective equipment by workers exposed to regulated carcinogens is considered a 'last resort' back-up procedure, whenever the primary methods of exposure control are inadequate.

DIFFICULT CASE

History

A 58-year-old man had worked intermittently as a general laborer and fork truck driver in a chemical manufacturing plant for 21 of the 28 years preceding his presentation in 1989. For 13 of these years he had worked in a facility manufacturing chloromethyl methyl ether (CMME) for use in the preparation of ion-exchange resins, and for his initial 4–6 years from 1961 (until he left the plant for a few years) the production process had not been fully enclosed. Evidence

arose that BCME was carcinogenic in laboratory animals and was a minor contaminant (1–3%) of industrial CMME. When an excess of lung cancer was detected in employees of a similar chemical manufacturing plant, his employer enclosed fully the production process and introduced a regular 3-yearly chest radiographic screening program for workers who had possibly sustained exposure.

He remained very well, smoking 5–10 cigarettes daily, but his most recent chest radiograph of 1989 proved to be unsatisfactory. A large round opacity was noted in each lung, with diameters of 5–6 cm. On direct questioning he admitted to a mild cough over the preceding 4 months, which was productive of a little mucoid sputum. He had been a little more short of breath when running or climbing hills than formerly, but he had attributed this to his increasing age. He had no other symptoms and recognized no disability.

There were raised serum levels of α-fetoprotein (12 µg/l) and carcinoembryonic antigen (176 µg/l), but no antineutrophil cytoplasmic antibody was detected, and an abdominal ultrasound examination revealed no abnormality. Fine needle aspiration of one lung nodule showed adenocarcinoma cells.

Issues

The major issues here are whether this man's intrapulmonary malignancy was a primary lung cancer and, if it was, whether it was attributable to his work with chloromethyl ethers.

Comment

The book's contributors were evenly divided, half concluding that his cancer probably had arisen primarily within the lung and half concluding that the pulmonary lesions were probably metastases from a primary site (probably intraabdominal) outside the chest. The second group considered the occupational exposures irrelevant, but the first group thought with a borderline to moderate degree of confidence that the cancer was occupational in origin.

An abdominal ultrasound examination showed no evidence of a primary cancer outside the lung, but the matter was not investigated exhaustively since the malignancy was considered to be incurable; no autopsy examination was carried out. The plant had used CMME to produce ion-exchange resins since 1956 only, and the production process became fully enclosed in the early 1970s as soon as the lung cancer risk became fully apparent. Occupational exposure in this man's case was consequently limited to a maximum of 4–6 years. An epidemiological study of lung cancer incidence involving 1196 plant employees up to 1980 showed less cases than expected compared with unexposed controls, but an excess was noted in a sister plant using CMME from about 1948, and in plants in two other countries [58–60]. The risks in these three plants were elevated well in excess of two-fold (though principally for small cell lung cancer), and so the crude balance of probabilities for an incident case of small cell lung cancer in any of them would lie clearly in favor of an occupational cause. For this Difficult Case, however, the relevance of occupational exposure is much less clear. He had not smoked heavily, but the plant was known to have produced lesser levels of exposure; the tumor was an adenocarcinoma, not small cell carcinoma; and there are no epidemiological data to assess the probability of an occupational cause in his plant for tumors arising after 1980.

SUMMARY POINTS

Recognition

- Occupational exposure is estimated to cause about 10% of lung cancers in men and 3–5% of those in women.
- Asbestos is estimated to account for about 60% of occupationally induced lung cancer.
- There is controversy as to whether asbestos causes lung cancer directly or by inducing asbestosis.
- The IARC has judged that occupational lung cancer is additionally associated with coal gasification; coke production; the mining of hematite, uranium, and gold; iron and steel founding; aluminum production; painting; and exposure to arsenic, beryllium, cadmium, chloromethyl ethers, chromium, mustard gas, nickel, radon, silica, soot, sulfuric acid mist, and tetrachlorodibenzo-*para*-dioxin.
- The IARC has judged that probable causes of occupational lung cancer include the application of some (non-arsenical) insecticides and pesticides; art glass manufacture; and exposure to diesel exhaust, chlorinated toluenes and benzoyl chloride, and epichlorhydrin.
- From an epidemiological viewpoint alone, the balance of probabilities lies in favor of an individual case of lung cancer being occupational in origin if relevant variables resemble on average those of an exposed study population shown to have a two-fold or greater risk compared with unexposed controls.

Management

- Management of occupationally induced lung cancer is that of lung cancer generally.
- In most countries the affected individual will be entitled to compensation, and the supervising physician should be familiar with local regulations governing the compensatory process.

Prevention

- The most effective means of prevention is the reduction of exposure to the minimum practical level.
- Emerging molecular techniques may detect early biologic markers of lung cancer (such as DNA adducts) so that individuals with undue susceptibility may be identified for close surveillance, and populations may be surveyed to determine a biologically safe level of exposure.
- No screening program has yet been shown to be effective for occupational lung cancer, but there is optimism that new surveillance techniques based on CT scanning may allow emerging lung cancers to be detected when there is a high probability of surgical cure.

REFERENCES

1. Tomatis L. The contribution of the IARC monographs to the identification of cancer risk factors. *Ann NY Acad Sci* 1988; 534: 31–38.

2. IARC Monographs. *Chemicals and Industrial Processes Associated with Cancer in Humans.* Lyon, France IARC, 1979.

3. Vineis P, Cantor P, Gonzales C *et al.* Occupational cancer in developed and developing countries. *Int J Cancer* 1995; 15: 655–660.

4. Hill AB, Fanning EL. Studies in the incidence of cancer in a factory handling inorganic compounds of arsenic: I. Mortality experience in the factory. *Br J Ind Med* 1948; 5: 1–6.

5. Lee AM, Fraumeni JF. Arsenic and respiratory cancers in man: An occupational study. *J Natl Cancer Inst* 1969; 42: 1045–1052.

6. Lee-Feldstein A. Cumulative exposure to arsenic and its relationship to respiratory cancer among copper smelter employees. *J Occup Med* 1986; 28: 296–302.

7. Mazumdar S, Redmond CK, Enterline PE *et al.* Multistage modeling of lung cancer mortality among arsenic-exposed copper-smelter workers. *Risk Analysis* 1989; 9: 551–563.

8. Tokudome S, Kuratsune M. A cohort study on mortality from cancer and other causes among workers at a metal refinery. *Int J Cancer* 1976; 17: 310–317.

9. Jarup L, Pershugen G, Wall S. Cumulative arsenic exposure and lung cancer in smelter workers: a dose–response study. *Am J Ind Med* 1989; 15: 31–41.

10. Xu ZY, Blot WJ, Li G *et al.* Environmental determinants of lung cancer in Shenyang, China. *IARC Sci Publ* 1991; 105: 460–465.

11. Welch K, Higgins I, Oh M, Burchfield C. Arsenic exposure, smoking, and respiratory cancer in copper smelter workers. *Arch Environ Health* 1982; 37: 325–335.

12. Taylor PR, Qiao YL, Schatzkin A, *et al.* Relation of arsenic exposure to lung cancer among tin miners in Yunnan Province, China. *Br J Ind Med* 1989; 46: 881–886.

13. Mabuchi K, Lilienfeld AM, Snell LM. Lung cancer among pesticide workers exposed to inorganic arsenicals. *Arch Environ Health* 1979; 34: 312–320.

14. Nordmann M. Der Berufskrebs der Asbestarbeiter. *Z Krebsforsch* 1938; 47: 288–302.

15. Steenland K, Loomis D, Shy C, Simonsen N. Review of occupational lung carcinogens. *Am J Ind Med* 1996; 29: 474–490.

16. Hughes J, Weill H. Asbestosis as a precursor of asbestos-related cancer: results of a prospective study. *Br J Ind Med* 1991; 48: 229–233.

17. Selikoff IJ, Hammond EC, Seidman H. Mortality experience of insulation workers in the US and Canada *Ann NY Acad Sci* 1979; 330: 91–116.

18. Neuberger M, Kundi M. Individual asbestos exposure: smoking and mortality – a cohort study in the asbestos cement industry. *Br J Ind Med* 1990; 47: 615–620.

19. McDonald JC, Lidell F, Gibbs G *et al.* The 1891–1929 birth cohort of Quebec chrysotile miners and millers: mortality to 1976–1988. *Br J Ind Med* 1993; 50: 1073–1081.

20. Jones RN, Hughes KM, Weill H. Asbestos exposure, asbestosis, and asbestos-attributable lung cancer. *Thorax* 1996; 51 (Suppl. 2); 9–15.

21. Weiss W. Asbestosis: a marker for the increased risk of lung cancer among workers exposed to asbestos. *Chest* 1999; 115: 536–549.

22. Abraham J. Asbestos inhalation, not asbestosis, causes lung cancer. *Am J Ind Med* 1994; 26: 839–842.

23. Roggli V, Hammer S, Pratt P *et al.* Does asbestos or asbestosis cause carcinoma of the lung? *Am J Ind Med* 1994; 26: 835–838.

24. Egilman D, Reinert A. Lung cancer and asbestos exposure: asbestosis is not necessary. *Am J Ind Med* 1996; 30: 394–406.

25. Wilkinson P, Hansell DM, Janssens J *et al.* Is lung cancer associated with asbestos exposure when there are no small opacities on the chest radiography? *Lancet* 1995; 345: 1074–1078.

26. Hillerdal G, Henderson DW. Asbestos, asbestosis, pleural plaques and lung cancer. *Scand J Work Environ Health* 1997; 23: 93–103.

27. Hillerdal G. Carcinoma and mesothelioma: a prospective study. *Chest* 1994; 104: 144–150.

28. Mossman BT, Marsh JP. Evidence supporting a role for active oxygen species in asbestos-induced toxicity and lung disease. *Environ Health Persp* 1989; 81: 91–94.

29. Kelsey KT, Yano E, Liber HL, Little JB. The in vitro effects of fibrous erionite and crocidolite asbestos. *Br J Cancer* 1986; 54: 107–114.

30. Hei TK, Piao CQ, He ZY *et al.* Chrysotile fiber is a strong mutagen in mammalian cells. *Cancer Res* 1992; 53: 6305–6309.

31. Wang X, Christiani DC, Wiencke JK *et al.* Mutations in the p53 gene in lung cancer are associated with cigarette smoking and asbestos exposure. *Cancer Epidem Biomarkers Prev* 1995; 4: 543–548.

32. Liddell FDK, McDonald AD, McDonald JC. Dust exposure and lung cancer in Quebec chrysotile miners and millers. *Ann Occup Hyg* 1998; 42: 7–20.

33. Stayner LT, Dankovic DA, Lemen RA. Occupational exposure to chrysotile asbestos and cancer risk: A review of the amphibole hypothesis. *Am J Public Health* 1996; 86: 179–186.

34. Pang ZC, Zhang Z, Wang Y *et al.* Mortality from a Chinese asbestos plant: overall cancer mortality. *Am J Ind Med* 1997; 32: 442–444.

35. Cheng W, Kong J. A retrospective mortality cohort of chrysotile asbestos products workers in Tianjin 1972–1987. *Environ Res* 1992; 59: 271–278.

36. Huilan Z, Zhiming W. Study of occupational lung cancer in asbestos factories in China. *Br J Ind Med* 1993; 50: 1039–1042.

37. Vaino H, Boffetta P. Mechanisms of the combined effect of asbestos and smoking in the etiology of lung cancer. *Scand J Work Environ Health* 1994; 20: 235–242.

38. Kjuus H, Skjaerven R, Langard S, *et al.* A case-referent study of lung cancer, occupational exposure and smoking: II Role of asbestos exposure. *Scand J Work Environ Health* 1986; 12: 203–209.

39. Kannerstein M, Churg J. Pathology of carcinoma of lung cancer associated with asbestos exposure. *Cancer* 1972; 30: 14–21.

40. Karjalainen A, Anttila S, Heikkila L *et al.* Lobe of origin of lung cancer among asbestos-exposed patients with or without diffuse interstitial fibrosis. *Scand J Work Environ Health* 1993; 19: 102–107.

41. Brodkin CA, McCullough J, Stover B *et al.* Lobe of origin and histologic type of lung cancer associated with asbestos exposure in the carotene and retinal efficacy trial. *Am J Ind Med* 1997; 32: 582–591.

42. Lee BW, Wain JC, Kelsey KT *et al.* Association of cigarette smoking and asbestos exposure with location and histology of lung cancer. *Am J Respir Crit Care Med* 1998; 157: 748–755.

43. IARC Monograph 23. *Some Metals and Metallic Compounds.* Lyon, France: IARC, 1980.

44. Steenland K, Ward E. Lung cancer incidence among patients with beryllium disease: a cohort mortality study. *J Natl Cancer Inst* 1991; 83: 1380–1385.

45. Ward E, Okan A, Ruder A *et al.* A mortality study of workers at seven beryllium processing plants. *Am J Ind Med* 1992; 22: 885–904.

46. IARC Mongraph 58. *Beryllium Cadmium, Mercury and Exposures in the Glass Manufacturing Industry.* Lyons, France: IARC, 1994.

47. IARC Monograph 16. *Cadmium, Nickel, some Epoxides. Miscellaneous Industrial Chemicals and General Considerations on Volatile Anaesthetics.* Lyon, France: IARC, 1976.

48. Heinrick U. Pulmonary carcinogenicity of cadmium by inhalation in animals. In: Nordberg G, Herber R, Alessio L. eds. *Cadmium in the Human Environment: Toxicity and Carcinogenicity,* pp. 405–414. Lyon, France: IARC, 1992.

49. Waalkes M, Rehm S, Perantoni A, Coogan T. Cadmium exposure in rats and tumors of the prostate. In: Nordberg G, Herber R, Alessio L, eds. *Cadmium in the Human Environment: Toxicity and Carcinogenicity,* pp. 391–400. Lyon, France: IARC, 1992.

50. Waalkes M, Rehm S, Sass B, Ward J. Induction of tumors of the hematopoietic system by cadmium in rats. In: Nordberg G, Herber R, Alessio L, eds. *Cadmium in the Human Environment: Toxicity and Carcinogenicity,* pp. 401–404. Lyon, France: IARC, 1992.

51. Boffetta P. Methodological aspects of the epidemiological association between cadmium and cancer in humans. In: Nordberg G, Herber R, Alessio L, eds. *Cadium in the Human Environment: Toxicity and Carcinogenicity,* pp. 425–434. Lyon, France, IARC, 1992.

52. Stayner L, Smith R, Thun M *et al.* A dose–response analysis and quantitative assessment of lung cancer risk and occupational cadmium exposure. *Ann Epidemiol* 1992; 2: 177–194.

53. Thun M, Schnort T, Halperin W. Mortality from lung and prostatic cancer in US cadmium workers. In: *Workshop on Cadmium and Cancer,* Oxford, UK, September: IARC, 1986.

54. Drew RT, Laskin S, Kuschner M *et al.* Inhalation carcinogenicity of alpha halo ethers. I. The acute inhalation toxicity of chloromethyl methyl ether and bis (chloromethylether). *Arch Environ Health* 1975; 30: 61–69.

55. Laskin S, Drew RT, Capiello V *et al.* Inhalation carcinogenicity of alpha halo ethers. II. Chronic inhalation studies with chloromethyl methyl ether. *Arch Environ Health* 1975; 30: 70–72.

56. Kuschner M, Laskin S, Drew RT *et al.* Inhalation carcinogenicity of alpha halo ethers. III. Lifetime and limited period inhalation studies with bis (chloromethylether) at 0.1 ppm. *Arch Environ Health* 1975; 30: 73–77.

57. McCallum RI, Woolley V, Petrie A. Lung cancer associated with chloromethyl methyl ether manufacture: an investigation at two factories in the United Kingdom. *Br J Ind Med* 1983; 40: 384–389.

58. Gowers DS, DeFonso LR, Schaffer T *et al.* Incidence of respiratory cancer among workers exposed to chloromethyl-ethers. *Am J Epidemiol* 1993; 137: 31–42.

59. Weiss W, Nash D. An epidemic of lung cancer due to chloromethyl ethers. *J Occup Environ Med* 1997; 39: 1003–1009.

60. IARC Monograph 49. *Chromium, Nickel and Welding.* Lyon, France: IARC, 1990.

61. Wu W. Occupational cancer in the People's Republic of China. *J Occup Med* 1988; 30: 968–974.

62. ICNCM (International Committee on Nickel Carcinogenesis in Man). Report of the International Committee on Nickel Carcinogenesis in Man. *Scand J Work Environ Health* 1990; 16: 1–84.

63. IARC Monograph 68. *Silica, some Silicates, Coal Dust and para-Aramid Fibrils,* Lyons, France IARC, 1997.

64. Muhle H, Takenadka S, Mohr U, *et al.* Lung tumor induction upon long-term low-level inhalation of crystalline silica. *Am J Ind Med* 1989; 15: 343–346.

65. McDonald JC. Silica, silicosis, and lung cancer. [Editorial] *Br J Ind Med* 1989; 46: 289–291.

66. Goldsmith D. Silica exposure and pulmonary cancer. In: Samet J ed. *Epidemiology of Lung Cancer,* pp. 245–298. New York: Marcel Dekker, 1994.

67. Dubrow R, Wegman DH. Cancer and occupation in Massachusetts: a death certificate study. *Am J Ind Med* 1984; 6: 207–230.

68. Siemiatycki J, Gerin M, Dewar R, Lakhani R. Silica and cancer associations from a multicenter occupational case-referent study. *IARC Sci Pub* 1990; 97: 29–42.

69. Mastrangelo G, Zambon P, Simonato L, Rizzi P. A case-referent study investigating the relationship between exposure to silica dust and lung cancer. *Int Arch Occup Environ Health* 1988; 60: 299–302.

70. Meijers JM, Swaen GM, van Vliet K, Borm PJ. Epidemiologic studies of inorganic dust-related lung diseases in the Netherlands. *Exp Lung Res* 1990; 16: 15–23.

71. Lynge E, Kurppa K, Kristogersen L *et al.* Silica dust and lung cancer: results from the Nordic occupational mortality and cancer incidence registers. *J Natl Cancer Inst* 1986; 77: 883–889.

72. Carta P, Cocco PL, Casula D. Mortality from lung cancer among Sardinian patients with silicosis. *Br J Ind Med* 1991; 48: 122–129.

73. Finkelstein M, Liss GM, Krammer F, Kusiak RA. Mortality among workers receiving compensation awards for silicosis in Ontario 1940–1985. *Br J Ind Med* 1987; 44: 588–594.

74. Infante Rivard C, Armstrong B, Petitclerc M *et al.* Lung cancer mortality and silicosis in Quebec, 1938–1985. *Lancet* 1989; ii: 1504–1507.

75. Merlo F, Doria M, Fontana L *et al.* Mortality from specific causes among silicotic subjects: a historical prospective study. *IARC Sci Publ* 1990; 105–111.

76. Ng TP, Chan SL, Lee J. Mortality of a cohort of men in a silicosis register: further evidence of an association with lung cancer. *Am J Ind Med* 1990; 17: 163–171.

77. Partanen T, Pukkala E, Vainio H *et al.* Increased incidence of lung and skin cancer in Finnish silicotic patients. *J Occup Med* 1994; 36: 616–622.

78. Finkelstein MM. Radiographic abnormalities and the risk of lung cancer among workers exposed to silica dust in Ontario. *Can Med Assoc J* 1995; 152: 37–43.

79. Chiyotani K, Saito K, Okubo T, Takahashi K. Lung cancer risk among pneumonoconiosis patients in Japan, with special reference to silicotics. *IARC Sci Publ* 1990; 97: 95–104.

80. Amandus H, Costello J. Silicosis and lung cancer in US metal miners. *Arch Environ Health* 1991; 46: 82–89.

81. Hodgson JT, Jones RD. Mortality of a cohort of tin miners 1941–1986. *Br J Ind Med* 1990; 47: 665–676.

82. Chen J, McLaughlin JK, Zhang JY. Mortality among dust-exposed Chinese mine and pottery workers. *J Occup Med* 1992; 34: 311–316.

83. McLaughlin J, Chen J, Mustafa D *et al*. A nested case-control study of lung cancer among silica-exposed workers in China. *Br J Ind Med* 1992; 49: 167–171.

84. Chen SY, Hayes RB, Liang SR *et al*. Mortality experience of haematite mine worker in China. *Br J Ind Med* 1990; 47: 175–181.

85. Hnizdo E, Sluis Cremer GK. Silica exposure, silicosis, and lung cancer: a mortality study of South African gold miners. *Br J Ind Med* 1991; 48: 53–60.

86. Hessel PA, Sluis-Cremer GK, Hnizdo E. Silica exposures, silicosis, and lung cancer: a necropsy study. *Br J Ind Med* 1990; 47: 4–9.

87. Carta P, Cocco P, Picchiri G. Lung cancer mortality and airways obstruction among metal miners exposed to silica and low levels of radon daughters. *Am J Ind Med* 1994; 25: 489–506.

88. Samet JM, Pthak DR, Morgan MV *et al*. Silicosis and lung cancer risk in underground uranium miners. *Health Phys* 1994; 66: 450–453.

89. Costello J, Graham WB. Vermont granite workers' mortality study. *Am J Ind Med* 1988; 13: 483–497.

90. Chia SE, Chia KS, Phoon WH, Lee HP. Silicosis and lung cancer among Chinese granite workers. *Scand J Work Environ Health* 1991; 17: 170–174.

91. Sherson D, Svane O, Lynge E. Cancer incidence among foundry workers in Denmark. *Arch Environ Health* 1991; 46: 75–81.

92. Mehnert WH, Staneczek W, Mohner M *et al*. A mortality study of a cohort of slate quarry workers in the German Democratic Republic. *IARC Sci Publ* 1990; 55–64.

93. Amandus HE, Catellan RM, Shy C *et al*. Reevaluation of silicosis and lung cancer in North Carolina dusty trades workers. *Am J Ind Med* 1992; 22: 147–153.

94. Checkoway H, Heyer NJ, Demers PA, Breslow NE. Mortality among workers in the diatomaceous earth industry. *Br J Ind Med* 1993; 50: 586–597.

95. Tornling G, Hogstedt C, Westerholm P. Lung cancer incidence among Swedish ceramic workers with silicosis. *IARC Sci Publ* 1990; 97: 113–119.

96. Lagorio S, Forastiere F, Michelozzi P *et al*. A case-referent study on lung cancer mortality among ceramic workers. *IARC Sci Publ* 1990; 21–28.

97. IARC Monograph 69. *Polychorinated dibenzo-para-dioxins and Polychorinated Dibenzofurans*. Lyons, France: IARC, 1997.

98. Manz A, Berger J, Flesch-Janys D *et al*. Cancer mortality among workers in chemical plant contaminated with dioxin. *Lancet* 1991; 338: 959–964.

99. Becher H, Flesch-Janys D, Kauppinen T *et al*. Cancer mortality in German male workers exposed to phenoxy herbicides and dioxins. *Cancer Causes Controls* 1996; 7: 312–321.

100. Fingerhut MA, Halperin WE, Marlow DA *et al*. Cancer mortality in workers exposed to 2,3,7,8-tetrachlorodibeno-para-dioxin. *N Engl J Med* 1991; 324: 212–218.

101. Saracci R, Kogevinas M, Bertazzi PA *et al*. Cancer mortality in workers exposed to chlorophenozy herbicides and chlorophenols. *Lancet* 1991; 338: 1027–1032.

102. IARC Monograph 34. *Polynuclear Aromatic Compounds, Part 3: Industrial Exposures in Aluminum Production, Coal Gasification, Coke Production and Iron and Steel Founding*. Lyon, France: IARC, 1984.

103. Redmond CK. Cancer mortality among coke-oven workers. *Environ Health Perspec* 1983; 52: 67–73.

104. Dong MH, Redmond CK, Mazumdar S, Constantino JP. A multi-stage approach to the cohort analysis of lifetime lung cancer risk among steelworkers exposed to coke-oven emissions. *Am J Epidemiol* 1988; 128: 860–873.

105. IARC Monograph 35. *Polynuclear Aromatic Componnds Part 4: Bitumens, Coal Tars, and Derived Products, Shale-Oils, Soots*. Lyons, France: IARC, 1985.

106. Silverstein M, Maizlish N, Park R, Mirer F. Mortality among workers exposed to coal-tar pitch volatiles and welding emissions. *Am J Public Health* 1985; 75: 1283–1287.

107. Armstrong B, Tremblay C, Baris D, Theriault G. Lung cancer mortality and polynuclear aromatic hydrocarbons: a case-cohort study of aluminum production workers in Arvida, Quebec, Canada. *Am J Epidemiol* 1994; 139: 250–262.

108. Situs F, Douglas AJ, Webster EC. Respiratory disease mortality patterns among South African iron moulders. *Br J Ind Med* 1989; 46: 310–315.

109. IARC Monograph Supplement 7. *Iron and Steel Founding*, p. 133. Lyons, France: IARC, 1987.

110. Fletcher AC, Ades A. Lung cancer mortality in a cohort of English foundry workers. *Scand J Work Environ Health* 1984; 10: 7–16.

111. Jahn I, Ahrens W, Bruske-Hohlfeld I. Occupational risk factors for lung cancer in women: results of a case-control study in Germany. *Am J Ind Med* 1999; 36: 90–100.

112. IARC Monograph 47. *Some Organic Solvents, Resin Monomers, and Related Compounds, Pigments and Occupational Exposures in Paint Manufacturing and Painting*. Lyon, France: IARC, 1989.

113. Steenland K, Palu S. Cohort mortality study of 57,000 painters and other union members: a 15 year update. *Occup Environ Med* 1999; 56: 315–321.

114. Stockwell J, Matanowski G. A case-control study of lung cancer in painters. *J Occup Med* 1985; 13: 1125–1126.

115. National Research Council BEIR VI, 1998. Committee on Health Risks of Exposure to Radon: BEIR VI, National Research Council. Health Effect of Exposure to Radon: BEIR VI. Washington DC: National Academy Press, 1999

116. Samet JM, Pathak DR *et al*. Lung cancer mortality and exosure to radon progeny in a cohort of New Mexico underground uranium miners. *Health Phys* 1991; 6: 745–752.

117. KusiakKusiak RA, Ritchie AC, Muller J, Springer J. Mortality from lung cancer in Ontario uranium miners. *Br J Ind Med* 1993; 50: 920–928.

118. Wu KG, FuH, Mo CZ, Yu LZ. Smelting, underground mining, smoking, and lung cancer: a case-control in a tin mine area. *Biomed Environ Sci* 1989; 2: 98–105.

119. Radford E, St-Clair Renard K. Lung cancer in Swedish iron miners exposed to low doses of radon daughters. *N Engl J Med* 1984; 310: 1485–1494.

120. Solli H, Andersen A, Straden E, Langard S. Cancer incidence among workers exposed to radon and thoron daughters at a niobium mine. *Scand J Work Environ Health* 1985; 11: 7–13.

121. Qiao YL, Taylor PR, Yao SX *et al*. Relation of radon exposure and tobacco use to lung cancer among tin

miners in Yunnan Province, China. *Am J Ind Med* 1989; 16: 511–521.

122. Fu H, Gu X, Jon X *et al.* Lung cancer among tin miners in southeast China: silica exposure, silicosis and cigarette smoking. *Am J Ind Med* 1994; 26: 373–381.

123. Wyndham CH, Bezuidenhout BN, Greenacre MJ, Sleeis–Cremer GK. Mortality of middle aged white South African gold miners. *Br J Ind Med* 1986; 43: 677–684.

124. Parkin DM, Vizcaino AP, Skinner ME, Ndhlovu AC. Cancer patterns and risk factors in the African population of southwestern Zimbabwe, 1963–1977. *Cancer Epidem Biomarkers Prev* 1994; 3: 537–547.

125. Emmelin A, Nystrom L, Wall S. Diesel exhaust exposure and smoking: a care-referent study of lung cancer among Swedish dock workers. Epidemiology. 1993; 4(3): 237–44.

126. Wong O. A cohort mortality study of employees exposed to chlorinated chemicals. *Am J Ind Med* 1988; 14: 417–431.

127. Ishinishi N, Koizumni A, McClellan R, Stober W (eds.). *Carcinogenic and Mutagenic Effects of Diesel Engine Exhaust.* New York: Elsevier, 1986.

128. Howe GR, Fraser D, Lindsay J, *et al.* Cancer mortality (1965–67) in relation to diesel fume and coal exposure in a cohort of retired railway workers. *J Natl Cancer Inst* 1983; 70: 1015–1019.

129. Garshick E, Schenker MB, Munoz A. A retrospective cohort study of lung cancer and diesel exhaust in railroad workers. *Am Rev Respir Dis* 1988; 137: 820–825.

130. Gustafsson L, Wall S, Larsson L, Skog B. Mortality and cancer incidence among Swedish dock workers: a retrospective cohort study. *Scan J Work Environ Health* 1986; 12: 22–26.

131. IARC Monograph 46. *Diesel and Gasoline Engine Exhausts and Some Nitroarenes.* Lyons, France: IARC, 1989.

132. Boffetta P, Stellman S, Garfinkel L. Diesel exhaust exposure and mortality among males in the American Cancer Society Prospective Study. *Am J Ind Med* 1988; 14: 403–415.

133. Gustafsson L, Reuterwall C. Mortality and incidence of cancer among Swedish gas workers. *Br J Ind Med* 1990; 47: 169–174.

134. Steenland K, Silverman D, Hornung R. Case-control study of lung cancer and truck driving in the Teamsters Union. *Am J Public Health* 1990; 80: 670–674.

135. Boffetta P, Harris R, Wyners E. Case-control study on occupational exposure to diesel exhaust and lung cancer risk. *Am J Ind Med* 1990; 17: 577–591.

136. Lipsett M, Campleman S. Occupational exposure to diesel exhaust and lung cancer: a meta-analysis. *J Public Health* 1999; 89: 1009–1017.

137. IARC Monograph 71. *Re-evaluation of Some Organic Chemicals, Hydrazine and Hydrogen Peroxide.* Lyon, France: IARC, 1999.

138. Delzell E, Macaluso M, Cole P. A follow-up study of workers at a dye and resin manufacturing plant. *J Occup Med* 1989; 31: 273–278.

139. Barbone F, Delzell E, Austin H *et al.* A case-control study of lung cancer at a dye and resin manufacturing plant. *Am J Ind Med* 1992; 22: 835–849.

140. Tsai SP, Gilstrap EL, Ross CE. Morality study of employees with potential exposure to epichlorohydrin: a 10 year update. *Occup Environ Med* 1996; 53: 299–304.

141. Wingren G, Englander V. Mortality and cancer morbidity in a cohort of Swedish glassworkers. *Occup Environ Health* 1990; 62: 253–257.

142. Pirastu R, Bartoli D, Se Santis M *et al.* Cancer mortality of art glass workers in Tuscany, Italy. *Scand J Work Environ Health* 1998; 24: 386–391.

143. IARC Monograph 53. *Occupational Exposures in Spraying and Application of Insecticides.* Lyon, France: IARC, 1991.

144. Thomas HF, Winter PD, Donaldson LJ. Cancer morality among local authority pest control officers in England and Wales. *Occup Environ Med* 1996; 53: 787–790.

145. Pesatori AC, Sontag JM, Lubin JH *et al.* Cohort mortality and nested case-control study of lung cancer among structural pest control workers in Florida (United States). *Cancer Causes Control* 1994; 5: 310–318.

146. Morabia A, Markowitz S, Garibaldi K, Wynder E. Lung cancer and occupation: results of a multicentre case-control study. *Br J Ind Med* 1992; 49: 721–727.

147. Vineis P, Thomas T, Hayes R *et al.* Proportion of lung cancers in males due to occupation in different areas of the US. *Int J Can* 1988; 42: 851–856.

148. Doll R, Peto R. The causes of cancer: quantitative estimates of avoidable risk of cancer in the US today. *J Natl Cancer Inst* 1981; 66: 1191–1308.

149. Kleinbaum D, Kupper L, Morgansten H. *Epidemiologic Research.* Belmont CA: Lifetime Learning, 1982.

150. van Loon AJM, Kant IJ, Swaen GMH *et al.* Occupational exposure to carcinogenes and risk of lung cancer: results from the Netherlands cohort study. *Occup Environ Med* 1997; 54: 817–824.

151. Magnani C, Leporati M. Mortality from lung cancer and population risk attributable to asbestos in an asbestos cement manufacturing town in Italy. *Occup Environ Med* 1998; 55: 111–114.

152. Christiani DC. Occupational health in the People's Republic of China. *Am J Public Health* 194; 74: 58–64.

153. Christiani DC. Modernization and Occupational Cancer. *J Occup Med* 1988; 30: 975–976.

154. Wiencke J, Varkonyi A, Semey K *et al.* Validation of blood mononuclear cell DNA-adducts as a marker of DNA damage in human lung. *Cancer Res* 1995; 55: 4910–4915.

155. Wogan GN, Gorelick NS. An overview of chemical and biochemical dosimetry of exposure to genotoxic chemicals. *Environ Health Perspect* 1985; 62: 5–18.

156. McFarlane MJ, Feinstein AR, Wells CK. Clinical features of lung cancers discovered as a postmortem surprise. *Chest* 1986; 90: 520.

157. McFarlane MJ, Feinstein AR, Wells CK. Necropsy evidence of detection bias in the diagnosis of lung cancer. *Arch Intern Med* 1986; 146: 1695.

158. Dufresne A, Begin R, Churg A *et al.* Mineral fibre content of lungs in mesthelioma cases seeking compensation in Quebec. *Am J Respair Crit Care Med* 1996; 153: 711–718.

159. Banks DE, Wang ML, Parker JE. Asbestos exposure, asbestosis and lung cancer. *Chest* 1999; 115: 536–549.

160. Hammond EC, Selikoff IJ, Seidman H. Asbestos exposure cigarette smoking and death rates. *Ann NY Acad Sci* 1979; 330: 473–490.

161. Berlin NI, Buncher CR, Fontana RS *et al.* The National Cancer Institute Cooperative early lung cancer detection program: results of the initial screen (prevalence). *Am Rev Respir Dis* 1984; 130: 545–549.

162. Frost JK, Ball WC, Levin ML *et al.* Early lung cancer detection: results of the initial (prevalence) radiologic and cytologic screening in the Johns Hopkins Study. *Am Rev Respir Dis* 1984; 130: 549–554.

163. Flehinger BJ, Malamed MR, Zaman MB *et al.* Early lung cancer detection: results of the initial (prevalence) radiologic and cytologic screening in the Memorial Sloan–Kettering Study. *Am Rev Respir Dis* 1984; 130: 555–560.

164. Fontana RS, Sanderson DR, Taylor WF, *et al.* Early lung cancer detection: results of the initial (prevalence) radiologic and cytologic screening in the Mayo Clinic study. *Am Rev Respir Dis* 1984; 130: 561–565.

165. NCI Early Lung Cancer Cooperative Study. Early lung cancer detection: summary and conclusions. *Am Rev Respir Dis* 1984; 130: 565–570.

166. Henschke CI, McCauley DI, Yankelevitz DF, *et al.* Early lung cancer action project: overall design and findings from baseline screening. *Lancet* 1999; 354: 99–105.

20 DISORDERS FROM ALTERED AMBIENT PRESSURE

Thomas A. Dillard and Richard E. Moon

INTRODUCTION

The term barotrauma derives from the Greek word *baros* which means 'weight' [1]. In this context weight refers to the mass of a column of air or water bearing upon a given point of reference. This weight, the barometric pressure, results from the gravitational attraction between the earth and the mass of atmospheric air or water, and other forces. Whereas weight usually connotes a static force, the term barotrauma usually implies dynamic conditions. Steadman's *Medical Dictionary* defines barotrauma as 'Injury . . . resulting from imbalance between ambient pressure and that within the affected cavity' [1]. This definition reflects non-equilibrium or dynamic conditions usually associated with barotrauma wherein traumatic tissue injury results from resolution of the imbalance.

An imbalance in pressure may result from the physical environment changing at a rate faster than normal tissues can reach equilibrium. Pressure imbalance may be amplified by delayed equilibration owing to abnormal tissues. For example, the normal ears 'popping' can become severely painful aerotitis or barotitis, terms for middle ear trauma during flight or diving respectively, in the presence of abnormal Eustachian tube function.

The term barotrauma also applies to injuries sustained in situations were pressure is applied selectively to a specific body part or region. An example would be positive pressure ventilation, where only the respiratory tract is subjected to increased pressure.

Pulmonary barotrauma

Pulmonary barotrauma typically refers to specific manifestations of injury associated with imbalances in the total pressure with the air spaces. These include pneumothorax, pneumomediastinum, subcutaneous emphysema, systemic arterial gas embolism (AGE), pneumopericardium, and pneumoperitoneum. These forms of barotrauma presumably have a common mechanism. Figure 20.1 shows a schematic in which pulmonary interstitial emphysema represents a

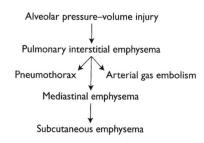

Fig. 20.1 The proposed sequence of events following a pressure and/or volume stress on the alveoli. The injury first produces interstitial emphysema before other manifestations of pulmonary barotrauma. Mediastinal emphysema is a common denominator for many manifestations.

common precursor to the manifestations of pulmonary barotrauma. In premature neonates with immature lung and respiratory distress syndrome, interstitial pulmonary emphysema can occur as the lone manifestation of barotrauma.

Non-pulmonary barotrauma

There are several conditions which might usually be considered non-pulmonary barotrauma. Decompression sickness (DCS), also known as caisson workers disease or 'the bends', is a classic hazard of diving and work in pressurized environments such as caissons and pressurized tunnels. This condition results from both a change in ambient pressure and from differences in solubility and equilibration times of dissolved gases within body compartments. In most cases, the lung's involvement in DCS is limited to its place in the pathway for gas equilibration between the local environment and the body; however, in some cases the lungs can become pathologically involved in DCS complicated by air emboli within the pulmonary arteries, the 'chokes'. Except for DCS, other forms of non-pulmonary barotrauma will be considered only in brief.

Disorders of altered partial pressure

A final group of disorders results from alterations of gas partial pressures that can occur in association with changes in total ambient barometric pressure. These disorders typically fall outside the usual scope of barotrauma defined in terms of traumatic injury resulting from change in total gas pressure. Examples of these disorders include hypoxia as a result of environmental causes, nitrogen narcosis, and high pressure syndrome.

The forms of pulmonary barotrauma, non-pulmonary barotrauma, and disorders resulting from alterations in gas partial pressure will be considered sequentially. The first section will address hyperbaric pathophysiology and diving accidents. The second section will consider hypobaric pathophysiology and altitude illnesses.

HYPERBARIC ENVIRONMENTS

Diving to significant depth involves pathophysiologic hazards that can produce a variety of injuries. The signs and symptoms of these injuries can afflict any part of the body. Emergency medical services may consult internists, pulmonologists, or intensivists to recommend acute management of divers with injuries or to attend divers after proper decompression.

Pulmonary and occupational practitioners also require expertise to evaluate fitness for diving. Exposure to rapid changes in ambient pressure is experienced by millions of recreational scuba divers in the USA alone, in addition to military and commercial divers, compressed air workers, and pilots. The occurrence of pulmonary conditions that may predispose to diving injuries, such as asthma or spontaneous pneumothorax, should be anticipated in the diving population.

The barometric pressure at sea level is 100 kPa (the equivalent of 1 atmosphere absolute, 760 mmHg, or 14.7 psi). Because pressure increases linearly underwater, every additional 10 m (33 ft) of descent adds 100 kPa (1 atmosphere) (Table 20.1). To make breathing possible for divers, the changing ambient pressure is balanced by a supply of air delivered at the pressure of the environment by a demand regulator from a gas diving apparatus.

Since most morbidity involving diving is related to the behavior of gases under changing conditions of pressure, a brief mention of the two most relevant gas laws is appropriate. Boyle's law states that at a constant temperature, the volume of gas varies inversely with the pressure applied. The physiologic ramifications of this law underlie the characteristics of pressure-related diving diseases (barotrauma). Henry's law states that the amount of a given gas that is dissolved in a liquid at a given temperature is directly proportional to the partial pressure of that

Table 20.1 Pressure equivalents of various depths in water below sea level

Feet	Meters	mmHg	kPa	ATA	PSIA	PSIG	P_{N_2}		P_{O_2}	
							mmHg	kPa	mmHg	kPa
0 (sea level)	0 (sea level)	760	100	1	14.7	0.0	600	78.9	160	21.1
33	10	1520	200	2	29.4	14.7	1200	157.9	320	42.1
66	20	2280	300	3	44.1	29.4	1800	236.8	480	63.2
99	30	3040	400	4	58.8	44.1	2400	315.8	640	84.2

kPa, kilopascales; ATA, pressure in absolute atmospheres; PSIA, pressure in pounds per square inch absolute pressure; PSIG, pressure in pounds per square inch gauge; P_{N_2}, nitrogen partial pressure in mmHg at standard temperature and pressure that contains no water vapor (STPD); P_{O_2}, Oxygen partial pressure in mmHg STPD.

gas. Henry's law provides the basic explanation of decompression sickness and nitrogen narcosis.

Barotrauma

Barotrauma refers to tissue injury resulting from the failure of a gas-filled body space (e.g. the lungs, the middle ear, and the sinuses) to equalize its internal pressure to correspond to changes in ambient pressure. During a diving descent, failure to equalize pressure leads to a decrease in the volume of these body spaces in accordance with Boyle's law. Since cavities located within a bone cannot collapse, the space they take up is filled by engorgement of the mucous membrane, often followed by hemorrhage. The risk of barotrauma is more pronounced near the surface of the water, where a small change in depth (of even a few meters) may lead to a large change in relative gas volume [2].

Recognition

Pulmonary barotrauma occurring during ascent is the most severe and life-threatening form of barotrauma. During a dive, the breathing apparatus delivers gas at the diver's ambient pressure. Therefore, compared with the surface, at the diver's depth there are increased numbers of molecules in the lung, in direct proportion to the absolute pressure. During ascent these excess gas molecules must be exhaled; otherwise, lung volume will increase, and barotrauma may occur [2]. During ascent, as the ambient pressure decreases, gas within the lungs expands. If through breath holding a diver does not permit expanding gas to escape from the lungs or the gas is trapped by localized airways obstruction caused by disease, than distention and rupture of the lungs may occur. Air escaping from the intraalveolar spaces may cause pneumothorax, pneumomediastinum, or subcutaneous emphysema of the neck and upper chest (Fig. 20.2) [2,3]. Air may also enter torn pulmonary veins, resulting in systemic arterial gas emboli (AGE) [4]. The most severe cases of pulmonary barotrauma are seen after an emergency ascent [4,5]. However, the condition may occasionally occur in healthy divers who have no detectable underlying pathologic conditions and who have carried out appropriate techniques of exhalation.

In this disorder, mediastinal and subcutaneous emphysema may produce changes in the voice, a feeling of fullness in the chest, dyspnea, dysphagia, supraclavicular crepitus, and typical radiographic findings on chest and neck films. Pneumothorax may cause sudden pleuritic pain and dyspnea. A rapidly developing large pneumothorax may impair cardiac function and in rare cases lead to shock and

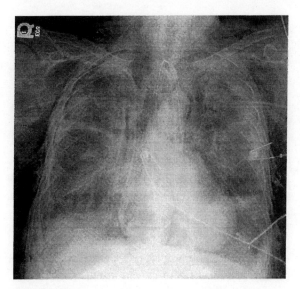

Fig. 20.2 The figure shows florid signs of barotrauma including subcutaneous emphysema in the soft tissues outlining the pectoral muscles. The figure also shows pneumomediastinum with para-aortic crescent and continuous diaphragm signs, pneumopericardium and pneumothorax.

death [2]. All the manifestations of pulmonary barotrauma may occur singly or in combination.

The most serious sequelae of pulmonary barotrauma is AGE as a result of the passage of gas into the pulmonary veins and from there into the systemic circulation [4]. Gas bubbles lodged in small arteries may occlude segments of the cerebral, coronary, and other systemic vascular beds. Small volumes of gas may occlude vessels only transiently, passing through into the venous blood within a few seconds or minutes. In the process, an incompletely understood process is triggered, causing a progressive decrease in cerebral blood flow. The clinical picture is usually that of a rapidly developing stroke-like syndrome, ranging from a focal neurologic deficit beginning hours after the dive to unconsciousness, collapse, and death immediately after the diver surfaces [2,4,5]. In some patients, myocardial ischemia or arrhythmias caused by coronary artery occlusion dominate the clinical picture [6]. There may also be skin marbling and gas bubbles in the retinal vessels [2]. Neurologic manifestations in a scuba diver surfacing from a deep dive can also be a result of DCS. This complication can occur either alone or in combination with air embolism, and it is discussed further below.

Management

The maintenance of respiration and adequate arterial oxygen tension is essential in all patients with pulmonary barotrauma. In those with mediastinal or subcutaneous emphysema, the administration of high concentrations of oxygen increases the rate of removal of nitrogen, enhancing the clearance of nitrogen from the emphysematous area. A large pneumothorax that interferes with pulmonary function requires tube thoracostomy. Most doctors specializing in diving problems recommend placement of a chest drain in most patients with pneumothorax and air embolism who are undergoing recompression therapy, since pneumothorax is likely to expand again during subsequent decompression.

Patients with air embolism should be transferred to the nearest hyperbaric oxygen facility for emergency therapy while breathing the highest available concentration of oxygen [2,4]. Older recommendations included placement of the patient in a head down position in order to decrease the risk of additional cerebral embolism and to increase the arterial pressure, hence reducing the volume of arterial gases. The head-down position may augment cerebral edema, however, and the current recommendation is the supine position unless the patient is hypotensive [7]. Recompression treatment is carried out in hyperbaric chambers, which are used to administer oxygen at high ambient pressures. Treatment with hyperbaric oxygen results in both a mechanical reduction of the volume of gas emboli (Boyle's law) and an increased nitrogen pressure gradient between emboli and blood, accelerating the absorption of the emboli. In addition, hyperbaric oxygen increases the oxygenation of hypoxic brain tissue and decreases postembolic brain edema. Although the optimal pressures and gas mixtures for this treatment are still under debate [8], most authorities use the protocol developed by the US Navy [9] (Fig. 20.3), which includes 100% oxygen at 280 kPa (2.8 atmospheres absolute). An option if clinical improvement does not occur at 280 kPa is to compress to 600 kPa and administer 21–50% oxygen.

Barotrauma of the middle ear during descent is the most common disorder in divers [10]. The symptoms of middle-ear barotrauma vary from a sensa-tion of pressure, followed by pain and conductive hearing loss, to rupture of the tympanic membrane, usually with an acute relief of pain, followed by whirling vertigo caused by uneven caloric stimulation [10]. The condition is caused by an inability to equalize the pressure in the middle ear because of faulty clearing techniques, upper respiratory infection, or anatomic variations in the nasal skeleton [11]. When a difference in pressure of 90 mmHg builds up between the middle-ear cleft and the nasopharynx, the Eustachian tube cannot be opened. In this situation, edema, exudation, and hematotympanum may occur [12,13]. A forceful Valsalva maneuver results in further locking forces, which may lead to rupture of the tympanic membrane or inner-ear barotrauma [12]. With the diver's deeper descent, the eardrum may rupture [14]. The failure of the expanding gas to vent through the Eustachian tube may occasionally lead to middle-ear barotrauma during ascent [10,12]. Barotrauma of ascent can cause facial nerve palsy [15].

The management of middle-ear barotrauma consists of topical nasal and systemic decongestants. If purulent otorrhea is observed, antibiotics should be prescribed. Most tympanic-membrane perforations heal spontaneously if infection is controlled and normal Eustachian-tube function is restored [10,12]. Concomitant inner-ear barotrauma should be ruled out in all cases of middle-ear barotrauma [12].

Inner-ear barotrauma may be a consequence of forceful efforts to equalize middle-ear pressure when the Eustachian tube is locked and blocked [12]. This increases intracranial pressure markedly and may cause the rupture of inner-ear membranes or the creation of labyrinthine window fistulae, with consequent impairment of cochlear and vestibular function. Inner-ear barotrauma may also occur independently of middle-ear barotrauma [16,17]. The main symptoms are persistent vertigo, sensorineural hearing loss, and loud tinnitus. The primary treatment is complete bed rest, with the patient's head ele-

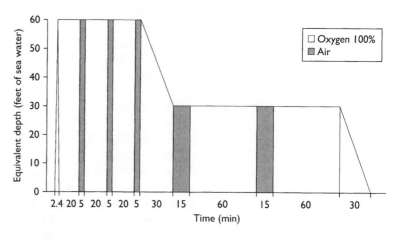

Fig. 20.3 The US Navy treatment table. This treatment table is the most commonly used algorithm for hyperbaric treatment of neurologic decompression illness and pain-only or mild cutaneous symptoms that are not relieved within 10 min of reaching an equivalent depth of 18 m (60 ft) breathing 100% oxygen. Periods of 100% oxygen breathing are interspersed with air breathing periods ('air breaks') to reduce oxygen toxicity. Additional oxygen breathing cycles can be administered at equivalent depths of 18 m (60 ft) and 9 m (30 ft) for persistent symptoms. Further details can be found in the US Navy Diving Manual [9].

vated and the avoidance of Valsalva maneuvers (e.g. during defecation). Such actions help to prevent an increase in the pressure of the cerebrospinal fluid that might aggravate a possible perilymphatic leak or the admixture of endolymph and perilymph, if there are tears in the labyrinthine membrane [16]. The deterioration of inner-ear function indicates a need for explorative tympanotomy and the patching of a round or oval window [10,12].

Alternobaric vertigo is a condition manifested by an asymmetric increase in pressure in the right and left middle ears that exceeds a threshold difference of 45 mmHg. This pressure difference is transferred to the labyrinth, resulting in nausea, vomiting, and disorientation. Although these symptoms are usually mild, when they occur underwater they may lead to aspiration of water and drowning [18].

Paranasal-sinus barotrauma, the second most common disease of divers [10], is frequently related to chronic dysfunction of the nasal or paranasal sinus, with blockage of the sinus ostia. Pain over the frontal sinus is the predominant symptom, often followed by epistaxis. The relatively long and tortuous course of the nasofrontal duct may explain the vulnerability of the frontal sinus [19]. Treatment for sinus barotrauma includes the use of topical and systemic decongestants or adrenergic agents, and of antibiotics if a purulent nasal discharge is present. Although recovery is usually uneventful with conservative therapy [19], the patient should be followed closely for the potential spread of infection to orbital and intracranial structures [20].

Decompression sickness

When a diver breathes air under increased pressure, the tissues are loaded with increased quantities of oxygen and nitrogen (Henry's law). Oxygen is used in tissue metabolism, whereas nitrogen, which is physiologically inert, is not. Thus, the nitrogen content of a tissue increases in proportion to the ambient pressure and also in relation to the tissue's fat content, since nitrogen is about five times more soluble in fat than in water [21].

When the ambient pressure decreases as the diver returns to the surface, the sum of the gas tensions in the tissue may exceed the absolute ambient pressure. At this point, a state of supersaturation is created that may lead to the liberation of free gas from the tissues and to the onset of DCS. The liberated gas can disturb organ function by blocking arteries, veins, and lymphatic vessels; in addition, its expansion can rupture or compress tissues. When gas is found in a space with rigid boundaries, as in a muscle enveloped by fascia, it may lead to a compartment syndrome. Gas may also form within cells,

causing the rupture of the cell membrane. Finally, reactions at the interface of blood and gas bubbles can activate the clotting cascade [21], and possibly other biochemical processes such as the complement system.

The probability of DCS has been reduced, but not eliminated, by the use of decompression schedules tables such as those of the US Navy [9], the Royal Navy [22], or a decompression computer. Moreover, 'silent' (asymptomatic) bubbles have been detected ultrasonically in the pulmonary circulation of divers during decompression from dives that do not require stops during ascent [23,24] or even from a series of dives made without equipment while the diver's breath is held ('breathhold dives') that do not require such stops [25]. Although mild transient reduction in pulmonary gas exchange has been described in professional divers in association with asymptomatic venous gas embolism, the long-term importance of silent bubbles is unclear. Risk factors that have been suggested to increase the probability of DCS (whether by increasing the accumulation of inert gases in tissues, slowing their release, or magnifying their secondary effects) include advanced age, female sex [26], obesity, low water temperature, poor physical fitness, a high level of physical activity during the dive, and altitude exposure after diving. Even the slight reduction in ambient pressure experienced during commercial airline flights can precipitate DCS, particularly within 18 hours after a dive. Dives repeated in a series can also be a major source of difficulty, since after one dive residual nitrogen may remain in the tissues [9].

Recognition

DCS has traditionally been classified into two types on the basis of clinical manifestations:

- type I includes skin bends and pain (usually around joints)
- type II is the more severe variety, which includes cardiorespiratory and neurologic manifestations.

Joint pain has been attributed to the supersaturation and separation of an inert gas within the poorly perfused periarticular tight connective tissues. The pain is usually not exacerbated by motion, and local tenderness or signs of inflammation are very uncommon [27,28]. Other manifestations of type I DCS include pruritus and skin rashes caused by the presence of gas bubbles in subcutaneous glands. Pruritus generally resolves within 10–30 min, even without treatment. Skin marbling may occur when subcutaneous microbubbles cause venous stasis. These mild symptoms signal possible systemic involvement, which may progress rapidly and require recompression treatment. Lymphatic obstruction can also occur, leading to lymphadenopathy, pain, and localized edema, which are only rarely alleviated by recompression.

Symptoms of type II DCS most commonly appear within 24 hours after the diver surfaces [27,28] and they can be preceded by joint pain or other symptoms of DCS. Central nervous system (CNS) involvement is most commonly characterized by damage to the spinal cord. Paresthesias that progress to numbness are the most common presenting symptoms [1]. In addition, the involvement of motor pathways may lead to paraparesis and paraplegia. Severe spinal lesions are usually associated with urinary and anal sphincter dysfunction. Referred abdominal pain, as well as girdle and back pain, is quite common in severe spinal cord DCS [29].

The symptoms of cerebral involvement include blurred vision, diplopia, tunnel vision or scotomas, dysarthria, dizziness, and vertigo, as well as mental and personality changes. Severe cerebral involvement may lead to convulsions and death [27,28]. In addition to the local separation of a free gas, neurologic manifestations of DCS may also be attributed to paradoxical gas embolization; that is, bubbles within the blood escape pulmonary filtration [30] by entering the arterial circulation through a patent foramen ovale or an atrial-septal defect [31]. These may occlude capillaries or damage the blood–brain barrier [32].

Poorly perfused areas of the nervous system with a high fat content are at a particularly high risk of decompression demage from underwater diving, which may in part explain the typical appearance of extensive demyelinating lesions in severe cases of CNS DCS [33,34].

Inner-ear DCS has been reported after recreational scuba diving, although most cases are the result of decompression with mixtures of helium and oxygen or of very deep air diving [35,36]. The pathophysiology of inner-ear DCS is not known with certainty, but has been suggested to be caused by bubble-induced rupture of lacunae, or bubble formation within the fluids of the cochlea or semicircular canals. Secondarily, osteoblastic differentiation can occur, leading to fibroosseous labyrinthitis. The main manifestations of this condition are severe sensorineural hearing loss, tinnitus, vertigo, and ataxia [37].

Pulmonary manifestations of type II DCS occur when excessive numbers of gas bubbles liberated during decompression are trapped in the pulmonary arteriolar circulation. Retrosternal discomfort, extreme fatigue, dry cough, and even severe respiratory distress caused by pulmonary edema (known among divers as 'the chokes') can occur [27,28].

Contrary to what was previously believed, type II DCS is more common among those engaging in recreational air diving than type I [27,38]. It should be emphasized that DCS can be a diffuse, multifocal disease, for which there is specific treatment. While most cases of DCS present within 24 hours following a dive, altitude exposure can occasionally precipitate symptoms even later.

Management

First aid for DCS includes the administration of inhaled oxygen at the highest possible concentration and hydration. Seriously ill patients should be resuscitated with intravenous fluids, preferably using either colloids or isotonic, glucose-free crystalloid solutions. Transportation to a recompression chamber should be as quick as feasible; the time to the administration of hyperbaric treatment is one of the main determinants of outcome [39]. However, even after a long delay (even several days), recompression treatment may still be beneficial [40].

The rationale for the use of hyperbaric oxygen to treat decompression sickness is similar to that described earlier to treat air emboli: namely, the need to eliminate gas bubbles and alleviate damage to hypoxic tissue. In principle, recompression protocols use oxygen at pressures sufficient to produce a therapeutic effect without causing oxygen toxicity. In most centers providing hyperbaric oxygen therapy, treatment is given according to the US Navy treatment tables (Fig. 20.3) [9]. A recompression protocol is selected according to the severity of illness (type I or II) and the patient's response during therapy. The most commonly used initial treatment regimen is shown in Figure 20.3. If this regimen fails, an extension of this protocol is possible. Other therapeutic regimens are available for severe cases [7]. Subsequently, the procedures described in Treatment Tables 5 or 6 of the US Navy diving manual [9], or short (90–120 min) treatments with hyperbaric oxygen at 2–2.5 atmospheres absolute, are usually given daily or twice daily until there is no further improvement in symptoms. Although severe neurologic disease may require multiple treatments to achieve a clinical 'plateau', the vast majority of patients with DCS are adequately treated with one or two hyperbaric exposures.

Because hemodynamic changes encountered during severe DCS may lead to hemoconcentration, intravenous fluids should be administered. Previous recommendations have included high doses of steroids and mannitol to reduce local edema in the CNS and maintain an intact blood–brain barrier, although there is no good evidence for either in this disorder. There is evidence that intravenous lidocaine (lignocaine) may be beneficial in animal models of AGE; a randomized study has demonstrated evidence of cerebral protection from its use during open heart surgery, and there is some anecdotal support for its use in DCS [41,42].

It is not always possible to differentiate the manifestations of DCS from those of AGE, and the two may coexist. Since the treatment of both conditions is the same, modern nomenclature describes the two diseases in one term: *decompression illness* (DCI).

Nitrogen narcosis

Recognition

A sufficiently raised partial pressure of nitrogen in the tissue of the CNS induces signs and symptoms of narcosis, which worsen in proportion to increases in the ambient partial pressure (the 'rapture of the depths') [43,44]. The clinical picture of nitrogen narcosis is similar to that of alcohol intoxication and is characterized by temporary impairment of intellectual and neuromuscular performance, and by changes in personality and behavior. The condition may occur at any depth exceeding 30 m (100 ft). At an extreme depth of 90–100 m (300–335 ft) it may lead to hallucinations, unconsciousness, or, if judgment and procedures are sufficiently impaired, death [43]. Alcohol, fatigue, cold, and increased arterial carbon dioxide tension all increase susceptibility to nitrogen narcosis [43,45]. The chief danger of this condition stems from the impairment of the diver's reactions to the environment, which severely diminishes the ability to function in an emergency. Nitrogen narcosis is therefore a common precipitant of diving accidents and drowning.

Management

Divers recover rapidly from nitrogen narcosis when they ascend to a shallower depth, where the narcotic effects of the gas are reduced [45]. It is easily prevented by avoiding air diving (with compressed air) to a depth of more than 30 to 50 m (100–170 ft).

Prevention

Because of the unique medical problems encountered in scuba diving, the importance of providing medical screening for applicants to diving courses cannot be overemphasized. In principle, diving is absolutely contraindicated in persons subjects to spontaneous pneumothorax, as well as in those with air-trapping pulmonary lesions or active bronchial asthma. The same applies to persons with conditions that impair the level of consciousness (e.g. epilepsy, diabetes mellitus, and drug addiction) or affect the person's ability to equalize pressure in the middle ear and the sinuses.

In view of the growing number of scuba divers and diving accidents, it is possible for any clinician working in general practice or in an emergency department to encounter patients requiring evaluations for fitness to dive or emergency treatment for decompression illness. In the USA, the Divers Alert Network (DAN) at Duke University Medical Center provides a 24-hour information and consultation service; the telephone number is (919) 684–8111. Similar service can be obtained from DAN centers in several other countries (the emergency number for DAN Europe is in Zurich, Switzerland: 383–1111). Basic knowledge, combined with a high index of suspicion, may prevent unnecessary delays in the diagnosis and proper treatment of potentially hazardous and irreversible conditions related to scuba diving.

In order to minimize the possibility of tissue bubble formation, caused by inert gas supersaturation, empirically developed decompression schedules (known as decompression tables) employ staged decompression, with 'stops' as needed to allow inert gas washout. The most widely promulgated decompression tables for air divers have been published by the US Navy [9]; other navies, commercial diving and compressed air work contractors, and recreational scuba agencies have developed tables tailored for different scenarios and breathing gases. Decompression computers using continuous ambient pressure monitors have been developed to monitor decompression in real time. Despite adherence to published decompression procedures, DCS may still occur: the disease cannot be excluded simply because the diver followed an accepted algorithm.

HYPOBARIC ENVIRONMENTS

As elevation above sea level increases, the ambient barometric pressure decreases in a curvilinear fashion. Table 20.2 shows the standard atmosphere in terms of elevation above sea level and barometric pressure [46]. As altitude increases the percentage of oxygen in the atmosphere remains constant at 20.9% but the partial pressure of inspired oxygen declines.

Terrestrial hypobaric exposures consist of breathing ambient air on the ground at some elevation above sea level. A variety of industries such as mining, transportation, logging, and others may require terrestrial hypobaric exposures for some operations or work sites. In addition, a variety of non-industrial occupations that support recreation or travel require terrestrial altitude exposures.

Aerospace hypobaric exposures occur during flight within an aircraft. Although the flight altitude may exceed 40 000 feet (12 000 m) above sea level in a commercial jet airliner, the cabin environment

Table 20.2 The International Standard Atmosphere in air above sea level

Feet	Meters	mmHg	kPa	PSIA	Temp (°C)
0	0	760	100	14.7	15.0
2000	610	706	92.9	13.7	11.0
4000	1219	656	86.3	12.69	7.1
6000	1829	609	80.1	11.78	3.1
8000	2438	565	74.3	10.92	−0.9
10 000	3048	523	68.8	10.11	−4.8
12 000	3658	483	63.6	9.35	−8.8
14 000	4267	447	58.8	8.63	−12.7
16 000	4879	412	54.2	7.97	−16.7
18 000	5486	380	50.0	7.34	−20.7
20 000	6096	349	45.9	6.75	−24.6
25 000	7620	282	37.1	5.45	−35.5
30 000	9144	228	30.0	4.36	−44.4
40 000	12 192	141	18.6	2.72	−56.4

PSIA, pressure in pounds per square inch absolute pressure.

usually remains equivalent to 8000 feet (2438 m) above sea level or less except in unusual situations [47]. In small aircraft, such as most propeller airplanes, the pilot and passengers breathe ambient air at the flight altitude and pressure of the aircraft.

Ascent from sea level or any ground position to a higher altitude constitutes a decompression event, and it carries with it some risk of decompression illness. The risk of altitude-induced barotrauma depends on the rate of decompression and the extent by which any preflight use of oxygen has depleted dissolved body nitrogen. During a mechanized ascent by means of jet engines or rocket power, barotrauma can result because of insufficient time for mass equilibration of nitrogen in body tissues with the outside environment. By contrast, during a slow ascent on foot, as in mountain climbing, mass equilibration occurs incrementally with ample time to dissipate the partial gas pressure of nitrogen in body tissues. Slow ascent usually prevents barotrauma during terrestrial hypobaric exposures, and it protects but does not prevent illness from exposure to hypoxia.

Acute hypoxemia is a constant threat of aerospace hypobaric exposures complicated by too high ascent, loss of internal air compression, or failure of supplemental oxygen. Depending on degree, acute hypoxemia can incapacitate within minutes and cause death. Other illnesses that result from the reduced partial pressure of oxygen in the ambient air at altitude include acute mountain sickness (AMS), high altitude pulmonary edema (HAPE), and high altitude cerebral edema (HACE). The last three manifestations of sustained hypoxia are usually associated with terrestrial hypobaric exposures.

Combinations of exposure scenarios can and do occur. They include deep sea diving followed by air travel, a common recreational theme. This poses a greater than usual risk for decompression sickness, as noted above. Another combination consists of air travel followed by terrestrial altitude exposure, as can occur with recreational mountain climbing, other recreational activities, and military maneuvers.

In the following sections we consider altitude-induced barotrauma causing pneumothorax and DCI. There is then a description of selected altitude illnesses, namely AMS, HACE, and HAPE.

Pneumothorax

As with diving ascents, altitude exposure alone sometimes causes pneumothorax, and it may markedly increase the severity of clinical manifestations if pneumothorax occurs for other reasons. The hypobaric environment causes hypoxia even in normal subjects and pneumothorax can only worsen gas exchange. It may produce a life-threatening situation, especially in aerospace settings. In subjects with preexisting underlying lung disease, the gas exchange derangement can become critically severe. Settings associated with altitude exposure may additionally prevent or delay definitive therapy for pneumothorax, thereby predisposing to a poor outcome.

Recognition

The diagnosis of pneumothorax is reached as in non-occupational settings, though the circumstances may not allow ready access to a stethoscope or radiographic imaging. A common situation is that of a subject at sea level engaging in airline travel with a preexisting pneumothorax. The air in the pleural space cannot equilibrate with the ambient barometric pressure but the remaining normal lung can. Without a chest tube to vent, the pneumothorax enlarges in inverse proportion to the change in barometric pressure. This obeys Boyle's law. A pneumothorax may expand by up to 34.5% of its initial volume in going from sea level to 8000 feet (2438 m) above sea level. This amount of change could tip the scales toward respiratory symptoms or tension physiology in the presence of a sizeable pneumothorax.

Rupture of a bulla results in interstitial pulmonary emphysema. Air then moves to the hilum, causing pneumomediastinum; as the mediastinal pressure rises relative to that in adjacent sites, rupture of the mediastinal parietal pleura occurs, causing pneumothorax [48]. Light and electron microscopy of tissue obtained at surgery have not shown defects in the visceral pleura through which air escapes directly from bullae into the pleural cavity [49].

Table 20.3 Causes of secondary spontaneous pneumothorax. Modified from Sahn and Heffner [50]

Systems	Causes
Airway diseases	Emphysema, chronic obstructive pulmonary disease, cystic fibrosis, status asthmaticus
Pulmonary infections	*Pneumocystis carinii*, anaerobes, Gram-negative bacteria, *Staphylococcus aureus*
Interstitial lung diseases	Sarcoidosis, idiopathic pulmonary fibrosis, eosinophilic granuloma, lymphangioleimyomatosis, tuberous sclerosis
Connective tissue diseases	Rheumatoid arthritis, dermatomyositis, scleroderma, Marfan's syndrome, Ehlers–Danlos syndrome
Neoplasms	Bronchogenic carcinoma, sarcoma
Other	Thoracic endometriosis

Primary spontaneous pneumothorax occurs in persons without clinically known preexisting lung disease whereas secondary spontaneous pneumothorax complicates preexisting lung disease [50]. Though not apparent at the time of diagnosis, primary spontaneous pneumothorax results from subpleural bullae in the vast majority of patients. Bullae do occur in non-smokers [51] often with a tall, thin body habitus [52], as well as smokers with subclinical respiratory bronchiolitis, interstitial disease, or emphysematous changes [53]. Secondary spontaneous pneumothorax occurs in patients with underlying pulmonary diseases (Table 20.3).

Management

The acute management of symptomatic or large pneumothorax calls for the administration of oxygen to promote nitrogen washout from the pleural cavity. Aspiration of the pleural space or insertion of a chest tube should follow depending on the size of the pneumothorax or the development of tension physiology. Following radiographic resolution, patients should delay air travel for 2 to 3 weeks [54]. Alternative options, which may also involve some added risk, include traveling by surface transportation or traveling with a chest tube in place.

The long-term management of pneumothorax, particularly if recurrent, may require a decision regarding occupation and recreation. In a review of 11 studies of primary spontaneous pneumothorax, the average rate of recurrence was 30%, with a range of 16–52% [55]. Radiographic evidence of pulmonary fibrosis, asthenic habitus, smoking, and younger age have been reported to be independent risk factors for recurrence [56].

Prevention

Because flying and diving increase the risk that complications will result from a pneumothorax, patients who intend to continue relevant occupa-

tions or pastimes should be considered for specific preventive treatment after the first episode [48]. Detailed counseling will be necessary because of the residual risk of a contralateral or ipsilateral pneumothorax [48]. Smoking cessation appears to reduce the risk of recurrence [57].

The intervention used for the prevention of recurrence depends on the techniques available. Concerns have been raised by reports of acute lung injury and respiratory failure following sclerotherapy with intrapleural talc [58]. Historic issues with talc also include purity with regard to infectious agents or asbestos fibers. At the present time, many centers prefer an approach that uses thoracoscopy through a single chest port, with patients found to have large apical bullae switched to video-assisted thoracoscopic surgery or a limited thoracotomy [48]. The array of techniques available for resection of bullae and achievement of pleural symphysis continues to evolve. Patients have been reported who have suffered AGE with further diving after pleurodesis. Therefore a history of a spontaneous pneumothorax should preclude diving even after surgical therapy designed to prevent recurrence.

Altitude decompression illness

Altitude DCS is a potential hazard encountered during high altitude flights or during extravehicular activity in space. Although less common than with deep sea diving, rapid ascent to over 18 000 ft (5500 m) can result in high altitude DCS [59,60]. The risk of altitude DCS appears to increase with the severity of hypobaric exposure, the duration of exposure, and exercise at altitude. It is decreased with the duration of pre-exposure oxygen treatment [61,62].

Recognition

Clinical manifestations of DCS at altitude do not differ significantly from those associated with deep sea diving. In aviation, monitoring of Doppler-detectable microbubbles can be done with relative ease in experimental and some operational settings. The Doppler test has greater utility in excluding DCS than confirming its presence [63], and a negative test has high specificity. In theory, the Doppler test could consequently be useful in making therapeutic decisions when confronted with non-specific symptoms at altitude [64]. In practice, symptoms that are consistent with DCS should receive treatment irrespective of the presence or absence of venous bubbles.

Instances of arterial gas embolism from barotrauma at altitude are relatively rare [65]. Investigation of patients with altitude gas embolism often reveals underlying pulmonary pathology as the primary attributable cause [66,67]. Clinical manifestations typically do not differ from diving events.

Management

Treatment of established altitude DCS requires immediate recompression to ground level and administration of 100% oxygen for 2 hours [68]. Most patients will respond with complete resolution of symptoms and require no further treatment. Some patients, especially those with neurologic symptoms or signs, require hyperbaric oxygen therapy as in diving incidents [69]. Patients with systemic gas embolism at altitude should receive hyperbaric oxygen as soon as possible.

Prevention

Prevention of altitude DCS centers on preflight administration of oxygen. This replaces nitrogen in body tissues, being both more soluble than nitrogen and available for tissue metabolism. Decompression tables for diving at altitude require modification; they are more conservative.

Acute mountain sickness

Recognition

AMS constitutes the commonest acute altitude illness, and it occurs in up to 20% of tourists to Colorado ski resorts (elevation 3000 m, 10 000 ft) [70]. The risk increases progressively at higher elevations. The symptoms of AMS, which include headache, fatigue, malaise, nausea, dizziness, anorexia, and sleep disturbance, occur with rapid ascent to 2500 m (8350 ft) or higher [71]. Untreated, AMS may be followed by HAPE and HACE. A thorough history and physical examination can exclude common conditions confused with AMS. The symptoms of AMS usually persist for 1 to 3 days while acclimatization occurs.

Management

Suspension of further ascent may be sufficient if symptoms are mild. Acetazolamide can be given in dosages of 125–250 mg twice a day, and symptomatic treatment should include analgesics, such as paracetamol (acetaminophen) or non-steroidal anti-inflammatory drugs, and antiemetics as needed [72]. A descent of 500 m (1600 ft) or more will usually reverse AMS and should be considered in mild cases refractory to these simple measures. With moderate symptoms of AMS, immediate descent is indicated. When available, acetazolamide and oxygen (1–2 min by nasal cannula) should be considered. Dexamethasone could also be used if evacuation is impossible. A portable hyperbaric chamber can be used if available (Table 20.4).

High-altitude pulmonary edema

Recognition

HAPE is life threatening because of the marked hypoxemia that results jointly from altitude condi-

Table 20.4 High altitude illnesses: prevention and treatment in adults. Modified from Klocke et al. [71]

Illness	Prevention	Treatment
Acute mountain sickness	Altitude limit of 2500 m (8350 ft) the first night; limit ascent to 600 m (2000 ft) per day; high carbohydrate diet; avoid heavy exercise; maintain hydration; avoid alcohol	Oxygen; non-narcotic pain relievers; phenothiazine antiemetics; acetazolamide 125–250 mg twice daily; descend if symptoms are severe
High–altitude pulmonary edema	Same as acute mountain sickness; also nifedipine 20 mg three times a day if known to be susceptible	Immediate descent; oxygen; acetazolamide orally 250 mg every 6 hours; nifedipine orally 10 mg every 4 hours; continuous positive airway pressure mask or Gamow bag
High–altitude cerebral edema	Same as acute mountain sickness; also acetazolamide 125 mg orally twice daily	Immediate descent; oxygen; dexamethasone 10 mg intravenous initially, then 4 mg intramuscular every 6 hours; Gamow bag

tions and impairment of gas exchange. The incidence of HAPE ranges from less than 1 in 10 000 skiers in Colorado (3000 m, 10 000 ft) to 1 in 50 climbers on Mount McKinley (6194 m, 20 650 ft) [73]. Many factors may contribute to HAPE, including individual susceptibility, rate of ascent, maximal altitude, cold ambient temperatures, level of exercise, and use of sleeping medications [69]. People with congenital unilateral absence of the pulmonary artery are highly susceptible to HAPE.

HAPE can occur at any elevation higher than 2500 m (8350 ft) and develops most often on the second night. Early symptoms include increased dyspnea on exertion, fatigue, weakness, and dry cough. Signs include tachycardia, tachypnea, rales, pink-tinged frothy sputum, and cyanosis as the disease progresses. A temperature up to 38.5°C may occur. Hemodynamic measurements and echocardiography reveal increased pulmonary artery pressure and normal left ventricular function [74]. The white blood cell count may increase to 14.0×10^9/l. Arterial blood gas measurements reveal respiratory alkalosis and severe hypoxemia, with a mean oxygen saturation of 56% before descent to a lower altitude. Chest radiographs of patients with HAPE show patchy infiltrates that may be unilateral or bilateral. Autopsy findings include extensive severe pulmonary edema; a protein-rich, permeability-type edema in the alveoli; and associated cerebral edema in more than half of HAPE victims [74].

Management

Immediate descent is indicated for persons with HAPE, even if this requires medical evacuation [71]. Minimizing exertion and avoiding hypothermia may help to slow the progression of symptoms. Oral nifedipine therapy, 10 mg every 4 hours, reduces symptoms [75]. Other measures include administration of oxygen (4–6 l/min) or hyperbaric therapy by means of a portable hyperbaric chamber until improvement is noted (Table 20.4).

High-altitude cerebral edema

Recognition

HACE may occur in 2 to 3% of travellers to altitudes of 5500 m (18 350 ft); however, symptoms may occur with lower frequency at any altitude higher than 2500 m (8350 ft). Clinical manifestations include severe headache, ataxia, severe lassitude, confusion, drowsiness, stupor, and coma (Table 20.4). Other signs and symptoms include vomiting, hallucinations, cranial nerve palsy, hemiparesis, hemiplegia, and seizures [71]. Without treatment death can occur. The skin may have cyanosis because some degree of pulmonary edema usually occurs with HACE, causing hypoxemia. Neurologic symptoms of altitude illness can progress from mild AMS to coma in 12 to 72 hours.

Management

Any evidence of HACE necessitates immediate descent with close supervision [71]. Progression of symptoms during descent creates the potential for fatal accidents. If descent cannot be immediately arranged, administration of oxygen and hyperbaric therapy using a portable chamber (Gamow bag or similar) should be used while waiting. Also, dexamethasone, 10 mg intravenously, followed by 4 mg intramuscularly every 6 hours benefits the patients if initiated early in the course of illness (Table 20.4).

Prevention

Gradual ascent is essential for prevention by avoiding abrupt changes to altitudes higher than 3000 m (10 000 ft). A period of 2 or 3 nights should be spent at 2500–3000 m (8350–10 000 ft) before further ascent. Increases in sleeping altitude greater than 600 m (2000 ft) in a day should be avoided. Moderate activity with day hikes to higher altitudes and a high-carbohydrate diet aid acclimatization. Severe exertion, alcohol, or sedatives predispose to altitude illness [72].

Acetazolamide, a carbonic anhydrase inhibitor, reduces the incidence of AMS when given as a preventive therapy. Bicarbonate diuresis speeds the metabolic compensation for hypoxemia, and allows increased nocturnal ventilation and the maintenance of oxygenation during sleep [76]. Acetazolamide, 125–250 mg twice a day, should be taken 24 hours before ascent and continued for 1 to 3 days, depending on clinical symptoms. Side-effects include paresthesias, polyuria, sulfonamide hypersensitivity, crystalluria, and bone marrow suppression.

The use of dexamethasone is controversial. It is generally not recommended for the prevention of AMS, but it has been used by rescue personnel involved in emergency ascents [72].

DIFFICULT CASE

History

The patient is a 39-year-old dive instructor, who runs a refrigerant/coolant business. He has made more than 3000 scuba dives. His initial complaint, 1 year previously, was waking up with sharp right-sided chest pain 1 week after completing three dives to 65 ft (20 m) with normal ascents. He described the pain as worse with breathing and rated it at 8/10 in intensity. Four days following onset, he sought medical attention. A chest radiograph revealed total right pulmonary collapse and attendant mediastinal shift (Fig. 20.4). Pulse oximetry at that time gave an oxygen saturation of 93%. A chest tube was placed, and at the time of removal 6 days later he was asymptomatic. One week after removal of the chest tube he underwent 10 mm thickness computed tomography (CT) scanning of the chest. A few areas of localized emphysema were seen (Fig. 20.5), but not bullae or blebs. At about this time he jogged for 1 mile, noting right upper chest discomfort (intensity 5/10) and a feeling as if air was trapped under the clavicle. He did not detect crepitus, and the discomfort resolved immediately with rest. Later that day he dived to 8–10 ft (2.5–3 m) to clean the bottom of his boat. He has dived four or five times to a maximum of 15 ft (4.5 m) over the ensuing year without incident.

He has intermittent exposure to freon and its combustion byproducts as a result of his work with coolant systems, and there was exposure to numerous chemicals up to 18 years ago during an earlier 5-year period of employment as a painter. He has a 20–40 pack-year smoking history, discontinued 9 years ago, and currently smokes marijuana daily. He uses alcohol only rarely, and he admits to using cocaine until 19 years ago. There is no history of thoracic trauma, rib or clavicular fracture, or thoracic penetrating wounds. He has normal exercise tolerance; he denies wheezing or cough, and he had never had a pneumothorax before this episode.

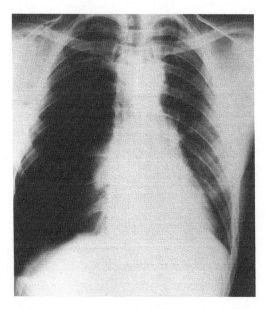

Fig. 20.4 Chest radiograph showing 100% pneumothorax on the right in the diver described in the difficult case.

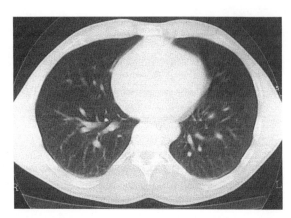

Fig. 20.5 Computed tomography scan showing small areas of focal emphysema in the diver described in the difficult case.

There were no abnormalities on physical examination, apart from a slightly prolonged forced expiratory time (6 s). Spirometry gave the data in Table 20.5.

Issues

The first major issue with this patient is the likely cause of the pneumothorax. In particular, was it related to barotrauma from his diving activities or not? If not, what is the likely cause? The second major issue is whether he should continue diving, and under what circumstances.

Comment

A minority (about 20%) of the book's contributors considered the pneumothorax to be a direct consequence of the last dive, but a clear majority considered it to be spontaneous and unrelated. A less clear majority advised against further diving in any circumstances. Some considered that the individual might reasonably choose to accept a mild increase in risk if pleurectomy was carried out and if there was no further marijuana smoking.

If a pneumothorax occurs during a diving ascent, its volume will increase as the ambient pressure is reduced. Such a situation could prove to be fatal, particularly if the pneumothorax comes under tension. Pneumothorax caused by decompression from a high pressure dry environment, such as a caisson, is less common probably because of the slower reduction in pressure and the absence of immersion-induced airway closure. Similarly, ascent to altitude is an uncommon precipitating cause of pneumothorax because of the smaller reduction in pressure, although the occurrence of spontaneous pneumothorax has been correlated with meteorologic reductions in barometric pressure [77,78].

Although this patient's symptoms did not begin until 1 week after his last dive, it is possible that his pneumothorax was related to diving. The fact that he waited 4 days before seeing a doctor suggests that he could have had a small pneumothorax shortly after the dive but he experienced minimal symptoms. It is impossible to be sure. Because a pneumothorax that occurs underwater could be fatal, and because spontaneous

Table 23.5 Spirometry readings for the diver described in the Difficult Case

Bronchodilator[a]	Forced vital capacity (l)	Forced expired volume in 1 s (l)	Forced expiratory flow at 25–75% of forced vital capacity (l/s)
Before treatment	4.03 (75.6%)	2.46 (56.8%)	1.35 (31.2%)
After treatment	4.34 (81.2%)	2.62 (60.7%)	1.37 (31.6%)

Values corrected to body temperature and ambient pressure saturated with water vapor (BTPS) with the percentage of predicted values in parentheses.
[a]Albuterol 2.5 mg in 2.5 ml 0.9% saline administered by nebulizer.

pneumothorax often recurs even in the absence of an increase in transpulmonary pressure, the recommendation of most doctors specializing in diving problems is that individuals with a history of diving-related pneumothorax that cannot be attributed to a procedural error (e.g. rapid ascent), or a history of spontaneous pneumothorax, should stop diving.

Epidemiological data that pertain to pleurodesis or pleurectomy for pneumothorax in divers do not exist. However, the authors have personal knowledge of two recreational scuba divers who underwent pleurodesis for recurrent pneumothorax, and who subsequently suffered AGE after diving. It appeared that in these individuals, who seemed to have a predisposition to pulmonary barotrauma, removal of the pleural space as an avenue for release of over-pressurized alveolar gas facilitated its entry into a pulmonary blood vessel. On the basis of this anecdotal experience, pleurodesis (or pleurectomy) is not to be recommended as means to allow continued diving after an episode of pneumothorax.

Irrespective of the history of pneumothorax, spirometry in this man's case indicates moderately severe diffuse airways obstruction, which is only partly reversible with bronchodilators. While many physicians consider asthma, even if well controlled, a contraindication to commercial diving, a consensus of experts felt that the risk of barotrauma in asthmatics is only minimally increased provided spirometry is normal [79]. In this case, however, spirometry was not normal, and CT scanning demonstrated that he also had emphysema. In addition to a likely predisposition to pulmonary barotrauma, this degree of reduction in pulmonary mechanical function, although minimally impairing at 1 atmosphere pressure, would be expected to produce a significant ventilatory deficit underwater. Airways resistance increases approximately in proportion to the square root of the gas density (which rises in proportion to absolute pressure). This is compounded by a mild restrictive deficit induced by immersion, largely because of the redistribution of blood from the extremities into the pulmonary circulation, causing a reduced pulmonary compliance. His ability to perform high-speed swimming at depth would therefore be reduced. On this basis alone, he should be disqualified from commercial diving (diving instructor).

SUMMARY POINTS

Recognition

- Barotrauma resulting from diving, high altitude flight, and work in pressurized (pneumatic) caissons may cause:
  - pneumothorax, pneumomediastinum, pneumopericardium, subcutaneous emphysema, systemic AGE (effects of tissue injury to the lung, i.e. 'pulmonary barotrauma')
  - DCS also known as caisson worker's disease or the bends (the effect of tissue injury in any organ resulting from dissolved gas, usually nitrogen, being released in the gaseous state' i.e. 'non-pulmonary barotrauma')
- Respiratory symptoms from barotrauma include dyspnea, chest pain, altered voice (because of air dissection into the larynx), and subcutaneous emphysema of overlying skin.
- Barotrauma symptoms resulting from dysfunction of organs other than the lung may arise through either AGE or DCS, and most commonly comprise periarticular joint pain, numbness, or paresthesias, generally within 24 hours after a dive.
- The CNS is principally affected in severe cases of DCS causing, typically, vertigo or hearing loss, urinary retention, confusion, altered consciousness, convulsions, paraparesis, or hemiparesis as a consequence of ischemia.
- The risk of barotrauma from diving ascents is most pronounced near the surface, where each meter of ascent is associated with the greatest increase in gas volume (a doubling from a depth of 10 m (33 ft) to the surface).
- Climbing, with a slow rate of decompression, may cause AMS, HAPE, and HACE even in the absence of barotrauma, through poorly understood mechanisms related to hypoxia and increased capillary permeability.
- Also unrelated to barotrauma is 'rapture of the depths': narcosis simulating alcohol intoxication that may arise from the raised partial pressure of nitrogen in nervous system tissue after diving to depths exceeding 30 m (100 ft).

Management

- In the absence of a significant pneumothorax or AGE, the effects of pulmonary barotrauma (e.g. pneumomediastinum or subcutaneous emphysema) will resolve spontaneously, although oxygen breathing may hasten resolution.

SUMMARY POINTS (contd.)

- Patients with evidence of pulmonary barotrauma should avoid diving (or a compressed air environment) for several weeks, to allow healing, and be evaluated for possible predisposing factors, such as obstructive lung disease or bullous disease.
- Pneumothorax should be managed conventionally with aspiration or tube drainage, as necessary, and it should preclude further diving even after a pleurodesis or other surgical procedure to reduce recurrence.
- DCS and AGE from diving should be treated initially (in addition to general resuscitative procedures) with supplemental oxygen and fluid administration, followed by transportation to a recompression facility; hyperbaric oxygen administration using a US Navy treatment table, or equivalent, can achieve resolution of symptoms and signs in a high percentage of cases.
- DCS from altitude exposure requires similar immediate treatment to that from diving (the administration of oxygen and recompression) but recompression is usually (but not always) satisfactorily achieved by a prompt return to lower altitude.
- AMS and HAPE should be treated, depending on severity, with oxygen, descent, acetazolamide, and appropriate palliative medications (analgesics,

antiemetics). HAPE patients may also benefit from nifedipine, positive airway pressure mask and portable hyperbaric therapy. HACE patients should be treated with oxygen, immediate descent, dexamethasone and portable hyperbaric therapy if available.

Prevention

- The main causes of pulmonary barotrauma from diving are breath holding or rapid ascent, bullous disease, and bronchial obstruction, and so prevention centers on assiduous training and screening for pulmonary disease.
- The prevention of DCS from diving involves training (so that the problem is quickly recognized), dive planning, the use of standard decompression procedures, and the maintenance of hydration.
- The prevention of DCS from flying also centres on training, and on the administration of preflight oxygen to displace dissolved nitrogen from the tissues.
- The prevention of AMS, HAPE, and HACE from climbing depends on gradual ascent; the avoidance of severe exertion, alcohol, and sedatives; the use of acetazolamide; and a high carbohydrate diet. Nifedipine may prevent HAPE in susception patients.

ACKNOWLEDGEMENTS

We are indebted to Dr Matthew Gilman of Tacoma, Washington, for advice and guidance; to Dr Philip James of the Wolfson Institute of Occupational Health at the University of Dundee, Scotland, for reviewing this article with his invaluable professional and critical expertise; and to Ms Julia Katz and Mr Richard Lincoln for expert assistance in the preparation of the manuscript. This article is dedicated to the memory of Jack C. Dillard and Mary S. Dillard.

REFERENCES

1. Steadman's *Medical Dictionary* 22nd edn, p. 144. Baltimore, MD: Williams & Wilkins, 1972.

2. Barotrauma. In: Edmonds C, Lowry C, Pennefather J eds. *Diving and Subaquatic Medicine*. 2nd edn, pp. 93–127. Mosman, Australia: Diving Medical Centre, 1983.

3. Boettger ML. Scuba diving emergencies: pulmonary overpressure accidents and decompression sickness. *Ann Emerg Med* 1983; 12: 563–567.

4. Dutka AJ. A review of the pathophysiology and potential application of experimental therapies for cerebral ischemia to the treatment of cerebral arterial gas embolism. *Undersea Biomed Res* 1985; 12: 403–421.

5. Greene KM. Causes of sudden death in submarine escape training casualties. In: Hallenbeck JM, Greenbaum LJ Jr eds. *Arterial Air Embolism and Acute Stroke: The Thirteenth Undersea Medical Society Workshop*, pp. 8–16. Bethesda, MD: Undersea Medical Society, 1977.

6. Evans DE, Hardenberg E, Hallenbeck JM. Cardiovascular effects of arterial air embolism. In: Hallenbeck JM, Greenbaum LJ Jr eds. *Arterial Air Embolism and Acute Stroke: The Thirteenth Undersea Medical Society Workshop*, pp. 20–33. Bethesda, MD: Undersea Medical Society, 1977.

7. Moon RE, Sheffield PJ. Guidelines for treatment of decompression illness. *Aviat Space Environ Med* 1997; 68: 234–243.

8. Leitch DR, Greenbaum LJ Jr, Hallenbeck JM. Cerebral arterial air embolism. I. Is there benefit in beginning HBO treatment at 6 bar? *Undersea Biomed Res* 1984; 11: 221–235.

9. Navy Department Naval Sea Systems Command. *US Navy Diving Manual*, Revision 4, Vol. 2: *Air Diving Operations*. NAVSEA 0910-LP-708-8000. Washington, DC: Naval Sea Systems Command, 1999.

10. Neblett LM. Otolaryngology and sport scuba diving: update and guidelines. *Ann Otol Rhinol Laryngol* 1985; 115 (Suppl): 1–12.

11. Farmer JC Jr. Eustachian tube function and otologic barotrauma. *Ann Otol Rhinol Laryngol Suppl* 1985; 120: 45–47.

12. Farmer JC Jr. Otologic and paranasal problems in diving. In: Bennett PB, Elliott DH, eds. *The Physiology and Medicine of Diving*, 3rd edn, pp. 507–536. San Pedro, CA: Best Publishing, 1982.

13. Miller JM, Axelsson A, Potter W. Chronic effects of phasic middle ear pressure changes. *Ann Otol Rhinol Laryngol* 1981; 90: 281–286.

14. Keller AP Jr. A study of the relationship of air pressure to myringopuncture. *Laryngoscope* 1958; 68: 2015–2029.

15. Eidsvik S, Molvaer OI. Facial baroparesis: a report of five cases. *Undersea Biomed Res* 1985; 12: 459–463.

16. Parell GJ, Becker GD. Conservative management of inner ear barotrauma resulting from scuba diving. *Otolaryngol Head Neck Surg* 1985; 93: 393–397.

17. Nakashima T, Itoh M, Watanabe Y *et al.* Auditory and vestibular disorders due to barotrauma. *Ann Otol Rhinol Laryngol* 1988; 97: 146–152.

18. Molvaer OI, Albrektsen G. Alternobaric vertigo in professional divers. *Undersea Biomed Res* 1988; 15: 271–282.

19. Fagan P, McKenzie B, Edmonds C. Sinus barotrauma in divers. *Ann Otol Rhinol Laryngol* 1976; 85: 61–64.

20. Bellini MJ. Blindness in a diver following sinus barotrauma. *J Laryngol Otol* 1987; 101: 386–389.

21. Edmonds C, Thomas RL. Medical aspects of diving – Part 3. *Med J Aust* 1972; 2: 1300–1304.

22. Ministry of Defence. *Royal Navy Diving Manual* (BR 2806) London: Ministry of Defence, 1987.

23. Evans A, Barnard EEP, Walder DN. Detection of gas bubbles in man at decompression. *Aerosp Med* 1972; 43: 1095–1096.

24. Spencer MP, Campbell SD. Development of bubbles in venous and arterial blood during hyperbaric decompression. *Bull Mason Clin* 1968; 22: 26–32.

25. Paulev P. Decompression sickness following repeated breath-hold dives. *J Appl Physiol* 1965; 20: 1028–1031.

26. Kizer KW. Women and diving. *Physician Sportsmed* 1981; 9: 84–92.

27. Hills BA. *Decompression Sickness. Vol. 1. The Biophysical Basis of Prevention and Treatment.* Chichester: John Wiley, 1977.

28. Elliott DH, Moon RE. Manifestations of the decompression disorders. In: Bennett PB, Elliot DH eds. *The Physiology and Medicine of Diving*, pp. 481–505. Philadelphia, PA: Saunders, 1993.

29. Melamed Y, Ohry A. The treatment and neurological aspects of diving accidents in Israel. *Paraplegia* 1980; 18: 127–132.

30. Butler BD, Hills BA. Transpulmonary passage of venous air emboli. *J Appl Physiol* 1985; 59: 543–547.

31. Moon RE, Camporesi EM, Kisslo JA. Patent foramen ovale and decompression sickness in divers. *Lancet* 1989; i: 513–514.

32. Hills BA, James PB. Microbubble damage to the blood–brain barrier: relevance to decompression sickness. *Undersea Biomed Res* 1991; 18: 111–116.

33. Palmer AC, Calder IM, Hughes JT. Spinal cord degeneration in divers. *Lancet* 1987; ii: 1365–1366.

34. Van Rensselaer H. The pathology of the caisson disease. *Med Rec* 1891; 40: 141–182.

35. Farmer JC, Thomas WG, Youngblood DG, Bennett PB. Inner ear decompression sickness. *Laryngoscope* 1976; 86: 1315–1327.

36. Shupak A, Doweck I, Greenberg E *et al.* Diving-related inner ear injuries. *Laryngoscope* 1991; 101: 173–179.

37. Landolt JP, Money KE, Topliff EDL *et al.* Pathophysiology of inner ear dysfunction in the squirrel monkey in rapid decompression. *J Appl Physical* 1980; 49: 1070–1082.

38. Melamed Y. Clinical aspects of spinal cord decompression sickness. In: Francis TJR, Smith DJ, eds. *Describing Decompression Illness: Proceedings of the 42nd Workshop of the Undersea and Hyperbaric Medical Society*, pp. 23–26. Bethesda, MD: Undersea and Hyperbaric Medical Society (UHMS publication no. 79(DECO) 5/15/91), 1991.

39. Melamed Y, Sherman D, Wiler-Ravell D, Kerem D. The transportable recompression rescue chamber as an alternative to delayed treatment in serious diving accidents. *Aviat Space Environ Med* 1981; 52: 480–484.

40. Halpern P, Greenstein A, Melamed Y *et al.* Spinal decompression sickness with delayed onset, delayed treatment, and full recovery. *Br Med J* 1982; 284: 1014.

41. Mitchell SJ, Pellett O, Gorman DF. Cerebral protection by lidocaine during cardiac operations. *Ann Thorac Surg* 1999; 67: 1117–1124.

42. Drewry A, Gorman DF. Lidocaine as an adjunct to hyperbaric therapy in decompression illness: a case report. *Undersea Biomed Res* 1992; 19: 187–190.

43. Bennett PB. Inert gas nacrcosis. In: Bennett PB, Elliott DH eds. *The physiology and medicine of diving.* 3rd edn, pp. 239–261. San Pedro, CA: Best Publishing, 1982.

44. Bennett PB, Simon S, Katz Y. High pressures of inert gas and anesthesia mechanism. In: Fink R ed. *Molecular Mechanisms of Anesthesia*, pp. 367–403. New York: Raven Press, 1975.

45. Bennett PB. The physiology of nitrogen narcosis and the high pressure nervous syndrome. In: Strauss RH ed. *Diving Medicine*, pp. 157–181. New York: Grune & Stratton, 1976.

46. Sharp GR. Chapter 1. The Earth's Atmosphere In: Dhenin G, ed. *Aviation Medicine: Physiology and Human Factors*, pp. 8–11. London: Tri-Med Books, 1978. 8–11.

47. Dillard TA, Berg BW, Rajagopal KR *et al.* Hypoxemia during air travel in patients with chronic obstructive pulmonary disease. *Ann Intern Med* 1989; 111: 362–367.

48. Macklin MT, Macklin CC. Malignant interstitial emphysema of the lungs and mediastinum as an important occult complication in many respiratory diseases and other conditions: an interpretation of the clinical literature in the light of laboratory experiment. *Medicine (Baltimore)* 1944; 23: 281–358.

49. Ohata M, Suzuki H. Pathogenesis of spontaneous pneumothorax: with special reference to the ultrastructure of emphysematous bullae. *Chest* 1980; 77: 771–776.

50. Sahn SA, Heffner JE. Primary care spontaneous pneumothorax the *N Engl J Med* 2000; 342: 868–874.

51. Bense L, Lewander R, Eklund G *et al.* Nonsmoking, non-alpha I-antitrypsin deficiency-induced emphysema in nonsmokers with healed spontaneous pneumothorax, identified by computed tomography of the lungs. *Chest* 1993; 103: 433–438.

52. Fujino S, Inoue S, Tezuka N *et al.* Physical development of surgically treated patients with primary spontaneous pneumothorax. *Chest* 1999; 116: 899–902.

53. Cottin V, Streichenberger N, Gamondes JP *et al.* Respiratory bronchiolitis in smokers with spontaneous pneumothorax. *Eur Resp J* 1998; 12: 702–704.

54. Cheatham ML, Safcsak K. Air travel following traumatic pneumothorax: when is it safe? *Am Surgeon* 1999; 65: 1160–1164.

55. Schramel FM, Postmus PE, Vanderschueren RG. Current aspects of spontaneous pneumothorax. *Eur Respir J* 1997; 10: 1372–1379.

56. Lippert HL, Lund O, Blegvad S, Larsen HV. Independent risk factors for cumulative recurrence rate after first spontaneous pneumothorax. *Eur Respir J* 1991; 4: 324–331.

57. Sadikot RT, Greene T, Meadows K, Arnold AG. Recurrence of primary spontaneous pneumothorax. *Thorax* 1997; 52: 805–809.

58. Campos JR, Werebe EC, Vargas FS et al. Respiratory failure due to insufflated talc. *Lancet* 1997; 349: 251–252.

59. Leach RM, Rees PJ, Wilmshurst P. ABC of oxygen: Hyperbaric oxygen therapy. *Br Med J* 1998; 317: 1140–1143.

60. Webb JT, Pilmanis AA, O'Connor RB. An abrupt zero-preoxygenation altitude threshold for decompression sickness symptoms. *Aviat Space Environ Med* 1998; 69: 335–340.

61. Kannan N, Raychaudhuri A, Pilmanis AA. A loglogistic model for altitude decompression sickness. *Aviat Space Environ Med* 1998; 69: 965–970.

62. Pilmanis AA, Olson RM, Fischer MD, et al. Exercise-induced altitude decompression sickness. *Aviat Space Environ Med* 1999; 70: 22–29.

63. Conkin J, Powell MR, Foster PP, Waligora JM. Information about venous gas emboli improves 1998 prediction of hypobaric decompression sickness. *Aviat Space Environ Med* 1998; 69: 8–16.

64. Kumar VK, Billica RD, Waligora JM. Utility of Doppler-detectable microbubbles in the diagnosis and treatment of decompression sickness. *Aviat Space Environ Med* 1997; 68: 151–158.

65. Rios-Tejada F, Azofra-Garcia J, Valle-Garrido J, Pujante Escudero A. Neurological manifestation of arterial gas embolism following standard altitude chamber flight: a case report. *Aviat Space Environ Med* 1997; 68: 1025–1028.

66. Cable GG, Keeble T, Wilson G. Pulmonary cyst and cerebral arterial gas embolism in a hypobaric chamber: a case report. *Aviat Space Environ Med* 2000; 71: 172–176.

67. Zaugg M, Kaplan V, Widmer U et al. Fatal air embolism in an airplane passenger with a giant intrapulmonary bronchogenic cyst. *Am J Resp Crit Care Med* 1998; 157: 1686–1689.

68. Krause KM, Pilmanis AA. The effectiveness of ground level oxygen treatment for altitude decompression sickness in human research subjects. *Aviat Space Environ Med* 2000; 71: 115–118.

69. Dart TS, Butler W. Towards new paradigms for the treatment of hypobaric decompression sickness. *Aviat Space Environ Med* 1998; 69: 403–409.

70. Honigman B, Theis MK, Koziol-McLain J et al. Acute mountain sickness in a general tourist population at moderate altitudes [published erratum appears in *Ann Intern Med* 1994; 120: 698]. *Ann Intern Med* 1993; 118: 587–592.

71. Klocke DL, Decker WW, Stepanek J Altitude-Related Illnesses. *Mayo Clin Proc* 1998; 73: 988–993.

72. Grissom CK, Roach RC, Sarnquist FH, Hackett PH. Acetazolamide in the treatment of acute mountain sickness: clinical efficacy and effect on gas exchange. *Ann Intern Med* 1992; 116: 461–465.

73. Hackett PH. The Denali Medical Research Project, 1982–1985. *Am Alpine J* 1986; 28: 129.

74. Schoene RB. Pulmonary edema at high altitude: review, pathophysiology, and update. *Clin Chest Med* 1985; 6: 491–507.

75. Bartsch P, Maggiorini M Ritter M et al. Prevention of high-altitude pulmonary edema by nifedipine. *N Engl J Med* 1991; 325: 1284–1289.

76. Arias-Stella J, Kryger H. Pathology of high altitude pulmonary edema. *Arch Pathol* 1963; 76: 147–157.

77. Bense L. Spontaneous pneumothorax related to falls in atmospheric pressure. *Eur J Respir Dis* 1984; 65: 544–546.

78. Scott GC, Berger R, McKean HE. The role of atmospheric pressure variation in the development of spontaneous pneumothoraces. [Published erratum appears in *Am Rev Respir Dis* 1989; 140: 862. *Am Rev Respir Dis* 1989; 139: 659–662.

79. Elliott DH (ed.) Are asthmatics fit to dive? Kensington, MD: Undersea and Hyperbaric Medical Society, 1996.

BENIGN PLEURAL DISEASE

Robin Rudd

INTRODUCTION

Pleural disease of occupational origin is almost exclusively a result of asbestos exposure, although other naturally occurring silicates are occasionally responsible, and there is a possible link between pleural plaques and ceramic fibers. Pleural thickening may accompany silicosis but the intrapulmonary changes dominate the picture. Rarely, pleural disease is a consequence of occupational injury or the occupational contraction of tuberculosis. Asbestos causes both benign and malignant pleural disease. The benign disorders are considered in this chapter; the malignant disease of mesothelioma is dealt with in Chapter 22.

Asbestos exposure causes several different types of benign pleural disease:

- plaque
- pleurisy without effusion
- pleurisy with effusion
- diffuse thickening
- entrapped 'folded (or enfolded) lung'.

Folded lung is also known as rounded atelectasis or Blesovsky's syndrome after the surgeon who first described it; it is closely associated with overlying diffuse pleural thickening. Although most cases of benign pleural disease are recognized from plain chest radiographs, there is greater diagnostic sensitivity from computed tomographic (CT) scans, and a few cases are identified initially at thoracotomy or autopsy. The frequency of each type of disease increases with increasing cumulative dose of asbestos inhaled. All types of asbestos may cause each type of disease, but there are some differences between fiber types in their propensity to cause different types of pleural disease. For example, in the anthophyllite exposed population of Northern Karelia in Finland, plaques are very common but pleurisy, diffuse pleural thickening, and mesothelioma are uncommon. By contrast, in areas of Turkey where there is exposure to erionite, pleurisy and diffuse thickening are relatively more common and the incidence of mesothelioma is extremely high [1].

PLEURAL PLAQUES

Background

Plaques are circumscribed areas of thickening of the parietal pleura of the chest wall and diaphragm. Occasionally they affect the visceral pleura, including that in the fissures.

Causes and epidemiology

Pleural plaques occur in members of the general population without identified exposure to asbestos, but they occur more frequently in subjects with known exposure [2] and are by far the most common respiratory effect of asbestos inhalation. Autopsy studies show a higher prevalence of plaques than do radiographic surveys, primarily because direct observation is diagnostically more sensitive than plain radiographs, but partly because a population studied at autopsy is generally older and more likely to have sustained occupational exposure than one undergoing chest radiography in life. For example, in a Swedish study, plaques were found in 6.8% of autopsies of which only 12.5% were detected by radiography [3]. In a UK study of a general urban population, plaques were reported from 4.2% of routine autopsies but this figure rose to 11.2% when a specific search for plaques was made in a subsequent series [4]. Plaques may occur after occupational exposure at a lower level than is required to cause asbestosis and are found in household contacts of asbestos workers and in persons exposed to environmental contamination with asbestos [2].

In certain areas, such as parts of Finland, Turkey, and Greece, plaques occur with much increased frequency. This has been attributed to the presence of asbestos in the soil and outcropping rocks [2]. In general, however, plaques are more common in urban than in rural dwellers [5]. Among an urban population, the frequency and extent of plaques at autopsy increases in relation to lung asbestos fiber content [6]. Similarly, among occupationally exposed persons, the prevalence of plaques increases in relation to the degree of asbestos exposure and in relation to the time elapsed since first exposure [7].

Pleural plaques are seldom apparent on plain chest radiographs less than 20 years after first exposure to asbestos; calcified plaques are rarely seen in this period. In a group of 624 asbestos workers from various industries, plaques were seen in none within 10 years, in 10% by 19 years, in 29% by 29 years, in 32% by 39 years and in 58% by 49 years [8]. In a study of 1117 insulation workers, pleural calcification was found in none of 346 men less than 10 years after first exposure, in only 1.1% of 379 men less than 20 years, in 10.4% up to 30 years, in 34.5% up to 40 years, and in 57.9% more than 40 years after first exposure. The extent of calcification also increased with time [9]. This pattern is probably largely a consequence of long latency and slow progression, though a contributory factor may be that the subjects with the longest periods since first exposure will tend to be the older subjects who were exposed historically to higher doses. There is conflicting evidence concerning the role of smoking. In a study of workers in an asbestos manufacturing plant, the prevalence of plaques was greater in smokers [10] but this relationship was not apparent among insulation workers [11].

Pleural plaques also occur in kaolin workers and talc workers, but in the latter the plaques are proba-

bly caused by contamination of commercial talc by asbestos since asbestos fibers can be identified in bronchoalveolar lavage samples from affected subjects [12,13]. There is some evidence that pleural plaques may be also caused by exposure to refractory ceramic fibers, which are amorphous silicates belonging to the man-made vitreous fibers group. They are used in industrial processes requiring high-temperature insulation. A retrospective cohort and nested case-control study of 652 workers involved in the manufacture of these fibers identified 19 (3.1%) with plaques, and one with diffuse pleural thickening [14]. Plaques were more common more than 20 years after first exposure and increased in frequency in relation to the cumulative level of exposure. This provides biologic plausibility of a causal relationship. A nested case-control study showed that asbestos exposure did not account for the observed association between ceramic fiber exposure and plaques.

Prognosis

Plaques may become more extensive and they may become more dense through increasing calcification, although they may be present for many years without calcifying. In a few patients, plaques may become confluent over large areas and lead to a restrictive ventilatory defect.

Pleural plaques are not thought to lead directly to any of the other benign varieties of asbestos-induced pleural disease, nor to pose any risk of malignant change leading to mesothelioma. Their presence may indicate, nevertheless, a cumulative level of asbestos exposure at which there is an increased risk of mesothelioma or other asbestos-related disorders. On average, in the absence of any other evidence about exposure, it is reasonable to assume that subjects with plaques will have had higher exposure to asbestos than subjects without plaques. The frequency of development of other complications of asbestos exposure in persons with plaques is not a function of the presence of the plaques but of the asbestos exposure that caused the plaques. Since plaques may occur after a wide range of different exposures, the risks of other asbestos-related conditions may differ widely between different populations and individuals with plaques.

Persons with plaques may develop other benign asbestos-induced conditions. A survey of 175 naval dockyard workers found that of 143 men who initially had plaques, 33 (23%) had diffuse pleural thickening at follow-up 10 years later or before death if this occurred within 10 years [15]. Among 155 living men with benign pleural lesions, mostly plaques, who were reexamined 10 years later, 16 (10.3%) had small opacities of category 1/1 pneumoconiosis or higher on the scale of the International Labor Office (ILO), representing radiologic evidence suggestive of asbestosis. In addition, 4.5% also had bilateral inspiratory basal crackles and impairment of the gas transfer factor below 75% of predicted, representing clinical evidence of asbestosis [15]. Comparable data were not provided for men who had no pleural abnormalities at the initial survey.

The presence of pleural plaques has been shown to be a risk factor for the development of malignancy. In a Swedish study of 1596 men with plaques followed for 16 369 person-years, there were nine mesotheliomas compared with 0.8 expected [16]. A necropsy-based Italian study found a higher frequency of plaques in subjects with mesothelioma than in other subjects and the odds ratio for mesothelioma increased with the size of the plaques, suggesting that larger plaques were associated with higher doses of asbestos [17].

The Swedish follow-up study of 1596 men found 50 bronchial carcinomas compared with 32.1 expected after correcting for smoking habits, indicating a 1.4-fold risk factor [16]. However, there have been conflicting reports as to whether or not patients with plaques are at increased risk of lung cancer. One review suggested that those studies that have supported an increased risk of lung cancer in subjects with plaques were the most subject to selection bias [18]. Each of the studies reviewed was unsatisfactory in one or more ways: they concerned populations with unknown or low level asbestos exposure, control for the effect of smoking was unsatisfactory, latency was ignored, follow-up was incomplete, and statistical power to detect small increases in risk was not estimated. The extent to which persons with plaques are at risk of cancer will depend upon the exposure experienced rather than the presence of the plaques and, therefore, the risk will vary between different populations with plaques. Unrealistically large population studies would be needed to demonstrate small increases in risk (e.g. of the order of 1.1) resulting from relatively low levels of environmental asbestos exposure, whereas studies of heavily exposed persons with plaques have demonstrated significantly increased risks factors of up to two- to threefold [19,20].

Recognition

Clinical features

Plaques are usually an incidental finding on a chest radiograph. They are not usually responsible for any symptoms, although rarely patients may be aware of an uncomfortable grating sensation associated with calcified plaques and ventilatory movement. Breathlessness is usually caused by a coexisting condition. Clinical examination reveals no abnormalities.

Investigation

Chest radiology

The diagnosis is usually obvious from the chest radiograph, which shows discrete areas of pleural thickening that may contain calcification. The plaques have well-circumscribed edges, which distinguish them from diffuse pleural thickening [21]. Calcification is not a reliable distinguishing feature as this may occur in areas of diffuse pleural thickening as well as in plaques, perhaps because the diffuse pleural thickening has developed in visceral pleura that has then fused with adjacent calcified parietal plaque. Plaques often follow the line of the ribs and may be elongated. Diaphragmatic plaques, by contrast, are more often symmetrical. The plaques usually have an irregular outline, and descriptive terms that have been applied include 'candle wax' and 'holly leaf' appearances.

If plaques are not apparent on a posteroanterior (PA) or lateral view and are being specifically sought, right and left 45 degree anterior oblique films increase diagnostic sensitivity since they occasionally reveal plaques that are not evident (or are partially obscured) on the conventional views, or which appear only as ill-defined hazy densities that are hard to discern and evaluate (Fig. 21.1) [22]. However, the incremental detection rate is low. In one study, 2.5% of 326 workers with normal PA films and 13% of 46 subjects with parenchymal but not pleural shadows on PA films had pleural abnormalities detectable only on oblique films [20]. Plaques are usually bilateral but unilateral plaques are not uncommon, particularly when few in number, constituting 19.3% of definite and 33.9% of probable plaques in one particular study [24]. Among subjects with unilateral plaques there is an unexplained left-sided predominance [24,25].

A high-resolution CT scan has slightly greater sensitivity for the detection of plaques than plain radiography and also assists in distinguishing between diffuse pleural thickening and multiple plaques. The latter on a plain chest radiograph may appear to overlap and hence mimic diffuse pleural thickening [26]. The plaques are then said to be confluent. However, CT is less useful than a plain chest radiograph in demonstrating diaphragmatic plaques since image and thin plaque are in the same plane [22].

Lung function

Surveys of groups of workers with plaques have shown that they are associated with small mean decrements in ventilatory capacity and total lung capacity (TLC) [27–30]. Elastic recoil pressure is increased and lung compliance is reduced in comparison with controls [31]. These alterations in lung function are probably a result of associated early

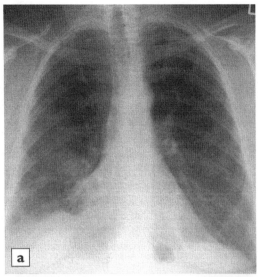

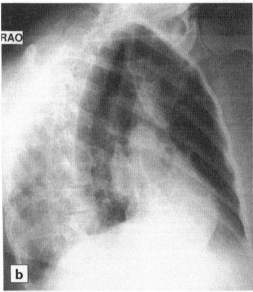

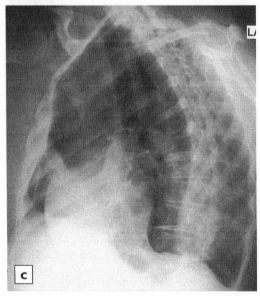

Fig. 21.1 Posteroanterior (a) and oblique (b,c) chest radiographs showing pleural plaques.

pathology in the underlying lung rather than the presence of the plaques themselves. Plaques are also associated with evidence of small airways dysfunction, which may be caused by an accompanying peribronchial reaction to asbestos fibers [32].

For an individual with plaques, lung function test results are usually within the normal range and breathlessness is usually absent; if it is present it is usually owing to coexisting respiratory or cardiac disease. Exceptionally extensive plaques that are fused (confluent) over a large area may be associated with sufficient restrictive impairment of ventilatory function to cause breathlessness, particularly if there is coexisting respiratory impairment from other causes, which produces an interactive adverse effect.

Further investigation is rarely required but occasionally the configuration of a plaque is atypical, leading to the suspicion of a malignant process. A pleural biopsy is then appropriate, either by means of a percutaneous cutting needle if the pleura is thick enough for this to be feasible, or by an open or thoracoscopic surgical procedure.

Pathology

Plaques may be situated within the parietal pleural overlying the chest wall, diaphragm, mediastinum, and pericardium. They rarely occur in the visceral pleura or in the peritoneum. They are smooth or coarsely nodular. Histology shows relatively acellular, avascular, hyalinized, collagenous bundles apparently arranged parallel to the surface in a 'basket weave' pattern, and a surface covering of mesothelial cells (Fig. 21.2). In nodular plaques the collagen bundles have a whorled arrangement [2]. Calcification may be evident.

There may be asbestosis of adjacent lung tissue but the frequency will depend upon the degree of exposure experienced. In a series of 56 cases selected on the basis that pleural plaques were identified at autopsy, there had been clinical evidence of asbestosis in 16 (29%). Histologic evidence of asbestosis was found in a further 8 (14%) [4]. Asbestos bodies are not found in plaques although they are commonly present in lung tissue. Subjects found to have plaques at autopsy have higher numbers of asbestos bodies in lung tissue than those without plaques, as might be expected since plaques are more likely to identify subjects with excessive exposure, and there is an excess of long amphibole fibers of commercial origin, but not of chrysotile [33]. Small numbers of asbestos fibers can be found by electron microscopy in plaques, but chrysotile is the predominant fiber type even if amphiboles predominate in lung tissue [34]. The reason for this is not known and many uncertainties remain concerning the pathogenesis of plaques [35]. The route by which asbestos fibers reach the parietal

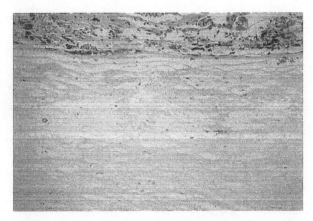

Fig. 21.2 Histologic appearances of pleural plaque.

pleura has not been fully elucidated. Alternative suggestions are via retrograde flow in the lymphatic system and direct penetration from the lung across the pleura. The distribution of asbestos fibers in the parietal pleura itself is heterogeneous. It has been recognized that anthracotic pigment, found in high concentrations in coal miners, accumulates preferentially in 'black spots' located near lymphatic vessels on the parietal pleura. Thoracoscopic biopsies of such areas, identified visually, contained higher concentrations of amphibole fibers than other areas of the parietal pleura, and in these areas chrysotile fibers were few or absent [36]. There was concordance between the amphibole content of the black spots and that of the lung tissue. The authors postulated that the black spots correspond to normal lymphatic stomata known as 'milky spots' and that amphibole fibers that have migrated directly through the visceral pleura are reabsorbed into the parietal pleura through the 'black spots'. The accumulation of amphiboles in such areas may explain the susceptibility of the parietal pleura to plaque formation and mesothelioma.

Management of the individual

The patient with plaques should be reassured that the condition itself is of no serious consequence and that the plaques are not likely to progress to cause symptoms in the future.

PLEURISY AND PLEURAL EFFUSION

Background

Asbestos may cause acute pleurisy, which is commonly but not invariably associated with an effusion. Pleural effusion is consequently the hallmark of asbestos-induced pleurisy. Although first described in

1962 [37], the condition did not become a widely recognized consequence of asbestos exposure until much later [38]. A causal relation was supported by a case-control study in which asbestos exposure was identified more frequently in persons with 'idiopathic' pleural effusion than in controls [39].

Epidemiology

Pleural effusion as a consequence of asbestos may develop earlier after first exposure than pleural plaque or asbestosis. It is the most common asbestos-related condition to occur during the immediately following 20 years, although in an exposed population effusions have been noted to appear up to 40 years after first exposure [8]. In a series of 20 insulation workers, the effusion occurred a mean of 26 years after first exposure, but in four it occurred within 10 years [40]. In a further series of 60 patients, the first effusion occurred a mean of 30 years after first exposure, with a range of 1 to 58 years [41]. The risk of benign effusion increases with the dose of asbestos [8].

Prognosis

The effusion commonly resolves to leave behind diffuse pleural thickening, which characteristically involves the costophrenic angle [40]. In some patients, however, there is complete reabsorption without sequelae. The effusion may recur on the same side, or more commonly on the contralateral side, after an interval of months or years (Fig. 21.3) [40,41]. In one series after a mean follow-up of 9.7 years, recurrent effusions occurred in 28.6% [8]. Ipsilateral recurrence is less common, probably because the pleural layers are frequently left fused together by diffuse pleural thickening. The risks of other asbestos-related conditions are related to the underlying level of exposure, the development of pleurisy with or without effusion providing clinical evidence of such exposure.

Recognition

Clinical features

The patient usually presents with pleuritic chest pain, though on occasions there are no symptoms and the condition is recognized only if there is a chance chest radiograph. There may also be breathlessness, depending on the quantity of associated pleural fluid. Mild fever and systemic disturbance are common, but not invariable, giving rise to the suspicion of infection. This is the initial diagnosis in many patients with asbestos pleurisy. Failure to identify any infective organism and lack of response to antibiotics point to the correct diagnosis. However, malignancy cannot be excluded without further investigation.

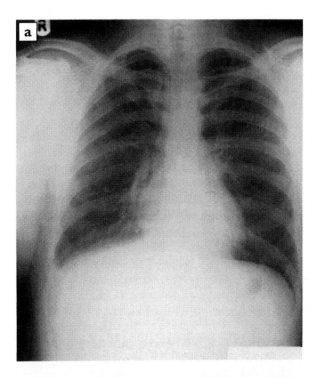

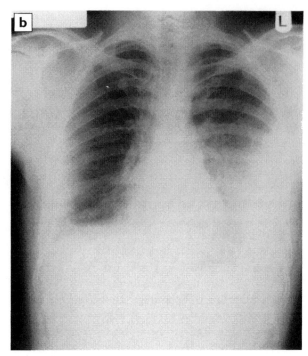

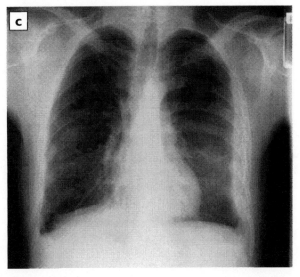

Fig. 21.3 Sequence of chest radiographs from an insulation worker showing asbestos-induced pleural effusions resolving to leave bilateral diffuse pleural thickening. The first shows a small right pleural effusion blunting the costophrenic angle. The second, 10 months later, shows a larger right pleural effusion and an even larger left pleural effusion. The third, after a further 7 months, shows bilateral diffuse pleural thickening.

Investigation

The chest radiograph and CT scan commonly show only a pleural effusion, but there may be coexisting pleural plaques. The effusion should be aspirated. The fluid is an inflammatory exudate, which may show neutrophils, mononuclear cells, and eosinophils [42]. Asbestos bodies are not seen. The effusion is commonly serosanguinous and may be frankly bloody. In the presence of fever, the alternative possibility of empyema or tuberculosis should be considered, and pleural fluid cultures are needed. The erythrocyte sedimentation rate (ESR) is usually elevated [43].

Pleural biopsies should be obtained in addition to fluid aspiration in order to exclude the possibility

of malignancy. Negative results from blind biopsies, such as are obtained by Abrams needle, and cytologic examination of aspirated fluid do not provide adequate reassurance that malignancy is not present since the diagnostic sensitivity of these procedures is low [44,45]. Video-assisted thoracoscopic pleural biopsy gives the most satisfactory outcome, and if this proves negative for malignancy a diagnosis of benign asbestos pleurisy can generally be accepted [45].

Differential diagnosis

The presence of blood in the pleural fluid gives rise to the suspicion of malignancy, which is appropriate, since mesothelioma and metastatic carcinoma figure prominently among the differential diagnoses. Nevertheless, benign asbestos-induced effusions are commonly blood stained, and this sometimes leads to the suspicion of pulmonary embolism. When the effusion is not blood stained, a parapneumonic effusion becomes the most probable alternative diagnosis. Parapneumonic effusions without empyema, and effusions consequent upon pulmonary embolism, usually resolve without leaving pleural thickening [42].

Empyema should be confirmed by pleural fluid culture, and a tuberculous effusion by culture or the typical histologic findings on biopsy of granulomatous inflammation. If the effusion is eosinophilic, parasitic infection should be considered if geographically appropriate, but the eosinophils may simply indicate chronicity. Drug-induced effusions (e.g. from amiodarone) should also be considered, and current medication should always be clarified. This may provide a valuable clue to the existence of an undisclosed, but relevant, additional disease.

Rheumatoid pleural disease, comprising effusions and visceral pleural thickening, shows a striking male predominance and occurs usually in patients with moderate to severe joint disease. Occasionally, pleural disease appears before joint disease. Biopsy of the pleural lesions occasionally shows the characteristic features of rheumatoid nodules, and rheumatoid factor is commonly present in both serum and pleural fluid. The latter characteristically has a low glucose content, a low pH, and may show diagnostic 'rheumatoid cells' (scavenger mononuclear cells with ingested immune complexes involving rheumatoid factor) [42]. Pleuritis associated with systemic lupus may present with small effusions, which may be blood stained. Other pulmonary and systemic manifestations of lupus are commonly present, lupus erythematus cells are often present in pleural fluid, and immunologic tests give the diagnosis [42].

Pathology

The pleura shows the non-specific features of an organising effusion, including reactive mesothelial cells, proliferating fibroblasts and capillaries, and, often, chronic inflammatory cells. Distinction from desmoplastic mesothelioma may be difficult but in the latter condition invasion of chest wall or lung, bland necrosis, or sarcomatoid areas can usually be identified [46]. Granulomas are not present and asbestos bodies and fibers are seldom found [38].

Management of the individual

It is important to complete diagnostic procedures before draining all the fluid from the chest. If this is done too early, it may make later thoracoscopy difficult

or impossible. Any residual fluid can be drained at the time of thoracoscopy. The effusion commonly does not recur and so it is not necessary to attempt pleurodesis routinely. In fact, pleurodesis is better avoided until a histologic diagnosis is available because if mesothelioma of epithelioid variety at an early stage is confirmed, which is potentially suitable for extrapleural pneumonectomy, a pleurodesis may make subsequent surgery more difficult. Pleurodesis may become appropriate, however, if the effusion recurs and is large enough to cause breathlessness and require drainage.

If the effusion is repeatedly recurrent over short periods and accompanied by systemic markers of inflammation such as raised ESR, it is reasonable to attempt corticosteroid therapy. Anecdotally such treatment may be useful although there are no randomized trials demonstrating efficacy.

DIFFUSE PLEURAL THICKENING

Background

The term diffuse pleural thickening relates to thickening that does not have well-circumscribed margins [21]. It principally involves the visceral pleura (and so is sometimes called visceral pleural thickening) though this is often adherent to the parietal pleura. It is believed to represent the outcome when the resolution of benign pleural effusion involves fibroblast infiltration and a fibrotic healing response. Hence the width is variable depending on how much fibrous tissue is laid down, and the process effectively glues parietal to visceral pleura, as occurs with the resolution of other inflammatory effusions.

Epidemiology

A study of asbestos cement workers found that the incidence of diffuse pleural thickening increased with dose of asbestos sustained, although the relationship was less strong than for parenchymal fibrosis [47]. Another study of asbestos cement workers found that the prevalence of pleural thickening increased with duration of exposure but not estimated cumulative dose [48]. A study of amosite workers found the prevalence increased with intensity of exposure and time since first exposure [49].

As with plaques, there has been conflicting evidence as to whether smoking affects the development of diffuse pleural thickening. A study of naval dockyard workers reported an increased prevalence of pleural lesions, including diffuse pleural thickening, in smokers [50], as did a study of sheet metal workers [51]; however a study of plumbers and pipefitters found no relation between smoking status and pleural thickening [52].

Prognosis

A study of asbestos cement workers found that 23% of subjects with diffuse pleural thickening showed radiologic progression over a 10-year period. The risk of progression was related to cumulative dust exposure [48]. An Australian study of Wittenoom crocidolite miners reported that the rate of radiologic progression of pleural thickening was greater in those with earlier onset of disease after first exposure to asbestos. The rate of progression decreased with time and there was no evidence of progression more than 15 years after first detection of pleural thickening [53]. A longitudinal study found no evidence that smoking affected progression [54]. Longitudinal lung function data over a mean period of 9 years in 36 subjects showed a significant decrement in forced expired volume in 1s (FEV_1) and forced vital capacity (FVC) in excess of that predicted from ageing alone [55]. Rarely diffuse pleural thickening may progress to the point of causing ventilatory failure and death [56].

The patient's risks of mesothelioma and other asbestos-related diseases are related to past asbestos exposure but are not additionally influenced directly by the presence or absence of diffuse pleural thickening [57]. As with the other manifestations of asbestos-induced benign pleural disease, however, the presence of diffuse pleural thickening provides crude surrogate evidence of such exposure.

Recognition

Clinical features

Diffuse pleural thickening of limited extent may be an asymptomatic incidental finding on a chest radiograph. More extensive disease commonly gives rise to symptoms. There is often a history of chest pain, which may have been pleuritic in nature. In a study of 64 affected patients, more than half reported chest pain of plausible relevance at some time [55]. A past history of diagnosed pleurisy is common, and the patient may be aware of an earlier pleural effusion for which no definite cause was identified. In a minority of cases there is persistent chest pain, which is commonly but not always of a pleuritic nature, and which may be quite disabling [58]. Breathlessness on exertion is the other principal symptom. Some patients, particularly in the early stages of the disorder when there is an active inflammatory process, have systemic symptoms such as mild fever, sweats, and malaise.

On physical examination chest expansion may be diminished, symmetrically if the condition is bilateral, but on one side only if it is predominantly uni-

lateral. On auscultation there may be fine mid to late inspiratory and fine early to mid expiratory crackles [59]. Their timing suggests that they are caused by friction between the pleural layers, which is maximal in mid-inspiration and mid-expiration. Clubbing is not a feature.

Rarely the clinical features of pericardial constriction may occur because of accompanying asbestos-induced pericardial thickening, which may occur in association with pleural disease [60]. An association between retroperitoneal fibrosis and asbestos exposure has been reported [61] and this may give rise to hydronephrosis.

Investigation

Chest radiology

A PA chest radiograph usually demonstrates the extent of the disease but, as with plaques, this is occasionally demonstrated much better by oblique views. Commonly, strands of fibrosis appear to extend across the lung fields from the thickened pleura and this has been described as a 'crow's foot' appearance (Fig. 21.4) [62].

High-resolution CT scanning is more sensitive and accurate for the detection of pleural disease. This results in greater interobserver agreement as to the extent and type of pleural disease than is possible by plain chest radiography [26]. The CT scan well demonstrates 'crow's feet' and its constituent parenchymal bands extending from thickened pleura, appearances that indicate involvement of the visceral pleura rather than parietal plaque [63].

The CT scan may also disclose the nature of rounded (rolled) atelectasis, otherwise known as folded (or enfolded) lung or Blesovsky's syndrome [64]. This has a characteristic appearance of vessels and bronchi radiating towards the hilum from a solid looking shadow contiguous with the pleura (Fig. 21.5). On the plain chest radiograph such lesions often suggest tumor, but if the characteristic features are present from CT scanning a confident diagnosis can be made and an unnecessary biopsy avoided.

In most cases, diffuse pleural thickening in asbestos-exposed workers involves the lower zones and middle zones, but in one series a minority showed pleural thickening that affected the apices – either predominantly or exclusively. Upper zone disease was observed in 40 of 1600 (2.5%) patients in one series [65]. Such appearances, sometimes associated with upper lobe parenchymal fibrosis, can be difficult to distinguish from those of tuberculosis [65,66] or other fibrosing diseases (for example that associated with ankylosing spondylitis and the HLA B27 genotype), and it is not universally accepted that such upper zone involvement is a consequence of asbestos exposure.

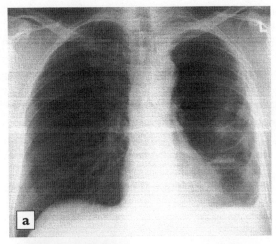

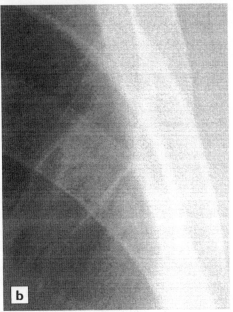

Fig. 21.4 Chest radiograph showing diffuse thickening (a) with 'crow's foot' (b).

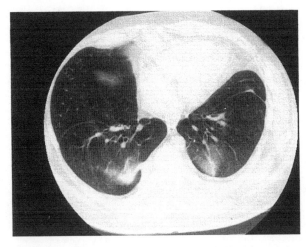

Fig. 21.5 High-resolution CT scan showing folded lung (rounded atelectasis).

Lung function

Diffuse pleural thickening reduces pulmonary compliance [67] and causes a restrictive ventilatory defect with reduction in total lung capacity [51,68,69]. The radiographic extent of pleural disease, as assessed by chest radiographs or CT scan, correlates with reduction in FEV_1, FVC, residual volume (RV), and TLC [26,69,70]. The FEV_1/FVC ratio is either normal or increased, unless there is coexisting airflow obstruction, which may obscure the characteristic pattern. Restrictive pleural disease is also associated with reduction in gas transfer factor (diffusing capacity) [26,71] but the gas transfer coefficient (diffusion constant) is normal or increased, reflecting the relative lack of impairment of parenchymal function and the reduction in alveolar volume. This pattern of impairment is sometimes described as 'constrictive', distinguishing it from the restrictive pattern associated with intrapulmonary fibrosis. Impairment of lung function is particularly associated with radiologic evidence of obliteration of the costophrenic angles [72]. This may be because obliteration of the costophrenic angles implies that the parietal pleura over the lower chest wall is stuck to the parietal pleura over the periphery of the diaphragm, thereby interfering with the diaphragm's descent and preventing the lung from expanding into this potential space on full inspiration. This does not happen with plaques and is possibly an important mechanism by which diffuse pleural thickening usually impairs ventilatory function but plaques usually do not [73].

The presence of rounded atelectasis is not independently associated with loss of lung function in excess of that resulting from the associated diffuse pleural thickening [71]. Respiratory muscle function is not adversely affected by asbestos-related pleural disease [74].

It is important to appreciate that if both asbestosis of lung tissue and diffuse pleural thickening are present, the gas transfer factor may be reduced but the gas transfer coefficient may be normal or even increased, reflecting a greater effect of pleural thickening on lung volume than of parenchymal disease on gas transfer. In this situation a normal or increased gas transfer coefficient does not imply that parenchymal function is normal or that asbestosis is not contributing to impairment of lung function [75].

Occasionally diffuse pleural thickening is accompanied by pericardial thickening and consequently restricted cardiac motion/function. This possibility should be considered in patients where breathlessness appears disproportionate to the observed impairment of lung function and can best be investigated by magnetic resonance imaging [76].

Pathology

The macroscopic findings indicate diffuse visceral pleural thickening, which may be very extensive and suggestive of mesothelioma. Pericardial thickening with pathologic features similar to those in the pleura may also occur [77]. The pericardial thickening occurs in association with pleural thickening but does not just reflect involvement of adjacent pleura. Rounded atelectasis on radiography corresponds to extensive wrinkling and folding of the visceral pleura with deep invaginations into pulmonary tissue, which is compressed and in some cases shows interstitial fibrosis [78]. It has been suggested that rounded atelectasis occurs either when diffuse fibrotic changes in the pleura contract, forcing part of the adjacent lung to become atelectatic, or when a pleural effusion causes a segment of lung to become atelectatic, causing its components to become adherent to each other and remain so after the effusion has been reabsorbed [78,79].

The histologic findings are of paucicellular collagen deposition. A basket weave appearance as seen in plaques has been described [80] but other authors do not report this [81]. Lung tissue immediately beneath the thickened pleura usually shows interstitial fibrosis up to 1 cm in depth [80]. This differs from the appearances in classical asbestosis, where changes are more diffuse rather than being confined to areas beneath pleural thickening [81], and it is a matter of controversy as to whether the fibrosis occurring only beneath diffuse pleural thickening should be taken as histologic evidence of asbestosis. There may be reactive mesothelial hyperplasia, which may be difficult to distinguish from mesothelioma. Immunohistochemical stains may be helpful: epithelial membrane antigen (EMA) is generally positive in mesothelioma but negative in benign mesothelial hyperplasia. Amphibole counts are usually raised in lung tissue whereas relatively few fibers, mainly chrysotile, are found in the pleural tissue [77]. The range of amphibole counts is broadly comparable to the ranges found in patients with pleural plaque, mesothelioma, and mild asbestosis [77].

Differential diagnosis

Patients with diffuse pleural thickening may have a raised ESR and a few have weakly positive antinuclear factor and rheumatoid factor in serum, consistent with the presence of systemic disturbance [82]. In the presence of such features, consideration should be given to the possibility of connective tissue disorders such as rheumatoid disease, systemic lupus erythematosus, and ankylosing spondylitis as the cause of the pleural disease.

The differential diagnosis should also include drug-induced pleural disease, and appropriate inquiries should be made concerning relevant agents, for example ergot drugs (known as ergolines; methysergide, bromocriptine, nicergoline, pergolide and dopergine), practolol, amiodarone, and nitrofurantoin. Useful distinguishing features of drug-induced pleural thickening are said to be more rapid development, absence of associated pleural calcification, and, most importantly, rapid diminution of chest discomfort and fall in ESR on drug withdrawal. Radiologic regression is, however, slower and incomplete [83].

Rounded atelectasis is usually caused by asbestos-induced diffuse pleural thickening, but it may occur with diffuse pleural thickening of other causes including chest traumal [79]. Cryptogenic fibrosing pleuritis is a label applied to bilateral diffuse pleural thickening in the absence of any identifiable extrinsic cause [84]. Like asbestos-induced disease, it may evolve by way of pleural effusions.

Management of the individual

Surgical resection of thickened visceral pleura (decortication) has been attempted in patients with folded lung but this more often leads to a further decline in lung function than to an improvement [85]. Parietal pleurectomy has been performed in an attempt to alleviate persistent pain, with occasional benefit in patients whose pain was of a pleuritic rather than neuropathic type [86]. Surgery should be considered as a last resort for relief of either severe ventilatory restriction, and ensuing breathlessness of disabling degree, or intractable pain. If there is clinical evidence of progressive pleural disease, often accompanied by systemic markers of inflammation such as raised ESR, it is reasonable to attempt to suppress this with corticosteroid therapy. Anecdotally, such treatment may be useful, although there are no randomized trials demonstrating efficacy.

GENERAL MANAGEMENT

Of the individual

As indicated above, the patient with plaques should be reassured that the condition itself is of no serious consequence and that the plaques are not likely to progress to cause symptoms in the future. The patient with asbestos pleurisy, effusion, or diffuse pleural thickening should be given realistic information about the chances of future progression.

Patients with any type of asbestos-induced pleural disease should be advised that its presence indicates that a clinically significant quantity of asbestos has been inhaled and that there are, therefore, risks of other asbestos-related diseases in future. Patients who are smokers should be firmly advised to quit the habit, with explicit explanation of the synergistic interaction between tobacco and asbestos in causing lung cancer.

The patient should also be advised of the possibility of claiming compensation if eligible under local jurisdiction. In the UK, Industrial Injuries Disablement Benefit is not payable in respect of plaques or effusion but it is payable in respect of diffuse pleural thickening that meets the following criteria as to minimum extent: at least half the length of one chest wall (or this length cumulatively from both chest walls) with a maximum thickness of at least 5 mm. In the UK, a patient with any type of asbestos-related pleural disease can pursue a claim at common (i.e. civil) law for damages, either on a final award basis, which takes account of all possible eventualities, or a provisional basis, which provides a lower award of damages but allows a return to court in the event of serious deterioration in the future. This may involve the progression of existing pleural disease or the development of a new condition (i.e. asbestosis, mesothelioma, or asbestos-related lung cancer).

Of the workforce

The discovery of an asbestos-related condition in a member of a workforce may create anxieties in other workers, particularly those who have worked in conditions similar to those encountered by the affected individual. Appropriate reassurance should be offered, but if there are individuals with a history of significant exposure during a period sufficiently distant to put them at risk of present disease, a screening program of exposed workers often helps to allay anxiety. There is increasing interest in the possibility that early detection of lung cancer by screening of high-risk subjects with helical CT may reduce mortality; asbestos-exposed smokers are an ideal group for study. The prospect of reducing mortality from mesothelioma by similar means appears more remote.

PREVENTION

Current legal requirements in the UK concerning exposure to airborne asbestos dust should, if properly enforced, prevent new cases of pleural disease. In some other parts of the world, protection remains inadequate. In the UK, control limits for exposure are as shown in Table 21.1. The full effects of current regulations are not likely to be seen for several decades in view of the long latencies involved.

Table 21.1 Control limits specified by the Control of Asbestos at Work Regulations (1987) in the UK

	Fibres per ml of air averaged over	
	4 h	10 min
Chrysotile	0.5	1.5
Crocidolite	0.2	0.6
Amosite	0.2	0.6

DIFFICULT CASE

History

A man born in the early 1930s worked as an electrician from leaving school for nearly 40 years. In the course of his work he sometimes used asbestos rings for electrical insulation. He did not cut them himself but simply put them in place. From time to time he also worked in the vicinity of other tradesmen who stripped asbestos lagging from pipes prior to repair work and who used asbestos materials to restore the lagging afterwards. In earlier years, he wore a simple dust mask, but in later years he was provided with a rubber mask with a filter. He smoked 10–15 cigarettes daily and was not known to have ever received medication for migraine.

In the course of a routine medical evaluation in the late 1980s, a chest radiograph showed slight diffuse pleural thickening in the left mid-zone, and further films 3 and 5 years later demonstrated mild progression. Thereafter the appearances were stable until a clinical evaluation in mid-1990s.

There was then a reduced FEV_1: FVC ratio, a reduction in TLC, a mild reduction in gas transfer factor, and an increased gas transfer coefficient; the picture overall suggested a mixed obstructive and restrictive impairment of ventilatory function of moderate degree.

About a year later, he developed abdominal pain and malaise, and was investigated. The ESR was 80. An ultrasound study of the abdomen showed left hydronephrosis, and a CT scan demonstrated a mass partially obstructing the left ureter. The appearances suggested retroperitoneal fibrosis. He was treated with corticosteroids and a left ureteric stent was inserted. The hydronephrosis resolved and his symptoms improved. The pleural disease persisted unchanged.

Issues

The chief issues of interest are whether the presumed retroperitoneal fibrosis and the unilateral diffuse pleural thickening shared the same cause or had different causes, whether the occupational exposure to asbestos was relevant to either, and whether any additional investigation would be useful.

Comment

A clear majority of the book's contributors thought the pleural fibrosis was an effect of asbestos exposure but that the peritoneal fibrosis was not. A small minority considered that a common cause was likely, whether or not this was asbestos, and a modest minority favored additional investigation. CT of the chest was suggested to evaluate the pleural shadowing, and an abdominal biopsy was suggested to confirm the diagnosis of retroperitoneal fibrosis and exclude the possibility of peritoneal mesothelioma.

DIFFICULT CASE

History

A 48-year-old man underwent a statutory medical examination for the purpose of assessing fitness for work as an asbestos removal operative. These examinations are required at 2-yearly intervals in the UK under the Control of Asbestos at Work Regulations 1987. The assessment includes a history of occupational exposures and respiratory symptoms, clinical examination of the chest, chest radiograph, and spirometry. The examining physician must be approved by the Health and Safety Executive as suitably experienced but need not be a specialist respiratory physician. He/she is not required by statute to give the employer specific advice as to fitness for work but may give advice to the subject according to his/her own judgement. In practice, employers' liability insurance requires that employers do obtain such advice, whether from the physician carrying out the statutory examination (with the examinee's consent) or from another physician.

The subject was asymptomatic and no abnormalities were revealed except that the chest radiograph showed a few small calcified pleural plaques on the chest walls and diaphragms. The occupational history revealed that after leaving school at the age of 16 he had worked for 2 years in the insulation trade using asbestos materials in various forms. He had been heavily exposed to asbestos without any respiratory protection. After that he had worked in a variety of other jobs, none of which had involved exposure to asbestos. He had been entirely well and had not had any chest radiographs prior to the current film obtained in the course of the statutory examination soon after he had been offered employment in the insulation trade. In this job, he would have been using asbestos-free materials but from time to time he might have been required to assist in asbestos removal work under strictly controlled conditions using all recommended precau-

tions to ensure that his exposure did not exceed currently permitted limits. The examining physician considered that as he had an asbestos-related disease he was not fit for asbestos removal work. This was communicated to the subject who informed his prospective employer of the advice. The job offer was consequently withdrawn with serious adverse economic consequences for the subject.

Issues

The issues are whether further exposure to asbestos within the limits permitted by current regulation is likely to make any difference to this man's existing pleural plaques or to his risks for the future development of other more serious asbestos-related disorders, and whether he should be regarded as unfit for asbestos removal work.

Comment

A small minority of the book's contributors considered that additional exposure, at what is likely to be a very low level (barring accidents), would materially increase the risk for asbestos-related malignancy, but a clear majority thought such exposure would have no meaningful effect. The latter view implies that there is no valid medical reason why he should not undertake asbestos removal work using all currently recommended precautions. However, this man had already sustained a heavy level of exposure, albeit briefly, some years earlier and so is at some risk of developing other asbestos-related disorders anyway. A new employer might reasonably be wary of offering employment in such circumstances because, in the unfortunate event that a further asbestos-related disorder does emerge, additional exposure during the period of employment (however trivial) might lead to the charge that it played a contributory role.

SUMMARY POINTS

Recognition

- Plain chest radiographs provide the means by which most cases of benign asbestos-induced pleural disease are recognized, oblique views enhancing the sensitivity of detection.
- CT scans have much greater sensitivity and diagnostic precision, and provide the best means of resolving doubt as to whether:
  - pleural shadowing is a consequence of plaque, diffuse pleural thickening, or both
  - pleural effusion is isolated or associated with probable mesothelioma
  - a pleural-based opacity is caused by folded lung or tumor.
- When circumscribed pleural shadows show calcification, they are almost pathognomonic of plaques caused by asbestos exposure.
- Blunting of the costophrenic angle favors a diagnosis of diffuse pleural thickening over one of plaque.
- Once parapneumonic effusion/empyema, tuberculosis, malignancy, and rheumatoid disease are excluded in a patient with an exudative pleural effusion, asbestos becomes the most likely cause if there has been regular occupational exposure – particularly if pleurisy has been recurrent.
- Bilateral diffuse pleural thickening is commonly a consequence of recurrent asbestos-induced pleurisy and seldom the result of other causes apart from bilateral parenchymal tuberculosis.
- Unilateral diffuse pleural thickening is more commonly a consequence of other causes but is nevertheless a common consequence of asbestos exposure.
- Folded lung is usually a consequence of asbestos exposure.

- Asbestos is the only common cause of a benign blood-stained pleural effusion apart from pulmonary embolism.
- A thoracoscopic pleural biopsy should be obtained to exclude mesothelioma or other malignancy before a diagnosis of benign pleurisy is accepted as the explanation for a blood-stained pleural effusion in an asbestos-exposed patient.

Management

- Inform the patient of the nature of the disease, including its cause, effects, and prognosis.
- Inform the patient of the possibility and methods of seeking compensation for occupational disease.
- Drug therapy is usually not indicated, but occasionally corticosteroid therapy may be employed for the treatment of active pleural inflammation.
- Routine follow-up is not currently of proven value but may provide psychologic support in selected individuals.
- Surveillance programs may prove to be of value in the future if emerging methods of early detection of lung cancer and mesothelioma lead to a reduction in mortality.

Prevention

- End use of asbestos.
- Identify asbestos already in place in buildings and elsewhere, assess its condition, and seal or remove where necessary.
- Ensure building maintenance personnel are aware of the presence and location of asbestos so they do not disturb it inadvertently.
- Enforce strict regulations to prevent dissemination and inhalation of dust during disturbance or removal of asbestos.

REFERENCES

1. Hillerdal G. Pleural changes and exposure to fibrous minerals. *Scand J Work Environ Health* 1984; 10: 473–479.
2. Craighead JE, Abraham JL, Churg A *et al.* The pathology of asbestos-associated diseases of the lungs and pleural cavities: diagnostic criteria and proposed grading schema. Report of the Pneumoconiosis Committee of the College of American Pathologists and the National Institute for Occupational Safety and Health. *Arch Pathol Lab Med* 1982; 106: 544–596.
3. Hillerdal G, Lindgren A. Pleural plaques: correlation of autopsy findings to radiographic findings and occupational history. *Eur J Respir Dis* 1980; 61: 315–319.
4. Hourihane DO'B, Lessof L and Richardson PC. Hyaline and calcified pleural plaques as an index of exposure to asbestos. A study of radiological and pathological features of 100 cases with a consideration of epidemiology. *Br Med J* 1966; 1: 1069–1074.
5. Zitting AJ, Karjalainen A, Impivaara O *et al.* Radiographic small lung opacities and pleural abnormalities in relation to smoking, urbanization status, and occupational asbestos exposure in Finland. *J Occup Environ Med* 1996; 38: 602–609.
6. Karjalainen A, Karhunen PJ, Lalu K *et al.* Pleural plaques and exposure to mineral fibres in a male urban necropsy population. *Occup Environ Med* 1994; 51: 456–460.
7. Harries PG, Mackenzie FA, Sheers G *et al.* Radiological survey of men exposed to asbestos in naval dockyards. *Br J Ind Med* 1972; 29: 274–279.
8. Epler GR, McLoud TC, Gaensler EA. Prevalence and incidence of benign asbestos pleural effusion in a working population. *JAMA* 1982; 247: 617–622.
9. Selikoff IJ. The occurrence of pleural calcification among asbestos insulation workers. *Ann NY Acad Sci* 1965; 132: 351–367.
10. Weiss W, Levin R, Goodman L. Pleural plaques and cigarette smoking in asbestos workers. *J Occup Med* 1981; 23: 427–430.

11. Lilis R, Selikoff IJ, Lerman Y et al. Asbestosis: interstitial pulmonary fibrosis and pleural fibrosis in a cohort of asbestos insulation workers: influence of cigarette smoking. Am J Ind Med 1986; 10: 459–470.

12. Chaudhary BA, Kanes GJ, Pool WH. Pleural thickening in mild kaolinosis. South Med J 1997; 90: 1106–1109.

13. Scancarello G, Romeo R, Sartorelli E. Respiratory disease as a result of talc inhalation. J Occup Environ Med 1996; 38: 610–614.

14. Lockey J, Lemasters G, Rice C et al. Refractory ceramic fiber exposure and pleural plaques. Am J Respir Crit Care Med 1996; 154: 1405–1410.

15. McMillan GHG, Rossiter CE. Development of radiological and clinical evidence of parenchymal fibrosis in men with non-malignant asbestos-related pleural lesions. Br J Ind Med 1982; 39: 54–59.

16. Hillerdal G. Pleural plaques and risk for bronchial carcinoma and mesothelioma. A prospective study. Chest 1994; 105: 144–150.

17. Bianchi C, Brollo A, Ramani L, Zuch C. Pleural plaques as risk indicators for malignant pleural mesothelioma: a necropsy-based study. Am J Ind Med 1997; 32: 445–449.

18. Weiss W. Asbestos-related pleural plaques and lung cancer. Chest 1993; 103: 1854–1859.

19. Nurminen M, Tossavainen A. Is there an association between pleural plaques and lung cancer without asbestosis? Scand J Work Environ Health 1994; 20: 62–64.

20. Hillerdal G, Henderson DW. Asbestos, asbestosis, pleural plaques and lung cancer. Scand J Work Environ Health 1997; 23: 93–103.

21. International Labour Office. Guidelines for the use of ILO International Classification of Radiographs of Pneumoconioses, revised edn. Occupational Health and Safety Series No 22 (Rev). General ILO, 1980.

22. Begin R, Boctor M, Bergeron D et al. Radiographic assessment of pleuropulmonary disease in asbestos workers: posteroanterior, four view films, and computed tomograms of the thorax. Br J Ind Med 1984; 41: 373–383.

23. Sherman CB, Barnhart S, Rosenstock L. Use of oblique chest roentgenograms in detecting pleural disease in asbestos-exposed workers. J Occup Med 1988; 30: 681–683.

24. Withers BF, Ducatman AM, Yang WN. Roentgenographic evidence for predominant left-sided location of unilateral pleural plaques. Chest 1989; 95: 1262–1264.

25. Hu H, Beckett L, Kelsey K, Christiani D. The left-sided predominance of asbestos-related pleural disease. Am Rev Respir Dis 1993; 148: 981–984.

26. Al Jarad N, Poulakis N, Pearson MC et al. Assessment of asbestos-induced pleural disease by computed tomography – correlation with chest radiograph and lung function. Respir Med 1991; 85: 203–208.

27. Jarvholm B, Sanden A. Pleural plaques and respiratory function. Am J Ind Med 1986; 10: 419–426.

28. Hjortsberg U, Orbaek P, Aborelius M Jr et al. Railroad workers with pleural plaques: I. Spirometric and nitrogen washout investigation on smoking and nonsmoking asbestos-exposed workers. Am J Ind Med 1988; 14: 635–641.

29. Bourbeau J, Ernst P, Chrome J et al. The relationship between respiratory impairment and asbestos-related pleural abnormality in an active work force. Am Rev Respir Dis 1990; 142: 837–842.

30. Oliver LC, Eisen EA, Greene R, Sprince NL. Asbestos-related pleural plaques and lung function. Am J Ind Med 1988; 14: 649–656.

31. Fridriksson HV, Hedenstrom H, Hillerdal G, Malmberg P. Increased lung stiffness of persons with pleural plaques. Eur J Respir Dis 1981; 62: 412–424.

32. Hjortsberg U, Orbaek P, Aborelius M Jr et al. Railroad workers with pleural plaques: II. Small airway dysfunction among asbestos-exposed workers. Am J Ind Med 1988; 14: 643–647.

33. Churg A. Asbestos fibers and pleural plaques in a general autopsy population. Am J Pathol 1982; 109: 88–96.

34. Dodson RF, Williams MG Jr, Corn CJ et al. Asbestos content of lung tissue, lymph nodes, and pleural plaques from former shipyard workers. Am Rev Respir Dis 1990; 142: 843–847.

35. Churg A. The pathogenesis of pleural plaques. Indoor Built Environ 1997; 6: 73–78.

36. Boutin C, Dumortier P, Rey F et al. Black spots concentrate oncogenic asbestos fibers in the parietal pleura. Thoracoscopic and mineralogic study. Am J Respir Crit Care Med 1996; 153: 444–449.

37. Eisenstadt HB. Pleural asbestosis. Am Pract 1962; 13: 573–578.

38. Gaensler EA, Kaplan AI. Asbestos pleural effusion. Ann Intern Med 1971; 74: 178–191.

39. Martensson G, Hagberg S, Pettersson K, Thiringer G. Asbestos pleural effusion: a clinical entity. Thorax 1987; 42: 646–651.

40. Lilis R, Lerman Y, Selikoff IJ. Symptomatic benign pleural effusions among asbestos insulation workers: residual radiographic abnormalities. Br J Ind Med 1988; 45: 443–449.

41. Hillerdal G, Ozesmi M. Benign asbestos pleural effusion: 73 exudates in 60 patients. Eur J Respir Dis 1987; 71: 113–121.

42. Sahn SA. The pleura. Am Rev Respir Dis 1988; 138: 184–234.

43. Renshaw AA, Dean BR, Antman KH et al. The role of cytologic evaluation of pleural fluid in the diagnosis of malignant mesothelioma. Chest 1997; 111: 106–109.

44. Whitaker D, Shilkin KB. Diagnosis of pleural malignant mesothelioma in life – a practical approach. J Pathol 1984; 143: 147–175.

45. Boutin C, Rey F. Thoracoscopy in pleural malignant mesothelioma: a prospective study of 188 consecutive patients. Part 1: Diagnosis. Cancer 1993; 72: 389–393.

46. Mangano WE, Cagle PT, Churg A et al. The diagnosis of desmoplastic malignant mesothelioma and its distinction from fibrous pleurisy: a histologic and immunohistochemical analysis of 31 cases including p53 immunostaining. Am J Clin Pathol 1998; 110: 191–199.

47. Finkelstein MM, Vingilis JJ. Radiographic abnormalities among asbestos-cement workers. An exposure–response study. Am Rev Respir Dis 1984; 129: 17–22.

48. Jones RN, Diem JE, Hughes JM et al. Progression of asbestos effects: a prospective longitudinal study of chest radiographs and lung function. Br J Ind Med 1989; 46: 97–105.

49. Shepherd JR, Hillerdal G, McLarty J. Progression of pleural and parenchymal disease on chest radiographs of workers exposed to amosite asbestos. Occup Environ Med 1997; 54: 410–415.

50. McMillan GH, Pethybridge RJ, Sheers G. Effect of smoking on attack rates of pulmonary and pleural lesions related to exposure to asbestos dust. Br J Ind Med 1980; 37: 268–272.

51. Schwartz DA, Fuortes LJ, Galvin JR et al. Asbestos-induced pleural fibrosis and impaired lung function. Am Rev Respir Dis 1990; 141: 321–326.

52. Rosenstock L, Barnhart S, Heyer NJ *et al*. The relation among pulmonary function, chest roentgenographic abnormalities, and smoking status in an asbestos-exposed cohort. *Am Rev Respir Dis* 1988; 138: 272–277.

53. de Klerk NH, Cookson WOC, Musk AW *et al*. Natural history of pleural thickening after exposure to crocidolite. *Br J Ind Med* 1989; 46: 461–467.

54. Yano E, Tanaka K, Funaki M *et al*. Effect of smoking on pleural thickening in asbestos workers. *Br J Ind Med* 1993; 50: 898–901.

55. Yates DH, Browne K, Stidolph PN, Neville E. Asbestos-related bilateral diffuse pleural thickening: natural history of radiographic and lung function abnormalities. *Am J Respir Crit Care Med* 1996; 153: 301–306.

56. Miller A, Teirstein AS, Selikoff IJ. Ventilatory failure due to asbestos pleurisy. *Am J Med* 1983; 75: 911–919.

57. de Klerk NH, Musk AW, Cookson WO *et al*. Radiographic abnormalities and mortality in subjects with exposure to crocidolite. *Br J Ind Med* 1993; 50: 902–906.

58. Miller A. Chronic pleuritic pain in four patients with asbestos induced pleural fibrosis. *Br J Ind Med* 1990; 47: 147–153.

59. Al Jarad N, Davies SW, Logan-Sinclair R, Rudd RM. Lung crackle characteristics in patients with asbestosis, asbestos-related pleural disease and left ventricular failure using a time-expanded waveform analysis – a comparative study. *Respir Med* 1994; 88: 37–46.

60. Davies D, Andrews MI, Jones JS. Asbestos induced pericardial effusion and constrictive pericarditis. *Thorax* 1991; 46: 429–432.

61. Sauni R, Oksa P, Jarvenpaa R *et al*. Asbestos exposure: a potential cause of retroperitoneal fibrosis. *Am J Ind Med* 1998; 33: 418–421.

62. Mackenzie FA, Harries PG. Changing attitudes to the diagnosis of asbestos disease. *J R Nav Med Serv* 1970; 56: 116–123.

63. Gevenois PA, de Maertelaer V, Madani A *et al*. Asbestosis, pleural plaques and diffuse pleural thickening: three distinct benign responses to asbestos exposure. *Eur Respir J* 1998; 11: 1021–1027.

64. Blesovsky A. The folded lung. *Br J Dis Chest* 1966; 60: 19–22.

65. Hillerdal G. Pleural and parenchymal fibrosis mainly affecting the upper lung lobes in persons exposed to asbestos. *Respir Med* 1990; 84: 129–134.

66. Oliver RM, Neville E. Progressive apical pleural fibrosis: a 'constrictive' ventilatory defect. *Br J Dis Chest* 1988; 82: 439–443.

67. Valkila EH, Nieminen MM, Moilanen AK *et al*. Asbestos-induced visceral pleural fibrosis reduces pulmonary compliance. *Am J Ind Med* 1995; 28: 363–372.

68. Schwartz DA, Galvin JR, Dayton CS *et al*. Determinants of restrictive lung function in asbestos-induced pleural fibrosis. *J Appl Physiol* 1990; 68: 1932–1937.

69. Schwartz DA, Galvin JR, Yagla SJ *et al*. Restrictive lung function and asbestos-induced pleural fibrosis: a quantitative approach. *J Clin Invest* 1993; 91: 2685–2692.

70. Al Jarad N, Wilkinson P, Pearson MC, Rudd RM. A new high resolution computed tomography scoring system for pulmonary fibrosis, pleural disease, and emphysema in patients with asbestos related disease. *Br J Ind Med* 1992; 49: 73–84.

71. Kee ST, Gamsu G, Blanc P. Causes of pulmonary impairment in asbestos-exposed individuals with diffuse pleural thickening. *Am J Respir Crit Care Med* 1996; 154: 789–793.

72. Lilis R, Miller A, Godbold J *et al*. Pulmonary function and pleural fibrosis: quantitative relationships with an integrative index of pleural abnormalities. *Am J Ind Med* 1991; 20: 145–161.

73. Singh B, Eastwood PR, Finucane KE *et al*. Effect of asbestos-related pleural fibrosis on excursion of the lower chest wall and diaphragm. *Am J Respir Crit Care Med* 1999; 160: 1507–1515.

74. Al Jarad N, Carroll MP, Laroche C *et al*. Respiratory muscle function in patients with asbestos-related pleural disease. *Respir Med* 1994; 88: 115–120.

75. Cookson WO, Musk AW, Glancy JJ. Pleural thickening and gas transfer in asbestosis. *Thorax* 1983; 38: 657–661.

76. Al Jarad N, Underwood SR, Rudd RM. Asbestos-related pericardial thickening detected by magnetic resonance imaging. *Respir Med* 1993; 87: 309–312.

77. Gibbs AR, Stephens M, Griffiths DM *et al*. Fibre distribution in the lungs and pleura of subjects with asbestos related diffuse pleural fibrosis. *Br J Ind Med* 1991; 48: 762–770.

78. Menzies R, Fraser R. Round atelectasis. Pathologic and pathogenetic features. *Am J Surg Pathol* 1987; 11: 674–681.

79. Hillerdal G. Rounded atelectasis. Clinical experience with 74 patients. *Chest* 1989; 95: 836–841.

80. Stephens M, Gibbs AR, Pooley FD, Wagner JC. Asbestos induced diffuse pleural fibrosis: pathology and mineralogy. *Thorax* 1987; 42: 583–588.

81. Churg A, Green FHY. *Pathology of Occupational Lung Disease*, p. 309. Lippincott, Williams & Wilkins, 1998.

82. Hillerdal G. Asbestos related pleuropulmonary lesions and the erythrocyte sedimentation rate. *Thorax* 1984; 39: 752–758.

83. de Vuyst P, Pfitzenmeyer P, Camus P. Asbestos, ergot drugs and the pleura. *Eur Respir J* 1997; 10: 2695–2698.

84. Buchanan DR, Johnston ID, Kerr IH *et al*. Cryptogenic bilateral fibrosing pleuritis. *Br J Dis Chest* 1988; 82: 186–193.

85. Dernevik L, Gatzinsky P. Long term results of operation for shrinking pleuritis with atelectasis. *Thorax* 1985; 40: 448–452.

86. Fielding DI, McKeon JL, Oliver WA *et al*. Pleurectomy for persistent pain in benign asbestos-related pleural disease. *Thorax* 1995; 50: 181–183.

22 MALIGNANT MESOTHELIOMA

Y. C. Gary Lee, Nicholas H. de Klerk, Douglas W. Henderson, and A. William Musk

BACKGROUND

Malignant mesothelioma is an incurable malignancy with unique characteristics with respect to etiology, diagnosis, management, and prevention that separate it from other cancers. Mesotheliomas typically arise from serosal membranes of body cavities, especially the pleura and peritoneum. Occasionally the pericardium or the tunica vaginalis testis provides the membrane of origin.

Historical considerations

It is now well accepted that the majority of cases of mesothelioma are a result of exposure to asbestos, especially the amphibole varieties. The earliest description of primary pleural malignancy was made before 1900, and several reports were published suggesting a causal effect from asbestos in the first half of the 20th century [1,2]. However, it was only after the seminal report of Wagner and colleagues in 1960 of 33 cases of mesothelioma in South African miners that mesothelioma became accepted as a disease in its own right, together with its association with asbestos [3].

Several reasons contributed to the delay in establishing mesothelioma as an asbestos-induced malignancy, the chief of which were the limited epidemiological data, the difficulty in making the diagnosis on histologic grounds, and an initial widespread belief that the great majority of reported cases were examples of serosal disease secondary to undiscovered primary tumors in neighboring viscera [3].

The association between asbestos exposure and the development of mesothelioma has subsequently been confirmed by numerous reports from around the world. It is now proven beyond doubt to be causal, but there is no relation to smoking.

Causes

Asbestos

There are two main families of asbestos fiber: the serpentine form (chrysotile) and the amphiboles (including crocidolite, amosite, and tremolite). They are discussed in more detail in Chapter 9. Amphiboles (Fig. 22.1) are more carcinogenic for the mesothelium than serpentine asbestos fibers. Recent studies on the exposure–response relationships confirm that crocidolite is by far the most potent fiber type for mesothelioma, apart from the non-commercial fibrous mineral erionite. The potency of crocidolite for mesothelioma induction is

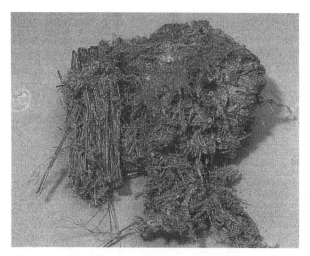

Fig. 22.1 Asbestos ore (crocidolite) from the Wittenoom mines of Western Australia.

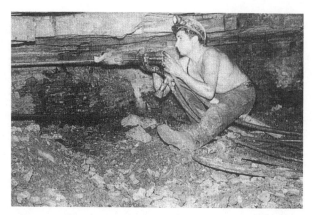

Fig. 22.2 Asbestos miner at work in former times in an underground mine without any respiratory protection.

substantially greater than amosite, which in turn is more potent than chrysotile [4].

While legislation has been implemented in most developed countries to minimize occupational and environmental asbestos exposure since the early 1970s, the use of asbestos worldwide has been under-regulated. Chrysotile now constitutes 99% of current global asbestos production, and sales remain strong in Asia and in developing nations worldwide [5].

Whether chrysotile per se causes mesothelioma is a topic of intense ongoing debate [6,7]. Some authorities maintain that chrysotile in its pure form does not cause mesothelioma and, thus, justify its continued commercial use in countries where the economic benefits may outweigh the risks. In reality, chrysotile very seldom exists in a pure form but is usually contaminated by other amphiboles, especially tremolite [8]. Also, chrysotile exposure has now been associated with increased risks of asbestosis as well as lung cancer [4]. In animal studies, intrapleural injection of pure chrysotile can induce mesothelioma. These concerns have been echoed by the International Program on Chemical Safety of the World Health Organization, which concluded that 'exposure to chrysotile poses increased risks for asbestosis, lung cancer and mesothelioma in a dose-dependent manner' and 'no threshold has been identified for carcinogenic risk' [9].

The majority of cases of mesothelioma arise in workers with direct occupational exposure to asbestos. Historically, the highest rates were experienced by those employed in the mining and milling of crocidolite asbestos materials (Fig. 22.2) [10]. Workers who handled the transport and shipment of asbestos were also at risk, as were those involved in the manufacture of asbestos products and those who used the end-products (e.g. construction and insulation workers). The types of direct occupational exposure have been well described [11].

Many of these occupational exposures could have been foreseen and potentially avoided. The use of leaky hessian bags instead of impermeable ones for transport of crocidolite from the Wittenoom mines in Western Australia was a typical example. As a result, asbestos exposure (and resultant high incidences of mesothelioma) occurred in workers on local wharves and ships used for transportation during the brief period of major exploitation 1943–66. In addition, the Aborigines in the Wittenoom area have developed one of the highest population-based mesothelioma rates in the world as a result of environmental exposure [12]. Bags previously used at Wittenoom were then reused at the chrysotile mine in Baryulgil of New South Wales, and this contributed to the cases of mesothelioma amongst workers there [13].

Environmental exposure to asbestos, especially amphiboles, is also associated with increased risks of mesothelioma [10]. It may arise from geological out-cropping of asbestos-containing rock or from environmental contamination (for example from local industries). Domestic and household exposure can result from living with asbestos workers, who bring contaminated clothing into the home [10].

The various types of asbestos fiber are cleared from the lung at different rates, presumably as a result of their different physical characteristics. This may account, in part, for the differences in carcino-genicity. Fibers that are long (>4 μm) and thin (<0.25 μm) are more stable in lung tissue and have a higher carcinogenicity for the mesothelium than short thick fibers [14]. Crocidolite, on the one hand, is cleared from the lungs at a rate of approximately 9% per year and has a long half life of over 7 years [15]. Chrysotile, on the other hand, has higher solubility and a greater propensity to break into smaller fibrils, which are eliminated from the lung more readily (half life less than a year) [14].

The incidence of mesothelioma increases linearly with intensity of exposure but exponentially (to the third or fourth power) with time from first asbestos exposure. This is from birth in some individuals. The incidence can be estimated from the following mathematical model:

$$I = KFT^p$$

where I is the incidence rate, F is the fiber density (fibers/ml), T is the time after first exposure, p is the exponent of time since first exposure (between 3 and 4), and K is a coefficient that depends on fiber size, type, mix, and other site-specific variables. The value of K is highest for crocidolite, followed by amosite and then chrysotile. The form of this exposure–response model is similar for all asbestos types and is discussed in more detail elsewhere [4,6,11].

The pathogenic mechanism by which asbestos induces the development of mesothelioma remains poorly understood but is likely to be a multistep process. Contributing factors may include chromosomal changes, abnormal immune responses, potential associations with prooncogenes and tumor-suppressor genes, as well as oxidant-mediated cell injury and growth factor amplifications [14]. Detailed review of the experimental evidence is outside the scope of this chapter.

While asbestos is the most common cause of mesothelioma, up to 20% of patients have no identifiable history of definite exposure, whether from occupational or other sources. The implications have been discussed extensively [17,18]. It had been feared that, because of the increasing amounts of asbestos in general use up to the 1970s, such cases would become more and more common. However, rates in Western Australia appear to have ceased increasing over the last few years, both in populations who are apparently unexposed and in the total population (Figs 22.3 and 22.4). This is true for

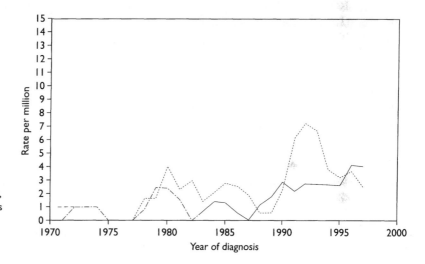

Fig. 22.3 Western Australian mesothelioma rates (cases per million population aged 15+), subjects with no known exposure to asbestos or unknown exposure status, 3-year moving averages, 1971–1998.

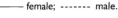 female; ------ male.

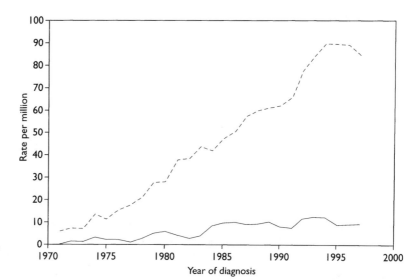

Fig. 22.4 Western Australian mesothelioma rates (cases per million population aged 15+), all cases, 3-year moving averages, 1971–1998.
——— female; ------ male.

both males and females, though a far greater increase was noted in males than females from 1970 to 1994. The female rate is often used as a surrogate when the rate in unexposed subjects is unavailable.

Erionite

Erionite is a non-asbestos fibrous zeolite that occurs naturally in the Cappadocian region of Turkey. It is used as a building material, especially for stucco, and is responsible for the very high local incidence of mesothelioma. It is associated additionally with pleural plaques, pulmonary fibrosis, and lung cancer. It causes significantly higher incidences of mesothelioma than crocidolite. The form of the exposure–response relationship derived from the Turkish studies of erionite is similar to that for crocidolite. However, the increase in rate with the third or fourth power of time from first exposure equates to an increase with the third or fourth power of age because the population involved was exposed from birth [17]. While the change in risk with time is very similar, the absolute risk is much higher after exposure to erionite; that is, the value of K in the equation above is over 100 times larger for Karain erionite than, for example, for Wittenoom crocidolite [11]. The same greater risk has been found in animal inhalation studies [19].

Other fibers

Concerns have been expressed over the potential risk for mesothelioma of different synthetic fibers. This is based on *in vitro* and *in vivo* evidence of carcinogenic potential, and on the similar sizes and shapes of some of these fibers to those of asbestos (e.g. refractory ceramic and glass fibers [20,21]). Workers in the synthetic fiber industries have, therefore, undergone extensive surveillance for many years, but no excess of mesothelioma has been detected that could not be attributed to concomitant exposure to asbestos [22].

Irradiation

Radiation [23], in particular previous use of the radiographic contrast material thorium oxide (Thorotrast), is an uncommon but established cause of mesothelioma [24]. Thoracic radiotherapy, however, has not been shown to increase the risk of pleural mesothelioma [25].

Genetic associations

Why some subjects exposed to asbestos go on to develop mesothelioma and most do not remains an unanswered question. While factors such as fiber type, the intensity of exposure, duration, and time from first exposure are each critically important, they predict poorly whether an individual will or will not develop mesothelioma. Although clusters of mesothelioma have been reported within families, it is difficult to establish whether they reflect common sources of environmental and/or occupational exposure or whether they represent a genetic predisposition.

Studies of migrants and of distinct ethnic groups may further the understanding of potential differences in genetic susceptibility to mesothelioma. For example, it has been suggested that Italian immigrants who worked at the Wittenoom mines have higher rates of mesothelioma than Australian-born workers with similar exposures, but the evidence is far from conclusive [26].

A number of chromosomal abnormalities have been described in association with mesothelioma, but no consistent abnormalities in oncogenes or suppressor genes have been found, and the molecular pathogenesis of mesothelioma remains poorly understood [14,27,28]. However, one interesting association between mesothelioma and a possible genetic aberration has been reported, that concerning simian virus 40. It is described in Box 21.1.

Epidemiology

Malignant mesothelioma can be considered to have caused a pandemic in the sense that it now occurs worldwide and has a prevalence that greatly exceeds that evident in the 1940s. Its incidence in most countries will continue to rise, at least until 2020 [29]. About 250 000 deaths from mesothelioma are expected in western Europe in the period to 2035 as a result of the continued use of amphibole asbestos in industry into the 1970s [30]. In developing countries, which imported crocidolite and amosite beyond the 1970s, a longer period of increasing incidence can be expected [31]. The mortality rates from mesothelioma in different countries are shown in Figures 22.5 and 22.6. The highest rates occur in countries that have produced amphiboles or made the most use of crocidolite and amosite, in particular with relation to the shipbuilding industry. In endemic regions such as Western Australia, the incidence was as high as 66 per million for men aged 35 or above in the 1980s [32]. In the USA approximately 3000 patients die each year from mesothelioma [33].

The steady increase in mortality rates from mesothelioma since the 1950s has slowed down in some parts of the world during recent years, and in the USA and Western Australia the rates even appear to be declining (Fig. 22.4). This can be attributed to decreases in production and use of crocidolite. It is now over 30 years since the closure of the Wittenoom mine in Western Australia in 1966, and the use of crocidolite has declined abruptly in

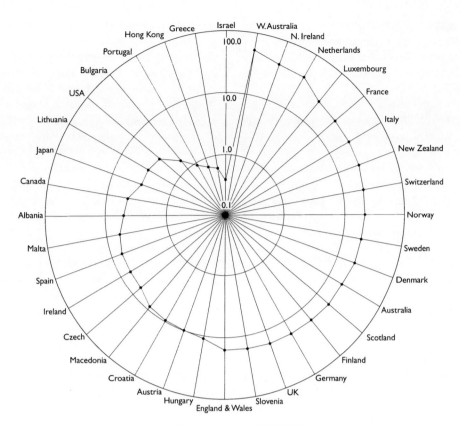

Fig. 22.5 Mortality rates (deaths per million population, all ages) for males, 1993, WHO-reported data.

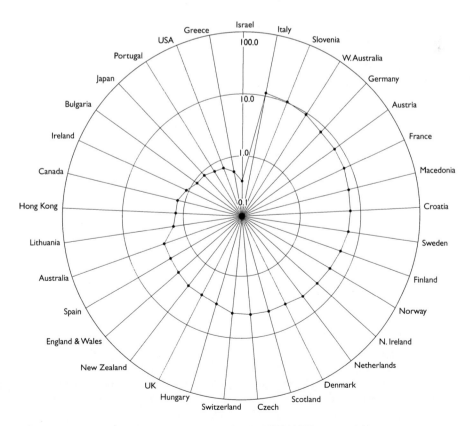

Fig. 22.6 Mortality rates (deaths per million population, all ages) for females, 1993, WHO-reported data.

Australia since then. However, the true incidence of mesothelioma may have been underestimated since mesotheliomas are difficult to diagnose and statistics derived from death certification have well-recognized inaccuracies [34].

The incidence of mesothelioma increases with age, consistent with the exponential shape of the relationship between risk and latency since first exposure, and two thirds present between the ages of 50 and 70 years. Up to 10% of asbestos-exposed workers may develop the disease, with an average latency of more than 30 years [2]. Although mesothelioma is two to nine times more common in males in many population studies, this is a result of differences in workplace exposure. Once there is adjustment for exposure, the incidence is similar in both sexes, and susceptibility appears uninfluenced by the age at which exposure occurs [10].

The pleura is the most common primary site of mesothelioma, followed by the peritoneum. In Australia, the pleura is involved in about 91–93% of cases, the peritoneum in about 7%, and the pericardium or tunica vaginalis of the testis in <1% [35]. The latent periods between exposure onset and disease onset are similar for both pleural and peritoneal sites, but primary peritoneal mesotheliomas are more generally associated with heavy asbestos exposures. They are unusual in non-occupationally exposed populations [36]. Reflecting this difference in exposure profile, pleural plaques and interstitial fibrosis have been detected in 50% of patients with peritoneal mesothelioma compared with 20% of those with pleural mesothelioma [36]. Mesothelioma of the tunica vaginalis testis is extremely rare, with less than 80 cases reported in the literature. The population incidence is unknown, but approximately one third of patients have documented asbestos exposure. While the median age of presentation is 60 years, 10% of those affected are under <25 years of age [37]. More detailed epidemiological information of malignant mesothelioma is available in other texts [4,11,17,38].

Prognosis

Mesothelioma remains an incurable malignancy. The average survival of patients in Western Australia is 9 months [39]. However, the disease in a small number of patients is known to follow an indolent course and most experienced clinicians have had patients who survived for many years without treatment [40]. The longest survival in our experience has been 9 years. In general, younger age, better performance status, less weight loss, and a shorter duration of symptoms before diagnosis are favorable prognostic factors [2,39]. Patients present-

ing with breathlessness survive longer than patients presenting with pain.

Patients with primary peritoneal mesothelioma have a poorer median survival than those with pleural mesothelioma (6 and 9 months, respectively), but mesothelioma of the tunica vaginalis testis has a reported median survival of 23 months [37].

The histologic subtype has an important prognostic influence, with epithelial mesothelioma predicting a significantly better survival than sarcomatous and biphasic subtypes [14]. Clinical staging (using the Butchart classification) also correlates with survival, the lesser the extent the greater the survival period.

Recent studies suggest that some biological factors, for example polysomy of chromosome 7, immunoreactivity for p21 *ras* oncogene, proliferating cell nuclear antigen (PCNA), and mitotic activity, may also carry prognostic significance. In a study of only 31 samples, patients whose mesothelioma tissues demonstrated high mitotic volume index and more PCNA immunoreactive cells had poorer survival [41]. Cytokeratin 19.1 and 19.21 (Cyfra 21–1) levels are elevated in pleural effusions of mesothelioma [42] and high serum levels of Cyfra 21–1 have been associated with poorer prognosis [43].

RECOGNITION

Clinical features

History

Malignant mesothelioma should be considered in any patient with pleural effusion or ascites, especially those with a history of asbestos exposure. A detailed occupational and environmental/residential history is essential whenever mesothelioma is suspected and may help the patient to pursue compensation issues promptly if the diagnosis is confirmed.

Pleural effusion affects most patients (95%) and for 40–70% there is breathlessness and non-pleuritic chest pain [14]. In contrast to many other malignancies, constitutional symptoms such as weight loss (in 30%), cough (in 10%), and fatigue are relatively uncommon at initial presentation, though weight loss is often prominent in advanced disease [64]. The presenting symptoms are usually nonspecific and of gradual onset, resulting in delay in seeking medical advice. The average time between symptom onset and diagnosis is 2–3 months, but 25% of patients may present more than 6 months after symptoms first began [65]. Most symptoms are a consequence of the local effects of the tumor, but hematogenous metastases do occur and are an occasional source of symptoms.

Box 22.1 Simian virus 40 (Douglas W. Henderson)

Over the last few years, an extensive literature has grown rapidly on the detection of simian virus (SV40) DNA in human mesotheliomas [44–48] and other tumors, such as osteosarcomas, brain tumors [44,49,50] and papillary thyroid carcinomas [51]. These observations followed an initial finding that SV40 induces mesothelioma in hamsters when injected intrapleurally [52]. It was shown later that SV40 can inactivate the tumor suppressor genes – p53 and the retinoblastoma gene (Rb) – via the large T antigen (TAG) [28,44,48]. Early poliomyelitis vaccines, which were raised from monkey kidney tissue and contaminated with SV40, were a potential source for the SV40 DNA in humans [44,45,53], though it is also possible that SV40 had entered the human genome before the development of polio vaccines.

It has been suggested that the presence of SV40 might explain why mesothelioma only develops in a relatively small proportion of asbestos-exposed individuals, and why no history of asbestos exposure is obtained in up to 20% of patients with mesothelioma [54]. However, the existing data on SV40 in human mesothelioma tissue do not adequately address either of these observations – for which there are alternative explanations – because almost all the mesotheliomas in which SV40 DNA has been found have been with associated asbestos. One small study by Mayall et al. [55] detected SV40 sequences in five of seven asbestos-associated mesotheliomas, but not in any of the four mesotheliomas that were not asbestos related. So far as we are aware, there is no reported

case-control analysis of SV40-associated mesothelioma where asbestos fiber counts were not elevated above reference values, except for the four cases that were not asbestos related in the study by Mayall et al. [55].

In other studies, neither SV40 nor TAG was detected within mesotheliomatous tissues [56–58]. Galateau-Salle et al. [59] found SV40 in benign inflammatory pleural diseases and in non-neoplastic lung tissue. We have also detected SV40 in non-neoplastic pleural lesions, normal tissues, and colon cancers, casting further doubt on the specificity of the association (Henderson DW, unpublished data).

Two epidemiological studies have shown no increase in the incidence of bone or brain tumors – or mesothelioma – 30 years after the use of polio vaccines contaminated with SV40 [60,61]. However, in a later study using data from the National Cancer Institute's Surveillance Epidemiology and End Results Programme (SEER), Fisher et al. [62] reported an increased frequency of these tumors in subjects who had received SV40-contaminated polio vaccines.

The evidence accumulated so far only points to SV40 as a possible cofactor for asbestos in the genesis of mesothelioma [55]. The evidence in favor remains inconclusive, and in humans SV40 may represent a bystander or passenger, or the tumour tissue may represent a favorable milieu for the replication of preexisting latent SV40: the criteria for causality [63] have not been fulfilled.

Mesothelioma frequently invades the neighboring structures, and direct invasion of the chest wall is common. This usually results in pain, often severe and debilitating. Malignant pericardial invasion may lead to pericardial effusion, cardiac tamponade and/or arrhythmias. Symptoms may also arise from esophageal compression, superior vena caval obstruction, and brachial plexus or spinal cord invasion. As the disease progresses, the tumor often extends to the serous membranes of the contralateral hemithorax or the peritoneal cavity, leading to bilateral pleural effusions or ascites. Tumor extension at sites of previous invasive procedures, such as thoracoscopy or percutaneous biopsy, is a characteristic feature of mesothelioma, with reported incidences ranging from 2 to 51% (mean 19%) [66].

The peritoneum may become involved either as a site of primary disease or from transdiaphragmatic invasion of disease arising primarily in the pleura. Ascites is the most common manifestation, but abdominal distension, small bowel obstruction, and (in advanced disease) palpable abdominal masses from omental deposits can occur. Scrotal enlargement of insidious onset is the most frequent pre-

senting complaint when the tunica vaginalis of the testis is the primary site, but local invasion and regional lymphatic spread are not uncommon [37].

Although generally regarded as a localized condition, bloodborne metastases of mesothelioma do occur and are often underrecognized. The nature of the symptoms that result depends on the site of involvement. At autopsy, extrathoracic spread may be found in up to 80% [14,67,68]; in one study there were hilar or mediastinal lymph node metastases in 44% [69]. Spread to intraabdominal organs, mostly liver, adrenals, and kidneys, is not uncommon, and intracranial metastases have been seen in 3%, usually of the sarcomatous type. 'Miliary mesothelioma', though rare, has also been described [70].

Physical signs

Evidence of pleural effusion is often the only abnormal feature on physical examination. Chest wall involvement may cause localized tenderness and/or a palpable mass (Fig. 22.7), and occasionally there is neurologic evidence of brachial plexus infiltration. Contralateral mediastinal shift can result from large pleural effusions or tumor masses, and occasionally

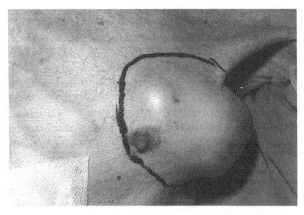

Fig. 22.7 Left chest wall invasion from malignant mesothelioma.

there are signs of compression or invasion of mediastinal structures. Signs of extrathoracic involvement are uncommon (11%), at least at the initial presentation [71]. Clubbing is not a feature and, if present, usually indicates coexisting asbestosis. Hypertrophic pulmonary osteoarthropathy and intermittent hypoglycemia are unusual and are more commonly associated with rare localized fibrous tumors of the pleura than with mesothelioma.

Investigation

Imaging

The typical findings on plain radiographs are a unilateral pleural effusion at presentation (Fig. 22.8). In advanced cases, diffuse pleural-based nodular opacification may be seen (Fig. 22.9). The mediastinum may be shifted contralaterally if the effusion is large, or ipsilaterally if there is extensive pleural thickening and tumor encasement of the underlying lung. Approximately 20% of patients have other radiographic evidence of asbestos expo-

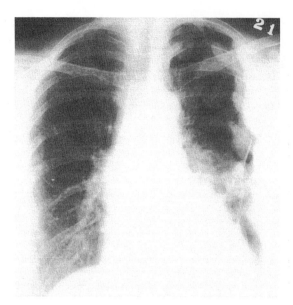

Fig. 22.9 Chest radiograph showing left pleural masses from malignant mesothelioma.

sure, particularly pleural plaques (with or without calcification) or interstitial fibrosis [36]. The demonstration of pleural plaques suggests previous asbestos exposure and should raise the suspicion of mesothelioma in the presence of an unexplained pleural effusion. Mesothelioma often arises in isolation, however, and so the absence of other asbestos-related disorders does not exclude the diagnosis.

Computed tomography (CT) has some success in distinguishing malignant from benign pleural disease (specificity 83% and sensitivity 72%) but is much less able to differentiate mesotheliomas from metastatic carcinomas [72]. In patients with mesothelioma, CT scanning may reveal thickening of the pleura (92%), interlobular fissures (86%), effusion (74%), pleural calcification (20%), chest wall invasion (18%), or occasionally, percardial or lymph node involvement (Fig. 22.10) [73]. High-resolution CT may additionally reveal other abnormalities associated with asbestos exposure (subpleural lines, parenchymal bands, interstitial fibrosis, diffuse pleural thickening, rolled atelectasis) that are masked by overlying pleural shadowing on the plain radiographs. Where a pleural-based tumor can be identified (Fig. 22.10), CT may be of further use in guiding percutaneous biopsy.

Magnetic resonance imaging (MRI) has similar diagnostic accuracy to CT imaging in assessing the extent of tumor involvement for the purpose of staging [14,74,75]. It is similarly no more than 50% accurate in determining hilar and mediastinal lymph node involvement [74], and it is unable to distinguish mesothelioma from secondary pleural malignancies. It is most useful when tumor extension into the spine or spinal cord is suspected, or in

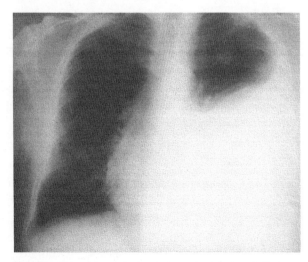

Fig. 22.8 Chest radiograph showing a massive left pleural effusion from malignant mesothelioma.

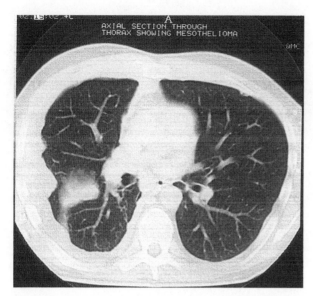

Fig. 22.10 Computed tomographic scan showing diffuse nodular thickening of the right pleura from malignant mesothelioma. Note that it extends to involve the mediastinal pleura.

research protocols involving novel therapies where accurate measurement of the tumor size is important to judge therapeutic response.

By contrast, positron emission tomography (PET) with 2-fluoro-2-deoxy-D-glucose (FDG) is a new imaging modality that has shown promise in aiding the differentiation of mesothelioma from benign pleural diseases, achieving a sensitivity of 91% and 100% specificity in a small series of highly selected patients [76]. However, its place in clinical practice remains to be established, and it awaits direct comparison with conventional modalities.

Lung function

Measurements of lung function have little to offer to assist the diagnosis of mesothelioma. Ventilatory restriction is to be expected, as a result of pleural effusion, tumor encasement of underlying lung and/or tumor invasion of the chest wall.

Cytology and biopsy procedures

A definitive diagnosis of mesothelioma can only be established with cytologic or histologic confirmation. Hence, the pathologic diagnosis of mesothelioma depends on material obtained by pleural biopsy or thoracentesis. Thoracentesis should be the first line of investigation for patients presenting with a pleural effusion. The pleural fluid is typically an exudate, but distinguishing between reactive mesothelial cells and malignant ones with certainty may be difficult, as may the differentiation between mesothelioma and metastatic adenocarcinomas. The diagnostic yield of aspirate cytology of pleural or peritoneal fluids varies from 33 to 84% and depends

on the experience of the cytologist [77]. Mesothelioma is not, therefore, excluded if the cytologic findings are negative.

Closed pleural biopsies with Abrams or Cope needles at the time of pleural aspiration can improve the diagnostic yield by 30–50%, and this is enhanced further if multiple biopsies are taken [14].

'Medical thoracoscopy' allows extensive inspection of the pleural cavity, and multiple biopsies can be taken under direct vision. This reduces sampling error and usually provides sufficient diagnostic material. Performed under sedation with adequate analgesia, it is usually safe and well tolerated. In experienced hands, the diagnosis of mesothelioma can be established in up to 98% of patients, as was shown in one prospective study of 188 patients [78]. A small portion of the biopsy tissues should be collected in glutaraldehyde in case electron microscopic examination is needed [36]. It has been suggested that patients seen to have involvement of only the parietal pleura have a better prognosis than those with both parietal and visceral disease [78]. If the diagnosis is established at the time of the thoracoscopy (i.e. with on-site cytology), chemical pleurodesis can be performed during the same procedure. An intercostal chest tube is usually left in situ for 24 to 36 hours after the procedure, and can be used to administer agents for chemical pleurodesis if the diagnosis is confirmed during that time.

Video-assisted thoracoscopy under general anesthesia is an alternative to medical thoracoscopy. Thoracoscopy is contraindicated if the pleural cavity is obliterated by tumor or adhesions. In such cases, an open biopsy may be necessary. However, open biopsy is more invasive, requires a longer hospital stay, carries a higher morbidity, and should only be performed if thoracoscopy is contraindicated or has failed to produce a diagnosis.

Blood tests

There are no specific hematologic or biochemical tests for diagnosing mesothelioma. While non-specific abnormalities such as anemia, thrombocytosis, and hyperimmunoglobulinemia occur often, they are of little diagnostic significance. Many serum tumor markers have been investigated but none can provide the sensitivity and specificity needed to be a sole diagnostic tool.

Molecular genetic studies

Various novel molecular techniques have been studied as potential tools to aid the diagnosis [79]. Though the methods are still experimental at present, it is likely that molecular biology will play an important part in the diagnosis and management of mesothelioma in the future.

Pathology

Epithelial (epithelioid), biphasic, and sarcomatoid mesotheliomas

The pathology of malignant mesothelioma has been described extensively in a plethora of specialized texts [80–85] and in more general texts on pulmonary pathology [35,86,87]. This chapter concentrates on selected salient gross and microscopic features likely to be of interest to the clinician. It sets these features into overall perspective as part of the diagnostic process and includes the changing role of immunohistochemistry and some unusual histologic variants of malignant mesothelioma.

An unknown proportion of pleural malignant mesothelioma appears to develop through a preliminary phase of mesothelioma in situ [88,89], with the subsequent development of multiple small foci of invasive mesothelioma, followed by diffuse spread along the pleura with encasement of the underlying lung (Fig. 22.11). Conversely, localized mesotheliomas are well described [80,90] and secondary neoplasms are capable of producing diffuse pleural disease.

At the level of histology, it is well known that mesothelioma can be epithelial (epithelioid) in character (about 60% of cases); about 10% represent sarcomatoid mesotheliomas and the remainder show biphasic (mixed) epithelioid and sarcomatoid differentiation [80]. For the diagnosis of biphasic mesotheliomas, 10% or more of either component should be present, by analogy with the proportions required for delineation of mixed carcinomas of lung [91]. Pleura-based diffuse anaplastic epithelial tumors represent a problem area of histologic diagnosis; some such tumors represent anaplastic epithelioid mesothelioma, as demonstrated by a transition to areas of more typical mesothelioma or by immunohistochemistry or electron microscopy, whereas others resist precise phenotypic characterization. The histologic appearances of sarcomatoid mesothelioma usually closely resemble fibrosarcoma or malignant fibrous histiocytoma [35,80], but heterologous patterns are sometimes encountered, including chondrosarcoma-like or osteosarcomatous differentiation [35,80].

Mucin histochemistry, immunohistochemistry, and electron microscopy

The identification of neutral (epithelial-type) mucin by stains such as diastase–periodic acid–Schiff base (PAS) or mucicarmine has long been used to discriminate between secondary adenocarcinoma (frequently positive) and epithelial mesothelioma [35,80]. About 20–55% of mesotheliomas stain for acidic mucosubstances, notably hyaluronic acid. Even so, epithelial mesotheliomas uncommonly produce mucin-like substances stainable by diastase–PAS or mucicarmine and are diagnosable as mesotheliomas by immunohistochemistry or, especially, electron microscopy [92].

To a large extent, immunohistochemistry has supplanted mucin histochemistry and electron microscopy for the diagnosis of most mesotheliomas and is now the mainstay of diagnosis. A detailed description lies beyond the scope of this chapter, and we present here a brief outline of our own current approach. We use the following probes for the diagnosis by immunohistochemistry: a label for low-molecular-weight cytokeratins, CK 5/6 [93], and epithelial membrane antigen (EMA). We also use three mesothelial cell markers, namely the mesothelial cell antibody HBME-1, thrombomodulin, and calretinin [35,94–97]. At present, calretinin is widely considered to be the most sensitive and specific positive marker for normal, hyperplastic and neoplastic mesothelial cells [96–98]. In addition, we use three markers for carcinoma, including carcinoembryonic antigen (CEA) and CD15 (Leu-M1 antigen). Characteristically, there is an absence of detectable labeling using these markers, although discordant positive findings are encountered occasionally.

We usually employ electron microscopy for the diagnosis of mesothelioma in the following circumstances: when the diagnostic sample is small (e.g. cytology cell-block preparations), when there are

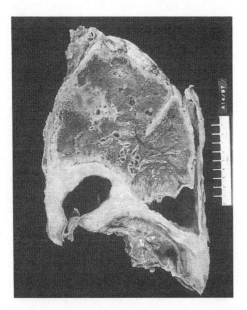

Fig. 22.11 Diffuse mesothelioma of the pleura (sagittal section). The tumor forms a confluent rind of tissue, with encasement of the lung, extensive obliteration of the pleural space, extension along the oblique interlobar fissure, and invasion into the upper lobe. The mesothelioma in this case invaded the posterior chest wall deep to the scapula (not shown), causing severe deformity of the thorax.

atypical histologic features, and when there are discordant findings on mucin histochemistry or immunohistochemistry [24].

A more restricted panel of antibodies can be used for the diagnosis of sarcomatoid mesotheliomas and desmoplastic mesotheliomas. Usually, we label for low-molecular-weight cytokeratins because most sarcomatoid mesotheliomas show strong positive labeling for these throughout the tumor [35,81]; positive labeling of this type is also valuable for the assessment of invasion, especially in desmoplastic mesotheliomas. In a smaller proportion of patients, expression of cytokeratins in sarcomatoid mesotheliomas is weak and focal, and cytokeratin-negative sarcomatoid mesotheliomas are encountered occasionally.

Variants of mesothelioma

In addition to mucin-positive epithelioid malignant mesothelioma, other recognized variants include mesothelioma in situ [88,89], desmoplastic mesothelioma [35,81,91], lymphohistiocytoid mesothelioma [35,81,91], small-cell mesothelioma [99,100], and deciduoid mesothelioma [101,102].

Mesothelioma in situ

Analogous to the concept of carcinoma in situ, mesothelioma in situ can be defined as the replacement of surface mesothelium by a layer of mesothelial cells that have cytoarchitectural features of malignancy [88]. In our experience, predominantly in situ mesothelioma is an uncommon lesion (about 3% of mesotheliomas). Because there is no distinctive marker for malignant mesothelial cells in situ, we require the presence of at least focal invasion in the same biopsy, a follow-up biopsy, or autopsy in order to make this diagnosis [88,89]. In the absence of invasion, a clear diagnosis of mesothelioma should not be made and a diagnosis of (non-invasive) atypical mesothelial proliferation is appropriate pending clarification.

Desmoplastic mesothelioma

Mesotheliomas are usually designated as desmoplastic when 50% or more of a tumor sample comprises hypocellular fibrous tissue [91,103,104]. Desmoplastic mesothelioma constitutes approximately 5–10% of mesotheliomas. These tumors are usually pleural in location [35,81,105,106], although rare peritoneal desmoplastic mesotheliomas do occur [107]. Because of its hypocellularity, desmoplastic mesothelioma is perhaps the most deceptive type of mesothelioma in a biopsy sample (Fig. 22.12): liable to misdiagnosis as either benign fibrous pleuritis or fibrous plaque. In fact, desmoplastic mesothelioma produces the poorest level of interobserver agreement on diagnosis, and follow-up sometimes fails to confirm the majority diagnosis from expert panels

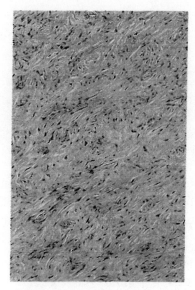

Fig. 22.12 Desmoplastic sarcomatous mesothelioma. The neoplastic tissue is paucicellular and collagen rich, with a disordered pattern of the collagenous tissue.

[108]. Accurate diagnosis of desmoplastic mesothelioma is often impossible with small core biopsies, and the diagnosis is most readily made on large tissue biopsies (e.g. wedge biopsies taken at video-assisted thoracoscopy). It is important for the biopsy to include the subpleural adipose tissue or deeper layers, for the all-important assessment of invasion (Fig. 22.13) [81]. Despite the seemingly innocent appearance of the tumor, desmoplastic mesothelioma represents an aggressive form of mesothelioma with a mean survival time of only 6 months after diagnosis [35,103,104].

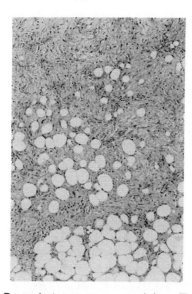

Fig. 22.13 Desmoplastic sarcomatous mesothelioma. The tissue was from the same patient as shown in Figure 22.12. In this sample, the most cellular tissue was found at the deep margin of the tumor, where there was an insinuative pattern of invasion into the subpleural fat, with splaying apart of individual adipocytes.

Lymphohistiocytoid mesothelioma

Lymphohistiocytoid mesothelioma is a rare subtype of predominantly sarcomatoid mesothelioma where the tumor comprises a background of atypical histiocytoid neoplastic cells suffused by intense lymphocytic infiltration, sometimes together with plasma cells and eosinophils. Consequently, this form of mesothelioma is liable to misdiagnosis as lymphoma [35,81,91,106,109–111].

Small-cell mesothelioma

Small-cell mesothelioma is another recently-recognised variant [99], with the potentiality for misdiagnosis as secondary small-cell carcinoma (conversely, small-cell carcinoma of the lung can spread into the pleura to produce a pseudomesotheliomatous pattern on rare occasions [100]).

Differential histologic diagnoses

The most problematical areas in the accurate diagnosis of mesothelioma include discrimination between reactive mesothelial hyperplasia and epithelial mesothelioma [35,89] and between benign fibrous pleuritis and sarcomatoid and desmoplastic mesothelioma [35,106]. In the first, atypical reactive hyperplasia versus epithelial mesothelioma, the extent and degree of cytologic atypia of the mesothelial proliferation are important, whereas identification of genuine neoplastic invasion – as opposed to benign displacement or sequestration of mesothelial cells as part of chronic inflammatory processes – is crucial to the diagnosis of mesothelioma [35,106]. In some cases, a clear distinction between these alternatives cannot be made, especially when the biopsy sample is small. Under these circumstances, either a repeat more adequate biopsy is necessary or, alternatively, close clinical and radiologic follow-up should be employed.

Two further malignant tumors may be confused with malignant mesothelioma. Pseudomesotheliomatous carcinoma of lung is defined by diffuse infiltration of the pleura in a pattern identical to mesothelioma, and its radiologic appearances on chest radiographs or CT scans are also identical to malignant mesothelioma. At present, pseudomesotheliomatous carcinoma of the lung is thought to originate from a small subpleural lung cancer that is engulfed and overgrown by its predominant pleural extension [112,113]. The diagnosis is usually achievable by mucin histochemistry or immunohistochemistry. Most pseudomesotheliomatous carcinomas represent adenocarcinomas, but other varieties of lung cancer can also produce this pattern of spread, including large-cell carcinoma [114], small-cell carcinoma [100] and spindle-cell carcinoma/carcinosar-

coma of lung [115]. Occupational exposure to asbestos has been recorded in some pseudomesotheliomatous carcinomas [113]. The prognosis is similar to that of mesothelioma, with a mean survival time of about 5 months after diagnosis [113].

Epithelioid hemangioendothelioma (EHAE) of the pleura represents a low-grade epithelioid angiosarcoma and is well described outside the pleura, including in somatic soft tissues, the liver, and the lung. Because of the epithelioid appearance of the neoplastic cells, epithelioid hemangioendothelioma infiltrating the pleura can be misdiagnosed as either secondary adenocarcinoma or mesothelioma [116–118]. These tumors are usually confluent along the pleura, and as a result the gross distribution is indistinguishable from mesothelioma. Epithelioid hemangioendothelioma of the pleura also carries a poor prognosis, analogous to mesothelioma, with a fatal outcome within 12 months in most instances [118]. At present there is no indication that asbestos is implicated in the induction of this tumor.

Differential diagnosis

The differential diagnosis of an exudative effusion is well described in standard texts [119]. The chief alternatives to mesothelioma are benign asbestos pleural effusion, malignant effusion from metastatic carcinoma, and other inflammatory pleural diseases. If the clinical suspicion of mesothelioma is high but repeated pleural biopsies are negative, an expectant course is usually justified, with close clinical and radiologic surveillance. Pleurodesis should be reserved until a firm diagnosis has been established.

Localized fibrous tumor of the pleura (also called benign fibrous mesothelioma) is a rare entity worth consideration. In its phenotype, this tumor is different from mesothelioma and is unrelated to asbestos exposure. It is usually (>80%) benign and is solitary rather than diffuse. Symptoms and effusions are uncommon, but hypertrophic pulmonary osteoarthropathy may occur and intermittent hypoglycemia is an interesting feature in 4–5% of patients [120]. It is usually resectable with good long-term prognosis [121].

Clinical staging

The Butchart classification (Table 22.1) and the Tumour–Node–Metastasis (TNM) system from the International Mesothelioma Interest Group are the two most commonly used clinical staging protocols for pleural mesothelioma [122,123]. Neither is easy to perform and both necessitate additional investigations not routinely required to determining treatment. Hence, staging is not routinely carried out in

Table 22.1 Butchart staging system for pleural mesothelioma. From Butchart *et al.* [122]

Stage	Clinicopathologic staging
I	Tumor confined to ipsilateral pleura, lung, and pericardium
II	Mediastinal or chest wall invasion
III	Tumor penetrating the diaphragm and invading peritoneum; extrathoracic lymph node involvement
IV	Distant hematogenous spread

day-to-day practice. However, staging is useful in the setting of clinical trials to categorize patients according to disease extent and to measure responses.

Monitoring disease progression

In general, mesothelioma develops locally before invading adjacent structures. Encasement of the ipsilateral lung and chest wall invasion are both common. Further direct or hematogenous spread usually occur late. Progressive dyspnea is common and is often multifactorial. Respiratory failure, cachexia, and muscle wasting soon follow [124].

The clinical evaluation of advancing malignancy or a possible response to any intervention should include measures of performance status, body weight/body mass index, and quality of life. MRI and CT scanning provide good overall assessment of the extent of the disease process but do not usually contribute to ongoing clinical management. These procedures should only be employed if there is a specific indication (e.g. measuring response in clinical trials).

MANAGEMENT

Of the individual

Mesothelioma remains a uniformly fatal disease. Various experimental treatment modalities have resulted in a large volume of conflicting literature, but there is little evidence to suggest any survival benefit over that from palliative management alone [125]. Even so, physicians often find themselves under pressure to 'do something' and those who use no more than 'best supportive palliation' are often considered nihilistic [2,126].

Several unique properties of mesothelioma render it resistant to conventional therapies [125]. It is usually diffuse, with a strong tendency to infiltrate the underlying lung, mediastinum, diaphragm, and chest wall. Complete surgical resection is, therefore, not feasible in most patients. Its diffuse nature also makes radiotherapy unsuitable [126,127], and it is addition-

ally resistant to most chemotherapy agents. Since most patients are elderly at presentation and comorbidity is common, the opportunity for aggressive therapeutic intervention is often limited further [36].

An additional problem is difficulty in assessing tumor burden, whether by serologic or radiologic markers, and hence difficulty in evaluating response in clinical trials. There is consequently no uniform use of a staging classification and this makes comparison of clinical studies difficult [128]. Most patients with early-stage disease have no measurable tumor on chest radiographs or CT scans, and radiologic assessment is especially difficult if there is extensive preexisting pleural disease or pleurodesis. Few trials of new treatment modalities have been conducted in a randomized controlled fashion, and selection bias is extremely common as fitter patients are more likely to volunteer or be selected for active experimental (but not placebo) treatments.

Best supportive care

A multidisciplinary approach generally offers the best outcome when management is focused to provide supportive care. It is important that advice on prognosis is consistent and that management plans are carried out in a coordinated fashion, thus maintaining trust and confidence between the patient, family, and the palliative care team of physicians, nurses, social workers, and psychologists [129]. All should understand the primary aims to provide care and support within the home, together with maximum symptom relief and a minimum of adverse effects. As pain and dyspnea are the commonest symptoms, adequate analgesia, including opioids, is important. Transcutaneous fentanyl patches and chronic indwelling epidural catheters have advantages in suitable patients, though neuropathic pain is better treated with anticonvulsants. Radiotherapy is useful for localized pain and for needle-tract metastases but should be avoided for treating nerve root pain [127].

Dyspnea from pleural effusions is common. Chemical or surgical pleurodesis is useful in preventing fluid reaccumulation and should be performed as early as possible. Talc offers the best rate of successful pleurodesis amongst commonly used agents but can cause pain/fever and, occasionally, acute respiratory distress syndrome [130]. Tetracycline and bleomycin are alternative agents. In patients with advanced disease, small catheter drainage may provide an alternative to hospital admission and pleurodesis [131], though needle-tract metastasis is a potential complication. Pleuroperitoneal shunting is not recommended because of the potential risk of enhancing intraperitoneal spread of the tumor [127]. A potential role of chemotherapy for symptom palliation has been suggested in two recent trials and warrants further investigation [132,133].

Surgery

Neither pleurectomy nor extrapleural pneumonectomy is curative, and neither has been shown to improve survival [2,40,44,124,134–136]. Extrapleural pneumonectomy involves *en block* removal of the lung, pleura, ipsilateral hemidiaphragm, and pericardium. The diaphragm and pericardium are then reconstructed [137]. It offers better local control than pleurectomy as it allows a more complete removal of tumor mass and the use of high-dose postoperative irradiation without concern for pneumonitis. Local recurrence is less common than with pleurectomy (10% versus 52% in one series) but extrapleural pneumonectomy carries a higher mortality than pleurectomy (5% versus 2%) and significant morbidity (25%) [44,126,128]. Cardiac arrhythmia is also a common problem, affecting 25–40% of the patients postoperatively.

Radiotherapy

Radiotherapy alone has no effect on survival (median 8–15 months) [138,139]. Despite modification to the techniques used, radiotherapy with curative intent is still limited by unacceptable toxicity [126]. The most established role of radiotherapy is in preventing needle tract metastases after invasive procedures into the pleural space. In a randomized controlled trial, 21 Gy (in three doses over 48 hours) was administered 10–12 days after invasive procedures. In the control group 8 of 20 patients developed malignant seeding while none of 20 in the treatment group did so [46]. Prophylactic local radiotherapy after thoracoscopy has consequently been recommended [124]. Radiotherapy may also be useful for the treatment of established needle tract metastases and in controlling localized pain. It can also palliate symptoms that arise from extrinsic compression or direct tumor invasion to the esophagus, superior vena cava, and spinal cord [129].

Radiotherapy is often used as an adjuvant in multimodality therapy to help to eradicate residual tumor, but its role in this setting has not been formally assessed. The use of radioactive colloids (e.g. [^{32}P]-chromatic phosphate) and brachytherapy as adjuvant agents are under investigation [140].

Chemotherapy

There is no proven role for chemotherapy. Objective response rates rarely exceed 40% and no regimen has been shown to provide cure or to impact survival [1,126,128,141]. Chemotherapy trials are often small (<15 patients) and not randomized, and when positive results were reported they could not be confirmed in larger investigations [1,126, 128,141,142]. Intrapleural chemotherapy has also been disappointing.

Interestingly, a recent phase II study in 21 patients using cisplatin with gemcitabine demonstrated a 48% response rate [132]. More importantly, 90% of the responders reported symptomatic improvement. Further studies are required to determine if this regimen offers any survival benefit.

Multimodality therapy

As single modality regimes are ineffective, various combinations have been used in an attempt to improve the outcome. Combinations of radiotherapy and chemotherapy are ineffective. Surgery, to reduce the tumor load, followed by other treatment modalities to maximize local clearance and eradicate occult systemic spread has been tried with little success. A critical review of the experimental therapies has been detailed by Lee *et al.* [125].

Surgery followed by radiotherapy and systemic chemotherapy is the most publicized multimodality treatment. Sugarbaker *et al.* [135] claimed some success using extrapleural pneumonectomy followed by three to six cycles of chemotherapy, then external beam radiotherapy to the hemithorax and mediastinum and, whenever possible, a bolus dose to sites of bulky disease. Although the outcome of this regimen attracted initial interest, important concerns remains regarding its usefulness.

The patients included in the study of Sugarbaker *et al.* were by far the most highly selected population when compared with other studies and carried the best prognostic parameters even before treatment [143]. Yet the median survival of 19 months was disappointing. The largest series to date of 183 patients was accumulated over 17 years in a tertiary referral center, attesting to the limited use of this regimen. The 30-day mortality from extrapleural pneumonectomy was 4% and the morbidity from the procedure was 50%. Relapses after trimodality treatment can manifest as local or distant recurrence, or both [144]. The median time to relapse was 19 months. Once tumor recurred, the patients followed a rapid downhill course with a median survival of only 3 months [144]. Concerns have been raised over whether this trimodality therapy has adversely affected the outcome of at least some of these patients, particularly if peri-operative mortality is included in the analysis [125]. From the available data, this treatment regimen cannot be recommended.

Experimental therapy

At present, gene therapy is still in its infancy but a recent phase I study has demonstrated its safety, and it may offer some hope for the future [33,145]. The rationale and basic delivery mechanisms are beyond the scope of this book but have been described elsewhere [33,126,145,146].

Intrapleural immunotherapy using interleukin 2 has shown some promise, but its usefulness has not yet been assessed in phase III trials [124]. A multicenter randomized controlled trial is underway using P-30 protein (Onconase): a novel ribonuclease with antitumor activity via degradation of RNA and induction of apoptosis in malignant cells [126]. The application of first-generation photodynamic therapy using hematoporphyrin derivatives as an adjunct to surgery and immunochemotherapy provided no benefit to survival (median 14 months) in a phase III trial [147]. Whether the use of a second-generation photosensitiser m-THPC (*meta*-tetrahydroxyphenylchlorin) is useful is now under study. Recent suggestions that SV40 may be pathogenic for mesothelioma have stimulated interests in strategies that abrogate SV40 expression (see Box 22.1) [148].

Of the workforce

There is no role for screening other asbestos-exposed subjects within the workforce for 'early mesothelioma' because of a lack of simple and effective screening procedures and because there is no effective treatment available. The pleural cavity is inaccessible for regular exfoliative cytology and routine thoracoscopy cannot be justified. The presence of benign asbestos-related lung or pleural diseases are common in individuals with known asbestos exposure and are not helpful in predicting mesothelioma. More importantly, screening cannot be justified even if this were to be practical until effective therapies for mesothelioma become available.

PREVENTION

In the workplace

The best prevention against mesothelioma is primary prevention against exposure to asbestos.

There is no practical threshold of exposure intensity or duration below which asbestos can be considered safe [36], but the risks should be seen in perspective. For example, de Klerk *et al.* [149] estimated that for a 70-year-old male in Western Australia, the risk of death from mesothelioma after no exposure was 4 per million person-years; the risk would increase to 325 per million person-years after 6 months of asbestos demolition work at age 24, and to about 25 000 per million person-years after 6 months work in the Wittenoom mill at age 24.

Secondary prevention using daily oral retinol (25 000 IU per day) in former asbestos workers has been studied recently, looking for protective effects of vitamin A with the same rationale as that for the CARET study [150]. Those who received retinol had significantly lower incidences of mesothelioma than workers who took daily β-carotene, or those who were not randomized into the study [151]. The relative rate of mesothelioma for those receiving retinol compared with those receiving β-carotene was 0.24 (95% confidence interval 0.07–0.86). The timing of this effect, if real, implied that the retinol was acting at a late stage of the disease and was consistent with the effective use of retinoids in treatment for example, of acute promyelocytic leukemia. This study is ongoing.

National regulatory strategies

The system for hazard control in Australia is based around individual legislation in each State. The legislation is usually written in general terms as Regulations and more specifically in Codes of Practice, which can be altered as current knowledge changes without the need for changing the legislation. Modern asbestos regulations were only adopted by the various states in the late 1970s and early 1980s. These now set exposure limits of 0.1 fiber/ml for crocidolite, amosite, and mixtures; and of 0.1–1.0 fiber/ml for chrysotile. In 1999, the National Occupational Health and Safety Commission agreed to support the phase-out of chrysotile use. Any impact of these regulations on the incidence of mesothelioma has yet to be seen.

DIFFICULT CASE

History

Malignant mesothelioma had been diagnosed in a 50-year-old Australian man who had no significant past medical history and had never smoked. He was seeking compensation through civil proceedings and was referred for an opinion concerning the probable cause. Over the 3 months that had elapsed following the initial diagnosis, he had noted worsening cough, malaise, anorexia, and had lost 16 kg in weight. A chest radiograph showed a pleural-based abnormality, and CT scans revealed extensive unilateral pleural thickening with a small effusion. Cytologic examination of a pleural aspirate confirmed the diagnosis of mesothelioma.

His father had died of lung cancer aged 50 years, and his mother had died of esophageal cancer in her 60s. His one sibling was well. He recalled frequent childhood exposure to asbestos, which had contaminated hessian bags that his father had acquired for use in his produce stall, and there had been probable occupational exposure to asbestos associated with his work as a cosmic ray physicist aged 21–25 years. His laboratory had been lined with asbestos, and during the period of 4 years he had used asbestos matting material to handle hot laboratory objects. He had additionally used radioactive thorium as a neutron source to calibrate neutron counters, on three or four occasions each month for about 10 min. He did not use monitoring badges to measure radiation exposure.

He worked as a science teacher without obvious exposure to asbestos for the following 20 years, and was a vocational counsellor for the 5 years preceding his presentation.

Issues

The critical issue here is whether the causal exposure was his childhood exposure to asbestos, his occupational exposure to asbestos, his occupational exposure to radiation, or some combination of these.

Comment

The book's contributors were almost equally divided between those who considered the childhood asbestos exposure alone to be responsible and those who thought both childhood and occupational exposures to asbestos had played a role. None considered the occupational exposure to radiation to be relevant.

The authors felt that the childhood exposure would be more important than the later occupational exposure to asbestos, since the risk of mesothelioma increases exponentially with time since first exposure. The exponent lies between 3 and 4, but the age at first exposure does not influence the risk independently of time. Also, his childhood exposure was more likely to have included crocidolite, which was mined and used extensively in Australia in that era, though not during his later period of occupational exposure. The radiation exposure was unlikely to have contributed significantly, although radiation from Thorotrast as a radiographic contrast agent has been associated with mesothelioma [152].

DIFFICULT CASE

History

An 83-year-old man was referred with increasing dyspnea over 3 months. During the preceding 6 months he had been investigated extensively for weight loss (10 kg) but no cause had been found. There was no other relevant medical history, apart from 20 pack-years of smoking completed 20 years previously. He had worked as a truck driver until he retired at age 65. For 1 year (aged 33–34) his work had involved loading/unloading asbestos, but there had been no apparent domestic or other occupational exposure to asbestos. There was no clinical evidence of connective tissue disease and he had not taken any medication associated with pleural disease.

A chest radiograph revealed a large right pleural effusion. Aspiration and closed biopsy on two occasions failed to give a cytologic or histologic diagnosis. The effusion was an exudate with 50% lymphocytes. Culture of the aspirate, Mantoux testing, and connective tissue screening tests were negative. Thoracoscopy and CT showed no obvious abnormality apart from residual fluid, and multiple biopsies from thoracoscopy showed non-specific inflammatory changes without malignant cells or asbestos bodies.

Issues

The diagnostic issues here are whether this man's effusion is malignant in nature or benign, and if malignant whether it is caused by mesothelioma. There are additionally issues of ongoing management; in particular what now should be done?

Comment

A small majority of the book's contributors thought that the effusion was most likely benign in nature, but an important minority favored a diagnosis of mesothelioma. None advocated any further immediate diagnostic procedure, but all recognized a need for ongoing surveillance with the possible need for repeated therapeutic aspiration of reaccumulating pleural fluid. Many favored the immediate instillation of a sclerosing agent in the hope that pleurodesis would prevent fluid reaccumulation.

There are no specific tests for the diagnosis of benign asbestos pleural effusion. The generally accepted diagnostic criteria are previous asbestos exposure, no other demonstrable cause, and eventual spontaneous resolution [153]. In experienced hands, thoracoscopy is very sensitive in detecting malignant pleural mesothelioma [78]. The absence of evidence of malignant mesothelioma on thoracoscopic biopsies makes a diagnosis of malignant mesothelioma unlikely in this case, though it is not fully excluded and the weight loss favours malignant over benign disease. The authors too would advise close clinical and radiologic follow-up of the patient's progress. Benign asbestos pleural effusion usually settles with time [153,154], with a mean duration of 3 months (range 1–10) in one series [154]. Some patients may eventually develop diffuse pleural thickening [155]. Pleurodesis is not usually necessary unless the effusion recurs rapidly and causes symptoms.

SUMMARY POINTS

Recognition

- Most patients with malignant mesothelioma present with a pleural effusion, the most common symptoms being breathlessness and chest pain.
- The absence of known exposure to asbestos does not exclude the diagnosis of mesothelioma, and this should be suspected in any patient with an unexplained exudative pleural effusion or ascites.
- A definitive diagnosis requires cytologic or histologic confirmation; CT or MRI scanning cannot reliably differentiate malignant mesothelioma from benign pleural disease or from metastatic carcinomas.
- Thoracentesis with or without pleural biopsy should be the first line of investigation, followed by thoracoscopy if these initial investigations are not diagnostic.

Management

- No treatment has been shown to prolong survival, and malignant mesothelioma remains an incurable malignancy.

- Best supportive care is the mainstay of treatment, with palliation provided by a multidisciplinary team.
- Randomized controlled trials are necessary to test new treatment modalities, and patients wishing to receive experimental treatment should do so within approved protocols.

Prevention

- Avoidance of asbestos exposure provides the best hope for prevention, either by using alternative materials within the workplace and the home or by using appropriate industrial controls (ventilation, extraction, personal protective equipment).
- There are no proven secondary prevention strategies in subjects who have been exposed to asbestos.
- Regular surveillance is not indicated in an exposed population; partly because of the lack of a simple, safe, and cost-effective method, and partly because there is currently no effective treatment.
- No threshold of exposure can be considered safe.

REFERENCES

1. Baas P, Schouwink H, Zoetmulder FAN. Malignant pleural mesothelioma. *Ann Oncol* 1998; 9: 139–149.
2. Pisani RJ, Colby TV, Williams DE. Malignant mesothelioma of the pleura. *Mayo Clin Proc* 1988; 63: 1234–1244.
3. Wagner JC, Sleggs CA, Marchand P. Diffuse pleural mesothelioma and asbestos exposure in the North Western Cape Province. *Br J Ind Med* 1960; 17: 260–271.
4. Hodgson J. The quantitative risks of mesothelioma and lung cancer in relation to asbestos exposure. *Ann Occup Hygiene* 2000; 44: 565–601.
5. Landrigan PJ, Nicholson WJ, Suzuki Y, Ladou J. The hazards of chrysotile asbestos: a critical review. *Ind Health* 1999; 37: 271–280.
6. Cullen MR. Chrysotile asbestos: enough is enough. Lancet 1998; 351: 1377–1378.
7. Smith AH, Wright CC. Chrysotile asbestos is the main cause of pleural mesothelioma. *Am J Ind Med* 1996; 30: 252–266.
8. Churg A, Wright JL, Vedal S. Fiber burden and patterns of asbestos-related disease in chrysotile miners and millers. *Am Rev Respir Dis* 1993; 148: 25–31.
9. Bonn D. Asbestos – the legacy lives on. *Lancet* 1999; 353: 1336.
10. Hansen J, de Klerk NH, Musk AW, Hobbs MST. Environmental exposure to crocidolite and mesothelioma: exposure–response relationships. *Am J Respir Crit Care Med* 1998; 157: 69–75.
11. de Klerk NH, Armstrong BK. The epidemiology of asbestos and mesothelioma. In: Henderson DW, Shilkin KB, Langlois SL, Whitaker D, eds. *Malignant Mesothelioma*, pp. 223–250. New York: Hemisphere, 1992.
12. Musk AW, de Klerk NH, Eccles JL *et al.* Malignant mesothelioma in Pilbara Aborigines. *Aust J Public Health* 1995; 19: 520–522.

13. House of Representatives Standing Committee on Aboriginal Affairs. *The Effects of Asbestos Mining on the Baryulgil Community*. Canberra: Australian Government Publishing Service, 1984.
14. Pass HI, Pogrebniak HW. Malignant pleural mesothelioma. *Curr Probl Surg* 1993; 30: 921–1012.
15. de Klerk NH, Musk AW, Williams VW *et al.* Comparison of measures of exposure to asbestos in former crocidolite workers from Wittenoom Gorge, W. Australia. *Am J Ind Med* 1996; 30: 579–587.
16. Peto J. The hygiene standard for chrysotile asbestos. *Lancet* 1978; i: 484–489.
17. de Klerk NH. Environmental mesothelioma. In: Bignon JJMC ed. *Mesothelial Cell and Mesothelioma*, pp. 19–36. New York: Marcel Dekker, 1994.
18. Hillerdal G. Mesothelioma: cases associated with non-occupational and low dose exposures. *Occup Environ Med* 1999; 56: 505–513.
19. Wagner JC, Skidmore JW, Hill RJ, Griffiths DM. Erionite exposure and mesothelioma in rats. *Br J Cancer* 1985; 51: 727–730.
20. Stanton MF, Wrench C. Mechanisms of mesothelioma induction with asbestos and fibrous glass. *J Natl Cancer Inst* 1972; 48: 797–821.
21. Wagner JC, Berry G, Timbrell V. Mesothelioma in rats after inoculation with asbestos and other materials. *Br J Cancer* 1973; 28: 173–185.
22. de Klerk NH. Malignant mesothelioma. In: Robinson BWS, Chahinian P eds. *Mesothelioma*. London. Taylor and Finch, in press.
23. Stock RJ, Fu YS, Carter JR. Malignant peritoneal mesothelioma following radiotherapy for seminoma of the testis. *Cancer* 1979; 44: 914–919.
24. Comin CE, de Klerk NH, Henderson DW. Malignant mesothelioma: current conundrums over risk

estimates, and whither electron microscopy for diagnosis? *Ultrastruct Pathol* 1997; 21: 315–320.

25. Neugut AI, Ahsan H, Antman KH. Incidence of malignant pleural mesothelioma after thoracic radiotherapy. *Cancer* 1997; 80: 948–950.

26. Merler E, Ercolanelli M, Cappelletto F *et al*. On 1126 Italian migrants to Australia who worked at the crocidolite mine of Wittenoom Gorge between 1946 and 1966. In: Grieco A, Iavicoli S, Berlinguer G eds. *Proceedings of the 1st International Conference of Occupational and Environmental Prevention*, Rome,1998.

27. Lee WC, Testa JR. Somatic genetic alterations in human malignant mesothelioma. *Int J Oncol* 1999; 14: 181–188.

28. Murthy SS, Testa JR. Asbestos, chromosomal deletions, and tumour suppressor gene alterations in human malignant mesothelioma. *J Cell Physiol* 1999; 180: 150–157.

29. Peto J, Hodgson JT, Matthews FE, Jones JR. Continuing increase in mesothelioma mortality in Britain. *Lancet* 1995; 345: 535–539.

30. Peto J, Decarli A, La Vecchia C *et al*. The European mesothelioma epidemic. *Br J Cancer* 1999; 79: 666–672.

31. Harington JS, McGlashan ND. South African asbestos: production, exports, and destinations, 1959–1993. *Am J Ind Med* 1998; 33: 321–326.

32. Armstrong BK, Musk AW, Baker JE *et al*. Epidemiology of malignant mesothelioma in Western Australia. *Med J Aust* 1984; 141: 86–88.

33. Sterman DH, Kaiser LR, Albelda SM. Gene therapy for malignant pleural mesothelioma. *Hematol/Oncol Clin North Am* 1998; 12: 553–568.

34. Lilienfeld DE, Gunderson PD. The 'missing cases' of pleural malignant mesothelioma in Minnesota, 1979–81; preliminary report. *Public Health Rep* 1996; 101: 395–399.

35. Henderson DW, Comin CE, Hammar SP *et al*. Malignant mesothelioma of the pleura: current surgical pathology. In: Corrin B ed. *Pathology of Lung Tumors* pp.240–280. New York: Churchill Livingstone, 1997.

36. Antman KH. Current concepts: malignant mesothelioma. *N Engl J Med*; 1980; 303: 200–202.

37. Plas E, Riedl CR, Pfluger H. Malignant mesothelioma of the tunica vaginalis testis. *Cancer* 1998; 83: 2437–2446.

38. MacDonald JC, MacDonald AD. The epidemiology of mesothelioma in historical context. *Eur Respir J* 1996; 9: 1932–1942.

39. Musk AW, Woodward SD. Conventional treatment and its effect on survival of malignant pleural mesothelioma in Western Australia. *Aust NZ J Med* 1982; 12: 229–232.

40. Law MR, Gregor A, Hodson ME *et al*. Malignant mesothelioma of the pleura: a study of 52 treated and 64 untreated patients. *Thorax* 1984; 39: 255–259.

41. Ramael M, Jacob W, Weyler J *et al*. Proliferation in malignant mesothelioma as determined by mitosis counts and immunoreactivity for proliferating cell nuclear antigen (PCNA). *J Pathol* 1994; 172: 247–253.

42. Lee YC, Knox BS, Garrett JE. Use of cytokeratin fragments 19.1 and 19.21 (Cyfra 21–1) in the differentiation of malignant and benign pleural effusions. *Aust NZ J Med* 1999; 29: 765–769.

43. Bonfrer JMG, Schouwink JH, Korse CM, Baas P. Cyfra 21–1 and TPA as markers in malignant mesothelioma. *Anticancer Res* 1997; 17: 2971–2974.

44. Carbone M, Rizzo P, Grimley PM *et al*. Simian virus-40 large T-antigen binds p53 in human mesotheliomas. *Nat Med* 1997; 3: 908–912.

45. Carbone M, Rizzo P, Pass HI. Simian virus 40, poliovaccines and human tumors: a review of recent developments. *Oncogene* 1997; 15: 1877–1888.

46. Carbone M, Fisher S, Powers A *et al*. New molecular and epidemiological issues in mesothelioma: role of SV40. *J Cell Physiol* 1999; 180: 167–172.

47. Stenton SC. Asbestos, simian virus 40 and malignant mesothelioma. *Thorax* 1997; 52(Suppl 3): S52–S57.

48. de Luca A, Baldi A, Esposito V *et al*. The retinoblastoma gene family pRb/p105, p07, pRb2/p130 and simian virus-40 large T-antigen in human mesotheliomas. *Nat Med* 1997; 3: 913–916.

49. Butel JS, Lednicky JA, Stewart AR *et al*. SV40 and human brain tumors. *J Neurovirol* 1997; 3(Suppl 1): S78–S79.

50. Huang H, Reis R, Yonekawa Y *et al*. Identification in human brain tumors of DNA sequences specific for SV40 large T antigen. *Brain Pathol* 1999; 9: 33–42.

51. Pacini F, Vivaldi A, Santoro M *et al*. Simian virus 40-like DNZ sequences in human papillary thyroid carcinomas. *Oncogene* 1998; 16: 665–669.

52. Cicala C, Pompetti F, Carbone M. SV40 induces mesotheliomas in hamsters. *Am J Pathol* 1993; 142: 1524–1533.

53. Kuska B. SV40: working the bugs out of the polio vaccine. *J Natl Cancer Inst* 1997; 89: 283–284.

54. Mutti L, Carbone M, Giordano GG, Giordano A. Simian virus 40 and human cancer. *Monaldi Arch Chest Dis* 1998; 53: 198–201.

55. Mayall FG, Jacobson G, Wilkins R: Mutations of p53 gene and SV40 sequences in asbestos associated and non-asbestos-associated mesotheliomas. *J Clin Pathol* 1999; 52: 291–293.

56. Dhaene K, Verhulst A, van Marck E. SV40 large T-antigen and human pleural mesothelioma. Screening by polymerase chain reaction and tyramine-amplified immunohistochemistry. *Virchow Archiv* 1999; 435: 1–7.

57. Strickler HD, Goedert JJ, Fleming M *et al*. Simian virus 40 and pleural mesothelioma in humans. *Cancer Epidemiol Biomarkers Prev* 1996; 5: 473–475.

58. Mulatero C, Surentheran T, Breuer J, Rudd RM. Simian virus 40 and human pleural mesothelioma. *Thorax* 1999; 54: 60–61.

59. Galateau-Salle F, Bidet P, Iwatsubo Y *et al*. SV40-like DNA sequences in pleural mesothelioma, bronchopulmonary carcinoma, and non-malignant pulmonary diseases. *J Pathol* 1998; 184: 252–257.

60. Olin P, Giesecke J. Potential exposure to SV40 in polio vaccines used in Sweden during 1957: no impact on cancer incidence rates 1960 to 1993. *Dev Biol Stand* 1998; 94: 227–233.

61. Strickler HD, Rosenberg PS, Devesa SS *et al*. Contamination of poliovirus vaccines with simian virus 40 (1955–1963) and subsequent cancer rates. *JAMA* 1998; 279: 292–295.

62. Fisher SG, Weber T, Carbone M. Cancer risk associated with simian virus 40 contaminated polio vaccine. *Anticancer Res* 1999; 19: 2173–2180.

63. Stolley PD, Lsaky T (eds.) *Investigating Disease Patterns: The Science of Epidemiology*. New York: Scientific American 1998.

64. Rusch VW, Piantadosi S, Homes EC. The role of extrapleural pneumonectomy in malignant pleural mesothelioma. A Lung Cancer Study Group trial. *J Thorac Cardiovasc Surg* 1991; 102: 1–9.

65. Chahinian AP, Pajak TF, Holland JF et al. Diffuse malignant mesothelioma: prospective evaluation of 69 patients. *Ann Intern Med* 1982; 96: 746–755.

66. Boutin C, Roy F, Viallat JR et al. Prevention of malignant seeding after invasive diagnostic procedures in patients with pleural mesothelioma. *Chest* 1996; 108: 754–758.

67. King JAC, Rucker JA, Wong SW. Mesothelioma: a study of 22 cases. *South Med J* 1997; 90: 199–205.

68. Hulks G, Thomas JSJ, Waclawski E. Malignant pleural mesothelioma in western Glasgow 1980–1986. *Thorax* 1989; 44: 496–500.

69. Kim SB, Varkey B, Choi H. Diagnosis of malignant pleural mesothelioma by axillary lymph node biopsy. *Chest* 1987; 91: 279–282.

70. Musk AW, Dewar J, Shilkin KB, Whitaker D. Miliary spread of malignant pleural mesothelioma without a clinical identifiable pleural tumour. *Aust NZ J Med* 1991; 32: 460–462.

71. Chailleux E, Dabouir G, Pioche D. Prognostic factors in diffuse malignant mesothelioma. *Chest* 1988; 93: 159–162.

72. Leung AN, Muller NL, Miller RR. CT in differential diagnosis of diffuse pleural disease. *Am J Roentgenol* 1990; 154: 487–492.

73. Muller NL. Imaging of the pleura. *Radiology* 1993; 186: 297–309.

74. Heelan RT, Rusch VW, Begg CB et al. Staging of malignant pleural mesothelioma: comparison of CT and MR imaging. *Am J Roentgenol* 1999; 172: 1039–1047.

75. Knuuttila A, Halme M, Kivisaari L et al. The clinical importance of magnetic resonance imaging versus computed tomography in malignant pleural mesothelioma. *Lung Cancer* 1998; 22: 215–225.

76. Benard F, Sterman DH, Smith RJ et al. Metabolic imaging of malignant pleural mesothelioma with fluorine-18-deoxyglucose positron emission tomography. *Chest* 1998; 114: 713–722.

77. Whitaker D, Sterrett G, Shilkin K. Early diagnosis of malignant mesothelioma: the contribution of effusion and fine needle aspiration cytology and ancillary techniques. In: Peters GA, Peters BJ eds. *Asbestos Disease Update, March 1989*, pp. 73–112. New York: Garland Law, 1989.

78. Boutin C, Rey F. Thoracoscopy in pleural malignant mesothelioma: a prospective study of 188 consecutive patients. Part 1: Diagnosis. *Cancer* 1993; 72: 389–393.

79. Sheibani K, Esteban JM, Bailey A et al. Immunopathologic and molecular studies as an aid to the diagnosis of malignant mesothelioma. *Hum Pathol* 1992; 23: 107–116.

80. Henderson DW, Shilkin KB, Whitaker D et al. The pathology of mesothelioma, including immunohistology and ultrastructure. In: Henderson DW, Shilkin KB, Langois SL, Whitaker D eds. *Malignant Mesothelioma*, pp. 69–139. New York: Hemisphere, 1992.

81. Henderson DW, Shilkin KB, Whitaker D et al. Unusual histological types and anatomic sites of mesothelioma. In: Henderson DW, Shilkin KB, Langlois SL, Whitaker D, eds. *Malignant Mesothelioma*, pp. 140–166. New York: Hemisphere, 1992.

82. Henderson DW, Whitaker D, Shilkin KB. The differential diagnosis of mesothelioma: a practical approach to diagnosis during life. In: Henderson DW, Shilkin KB, Langlois SL, Whitaker D eds. *Malignant Mesothelioma*, pp. 183–197. New York: Hemisphere, 1992.

83. Churg A. Neoplastic asbestos-induced disease. In: Churg A, Green FHY eds. *Pathology of Occupational Lung Disease*. 2nd edn. Baltimore, MD: Williams & Wilkins, 1998; 279–325.

84. Chretien J, Bignon J, Hirsch A (eds.). *The Pleura in Health and Disease*. New York: Marcel Dekker, 1985.

85. Roggli VL, Sanfilippo F, Shelburne JD. Mesothelioma. In: Roggli VL, Greenberg SD, Pratt PC eds. *Pathology of Asbestos-associated Diseases*. Boston, MA: Little Brown 1992; 109–64.

86. Hammar SP. Pleural diseases. In: Dail DH, Hammar SP eds. *Pulmonary Pathology*. New York: Springer-Verlag, 1994; 1463–1579.

87. Churg A. Diseases of the pleura. In: Thrulbeck WM, Churg AM eds. *Pathology of the Lung*, 2nd ed. New York: Thieme, 1995; 1080–1090.

88. Whitaker D, Henderson DW, Shilkin KB. The concept of mesothelioma in situ: implications for diagnosis and histogenesis. *Semin Diagn Pathol* 1992; 9: 151–161.

89. Henderson DW, Shilkin KB, Whitaker D. Reactive mesothelial hyperplasia vs mesothelioma, including mesothelioma in situ: a brief review. *Am J Clin Pathol* 1998; 110: 397–404.

90. Crotty TB, Myers JL, Katzenstein A-A et al. Localized malignant mesothelioma: a clinicopathologic and flow cytometric study. *Am J Surg Pathol* 1994; 18: 357–363.

91. Travis WD, Colby TV, Corrin B. Histological typing of lung and pleural tumours. In: *World Health Organization International Histological Classification of Tumours*, 3rd edn. Berlin: Springer, 1999.

92. Hammar SP, Bockus DE, Remington FL, Rohrback KA. Mucin-positive epithelial mesotheliomas: a histochemical, immunohistochemical and ultrastructural comparison with mucin-producing pulmonary adenocarcinomas. *Ultrastruct Pathol* 1996; 20: 292–325.

93. Clover J, Oates J, Edwards C. Anti-cytokeratin 5/6: a positive marker for epitheliod mesothelioma. *Histopathology* 1997; 31: 140–143.

94. Ordonez NG. The value of antibodies 44-3A6, SM3, HBME-1, and thrombomodulin in differentiating epithelial pleural mesothelioma from lung adenocarcinoma: a comparative study with other commonly used antibodies. *Am J Surg Pathol* 1997; 21: 1399–1408.

95. Ordonez NG. Value of thrombomodulin in the diagnosis of mesothelioma. *Histopathology* 1997; 31: 25–30.

96. Doglioni C, Tos AP, Laurino L et al. Calretinin: a novel immunocytochemical marker for mesothelioma. *Am J Surg Pathol* 1996; 20: 1037–1046.

97. Leers MP, Aarts MM, Theunissen PH. E-cadherin and calretinin: a useful combination of immunochemical markers for differentiation between mesothelioma and metastatic adenocarcinoma. *Histopathology* 1998; 32: 209–216.

98. Barberis MC, Faleri M, Veronese S et al. Calretinin: a selective marker of normal and neoplastic mesothelial cells in serous effusions. *Acta Cytol* 1997; 41: 1757–1761.

99. Mayall FG, Gibbs AR. The histology and immunohistochemistry of small cell mesothelioma. *Histopathology* 1992; 20: 47–51.

100. Falconieri G, Zanconati F, Bussani R, Di Bonito L. Small cell carcinoma of lung simulating pleural mesothelioma: report of 4 cases with autopsy confirmation. *Pathol Res Pract* 1995; 191: 1147–1152.

101. Nascimento AG, Keeney GL, Fletcher CDM. Deciduoid peritoneal mesothelioma: an unusual phenotype affecting young females. *Am J Surg Pathol* 1994; 18: 439–445.

102. Orosz N, Nagy P, Szentirmay Z et al. Epithelial mesothelioma with deciduoid features. *Virchow Archiv* 1999; 434: 263–266.

103. Cantin R, Al-Jabi M, McCaughey WT. Desmoplastic diffuse mesothelioma. *Am J Surg Pathol* 1982; 6: 215–222.

104. Wilson GE, Hasleton PS, Chatterjee AK. Desmoplastic malignant mesothelioma: a review of 17 cases. *J Clin Pathol* 1992; 45: 295–298.

105. Colby TV. The diagnosis of desmoplastic malignant mesothelioma. *Am J Clin Pathol* 1998; 110: 135–136.

106. Mangano WE, Cagle PT, Churg A et al. The diagnosis of desmoplastic malignant mesothelioma and its distinction from fibrous pleurisy: a histologic and immunohistochemical analysis of 31 cases including p53 immunostaining. *Am J Clin Pathol* 1998; 110: 191–199.

107. Roggli VL. Case 7: desmoplastic mesothelioma of the peritoneum. Short course 10: Tumors and tumor-like disorders of serosal membranes. In: *Proceedings of the XXI International Congress of the International Academy of Pathology*, 1996.

108. McCaughey WTE, Colby TV, Battifora H et al. Diagnosis of diffuse malignant mesothelioma: experience of a US/Canadian mesothelioma panel. *Mod Pathol* 1991; 4: 342–353.

109. Henderson DW, Attwood HD, Constance TJ et al. Lymphohistiocytoid mesothelioma: a rare lymphomatoid variant of predominantly sarcomatoid mesothelioma. *Ultrastruct Pathol* 1988; 12: 367–384.

110. Khalidi HS, Medeiros LJ, Battifora H. Lymphohistiocytoid mesothelioma: an often misdiagnosed variant of sarcomatoid mesothelioma. *Am J Clin Pathol* 2000; 113: 649–654.

111. Wick MR, Mills SE. Mesothelial proliferations: an increasing morphologic spectrum. *Am J Clin Pathol* 2000; 113: 619–622.

112. Harwood TR, Gracey DR, Yokoo H. Psedomesotheliomatous carcinoma of the lung: a variant of peripheral lung cancer. *Am J Clin Pathol* 1976; 65: 159–167.

113. Koss M, Travis W, Moran C, Hochholzer L. Pseudomesotheliomatous adenocarcinoma: a reappraisal. *Semin Diagn Pathol* 1992; 9: 117–123.

114. Brunner-La Rocca HP, Schlossberg D, Vogt P. Pseudomesotheliomatous carcinoma of HIV infection. In: [German] *Deut Med Wschrift* 1995; 120: 1312–1317.

115. Mayall FG, Gibbs AR. 'Pleural' and pulmonary carcinosarcomas. *J Pathol* 1992; 167: 305–311.

116. Battifora H, McCaughey WTE (eds.). *Tumour of the Serosal Membranes*, Tumors of Serosal Membranes Atlas of Tumor Pathology, 3rd series, fasc 15. Washington DC: Armed Forces Institute of Pathology; 1995.

117. Lin B-Y, Colby T, Gown AM et al. Malignant vascular tumors of the serous membranes mimicking mesothelioma. *Am J Surg Pathol* 1996; 20: 1431–1439.

118. Zhang PJ, Livolsi VA, Brooks JJ. Malignant epithelioid vascular tumors of the pleura: report of a series and literature review. *Hum Pathol* 2000; 31: 29–34.

119. Light RW. *Pleural Disease*, 3rd edn. Baltimore, MD: Williams & Wilkins, 1995.

120. Briselli M, Mark EJ, Dickersin GR. Solitary fibrous tumours of the pleura: eight new cases and review of 360 cases in the literature. *Cancer* 1981; 47: 2678–2689.

121. Suter M, Gebhard S, Boumghar M et al. Localized fibrous tumours of the pleura: 15 new cases and review of the literature. *Eur J Cardiothorac Surg* 1998; 14: 453–459.

122. Butchart EG, Ashcroft T, Barnsley WC, Holden M. The role of surgery in diffuse malignant mesothelioma of the pleura. *Semin Oncol* 1981; 8: 321–328.

123. International Mesothelioma Interest Group. A new staging system for malignant mesothelioma. *Chest* 1995; 108: 1122–1126.

124. Boutin C, Schlesser M, Frenay C, Astoul P. Malignant pleural mesothelioma. *Eur Respir J* 1998; 12: 972–981.

125. Lee YC, Light RW, Musk AW. Management of malignant pleural mesothelioma: a critical review. *Curr Opin Pulmon Med* 2000; 6: 267–274.

126. Sterman DH, Kaiser LR, Albelda SM. Advances in the treatment of malignant pleural mesothelioma. *Chest* 1999; 116: 504–520.

127. Astoul P. Pleural mesothelioma. *Curr Opin Pulm Med* 1999; 5: 259–68.

128. Aisner J. Current approach to malignant mesothelioma of the pleura. *Chest* 1995; 107: 332S–344S.

129. Lee YC, Musk AW, Dean A et al. Clinical aspects of mesothelioma. In: Robinson BWS, Chahinian P eds. *Mesothelioma*. London. Taylor and Finch, in press.

130. Rehse DH, Aye RW, Florence MG. Respiratory failure following talc pleurodesis. *Am J Surg* 1999; 177: 437–440.

131. Putnam JB, Light RW, Rodriguez RM et al. A randomized comparison of indwelling pleural catheter and doxycycline pleurodesis in the management of malignant pleural effusions. *Cancer* 1999; 86: 1992–1999.

132. Bryne MJ, Davidson JA, Musk AW et al. Cisplatin and gemcitabine treatment for malignant mesothelioma: a phase II study. *J Clin Oncol* 1999; 17: 25–30.

133. Middleton GW, Smith IE, O'Brien MER et al. Good symptom relief with palliative MVP (mitomycin C, vinblastine, cisplatin) chemotherapy in malignant mesothelioma. *Ann Oncol* 1998; 9: 269–273.

134. Rusch VW. Indications for pneumonectomy. Extrapleural pneumonectomy. *Chest Surg Clin North Am* 1999; 9: 327–338.

135. Sugarbaker DJ, Jaklittsch MT, Liptay MJ. Mesothelioma and radical multimodality therapy: who benefits? *Chest* 1995; 107: 345S–350S.

136. Worn H. Moglichkeiten und Ergebnisse der chirurgischen Behandlung des malignen Pleuramesothelioms. *Thorax-Chirurgie* 1974; 22: 391–393.

137. Sugarbaker DJ, Richards WG, Garcia JP. Extrapleural pneumonectomy for malignant mesothelioma. *Adv Surg* 1998; 31: 252–270.

138. Alberts AS, Falkson G, Goedhals L et al. Malignant pleural mesothelioma: a disease unaffected by current therapeutic maneuvers. *J Clin Oncol* 1988; 6: 527–535.

139. Gordon W, Antman KH, Greenberger JS et al. Radiation therapy in the management of patients with mesothelioma. *Int J Radiat Oncol* 1982; 8: 19–25.

140. Brady LW. Mesothelioma, the role for radiation therapy. *Semin Oncol* 1981; 8: 329–334.

141. Ryan CW, Herndon J, Vogelzand NJ. A review of chemotherapy trials for malignant mesothelioma. *Chest* 1998; 113: 66S–73S.

142. Krarup-Hansen A, Hansen HH. Chemotherapy in malignant mesothelioma: a review. *Cancer Chemother Pharmacol* 1991; 28: 319–330.

143. Sugarbaker DJ, Flores RM, Jakiltsch MT *et al*. Resection margins, extrapleural nodal status, and cell type determine postoperative long-term survival in trimodality therapy of malignant pleural mesothelioma. Results in 183 patients. *J Thorac Cardiovasc Surg* 1999; 117: 54–65.

144. Baldini EH, Recht A, Strauss GM *et al*. Patterns of failure after trimodality therapy for malignant pleural mesothelioma. *Ann Thorac Surg* 1997; 63: 334–338.

145. Albelda SM. Gene therapy for lung cancer and mesothelioma. *Chest* 1997; 111: 144S–149S.

146. Schwarzenberger P, Harrison L, Weinacker A *et al*. Gene therapy for malignant mesothelioma: a novel approach for an incurable cancer with increased incidence in Louisiana. *J LA State Med Soc* 1998; 150: 168–174.

147. Pass HI, Temeck BK, Kranda K *et al*. Phase III randomized trial of surgery with or without intraoperative photodynamic therapy and postoperative immunochemotherapy for malignant pleural mesothelioma. *Ann Surg Oncol* 1997; 4: 628–633.

148. Waheed I, Guo ZS, Chen GA *et al*. Antisense to SV40 early gene region induces growth arrest and apoptosis in T-antigen-positive human pleural mesothelioma cells. *Cancer Res* 1999; 59: 6068–6073.

149. de Klerk NH, Musk AW, Eccles JL *et al*. Risk of mesothelioma after environmental exposure to asbestos. *Eur Resp Rev* 1993; 3: 108–110.

150. Omenn GS, Goodman GE, Thornquist MD *et al*. Effects of a combination of beta-carotene and vitamin A on lung cancer and cardiovascular disease. *N Engl J Med* 1996; 334: 1150–1155.

151. Musk AW, de Klerk NH, Ambrosini GL *et al*. Vitamin A and cancer prevention I: Observations in workers previously exposed to asbestos at Wittenoom, Western Australia. *Int J Cancer* 1998; 75: 355–361.

152. Andersson M, Wallin H, Jonsson M *et al*. Lung carcinoma and malignant mesothelioma in patients exposed to Thorotrast: incidence, histology and p53 status. *Int J Cancer* 1995; 63: 330–336.

153. Robinson BWS, Musk AW. Benign asbestos pleural effusion: diagnosis and course. *Thorax* 1981; 36: 896–900.

154. Hillerdal G, Ozesmi M. Benign asbestos pleural effusion: 73 exudates in 60 patients. *Eur J Respir Dis* 1987; 71: 113–121.

155. Cookson WOC, de Klerk NH, Musk AW *et al*. Benign and malignant pleural effusions in former Wittenoom crocidolite millers and miners. *Aust NZ J Med* 1985; 15: 731–737.

23 MISCELLANEOUS DISORDERS

Daniel E. Banks and David J. Hendrick

INTRODUCTION

The lung has several important functions. At perhaps its most elementary level, it behaves as a bellows, allowing for the balanced exchange of oxygen and carbon dioxide. Because it is at the interface with the external environment, a second critical role is to protect the body from adverse environmental challenges. A large area of interface surface is involved (estimated to be approximately $100 \, m^2$); this implies that the protective mechanisms have to be particularly effective and that the lung itself is particularly vulnerable to injury. When the lung is injured, its ability to protect the body is often impaired, and infection (in particular) is a common consequence.

In this chapter concerning miscellaneous disorders and their causes, we consider occupational origins of lung injury that are not addressed directly in other chapters because they involve exposure routes other than inhalation, or because the disorder (or the exposure) is unusual and is not readily covered elsewhere.

IONIZING IRRADIATION

Matter is made up of atoms, the building blocks of molecules. The atom is electrically neutral ('matter in balance') and is structured so that in all atoms of the same element the number of electrons circling the nucleus is the same as the number of protons (but not necessarily neutrons) in the center of the atom. The atomic number identifying a particular element is determined by the number of protons, and the mass number is determined by the number of protons and neutrons. When the number of neutrons vary, the mass number varies, and these variants of a particular element are known as isotopes. Such isotopes may be unstable and may change into other elements with the release of radioactive particles (alpha-, beta-, or gamma-particles, X-rays, or neutrons depending on the element) in a process described as radiation. Change within the atom is described as radioactive decay, with the unstable atom described as a radionuclide.

Ionizing radiation is just that, radiation that dissipates energy within the cell resulting in the production of two ions from an atom; one being a negatively charged electron and the other a positively charged residual atom. Fracturing the atom causes the electron to rest a distance away from the original atom, making original recombination impossible, and leading to the adhesion of molecules with a negative charge (i.e. free radicals) to healthy molecules. These free ions exist for just a moment before reacting with ions of opposite charge, and they have a long-term potential to cause further biochemical damage including cell death, reproductive effects, and cancer.

Ionizing radiation may be attributed to exposure to higher energy particles (such as X-rays or gamma-rays) or to energetic subatomic particles such as alpha- or beta-particles and neutrons. The different radiations penetrate matter in different ways, as determined by the size, charge, and energy of each type. Alpha-particles (typically not a significant health hazard when exposure is delivered externally, but dangerous if internal exposure occurs) can be stopped by a thin piece of paper or dead layer of skin; by comparison, beta-particles can penetrate the hand but can be stopped by an aluminum shield. X- and gamma-rays require a lead shield to stop them from penetrating into the body. Neutrons are most potent (and tend to be the most penetrating because of the absence of electrical charge). They require concrete to halt penetration.

In addition, irradiation induces 'excitation' of the electrons within the residual atom, resulting in incomplete separation, but the generation of heat. This is also the end result of non-ionizing radiation, a term used to describe radiation that is insufficient to ionize but energizes and generates heat. Ionization and excitation may occur in all kinds of molecule within irradiated cells, and they can damage molecules through direct action. Cell death or serious mutation can occur if there is molecular damage such as the induction of double-bond breakage in the DNA molecule or damage to proteins responsible for vital cell function, such as cell division and growth, protein synthesis, or enzymatic reactions. Alternatively, an indirect action, possibly accounting for about two thirds of the damage attributable overall to irradiation, occurs through the irradiation of water in the cell (most effectively in the segment of the cell in close proximity to the genome) with the production of small, highly reactive water products such as hydroxyl radicals (OH·), hydrogen peroxide (H_2O_2), superoxide anions (O_2^-), and 'hydrated electrons'. Both direct and indirect actions induce chemical changes of biologic importance within the cell. Although full recovery of the cell may occur, a more likely result is cell death (the immediate effect of DNA injury), mutant offspring

(attributable to DNA and chromosomal damage), or clinically important late effects (such as the development of cancer following a latency period).

Yet, unlike other physical agents (e.g. heat or cold) that cause cellular injury, the amount of energy released within a cell involved in lethal radiation injury is very small (thought to be less than one millionth of the amount of energy needed for normal metabolic processes in the same cell over the same time period) with a very small fraction of the total number of available molecules exposed. This implies that the events induced by radiation injury must be amplified many times by intracellular mechanisms specific to radiation damage [1].

The damaging actions of irradiation can be modified by both physical and biologic factors. Physical ameliorating factors include shielding, less-intense ionizing radiation, lower doses, and diminished oxygen concentration within the tissues. Relevant biologic factors may include age, genetic make-up, gender, underlying state of health, diet, and endocrinologic state. Such variables have been assembled into a model which, for a given exposure, the size of the dose, the age and gender of the individual involved, and the elapsed time, can, for example, predict the excess relative risk for cancer [2].

There are three main occupational settings associated with recognized radiation risk: uranium mining and processing, the nuclear power industry, and healthcare work using ionizing radiation diagnostically or therapeutically.

Uranium mining and processing

Isotopes of radium occur naturally in the earth's crust and decompose to produce the radioactive gas radon (^{219}Rn, ^{220}Rn, ^{222}Rn); this diffuses from the soil into the atmosphere. Uranium ores release radon gas, and those employed in uranium mining and milling are at greatest risk of excessive exposure. The mining of other minerals from the earth's crust may pose a risk of lesser degree. Radon undergoes rapid radioactive decay (on average, an equilibrium between radon and its daughters is reached after about 3 hours). As radon particles breakdown within tissue into radon daughters, more radioactivity is released than from radon itself. These daughters are easily absorbed on solid surfaces, especially dust particles in the context of uranium milling and mining; they are inhaled, ingested, and absorbed through the skin. In miners, the lung is the primary port of entry into the body and radon absorbed to particles is retained in lung tissue, leading to the release of alpha-particles on the alveolar lining cells, as well as their absorption into the blood (with important subsequent localization in the kidney and in fatty tissues). In addition to lung cancer, associations have been suggested between exposure to radon progeny and other cancers, including leukemia, non-Hodgkin's lymphoma, malignant melanoma, and kidney cancer [3–6].

Radon is primarily excreted by exhalation, while radon daughters are eliminated mainly in feces and urine. Within mines and mills, the best approach to minimizing radon exposure to the worker is optimal ventilation, with the trapping of exhaust ventilation by filters to protect the ambient environment. Within the mine, important specific measures to minimize risk include rapid drilling and transport of ore, appropriate ventilation, and the sealing of sections without activity. If a safe-level ambient exposure cannot be achieved through engineering controls, personal protective measures will be needed.

The chief risk for those exposed to radon and its decay products is recognized to be lung cancer, and there is now considerable epidemiological evidence worldwide that uranium miners are at increased risk for the development of lung cancer after taking account of the effects of cigarette smoking. The use of radiation therapeutically has demonstrated additional risks for the development of pneumonitis and pulmonary fibrosis. Although occupational exposures, unless there is an accident, should generally be insufficient to cause such effects, Archer *et al.* have recently described five uranium miners in whom chronic interstitial pulmonary fibrosis with end-stage (honeycomb) lung was attributed more to occupational radiation than silicosis [7]. Uranium miners also appear to have increased risks for other lung diseases, though the contributions of ionizing radiation are not always readily separated from those of siliceous mine dust and smoking.

In the western USA, a number of mortality studies of Caucasian male (typically heavy smoking) uranium miners have revealed not only an increased incidence of lung cancer but also an increased mortality attributable to pneumoconiosis, tuberculosis, and renal failure [8–10]. A cohort mortality study on a second population of American uranium miners, all members of the Navajo nation, has also been serially reported [11,12]. In this group nearly 60% were never-smokers. The most recent study included all miners with one or more months of underground uranium mining and showed elevated standardized mortality ratios (SMR) for lung cancer (3.2), tuberculosis (2.6), and pneumoconiosis plus other respiratory diseases (2.6) [13]. When those with a longer duration of mining work were selected (400–1000 months), the SMR increased to 6.9 compared with the local non-White population. Intriguingly, a recent mortality report of Navajo men who died from lung cancer and resided in New

Mexico and Arizona from 1969 to 1993 showed that 63 of 94 (67%) were former uranium miners [14]. The relative risk for a history of uranium mining was 28.6. Smoking could not account for the strong relationship between lung cancer and uranium mining. This is a unique example where exposure occurring within a single occupation appears to have driven the mortality rate for lung cancer in the entire population. However, most underground uranium mines in the USA had shut by the late 1980s [15].

In one of the oldest studied cohorts, the mortality of more than 4000 Czech uranium miners who began work between 1948 and 1957 and had at least 4 years of underground mining was followed to 1985. The SMR compared with the mortality of men in the national population was increased approximately 4.5-fold [16]. In uranium miners from West Bohemia, where there was a fourfold increase in lung cancer incidence, there were additionally increases in incidence of liver and gall bladder cancers, but mortality did not increase with duration of employment or cumulative exposure to radon, and there has not been clear and consistent evidence that the risk for other cancers is increased [17].

In a mortality report of Chinese tin miners exposed to radon and radon products, the excess relative risk for lung cancer increased linearly by 0.2% per month of radon exposure at a specific working level, after adjusting for arsenic exposure, a recognized carcinogen found in relatively high amounts in this mining environment [18]. There have been two mortality studies of uranium miners from Ontario, Canada. The first showed a lung cancer SMR of 225 compared with that of the general Ontario population, but it attributed part of the excess to cigarette smoking and concomitant occupational exposure to arsenic. Lung cancer mortality in younger members of this population involved an unusually high percentage of small cell carcinomas [19]. The second study reported an increase in lung cancer mortality of approximately threefold among uranium miners. In this population, the risk for lung cancer was dramatically diminished by ceasing cigarette smoking [20]. In a final group, one of French uranium miners who had relatively low radon exposures while working for at least 2 years underground from 1946 to 1972, there was an excess of lung (and laryngeal cancer) with an increase in the SMR for lung cancer of 0.6% for each 'working level month' [21].

Nuclear power industry

A number of studies have addressed the mortality of workers employed in atomic energy workplaces. The first report showed no clear evidence of an increase in lung cancer in 4563 workers exposed to external radiation from 1950 to 1993 in a research and production facility in southern California. Of the 875 deaths, there was no increase in total cancers compared with the gender-adjusted US population, but there was an increase in the number of workers dying from leukemia [22]. In a larger study, a total of 22 552 workers employed between 1951 and 1982 by the UK Atomic Weapons Establishment were followed for an average of 18.6 years [23]. Of 3115 deaths, 865 (28%) were attributed to cancer. Mortality rates were 23% lower than the national average for all causes of death and 18% lower for cancer. Among the cancer deaths, only that of prostate cancer showed a clearly increased SMR (2.23). The outcome was attributed to selection biases, and the disproportionate recruitment of healthy individuals from the higher social classes. A similar conclusion can be drawn for US Los Alamos National Laboratory workers. The mortality of 15 727 white men employed from 1943 to 1977 was determined at the end of 1991. Again, there were fewer than expected deaths in this population as a whole and no increase incidence of any malignancy. However, among those who had measurable exposure to plutonium there was an SMR for lung cancer of 1.78 [24].

The importance of plutonium (^{239}Pu) exposure in the development of lung cancer was studied by a case-control methodology in workers at the Mayak nuclear enterprise in Russia [25]. Increasing absorption of ^{239}Pu (determined by urine assessment) was associated with an increasing risk for lung cancer (chiefly adenocarcinoma). Smoking proved to be more important, and a 5 pack-year cigarette smoking history (identified by questionnaire) doubled the lung cancer risk (chiefly for squamous cell carcinoma). No clear association was found with external gamma irradiation (determined by dosimetry badge measurements).

Healthcare services

Little information is available regarding the risk of radiation exposure in the healthcare industry. A mortality study of 143 517 US certified radiologic technologists who had worked with low-level ionizing radiation within the period 1926 to 1980 ended in 1990 [26]. For the group as a whole, the 7345 recorded deaths (73% in women) did not exceed the number expected, but for those employed prior to 1940 and for those employed for more than 30 years the SMR values for breast cancer were increased to 1.5 and 1.4, respectively. There was no excess of respiratory disease.

Determinants of disease

Several issues must be considered when addressing the risk from various types of radiation exposure. The latency period (time from first exposure to development of disease), age, and dose are all critical, and it is likely that smoking exerts a multiplicative interactive effect. Ritz [27] addressed mortality in 4014 radium processing workers and showed increased relative risks for all cancer mortality (1.92) and lung cancer mortality (2.77) per 100 mSv of external (gamma) radiation. The effects were strongest after long periods of surveillance and when exposure occurred at older ages. The estimated relative risk for lung cancer mortality from internal (alpha) radiation was somewhat less, being 1.92 from exposures of ≥200 mSv.

A study of 14 095 workers employed at the US Oak Ridge National Laboratory during the years 1943 to 1972 evaluated the cause of death up to 1990. All cancer mortality was associated with low-level ionizing radiation, similarly to lung cancer mortality, and increased by 4.98% per 10 mSv using a 10-year lag, but by 7.31% using a 20-year lag for doses received after age 45 years [28]. The associations were less strong for doses received before the age of 45 years.

The importance of exposure dose (and by implication threshold) is illustrated further by a mortality study among 5413 men who were employed for at least 2 years at a US plutonium weapons facility and had sustained low level exposures to plutonium and external radiation [29]. When compared to national US death rates, fewer deaths than expected were found for all causes of death, all cancers, and lung cancer. However, in those with plutonium body burdens greater than 2 nCi, an increase in all causes of death, all lymphopoietic neoplasms, gastrointestinal malignancies (esophageal, stomach, and colon), prostate cancers, and lymphosarcomas and reticulum cell sarcomas was recognized compared with fellow workers with lesser body burdens.

PARAQUAT POISONING

The best known bipyridyl pesticide is paraquat (1,1′-dimethyl-4,4′-bipyridilium dichloride), a nonselective plant-killing agent. Although recognized to be potentially highly toxic to both humans and animals if ingested in concentrated form, its use in agriculture has certain advantages because it is not only an effective pesticide but it also binds tightly to clay in the soil and is quickly inactivated.

Despite paraquat's well-recognized life-threatening toxicity following even small levels of exposure to the concentrated form, it has an otherwise remarkably safe track record after nearly 40 years of widespread use around the world [30,31]. Two studies of Malaysian rubber plantation workers engaged in spraying paraquat showed no ill effects after periods of, respectively, several weeks and 5 years [32,33]. The extensive investigation by Senanayake et al. of lung, renal, and hepatic function among tea plantation paraquat sprayers (mean employment of 12 years), general employees and tea factory workers on a tea plantation (a group without paraquat exposure), and local factory workers (also without paraquat exposure) showed no difference in measured parameters among these three groups [34].

Clinical features

Paraquat poisoning is characterized by multiorgan failure, most frequently kidney, liver, and lung. After oral ingestion, paraquat is rapidly absorbed by the gut. The peak serum level then declines over a period of hours, partly because the kidney filters and actively secretes paraquat from the blood and partly because it is absorbed by the kidney and other organs. As renal failure develops, an increasing proportion of blood-borne paraquat is taken up by perfused organs, and multiorgan failure accelerates. At the end of 24 hours, tissue paraquat levels are high and most is concentrated in the liver, kidney, and lung. Although paraquat injury is often thought to be lung-specific and to comprise a unique accelerated fibrosis, there are occasional reports where toxicity dominantly involved the kidney [35,36]. and resulted in acute renal failure [37,38]. Paraquat may similarly induce lethal liver disease. Kuo analyzed 189 cases of paraquat toxicity and showed that patients uniformly died if the total bilirubin level exceeded 3 mg/dl (30 mg/l) during the first week following ingestion [39].

Lung damage caused by paraquat was initially thought, incorrectly, to have a uniformly fatal outcome, and thousands have indeed died from ingestion of this agent since its introduction in 1962 [40,41]. Pulmonary death in the first few days is primarily the result of respiratory failure associated with hemorrhagic alveolitis and non-cardiogenic pulmonary edema (adult respiratory distress syndrome; ARDS). There may also be transient pleural effusions. Survivors of the initial acute injury are left with varying degrees of lung damage.

In 1991, Im et al. reported chest radiographic features of 42 individuals with paraquat poisoning [42]. Many features were non-specific, typically beginning with air space consolidation, and inevitably leading to end-stage pulmonary failure. The most common pattern on computed tomography

(CT) scans performed within the first 10 days after the initial exposure was a ground glass attenuation, typically bilateral and diffuse (likely correlating to areas of hemorrhage), inflammatory cell influx, and edema. This feature, often in combination with local areas of consolidation and/or irregular markings, was also recognized in scans performed during days 10 to 16 postexposure. It is consistent with the histologic development of patchy alveolar fibrosis. No definite relationship was recognized between the amount of paraquat ingested and the pattern, distribution, or extent of CT findings. On follow-up scans, many of the areas of ground glass appearance changed to consolidation with bronchiectasis and irregular lines [43], features reflecting the development of continuing fibrosis.

Exposure pathway

Paraquat is poorly absorbed through intact skin or the respiratory tract: less than 10% is absorbed. When ingested, the peak plasma concentration occurs in approximately 2 hours, and absorbed paraquat is sequestered in the lungs, by an energy-dependent active adenosine trisphosphate (ATP)-dependent transport system. Paraquat is not extensively metabolized, and much of the drug is excreted unchanged in the urine in the first 24 hours after exposure. If renal function is preserved, urinary excretion may continue for days or weeks after exposure, as paraquat stored in lung and muscle is slowly released in the blood.

There is, nevertheless, some potential for lethal lung injury whatever the pathway of exposure, be it ingestion, dermal contact, aerosol inhalation, or even intravenous injection [44]. When unintentional paraquat poisoning leads to death, the exposure (or exposures) may be considered trivial. Although paraquat may cause death by suicide or homicide, in many instances ingestion is accidental and the typically affected individual is the unknowing farm worker. In a summary of worldwide reported deaths occurring between 1964 and 1975, approximately two thirds were suicides, approximately 10% were homicides, and the rest were caused by accidental exposures [45]. Accidents are best recognized in agricultural workers and may involve confusion of bottle labels and contents (with the worker taking just a taste of concentrated paraquat); drinking water from a measuring cup which had contained paraquat; eating with hands contaminated with paraquat following preparation of pesticide spray; transferring paraquat between containers by sucking it through a hose; spilling paraquat on the mouth or skin, or spraying dilutions into the wind thereby contaminating open sores or wounds [46]. Although inhalation injuries are possible, they rarely cause serious toxicity, perhaps because most spraying equipment produces droplets that are too large to be respirable.

Fatal paraquat poisoning through skin absorption from a concentrated solution was first described by Jaros [47]. Levin *et al.* subsequently [48] described a farm laborer who held a container of paraquat in such a manner that the solution dripped to cause an open sore on his skin and progressive disease leading to respiratory failure and death. In nine coworkers, two had impaired diffusion capacity and underwent open lung biopsy. This showed pulmonary fibrosis and pulmonary artery muscular hypertrophy in one, and pulmonary artery muscular hypertrophy alone in the other. The changes in the pulmonary arteries were consistent with thrombotic disease, and they were thought to be attributable to paraquat exposure. Similar vascular changes were induced in rats who received daily topical applications of paraquat.

Paraquat poisoning in a pregnant woman has showed that paraquat crosses the placenta and is concentrated to a level four to six times that of the mother. Although typically fatal for the fetus, this is not uniformly the case. It has been suggested that survival is better at an early fetal age, but if the fetus is more than 30 weeks of gestation, there are rapid pulmonary manifestations of paraquat poisoning. As the fetus ages, the fetal lung appears to behave as a reservoir for paraquat, allowing slow paraquat excretion back into the maternal circulation [49].

Exposure dose

As a general rule, lung disease caused by paraquat ingestion is dose related [50–52]. Serum paraquat levels can be measured and survival correlates well with these levels. A large ingested dose of paraquat ion (over 40 mg/kg) is invariably fatal, while ingestion of lesser doses (20–40 mg/kg) may be fatal. Death is usually the result of progressive pulmonary fibrosis but can be delayed for several weeks [53,54]. It can follow the ingestion of as little as 10 ml of a commercially available 20% solution. With lesser exposures there may be acute, yet potentially reversible, lung injury. The overall death rates of paraquat poisoned individuals have ranged from 20 to 75% in different reported series [55], and development of renal failure is a poor prognostic sign [56]. In those who survived as long as 3 weeks after ingestion, measurable amounts of paraquat have been identified in the serum, lungs, liver, brain, kidney, spleen, and muscle. Myopathy is a recognized complication and muscle is a recognized source for the long-term release of paraquat in those who survive the acute period of injury.

Pathogenic mechanisms

Age, ingested dose, and the white blood cell count at the time of initial hospitalization have been shown to be correlated positively with mortality [57]. In those who survive the first few days of paraquat ingestion, there are persisting features of ARDS with fibrosis and distortion of the pulmonary architecture, dilatation of bronchioles and alveolar ducts, and local alveolar collapse. Increased deposition of collagen is clearly measurable in those who survive to day 20 [58], consistent with alveolar obliteration and progressive thickening of the alveolar septae because of deposition of protein-rich ground substance [59]. At about this time, there are two discrete areas of change in the lung. First, the lung structure is very disorganized with fibrosis. Second, some alveolar spaces are replaced by microcysts lined by fibrous tissue or filled with loose fibrous tissue [60,61]. Some areas of the lung nevertheless remain apparently unaffected and without measurably increased levels of collagen.

Paraquat is selectively concentrated in the lung and is enzymatically reduced continuously to a paraquat radical which reacts with oxygen and produces reactive oxygen species, hydrogen peroxide (H_2O_2), hydroxyl radicals (OH·), and superoxide $(O_2^-$ anions). Paradoxically, the use of supplemental oxygen, typically essential to prolong survival in those with serious lung injury attributable to paraquat, may further increase the concentration of O_2^- and potentiate lung injury [62]. These free radicals cause peroxidation of lipids within the cell membrane. Neutrophil influx into the lung following paraquat injury provides a further source of toxic oxidant radicals, which contribute to cellular damage, and additionally release potent proteases, which can damage connective tissue.

Schoenberger *et al.* [63] reported the effects of sublethal subcutaneous doses of paraquat given for 2 consecutive weeks to cynomolgous monkeys who underwent weekly bronchoalveolar lavage and were sacrificed at biweekly intervals over 8 weeks. Over time typical pulmonary fibrosis developed. Within 2 weeks, there was widespread alveolitis, characterized by inflammatory cells (macrophages and neutrophils) and fibrin accumulation with formation of hyaline membranes in the alveolar lumen. The neutrophil component of alveolitis ceased after 2 weeks. At 4 weeks, septal fibrosis with progressive inflammation was defined, with intact airways and blood vessels; at 8 weeks, there were severe interstitial changes with fibroblast infiltration and deposition of interstitial collagen with further lining of the fibrotic alveoli by cuboidal cells. Bronchoalveolar lavage showed that the collected macrophages produced fibronectin (a chemoattractant for fibroblasts) and alveolar macrophage-derived growth factor. This cytokine, with fibronectin, provides a stimulus for fibroblasts to duplicate and helps to explain the accumulation of these cells in the alveolar spaces.

In a second animal model, Shinozaki *et al.* [64] addressed sublethal paraquat effects on hemodynamics and lung mechanics in sheep given a 5 mg/kg intramuscular dose of paraquat. All sheep developed a transiently decreased hypoxic pressor response, progressive gas-exchange abnormalities, decreased dynamic compliance, and histologic evidence of fibrosis. The authors indirectly confirmed the role of free radical injury, showing that levels of superoxide dismutase (an enzyme which converts O_2^- to H_2O_2 in the lung, thereby lessening the free radical effect) were diminished, and levels of malondialdehyde (a marker of lipid peroxidation) increased within the first 3 weeks of exposure. In a similar approach in a rat model, Minakata *et al.* showed that there was an increase in the ascorbate radical, another marker of free radical injury, after paraquat intoxication [65].

As noted, the lung is a particularly vulnerable organ. Kinetic studies in dogs have shown higher paraquat concentrations in blood entering the pulmonary circulation compared with that in the pulmonary veins, and human investigations have shown an energy-dependent accumulation of paraquat in lung. The paraquat that is stored in this way may be released subsequently as the clinical course of the poisoned individual progresses [66–68]. Overall, it appears that the best chance to effect meaningful effective therapy is intervention during the very short time period in the initial phase prior to significant organ uptake.

Management

There have been a number of experimental therapies for paraquat-induced lung toxicity, all of which appear to have a reasonably sound physiologic basis, but their effectiveness has not been proven in any structured clinical trial. Although none can yet be recommended, anecdotal reports suggest that some may be effective. It remains unclear whether these interventions alter the natural history or change the frequently dismal outcome.

Once toxic levels of paraquat result in renal failure, there is diminished excretion in the urine. The key initial aim is, therefore, to minimize serum levels. This can be addressed first by lessening paraquat absorption from the gut. Since paraquat is readily bound to soil and clay, ingested Fuller's Earth (calcium montmorillonite) has been traditionally recommended. However, in a rabbit model of oral paraquat intoxication, activated charcoal was equally successful in lessening blood paraquat levels if given within the first hour of ingestion [69]. Thereafter neither agent had much effect. In a mouse model, activated charcoal's absorbing capacity for paraquat significantly exceeded that for Fuller's Earth when the charcoal was first suspended in magnesium citrate [70].

A second approach is to lessen blood paraquat levels following absorption. Forced diuresis, hemodialysis, peritoneal dialysis, hemoperfusion, and chronic arteriovenous hemofiltration (CAVH) have all been used. Large amounts of paraquat can be removed by both hemodialysis and forced diuresis, but forced diuresis has the lesser effect and becomes useless if renal failure supervenes. Even so, measurable levels of paraquat persist despite aggressive therapy, and after the first day little more paraquat can be removed by either approach [71]. Hemoperfusion has had mixed success. In several instances it gave no clear benefit in ultimate outcome when performed just once or twice [72–74] but when performed serially considerable amounts of paraquat were removed [75]. Pond performed initial hemoperfusion, followed by CAVH, on a man who died on day 12 after a paraquat ingestion suicide attempt, and showed that paraquat can be removed continuously using this approach [76].

The results of adding nitric oxide (NO) to the ventilator circuitry or bilevel airway pressure mask have been reported for two patients with paraquat-induced respiratory failure. In one, inhaled NO therapy was used for 25 days and the paraquat-poisoned individual survived [77,78]. During the course of this illness, clinical parameters of lung function declined whenever the NO was tapered or stopped, only to improve when NO inhalation was re-started. NO has been shown to inactivate directly O_2^- and oxidant-producing enzymes [79,80]. NO is thought to play a role in lowering pulmonary hypertension that may develop because O_2^- produced in the endothelium impairs the relaxation response of the blood vessel.

In 16 patients with paraquat intoxication (the largest series where a consistent approach to therapy has been reported), cyclophosphamide (1 g/day for 2 days) and methylprednisolone (1 g/day for 3 days) resulted in lower mortality (4; 25%) compared with that in 17 individuals in an historical control population (12; 71%) [81]. Although a second report showed similarly encouraging results [82], such benefit was not confirmed by prospective trials [83,84].

There is a suggestion that the addition of free radical scavengers might lessen the injury caused by paraquat by countering oxidative damage. MnTBAP, a low-molecular-weight metalloporphyrin that mimics superoxide dismutase, has been shown to protect against paraquat-induced lung injury in an animal model, as have other antioxidants, notably vitamin E in association with colchicine [85,86]. N-Acetylcysteine has been shown to have similar effects in an animal model [87,88] and in one human case of paraquat toxicity [89].

Outcome

There have been a number of studies reporting survivors of paraquat ingestion, but relatively few reports describing lung function in these individuals. Over the short term (assessment of lung function of survivors 3 months after paraquat exposure), there was significant recovery but without return to normal. This improvement was thought to be because of lessening or resolution of acute or subacute inflammatory and fibrotic changes in the lung, or resolution of pleural effusion [90]. Over the long term, there is evidence that an initial restrictive loss of ventilatory function may slowly improve over as long a period as 10 years, with lung function eventually approaching (but not achieving) base-line values [91].

Although there are reports of survival following lung irradiation after a potentially lethal paraquat ingestion [92], performed in an attempt to lessen the very exudative fibroblastic response post injury, this has not been proven to be an effective therapy [93]. Lung transplantation has been attempted, but because of the reservoir of paraquat in a number of the organs, most notably the muscle, the transplanted organ has been sufficiently damaged by paraquat released from stored organs that this approach was not successful [94,95].

LIPOID PNEUMONIA

Lipids, fat-like compounds of mineral, animal, or vegetable origin, contain long-chain fatty acids combined with an alcohol. They are oils at room temperature. The word lipoid is often used as a synonym for 'lipid', but more precisely refers to fat-like particles in the lung that look like lipids on histologic section. The clinical illness described as lipoid pneumonia reflects the lung's response to the accumulation of these lipids.

Endogenous lipoid pneumonia

There are two pathways by which lipids can accumulate in the lung. The endogenous pathway is of no relevance to occupation and results from the accumulation of cholesterol and its esters from the degradation of cells trapped distally in segments of obstructed lung. Such accumulations may be associated with malignancy, bronchiectasis, lung abscess,

fat emboli, pulmonary alveolar proteinosis, and glycogen storage disorders [96,97]. Macroscopically the lung in endogenous lipoid pneumonia has as a golden or yellowish appearance distal to an obstructing mass and is sometimes referred to as a cholesterol or golden pneumonia. Histologically, the airspaces are filled with macrophages with a foamy cytoplasm. As these degenerate, cholesterol and other lipids are released, and cholesterol clefts are formed [98].

Exogenous lipoid pneumonia

Most exogenous lipoid pneumonia is caused by the inhalation or aspiration of oil, a generally inert substance of pure hydrocarbon content [99]. Such agents do not readily elicit a cough reflex and so are not readily expectorated. Nor are they readily digested within the lung and they may illicit no more than a minimal response (a foreign-body-like reaction with local fibrosis) once emulsified and ingested by macrophages. Mineral and most vegetable oils do not undergo lipolysis and are therefore less fibrogenic, but when the exogenous lipid is of animal origin, lung lipase digestion may produce irritating fatty acids, and a pneumonitis results [100]. Most exogenous lipids will, however, induce an inflammatory reaction and subsequent pulmonary fibrosis eventually if present in the alveolar spaces for a sufficient amount of time [101,102]. A proliferative fibrotic response develops, the normal underlying architecture is lost, and an enlarging nodular mass (sometimes called a paraffinoma) may come to simulate a peripheral tumor (Fig. 23.1). By contrast, if lipid material is inhaled as an aerosol over a prolonged period, there may be a widespread pneumonitis and acute respiratory distress.

The natural history of the illness has been gleaned from serial evaluation of anecdotal cases, rather than formal epidemiological study. It is most frequently

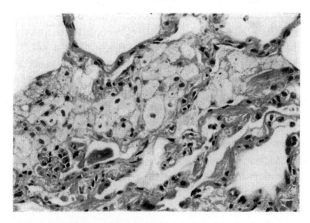

Fig. 23.1 Lung biopsy of a peripheral lung 'tumor' showing lipoid pneumonia. There is a proliferative fibrotic response disrupting the normal underlying pulmonary architecture.

an indolent process with a benign clinical course, although rarely an aggressive illness is seen and with continued exposure there may be progressive debility [103]. Recurrent pneumonias have been recognized in some cases, including infection and/or colonization with atypical mycobacteria, *Cryptococcus neoformans*, and *Aspergillus fumigatus* [104–106]. In an animal model, typically non-pathogenic rapid growing atypical mycobacteria caused progressive disease when injected in an oil suspension [107].

Diagnosis

The diagnosis of lipoid pneumonia is usually made by lung biopsy, but the finding of oil or lipid-laden macrophages (lipophages) in sputum, bronchoalveolar lavage (BAL) fluid, or fine needle aspirates may provide sufficient confirmatory evidence if the clinical features are already typical [108–111]. The specific identities of fats and oils recovered from BAL can be investigated by high performance thin-layer chromatographic purification, extraction, and infrared spectroscopic analysis [112].

Radiographically, the picture is variable. Ill-defined opacities are common, but more discrete lesions may be recognized and occasionally there is a discrete mass. The presence of air bronchograms suggests benign disease. High-resolution CT scans in subjects with proven lipoid pneumonia have given different appearances depending generally on the volume of retained oil and its residence time within the lung [113]. While the oil persists in the alveolar spaces following the briefest exposures, there are ground-glass opacities most often located in the dependent part of the lung that can mimic the 'crazy paving' of alveolar proteinosis [114]. When there are heavier exposures, a combination of alveolar and interstitial opacities may be seen as the emulsified oil is engulfed and transported from the alveoli by macrophages. With more marked exposures, lobar or segmental consolidation results, obliterating the vascular markings.

Occupational causes

In 1961, Jones reported a series of workers exposed to oil mists employed in a large UK steel rolling plant. Although radiologic abnormalities were noted, the workers did not report dyspnea and there was no detailed physiologic assessment [115]. Subsequent investigations of similar worker groups have demonstrated that aerosolized hydrocarbons may cause lipoid pneumonia and progressive respiratory impairment [116]. 'Machine oils' when aerosolized are also recognized to pose a risk for occupational asthma, but in general the inhalation

or aspiration of lipid material is not a common cause occupational lung disease. Most reported cases refer to sporadic episodes, often accidents or fires (shipwrecked sailors occasionally aspirate floating oil, and burning fats may release aerosols of lipid material), but their disparate nature suggests lipoid pneumonia of occupational origin can occur in diverse circumstances. This can be illustrated by three individual cases.

A 'fire-eater' in training inadvertently inhaled ignition fluids that contained paraffins. Acute chest pain, cough, and dyspnea were associated with a chest infiltrate, which resolved after several months [117]. A second case developed in a diver who breathed unfiltered air from an oil-contaminated surface compressor, and a third case arose in a 24-year-old man who was employed testing the effectiveness of 'restaurant fire control systems' in eradicating flash fires of vegetable oils, commercial lards, wood, and charcoals. He used a fire extinguisher containing sodium bicarbonate or mono-ammonium bicarbonate in an unventilated space in the absence of personal respiratory protection. He developed severe dyspnea, and showed a moderately severe restrictive loss of ventilatory function. A chest radiograph showed diffuse irregular markings at the bases and midzones, and a lung biopsy showed lipoid pneumonitis. He was given steroid therapy and improved [118].

Management

The treatment of lipoid pneumonia involves discontinuing exposure to the offending agent, identifying and treating complications, and providing supportive care. A number of methods have been tried, but no clinical trials have been attempted to define the best therapy. High doses of corticosteroids in an attempt to lessen inflammation is the most frequently reported approach [119,120], but oil removal using whole lung lavage [121] or repeated BAL [122] may also be effective.

PULMONARY ALVEOLAR PROTEINOSIS

First described in 1958, pulmonary alveolar proteinosis (PAP) is a rare disorder that exerts its primary effects in the alveolar spaces [123]. Over a period ranging from months to years, these become filled with an amorphous, largely cell-free, lipoproteinaceous material which is not readily expectorated. Inflammation and fibrosis are conspicuously absent and there are two major consequences. First, depending on the number of alveoli involved, the lungs become stiff, ventilatory function becomes restricted, and shunting occurs at the alveolar capillary level causing hypoxemia. The outcome is breathlessness, reduced exercise tolerance, and in some cases death from respiratory failure. The second major consequence, and a not uncommon cause of death, is secondary infection. The responsible organisms are generally those that are associated with intracellular infection and impaired T lymphocyte function, nocardia being particularly prominent. In many cases, however, extensive involvement does not occur, there being little or no progression, or even spontaneous remission. Epidemiological data are scarce but one estimate suggests an annual incidence of the order 2–5/million.

Pathogenesis

The cause in most cases is unknown, but an apparently identical (though steadily progressive) disorder can arise within months of massive exposure to respirable mineral dust, especially silica: both in the unfortunate worker exposed negligently without adequate respiratory protection and in experimental animal models. This has been called acute silicoproteinosis or silicolipoproteinosis. Less commonly aluminum dust may be responsible, and there have been reports inditing titanium and insecticides. A few reports describe affected sibships, implying a possible hereditary factor, and some associate PAP with hematological disorders (usually malignant and often after the use of cytotoxic agents) or immunodeficiency disorders.

The secreted material is rich in protein and phospholipid, and it stains strongly with periodic acid–Schiff (PAS) and eosin. The secretions are chiefly the product of surfactant-producing type II pneumocytes, and the chief phospholipid is dipalmitoyl phosphatidylcholine: the dominant phospholipid of normal surfactant. The secretion may also contain structures resembling tubular myelin that are derived from lamellar bodies of the type II pneumocytes. It is unclear whether the accumulation of these secretions results from an abnormality of the type II pneumocytes (excessive or abnormal production) or from impaired resorption by alveolar macrophages. Recent research suggests that both mechanistic avenues may be relevant, and it seems likely that the PAP phenotype can arise through a number of different mechanisms.

The vulnerability to infection with opportunistic organisms and the in vitro demonstration of a number of abnormalities of macrophage function possibly incriminate the macrophage more than the pneumocyte. This is consistent with PAP arising after macrophage function has been disrupted by massive exposure to silica, and with silicosis posing vulnerability to mycobacterial infection. It has been shown, however, that ingestion of PAP material may itself cause impairment of phagocytic function in macrophages harvested from normal controls, and so in some cases the primary abnormality could still lie with the type II pneumocyte and its alveolar secretions. This would be consistent with the belief that chemotherapeutic agents associated with the later development of PAP (e.g. bleomycin) are more likely to damage pneumocytes than macrophages. Support for this view comes from the recent demonstration of an inhibitory factor for granulocyte-macrophage colony-stimulating factor (GM-CSF) within the bronchoalveolar secretions of PAP to which GM-CSF binds more avidly than it does to the cells it should stimulate [124]. Its source of origin, however, has not yet been shown to be the type II pneumocyte.

Clinical features

The affected individual usually presents with progressive shortness of breath caused by the disease itself or with a pneumonic illness caused by superimposed infection [125]. Occasionally, the disease is without symptoms when it is first recognized from the appearances of an incidental chest radiograph. Cough is common but is rarely productive unless there is infection. There may be crackles and clubbing in advanced stages, and fever becomes characteristic when infection supervenes. When nocardia is not responsible for this, aspergillus, candida, cryptococcus, cytomegalovirus, histoplasma, human immunodeficiency virus (HIV), mucor, mycobacteria, pneumocystis, and viruses are the most common culprits.

Diagnosis

The chest radiograph characteristically shows an alveolar filling pattern, which radiates from the hila and simulates pulmonary edema. There is no other evidence of heart failure, however, and the appearances may be somewhat patchy and asymmetrical. Diffuse pulmonary fibrosis is very rare, unless provoked by complicating infection or when PAP is the consequence of exposure to fibrogenic dust. A micronodular infiltration is occasionally seen, but lymphadenopathy is characteristically absent. CT scanning, particularly with high resolution, shows the non-specific features of air space filling (ground-glass attenuation or consolidation) and commonly a patchiness, which distinguishes affected from unaffected lobules. There may also be septal thickening and hence the 'crazy paving' appearance typical of combined alveolar and interstitial disease.

Pneumonia or aspiration is often suspected initially, but the cough produces little or no sputum and no organisms are isolated if the disease remains uncomplicated. Occasionally white gelatinous material is expectorated, and bronchoalveolar lavage fluid is typically milky in color. Gallium scanning may be useful in showing negligible pulmonary uptake in contrast to the outcome seen in pneumonia. In established PAP, a positive gallium scan may be invaluable in suggesting the development of superimposed infection.

The key to the diagnosis of uncomplicated PAP rests with the demonstration that the alveolar secretions are strongly PAS-positive but contain no organisms and no excessive cellular response [126]. Indeed the macrophages appear to be deficient in numbers as well as function. Biochemical and immunochemical tests may be used to show that phospholipids and specific surfactant proteins are present in excess. Occasionally the sputum provides diagnostic material, identification of lamellar bodies or their debris by electron microscopy being particularly useful. These may be found within macrophages or pneumocytes or may lie free within the secretions. More commonly BAL [127] or lung biopsy is required, though the former may suffice since PAS-positive amorphous globules demonstrated by cytologic smears have high diagnostic specificity. Ultrastructural examination shows that these too generally contain multilaminated structures derived from lamellar bodies.

Management

In perhaps a third to a half of 'idiopathic' cases, no appreciable disability develops and the disease remits spontaneously or fails to progress, but when PAP is the result of massive exposure to silica there is unremitting progression. This may, however, be more a consequence of rapidly progressive silicosis than of PAP. Corticosteroids are of no value and may increase the risk of infection. Prolonged periods of inhalation therapy with expectorants (potassium iodide) or proteolytic enzymes (trypsin) have been claimed to offer some benefit but have caused frequent irritative responses in the airways. Furthermore, trypsin does not digest PAP material in vitro. Neither form of treatment is currently recommended, though the addition of trypsin to therapeutic BAL fluid has been reported to be both effective and well tolerated.

The most effective measure for PAP has been physical removal of the secretions by BAL, a procedure that may additionally be of value in limiting the rate of progression of silicosis. This is usually performed under general anesthesia using a double lumen endotracheal tube, one lung being repeatedly lavaged with a total of 20–50 liters warm sterile buffered saline while the other is mechanically ventilated (see Box 7.1). The procedure is then reversed so that the other lung is treated. When severe respiratory failure has already supervened despite ventilatory support, cardiopulmonary bypass has been used successfully to maintain gas exchange during the lavage procedure. An alternative is sequential lobar lavage using a fiberoptic bronchoscope and a cuffed catheter. Further lavage is usually necessary every few weeks or months, but the activity of the non-occupational disease may lessen and the frequency of this need may diminish.

The risk of premature death in non-occupational causes of PAP has been low in most series (mostly <10%), but a considerable threat to life is associated with complicating infection, and when massive exposure to silica is the cause, death is usually inevitable within a few years. It has been argued that regular BAL may limit the degree of immunosuppression and provide valuable prophylaxis against life-threatening infections [128].

DIFFUSE ALVEOLAR HEMORRHAGE

Pulmonary capillary (i.e. alveolar) hemorrhage is not a disease entity of itself, merely a clinical feature of several diseases. Most are not occupational in origin, but there is one well-documented occupational cause: exposure to the acid anhydride trimellitic anhydride.

While the lung can accommodate only small quantities of blood in the major airways without threatening life from asphyxiation, it can sequester surprisingly large amounts (liters) at alveolar level. This leads to a curious characteristic that is unique among diffuse parenchymal diseases of the lung, and which is of considerable diagnostic value: the carbon monoxide gas transfer (T_LCO) is elevated significantly above normal. Not only are physiologically useful red cells within the alveolar capillaries able to absorb the inhaled carbon monoxide, but so too are those lost from the circulation into the alveolar spaces.

Clinical features

Pulmonary capillary hemorrhage is characterized by hemoptysis, breathlessness, diffuse air space shadowing on the chest radiograph, anemia (normochromic normocytic if acute, iron deficient with chronicity), and an elevated T_LCO. The extravasated red cells are not readily expectorated, though enough generally escape to cause hemoptysis; consequently, hemosiderin accumulates within alveolar macrophages as the red cells and their debris are engulfed. When hemosiderin-laden macrophages are identified in sputum, the diagnosis is largely confirmed, but if sputum is not expectorated or hemoptysis is absent, minimal, or otherwise explained, BAL and/or lung biopsy is often necessary. An alternative approach is CT and magnetic resonance imaging, which may alone provide convincing evidence of blood sited diffusely within the alveoli [129]. Serial measurement of T_{LCO} can be used to monitor progression.

Causes

Diffuse pulmonary capillary hemorrhage is the principal clinical feature of Goodpasture's syndrome and idiopathic pulmonary hemosiderosis, but it may complicate a wide variety of disorders with immunologic, vasculitic, vascular, hemostatic, toxic, or unknown origins. Environmental factors are increasingly implicated, domestic exposure to the mold *Stachybotrys* having incited particularly interest in recent years. This may contaminate wet or damp accommodation, releasing a particularly potent toxin with hemorrhagic properties. This is now thought to have etiologic significance in some childhood cases of 'idiopathic' pulmonary hemosiderosis, perhaps in synergy with environmental tobacco smoke [130]. The toxic or allergic effects of other molds, bacteria and viruses, and hymenoptera stings have also been cited.

Acid anhydrides

Diffuse alveolar hemorrhage in the occupational setting was first reported in 1977 when airborne exposure to the manufactured powder of trimellitic anhydride (TMA) or fume from its use was recognized to cause a variety of respiratory problems [131–133]. TMA and other acid anhydrides are used as hardening agents in alkyd and epoxy resin systems. They are particularly valuable in producing durable coatings of paints, varnishes, and plastics and, like other epoxy resins, may cause occupational asthma and rhinitis. The clinical picture is very similar to that of other types of occupational asthma, suggesting that hypersensitivity mechanisms are responsible, and both IgE

and IgG antibodies to hapten–protein complexes (trimellityl human serum albumin and trimellityl human erythrocytes) have been demonstrated [134].

The ability of TMA to induce a diffuse pneumonitis with alveolar hemorrhage is, however, almost unique among occupational agents in general and occupational allergens in particular. Although severe pneumonitis of toxic origin may sometimes be associated with alveolar hemorrhage and TMA is thought to provoke toxic/irritant effects on the lung, when it is responsible for diffuse alveolar hemorrhage the mechanistic pathway appears to be primarily one of immunologic hypersensitivity [134,135]. Thus, recurrent hemorrhage may occur in the absence of evident toxicity, and anemia may become prominent. The term pulmonary disease anemia syndrome is sometimes used in consequence. In an early report of seven affected young men, all had a normochromic anemia [131]. Cough, hemoptysis, breathlessness, fever and weakness were further characteristic features together with ventilatory restriction, hypoxemia, and unilateral or bilateral pulmonary infiltrates. Biopsy tissue revealed extensive hemorrhage into alveoli, but no antibasement-membrane antibodies. Rapid improvement followed cessation of exposure without any other therapeutic intervention. A later survey of all 29 current workers identified five further cases.

Several subsequent studies have confirmed this curious property of TMA exposure. More recently a further acid anhydride has been cited as a cause of diffuse pulmonary hemorrhage, pyromellitic dianhydride [136], but further surveys of TMA workers have shown decreasing levels of exposure and fewer incident cases.

Management

Symptoms generally resolve within a matter of days or weeks following cessation of exposure, and so it is rarely necessary to provide palliative support. Corticosteroids may, however, be expected to speed recovery, and medication for asthma may be useful if there are associated asthmatic symptoms. Anemia is generally not of a degree to demand transfusion.

DIFFICULT CASE

History

A 34-year-old man had operated a rotary drill for 5 years in preparation for surface coal mining [137]. He and other members of the drill crews used large mobile rigs and a dry drilling technique to make bore holes for explosive charges.

Following detonation, the fractured rock strata overlying the coal seam together with soil and any vegetation (the overburden) was removed by other workers with heavy earth-moving equipment. The drill crews consequently worked in isolation, the drill operator sitting in a cab close to the drill.

He had been well for the initial $4\frac{1}{2}$ years, but over the following 6 months developed progressive undue breathlessness, dry cough, and weight loss (13 kg), leading to hospital admission. Examination revealed a slender man with tachypnea, coarse crackles at both lung bases, healed ulceration on several fingertips, and sclerodactyly, but no fever.

There was a restrictive loss of ventilatory function with a forced vital capacity (FVC) of 63% of predicted, and marked impairment of parenchymal function (T_LCO 18% predicted). Arterial blood gas analysis at rest breathing air showed hypoxemia (arterial oxygen tension, PaO_2, 63 mmHg (8.4 kPa)) with an arterial carbon dioxide tension ($PaCO_2$) of 32 mmHg (4.3 kPa) and pH 7.44. A chest radiograph showed a patchy bilateral basal air space filling abnormality. There were no hematological abnormalities, but microscopic hematuria was detected with mild proteinuria and occasional hyaline casts. The levels of blood urea and creatinine were 20 mg/ml (7.7 mmol/l) and 1.5 mg/100 ml (130 μmol/l), respectively, and the serum albumin was 21 g/l. The creatinine clearance was 2 ml/min and the urinary excretion of protein was 0.75 g/24 h. Serologic tests for cryoglobulins, antinuclear antibodies, and rheumatoid factor were negative and the level of the C3 component of complement was normal, though circulating immune complexes were noted. A tuberculin skin test was negative, but there was skin reactivity to mumps antigen.

Issues

The chief issue here is whether this man's respiratory illness could have arisen as a consequence (at least in part) of his occupational exposures to dust while drilling surface rock, an earlier regional survey having concluded that 'current surface mining techniques are not likely to lead to the development of pneumoconiosis'. Associated issues, before those of management and prognosis can be considered, relate to the differential diagnosis, and the need for further investigation.

Comment

An open lung biopsy was performed which showed that many alveolar spaces were filled with PAS-staining material, consistent with pulmonary alveolar proteinosis. There was additionally gross distortion of the pulmonary architecture with extensive interstitial fibrosis and scattered small non-caseating granulomas. Light microscopy under polarized light demonstrated weakly birefringent particles within the fibrotic tissue, and scanning electron microscopy with back-scattered electron imaging and energy dispersive X-ray analysis showed the particles to be quartz. Some granulomas were necrotic and packed with this crystalline material, and so the appearances were interpreted to indicate silicoproteinosis. Silica was additionally considered to be the cause of his renal disease [138].

Cyclophosphamide was used in the hope this might ameliorate any adverse effect of the circulating immune complexes, but there was relentless progression, and 14 months later a chest radiograph showed the appearances of progressive massive fibrosis (complicated pneumoconiosis) with conglomerate mass lesions in both lungs, right upper lobe volume loss, and tracheal deviation. There was additionally mild diffuse pleural thickening bilaterally. Antinuclear antibodies (homogeneous and peripheral pattern, titer 1/640) were then identified, and the FVC fell to 33% of predicted. Death followed 26 months after the initial presentation.

The chest radiographs of 9 of 10 fellow drill operators were examined, and two (of men aged 28 and 31 years with 4–6 years drilling experience) were considered to show simple pneumoconiosis, category 1/2q ILO classification. It proved possible also to review 20 personal dust samples that had been obtained routinely during work from both drillers and the subject of the Difficult Case. Only one of the 20 exceeded the allowable respirable coal limit of 2.0 mg/m^3, but there was no assessment of silica content. The overburden rock within the mining area was, however, sandstone.

🔑 SUMMARY POINTS

IONIZING RADIATION
Recognition
- Low-level ionizing radiation is an occupational hazard in the uranium mining and processing industry, the nuclear power industry, and healthcare services.
- The principal respiratory risk is lung cancer.
- The principal determinants for lung cancer are exposure dose, latency (lag time), worker age, and concomitant smoking.
- There is some evidence that low-level ionizing radiation may also contribute to diffuse interstitial pulmonary fibrosis in uranium miners (but there are confounding issues with related exposures) and breast cancer in healthcare workers.
- The adverse effects of high-dose therapeutic radiotherapy (acute pneumonitis, radiation fibrosis, infection) are not likely to occur in the occupational setting.

Management
- The management of lung cancer from occupational exposure to low-level ionizing radiation does not differ from that of lung cancer in general.
- There may be benefit from regular surveillance of exposed workers so that emerging lung cancer may be detected and treated at the earliest possible opportunity, thereby increasing the chances of curative surgery (Chapter 20).

Prevention
- Prevention requires the establishment of adequate exposure limits and compliance with them.
- Since current exposure limits may not be fully adequate, there is likely to be benefit from minimizing the levels of exposure and from limiting the employment of smokers and older workers.

SUMMARY POINTS (*contd.*)

PARAQUAT POISONING
Recognition

- Paraquat is a bipyridyl pesticide that causes marked, usually fatal, multiple organ toxicity (principally lung, kidney, and liver) after the ingestion of small doses of concentrated solutions.
- In the occupational setting (farming and horticulture) it may be ingested inadvertently, absorbed through the skin after spills, or inhaled unavoidably after diluted solutions are sprayed.
- Absorption through intact skin and healthy lung is poor, and death (even ill effect) is uncommon following exposure by non-oral routes.
- Fulminant pulmonary toxicity is manifested by non-cardiogenic pulmonary edema followed by relentlessly progressive pulmonary fibrosis; it is enhanced by renal toxicity and a consequent failure to excrete paraquat absorbed into the blood.

Management

- Ingested Fuller's earth or activated charcoal are recommended to minimize further gastrointestinal absorption, but their use more than an hour after ingestion may be disappointing.
- Forced diuresis, hemodialysis, peritoneal dialysis, hemoperfusion, and chronic arteriovenous hemofiltration may all remove paraquat from circulating blood, but benefit (if any) is likely to be limited to the first 24 hours after ingestion.
- Experimental treatment has included the use of nitric oxide inhalation, cyclophosphamide, and free radical scavengers, with some (anecdotal) evidence of success.

Prevention

- Accidental ingestion is the major threat to life from paraquat, and it should be countered by clear warning to users of the hazard involved, by clear labeling of any paraquat-containing (or contaminated) receptacle, and by cleaning or disposal of used containers.
- Particular care should be exercised when concentrated solutions are handled:
  - open skin wounds need protecting
  - spills should be washed thoroughly from the skin
  - food should never be consumed until contaminated hands have been washed
  - paraquat solutions should never be siphoned using negative pressure generated at the mouth.

LIPOID PNEUMONIA
Recognition

- Exogenous lipoid pneumonia generally results from the aspiration or inhalation of oily hydrocarbons that do not readily illicit a cough response.
- If, rarely, it is occupational in origin, it usually results from exposure to hydrocarbon aerosols.
- The radiologic appearances often suggest a localized pneumonia or tumor.
- The diagnosis is suggested by lipid-laden macrophages in sputum, BAL fluid, or lung biopsy material.

- Secondary infection may follow.

Management

- The causal exposure should be discontinued.
- If severe, therapeutic BAL may be useful.
- Complicating infection may require antibiotics.

Prevention

- The generation of oily aerosols should be avoided, controlled, or locally exhausted.

PULMONARY ALVEOLAR PROTEINOSIS
Recognition

- PAP is a rare disorder characterized by progressive breathlessness and the accumulation within alveolar spaces of lipoproteinaceous material derived from surfactant-producing type II pneumocytes.
- It is mostly idiopathic in origin, but it is occasionally a consequence of massive exposure to mineral dust, principally silica.
- It is often complicated in its advanced stages by infection.

Management

Patients with PAP of non-occupational origin generally respond well to lung lavage procedures and may cease to progress spontaneously, but in those with occupational PAP the disease is generally less responsive and more relentlessly progressive.

Prevention

The disorder is entirely preventable with adequate control of occupational exposures to mineral dust.

DIFFUSE ALVEOLAR HEMORRHAGE
Recognition

- Diffuse alveolar (capillary) hemorrhage simulating pulmonary hemosiderosis has been described in workers exposed to powder or fume arising from the manufacture or use of the acid anhydrides, TMA and pyromellitic dianhydride.
- The underlying mechanism appears to be one of immunological hypersensitivity (with demonstrable IgE and IgG antibodies), and the exposures may additionally induce occupational asthma.
- The most characteristic features of diagnostic relevance are the finding of hemosiderin-laden macrophages in pulmonary secretions, an increase in the gas transfer factor for carbon monoxide (reflecting the presence of red blood cells in alveolar spaces), and the demonstration of alveolar blood by CT scanning.

Management

The syndrome generally resolves within a matter of days or weeks following cessation of exposure.

Prevention

The disorder is preventable with adequate control of occupational of the relevant exposures.

REFERENCES

1. International labour office (Parmeggiani L (tech. ed.)). Encyclopedia of Occupational Safety and Health, 3rd edn, vol 2, pp. 1840–1897. 1989

2. National Research Council Committee on the biological effects of ionizing radiation. Health effects of exposure to low levels of ionizing radiation (BEIR V). Washington, DC: National Academic Press, 1990.

3. Hodgson JT, Jones RD. Mortality of a cohort of tin miners. Br J Ind Med 1990; 47: 665–676.

4. Henshaw DL, Eatough JP, Richardson RB. Radon as a causative factor in induction of myeloid leukemia and other cancers. Lancet 1990; i: 1008–1112.

5. Morrison HI, Semenciw RM, Mao Y et al. Cancer mortality among a group of fluorspar miners exposed to radon progeny. Am J Epidemiol 1988; 128: 1266–1275.

6. Radford EP, Renard KGSC. Lung cancer in Swedish iron workers exposed to low doses of radon daughters. N Engl J Med 1984; 310: 1485–1494.

7. Archer VE, Renzetti AD, Doggett RS et al. Chronic diffuse interstitial fibrosis of the lung in uranium miners. J Occup Environ Med 1998; 40: 460–474.

8. Archer VE, Gillam JD, Wagoner JK. Respiratory disease mortality among uranium miners. Ann NY Acad Sci 1976; 271: 280–293.

9. Hornung RW, Meinhardt JT. Quantitative risk assessment of lung cancer in US uranium miners. Health Phys 1987; 52: 417–430.

10. Roscoe RJ, Steenland K, Halperin WE et al. Lung cancer mortality among nonsmoking uranium miners exposed to radon daughters. JAMA 1989; 262: 629–633.

11. Gottleib LS. Lung cancer among Navajo uranium miners. Chest 1982; 81: 449–452.

12. Samet JM, Kutvirt DM, Waxweiler RJ et al. Uranium mining and lung cancer in Navajo men. N Engl J Med 1984; 310: 1481–1484.

13. Roscoe RJ, Deddens JA, Salvan A et al. Mortality among Navajo uranium miners. Am J Public Health 1995; 85: 535–540.

14. Gilliland FD, Hunt WC, Pardilla M et al. Uranium mining and lung cancer among Navajo men in New Mexico and Arizona, 1969 to 1993. J Occup Environ Med 2000; 42: 278–283.

15. Samet JM. Diseases of uranium miners and other underground miners exposed to radon. J Occup Med 1991; 6: 629–639.

16. Svec J, Tomasek L, Kunz E et al. A survey of the Czechoslovak follow-up of lung cancer mortality in uranium miners. Health Phys 1993; 64: 355–369.

17. Tomasek L, Darby SC, Swerdlow AJ et al. Radon exposure and cancers other than lung cancer among uranium miners in West Bohemia. Lancet 1993; 341: 919–23.

18. Xiang-Zhen X, Lubin JH, Lin-Yao L et al. A cohort study in Southern China of tin miners exposed to radon and radon decay products. Health Phys 1993; 64: 120–131.

19. Kusiak RA, Ritchie AC, Muller J et al. Mortality from lung cancer in Ontario uranium miners. Br J Ind Med 1993; 50: 920–928.

20. Finkelstein MM. Clinical measures, smoking, radon exposure, and risk of lung cancer in uranium miners. J Occup Environ Med 1996; 53: 697–702.

21. Tirmarche M, Raphalen A, Allin F et al. Mortality of a cohort of French uranium miners exposed to relatively low radon concentrations. Br J Cancer 1993; 67: 1090–1097.

22. Ritz B, Morganstern H, Froines J et al. Effects of exposure to external ionizing radiation on cancer mortality in nuclear workers at Rocketdyne/Atomics International. Am J Ind Med 1999; 35: 21–31.

23. Beral V, Fraser P, Carpenter L et al. Mortality of employees of the Atomic Weapons Establishment, 1951–81. Br Med J 1988; 297: 757–770.

24. Wiggs LD, Johnson ER, Cox-DeVore CA et al. Mortality through 1990 among white male workers at the Los Alamos National Laboratory: considering exposures to plutonium and external ionizing radiation. Health Phys 1994; 67: 577–588.

25. Tokarskaya ZB, Okladnikova ND, Belyaeva ZD et al. Multifactorial analysis of lung cancer dose-response relationships for workers at the Mayak Nuclear Enterprise. Health Phy 1997; 73: 899–905.

26. Doody MM, Mandel JS, Lubin JH et al. Mortality among United States radiologic technologists, 1926–1990. Cancer Causes Control 1998; 9: 67–75.

27. Ritz B. Radiation exposure and cancer mortality in uranium processing workers. Epidemiology 1999; 10: 531–538.

28. Richardson DB, Wing S. Radiation and mortality of workers at Oaklidge National Laboratory: positive associations for doses received at older ages. Health Perspectives 1999; 107: 649–656

29. Wilkinson GS, Tietjen GL, Wiggs LD et al. Mortality among plutonium and other radiation workers at a plutonium production facility. Am J Epidemiol 1987; 125: 231–250.

30. Howard JK. Paraquat: a review of worker exposure in normal usage. J Soc Occup Med 1990; 30: 6–11.

31. Hart TB. Paraquat: a review of safety and in agricultural and horticultural use. Hum Toxicol 1987; 6: 13–18.

32. Swan AAB. Exposure of spray operators to paraquat. Br J Ind Med 1969; 26: 322–329.

33. Howard JK, Sabapathy NN, Whitehead AP. A study of the health of Malaysian plantation workers with particular reference to paraquat spraymen. Br J Ind Med 1981; 38: 110–116.

34. Senanayake N, Gurunathan G, Hart TB et al. An epidemiological study of the health of Sri Lankan tea plantation workers associated with long term exposure to paraquat. Br J Ind Med 1993; 50: 257–283.

35. Florowski CM, Bradberry SM, Ching GWK et al. Acute renal failure in a case of paraquat poisoning with relative absence of pulmonary toxicity. Postgrad Med J 1992; 68: 660–662.

36. Sobha H, Pushpakumari P, Nampoori MR et al. Paraquat poisoning with acute renal failure – a case report. J Assoc Physicians India 1989; 37: 34111–342.

37. Bullivant CM. Accidental poisoning by paraquat: Report of two cases in man. Br Med J 1996; i: 1272–1273.

38. Vaziri ND, Ness RL, Fairshter RD et al. Nephrotoxicity of paraquat in man. Toxicol Appl Pharmacol 1979; 34: 178–1186.

39. Kuo CH, Sheen IS, Huang CC et al. Liver biochemical tests in paraquat intoxication. Chang Gung Med 1988; 11: 160–166.

40. Cooke NJ, Flenley CD, Matthew H. Paraquat poisoning. Q J Med 1973; 42: 683–692.

41. Onyon L, Volans G. The epidemiology and prevention of paraquat poisoning. Hum Toxicol 1987; 6: 19–26.

42. Im JG, Lee KS, Han MC et al. Paraquat poisoning: findings on chest radiography and CT in 42 patients. AIR 1991; 157: 697–701.

43. Lee SH, Lee KS, Ahn JM et al. Paraquat poisoning of the lung: thin-section CT findings. *Radiology* 1995; 195: 271–274.

44. Pedrazzini GB, Saglini V, Pedrinis E et al. Fatal voluntary poisoning by parenteral paraquat. *Schweiz Med Wochenschr* 1991; 121: 1293–1297.

45. Rebello G, Mason JK. Pulmonary histological appearances in fatal paraquat poisoning. *Histopathology* 1978; 2: 53–66.

46. Wesseling C, Hogstedt C, Picado A et al. Unintentional fatal paraquat poisonings among agricultural workers in Costa Rico: report of 15 cases. *Am J Industr Med* 1997; 32: 433–441.

47. Jaros F. Acute percutaneous paraquat poisoning. *Lancet* 1978; i: 275–277.

48. Levin PJ, Klaff LJ, Rose AG et al. Pulmonary effects of contact exposure to paraquat: a clinical and experimental study. *Thorax* 1979; 34: 150–160.

49. Tsatsakis AM, Perakis K, Koumantakis E. Experience with acute paraquat poisoning in Crete. *Vet Human Toxicol* 1996; 38: 113–117.

50. Higenbottam T, Crome P, Parkinson C et al. Further clinical observations on the pulmonary effects of paraquat ingestion. *Thorax* 1979; 34: 161–165.

51. George M, Hedworth-Whitty RB. Non-fatal lung disease due to inhalation of nebulized paraquat. *Br Med J* 1980; 280: 902.

52. Hendy MS, Williams PS, Ackrill P. Recovery from severe pulmonary damage due to paraquat administered intravenously and orally. *Thorax* 1984; 39: 874–875.

53. Hudson M, Patel SB, Ewen SWB et al. Paraquat induced pulmonary fibrosis in three survivors. *Thorax* 1991; 46: 201–204.

54. Fock KM, Chan HC. Paraquat poisoning is not always fatal. *Singapore Med J* 1980; 5: 703–707.

55. Onyon LJ, Volans GN. The epidemiology and prevention of paraquat poisoning. *Hum Toxicol* 1987; 6: 19–29.

56. Bismuth C, Garnier R, Dally S et al. Prognosis and treatment of paraquat poisoning: a review of 28 cases. *J Toxicol Clin Toxicol* 1982; 19: 461–474.

57. Kaojaren S, Ongphiphadhanakul B. Predicting outcomes in paraquat poisonings. *Vet Hum Toxicol* 199; 33: 115–8.

58. Yamaguchi M, Takahashi T, Togashi H et al. The corrected collagen content in paraquat lungs. *Chest* 1986; 90: 251–257.

59. Takahashi T, Takahashi Y, Yamaguchi M et al. Morphologic and morphometric analysis of human paraquat lungs. *Pathol Clin Med* 1984; 2: 1343–1353.

60. Thurlbeck WM, Thurlbeck SM. Pulmonary effects of paraquat poisoning. *Chest* 1976; 69(Suppl.): 276–280.

61. Takahashi T, Takahashi Y, Nio M. Remodeling of the alveolar structure in the paraquat lung of humans: a morphometric study. *Hum Pathol* 1994; 25: 702–708.

62. Fisher HK, Clements JA, Wright RR. Enhancement of oxygen toxicity by the herbicide paraquat. *Am Rev Respir Dis* 1973; 107: 246–253.

63. Schoenberger CI, Rennard SI, Bitterman PB et al. Paraquat-induced pulmonary fibrosis: role of alveolitis in modulating the development of fibrosis. *Am Rev Respir Dis* 1984; 1229: 168–173.

64. Shinozaki S, Kobayashi T, Kubo K et al. Pulmonary hemodynamics and lung function during chronic paraquat poisoning in sheep. *Am Rev Respir Dis* 1992; 146: 775–780.

65. Minakata K, Suzuki O, Saito S-i et al. Ascorbate radical levels in human sera and rat plasma intoxicated with paraquat and diquat. *Arch Toxicol* 1993; 67: 126–130.

66. Brooke-Taylor S, Smith LL, Cohen GM. The accumulation of polyamines and paraquat by human peripheral lung. *Biochem Pharmacol* 1983; 32: 717–720.

67. Hawksworth GM, Bennett PN, Davies DS. Kinetics of paraquat elimination in the dog. *Toxicol Appl Pharmacol* 1981; 57: 139–145.

68. Baud FJ, Jaeger A, Keyes C. Toxicokinetics of paraquat through the heart–lung block: six cases of acute human poisoning. *Clin Toxicol* 1988; 26: 35–50.

69. Idid SZ, Lee CY. Effects of Fuller's Earth and activated charcoal on oral absorption of paraquat in rabbits. *Clin Exp Pharmacol Physiol* 1996; 23: 679–81.

70. Gaudreault P, Friedman PA, Lovejoy FH Jr. Efficacy of activated charcoal and magnesium citrate in the treatment of oral paraquat intoxication. *Ann Emerg Med* 1985; 14: 123–5.

71. Fairshter RD, Dabir-Vaziri N, Smith WR et al. Paraquat poisoning: an analytical toxicologic study of three cases. *Toxicology* 1979; 12: 259–266.

72. Mascie-Taylor BH, Thompson J, Davidson AM. Haemoperfusion ineffective for paraquat removal in life-threatening poisoning. *Lancet* 1983; ii: 1376–1377.

73. Bismuth C, Scherrmann JM, Garnier R et al. Elimination of paraquat. *Hum Toxicol* 1987; 6: 63-67

74. Van de Vyver FL, Guiliano RA, Paulus GJ et al. Hemoperfusion–hemodialysis ineffective for paraquat removal in life-threatening poisoning? *J Toxicol Clin Toxicol* 1985; 23: 117–131.

75. Okonek S, Weilemann LS, Majdandzic J et al. Successful treatment of paraquat poisoning by activated charcoal per os and continuous hemoperfusion. *J Toxicol Clin Toxicol* 1982–8; 19: 807–819.

76. Pond SM, Johnston SC, Schoof DD et al. Repeated hemoperfusion and continuous arteriovenous hemofiltration in a paraquat poisoned patient. *Clin Toxicol* 1987; 25: 305–316.

77. Eisenman A, Armali Z, Raikhlin-Eisenkraft B et al. Nitric oxide inhalation for paraquat-induced lung injury. *Clin Toxicol* 1998; 36: 575–584.

78. Koppel C, Wissman CV, Barckow D et al. Inhaled nitric oxide in advanced paraquat intoxication. *Clin Toxicol* 1994; 32: 205–214.

79. Fukahori M, Ichimori K, Ishida H et al. Nitric oxide reversibly suppresses xanthine oxidase activity. *Free Radical Res* 1994; 21: 203–212.

80. Rubanyi GM, Ho EH, Cantor EH et al. Cytoprotective function of nitric oxide: inactivation of superoxide radicals produced by human leucocytes. *Biochem Biophys Res Commun* 1991; 181: 1392–1397.

81. Lin JL, Wei MC, Liu YC. Pulse therapy with cyclophosphamide and methylprednisolone in patients with moderate to severe paraquat poisoning: A preliminary study. *Thorax* 1996; 51: 661–663.

82. Addo E, Poon-King T. Leukocyte suppression in treatment of 72 patients with paraquat poisoning. *Lancet* 1986; 1: 1117–1120.

83. Perriens JH, Benimadho S, Kiauw IL et al. High-dose cyclophosphamide and dexamethasone in paraquat poisoning: a prospective study. *Hum Exp Toxicol* 1992; 11: 129–134.

84. Nogue S, Munne P, Campana E et al. Failure of a cyclophosphamide–dexamethasone combination in

paraquat poisoning. *Med Clin (Barcelona)* 1989; 93: 61–63.

85. Day BJ, Crapo JD. A metalloporphyrin superoxide dismutase mimetic protects against paraquat-induced lung injury *in vivo*. *Toxicol Appl Pharmacol* 1996; 99: 77–88.

86. Shahar E, Keidar I, Herzog E *et al*. Effectiveness of vitamin E and colchicine in amelioration of paraquat lung injuries using an animal model. *Isr J Med Sci* 1989; 25: 92–94.

87. Wegener T, Sandhagen B, Chan KW, *et al*. N-Acetyl-cysteine in paraquat toxicity: toxicological and histological evaluation in rats. *Uppsala J Med Sci* 1988; 93: 81–89.

88. Hoffer E, Avidor I, Benjamin O *et al*. N-Acetyl cysteine delays the infiltration of inflammatory cells into the lungs of paraquat-intoxicated rats. *Appl Pharmacol* 1993; 120: 8–12.

89. Lheureux P, Leduc D, Vanbinst R *et al*. Survival in a case of massive paraquat ingestion. *Chest* 1995; 107: 285–289.

90. Lin J-L, Liu L, Leu M-L. Recovery of respiratory function in survivors with paraquat intoxication. *Arch Environ Health* 1995; 50: 432–439.

91. Bismuth C, Hall AH, Baud FJ. Pulmonary dysfunction in survivors of acute paraquat poisoning. *Vet Hum Toxicol* 1996; 38: 220–222.

92. Webb DB, Williams MV, Davies BH *et al*. Resolution after radiotherapy of severe pulmonary damage due to paraquat poisoning. *Br Med J* 1984; 288: 1259–1260.

93. Franzen D, Baer F, Heitz W *et al*. Failure of radiotherapy to resolve fatal lung damage due to paraquat poisoning. *Chest* 1991; 100: 1164–1165.

94. Matthews H, Logan A, Woodruff MFA *et al*. Paraquat poisoning – lung transplantation. *Br Med J* 1968; 3: 759–763.

95. The Toronto Lung Transplant Group. Sequential bilateral lung transplantation for paraquat poisoning. *J Thorac Cardiovasc Surg* 1985; 89: 734–742.

96. DeNavasquez S, Haslewood GAD. Endogenous lipoid pneumonia with special reference to carcinoma of the lung. *Thorax* 1954; 9: 35–37.

97. Genereux GP. Lipids in the lung: radiologic–pathologic correlation. *J Can Assoc Radiol* 1970; 21: 2–15.

98. Katzenstien A–LA. Miscellaneous II. Nonspecific inflammatory and destructive diseases of the lung. In: Katzenstein A-LA, Askin FB, eds. *Surgical Pathology of Non-neoplastic Lung Disease*, Volume 3 in series *Major problems in Pathology*: consulting ed.: Bennington JL . Philadelphia, PA: Saunders, 1985: 382–387

99. Wright BA, Jeffrey PH. Lipoid pneumonia. *Semin resp infect* 1990; 5: 314–321.

100. Antico A, Gabrielli M, D'Aversa C *et al*. Lipoid pneumonia: a case of cavitary bilateral nodular opacity. *Monalid Arch Chest Dis* 1996; 51: 296–298.

101. Lipinski JK, Weisbord GL, Sanders DE. Exogenous lipoid pneumonitis. *J Can Assoc Radiol* 1980; 31: 92–98.

102. Brody JS, Levin B. Interlobular septal thickening in lipid pneumonia. *Am J Roentgenol* 1962; 88: 1061–1069.

103. Spickard III A, Hirschmann JV. Exogenous lipoid pneumonia. *Arch Intern Med* 1994; 154: 686–692.

104. Jouannic I, Desrues B, Lena H *et al*. Exogenous lipoid pneumonia complicated by *Mycobacterium fortuitum* and *Aspergillus fumigatus* infections. *Eur Respir J* 1996; 9: 172–174.

105. Subramanian S, Kherdekar SS, Babu PGV *et al*. Lipoid pneumonia with *Cryptococcus neoformans* pneumonia. *Thorax* 1982; 37: 319–320.

106. Dreisin RB, Scoggin C, Davidson PT. The pathogenicity of *Mycobacterium fortuitum* and *M. chelonei* in man: a report of seven cases. *Tubercule* 1976; 57: 49–57.

107. Kudoh S. The virulence of saprophytic acid-fast bacteria coated with oil or fat: I. Intrapulmonary and subcutaneous inoculation of saprophytic acid-fast bacteria coated with liquid paraffin. *Jpn J Bacteriol* 1962; 17: 154–162.

108. Wheeler PB, Stitik FP, Hutchins G *et al*. Diagnosis of lipoid pneumonia by computed tomography. *JAMA* 1981; 245: 65–66.

109. Weill H, Ferrans VJ, Gay RM. Early lipoid pneumonia: roentgenologic, anatomic, and physiologic characteristics. *Am J Med* 1964; 36: 370–376.

110. Keshishian JM, Abad JM, Fuchs M. Lipoid pneumonia. *Ann Thorac Surg* 1996; 7: 231–234.

111. Silverman JF, Turner RC, West RL *et al*. Bronchoalveolar lavage in the diagnosis of lipoid pneumonia. *Diag Cytol* 1989; 5: 3–8.

112. Penes MC, Valion JJ, Sabot JF *et al*. GC/MS detection of paraffins in a case of lipoid pneumonia following occupational exposure to oil spray. *J Anal Toxicol* 1990; 14: 372–374.

113. Lee JS, Im J-G, Song KM *et al*. Exogeneous lipoid pneumonia: high resolution CT findings. *Eur Radiol* 1999; 9: 287–291.

114. Franquet T, Gimenez A, Bordes R *et al*. The crazy paving pattern in exogenous lipoid pneumonia: CY–pathologic correlation. *Am J Roentgenol* 1998; 170: 315–317.

115. Jones JG. An investigation into the effects of exposure to an oil mist in a mill for the cold reduction of steel strip. *Ann Occup Hyg* 1961; 3: 264–271.

116. Cullen MR, Balmes JR, Robins JM *et al*. Lipoid pneumonitis caused by oil mist exposure from a steel rolling tandem mill. *Am J Industr Med* 1981; 2: 51–58.

117. Beerman B, Christensson T, Moller P, *et al*. Lipoid pneumonia: an occupational hazard of fire eaters. *BMJ* 1984; 289: 1728–1729.

118. Oldenburger D, Maurer WJ, Beltaos E *et al*. Inhalation lipoid pneumonia from burning fats. *JAMA* 1972; 222: 1288–1289.

119. Ayvazian LF, Steward DS, Merkel CG *et al*. Diffuse lipoid pneumonitis successfully treated with prednisone. *Am J Med* 1967; 43: 930–934.

120. Nagrath SP, Sapru. Lipoid pneumonia: review of the literature with a case report. *J Ind Med Assoc* 1964; 42: 453–456.

121. Chang H-Y, Chen C-W, Chen C-Y *et al*. Successful treatment of diffuse lipoid pneumonitis with whole lung lavage. *Thorax* 1993; 48: 947–948.

122. Levade, Salvayre R, Dongay G *et al*. Chemical analysis of the bronchoalveolar lavage washing fluid in the diagnosis of liquid paraffin pneumonia. *J Clin Chem Biochem* 1987; 25: 45–48.

123. Wang BM, Stern EJ, Schmidt RA, Pierson DJ. Diagnosing pulmonary alveolar proteinosis: a review and an update. *Chest* 1997; 111: 460–466.

124. Tanaka N, Watanabe J, Kitamura T *et al*. Lungs of patients with idiopathic pulmonary alveolar proteinosis express a factor which neutralizes granulocyte-macrophage stimulating factor. *FEBS Lett* 1999; 442: 246–250.

125. Goldstein LS, Kavuru MS, Curtis-McCarthy P *et al.* Pulmonary alveolar proteinosis: clinical features and outcomes. *Chest* 1998; 114: 1357–1362.

126. Burkhalter A, Silverman JF, Hopkins MB, Geisinger KR. Bronchoalveolar lavage cytology in pulmonary alveolar proteinosis. *Am J Clin Pathol* 1996; 106: 504–510.

127. Mikami T, Yamamoto Y, Yokoyama M, Okayasu I. Pulmonary alveolar proteinosis: diagnosis using routinely processed smears of bronchoalveolar lavage fluid. *J Clin Pathol* 1997; 50: 981–984.

128. Hoffman RM, Dauber JH, Rogers RM. Improvement in alveolar macrophage migration after therapeutic whole lung lavage in pulmonary alveolar proteinosis. *Am Rev Respir Dis* 1989; 139: 1030–1032.

129. Weishaupt D, Hilfiker PR, Schmidt M, Debatin JF. Pulmonary hemorrhage: imaging with a new magnetic resonance blood pool agent in conjunction with breathheld three-dimensional magnetic resonance angiography. *Cardiovasc Intervent Radiol* 1999; 22: 321–325.

130. Anonymous. From the Centers for Disease Control and Prevention. Update: pulmonary hemorrhage/hemosiderosis among infants – Cleveland, Ohio, 1993–1996. *JAMA* 2000; 283: 1951–1955.

131. Herbert FA, Oxford R. Pulmonary hemorrhage and edema due to inhalation of resins containing tri-mellitic anhydride. *Chest* 1979; 6: 546–551.

132. Rice DL, Jenkins DE, Gray JM. Chemical pneumonitis secondary to inhalation of epoxy pipe coating. *Arch Environ Health* 1977; 32: 173–178.

133. Zeiss CR, Patterson R, Pruzansky JJ *et al.* Trimellitic anhydride-induced airway syndromes: clinical and immunologic studies. *J Allergy Clin Immunol* 1977; 60: 96–103.

134. Patterson R, Addington W, Banner AS *et al.* Antihapten antibodies in workers exposed to trimellitic anhydride fumes: a potential immunopathogenetic mechanism for the trimellitic anhydride pulmonary disease – anemia syndrome. *Am Rev Respir Dis* 1979; 120: 1259–1267.

135. Grammer LC, Shaughnessy MA, Zeiss CR *et al.* Review of trimellitic anhydride (TMA) induced respiratory response. *Allergy Asthma Proc* 1997; 18: 235–237.

136. Kaplan V, Baur X, Czuppon A *et al.* Pulmonary hemorrhage due to inhalation of vapor containing pyromellitic dianhydride. *Chest* 1993; 104: 644–645.

137. Banks DE, Bauer MA, Castellan RM, Lapp NL. Silicosis in surface coal mine drillers. *Thorax* 1983; 38: 275–278.

138. Banks DE, Milutinovic J, Desnick RJ *et al.* Silicon nephropathy mimicking Fabry's disease. *Am J Nephrol* 1983; 3: 279–284.

PARTICULAR INDUSTRIES
AND ASSOCIATED DISORDERS

24 AUTOMOTIVE INDUSTRY

Gianna Moscato, Aurelia Carosso, and Canzio Romano

INTRODUCTION

The automotive industry is engaged in the manufacture of automobiles, industrial and agricultural vehicles, and motorcycles. Technologies, and consequently health risk factors, are quite similar in these different settings, but in the manufacture of trucks, buses, and farm and construction equipment production rates are slower and processes less mechanized [1]. Major changes have occurred since the early 1980s in both the end-products and in production technologies. On the one hand, vehicles are progressively less 'ferrous' and progressively more 'plastic', which is probably shifting the spectrum of related lung diseases from pneumoconiosis to asthma [2,3]. On the other hand, the automotive (mainly the automobile) industry has been subject to much mechanization and automation. Transfer lines are increasingly taking the place of single machines, machines are frequently controlled by computer, and robots are being substituted for men in the more dangerous operations. This has led to a reduction (and frequently to a lack) of direct contact of the worker with the industrial process, and with a reduction of the related risks to the lungs.

The processes involved in the production of vehicles are numerous, complex, and varied. They, and the related hazards, will, therefore, be dealt with according to the sequence of the production cycle. Separate manufacturing plants producing necessary components support the 'core' assembly line for the production of vehicles. Traditionally, vehicle producers themselves manufacture the iron and steel components necessary for the construction of the 'bodies' and engines, and most have both ferrous and aluminum foundries in their production cycle. In Figure 24.1, shaded areas indicate the main processes and final products that are directly related to the automotive industry; the unshaded areas address the 'external' production of components. In Figure 24.2 the principal respiratory diseases associated with each process are identified.

The automotive industry is traditionally a large-scale industry, and production managers have focused on work safety and hygiene for a long time. It is important to realize that although many hazardous agents are used together with potentially hazardous processes, the level of risk has generally been brought to very low levels. The risks identified in this chapter may consequently be more theoretical than real in most sections of this particular industry.

FOUNDRY PROCESSES

Ferrous and steel foundries are used in the automobile industry to produce engine blocks, heads, and other parts. There are two basic types of ferrous foundry: grey iron foundries use scrap iron or pig iron (new ingots) to make standard iron castings, mainly used for crankcases; ductile iron foundries add magnesium, cerium, or other additives (often called ladle additives) to the ladles of molten metal before pouring to make nodular or malleable iron castings, mainly used for drive shafts, axles, and

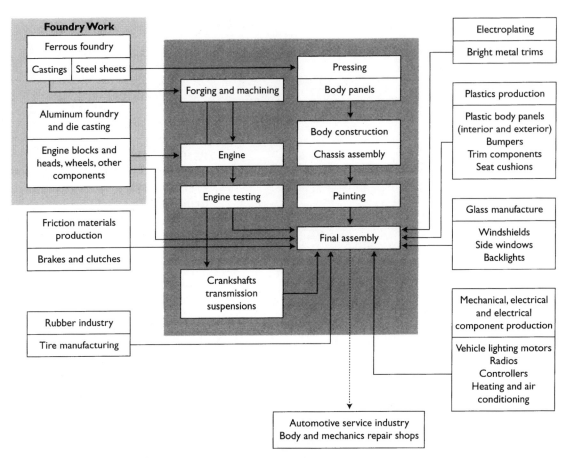

Fig. 24.1 Processes and final products of the automotive industry. The shaded areas indicate processes directly incorporated into the automotive industry, unshaded areas cover the external production of components. Foundry work is often managed directly by automotive companies, though generally on sites separate from the main production and assembly plant.

joints. The purpose of the steel foundries is to convert pig iron into a more elastic steel that can be forged and fabricated. This is obtained by a reduction of the carbon content and by the oxidation and removal of the impurities contained in pig iron. The incorporation of other metals produces special steel alloys with particular resistance to rust (chromium), hardness and toughness at high temperature (tungsten), strength, ductility and corrosion resistance (nickel). Molten metal is poured into molds or continuous-casting machines to form ingots or billets, which subsequently pass to the rolling mills or other processing.

The technology has changed over the years and the processes are presently more mechanized and automatic; wooden patterns have been replaced by patterns of metal and plastic, new substances have been developed for producing cores and molds, and a wide range of alloys are used. Prior to the 1960s, core mixtures comprised sand and binders, such as linseed oil, molasses or dextrin (oil sand), and molds were made from silica sand bound with clay. Now molding sand is usually damp or mixed with liquid resin; it is, therefore, less likely to be a significant

source of respirable dust. A 'parting' (or 'releasing') agent is sometimes added to promote the ready removal of the pattern from the mold. Chemical agents suspended or dissolved in isopropyl alcohol (isopropanol) have largely replaced talc for this purpose, and are sprayed onto the mold surface. The deposited carrier is then burned off to leave the parting agent (usually a type of graphite).

Thermosetting processes use furan-based resins (hot box) or urea- or phenol-formaldehyde resins (shell molding). Cold-setting (no-bake) hardening systems include acid-catalyzed urea- and phenol-formaldehyde resin with and without furfuryl alcohol, alkyd and phenolic isocyanates, self-adhesive siloxanes, and various types of sand. A 'lost foam' process allows particles of polystyrene foam to be vaporized by the molten metal. The isocyanates employed in binders are normally based on methylene diphenylisocyanate (MDI). In recent years, titanium, nickel, chromium, magnesium, and even more toxic metals such as beryllium, cadmium, and thorium have been used in foundry products. In particular, beryllium may be used for the production of high-performance racing car engines.

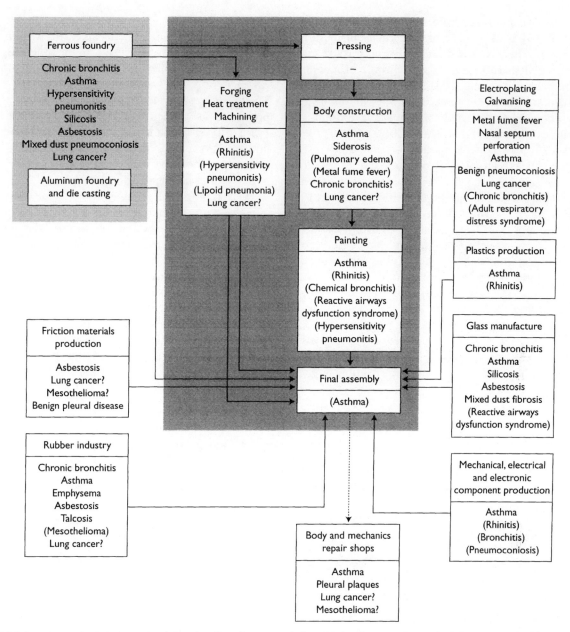

Fig. 24.2 Processes and principal associated disorders. Rare diseases are indicated in brackets, question marks indicate uncertain risks.

In non-ferrous foundries, aluminum casting is used to produce cylinder heads, transmission cases, engine blocks, and other automotive parts. These facilities cast the products in permanent molds with or without sand cores. Hazards can arise from pyrolysis of the core.

Workers in these foundries are exposed to a wide range of respirable hazards including silica, iron oxides, fumes, and gases from molten metals and bonding resins. Dust inhalation still poses an important risk. Pneumoconiosis is the dominant occupational respiratory disease in the steel fettling shop, though true silicosis is now rare except when sandblasting is used; a mixed pneumoconiosis (silica, silicates, iron) is more prevalent in iron fettling [4].

Besides fettling (the abrasive removal of surface impurities, largely sand, from metal castings) and work with furnace linings, other possible sources of silica exposure include the cleaning and repairing of furnaces, and the general contamination of the workplace by dusty processes. A further long reported silica-associated risk in foundry workers is tuberculosis. Where the prevalence of silicosis has declined, there has been a parallel fall in tuberculosis incidence, but it has not been completely eradicated. In countries where dust levels have remained high, where dusty processes are labor intensive, and where tuberculosis is endemic, tuberculosis remains an important cause of death among foundry workers.

Increased mortality from non-malignant respiratory disease was found in several studies of foundry workers. Whenever silicosis is common, it is likely to be associated with an excess of chronic bronchitis, often with emphysema. Asbestos is a further well-known, although overlooked, hazard in foundries [5], and may cause both malignant and non-malignant disorders (Chapters 9, 20–22).

Since the 1950s, a variety of synthetic resin systems have been introduced into foundries to bind sand in cores and molds. These generally comprise a base material and a catalyst or hardener (activator), which causes polymerization. Many of these chemicals are sensitizers (e.g. isocyanates, furfuryl alcohol, aliphatic amines, formaldehyde) and can cause occupational asthma and, occasionally, hypersensitivity pneumonitis. Formaldehyde exposure increases the risks of respiratory irritation, lung function abnormalities, and (in rodents at high dose levels) nasal cancer, but it is a much less potent sensitizer.

Compared with suitable reference populations, workers in dusty trades have an increased prevalence of chronic bronchitis. Acute irritation of the airways, adult respiratory distress syndrome (ARDS), and chemical pneumonia are also described. Over 1000 chemicals with well-known acute or chronic adverse effects on the lung are used or encountered in iron casting and steel making as raw materials, or as contaminants in scrap or fuels. They may be used additionally as additives in special processes, as refractories, as hydraulic fluids and solvents used in plant operation and maintenance, and as byproducts such as tar, benzene and ammonia. The most important groups for the respiratory tract are reported in Table 24.1.

There is sufficient evidence to conclude that iron and steel foundry environments are carcinogenic to human lung (International Agency for Research on Cancer (IARC) group 1). Despite a failure to identify the specific causal agent or agents (possibly polycyclic aromatic hydrocarbons, silica, metal fumes, or interactions between them) there has been a consistent excess of lung cancer in studies from around the world among workers in iron and steel foundries. The limited evidence available suggests that any silica-related cancer risk may be confined to subjects with silicosis. It is unclear whether crystalline silica is itself carcinogenic [6,7].

Table 24.1 Chemicals used or encountered in iron casting and steel making, and related hazards for the respiratory system

Substance	Possible Effect
Sulfur compounds (from high-sulfur fossil fuels and blast furnace slag)	Dryness and irritation of the nose and the upper respiratory tract, coughing, shortness of breath
Oil mists from tempering processes	Asthma, lipoid pneumonia. Polycyclic aromatic hydrocarbons (PAHs) can be formed, which have some risk of lung cancer
Metals (e.g. chromium, zinc, nickel, manganese, cadmium, aluminum, copper) in the form of particulates, fumes, and adsorbates on inert dust particles.	Short-term exposure to high levels of zinc and other vaporized metals (particularly magnesium, antimony) can cause 'metal fume fever' (fever, chills, nausea, respiratory difficulty and fatigue)
Acid mists from pickling areas	Respiratory irritation
Polycyclic aromatic hydrocarbons (from coal dust and combustion process): may be present as vapors, aerosols or adsorbates on fine particulates	Long-term exposure has been associated with carcinogenesis
Vanadium, cadmium and other alloy additions	Chemical pneumonitis. There is limited evidence of cadmium and cadmium carcinogenicity in humans (group 2A in IARC classification). Exposure is associated with increased risks of prostatic and respiratory cancers
Beryllium (high-performance special alloys)	Acute lung injury can occur with high concentrations (tracheitis, bronchitis, chemical pneumonia) and production of granulomata throughout the body but particularly in the lungs for chronic exposure, with possible evolution to lung fibrosis. Sufficient evidence for carcinogenicity for respiratory cancers
Nitrogen oxides from combustion processes	Airways irritation
Styrene (released as molten metal fills polystyrene molds)	Asthma and rhinitis
Asbestos used for insulation	Pleural plaques, malignant mesothelioma, mixed dust fibrosis

FORGING, MACHINING, PRESSING

Hot forging and cold forging followed by heat treatment are used to produce engine crankshafts, transmissions, and suspensions, and other vehicle components from metals coming from foundries. Today, the processes are mainly based on induction heating of billets that are then worked in forging presses using pressure instead of impact. The main dangers for the respiratory system (asthma and lipoid pneumonia) are from the possible inhalation of oil mists as mineral oil can be present on metals undergoing hot forging, or it can be used in the cooling process after heat treatment. In addition, polycyclic aromatic hydrocarbons (PAH) can be formed, by pyrolysis, and these may pose some risk of lung cancer.

Machining of engine blocks, crankshafts, gears, transmissions and other components is a characteristic task within the automotive industry. Machine lubricants (e.g. metal working fluids; MWF) are used to remove metal turnings, lubricate, and cool both the tool and the working surface. There are three major types: straight, soluble, and synthetic fluids. Straight oils (insoluble or cutting oils) are naphthenic or paraffinic mineral oil with additives such as polar lubricants and, occasionally, chlorine-, sulfur-, or phosphorus-based lubricants. Soluble oils (water-miscible or emulsified oils) and semisynthetic coolants are similar as they are emulsions of oil in water made with petroleum sulfonates and alkanolamines. Because of the presence of mineral oil they retain some of the lubrication advantages of straight oils but they also have excellent cooling capacity because of the water content. Additives include chlorine-, sulfur-, or phosphorus-based lubricants, corrosion inhibitors (e.g. polar organic compounds), and a number of other agents (odorants, antifoam agents, emulsifiers, antioxidants, detergents, viscosity index improvers, antiwear agents, extreme pressure agents such as non-corrosive sulfurized fatty compounds, zinc dithiophosphate and lead naphthenate, biocides such as phenol, triazinic compounds, formaldehyde donors, and pine oil). The addition of nitrite to amine-containing fluids is prohibited because of the risk of nitrosamine production. Synthetic oils are water-based alkaline solutions without mineral oil and are considered the fluid of choice for cooling and lubricating high-speed machining operations.

During use, MWF may be transformed by heat, with possible increase of PAH, or by chemical action. MWF may be contaminated with hydraulic fluids, gear oil that leaks past the seal of a machining tool, and microbial growth. Grinding and tool sharpening may present the further danger of hard metal disease because of dissolved cobalt and its consequent dispersal in the aerosolized fluids.

Studies concerning the respiratory effects of lubricant aerosols of respirable size are sparse and contradictory. Occupational exposure to MWF is common in automobile parts manufacturing, since mists or splashes generated during operations may be inhaled and ingested, or may settle directly on the skin. MWF may have irritant or sensitizing properties because of contamination with trace quantities of metals, additives, and bactericidal agents. Possibly as a consequence, a number of disorders have been reported among exposed workers: rhinitis, occupational asthma, hypersensitivity pneumonitis, lipoid pneumonia, industrial bronchitis, nasal mucosa dysplasia, and cancer of the nose, larynx, and lung [8–10]. A subclinical airway response to MWF, characterized by an increased prevalence of Monday across-shift declines in FEV_1 (forced expired volume in 1 s), has been reported among machine operators compared with assembly workers [11]. Respiratory effects are more prominent with synthetic and soluble oils than straight oil, which has been attributed to their content of chemical irritants such as petroleum sulfonates, tall oils, ethanolamines, formaldehyde donors, and microbial products.

A risk of hypersensitivity pneumonitis (machining operator's lung) may exist in machining plants where water-based fluids are used and unusual microbial contaminants predominate. The suspected etiological agents are generally non-tuberculous mycobacteria, fungi, Gram-negative bacteria (*Acinetobacter*, *Pseudomonas*, *Enterobacter*, *Escherichia coli*), and thermophiles [12]. A further risk from microbial contamination has been legionnaires' disease, though only one case had been described.

Although the causal agents specifically responsible for each reported case could not be identified, it is likely that both specific sensitizing agents and non-specific irritants (additives and contaminants) have played contributory roles to this spectrum of occupational respiratory illness. Asthma and hypersensitivity pneumonitis appear to be the most common manifestations of MWF-related disease, but in an absolute sense they occur only rarely among exposed populations. Studies addressing the risk for lung cancer have found both positive and negative associations with exposure to MWF. A recent case-control study of automotive workers demonstrated a negative, not positive, relationship between the highest level of lifetime cumulative exposure to synthetic MWF and lung cancer mortality (odds ratio, 0.6; 95% confidence interval 0.4–0.8). There was little evidence of any association with soluble or straight oil machining [13].

Pressing metal sheets, strips, or coils into body panels and other components (often combined with subassembly by welding) is carried out in large facilities with mechanical power presses. The operations are becoming increasingly mechanized, thereby limiting the respiratory risks, but they may occasionally produce aerosols similar in composition to those of MWF.

BODY CONSTRUCTION

After the metal pieces are pressed, they are assembled into subgroups, such as hoods and doors, mainly with electric welding presses. This process is increasingly performed in cells with robot transfer of parts. Small components are welded by flux-shielded or gas-shielded arc welding. Gas welding is exceedingly rare. The main respiratory hazards associated with the various welding processes are metal fumes, fluorides, ozone, and nitrogen dioxide. Thermal decomposition products of materials involved indirectly in the welding process may produce less obvious hazards. For example, epoxy resin sealants or paint coatings may provide an additional source of hazardous fume or gas. In practice, asthma attributable to such compounds is not commonly recognized in welders, though contact dermatitis has occasionally been described.

The hazards associated with welding are described more fully in Chapter 30. In brief, acute effects include metal fume fever (especially if the metal is galvanized (zinc coated)), asthmatic reactions in subjects who are already asthmatic, and pulmonary edema. The last is usually attributable to ozone and nitrogen dioxide toxicity. Such effects are exceedingly rare in the automotive industry. Among the chronic effects, siderosis from the inhalation of iron oxide is the most common. Asthma arising from metal hypersensitivity (mainly chromium) has been reported occasionally in welders [14,15], especially if welding stainless steel, and there is a distant risk of berylliosis in some settings [16]. Some studies have shown an increased prevalence of chronic bronchitis, but others have not. Some mortality studies have shown an increased risk from lung cancer (related to asbestos, mainly in shipyards, or to hexavalent chromium and nickel during stainless steel welding), but other studies have not confirmed such findings. IARC has deemed welding fumes and gases to be 'possibly carcinogenic to humans' (group 2B).

Such inconsistencies within the literature are not surprising since welders use a great variety of techniques and experience many exposure conditions. Welding in the automotive industry is not usually performed in confined environments, and a study of automotive welders performed by one of the authors failed to show significant abnormalities in lung function despite a significantly higher prevalence of airway symptoms compared to vehicle fitters [17]. The welding technology used in the automotive industry gives rise to limited exposure to metal, fume and nitrogen dioxide, as can be illustrated by our own measurements from the respiratory zones of workers (Table 24.2).

PAINTING

Automobile bodies from the body shop enter the paint shop on a conveyor where they are degreased, often by the manual application of solvents, cleaned in a closed tunnel, and undercoated. The undercoat is then rubbed down by hand with an oscillating tool using wet abrasive paper, prior to the application of the final layers of paint, and oven curing [1].

In the traditional painting process the potential risks are related to the level of volatile organic compounds (VOCs) released into the atmosphere by solvent-based paints. When two-component polyurethane spray paints are employed (as they still are for the painting of industrial vehicles and for the retouching of automobiles), a further important respiratory risk is represented by the isocyanate used as a hardener. In recent decades, much progress has been made to reduce emissions of VOCs by introducing 'high-solid' paints with lower solvent content, water-based paints (in which the solvents are replaced to a greater or lesser extent by water), and powdered paints, which contain no solvent at all. Moreover, the use of polyurethane paints has been greatly reduced.

High-solid paints with lower solvent content have the advantage that they can be used in existing painting processes, whereas powdered and water-based paints require important changes in technology. The new water-based formulations (based on

Table 24.2 Exposure to metal, fume and nitrogen dioxide from welding

Substance	Exposure	Percentage of current ACGIH TLV-TWA
Nitrogen dioxide	0.05–0.15 ppm	1.5–5
Fume	1.05–2 mg/m³	20–40
Iron oxide	0.20–0.40 mg/m³	4–8
Nickel	trace levels only	(<0.0025 mg/m³)

ACGIH TLV-TWA, American Conference of Governmental Industrial Hygienists threshold limit values as time-weighted averages.

melaminic resins) may generate substantial formaldehyde exposure. Water-based synthetic resins can achieve the desired paint quality even though they contain much smaller quantities of organic solvents [18], but they contain more reactive compounds, such as biocides, surfactants, pigments, binders, amines, monomers, and glycol ethers. This chemical complexity may introduce new hazards. Binders are usually represented by polyester, polyester–urethane acrylic, and styrene–acrylic resins. In polyester–urethane resin, the isocyanates are almost exclusively of the aliphatic type (hexamethylene diisocyanate (HDI) or isophorone diisocyanate (IPDI), because the presence of the aliphatic radical provides excellent light and weather resistance in the end-product.

Powdered paints consist of pulverized resins, pigments, and additives; their usual method of application is electrostatic spraying [19]. The most commonly used type in industry contains polyester resin, synthesized from polyvalent alcohol and organic acids, and/or acid anhydrides. The latter include maleic, phthalic, and trimellitic anhydride, and pyromellitic dianhydride. The curing agent is either epoxy resin or triglycidyl isocyanurate (TGIC), which is also an epoxy compound.

Coating for acoustic insulation no longer involves asbestos, but a number of resins are used (e.g. polyvinyl chloride (PVC), polyamide) and inert fillers (e.g. calcium carbonate and oxide).

Inhalation of diisocynate monomer is recognised as a leading cause of occupational asthma in a proportion of exposed workers, generally about 5% [3]. Apart from allergic asthma, which is the most commonly encountered effect, the spectrum of lung diseases that could be induced by diisocyanates also includes asthma caused by the reactive airways dysfunction syndrome (RADS), hypersensivity pneumonitis, chemical bronchitis, a dose-dependent excess annual decline in FEV_1, chronic obstructive pulmonary disease (COPD) and pulmonary edema (toxic pneumonitis) [3,20], though they are far less common than asthma.

Formaldehyde exposure can also cause allergic sensitization, and hence asthma and rhinitis, in exposed workers, though it is far less potent than diisocyanates [21]. Water-based paints are not as harmless as might be supposed. Both airway irritation and skin sensitization have been described in house painters in association with their use. Some studies indicate, in particular, a high prevalence of contact dermatitis to preservatives such as benzisothiazolinone and to the hardener aziridine [22]. Isothiazolinones have also been described as a cause of occupational asthma in chemical factories producing detergents [23] and biocides [24].

Although powder paints contain no organic solvents, they are potentially allergenic, mainly because of the presence of acid anhydrides, which can induce sensitization even at low levels of exposure [3]. Standard curing temperatures are in the range 160–180°C. When the paints are unduly overheated at 200–240°C the resins begin to disintegrate, releasing acid anhydrides in sufficient quantity to provoke symptoms of immunoglobulin E (IgE) mediated rhinitis, asthma, and urticaria in sensitized workers. Recently, two cases of allergic alveolitis following exposure to epoxy polyester powder paint containing low amounts of acid anhydrides have been described [25]. Epoxy resins and, particularly, the compound TGIC can cause respiratory and cutaneous manifestations, such as asthma and contact dermatitis [26], and a combined respiratory and systemic reaction following exposure to heated electrostatic polyester paint has recently been reported [27].

PLASTIC BODY PANELS AND TRIMS

Metal trim parts such as chrome strips, bumpers, and handles are being increasingly replaced by polymer materials. Hard body parts may be made by fiberglass-reinforced polyester–polystyrene systems, acrylonitrile–butadiene–styrene thermosetting systems, polyethylene, polypropylene, polycarbonates, PVC, and nylon. Talc, glass fibers, and kaolin can be used as fillers. The molding of thermosetting systems is a heat consuming process, but at normal operating temperatures only the physical properties of the compounds are modified. There is no chemical reactivity nor chemical decomposition. As a consequence, monomers and pyrolysis byproducts are not released. These can, however, be generated during subsequent maintenance and cleaning operations on the injectors. The respirable hazards are aldehydes (formaldehyde, acrolein), acid anhydrides, phthalates, and bisphenol A, which may cause irritative and allergic responses in both the airways and the lung parenchyma.

Polyurethane systems may require high density for body parts, but low density for foam in seats and interior padding. Prepolymerized toluene diisocyanate (TDI) is usually employed for the latter, prepolymerized MDI for the former. Prepolymerization greatly reduces volatility and sensitizing potency, whereas the inhalation of diisocyanate monomers carries high risks of respiratory sensitization [3,20]. Styrene exposure from fibrous glass compositions may also pose some risk of respiratory sensitization but potency is substantially less than with diisocyanates, and in practice very few cases of styrene-induced asthma have been reported despite its widespread use in many industries [28]. Acid anhydrides pose a more real threat of mucosal irritation and hypersensitivity (essentially causing asthma and rhinitis) [3]. Over the years there have been isolated and rather unconvincing case reports of PVC or fumes derived from it causing, respectively, pneumoconiosis and asthma.

Interior acoustic insulating panels are commonly made by heat pressing mixtures of shredded rags and phenolic resins at about 200°C. Several layers can be joined with water vynilic glue. Thermal byproducts (e.g. the respiratory sensitizer hexamethylenetetramine) may pose some risk of low-grade irritation or sensitization.

FRICTION MATERIALS

Brake linings, brake pads, and clutch facings are the major friction products used in motor vehicles. Until recently chrysotile asbestos formed 40–60% of drum brakes and clutches, and 20% of disc brakes. With many other components, the asbestos was weighed, mixed, pressed, and heat polymerized to produce the friction material, which was then ground, painted, and glued onto a metal mounting. Compressed asbestos was additionally used in gaskets in engines. Because of concern about the risks of adverse effects, several countries have banned any further use of asbestos of any type, and an EU ban is currently under consideration. Friction materials have consequently come to be made largely with asbestos substitutes, both natural (e.g. wollastonite, attapulgite, vermiculite, mica, basalt fibers) and synthetic. The latter include artificial mineral fibers (e.g. rockwool, ceramic fibers, and glass fibers) and organic fibers (e.g. aramid, polyacrylonitrile, polyester, and cellulose fibers). Aramid fibers, in particular, have proved to be popular substitutes for asbestos fibers.

Several of the substances used in the production of these friction materials may exert an irritating or sensitizing effect on the respiratory system; some may even have fibrogenic effects and a few are known or suspected pulmonary carcinogens. Whether plausible cumulative levels of exposure in the automotive industry will pose any real risk remains to be seen. Greater concern lies with the risk from past exposures to asbestos. Work with friction materials has never been associated with much parenchymal asbestosis, and even the carcinogenic effects of asbestos are questionable since there is a lack of evidence of increased mortality owing to lung or pleural cancer [29].

Although the substitute fibers of natural origin are certainly much less hazardous than chrysotile asbestos, only epidemiological study and the passage of time will show whether the newly adopted synthetic substitutes have negligible risk. Studies in experimental animals do raise concerns for the safety of artificial mineral fiber (Chapter 11), but extrapolation to humans of experimental animal data demands considerable caution [30]. At present it is prudent to be cautions and to minimize exposure levels. The new friction products do, however, have one clear advantage over earlier asbestos-based products: the content of potentially hazardous fiber is substantially less (between 1 and 5%). Moreover, granular alternatives are now being introduced to replace (partially) the fibers.

RUBBER MANUFACTURE

Rubber is needed for tire and gasket production. In addition to natural and synthetic rubber, over 250 materials are required to produce a single tire (Table 24.3). Natural rubber (polyterpene or 1–4-polyisoprene) derives from the milky fluid produced by the lacticifers of the tropical rubber tree *Hevea braziliensis* (Euphorbiaceae). The latex contains approximately 35% polyisoprene along with 5% plant proteins, sugars and other organic substances. Synthetic rubbers used within the automotive industry include, 1,4-*cis*-polyisoprene, with similar composition of natural rubber, but without sensitization properties; styrene–butadiene rubber; neoprene (polychloroprene); nitrile rubber (acrylonitrile–butadiene–styrene); and butyl-rubber (polybutadiene). In tire production, the ratio of synthetic to natural rubber is normally about 2:1.

Tire production involves the following steps:

- raw material handling, compounding, and mixing
- milling
- extruding, calendering, and component assembly
- tire building
- curing and vulcanizing
- inspection and final finishing
- storage.

Potential hazards in the rubber industry include the inhalation of rubber monomers, dusts, and vapors of both inorganic and organic origin. Historic exposures to potentially hazardous monomer in synthetic rubber production were much higher than they are today because of incomplete polymerization. Workers were particularly exposed during drying

Table 24.3 Chemical components of tires, in addition to natural and synthetic rubber

Use	Examples
Vulcanizing agents	Sulfur[a] or sulfur-containing materials, zinc oxide[a], stearic acid[a]
Accelerators	Hexamethyleneteramine[b], thiourea derivatives, sulfonamides, diphenylguanidine, mercaptobenzothiazol, thiurams[a], dithiocarbamates[a], thiophosphates
Activators	Zinc oxide[a], magnesium oxide, sodium carbamate
Antioxidants	Phenyl naphthylamine[a], quinoline[a], thioesters, arylamines, p-phenylendiamine derivatives
Softeners	Naphthenic and aromatic oils
Fillers	Talc in the past, zinc stearate, kaolin, barium carbonate
Reinforcing agents	Carbon black, amorphous silica
Emulsifiers	Stearic acid[a] or lauric acid, sodium bicarbonate, azodicarbonamide[b]
Retarders	Salicilic acid[a], phthalic anhydride[a,b]
Plasticizers	Phthalates[a], diethil sebacate[a], trixylyl phosphate[a]
Pigments	Organic and inorganic pigments

[a] Indicates a known irritant effect.
[b] Indicates a sensitizing action on the respiratory system, considering in particular the EC labeling for chemical products.

and compounding. Several studies have reported an excess of respiratory symptoms (mucous hypersecretion, chest tightness, shortness of breath, wheezing) and pulmonary function abnormalities (mild airways obstruction or decrements in flow rates with preservation of lung volumes) in rubber workers. Emphysema has been shown to be a common reason for early retirement. These disorders are thought to be associated with curing, processing (premixing, weighing, mixing, and heating of raw ingredients), and final finishing (inspections) areas of manufacturing plants. Many of the ingredients used in the tire manufacturing industry are potential respiratory irritants or sensitizers with well-known acute or chronic effects on the lung [31]. For example, sulfur dioxide is a common byproduct (deriving from accelerators) with marked irritant properties at sufficient concentration. Natural latex represents an increasing sensitization problem for other categories of workers (e.g. healthcare workers), since it can cause rhinoconjunctivitis, asthma, and dermatitis through systemic IgE-mediation [3]. However, no data have yet been published to suggest any excess risk of respiratory allergic diseases in the tire manufacturing industry. Work in the rubber industry was deemed to carry an increased risk of cancer (but not respiratory cancer) by IARC in 1987 [32].

GLASS MANUFACTURE

Glass is made by heating (and melting) naturally occurring raw materials prepared in powder or fine particulate form. Different types of glass require different mixes of raw materials of which the principal components are silica and silicates, clay, sand, alumina, limestone, alkaline dust as sodium and potassium carbonate, metal oxides, heavy metals, borax, boric acid, barium carbonate, feldspars, dolomite, pyrolusite, arsenic trioxide, pigments, and broken glass. Stratified laminated glass is used in the automotive industry to produce windshields, side windows, and backlights. The bonding agent usually is hexamethylene diisocyanate (HDI). Lead glass can be used for armor-plated cars [1,2,33].

The respiratory hazards include airborne particulate matter from the raw materials (silica and silicates), particularly in mixing and finishing operations, and fumes and gases from the firing and melting processes (sulfur and arsenic dioxide, nitrogen oxides, carbon dioxide and monoxide, hydrofluoric acid, and heavy metals). The potential acute effects are mucosal irritation (nuisance particulate) and, possibly, with accidents and severe respiratory insults, RADS; the chronic effects range from chronic bronchitis and COPD to silicosis and mixed dust fibrosis. Intense heating processes may lead to respirable exposure to the most hazardous forms of silica (cristobalite or tridymite). In addition, potential respiratory sensitizers may be present in binders, coating agents, or preservatives (e.g. polyurethanes), and exposure to silica, asbestos, and refractory ceramic fibers may be encountered during periodic major reconstruction activities, repairs to furnace and kilns, and demolition.

ELECTROPLATING, GALVANIZING AND METAL DUST

Electroplating is the process by which one metal is deposited onto another electrochemically to improve the surface properties. Certain pressed steel components and castings (bumpers, moldings, handles, metal trims, etc.) are electroplated mainly with copper, chrome, and nickel, and then buffed and polished. The parts to be treated first undergo a thorough cleaning, either by mechanical grinding, brushing, and polishing, or by solvent washing (acid or alkaline 'pickling') and electrolytic degreasing. Subsequently, they are immersed in an electrolyte solution (which can be acidic or alkaline, sometimes with added cyanide salts) for the electroplating process. Bright metal parts are being replaced increasingly by painted metal and painted plastic, and the importance of electroplating is decreasing in the automotive industry.

Steel sheeting for body manufacture is sometimes protected against corrosion prior to use by zinc coating. The galvanizing process, after a number of cleaning, rinsing, and drying processes, involves either a 'hot' passage in a bath of molten zinc or a cold process that is identical to electroplating. An ammonium chloride flux can be employed, which, on decomposition, can give rise to hydrogen chloride and ammonia gas, and the risk of inhalation injury.

Grinding and polishing operations that give rise to metallic and oxide dusts may cause benign pneumoconiosis, and solvents can cause mucosal irritation, mainly for the upper airways. In electroplating, respiratory hazards can derive from caustic and corrosive chemicals (acidic and alkaline vapors or aerosols), which can induce acute or chronic airways irritation. If nitric or hydrofluoric acid are used and there is accidental heavy exposures, ARDS may occur.

Metals (mainly chromium and nickel) are a greater cause of concern because of their irritating, carcinogenic, and sensitizing properties. Chromium compounds can cause a characteristic perforation of the nasal septum. Although benign, it provides a useful clinical warning of inappropriately high levels of exposure. An increased incidence of lung cancer has been associated in particular with chromic acid classified A1 by ACGIH and in group 1 by IARC. Epidemiological studies have suggested increased respiratory morbidity in electroplaters, compared with galvanizers, that is related to exposure to chromium. Although rare, chromium- and nickel-induced asthma (apparently not IgE-mediated) is a well-recognized occupational disease [3,34] that may occur in situations where exposure levels are likely to be within the current exposure standards. Metal fume fever constitutes a further risk and can arise from 'hot dip' galvanizing and the inhalation of zinc.

VEHICLE ASSEMBLY

In the final assembly shop, body, engine, and other components are joined together; electric and electronic components are installed; windshields, side windows and backlights are mounted; bumpers, internal and external panels and trims, and upholstery are fitted. Chemical products in use in this phase of production are essentially confined to adhesives and various technical fluids (brake circuit, air conditioning, antifreeze, etc.). The mounting of windscreens and backlights often involves polyurethane systems, currently based on MDI. For other mounting procedures epoxy adhesives and cyanoacrylates are used.

Respiratory hazards are quite limited in this production phase, and the important risks are confined to diisocyanates and cyanoacrylate inhalation. Like diisocyanates, cyanoacrylate and methacrylate are respiratory sensitizers and may cause asthma, albeit rarely [35]. Cyanoacrylate can also cause contact eczema and rhinitis. Recently, asthma caused by diacrylate contained in a primer used in an auto body shop has been reported for the first time, without evidence of cross-reactivity with methacrylate or cyanoacrylate [36]. Because of the ambient temperature of use, epoxy resins are not a consistent cause of respiratory ailments as they are extremely unlike to become airborne.

AUTOMOTIVE SERVICE AND REPAIR

Used vehicles need various interventions on both the mechanical parts and the bodywork. Clutch and, above all, brake repair are critical activities for car mechanics as they can be a source of significant asbestos exposure. In recent years, the need for drilling, facing, or grinding operations during installation has decreased considerably, and gasket processing remains hazardous only when older vehicles are repaired.

Auto body repair is likely to involve fiber glass, polystyrene, epoxy resins, and body filling compounds; sanding is needed to remove surface paint and smooth repaired body panels, and finally the repairs require painting. Airborne dusts may contain a variety of hazardous substances, such as lead and chromium from surface coatings and abrasives from sanding discs. Painting involves the use of polyurethane products much more extensively than in the production body shop.

Epidemiological data assessing the magnitude of risk in automotive servicing and repair are scanty and contradictory. Asbestos exposure, though possibly a cause of pleural plaques, has not been related consistently to any decrease in lung function [37,38]. An increased mortality from lung cancer has been described, but this could be explained by several confounders: heavier smoking habits than those of the general population, and exposure to air pollutants other than asbestos (exhaust gases, chromate-containing paints, lubricants) [39]. There is no clear evidence that car mechanics have an increased risk of mesothelioma, although a suggestive trend has been reported in recent years [40].

Exposure to body repair resins and spray paints constitutes the greatest current risk, and occupational asthma is a not uncommon consequence [3]. An increased longitudinal loss of ventilatory function has also been observed, though mainly in smokers. It was correlated with the frequency of high peak exposures to HDI-BT (a polycondensation product of HDI and water), but not with the mean exposure to diisocyanates [41].

ELECTRIC AND ELECTRONIC COMPONENTS

Since the very beginning of their history, motor vehicles have always included some electrical component. However, the most recent technologic developments have resulted in a tremendous increase in electrical and, especially, electronic equipment. A comprehensive treatment of the technology and of the potential respiratory hazards is beyond the scope of this chapter. Therefore, only a few typical and representative aspects will be covered.

The electrical equipment industry has developed rapidly in the last few decades and production has become highly automated. The range of materials used is wide, including metals (e.g. steel, aluminum, copper, magnesium, beryllium, lead, cadmium, mercury, selenium, zirconium), insulating materials (plastic tapes, resins, dielectric fluids), paints and varnishes, solvents, acids, alkalis, and an increasing amount of plastics.

The manufacture of lead-acid batteries involves the use of sulfuric acid. Separators used in such batteries are increasingly made of glass fiber materials.

The manufacture of electric cables entails the use of metals (copper, aluminum, steel) and insulating materials, such as polyvinyl chloride, polyethylene, polyamides, natural and synthetic rubber. Talc as a lubricating agent is still in use, even though to a much lesser extent.

Incandescent lamps (with or without a halogen added to reduce the evaporation of tungsten during use) consist of a glass envelope sealed to a mount holding two supporting wires that carry the coiled tungsten filament. Manufacture is largely mechanized. Sulfur dioxide is frequently used as a lubricant during high-speed lamp assembly.

Headlights are becoming progressively more plastic than metallic; epoxy and cyanoacrylate adhesives are commonly used.

The electronic industry employs both the conventional materials of precision engineering, such as steel, copper, aluminum, glass and plastics, and also very special materials such as silicon and germanium (used for the semiconductor manufacture). Circuit components and complete circuits are usually joined together by soldering with special alloys. Polyester and epoxy resin systems are widely used as insulating materials; quartz flour is sometimes added to the system to improve strength and appearance. The preparation of printed circuit cards from offset plates is basically an etching process.

Respiratory health damage could be due to the irritant effects of the inhalation of solvent vapours, sulfur dioxide, or acids.

The manufacture of lead-acid batteries can generate sulfuric acid mists, which used to be so concentrated that tooth erosion was, at one time, a common feature amongst the workers in formation areas. Exposure levels are today much less relevant, although irritation of the airways cannot be completely ruled out: some studies have suggested a possible link between exposures to inorganic acid mists (including sulfuric acid) and cancer of the larynx; further research is needed in this area. The use of glass fiber separators in the batteries could further increase the risk due to the inhalation of man-made mineral fibers.

Particular risks lie with nitrogen oxides that can be liberated by the mixture of concentrated nitric acid and sulfuric acid used in the manufacture of tungsten for the coiled filaments of incandescent lamps, and with the use of quartz flour. There is also growing evidence of asthma due to cyanoacrylates, but nowadays the incidence of occupational diseases in the electrical equipment industry is overall very low, due to high automation and the usually high standards of hygiene.

The fumes from electronic soldering may contain, besides the various metals employed, rosin. Rosin (colophony) is a resin obtained from pine trees, which is widely used as a 'flux' in the electronics industry to prevent corrosion. Asthma due to the inhalation of this agent has been repeatedly described [42] and represents one of the more 'classic' examples of occupational asthma. Rhinitis is also possible. The mechanism of reaction of colophony remains unknown; some arguments seem to support an immunologic pathway, but specific IgE have not been found, and some authors favour an irritating mechanism [43]. Other types of soldering flux, containing zinc chloride and ammonium chloride or alcohol-polypropylene glycol, have been reported to cause occupational asthma.

DIFFICULT CASE

History

A 35-year-old non-smoking man worked as a machinist in an automobile manufacturing plant. After about 18 months he noticed shortness of breath, chest tightness, wheezing, persistent cough (sometimes productive), and a stuffy nose, but there were no other symptoms. He came to believe that all these symptoms were related to his work because they improved, though not substantially, during weekends away from work. They resolved more fully during long holidays. He worked closely with machine fluids, used as lubricants and coolants for the rapidly moving parts of some of the machines, and it is likely that aerosols were formed as a result. He had no history of allergy or asthma, and he had not previously been troubled by respiratory symptoms.

There was mild airway obstruction (FEV$_1$ 84% predicted, vital capacity 100% predicted, FEV$_1$/FVC 67%) when he was first examined, but inhaled β$_2$-agonist and corticosteroid medication reversed this fully. A methacholine test gave a PD$_{20}$ (dose that caused a 20% change for FEV$_1$) of 149 μg (within the asthmatic range), and skin prick tests with common inhalant allergens were negative.

Peak expiratory flow (PEF) monitoring over a month revealed high variability (>40%), with a suggestive relationship between decreased values and periods at work (Fig. 24.3).

Occupational asthma was considered likely, and he was relocated within the factory to prevent ongoing exposure to MWF. His inhaler medication was continued, and he improved.

A year later specific bronchial provocation tests (sBPT) were carried out at the request of the local compensation board. An exposure chamber was used in which MWF and solutions of its principal constituents (cobalt chloride and nickel chloride) were nebulized. The tests did not provoke respiratory or other symptoms, and the results (summarized in Table 24.4) were considered to be negative. Serial methacholine tests were used to monitor airway responsiveness for 2–3 years from the time of his first evaluation, and the results are shown in Figure 24.4.

Issues

The chief issues in this case are, first, whether this man's respiratory disease was truly occupational in origin; if so what was its nature? Second, how should the investigations be interpreted?

Comments

There was, unusually, full agreement among the book's contributors that the respiratory disorder was asthma (the con-

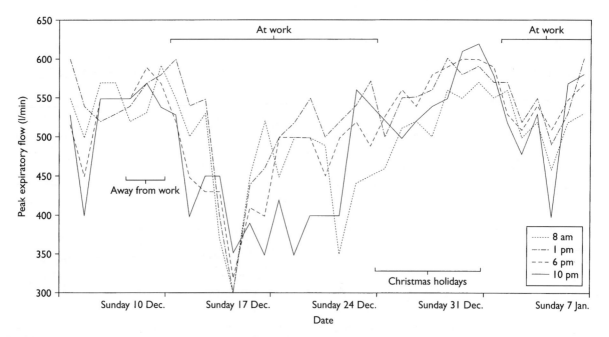

Fig. 24.3 Difficult Case: peak expiratory flow monitoring. The time scale is not linear.

Table 24.4 Difficult Case: results of specific bronchial provocation tests

Specific bronchial provocation test compounds	FEV_1 (% decrease)	MEF_{50} (% decrease)	MEF_{25} (% decrease)	VC (% decrease)	Methacholine PD_{20} for FEV_1 after test (µg)
Metal working fluids	8	20	15	3	>3200
Cobalt chloride 30 min at mean concentration 0.175 mg/m³	9	18	57	11 (9 h after challenge onset)	>3200
Cobalt chloride >1 h at mean concentration 0.151 mg/m³	14	29	77	13 (after 9 h)	2700
Nickel chloride 30 min at mean concentration 1.109 mg/m³	9 (after 9 h)	6	59 (after 9 h)	13	990

FEV_1, Forced expired volume in 1s; MEF, maximum expiratory flow during a forced vital capacity maneuver; MEF_{50}, MEP at 50% of FVC; MEF_{25}, MEF at 25% of FVC; VC, vital capacity; PD_{20}, dose giving a 20% change. Threshold limit value (time-weighted average is 0.02 mg/m³ for cobalt ion, 1.5 mg/m³ for elemental nickel and 0.1 mg/m³ for nickel ions in soluble compounds [44].

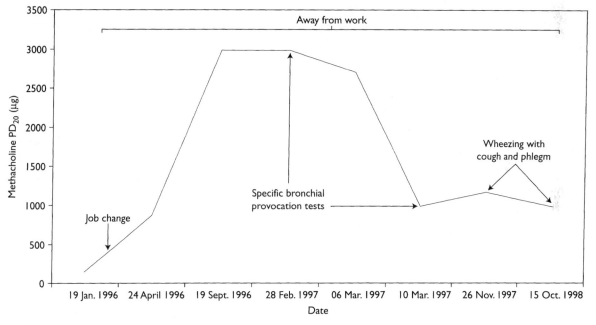

Fig. 24.4 Difficult Case: serial measurements of airway responsiveness by methacholine tests. The PD_{20} is the dose causing a 20% change in the FEV_1 (forced expired volume in 1 s).

sistent evidence from spirometry, bronchodilator effect, the methacholine test, and peak expiratory flow (PEF) variability) and that it was primarily occupational in origin. The PEF data were reanalysed using OASYS (Chapter 4), which produced conclusions of both asthma and 'work-relatedness' at the highest level of confidence. The case, therefore, illustrates an apparent failure of specific inhalation provocation tests to confirm a diagnosis of occupational asthma. Several contributors challenged the conclusion that the inhalation provocation tests were in fact negative, noting that FEV_1 measurements had declined variously by 8–14% and the PD_{20} from 2700 to 990 µg following nickel challenge. The significance of these changes has to be assessed against sponta-

neous change following, for example, control tests with 'dummy' challenge agents. These contributors considered the results 'equivocal' and would have administered an additional challenge with nickel. There was more general agreement that the challenge tests could have given false-negative results because the level of specific hypersensitivity might have declined during the intervening year without exposure, or because the true causal agent (perhaps a microbial contaminant or a protective biocide) had not been included in the challenge exposures.

The investigators were not able to obtain any further information of relevance, but they too concluded that occupational asthma was the correct diagnosis. In their opinion, the most likely explanation for the negative responses to bronchial challenges is that the causal agent had not been included in the exposures. They speculated, alternatively, that

the case could have been one of 'low-dose-irritant asthma' since no information was available concerning the level of exposure at the workplace [45].

ACKNOWLEDGEMENT

The authors would like to thank Dr Ivo Pavan, Head of the Epidemiology and the Industrial Toxicology Unit of the Dipartimento di Traumatologia, Ortopedia e Medicina del Lavoro, Università di Torino for his assistance in the technical field.

REFERENCES

1. Stellman JM (chief ed.). *Encyclopaedia of occupational health and safety*, 4th edn, Chs 73, 77, 80, 82, 84, 91. Geneva: International Labour Office, 1999.

2. Candura F. *Elementi di Tecnologia Industriale a uso dei Cultori di Medicina del Lavoro*. Pavia: Comet Editore, 1991.

3. Bernstein IL, Chan-Yeung M, Malo J-L, Bernstein DI. Asthma in the Workplace, 2nd edn, Chs 23, 25, 26, 35. New York: Marcel Dekker, 1999.

4. Rosenman KD, Reilly MJ, Kalinowski DJ, Watt FC. Silicosis in the 1990s. *Chest* 1997; 111: 779–786.

5. Rosenman KD, Reilly MJ. Asbestos-related X-ray changes in foundry workers. *Am J Ind Med* 1998; 34: 197–201.

6. Soutar CA, Robertson B, Miller BG et al. Epidemiological evidence on the carcinogenicity of silica: factors in scientific judgement. *Ann Occup Hyg* 2000; 44: 3–14.

7. International Agency for Research on Cancer (IARC). *Silica and some Silicates*. (IARC Monographs on the Evaluation of The Carcinogenic Risk of Chemicals to Humans, Vol. 42.) Lyon, 1997.

8. Sprince N, Thorne PS, Cullen MR. Oils and related petroleum derivatives. In: Rosenstock L, Cullen MR, eds. *Textbook of clinical occupational and environmental medicine*, pp. 814–824. Philadelphia, PA: Saunders, 1994.

9. Hendy MS, Beattie BE, Burge PS. Occupational asthma due to an emulsified oil mist. *Br J Ind Med* 1985; 42: 51–54.

10. Rosenman KD, Reilly MJ, Kalinowski D. Work related asthma and respiratory symptoms among workers exposed to metal-working fluids. *Am J Ind Med* 1997; 32: 325–331.

11. Kennedy SM, Greaves IA, Kriebel D et al. Acute pulmonary responses among automobile workers exposed to aerosols of machining fluids. *Am J Ind Med* 1989; 15: 627–641.

12. Kreiss K, Cox-Ganser J. Metalworking fluid-associated hypersensitivity pneumonitis: a workshop summary. *Am J Ind Med* 1997; 32: 423–432.

13. Schroeder JC, Tolbert PE, Eisen EA et al. Mortality studies of machining fluid exposure in the automobile industry. IV: A case-control study of lung cancer. *Am J Ind Med* 1997; 31: 525–533.

14. Lee HS, Chia SE, Yap JC et al. Occupational asthma due to spot-welding. *Singapore Med J* 1990; 31: 506–508.

15. Wang ZP, Larsson K, Malmberg P et al. Asthma, lung function, and bronchial responsiveness in welders. *Am J Ind Med* 1994; 26: 741–754.

16. Monie RD, Roberts GH. Chronic beryllium pneumonitis: first case accepted by UK register from Scotland. *Scot Med J* 1991; 36: 185–186.

17. Sulotto F, Romano C, Piolatto G et al. Compromissione respiratoria ed esposizione a metalli in un gruppo di 68 saldatori al lavoro. *Med Lav* 1989; 80: 201–210.

18. Jargot D, Dieudonné M, Hecht C et al. Peintures en Phase Aqueuse pour l'industrie Automobile. Cahiers de notes documentaires. *Hygiène et sécurité du travail* 1999; 177; 2115–2125.

19. Leleu J. Peintures en poudre. Composition et risques toxicologique. Cahiers de notes documentaires. *Hygiène et sécurité du travail* 1981; 102: 51–53.

20. Vandenplas O, Malo J-L, Saetta M et al. Occupational asthma and alveolitis due to isocyanates: current status and perspectives. *Br J Ind Med* 1993; 50: 213–228.

21. Burge PS, Harries MG, Lam WK et al. Occupational asthma due to formaldehyde. *Thorax* 1985; 40: 255–260.

22. Wieslander G, Norback D, Edling C. Airway symptoms among house painters in relation to exposure to volatile organic compounds (VOCS) – a longitudinal study. *Ann Occup Hyg* 1997; 41: 155–166.

23. Moscato G, Omodeo P, Dellabianca A et al. Occupational asthma caused by 1,2-benzisothiazolin-3-one in a chemical worker. *Occup Med* 1997; 47: 249–251.

24. Bourke SJ, Convery RP, Stenton SC et al. Occupational asthma in an isothiazolinone manufacturing plant. *Thorax* 1997; 52: 746–748.

25. Piirila P, Keskinen H, Anttila S et al. Allergic alveolitis following exposure to epoxy polyester powder paint containing low amounts (<1%) of acid anhydrides. *Eur Respir J* 1997; 10: 948–951.

26. Meuleman L, Goossens A, Linders C et al. Sensitization to triglycidylisocyanurate (TGIC) with cutaneous and respiratory manifestations. *Allergy* 1999; 54: 752–756.

27. Cartier A, Vandenplas O, Grammer LC et al. Respiratory and systemic reaction following exposure to heated electrostatic polyester paint. *Eur Respir J* 1994; 7: 608–611.

28. Moscato G, Biscaldi GP, Cottica D et al. Occupational asthma due to styrene: two case reports. *J Occup Med* 1987; 29: 957–960.

29. Berry G. Mortality and cancer incidence of workers exposed to chrysotile asbestos in the friction-products industry. *Ann Occup Hyg* 1994; 38: 539–546.

30. Harrison PTC, Levy LS, Patrick G et al. Comparative hazards of chrysotile asbestos and its substitutes: a European perspective. *Environ Health Perspect* 1999; 107: 607–611.

31. Roth VS. Rubber industry epidemiology. *Occup Med (Phil.)* 1999; 14: 849–54.

32. Kogevinas M, Sal M, Boffetta P. Cancer risk in the rubber industry: a review of the recent epidemiological evidence. *Occup Environ Med* 1998; 55: 1–12.

33. Scansetti G, Piolatto PG, Perrelli G. *Medicina del Lavoro*. Torino: Minerva medica, 2000.

34. Bright P, Burge PS, O'Hickey SP *et al.* Occupational asthma due to chrome and nickel electroplating. *Thorax* 1997; 52: 28–32.

35. Savonius B, Keskinen H, Tuppurainen M, Kanerva L. Occupational respiratory disease caused by acrylates. *Clin Exp Allergy* 1993; 23: 416–424.

36. Weytjens K, Cartier A, Lemière C, Malo J-L. Occupational asthma to diacrylate. *Allergy* 1999; 54: 287–296.

37. Plato N, Tornling G, Hogstedt C, Krantz S. An index of past asbestos exposure as applied to car and bus mechanics. *Ann Occup Hyg* 1995; 29: 441–454.

38. Dahlqvist M, Alexandersson R, Hedenstierna G. Lung function and exposure to asbestos among vehicle mechanics. *Am J Ind Med* 1992; 22: 59–68.

39. Järvholm B, Brisman J. Asbestos associated tumours in car mechanics. *Br J Ind Med* 1988; 45: 645–646.

40. Yeung P, Patience K, Apthorpe L, Willcocks D. An Australian study to evaluate worker exposure to chrysotile in the automotive service industry. *Appl Occup Environ Hyg* 1999; 14: 448–457.

41. Tornling G, Alexandersson R, Hedenstierna G, Plato N. Decreased lung function and exposure to diisocyanates (HDI and HDI-BT) in car repair painters: observations on re-examination 6 years after initial study. *Am J Ind Med* 1990; 17: 299–310.

42. Burge PS. Occupational asthma due to soft soldering fluxes containing colophony (rosin, pine resin). *Eur J Respir Dis* 1982; 63 (Suppl. 123): 65–67.

43. Bessot JC, Pauli G. *L'Asthme Professional*. Paris, Editions Margaux Orange, 1999.

44. American Conference of Govermental industrial Hygienists (ACGIH) *1998 TLVS and BEls. Threshold Limit Values for Chemical Substances and Physical Agents. Biological Exposure Indices*. Cincinnati, 1998.

45. Brooks SM, Hammad Y, Richards I *et al.* The spectrum of irritant-induced asthma. Sudden and not-so sudden onset and the role of allergy. *Chest* 1998; 113: 42–49.

25 CHEMICALS AND PLASTICS

Paul F. G. Gannon

INTRODUCTION

Chemicals used within the chemicals and plastics industries pose respiratory risks of sensitization at low levels of exposure and irritancy or toxicity at higher levels of exposure. For the former, the principal respiratory manifestation is occupational asthma, the level of risk depending mostly on the sensitizing potency of particular chemicals (Chapter 4). For the latter, irritant airborne concentrations of many chemicals may contribute to worsening symptoms in subjects who are already asthmatic, or even to sick building syndrome, though this is not generally considered an important occupational risk in the chemicals and plastics industries. Toxic concentrations that pose a potentially major threat of injury to the lungs and upper respiratory tract are the consequence of accidents (Chapters 6 and 12).

ALLERGIC ASTHMA

The chemicals and plastics industries have an excess of workers developing occupational asthma according to the Shield surveillance scheme in the West Midlands, UK [1]. Rubber and plastics workers had an annual incidence of 1054 new cases per million workers and those working in chemical processing 143 cases per million. These can be compared with an average incidence across all industries of 43 cases per million, and with eight cases per million in office-based clerks. The causal chemicals were most commonly isocyanates followed by acid anhydrides.

The European Union (EU) has identified the following criteria for the classification of respiratory sensitizers.

- Evidence that the substance can induce specific respiratory hypersensitivity (e.g. clinical history and data from appropriate lung function tests related to exposure to the substance, confirmed by other supportive evidence, which may include (i) a chemical structure related to substances known to cause respiratory hypersensitivity; (ii) in vivo immunologic tests (e.g. skin prick tests); (iii) in vitro immunologic tests (e.g. serologic analysis); (iv) studies that may indicate other specific but non-immunologic mechanisms of action (e.g. repeated low-level irritation, pharmacologically mediated effects); (v) data from positive bronchial challenge tests with the substance conducted according to accepted guidelines for the determination of a specific hypersensitivity reactions.

- Positive results obtained from appropriate animal tests.

- The substance is an isocyanate, unless there is evidence that the substance does not cause respiratory hypersensitivity.

Industrial agents that meet these criteria require labeling with the R42 risk phrase 'may cause sensitization by inhalation'. The following agents are used in the chemicals and plastics industries and are considered by the UK Government to meet the EU criteria [2]:

isocyanates

maleic anhydride

methyl-tetrahydrophthalic anhydride (MTHPA)

phthalic anhydride (TCPA)

tetrachlorophthalic anhydride (TCPA)

trimellitic anhydride

azodicarbonamide

diazonium salts

ethylenediamine

reactive dyes.

Industrial chemicals

Isocyanates

Isocyanates are widely used in the manufacture of polyurethane foams, plastics, coatings and adhesives, with an estimated global production of 5 million tons in 1990. Three diisocyanates, diphenylmethane-4,4′-diisocyanate (MDI), toluene diisocyanate (2,4-TDI and 2,6-TDI), and hexamethylene diisocyanate (HDI), account for greater than 90% of the commercial use. The use of monoisocyanates is limited. Isocyanates are very reactive, binding readily to proteins, they are irritant, and at high exposure levels they cause damage to airway epithelia [3,4].

Isocyanates may cause occupational asthma in a high proportion of exposed workers. An immunologic response appears to be involved in at least some, although a direct effect on the airways has also been postulated. A smaller proportion of exposed workers suffer from rhinitis, conjunctivitis, bronchitis, or obstructive airway disease [3]. Urticaria, fever and extrinsic allergic alveolitis can also occur, but rarely. The estimated prevalence for asthma has most commonly been reported in the range 5–10%, although 30% has been found in some studies. There is a latent period, with 60% of affected workers developing asthma within 5 years. There is no evidence that atopy or smoking influences susceptibility. It is clear that isocyanates can trigger asthmatic responses at relatively low concentrations, with some individuals responding to extremely low concentrations once sensitization has occurred. Respiratory sensitisation to isocyanates also appears to be life long but may not be obvious on initial reexposure [5].

Specific immunoglobulin E (IgE) antibodies have been detected in some workers exposed to isocyanates. In one review, 148 (14%) of 1095 workers who had asthmatic symptoms also had specific IgE to at least one of the three common isocyanates [3]. Only one of 685 workers without symptoms had such antibodies. There was an association between the presence of specific IgE and positive skin prick tests. It has also been suggested that the prevalence of specific IgE may be underestimated, since the detection assay, which usually uses 2,4-TDI isomer, may not adequately pick up antibodies to the 2,6-TDI isomer [6]. Using a reportedly more sensitive assay, 27% (6 out of 22) of symptomatic workers were found to have specific IgE to TDI, and 83% (5 out of 6) to MDI; three of the latter had been exposed to accidental 'high' concentrations of MDI [7]. Those developing occupational asthma within 6 years of first exposure were more likely to have specific IgE antibodies than those developing it later. In contrast to the results for IgE, similar levels of IgG were reported for exposed workers whether (24%) or not (17%) they had symptoms [3].

In addition to producing an immunologic response in some individuals, isocyanates have a direct constrictive effect on bronchial smooth muscle, as detected both in vitro and in animals, resulting in hyperresponsiveness to acetylcholine. There are indications that neuropeptides and tachykinins play a part in this response [3,8]. However, the high concentrations of isocyanates used in some of the animal studies could have caused airway damage.

Maleic anhydride

Maleic anhydride is a versatile chemical intermediate that has applications in a wide range of commercial products. The principal use of the substance is in the manufacture of unsaturated polyester resins. Other uses include the manufacture of oil additives and maleic acid. Evidence that maleic anhydride can cause work-related asthma is provided by six cases in which bronchial challenge testing demonstrated that it was likely to have been the inducing agent [9–11]. Supporting evidence is provided by its close structural relationship to other asthmagenic acid anhydrides, phthalic anhydride and trimellitic anhydride.

Methyl-tetrahydrophthalic anhydride

MTHPA is irritant to eyes, skin, and respiratory mucosa [12]. It acts as a cross-linking agent in the production of the epoxy resins used in the manufacture of plastics with special applications, such as the barrels of grenade launchers. Several studies on MTHPA indicate that it can induce occupational asthma, although the findings of the reported bronchial challenge tests are of limited value [13,14]. Immunologic data suggest an allergic mechanism for induction of the asthma, although antibody responses often correspond to exposure rather than symptoms. Supporting evidence is provided by the close structural relationship to phthalic anhydride.

Phthalic anhydride

Phthalic anhydride is a chemical intermediate that has applications in the manufacture of a wide range of commercial products, including plasticizers, resins, dyes, pesticides, and pharmaceuticals. The results of chemical factory health surveys in several countries provide convincing evidence that phthalic anhydride can cause asthma and rhinitis in a proportion of exposed individuals [15,16]. This conclusion is backed up by occasional reports of phthalic anhydride-associated asthma in earlier literature and a number of recent case reports. Positive bronchial challenge test results are also available. Immunologic data are too limited to allow firm conclusions to be made regarding mechanism of action.

Tetrachlorophthalic anhydride

Tetrachlorophthalic anhydride (TCPA) is irritant to eyes, skin, and respiratory mucosa [12]. It acts as a cross-linking agent in the production of epoxy resins used in the manufacture of plastics, paints, and electronic components. A number of positive bronchial challenge tests indicate that TCPA can induce occupational asthma. The immunologic data suggest an allergic mechanism for induction of the asthma, although in one study antibody responses corresponded to exposure rather than to symptoms. Supporting evidence is provided by the close structural relationship to phthalic anhydride.

Trimellitic anhydride

Trimellitic anhydride is a chemical intermediate with principal uses in the production of plasticisers, wire enamels, surface coatings, and wall and floor coverings. A number of allergic or toxic syndromes involving respiratory reactions have been identified in workers exposed to trimellitic anhydride dust or fume. Trimellitic anhydride-related respiratory illness was first observed in exposed workers at a US chemical plant in 1977 [17]. Three clinical syndromes believed to involve the immune system (together with a fourth, irritant, condition) have since been described [18,19].

The first syndrome is characterized by asthma and rhinitis and begins after a latent period varying from 2 weeks to 4 years; symptoms then occur immediately after exposure. For some affected individuals exposure to very low concentrations can provoke symptoms. The second condition (late-onset respiratory systemic syndrome or 'trimellitic anhydride-flu') involves a local respiratory reaction and systemic effects; coughing, wheezing, and dyspnea are generally observed 4 to 8 hours after a work shift, often accompanied by malaise, chills, fever, myalgia, and arthralgia. Third, there is a pulmonary disease/anemia syndrome, a potentially fatal illness involving both respiratory and systemic effects. It has been observed only in a small number of workers exposed to fume produced by spraying hot pipes with a resin containing trimellitic anhydride. The effects, observed after a latent period of several weeks, include dyspnea, pulmonary infiltrates, and anemia (Chapter 23).

There is strong evidence that the immune system is involved in trimellitic anhydride-related illness. The asthma and rhinitis syndrome is associated with a positive skin prick test to trimellitic anhydride–human serum albumin (HSA) conjugate and with the presence of serum IgE antibodies specific to trimellitic anhydride–HSA. The late-onset respiratory systemic syndrome is associated with the presence of elevated serum levels of specific IgG and IgA antibodies. However, skin prick tests with trimellitic anhydride–HSA are negative and the presence of serum specific IgE antibodies cannot be demonstrated.

Azodicarbonamide

Azodicarbonamide is primarily used as a blowing agent in the rubber and plastics industries. It is used in the expansion of a wide range of polymers including polyvinyl chloride, polyolefins, and natural and synthetic rubbers. It is estimated that several thousand workers are exposed to azodicarbonamide. Of this total, only a few hundred persons sustain exposure as part of their main work activity (i.e. those involved in compounding, mixing, or handling the raw material). The results of worker surveys and investigations of individuals show that occupational asthma develops in a substantial proportion of exposed workers [20]. The mechanism underlying the induction of asthma remains to be elucidated since there is currently no evidence that an immunologic or an irritant reaction is involved.

Diazonium salts

Diazonium salts are intermediates used in the manufacture of some reactive dyes, photocopier paper, and fluorine polymers. It has been reported that most workers exposed to the dust experience respiratory and mucosal irritation [21–23]. The available data are limited but they indicate that diazonium salts are capable of causing occupational asthma. Similarly, mechanistic information is sparse, but it is clear that an immunologic response occurs in a proportion of exposed, symptomatic workers [24].

Ethylenediamine

Ethylenediamine is used as an intermediate in the manufacture of various industrial chemicals, organic flocculants, urea resins, and fatty bisamides. It is also used in the production of formulations for use in the printed circuit board and metal finishing industries, as an accelerator or curing agent in epoxy coatings/resins, and in the manufacture of pharmaceuticals. It is classified as corrosive, and the vapor is likely to be irritating to the respiratory tract. Its potential as a skin sensitizer is well-known in animals and humans; in the latter from its clinical use in aminophylline. A number of reports indicate that exposure of workers to ethylenediamine can produce occupational asthma and a hypersensitive state [25]. The mechanism underlying the induction of asthma has not been established.

Reactive dyes

Reactive dyes have become used widely since their introduction in 1956. Each dye is made up of three moieties: the chromophore (dye), hydrophilic groups to improve water solubility, and a reactive group that will react directly with the substrate, usually a protein or cellulose fiber. The chemical class of the chromophore can be azo, anthraquinone, phthalocyanine, or oxazine. The reactive groups in use include vinylsulfonyl, halogenated triazinyl, bromoacrylamide, halogenated pyrimidine, and pyrazolone. When the dyes are supplied, they may contain unspecified additives [24,26–29].

A number of reports indicate that workers who have been exposed to reactive dyes can develop asthma. Although the available bronchial challenge data have not been generated under the most stringent conditions, they do suggest that the asthma is induced by specific immunologic hypersensitivity. There is evidence for an immune response occurring in workers with symptoms, specific IgE in particular showing a good correlation with bronchial challenge responses. Surveys indicate that the prevalence of occupational asthma amongst current workers is about 4%, with the suggestion of a higher incidence in leavers. It should be noted that the term 'reactive dye' covers a range of chemical classes, and not all may be responsible for causing occupational asthma.

Other causal agents

A number of other materials known to cause occupational asthma are manufactured within the chemicals and plastics industries, but their main use is outside these industries. They are not discussed here, though they are mentioned in Chapter 4. There are a myriad of other substances used in the chemicals and plastics industries. Some will be capable of causing occupational asthma, though the evidence at present may be inconclusive or nonexistent; consequently, the list of agents discussed above should not be considered exhaustive.

Investigation and management

Asthma of possible occupational origin within the chemicals and plastics industries requires investigation and management along standard lines (Chapter 4), though the consulted physician should be particularly sensitive to the possibility of a respirable chemical being the causal agent. A detailed occupational history is essential. The worker should be asked what he or she feels is the cause, but this should not prevent further enquiries as often workers identify mistakenly the most commonly used or most odorous agent: for example, strongly smelling solvents in a paint factory rather than odorless isocyanate used in small quantities. Previous jobs with the current and any previous employer should also be considered, as should the possibility of there being similarly affected workmates.

Workers often refer to chemicals by 'nicknames' or trade names, and so the physician should always ask for a Safety Data Sheet (SDS), which suppliers of chemicals in most countries are obliged to provide with the products they supply. In the UK, this is required under the Chemicals (Hazard Information and Packaging for Supply) Regulations 1994. Assuming the worker is agreeable to his/her employer being approached, these are usually easily available. SDSs vary in quality from those listing detail of all constituents and health effects to those supplying only generic information about constituents (e.g. 'binders' or 'active ingredient' rather than actual chemical names). Constituents are sometimes not listed unless they are present in the product above a particular concentration. It may consequently be necessary to seek more detailed information from the supplying company.

If no obvious causal agent is identified it may be appropriate to visit the workplace. If this is refused, the consulted physician may need to involve government inspection agencies. Information on exposure levels within the workplace may be useful, but measured exposures below any recommended limits may not exonerate a particular chemical agent as the results are not always representative; an earlier accident with transitorily high levels of exposure may have been critical in causing sensitization, and sensitization might have occurred within regulatory limits.

The most useful initial investigation, once asthma is confirmed, is serial peak expiratory flow (PEF) measurement. This may be complicated in the chemicals and plastics industries by many workers working rotating shift patterns, since this tends to make analysis difficult. However, many shift patterns include periods of up to 4 days off on a regular basis which may assist in identifying improvements in PEF away from work.

If no obvious cause has been found or multiple potential agents have been identified, then specific bronchial provocation tests may need to be undertaken at a specialist referral center. Most employers will be prepared to provide samples of chemicals that are suspected causal agents for use in this investigation since a confident diagnosis (whether occupational asthma is confirmed or excluded) is in their best interests also. If the employer is not willing, samples can usually be obtained readily from the supplier identified by the SDS sheet.

Once a diagnosis of occupational asthma has been made, the management plan should include removing the worker from further exposure. Ideally this will involve substituting the agent with alternative non-sensitizing agent; more commonly the worker is relocated. This is more easily undertaken if the employer has access to occupational health advice. When this is not the case it is important that the investigating physician gives clear instructions on which exposures the worker should avoid and it is explained that even low levels or short lived exposures to the sensitizing agent may lead to a further deterioration of work-related symptoms. It is also important to remind an employer of any legislative duty to report an occupational disease (e.g. Reporting on Injuries, Disease, and Dangerous Occurrence Regulations (RIDDOR) in the UK). The physician should also report the case to any reporting scheme in operation to ensure that, if other cases from the same factory are seen at different clinics, the cluster is identified at an early stage.

When considering a diagnosis of occupational asthma in the chemicals and plastics industries it is important to differentiate from 'constitutional' asthma, which is made worse non-specifically by exposure to irritant substances in the workplace, of which there are many (e.g. acids, alkali, oxides of nitrogen, chlorine). Key indicators of this will be asthma predating employment, reactions to irritants outside the workplace (e.g. perfumes, hairsprays, or smoky environments), and symptoms that are less consistent at work.

Health surveillance

Many countries have health and safety regulations that require health surveillance when, for example, workers are exposed to respiratory sensitizers (e.g. the UK Control of Substance Hazardous to Health [COSHH] 1999 Regulations), unless there is known to be no occupational risk. Health surveillance should start at the preplacement stage with questions about preexisting asthma and current symptoms of asthma, plus lung function testing. It is often normal practice to exclude workers with active asthma from working with respiratory sensitizers, because of the probable greater risk of developing occupational asthma, the ensuing risk of greater disability, and the difficulty that might occur later in determining whether true occupational asthma has arisen. Lung function testing (usually forced expired volume in 1 s (FEV_1) and forced vital capacity (FVC) may detect not only preexisting asthma but undisclosed lung problems; it also establishes a baseline for future measurements.

Workers with a past history of asthma, which is currently quiescent and not requiring treatment, will normally be allowed to work with respiratory sensitizers if lung function is well preserved, but more frequent surveillance is prudent in these circumstances. Atopy without asthma is not usually seen as an impediment to employment in the chemicals and plastics industries; to exclude atopic workers would exclude a large percentage of the workforce and may contravene national disability legislation, such as the Disability Discrimination Act in the UK.

The health surveillance procedure should normally involve a questionnaire on asthmatic symptoms and spirometric tests. Once work with respiratory sensitizers has commenced, health surveillance should initially be frequent since most of the workers who become affected will develop asthma after relatively short latent periods. In the UK, the recommended regimen involves testing at 6 weeks, 3 months, and annually thereafter [30]. It is useful to plot an individual's lung function results serially on a graph so that any deterioration can be easily detected.

Health surveillance should also include training the worker about relevant symptoms and minimizing exposure. He/she should be encouraged to report symptoms as soon as they develop, as opposed to waiting for the next round of surveillance tests. In addition, sickness absence records should be scrutinized for workers taking recurrent periods off work because of chest-related complaints.

This intensive program of health surveillance should always be undertaken for the agents listed above. For chemicals for which there is less good evidence of asthmagenic potential, a questionnaire alone could be used. When the risk is considered very low, a simple mechanism to report symptoms of possible occupational origin may be sufficient.

INHALATION ACCIDENTS AND REACTIVE AIRWAYS DYSFUNCTION SYNDROME

Exposure to toxic or irritant liquids, vapors, or gases in the chemicals and plastics industries is usually well controlled by either containment or the provision of personal protective equipment including respiratory protective equipment. Sudden loss of containment caused by leaks or spillages may lead to exposure many times above the occupational exposure limit for unprotected workers. These exposures may have direct effects on the upper and lower respiratory tract, including severe mucosal irritation or structural damage caused by chemicals such as acids, alkalis, oxides of nitrogen, or chlorine (see Chapters 6 and 12). These effects may lead acutely to pulmonary edema (toxic pneumonitis), although symptom onset may be delayed by up to 24 hours. Between 5 and 13% of reports to the Surveillance of Work-related and Occupational Respiratory Disease (SWORD) scheme in the UK have been for inhalation accidents.

Such exposures may lead immediately to increased non-specific responsiveness of the airways, and hence asthmatic symptoms, which may persist for some time after the incident, even in workers who had no previous history of asthma. This has been termed reactive airways dysfunction syndrome (RADS) or irritant asthma; it provides an alternative pathway for the development of occupational asthma (Chapter 4).

When inhalation accidents involve exposure to respiratory sensitizers, a single large exposure may be sufficient to lead to sensitization. Symptoms of occupational asthma can then be provoked at much lower levels, well below occupational exposure limits.

Not to be forgotten are the potential lethal systemic effects that uncontrolled exposure to some toxic gases can produce, for example, carbon monoxide, hydrogen cyanide, hydrogen sulphide, hydrogen fluoride, and organophosphates. Some of these require specific treatment with antidotes, for example amyl nitrite and dicobalt edetate (EDTA) for hydrogen cyanide. It is, therefore, always important when dealing with such exposures to know exactly what the exposure was and what the effects might be. This information will be provided by the SDS, which should accompany the injured worker(s) to hospital. This information can also be found from the national poisons information schemes. The topic is discussed more fully in Chapter 18.

POLYMER FUME FEVER

Polymer fume fever is a self-limiting condition with influenza-like symptoms (fever, headache, dry cough, dyspnea, and myalgia). It is caused by the inhalation of toxic products released by combustion of fluorocarbon polymers [31,32]. The fever usually occurs as a self-limited systemic illness with only minor pulmonary symptoms. Like metal fume fever, constitutional signs and symptoms typically develop several hours after initial exposure, often giving rise to a misdiagnosis of viral influenza. Compared with metal fume fever, polymer fume fever has a more varied clinical presentation, the severity of which depends upon the specific conditions of exposure. When higher temperatures and/or longer durations of exposure are involved, significant pulmonary involvement, including radiographic consolidation, is a potential complication. Although a number of industrial outbreaks have implicated the smoking of contaminated cigarettes as a vehicle of exposure, any industrial (or household) activity in which fluorocarbon polymers are heated above 350–400°C puts nearby workers or residents at risk of illness. Such activity should be avoided without strict industrial hygiene controls. There is no specific treatment, and the symptoms usually clear up spontaneously within 24 hours.

ASBESTOS-INDUCED RESPIRATORY DISORDERS

Many older chemicals and plastics factories have much of the pipework lagged by asbestos insulation, since they are often used to transport chemicals at high temperature. Asbestos was also used extensively in fire protection of structural supports in many buildings. If this is not damaged, airborne exposure levels should be minimal. However, damaged asbestos insulation may lead to significant exposure, and with it the risk of asbestos-induced diseases (Chapters 9, 19, 21 and 22). Any current work to repair or remove asbestos insulation will normally be contracted out to specialist insulation engineers, who will use appropriate protective equipment to protect themselves and appropriate enclosures to protect other employees. Such care may not always have been exercised in the past; therefore, a detailed occupational history is indicated if a worker appears to be suffering from asbestos related lung disease.

Asbestos is sometimes still used in filters or gaskets used on chemical plants. Such use is gradually being phased out. If the materials are not damaged, they are used correctly, and any debris is disposed of adequately, exposure risks should be minimal.

History

A 27-year-old man presented with an 18-month history of breathlessness, cough, and wheeze improving on days away from work. There was no personal or family history of asthma or atopy. He was a non-smoker and took no regular medication. For 3 years he had worked as an injection molder in an area housing 20 injection molding machines using a poly-oxymethane copolymer; the area had general, but no local exhaust ventilation. The machines were 10 years old and suffered from a thermostat problem that caused intermittent overheating. This resulted in the release of fumes produced from the thermal degradation of the polymer. Exposure to these fumes appeared to produce severe asthmatic attacks, and

on one occasion this resulted in a PEF reading of 230 l/min (predicted PEF 620 l/min) and hospitalization. This improved to 550 l/min following nebulized β_2 agonist treatment. At least two machines would overheat in any month.

Review of the Safety Data Sheet for the polymer, provided by the supplier, revealed no evidence of it having properties that could cause respiratory irritation or sensitization. Similarly no evidence of such an effect was found on a literature search. A visit to the workplace showed no other likely cause of his symptoms.

Serial PEF measurements were carried out over a 3-week period including a 1-week holiday away from work. The results plotted as maximum, mean, and minimum are shown in Figure 25.1.

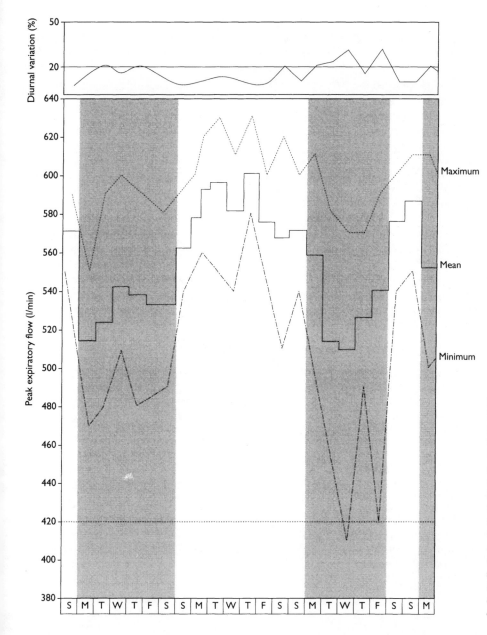

Fig. 25.1 Serial peak expiratory flow (PEF) measurements plotted as maximum, minimum, and mean against time in days. Days at work are shaded and the predicted PEF of 420 l/min is represented by the dashed line. Diurnal variation shown at the top of the figure exceeds 20% during work periods and as such is suggestive of asthma. The mean PEF shows a deterioration on work days with recovery away from work over the 8-day holiday and 2-day weekend. The changes are typical for occupational asthma.

Issues

The first issues for consideration are whether this man has developed occupational asthma or whether additional investigation is required before a diagnosis could reasonably be reached. Secondary issues are how he and the plant should be managed.

Comment

The book's contributors did consider this man to have occupational asthma, mostly with a high degree of confidence. Most additionally thought no further investigation was necessary. Since the working environment had not previously been associated with occupational asthma, a minority recommended industrial hygiene measurements to characterize the nature of any respirable chemicals and subsequent inhalation provocation tests to identify the causal agent.

The supervising physician contacted the supplier of the polyoxymethane copolymer to discuss the likely thermal degradation products of the polymer. Initially it was said that the product did not decompose on the normal heating experienced during injection molding. After discussion of the actual situation of use, where the polymer was exposed to temperatures much higher than normal because of the thermostat problem, the supplying company described a number of degradation products, including formaldehyde. This is a less well-known, but nevertheless recognized, cause of occupational asthma [33]. Whether it was responsible, in this case, is unclear.

A diagnosis of occupational asthma was made, and the worker was relocated to another area of the factory where a different polymer was used. There was complete resolution of his symptoms, and the abolition of asthma was confirmed by a normal serial PEF record. The company replaced the faulty thermostats on all the machines and no further cases of occupational asthma were reported.

 SUMMARY POINTS

Recognition

- Occupational asthma is the most common work-related respiratory disease in the chemicals and plastics industries: usually through the sensitization pathway, occasionally through the RADS pathway.
- Occupational asthma is more common in workers in these industries than in workers in general.
- A small number of agents cause most of the occupational asthma in these industries, but the possibility of less well-known causes should not be dismissed.
- Other important occupational respiratory disorders within the chemicals and plastics industries include inhalation accidents, polymer fume fever, and asbestos-induced lung and pleural disease.

Management

- Serial PEF measurement is the most appropriate investigation for occupational asthma and can be carried out effectively in the workplace.
- Lifelong removal from exposure is the most appropriate management for occupational asthma.

Prevention

- Information on chemicals should be obtained from Safety Data Sheets.
- Accidental exposure to certain toxic chemicals (e.g. chlorine fumes, oxides or nitrogen) may have delayed a potentially fatal respiratory (or systemic) effects, such as pulmonary edema, and so subjects encountering such exposures require appropriate close observation.

REFERENCES

1. Gannon PFG, Burge PS. The Shield scheme in the West Midlands Region, United Kingdom. *Br J Ind Med* 1993; 50: 791–796.
2. Health and Safety Executive. *Asthmagen? Critical assessments of the evidence for agents implicated in occupational asthma.* Sudbury, UK: HSE Books, 1997.
3. Baur X, Marek W, Ammon J *et al.* Respiratory and other hazards of isocyanates. *Int Arch Occup Environ Health* 1994; 66: 141–152.
4. Kennedy AL, Brown WE. Isocyanates and lung disease: experimental approaches and molecular mechanisms. *Occup Med* 1992; 7: 301–329.
5. Banks DE, Rando RI. Recurrent asthma induced by toluene diisocyanate. *Thorax* 1988; 43: 660–662.
6. Karol MH, Jin R. Mechanisms of immunotoxicity to isocyanates. *Chem Res Toxicol* 1991; 4: 503–509.
7. Pezzini A, Riviera A, Paggiaro P *et al.* Specific Ig E antibodies in twenty eight workers with diisocyante-induced bronchial asthma. *Clin Allergy* 1984; 14: 453–461.

8. Hayes JP, Newman Taylor AJ. In vivo models of occupational asthma due to low molecular weight chemicals. *Occup Environ Med* 1995; 52: 539–543.
9. Graneek BJ, Durham SR, Topping M *et al.* Occupational asthma caused by maleic anhydride: bronchial provocation testing and immunolgical data. *Thorax* 1986; 41: 251.
10. Durham SR, Graneek BJ, Hawkins R, Newman Taylor AJ. The temporal relationship between increases in airway responsiveness to histamine and late asthmatic responses induced by occupational agents. *Allergy Clin Immunol* 1987; 79: 398–406.
11. Graneek BJ, Durham SR, Newman Taylor AJ. Late asthmatic reactions and changes in histamine responsiveness provoked by occupational agents. *Clin Resp Physiol* 1987; 23: 577–581.
12. Venables KM. Low molecular weight chemicals, hypersensitivity, and direct toxicity: the acid anhydrides. *Br J Ind Med* 1989; 46: 222–232.
13. Drexler H, Weber A, Letzel S *et al.* Detection and clinical relevance of a type I allergy with

occupational exposure to hexahydrophthalic anhydride and methyl-tetrahydrophthalic anhydride. *Int Arch Occup Environ Health* 1994; 65: 279–283.

14. Nielsen J, Welinder H, Bensryd I *et al.* Symptoms and immunolgical markers induced by exposure to methyltetrahydrophthalic anhydride. *Allergy* 1994; 49: 281–286.

15. Wernfors M, Nielson J, Schutz A, Skerfving S. Phthalic anhydride induced occupational asthma. *Int Arch Allergy Appl Immunol* 1986; 79: 77–82.

16. Ahlberg RW, Keskinen H. Respiratory tract allergy caused by phthalic anhydride; degree of exposure and specific antibodies. *Hygiea* 1984; 93: 123–124.

17. Zeiss CR, Patterson R, Pruzansky JJ *et al.* Trimellitic anhydride induced airways syndromes: clinical and immunological studies. *J Allergy Clin Immunol* 1977; 60: 96–103.

18. Ahmad D, Morgan WKC, Patterson R *et al.* Pulmonary Haemorrhage and haemolytic anaemia due to trimellitic anhydride. *Lancet* 1979; 2: 328–330.

19. Zeiss CR, Mitchell JH, van Peenan PFD *et al.* A clinical and immunolgic study of employees in a facility manufacturing trimellitic anhydride. *Allergy Proc* 1992; 13: 193–198.

20. Slovak AJM. Occupational asthma caused by a plastics blowing agent, azodicarbonamide. *Thorax* 1981; 36: 906–909.

21. Armeli G. Bronchial asthma from diazonium salts. *Med Lav* 1968; 59: 463–466.

22. Graham V, Coe MJS, Davies RJ. Occupational asthma after exposure to diazonimum salts. *Thorax* 1981; 36: 950–951.

23. Luczynska CM, Hutchcroft BJ, Harrison MA *et al.* Occupational asthma and specific IgE to diazonium salt intermediate used in the polymer industry. *J Allerg Clin Immunol* 1990; 85: 1076–1082.

24. Luczynska CM, Topping MD. Specifc IgE antibodies to reactive dye-albumin conjugates. *J Immunol Meth* 1986; 95: 177–186.

25. Popa V, Teculescu D, Stanescu D, Gavrilescu N. Bronchial asthma and asthmatic bronchitis determined by simple chemicals. *Dis Chest* 1969; 56: 395–404.

26. Stern MA. Occupational asthma from reactive dyes. *Ann Allergy* 1985; 55: 264.

27. Wattie JM. A study into respiratory disease in dyehouse operatives exposed to reactive dyes. *J Soc Dyers Col* 1987; 103: 304–308.

28. Rosenberg N, Rousselin X, Gervais P. Occupational rhinitis and asthma due to reactive dyes. *Docs Med Trav* 1988; 34: 111–114.

29. Romano C, Sulotto F, Pavan I *et al.* A new case of occupational asthma from reactive dyes with severe anaphylactic response to the specific challenge. *Am J Ind Med* 1992; 21: 111–114.

30. UK Health and Safety Executive. *HSE Guidance Note MS 25: Medical Aspects of Occupational Asthma*. London: HSE.

31. Barnes R, Jones AT. Polymer fume fever. *Med J Aust* 1967; 2: 60–61.

32. Shusterman DJ. Polymer fume fever and other fluorocarbon pyrolysis-related syndromes. *Occup Med* 1993; 8: 519–531.

33. Nordman H, Keskinen H, Tuppurainen M. Formaldehyde asthma – rare or overlooked? *J Allergy Clin Immunol* 1985; 75: 91–99.

26 | FARMING

Katja Radon and Dennis Nowak

INTRODUCTION

Farmers (farm owners and farm workers) have traditionally been described as having one of the most dangerous occupations; the hazards from grain dusts were noted as early as 1555 by Olaus Magnus [1]. In particular, epidemiological studies have indicated a greater risk of respiratory disorders in farming than non-farming occupations. Workers on farms have a wide variety of different tasks depending on the type of produce. Agriculture has been defined by the World Health Organization (WHO) as all forms of activity connected with growing, harvesting, and primary processing of all types of crops; with breeding, raising, and caring for animals; and with tending gardens and nurseries [2].

Different types of exposure on farms may affect one or more regions in the respiratory system, and it may be useful to distinguish the risks from producing plant crops from those from raising animals. Some risks are, nevertheless, common to both types of farming. With plant crops, especially in greenhouses, workers are at particular risk because of pollen, fungal spores, pesticides and other chemicals, high temperature, and high humidity. Allergic sensitization of the intrathoracic airways (asthma) or the lung parenchyma (hypersensitivity pneumonitis) may be a major health problem, and there is

concern in the long term for exposure to inhaled organophosphate pesticides [3].

In animal farmers by contrast, endotoxins and ammonia may pose a greater threat, leading to non-allergic rhinitis or organic dust toxic syndrome (ODTS). In the conducting airways these substances, like insect antigens, aeroallergens, bacteria, fungi, mycotoxins, nitrogen oxides, paraquat, and hydrogen sulfide, may additionally induce bronchitis or asthma; more distally they may induce pulmonary edema, adult respiratory distress syndrome (ARDS), bronchiolitis obliterans, hypersensitivity pneumonitis, or interstitial fibrosis.

The evaluation of adverse respiratory effects in farmers compared with other occupational groups carries certain unusual difficulties: the percentage of smokers is generally low [4]; the healthy worker effect is often less influential [5]; farmers usually start working in childhood and often continue to work well beyond the age of 65; they often live in their occupational environments, thereby enhancing relevant exposures; and in small family-based farms the types of hazardous exposure may vary over a wide range. However, farm workers are more likely to leave their jobs than the general population, and in the case of migrant workers they are likely to be younger and lack basic healthcare services, at least in some countries [5].

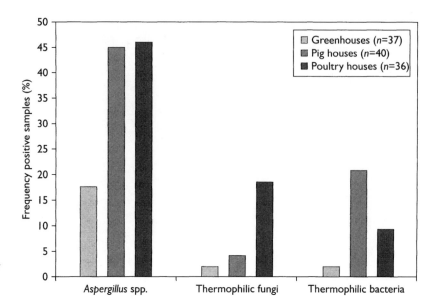

Fig. 26.1 Frequency of positive samples for fungi and bacteria in pig and poultry houses and in greenhouses [7].

The principal occupational respiratory disorders of farmers are asthma, chronic obstructive pulmonary disease (COPD), hypersensitivity pneumonitis, and ODTS. They provide the focus for this chapter and are outlined in Table 26.1 together with their most characteristic features.

EXPOSURES IN FARMING ENVIRONMENTS

Animal confinement buildings

Manure pits, which collect waste material as liquid or slurry under animal confinement units for fertilizer application, are a major source of toxic gases. High levels are found especially in confinement units with slatted floors. The most important gases inside the buildings are ammonia, methane, and hydrogen sulfide. Ammonia levels in swine confinement buildings frequently exceed threshold limit values (TLV) of, depending on the country, 20–40 ppm. Carbon dioxide may also occur at high levels in tightly closed areas. These gases may then be absorbed onto respirable particles. Dust inside animal confinement houses is mainly respirable. The main sources are the animals themselves (e.g. dander, dried fecal material), animal feed (e.g. grain, soy beans, fish meal), and bedding [6].

Many confinement houses have a warm and humid climate resulting in an increased growth of bacteria and fungi. The frequencies of common microorganisms in swine and poultry confinement

houses are given in Figure 26.1. Gram-negative bacteria produce endotoxin, resulting often in high indoor levels.

Crop farming environments

With the exception of storage silos, gases pose a minor risk in crop farming environments. Potential exposure hazards include pesticides and the dust emitted whenever grain is moved. In certain crop farming settings, such as greenhouses, dust levels are very low [7], and in these environments fungi, bacteria, and other allergens may pose the principal threats to the respiratory tract of the farmer (Tables 26.2–26.5) [8].

ASTHMA

Asthmatic symptoms in agricultural settings can be caused by immunologic responses to sensitizing agents, by direct irritant effects, or by other non-immunologic mechanisms. Many are not IgE mediated but are related to chronic exposure to irritants. This may aggravate preexisting asthma but does not often cause asthma [1,17]. Some authors define such work-related symptoms as an asthma-like syndrome, which is distinguished from asthma as a self-limited inflammatory event that does not involve persistent airway hyperresponsiveness [1].

Important examples of sensitizing agents causing occupational asthma through immunologic mechanisms are pollens from cereal grain, other grain

Table 26.1 Respiratory disease in farmers

Characteristics	Asthma	Chronic obstructive pulmonary disease	Hypersensitivity pneumonitis	Organic dust toxic syndrome
Symptoms	Shortness of breath, wheezing, cough	Cough with phlegm, shortness of breath	Fever, shortness of breath, cough	Fever, malaise, cough, chest tightness
Lung function	Obstruction	Obstruction	Restriction	Normal or mild restriction
Bronchoalveolar lavage	Eosinophils	Neutrophils	Neutrophils, lymphocytes	Neutrophils
Trigger	Type I allergens, irritating agents	Organic dusts	Type III allergens	Endotoxins?, beta-1,3 glucans?
Pathogenesis	Inflammation, obstruction	Inflammation, particle deposition, obstruction	Inflammation of the interstitium	Inflammation of the airways and alveoli
Mechanism	IgE, mast cells, histamine, muscle contraction	Destruction of cilia, production of phlegm emphysema	Macrophages, fibroblasts, fibrosis	Systemic cytokine response
Time course	Chronic	Chronic	Chronic	Acute

Table 26.2 Causes of asthma in farming

Trigger	Typical levels of exposure in the farming environment	Threshold levels
Sensitizing agents		
Storage mites: most common *Lepidoglyphus, Acarus, Tyrophagus, Tydeus, Tarsonemus*	Swine confinement houses: 0.0–54.1 µg/g dust of *Lepidoglyphus* sp. [9] Grain: 1.8 living storage mites/g grain [10]	No data available
Dander (mainly cow and horse dander)	No data available	No data available
Pollen (grain, grass)	No data available	
Soy beans	No data available	
Chemical irritants		
Ammonia	Median swine confinement houses: 6 ppm [16] Median poultry confinement houses: 12 ppm	US short-term exposure limit (STEL): 35 ppm
Pesticides (insecticides, herbicides)	Swine confinement houses: 0.2 µg/m³ [11] Greenhouses during pesticide application: 86–4300 µg/m³ [12]	Exposure limits in the USA (OSHA PELs) do not apply to agricultural field operations

OSHA PELs, US Occupational Safety and Health Administration permissible exposure levels.

Table 26.3 Causes of chronic bronchitis and chronic obstructive pulmonary disease

Trigger	Typical levels of exposure in the farming environment (mean values, mg/m³)	Threshold levels
Organic dust (plants, soil, bacteria, endotoxin, beta-1,3-glucans, fungi, mycotoxins) [7,13,14]		
Inhalable dust	Cattle buildings: 0.38 Pig buildings: 2.19 Poultry buildings: 3.60 Greenhouses: 0.14 Grain handling: 72.5	No special reference values for organic dust given; OSHA non-specific dust standards for particulates not otherwise regulated (PNOR): total dust 15 mg/m³, respirable dust 5 mg/m³
Respiratory dust	Cattle buildings: 0.07 Pig buildings: 0.23 Poultry buildings: 0.45	

OSHA, US Occupational Safety and Health Administration.

Table 26.4 Causes of hypersensitivity pneumonitis

Trigger	Typical levels of exposure in the farming environment (cfu/m³)	Threshold levels
Microorganisms: thermophilic actinomycetes Aspergillus spp. [7]		No data available
Fungus	Pig buildings: 383 333 Poultry buildings: 5 069 069 Greenhouses: 83 333	
Bacteria	Pig buildings: 5 833 333 Poultry buildings: 194 119 712 Greenhouses: 40 983	
Bird droppings	No data available	No data available

Table 26.5 Causes of organic dust toxic syndrome

Trigger	Typical levels of exposure in the farming environment (mean ng/m³)	Threshold levels
Endotoxin [7,15] Inhalable	Cattle buildings: 15 Pig buildings: 67 Poultry buildings: 200 Greenhouses: 1	Recent proposal of the National Health Council of the Netherlands [16]: 4.5 ng/m³ inhalable endotoxin
Respirable	Cattle buildings: 1 Pig buildings: 7 Poultry buildings: 21	
Beta-1,3 glucans	No data available	No data available

antigens, animal dander (in particular cow epithelia), fungal antigens, and dust mites [9,18]. Additionally, organic phosphates used as insecticides may induce asthma attacks by inhibition of cholinesterase. Bronchospasm in farmers with asthma, or with high levels of airway responsiveness, may be induced by various dusts, fumes, vegetable matters, and gases in the farming environment. Typical levels of exposure in farming environments are given in Tables 26.2–26.5. Examples of agriculture-specific activities and related exposures associated with an increased risk of developing occupational asthma include handling and harvesting grain, working in a barn, and raising animals.

The global prevalence of asthma in adults of working age is of the order of 5–10%. The prevalence of self-reported asthmatic symptoms in several populations of farm workers has ranged more widely from 3.3% to 13% [1,8]. Recent studies comparing asthma and allergy between the general population and farmers have shown a similar or even lower prevalence among farmers [19–21]. They reflect, additionally, a lower risk for the development of allergies among children living on farms [22,23]. Living on farms may consequently exert a protective effect for the development of allergies [24]. Responsible factors might be dietary habits, environmental influences such as endotoxin exposure, or 'lifestyle' factors such as spending less time in well-insulated buildings compared with the non-farming population. Another but less convincing explanation could be a long-term healthy worker effect over multiple generations. Therefore, IgE-mediated asthma seems not to be increased in farmers as a group. Nevertheless, European poultry farmers (odds ratio [OR] 1.9; 95% confidence interval [CI] 1.3–3.0) and flower farmers (OR 2.2; 95% CI 1.2–4.2) have been reported to be at higher risk for the development of asthma compared with other farmers [8,25], and reversible airway constriction may be seen in up to 25% of confinement livestock or grain workers [17].

Recognition

After asthma has been diagnosed, the occupational etiology has to be identified (Table 26.2). The following information from the patient may be useful:

- presence of asthma-inducing agents in the workplace

■ worsening of symptoms during the work week, improving on weekends and holidays

■ exposure to a high concentration of an irritant gas (e.g. ammonia).

An overwhelming exposure to a toxic gas may lead to the reactive airways dysfunction syndrome (RADS; Chapter 4), but lower levels of 'irritancy' may also provoke symptoms depending on the pre-existing levels of airway responsiveness. In agricultural settings a temporal relationship between exposure and symptoms may be difficult to find because many farmers live on their farms and/or work seven days a week.

Serial monitoring of ventilatory function in the workplace, especially using computer-linked meters, provides a very useful means of evaluating the temporal relationship between occupational exposure and airway obstruction (characteristic drops in peak expiratory flow (PEF) or forced expired volume in 1s (FEV_1) over the workshift).

Specific inhalation testing is generally the most definitive method to evaluate occupational asthma in the laboratory. False-positive results may be obtained if a patient with non-occupational asthma responds non-specifically to the irritative potency of agricultural dusts or gases. Conversely, it may be difficult to obtain a clear-cut positive acute bronchial response in a farmer with longstanding moderate obstruction that is likely to be a result of agricultural exposure. Therefore, the results of bronchial challenge tests have to be seen in the context of the clinical history and the markers of disease. In difficult cases, lung function monitoring with and without workplace exposure on the farm may be helpful.

Serologic or skin tests may help to determine the atopic status of the patient, but in most investigations IgE antibody levels did not correlate with pulmonary function [9,17]. Together with other tests and a careful patient history, allergy tests may nevertheless help to clarify a specific etiology. There is considerable variability in the sensitizing potential of animal dander. Whereas cow epithelium is highly allergenic, pig epithelium causes sensitization infrequently. When investigating storage mite allergy, partial cross-reactivity with house dust mite antigens has to be kept in mind.

Management

Standard treatment of asthma (inhaled steroids, bronchodilators) should be recommended also for asthma in agricultural settings [1]. Additional prophylactic doses may be useful prior to unavoidable heavy exposures [17].

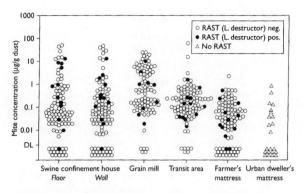

Fig. 26.2 Levels of *Lepidoglyphus destructor* 2 in dust from five sampling sites in pig farming and other environments. DL, detection limit.

As in other forms of asthma, the avoidance of recognized environmental triggers in affected agricultural workers is the best way to improve current control and future prognosis. For example, farmers with sensitization to cow epithelium should avoid contact with cattle, but they may still work with grain. Additionally, exposure reduction should be recommended not only for the workplace but also for the farmer's home (Fig. 26.2). It has been shown that the concentration of storage mites in animal confinement buildings correlated with the concentration of storage mites in farmers' beds [9], and high concentrations of cow allergen have been found in beds of farmers living on cattle farms [26].

The effectiveness of respiratory protection devices has proved disappointing, partly because compliance with their correct use is often poor. Müller-Wening and Neuhauss [27] could only show a partial reduction in the development of bronchial obstruction with a 'P2' filter. Therefore, dust masks may be of only limited value in asthmatic farmers, and their effectiveness should be checked individually. In some cases of occupational asthma in farmers, removal from the workplace offers the only possibility of adequate protection. This may be particularly difficult if the farmer is the owner.

CHRONIC OBSTRUCTIVE PULMONARY DISEASE AND CHRONIC BRONCHITIS

The main cause of COPD in the general population is smoking. Compared with other occupational groups the percentage of smokers is known to be low in farmers [4]. However, farmers are exposed to high levels of irritant gases and organic dusts, which include grain dusts, aeroallergens, endotoxins, insect antigens, beta-1,3-glucans, fungi, and mycotoxins.

Endotoxin and beta-1,3-glucans especially are thought to mediate macrophage activity and, therefore, may induce neutrophilic inflammation of the respiratory tract [28] (Table 26.3). These products of Gram-negative bacteria and fungi are present not only in grain dust but also in confinement buildings, especially those for poultry and swine. Additionally, differences in individual susceptibility are recognized. COPD [29] and the expectoration of phlegm are increased two to four-fold in prevalence in atopic compared with non-atopic farmers. Immunologic factors may consequently play a role in the development of COPD and chronic bronchitis in farmers. Acute symptoms during work may also predict these more chronic airway effects [30]. In a study of 4218 European animal farmers [25], nasal irritation during work was associated with a four-fold rise in the prevalence of phlegm expectoration.

Among grain workers, the prevalence of COPD has been found to be 25–30%. A high prevalence of chronic expectoration of phlegm (chronic bronchitis) among farmers compared with controls has also been reported. It has ranged between 3 and 30% in non-smoking farmers [17]. In the European Community Respiratory Health Survey [31], the prevalence of chronic bronchitis in winter in the general population aged 20–44 years was shown to be 7.5% compared with 9.4% of animal farmers within this age group in the study of European farmers [25] ($p < 0.001$). This prevalence did not differ significantly between different groups of animal farmers. Among crop farmers, those cultivating oil plants (OR 1.3; 95% CI 1.0–1.6) or flowers (OR 1.4; 95% CI 1.0–2.0) showed a greater risk for chronic bronchitis than other crop farmers. The prevalence of COPD in animal and grain farmers is related to exposure to large amounts of organic dust [32]. In pig farmers, it has been shown that the prevalence of COPD is significantly related to the time spent daily inside swine confinement buildings [25].

Recognition

Chronic bronchitis is defined by the British Medical Research Council as cough with phlegm for at least 3 months per year for no less than 2 years. In farmers, these symptoms often worsen at work after 2 or more hours, for example in animal confinement buildings. If there is also airway obstruction, affected farmers may additionally complain of dyspnea, chest tightness, and wheezing. All these symptoms may improve on vacations away from work, only to worsen on returning to work [33].

Several studies have shown that the expectoration of phlegm among farmers does not correlate with airway obstruction [34,35] and pulmonary function often shows no clear abnormality despite the high prevalence of chronic bronchitis.

Management

Patients with chronic bronchitis without obstruction may benefit from low-dose sympathomimetic agents or anticholinergics, possibly through improvement of mucociliary clearance. Few investigations have been carried out to identify effective pharmacologic treatment specific to chronic obstructive bronchitis in agricultural workers. Standard pharmacologic treatment is recommended [36].

Little is known on the prognostic factors of COPD and chronic bronchitis among farmers. The prognosis of COPD depends mainly on the degree of airflow obstruction, and its rate of progression. It can be assumed that smoking cessation is beneficial because of its probable additive or synergistic effect with that of agricultural dust, but no studies have specifically addressed this particular issue [33]. High levels of dust exposure and longer durations of employment are likely to pose greater risks [34], and so dust reduction and the avoidance of peak levels of exposure are suggested to improve the prognosis of affected farmers [37]. Limited data are available to support these assumptions. The topic is discussed more fully in Chapter 5.

HYPERSENSITIVITY PNEUMONITIS

Hypersensitivity pneumonitis, also called extrinsic allergic alveolitis or, in farmers, farmer's lung, is a type III and IV allergy following inhalation of organic dusts. Causative agents in the farming environment are *Micropolyspora faeni*, *Thermophilic actinomycetes* and *Aspergillus* species growing in moldy hay, grain, and other vegetable matter, as well as proteins derived from bird droppings or feather bloom. After sensitization, low levels of exposure may trigger an attack of hypersensitivity pneumonitis. Typical levels of microbiologic exposure in randomly selected farming environments are given in Table 26.4. There are some indications that cofactors are needed to induce the disorder in farmers, for example bacterial endotoxin or fungal beta-1,3-glucan [1].

The prevalence of hypersensitivity pneumonitis in agricultural populations remains uncertain because of diagnostic limitations in epidemiologic studies. Representative surveys conducted in various populations and geographic regions indicate prevalence rates between 1 and 10%. Prevalence appears much lower if the diagnosis was verified by chest radiography [38]. The incidence of clinically confirmed cases has been estimated at 0.2–0.5/1000 per year among those at risk [38]. The incidence and prevalence of farmer's lung depend considerably on climatic conditions and farming practices, which in turn determine the likely degree of microbial contamination. Therefore farmers working in climates with relatively high rainfalls where dairy farming is practiced (e.g. Finland) seem to be at high risk [1].

Recognition

In farmers, acute symptoms of hypersensitivity pneumonitis may resemble those of ODTS. The following diagnostic criteria, which partially overlap those of ODTS, have been advocated by several authors [1,39] (Table 26.6):

- previous (potentially sensitizing) exposure to organic dust
- febrile episodes some hours after antigen exposure
- dyspnea on exertion
- basal crepitant rales on auscultation
- restrictive lung function impairment
- decreased diffusing capacity for carbon monoxide in the lung (T_LCO)

- radiographic interstitial infiltration
- serum precipitating antibodies to the causal allergen (its identification may be facilitated by environmental assessment)
- improvement with avoidance of the causal allergen.

The demonstration of a decreased $CD4^+$ to $CD8^+$ T lymphocyte ratio in bronchoalveolar lavage fluid provides a valuable diagnostic sign of chronic hypersensitivity pneumonitis. Transbronchial biopsy reveals an alveolar and interstitial infiltrate consisting of plasma cells, lymphocytes, and occasionally eosinophils, in all affected subjects, and a granulomatous interstitial reaction in 50–70% of affected subjects.

Visiting the workplace of the farmer, taking microbial samples, and checking whether he/she has IgG antibodies to antigens of these particular microorganisms is often helpful, though an antibody response is generally more indicative of relevant exposure than of active disease. The diagnosis of residual fibrotic disease long after exposure has ceased can be made only from an appropriate history and compatible clinical features (Chapter 14).

Management

Acute and severe episodes of hypersensitivity pneumonitis are best treated with high-dose corticosteroids, but the long-term prognosis of farmer's lung

Table 26.6 Comparison of the epidemiology and clinical patterns of hypersensitivity pneumonitis with organic dust toxic syndrome

	Organic dust toxic syndrome	Hypersensitivity pneumonitis (acute farmers' lung)
Incidence (per 10 000 per year)	20–190	2–30
Clustering	Yes	Uncommon
Smoking history	Non-smokers > smokers	Non-smokers > smokers
Exposure history	Organic dust, 'moldy' grain, silage, hay, ,woodchips, may occur with first exposure	Repeated exposure to causative agent
Causative agent	Endotoxin? Fungal toxins? Other?	Antigens in thermophilic actinomycetes, aspergillus sp. etc.
Latency (h)	4–12	4–8
Symptoms	Cough, chills, fever, malaise, myalgia, chest tightness, headache	Fever, chills, malaise, cough, shortness of breath
Chest examination	Normal or scattered rales	End-inspiratory basal rales
Blood gas analysis	Normal, sometimes mild hypoxemia	Hypoxemia
Lung function	Normal, sometimes mild restriction	Restriction, reduced diffusing capacity for carbon monoxide (T_LCO), obstruction
Precipitins	Mostly negative	Mostly positive
Bronchoalveolar lavage	Neutrophils	Neutrophils, lymphocytes

is probably not affected by this [1]. Hay, grain, silage, and bedding are the principal and largely unavoidable sources of moldy dust in agriculture. Therefore, it has been common practice to recommend cessation of farm work for affected workers. However, several longitudinal studies have shown that the prognosis of hypersensitivity pneumonitis in farmers did not differ significantly between those who continued to work and those who did not [40,41]. As a consequence, greater emphasis is now directed to the avoidance of high levels of airborne microbial contamination. Reduced occupational exposure may be achieved by automatic feeding equipment and by diminishing airborne dust levels by the use of pelleted feed material or silage. It is helpful additionally to encourage the use of appropriate respiratory protection equipment (RPE). This should be properly selected for the type of task and the nature of the exposure, but the use of RPEs with physical work may pose difficulties, and compliance is not always satisfactory. Ideally, its use should be carefully supervised by a specialized respiratory or occupational physician.

ORGANIC DUST TOXIC SYNDROME

ODTS is an acute inflammatory condition affecting airways and alveoli that simulates influenza with or without additional respiratory symptoms. It may occur even in the absence of exposure to antigens known to cause hypersensitivity pneumonitis. After particularly high levels of exposure to organic dust, all involved workers may develop the syndrome, implying toxicity rather than hypersensitivity mechanisms [42]. Typical working tasks associated with ODTS are handling moldy grain in confined environments and mucking out animal confinement buildings. The causal agents have not yet been fully identified, but endotoxin is obviously and importantly involved in pathogenesis [1]. Typical levels of exposure to endotoxin in different farming environments are given in Table 26.5. Other agents possibly involved in the development of ODTS in agriculture are mycotoxins and proteinase enzymes [28].

In the study of European farmers, the overall prevalence of influenza-like illness after exposure to organic dust was 16.0% among 5685 farmers [25]. Other studies have shown similar or slightly lower prevalences of ODTS [1]. The incidence has been estimated at between 20 and 190 per 10 000 farmers per year [1,42]. Reports have particularly addressed ODTS in dairy, pig, and grain farmers [43]. Vogelzang and colleagues [44] reported a higher risk of ODTS among pig farmers compared with rural controls, and in the study of European farmers pig

farmers were shown to have a risk for the development of influenza-like illness slightly in excess of other farmers. Work in confined environments has been shown to be an important risk factor, particularly work in enclosed buildings (e.g. silos) with grain (whether moldy or not) or animals [44].

Recognition

The principal difficulty in defining the clinical characteristics of ODTS is to distinguish it from farmer's lung. The following features may be useful (Table 26.6):

- the extra-pulmonary symptoms of chills, fever, malaise, myalgia, and headache are more dominant than the respiratory symptoms of dry cough, chest tightness, and dyspnea
- there was a recognized exposure to high rather than 'usual' levels of organic dust (unloading silos, cleaning animal confinement houses) 4 to 12 hours before the start of the symptoms
- there was no sensitization period
- clusters of similarly exposed coworkers became ill also
- examination of the chest is normal or (rarely) there are scattered rales
- chest radiographs are normal or show no more than minimal infiltration
- leukocytosis is marked
- symptoms decrease in severity with repeated exposure (tachyphylaxis).

ODTS is most likely if the patient was in good health prior to the incident and recovers completely within a few days, though this pattern may be seen also in acute hypersensitivity pneumonitis of mild severity. The topic is discussed more fully in Chapter 13.

Management

In most patients with ODTS there is no need for specific pharmacologic treatment, though symptomatic medication is sometimes helpful. Symptoms will disappear spontaneously, mostly within 36 hours. While the prognosis of a single attack is very good [42] less is known about long-time sequelae after repeated exposures and repeated episodes.

PREVENTION

Environmental hygiene

The key to preventing respiratory disease among farmers, and particularly animal confinement workers, is improving the characteristics and management of the confinement buildings. Adequate ventilation is the single most effective measure in reducing the prevalence of work-related respiratory symptoms and the irreversible loss of lung function [34,45]. The higher the ventilation rate, the lower is the prevalence of symptoms. By contrast the use of wood-shavings as bedding, disinfectants, and non-slatted floors may increase the risk [46]. Some of these measures, especially increasing the ventilation rate, may prove to be expensive and the affected farmer may be unable (or unwilling) to adopt them. The use of silage, instead of hay and other fodder that dries following microbial contamination to produce respirable dust, should be encouraged wherever possible.

Exposure limits

In most countries, few exposure limits are applied in agricultural settings. While time weighted average (TWA) values exist for ammonia (but are frequently exceeded), the reference values for carbon monoxide, carbon dioxide, and hydrogen sulfide are seldom reached in farming environments. In general, there are no exposure limits specific for organic dust, endotoxin, bacteria, and fungi in the working environment, though many countries legislate to limit total and respirable exposure to 'nuisance' dust. Reference values are in most instances applicable for exposure to single agents only, since there are obvious difficulties in legislating for mixed dusts of variable composition. Adverse synergistic effects may nevertheless occur between respirable agents in agricultural settings, and there is need to define threshold levels appropriate to certain mixed dusts. An overview of the existing threshold levels in farming environments is given in Tables 26.2–26.5.

Personal protection equipment

Because job changes may be more difficult for farm owners than for workers in other occupations, additional means of prevention may be required, particularly the use of respirators in animal confinement buildings and during work with grain. Half-face respirators with an ammonia cartridge and a dust prefilter or positive-pressure full-face respirators are most suitable [6]. The efficiency of respiratory protection should always be assessed individually on a longitudinal basis. Gjerde and colleagues [47] found a higher rate of dust mask use when farmers had been introduced to them during a health education program.

DIFFICULT CASE

History

For 7 years, a 48-year-old non-smoking fruit farmer had experienced non-productive cough, that occurred principally during exercise and prolonged speaking. The problem was most troublesome in September and October of each year and tended to worsen in the evenings. At such times he reported sweating at nighttime, and temperature measurements gave values between 38.1 and 39.0°C. Non-specific pneumonia had been diagnosed on a number of occasions, and he had received several courses of antibiotic treatment.

Auscultation at the time of one presentation revealed inspiratory rales. A chest radiograph showed a middle lobe infiltrate and the erythrocyte sedimentation rate (ESR) was 37 mm in the first hour. Normal values were obtained for differential blood count, spirometry, D_LCO, and whole body plethysmography. Skin prick tests with ubiquitous allergens were negative, but serum IgG antibodies were demonstrated against *Alternaria* and *Penicillium* spp. Bronchoalveolar lavage revealed a CD8+T cell-dominant lymphocytosis, and transbronchial biopsy showed mesenchymal proliferation with thickening of alveolar membranes and lymphohistiocytic infiltration (Figure 26.3).

Issues

The issues here are what diagnostic possibilities should be considered and what further investigations should be undertaken?

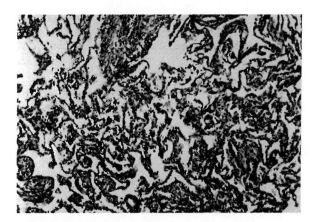

Fig. 26.3 Histopathologic findings of the transbronchial biopsy of the Difficult Case. (Courtesy RF Kroidl and M Amthor.)

Comment

The book's contributors strongly favored a diagnosis of hypersensitivity pneumonitis, though recognized that this was not necessarily occupational in origin. They consequently recommended a more detailed occupational and domestic history (was there a bird in the home, was the home contaminated with mold, were relevant medications being used?), and an inspection of the occupational environment. Culture of bronchoalveolar lavage fluid was also recommended in case there was an indolent infection, together with computed tomography and more detailed tests of lung function (were volumes increased or decreased, and how did spirometry change in association with work activity?).

In fact there was an inspection of the workplace. The ceiling of the apple storage building was seen to be covered with grey mold. Cultures revealed a predominant growth of *Penicillium* spp., but also *Alternaria tenuis* and *Aspergillus fumigatus*. A more detailed occupational history revealed that the apples were stored every year from September to be sold continuously until the supply was exhausted, generally by April of the

subsequent year. Within the storage building, a cooling and humidifying system provided optimal climatic conditions for preserving apples (temperature 5°C, humidity >90%).

The farmer was consequently diagnosed to have hypersensitivity pneumonitis, with a somewhat unusual radiologic presentation suggesting atelectasis within the middle lobe. The fungi, specifically *Penicillium* spp., are present during the whole year in the storage house, sporulation increasing during the spring and summertime when temperature is >12°C. However, during spring and summer little work is needed inside the storage house and exposure is limited. By contrast, during September and October, sporulation is still active within the storage building, and so is work.

SUMMARY POINTS

Recognition

- Even in modern agricultural settings farmers are at risk for the development of respiratory disease – principally asthma, COPD, chronic bronchitis, hypersensitivity pneumonitis, and ODTS.
- The most prevalent problem is chronic bronchitis (productive cough), which occurs in both smoking and non-smoking farmers.
- Chronic bronchitis may be associated additionally, but not necessarily, with fixed and progressive airway obstruction (COPD).
- Hypersensitivity disorders (asthma and hypersensitivity pneumonitis) are less common but not rare problems in both crop farmers and animal farmers.
- ODTS occurs in circumstances of high exposure to microbially (and hence endotoxin) contaminated

organic dust, most commonly in swine confinement buildings and grain silos.

Management

- Standard treatments for asthma can be used and sensitizing allergens identified and avoided.
- Chronic bronchitis may benefit from low-dose sympathomimetic or anticholinergic agents.
- Acute hypersensitivity pneumonitis is best treated with high-dose corticosteroids.
- Avoidance of the precipitating allergen is most effective.
- Respiratory protection devices exist but compliance is poor.

Prevention

- Control of these disorders depends primarily on reducing the prevailing levels of exposure.

REFERENCES

1. Schenker MB for the American Thoracic Society. Respiratory health hazards in agriculture. *Am J Respir Crit Care Med* 1998; 158: S1–S76.

2. World Health Organization. *Occupational Health Problems in Agriculture: Fourth Report of the Joint ILO/WHO Committee on Occupational Health*. Geneva: World Health Organization, 1962.

3. Senthilselvan A, McDuffic HH, Dosman JA. Association of asthma with use of pesticides: results of a cross-sectional survey of farmers. *Am Rev Respir Dis* 1992; 146: 884–887.

4. Stellmann SD, Boffetta P, Garfinkel L. Smoking habits of 800 000 American men and women in relation to their occupations. *Am J Ind Med* 1988; 13: 43–58.

5. Thelin A, Hoglund S. Change of occupation and retirement among Swedish farmers and farm workers in relation to those in other occupations: a study of 'elimination' from farming during the period 1970–1988. *Soc Sci Med* 1994; 38: 147–151.

6. Merchant JA, Donham KJ. Health risks from animal confinement units. In: Dosman JA, Cockcroft DW eds. *Principles of Health and Safety in Agriculture*, pp. 58–61. Boca Raton, FL: CRC Press, 1989.

7. Radon K, Danuser B, Iversen M *et al.* Air contaminants in different European farming environments. Submitted.

8. Monsó E, Radon K, Danuser B *et al.* Respiratory symptoms in European crop farmers. *Am J Respir Crit Care Med* 2000; 162: 1246–1250.

9. Radon K, Schottky A, Garz S *et al.* Distribution of dust-mite allergens (*Lep* d 2, *Der* p 1, *Der* f 1, *Der* 2) in pig-farming environments and sensitization of the respective farmers. *Allergy* 2000; 55: 219–225.

10. Iversen M, KJ, Hallas T, Dahl R. Mite allergy and exposure to storage mites and house dust mites in farmers. *Clin Exp Allergy* 1990; 20: 211–219.

11. Stewart PA, Fears T, Kross B *et al.* Exposure of farmers to phosmet, a swine insecticide. *Scand J Work Environ Health* 1999; 25: 33–38.

12. Archibald BA, Solomon KR, Stephenson GR. Estimation of pesticide exposure to greenhouse applicators using video imaging and other assessment techniques. *Am Ind Hyg Assoc J* 1995; 56: 226–235.

13. Takai H, Pedersen S, Johnsen JO *et al.* Concentrations and emissions of airborne dust in livestock buildings in Northern Europe. *J Agric Eng Res* 1998; 70: 59–77.

14. Simpson JC, Niven RM, Pickering CA *et al.* Comparative personal exposures to organic dusts and endotoxin. *Ann Occup Hyg* 1999; 43: 107–115.

15. Seedorf J, Hartung J, Schröder M *et al.* Concentrations and emissions of airborne endotoxins and microorganisms in livestock buildings in Northern Europe. *J Agric Eng Res* 1998; 70: 97–109.

16. Dutch Expert Committee on Occupational Standards. Health-based Recommended Occupational Exposure Limit for Endotoxins. Rijswijk: Health Council of the Netherlands, 1997.

17. von Essen SG. Respiratory diseases related to work in agriculture, in safety and health. In: Langley RL, Meggs WJ, Roberson GT eds. *Agriculture, Forestry, and Fisheries'* pp. 353–384. Rockville, MD: US Government Print Office, 1997.

18. Dosman JA, Graham BL, Hall D *et al.* Respiratory symptoms and pulmonary function in farmers. *J Occup Med* 1987; 29: 38–43.

19. Kimbell-Dunn M, Bradshaw L, Slater T *et al.* Asthma and allergy in New Zealand farmers. *Am J Ind Med* 1999; 35: 51–57.

20. Susitaival P. Farming and occupational health in Finland in 1992. *Pub Social Insurance Inst M* 1994; 133: 228.

21. Choudat D, Goehen M, Korobaeff M *et al.* Respiratory symptoms and bronchial reactivity among pig and dairy farmers. *Scand J Work Environ Health* 1994; 20: 48–54.

22. von Ehrenstein OS, von Mutius E, Illi S *et al.* Reduced risk of hay fever and asthma among children of farmers. *Clin Exp Allergy* 2000; 30: 187–193.

23. Braun-Fahrländer C, Gassner M, Grize L *et al.* Prevalence of hay fever and allergic sensitization in farmer's children and their peers living in the same rural community. SCARPOL team. *Clin Exp Allergy* 1999; 29: 28–34.

24. Von Mutius E, Braun-Fahrländer Ch, Schierl R *et al.* Exposure to endotoxin or other bacterial components might protect against the development of atopy. *Clin Exp Allergy* 2000; 30: 1230–1234.

25. Radon K, Danuser B, Iversen M *et al.* Respiratory symptoms in European animal farmers. *Eur Respir J,* 2001; in press.

26. Hinze S, Bergmann KC, Lowenstein H, Hansen GN. Cow hair allergen (*Bos* d 2) content in house dust: correlation with sensitization in farmers with cow hair asthma. *Int Arch Allergy Immunol* 1997; 112: 231–237.

27. Müller-Wening D, Neuhauss M. Protective effect of respiratory devices in farmers with occupational asthma. *Eur Respir J* 1998; 12: 569–572.

28. Zejda JE, Dosman JA. Respiratory disorders in agriculture. *Tubercle Lung Dis* 1993; 74: 74–86.

29. Vohlonen I, Terho EO, Hosmanheimo M *et al.* Prevalence of chronic bronchitis in farmers according to smoking and atopic skin sensitization. *Eur J Respir Dis* 1987; 71(Suppl 152): 175–180.

30. Dalphin JCH, Pernet D, Dubiez A *et al.* Etiologic factors of chronic bronchitis in dairy farmers. *Chest* 1993; 103: 417–421.

31. Burney PG, Luczynska C, Chinn S, Jarvis D. The European Community Respiratory Health Survey. *Eur Respir J* 1994; 7: 954–960.

32. Cormier Y, Boulet LP, Bedard G, Tremblay G. Respiratory health of workers exposed to swine confinement buildings only or to both swine confinement buildings and dairy barns. *Scand J Work Environ Health* 1991; 17: 269–275.

33. Donham KJ, Merchant JA, Lassise D *et al.* Preventing respiratory disease in swine confinement workers: intervention through applied epidemiology, education, and consultation. *Am J Ind Med* 1990; 18: 241–261.

34. Radon K, Schottky A, Garz S *et al.* Lung function and work-related exposure in pig farmers with respiratory symptoms. *J Occup Environ Med* 2000, 42 : 814–820.

35. von Essen S. Bronchitis in agricultural workers. *Sem Respir Med* 1993; 14: 60–72.

36. Senior RM, Anthonisen NR. Chronic obstructive pulmonary disease. *Am J Respir Crit Care Med* 1998; 157: 139–147.

37. Holness D. What actually happens to the farmers? Clinical results of a follow-up study of hog confinement farmers. In: Dosman JA, Semchok KH, McDuffie HH, eds. *Agricultural Health and Safety: Workplace, Environment, Sustainability.* Boca Raton, FL: Lewis Publishers, 1995, pp 49–52.

38. Malmberg PR-AA, Höglund S, Kolmodin-Hedman B, Read Guernsey J. Incidence of organic dust toxic syndrome and allergic alveolitis in Swedish farmers. *Int Arch Allergy Appl Immunol* 1988; 87: 47–54.

39. Terho E. Diagnostic criteria for famer's lung disease. *Am J Ind Med* 1986; 10: 329.

40. Cormier Y, Belanger J, Laviolette M. Prognostic significance of bronchoalveolar lymphocytosis in farmer's lung. *Am Rev Respir Dis* 1987; 135: 692–695.

41. Mönkäre S, Haahtela T. Farmer's lung – a 5-year follow-up of eighty-six patients. *Clin Allergy* 1987; 17: 143–151.

42. von Essen S, Thompson AB, Rennard SI. Organic dust toxic syndrome: an acute febrile reaction to organic dust exposure distinct from hypersensitivity pneumonitis. *Clin Tox* 1990; 28: 389–420.

43. Rask-Andersen A, Malmberg P. The organic dust toxic syndrome in Swedish farmers: symptoms, clinical findings and exposure in 98 cases. *Am J Ind Med* 1990; 17: 116–117.

44. Vogelzang PFJ, van der Gulden JWJ, Folgering H, van Schayck CP. Organic dust toxic syndrome in swine confinement farming. *Am J Ind Med* 1999; 35: 332–334.

45. Radon K, Opravil U, Hartung J *et al.* Work-related respiratory disorders and farming characteristics among cattle farmers in Northern Germany. *Am J Ind Med* 1999; 36: 444–449.

46. Vogelzang PFJ, van der Gulden JWJ, Preller L *et al.* Respiratory morbidity in relationship to farm characteristics in swine confinement work: possible preventive measures. *Am J Ind Med* 1996; 30: 212–218.

47. Gjerde C, Ferguson K, Mutel C *et al.* Results of an educational intervention to improve the health knowledge, attitudes and self-reported behaviors of swine confinement workers. *J Rural Health* 1991; 7: 278–286.

27 | FORESTRY, WOOD, PAPER, AND PRINTING

David J. Hendrick and Kjell Torén

INTRODUCTION

Forests provide the most efficient means on land for producing and storing organic matter, a resource that is fortunately renewable. Trees are harvested for two principal reasons: to provide timber and to produce wood pulp. Both have an almost endless variety of uses. Timber has traditionally provided building and construction material, and continues to be used widely in the building and construction industry. It is also the dominant material in the furniture industry, carpentry, and joinery work. Straight stems (round wood) provide poles for many purposes, and rotary cuts, bark, branches, chippings, sawdust, and other 'waste products' are used to produce variously veneer, plywood, composite panels (chipboard, fiberboard, particle board), mulch, and compost. Wood pulp is the starting point for paper making and for the extraction of cellulose – itself a major starting point for the production of organic chemicals that rivals closely the versatility of the petroleum industry. There are additional conservation and recreational benefits from forests, which for some continue to provide a renewable source of heating and cooking fuel. Overall, about an eighth of working men report occupational exposure to wood dust [1].

Of the world's annual harvest, some 5–10% is devoted to the production of composite board products with chemical bonding resins (chiefly urea-formaldehyde or phenol-formaldehyde, but also epoxy or polyurethane-based compounds). The obvious advantages to the user are convenient size, resistance to microbial decay and insect infestation,

and modest cost (the wood component is largely 'scrap'). The remainder of the current harvest, the bulk of it, is divided in proportions of about 2:1 to sawn lumber and wood pulp, paper making and cellulose extraction being almost equally important end uses of wood pulp.

The wide spectrum of occupations that depend on forestry, woodworking, paper making, and printing involve, in turn, a wide spectrum of hazardous exposures and some risk for almost all the respiratory disorders described in this book. The mechanisms involve a wide spectrum also, and include (aside from trauma to the thorax) infection, allergy, toxicity, and malignancy.

FORESTRY AND WOODWORKING

Epidemiology

Morbidity

Perhaps the most obvious exposure of forest workers, sawmill workers, carpenters, joiners, and other wood workers is dust derived from wood itself. Wood dust, in a generic sense, has proved to be an important cause of occupational asthma, and asthma has proved to be the most prominent occupational respiratory disorder within the forestry and woodworking industries, just as it has among employed adults generally in industrially developed countries. It is clear, however, that different species pose different levels of risk, and it may be that some species (particularly softwoods) have relatively little potential to cause asthma. In areas where forestry of western red cedar (*Thuja plicata*) provides a major source of employment (for example, in British Columbia in Canada), wood dust is the leading cause of occupational asthma [2]. At a national level in Canada, wood dust is the third leading reported causal agent (after isocyanates and flour), and wood-centered industries comprise the leading causal occupational environment. In the UK, wood dust accounts for about 5% of newly recognized cases and those who work with wood have an annual incidence of occupational asthma of about 150 per million [3–7]. This is three to four times the average incidence among all those who are employed, but concomitant exposure to isocyanates and other reactive chemicals within the industry may have confounded the matter. Two Swedish population-based case–control studies of asthma failed to show any association with wood dust exposure [8,9].

The most potent allergenic species are not necessarily the most important in an epidemiologic sense, since the species that grow most quickly tend to be the most economic and the most widely used. Among these, western red cedar has attracted particular attention, partly because of its potency and widespread use, and partly because of the pioneering investigations of affected workers by Chan-Yeung and colleagues in Vancouver [10,12]. In their study comparing 619 western red cedar sawmill workers with 1127 unexposed controls, the prevalence of asthma after commencing work in the current employment (a surrogate for occupational asthma) was 3.9 times greater in the cedar workers [11]. Atopy was not a risk factor, and smoking appeared to exert a protective effect. Among various groups of western red cedar workers the prevalence of occupational asthma has varied from 4% to 13.5% [12].

Wood dust is not the only respiratory hazard within wood-centered industries, however, nor is asthma the only respirable disorder for which there is risk. Wood is readily contaminated with various undesired infectious, allergenic, or toxic agents, and is often treated with potentially hazardous preservatives. There is some risk of malignancy for which the causal agent is not clearly identified, and mucosal irritation, infection, chronic bronchitis, chronic obstructive pulmonary disease (COPD), hypersensitivity pneumonitis, inhalation fever, toxic pneumonitis, and the organic dust toxic syndrome (ODTS) may all occur.

This wide range of potential effects and the many levels of the respiratory tract at risk are partly consequences of the wide range of particle size within dust derived from wood. Sawmills often produce dust of relatively large and non-respirable particle size, but there is considerable variability, and so the upper airway and major intrathoracic airways provide the chief targets for deposition. For example, a Taiwanese study in sawmills revealed total dust concentrations in ambient air ranging from 4.4 to 22.4 mg/m³, of which the respirable component ranged widely between 2% and 50% [13]. In the UK, exposure should be limited 5 mg/m³ as an 8-hour time-weighted average (TWA) for total dust. Rhinitis, asthma, and chronic bronchitis could therefore be expected to be the most common consequences of prolonged occupational exposure to wood dust. When wood has become contaminated with molds and spore-forming bacteria, however, small respirable particles are also present, as are respirable aerosols of saps, gums, and wood tars; these pose additional risks for hypersensitivity pneumonitis, inhalation fever, ODTS and (possibly) lung cancer.

This is not to say that small respirable particles pose no risk for the mucous membranes of the upper respiratory tract or the large intrathoracic airways. Norwegian wood trimmers ($n = 303$) and planing operators ($n = 170$) completed questionnaires related to handling moldy timber, and underwent serum immunoglobulin G (IgG) assays to molds by enzyme-linked immunosorbent assay (ELISA) [14]. The most common antibody response was to *Rhizopus microsporus*. The trimmers had greater exposure to dust and higher antibody titers than the planers, and more symptoms of mucous membrane irritation as well as ODTS and alveolitis. In both groups IgG to *R. microsporus* was the best predictor of symptoms, suggesting that this contaminating microbe might play a causal role at all the relevant levels of the respiratory tract.

Mortality

There is no clear evidence of an excess mortality attributable to working directly with wood, but Swedish sawmill workers experienced an increased mortality rate due to asthma [15]. In addition, a study among 27 362 members of the US Carpenters' Union over the period 1987–1990 showed increased mortality from asbestos-related disorders (asbestosis, lung cancer, and mesothelioma) among those employed in the construction industry but not those working with wood in other industries [16]. Similarly, a US study of 34 081 furniture workers involving 411 000 person-years showed a significant excess of mesotheliomas (standardized mortality ratio (SMR) 3.7) among the dominant subgroup of white men, but this could not be linked to furniture plants using wood rather than metal [17].

Malignancy

The International Agency for Research on Cancer (IARC) reanalyzed data from five cohorts of wood workers (furniture makers, plywood workers, and wood model makers) that involved 28 704 subjects and 7665 deaths. There was no excess of lung cancer, but 11 nasal cancers were noted and nine nasopharyngeal cancers (SMRs 3.1 and 2.4 respectively), the excess nasal cancer being confined to only one of the five cohorts (UK furniture makers) [18]. Wood dust has consequently been classified by IARC as a human carcinogen, the evidence being stronger for hardwoods than softwoods. Hardwoods appear to be associated particularly with adenocarcinoma even in the absence of chemical additives, but latency from first exposure is long – an average of 40 years in one study [19]. Hardwoods are distinguished from softwoods by their botanical structure, not by density, and balsa is actually a hardwood.

An excess risk for cancer of the upper respiratory tract has been reported from several other studies and from several countries. Data from 12 case–control studies were pooled, and showed a strong association between nasal adenocarcinoma and work in wood-related occupations (odds ratio, OR 13.5, 95% CI 9.0–20.0). Exposure was assessed using a job exposure matrix and industry titles. There was additionally an ambiguous increase in risk for squamous carcinoma [20]. In a French case–control study of sinonasal cancer (207 cases versus 409 controls) the risk for squamous carcinoma was increased 2-fold if wood dust exposure first occurred before 1945 [21], and a study in Nordic countries found that woodworkers had the highest incidence of nasal cancer during 20 years of surveillance of cancer incidence from 1970 among a working population of 10 million aged 25–64 initially [22]. Similarly in Spain, a case–control study of 50 incident cases of laryngeal carcinoma during 1982–1985 and 89 controls showed that woodworkers had the greatest OR among occupational groupings, after adjusting for alcohol and smoking. The risk increased with duration of exposure, the OR reaching 5.6 for more than 20 years' work, especially in the subgroup of furniture workers (OR 6.7) [23].

There have, however, been discrepancies, raising suspicion that contaminants (particularly preservatives) present in varying degree might be primarily responsible rather than any intrinsic constituent of wood itself. One report suggested that three of eight studied wood perservatives were genotoxic, as were five of 16 wood stains, and two of 11 paints [24]. So, too, were certain substances extracted from wood itself (e.g. oak and beech), and the authors suggested that the carcinogenic effect might depend on interactive effects from several exposures (especially involving hardwoods) since the risk appeared greater in workers in small companies exposed generally to multiple agents than in large companies where single agents were more often used.

Polyaromatic hydrocarbons (PAHs) have attracted particular attention, not only for upper respiratory tract cancer, but also for lung cancer. High exposure to some of these compounds is recognized by IARC to be a cause of lung cancer (e.g. in coal gasification and coke production; Chapter 19) [25]. In a Montreal population of workers exposed to various PAHs in the wood, petroleum, coal, and other industries, an increased risk of lung cancer was noted overall in non-smokers and light smokers, but not in heavy smokers [26]. A further Canadian study studied a specific group of PAHs used for wood preservation – chlorophenates – by comparing lung cancer incidence in sawmills in which they were used with those in which they were not. No excess of lung cancer was found [27]. A Finnish nested case–control study of cancer of the lung and upper respiratory tract ($n = 136$) among 7307 workers in 35 plants of woodworkers did, however, show an increasing risk in association with increasing exposure to petrol and diesel exhaust (hence PAHs), and with pesticides [28]. Slightly increased risks were noted for terpene (a wood tar constituent) and mold spore exposure, which may have been a consequence of chance, but there was no increased risk from wood dust exposure (principally pine, spruce, birch).

There have been other studies identifying more generally a possible increase in risk of lung cancer from work with wood. The US Cancer Society's Cancer Prevention Study involving 362 823 men showed that about one in eight (45 399) reported occupational wood dust exposure. Their relative risk for lung cancer was mildly increased at 1.17 (1.04–1.31), and there was a significant trend of increasing lung cancer risk with increasing duration of exposure [1]. A Chinese study among different industries took account of smoking and found increased risks for lung cancer in textile, wood, metal, and construction industries [29]. In Spain, wood dust has been considered one of the four most common occupational carcinogens, along with solar radiation, environmental tobacco smoke, and silica [30]. A case–control study of lung cancer in Argentina attributed 85% of cases to smoking with an additional significant association with work in sawmills or wood mills (OR 4.6) [31].

Injury

The risk of occupational injury is high among forestry workers; a New Zealand study demonstrated the annual mortality rate from work-related injury (principally from chainsaw accidents, falling trees, rolling logs, and falls) to be 2.03 per 1000 loggers.

This can be compared with 0.15 per 1000 silviculture workers, and only 0.07 per 1000 in the working population at large [32].

Wood dust

In individual cases, a diagnosis of occupational asthma attributable to wood dust is most convincingly made with inhalation provocation tests. These may be carried out with pure extracts, such as plicatic acid from western red cedar, in which case the allergen is conveniently administered by nebulizer, or with samples of the wood dust (sawdust) itself simulating occupational exposure [33,34]. Fig. 27.1 provides an example. The subject was a carpenter who worked with many different woods and noted irregular episodes of occupationally related symptoms. In a laboratory-based challenge test he tipped sawdust to and fro between trays for an hour. Sawdust from western red cedar reproduced his symptoms and gave a typical late asthmatic reaction, but mixed sawdust derived from woods other than western red cedar gave no reaction.

As with other allergenic types of occupational asthma, the level of specific sensitization to wood dust may decline in the affected individual with the passage of time after exposure ceases, and with this there may be a reduction of asthmatic activity (airway responsiveness) and asthmatic symptoms. With renewed exposure, however, the level of sensitization generally rises quickly, and an increasing level of airway responsiveness may be the first manifestation. Thus, specific inhalation provocation tests may need more challenge doses than are usually required before positive results are obtained [35].

Chan-Yeung and colleagues followed 280 men with western red cedar asthma for a minimum of 1 year, and compared the longitudinal loss of ventilatory function with that of 399 sawmill workers unaffected by asthma [36]. Multiple regression analysis showed that continuing exposure to western red cedar in the asthmatic group was associated with an excess mean annual loss of forced expiratory volume in 1 s (FEV_1) of 26 ml, while smoking was associated with a mean annual loss of 43 ml. This suggests that the asthmatic effect of western red cedar may be associated with an additional COPD effect, as has been demonstrated with a number of other occupational asthmagens.

There is increasing evidence that cryptogenic fibrosing alveolitis (CFA), often known as idiopathic pulmonary fibrosis, occurs more often in subjects who have previous occupational exposure to dusts, particularly wood and metal dusts. A postal questionnaire was used in a UK study to evaluate the lifetime occupational history of 218 subjects with CFA (the cases of a case–control study) and 569 controls matched by age, sex, and living community [37]. The risk of CFA was significantly increased (OR 1.7, 95% Cl 1.01–2.92) in those reporting occupational exposure to wood dust, and a significant exposure–response relation was noted. Similar observations were noted with metal dust exposure; overall about 20% of the cases were thought to be occupational in origin.

Intrinsic agents

The causal asthmagenic agent in western red cedar is predominantly a component of the sap (plicatic acid) and so the risk of asthma will be present for anyone working with western red cedar, whether or not the wood is microbially contaminated, infested with insects, treated with preservatives, painted, or bonded with chemical resins. Many other species of wood are similarly believed to have

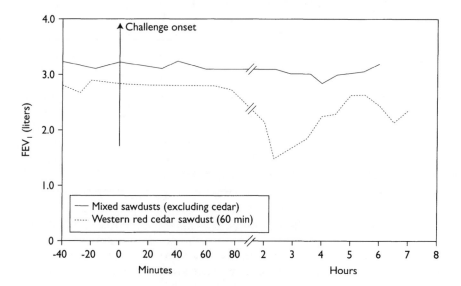

Fig. 27.1 Late asthmatic reaction to western red cedar sawdust but not other wood species. The carpenter tipped sawdust to and fro between trays for 1 hour. He had worked with a number of different woods, and noted irregular episodes of occupationally related asthmatic symptoms. Adapted from Hendrick et al. [85].

intrinsic sensitizing and asthmagenic properties, and are listed in Chapter 4. Plicatic acid can be conjugated with human serum albumin (HSA) to produce a hapten–protein complex for immunologic studies. This complex has been shown to release histamine from basophils and bronchial biopsy specimens of subjects with western red cedar asthma but not from non-asthmatic subjects nor subjects with atopic asthma, thereby inferring an aetiologic role for plicatic acid. IgE antibodies to plicatic acid–HSA conjugates are not, however, detectable in most subjects with western red cedar asthma and so plicatic acid may have specific and non-specific effects on these cells, and western red cedar asthma may not be solely an IgE-mediated disease [38]. Western red cedar asthma might also be induced in some cases by components other than plicatic acid.

Plicatic acid is also present in eastern white cedar, although at approximately half the concentration of that in western red cedar, but the prevalence of occupational asthma among exposed workers appears roughly comparable to that associated with western red cedar [39]. Among 164 Swedish sawmill workers who were not exposed to western red cedar, there was a significantly greater level of airway responsiveness in those most heavily exposed to wood dust as sawyers than those least heavily exposed, and there was no association with precipitating antibodies to contaminating fungi. This implies an asthmagenic effect attributable to intrinsic wood antigens other than plicatic acid [40].

Microbial contaminants

Respiratory infection in forestry and wood workers is very rarely occupational in origin, but one or two particular pathogens occur in forest environments, and some fungi contaminating stored wood or (less commonly) growing trees cause infection when inhaled, especially if the worker is immunocompromised.

Sporotrichosis is a well described occupational infection associated with work with contaminated sphagnum moss, but similar contamination in stored wood (and hay) may also pose an occupational risk [41]. Infection is usually confined to the skin and local lymphatics, although systemic spread can occur and isolated respiratory infection is sometimes seen. This probably results from inhalation, and simulates other indolent fungal infections.

Contamination with allergenic material provides a much greater cause of respiratory disease in forestry and woodworkers than infection. The responsible agents are both naturally occurring microbial contaminants and chemicals introduced by humans for

preservation or for the bonding of composite boards [42]. The principal effects are rhinitis, asthma, and, very occasionally, hypersensitivity pneumonitis.

Microbial contamination is also associated with occupational exposure to fungal toxins and bacterial endotoxin, and these may produce episodes of inhalation fever and ODTS. Inhalation fever is common, and was reported in questionnaires by as many as one fifth of 2052 trimmers in 233 Swedish sawmills [43]. By contrast, investigation showed only one case of hypersensitivity pneumonitis. Other studies from Sweden have suggested a much higher prevalence for hypersensitivity pneumonitis (of the order 5–10%), but this risk has been reported only rarely from other countries. The detailed investigation of one affected subject in the UK suggested that hypersensitivity to the fungus *Trichoderma koningii* was responsible [44].

Chemical contaminants

Chemicals may contaminate wood dust because of their use in preservation (e.g. arsenic compounds against termite attack) or in the bonding of composite boards (e.g. epoxy resins, phenol- and urea-formaldehyde resins, and polyurethane). A number of chemicals are additionally used to protect young saplings from disease at the time of planting. All may pose a threat of ill health to exposed workers, although the attribution of a causal role to one rather than another is usually a matter of considerable difficulty, especially as there is generally additional, and potentially confounding, contamination with microbial toxins. Furthermore, certain potentially toxic chemicals are produced by the tree itself during normal growth (e.g. terpenes), and metal contamination (chromium, cobalt, tungsten carbide) of ambient air or wood dust may be associated with sawing, milling, and chipping.

Dust released from working with wood and composite board products in joineries is more likely to be contaminated with chemical preservatives and chemical bonding agents than dust released in sawmill or chipping work. Conversely, exposure to microbial contaminants is generally greater in sawmill and chipping mill workers than in joinery workers. An interesting Australian study assessed personal exposure levels of workers in all three sites to wood dust, Gram-negative bacteria (and their endotoxin), and fungi (and β-D-glucans from their cell walls), and measured across shift changes in ventilatory function [45,46]. The relationships linking across shift change to exposure were stronger and more clearly significant in the joinery workers than in the sawmill and chipping mill workers, and the joinery workers had a higher prevalence of regular productive cough. This was so whether exposure was measured as total or respirable dust, or as the endotoxin and glycan levels, the latter being correlated with the respective concentrations of colony-forming Gram-negative bacteria and fungi. This raises the possibility of an interactive effect of the chemical contaminants to which the joinery workers were additionally exposed, although other factors may also have been relevant. For example, the joinery workers worked with many different wood species, both hard and soft, whereas the sawmill and chipping workers worked exclusively with eucalyptus (a hardwood). In general, hardwoods are thought to carry greater risks of respiratory disease than softwoods [47].

More importantly, the woodworkers as a group reported more than twice the prevalence of cough, whether dry or productive, than unexposed controls, and the joinery workers reported more than twice the prevalence of wheezing and nasal blockage. This was associated with significantly lower ventilatory function in the woodworkers than in the controls, although the impairment appeared more restrictive than obstructive in nature.

Airway obstruction was more clearly associated with the respiratory symptoms of a cluster of 18 workers in a single US wood products plant during its first 2.5 years of operation [48]. All developed asthma from sensitization to steam-heated methylene diisocyanate (MDI), which was used to make a synthetic wood board product. The high temperature evidently increased substantially the risk of MDI vaporization and sensitization.

Smoke

Smoke poses an unpredictable risk to forestry workers, although its adverse respiratory effects are well known in other settings. A longitudinal study across the 1992 summer season in the USA provided across-shift measurements of spirometry for 76 firefighting forestry workers, and across-season measurements for 53 [49]. For the former, the greatest change was noted at the midpoint of each shift (mean declines in FEV_1 and forced vital capacity (FVC) of 190 and 89 ml respectively), following which there was a mild improvement, leaving overall declines across the whole shift of 150 and 65 ml. Across the season the mean FEV_1 declined significantly, by 104 ml. An obstructive effect was therefore demonstrated, much of it reversible. The effect proved to be fully reversible in a small subset studied annually. An excess decline in FEV_1 was also demonstrated in association with the use of wood for heating.

A unique case–control study in Mexico assessed the role of wood smoke from cooking with traditional wood stoves on the development of chronic productive cough (chronic bronchitis) and COPD in 127 women aged over 40 years who were attending a hospital chest clinic [50]. Four groups of controls were used: patients with tuberculosis ($n = 83$), interstitial lung disease ($n = 100$), ear, nose, and throat disease ($n = 97$), and healthy visitors to the hospital ($n = 95$). Crude ORs for exposure to wood smoke were significantly increased for chronic bronchitis without COPD (3.9), chronic bronchitis with COPD (9.7), and COPD without chronic bronchitis (1.8). The associations remained significant after adjusting for age, income, education, smoking, place of residence, and place of birth, and were strengthened with increasing periods of estimated exposure. When the women with the highest levels of exposure were compared with those who were unexposed, the OR for chronic bronchitis without COPD rose to 15.0 (95% CI 5.6–40), and that for chronic bronchitis with COPD to 75 (18–306). The results suggest a causal role of wood smoke for both chronic bronchitis and COPD.

In a further, but independent, Mexican study of 30 non-smoking patients with extensive indoor exposure to wood smoke, detailed investigation indicated both obstructive and restrictive abnormalities of ventilatory function, and reticulonodular radiographic abnormalities [51]. Endoscopic examination revealed inflammatory abnormalities of the airways and an intense anthracotic staining which the investigators considered characteristic. There was unusually severe pulmonary hypertension complicating these abnormalities, but selection bias for participation in the investigation may have accounted for this.

Other environmental agents

Some occupational disorders of forestry workers arise from environmental factors that are not directly related to wood. A celebrated example over recent years has been the tickborne transmission of the spirochetal infection, lyme disease (borreliosis). The chief hosts for this zoonosis are deer and other forest animals. The infecting microorganism, *Borrelia burgdorferi*, does not characteristically involve the lung, however, but it may involve the heart and so produce breathlessness. Serologic testing suggests that infection is common in forestry workers, although clinical disease is rare [52–54].

Respiratory disease is more obviously responsible for breathlessness if bronchospasm follows hymenoptera stings (common in forestry workers), and there is some risk of systemic reactions [55]. More remarkably, complicated silicosis has been reported in a forestry worker who worked for some years driving roadways through forested land. He had hand drilled and blasted dry granite and sandstone without respiratory protection.

PAPER MAKING

Wood is pulped either mechanically or chemically (or both) and heated in water, often with alkali or sulfite, to release its cellulose content (about 50% by weight). The freed cellulose, a fibrous polysaccharide polymer, is used principally in paper making or plastics manufacture. Wood pulp additionally contains lignin, the natural binding agent for the cellulose, which discolors the pulp and so has to be bleached before the pulp can be processed to make paper. This poses the greatest risk to pulp workers, although some exposure to wood dust and other wood products is also inevitable. Bleaching is most commonly achieved with chlorine, although ozone, peroxides, and fungal enzymes are finding an increasing role as they pose a lower risk of pulmonary toxicity to exposed workers. Although ozone is less potent, it nevertheless has similar irritant and toxic effects on both airway (bronchitis, asthma) and parenchyma (pneumonitis), and fungal enzymes have well recognized risks for sensitization (asthma, alveolitis). Historically, death from chlorine exposure has not been a rare occurrence [56], and in modern times airway disease (COPD, asthma) has proved to be a common effect with occasional episodes of inhalation accidents causing pneumonitis [57–59].

The most important exposures in paper making consequently include chlorine dioxide, other bleaching agents, sulfur dioxide, and to some extent wood dust and paper dust. Some epidemiological studies have shown an increased prevalence of wheeze and decreased lung function among pulp mill workers, especially among the bleach workers [60–62]. A history of gassing events seems to be a major risk factor [60], especially for smokers [62].

In a study by Chan-Yeung and colleagues that compared 399 pulp mill workers with 1127 unexposed controls, the prevalence of asthma after commencing work in the current employment (a surrogate for occupational asthma) was 2.2 times greater in the pulp mill workers, and atopy appeared to be a risk factor [11]. An asthmagenic risk from paper manufacture was also suggested among 83 Swedish paper workers who were compared with 44 controls to assess the relation between, on the one hand, reported symptoms, spirometry, airway responsiveness (methacholine tests), and eosinophilic cationic protein (ECP) and, on the other hand, measured exposure levels to Gram-negative endotoxin and fungal β-D-glucan. The paper workers reported more asthmatic symptoms, and showed greater levels of airway obstruction, airway responsiveness, and serum ECP. Furthermore, the levels of airway responsiveness and ECP were positively related to endotoxin and β-D-glucan, after controlling for appropriate confounders [59].

Hypersensitivity pneumonitis is a much less common occupational allergic disorder of wood pulp workers, but may occur as a consequence of fungal contamination of wood, as it may in forestry workers. Inhalation provocation tests in one affected wood pulp worker confirmed that an acute alveolar response could be reproduced by an extract of *Alternaria* [63].

Cough, sputum expectoration, and airways obstruction may also have an increased prevalence in the paper industry [57,59], in keeping with forestry work, and these are seen additionally in workers exposed to paper dust in recycling plants [58].

A recent literature review of malignant diseases associated with pulp and paper mills concluded that among maintenance workers there was an increased risk of lung cancer and mesothelioma, implying asbestos exposure. Lung cancer was additionally associated with exposure to chorine compounds, while an excess of lymphoma was associated with wood pulp work. The causal agent was speculated to be wood dust itself (perhaps terpenes from wood tars) or preservatives [64]. A Norwegian study of 23 718 pulp and paper workers also found an excess incidence of lung cancer (standardized incidence ratio 1.5). Asbestos was again considered to be the major occupational factor of relevance, smoking habit being highly relevant also. The mesothelioma incidence was increased 2.4-fold, more obviously among maintenance workers [65].

There is, nevertheless, considerable concern throughout the wood, paper, and printing industries that there may be an excess risk of lung cancer irrespective of any asbestos exposure, and several studies have suggested an increased risk for cancer in organs other than the lung (notably stomach, nasopharynx, lymphoma, and leukemia) [64,66–69]. As a consequence many investigations have addressed the matter in many countries. There has not been a consistent outcome, which possibly provides reassurance that any excess risk cannot be marked. Thus, investigations of wood pulp and paper workers in the USA [70], Scotland [71], and Spain [72] revealed less death from lung cancer than expected, but an excess of deaths from lung cancer, although not mesothelioma, was noted among similar workers in New Hampshire (hazard ratio 2.5), Michigan (proportionate mortality ratio 1.51), and Poland (SMR 122) [73–75]. The latter was said to be confounded only weakly by smoking. Whether adequate adjustment is always possible for potential confounders is an inevitable issue with studies of this nature, and many have suffered from inadequate numbers for the identification of small risks. Several 'negative' studies (i.e. those that failed to show any significant excess risk for lung cancer) gave risk ratios or odds ratios between 1 and 2. It seems likely, therefore, that, if there is any increase in risk of lung cancer associated with wood pulping and paper making, it does not exceed two-fold, and it may not be meaningful in the absence of concomitant exposure to asbestos.

PRINTING

A historically notable example of occupational asthma was 'printers' asthma'. This arose from the use of powdered gum arabic as a drying agent for newly printed paper, although this form of occupational allergy is now seen only rarely. Some risk of asthma nevertheless remains from more modern printing techniques and the use of various dyes. Some printing procedures require closely controlled conditions of humidity, and hence the use of humidifiers. The water reservoirs that are involved may, of course, become contaminated with a variety of microorganisms (even protozoa) and these may lead to asthma also [76]. Microbially contaminated humidifiers may additionally lead to 'humidifier fever' (an example of inhalation fever) [77] or 'humidifier lung' (an example of hypersensitivity pneumonitis) [78].

Current printing processes produce some exposure to volatile organic solvents, and a study of newspaper

pressroom workers demonstrated exposure–response relationships between organic solvents and symptoms of upper respiratory tract mucous membrane irritation, after adjustments were made for potential confounders. There were no differences in spirometric indices, however, between the solvent-exposed pressroom workers and unexposed controls [79].

In view of cancer concerns among wood and paper workers, it is not surprising that concern also exists among print industry workers. A UK study of 9500 such men failed to confirm earlier fears of an excess of bladder cancer, but showed that men involved in newspaper letterpress printing had an SMR for lung cancer of 179 (95% CI 144–218) [80]. Confounding was thought to have exaggerated the observed risk, but a nested case–control study provided further evidence that exposure to ink mist (which contained the recognized carcinogen, benzo[a]pyrene) may have played a causal role [81]. In addition, there was a greater SMR among the various employment groups for oropharyngeal cancer. Further support for an excess lung cancer risk among print workers was reported subsequently from Denmark and France [82,83]. Among German women with lung cancer, a case–control study showed a significant association with work in the printing, paper, or wood industries (OR 1.9) [84].

DIFFICULT CASE

History

A 59-year-old female gardener spent a spring day working with a pile of chipped and shredded tree branches that had come from a copse in the garden in which she was working. The copse itself had been cut down a day or two earlier, and she worked with a wheelbarrow distributing some of the debris as a surface mulch. By the end of her shift she was physically tired and exhausted, although otherwise fine, and she recalled sleeping particularly well during the following night. She had previously been well without any suspicion of respiratory disease, although had smoked 20 cigarettes daily for about 45 years.

Three weeks later she did very similar work, again all day, but by then the remaining pile of shredded and chipped wood was 'steaming'. At the end of this shift she was even more tired and exhausted, but this time all her muscles ached and she felt unwell – as if she had 'flu'. By 5pm she began to feel uncomfortable in the chest, and over next the 2 hours developed a dry cough; she then became breathless and wheezy. Her chest began to ache and feel under pressure, and she was unable to sleep at all during the following night. She passed loose stools, and by morning was quite distressed. She called an emergency ambulance and was admitted to hospital.

Wheezing was then obvious, and mild to moderate respiratory distress at rest was evident. Auscultation revealed wheezing not crackles, although paramedics had reported crackles when she was first examined. The respiratory rate was 22 per minute, and the pulse 100 per minute. Her body temperature was normal and no other abnormal physical signs were detected. A chest radiograph showed possible overinflation, but otherwise appeared normal. Arterial blood gas analysis while breathing air showed: pH 7.39, PaO_2 7.6 kPa (57 mmHg), PCO_2 5.5 kPa (41 mmHg), base excess 0, oxygen saturation 89%. The hemoglobin was 12.0 g/dl, the white cell count 8.4 x 10^9/L, and the erythrocyte sedimentation rate (ESR) 32 mm/hr. A sputum sample failed to grow any pathogens.

She was treated with oxygen and nebulized bronchodilators, and improved slowly but steadily over the following hours. Corticosteroids were withheld pending an assessment of her progress, lest they should encourage fungal invasion. Spirometry during the first hospital day (April 4th 2000) showed severe airway obstruction with only minimal immediate responses to further doses of bronchodilators, and gas transfer was impaired by similar degree (Table 27.1).

Although sleep was impaired over the following 2 nights, she felt much improved within 24–48 hours, and so neither

Table 27.1 Serial lung function test results of the gardener in the Difficult Case

	Predicted	11/4	13/4	17/4	28/4
FEV₁ (liters)					
Pre*	1.91	0.57 (30)	0.81 (42)	0.90 (47)	1.70 (89)
Post*		0.64 (34)	0.80 (42)	1.12 (59)	1.78 (93)
FVC					
Pre	2.29	1.24 (54)	1.95 (85)	2.05 (90)	2.58 (113)
Post		1.61 (70)	2.15 (94)	2.24 (98)	2.77 (121)
FEV₁/FVC					
Pre		46%	42%	44%	66%
Post		40%	37%	50%	64%
TLC	4.22	4.12 (98)			
RV	1.68	2.64 (157)			
TₗCO	6.76	2.32 (34)	3.59 (53)	3.92 (58)	5.03 (74)
Kco	1.60	1.09 (68)	1.18 (74)	1.23 (77)	1.22 (76)
SaO₂		92%	92%	93%	96%

SaO₂, oxygen saturation. Values in parentheses are percentages of predicted.
*Bronchodilator inhalation

corticosteroids nor antibiotics were ever administered. Lung function improved less quickly (Table 27.1), but after 6 days she appeared entirely comfortable and was discharged from hospital.

Issues

The major issue here is the nature of this woman's acute and severe respiratory illness. Was it fundamentally an airway or parenchymal disorder (or both), and was it allergic, infectious, or toxic in etiology? Finally, was it occupational or coincidental to her work in the garden?

Comment

No evidence of infection was found, and the woman recovered steadily without any need for antibiotic therapy. The protracted period of recovery was unusual for an allergic etiology if the allergen was indeed released from the pile of wood chippings, and it was unusual also for ODTS (Chapters 13 and 26). Nevertheless, the circumstances of the episode leave little room to doubt that the illness was a consequence of her work with the pile of wood chippings, and there can be little doubt that substantial microbial contamination would have occurred by the time of her second (but not first) day working with it. She had noted on the second occasion that the pile was 'steaming' – heat from fungal growth vaporizing water which then condensed on meeting cold environmental air. Such accumulations of harvested vegetable matter that are damp or wet are well recognized to undergo microbial decomposition with the production of fungal mycotoxins and bacterial endotoxin, and situations such as the one she encountered are well recognized causes of ODTS.

Pyrexia was not recorded, but the woman had both feverish symptoms and the systemic symptoms of an influenza-like illness. The respiratory disorder was characterized most by airway obstruction, which resolved slowly, but the possibility cannot be excluded that there was additionally an alveolar component. There probably was. The airway component simulated that which characterizes the reactive airways dysfunction syndrome (RADS) in its initial stages, but once recovery appeared complete after 2–3 weeks there was no ongoing evidence of active asthma. There was then a mild degree of persisting and apparently fixed airway obstruction together with a mild loss of parenchymal function – probably a long-standing effect of her smoking habit (Table 27.1). Occupational environments associated with ODTS, inhalation fevers, RADS, and chemical pneumonitis produce a variety of overlapping effects at both airway and parenchymal levels, and this case is nicely illustrative of this.

SUMMARY POINTS

- Forestry work, like work with wood, wood pulp, paper, and printing, is associated with several respiratory disorders:
  — mucosal irritation
  — rhinitis
  — asthma
  — chronic productive cough (chronic bronchitis)
  — COPD
  — hypersensitivity pneumonitis
  — inhalation fever
  — toxic pneumonitis
  — ODTS
  — nasopharyngeal cancer
  — lung cancer
  — mesothelioma
- Mesothelioma can be attributed to asbestos, which is likely to be the major cause of any excess lung cancer.

- Nasopharyngeal cancer (including cancer of the nasal sinuses) cannot be attributed to asbestos, but it is unclear whether the carcinogen is derived primarily from wood (especially hardwood) or from chemical preservatives or coatings – both may be relevant and there may be an interactive mechanism.
- There is concern that there may be an excess risk of lung cancer unrelated to asbestos.
- The non-malignant disorders are mostly the result of allergic and toxic reactions to intrinsic constituents of wood, bacterial and fungal contaminants, chemical preservatives or bonding agents, or smoke.
- Chest trauma is common in forestry workers as a result of accidents with chain-saws, logs, or falling trees.
- Exceptionally rare cases of infection (e.g sporotrichosis), bronchospasm with anaphylaxis, asbestosis, and even silicosis have been reported.

REFERENCES

1. Stellman SD, Demers PA, Colin D, Boffetta P. Cancer mortality and wood dust exposure among participants in the American Cancer Society Cancer Prevention Study-II. *Am J Indust Med* 1998; 34: 229–237.
2. Provencher S, Labreche FR, De Guire L. Physician based surveillance system for occupational respiratory diseases: the experience of PROPULSE, Quebec, Canada. *Occup Environ Med* 1997; 54: 272–276.
3. Meredith SK, McDonald JC. Work-related respiratory disease in the United Kingdom 1989–92: report on the SWORD project. *Occup Med* 1994; 44: 183–189.
4. Ross DJ, Keynes HL, McDonald JC. SWORD '96: surveillance of work-related and occupational respiratory disease in the UK. *Occup Med* 1997; 47: 377–381.
5. Ross DJ, Keynes HL, McDonald JC. SWORD '97: surveillance of work-related and occupational respiratory disease in the UK. *Occup Med* 1998; 48: 481–485.
6. Meyer JD, Holt DL, Cherry NM, McDonald JC. SWORD '98: surveillance of work-related and occupational respiratory disease in the UK. *Occup Med* 1999; 47: 485–489.
7. Newman Taylor A. Non-malignant diseases. In: McDonald JC, ed. *Epidemiology of Work Related Diseases*, 2nd edn, pp. 149–174. London: BMJ Books, 1999.
8. Torén K, Balder B, Brisman J *et al*. The risk of asthma in relation to occupational exposures: a case–control study from a Swedish city. *Eur Respir J* 1999; 13: 496–501.
9. Torén K, Järvholm B, Brisman J *et al*. Adult-onset asthma and occupational exposures. *Scand J Work Environ Health* 1999; 25: 430–435.
10. Chan-Yeung M, Lam S, Koener S. Clinical features and natural history of occupational asthma due to western red cedar (*Thuja plicata*). *Am Rev Respir Dis* 1982; 72: 411–415.
11. Siracusa A, Kennedy SM, DyBuncio A *et al*. Prevalence and predictors of asthma in working groups in British Columbia. *Am J Indust Med* 1995; 28: 411–423.

12. Chan-Yeung M. Mechanism of occupational asthma due to western red cedar. *Am J Indust Med* 1994; 25: 13–18.
13. Liou SH, Cheng SY, Lai FM, Yang JL. Respiratory symptoms and pulmonary function in mill workers exposed to wood dust. *Am J Indust Med* 1996; 30: 293–299.
14. Eduard W, Sandven P, Levy F. Serum IgG antibodies to mold spores in two Norwegian sawmill populations: relationship to respiratory and other work-related symptoms. *Am J Indust Med* 1993; 24: 207–222.
15. Torén K, Hörte L-G, Järvholm B. Occupation and smoking adjusted mortality due to asthma among Swedish men. *Br J Indust Med* 1991; 48: 323–326.
16. Robinson CF, Petersen M, Sieber WK *et al*. Mortality of Carpenters' Union members employed in the US construction or wood products industries. *Am J Indust Med* 1996; 30: 674–694.
17. Miller BA, Blair A, Reed EJ. Extended mortality follow-up among men and women in a US furniture workers union. *Am J Indust Med* 1994; 25: 537–549.
18. Demers PA, Boffetta P, Kogevinas M *et al*. Pooled renalysis of cancer mortality among five cohorts of workers in wood-related industries. *Scand J Work Environ Health* 1995; 21: 179–190.
19. Nylander LA, Dement JM. Carcinogenic effects of wood dust: review and discussion. *Am J Indust Med* 1993; 24: 619–647.
20. Demers PA, Kogevinas M, Boffetta P *et al*. Wood dust and sino-nasal cancer: pooled re-analysis of twelve case–control studies. *Am J Indust Med* 1995; 28: 151–166.
21. Leclerc A, Martinez Cortes M, Gerin M *et al*. Sinonasal cancer and wood dust exposure: results from a case–control study. *Am J Epidemiol* 1994; 140: 340–349.
22. Andersen A, Barlow L, Engeland A *et al*. Work-related cancer in the Nordic countries. *Scand J Work Environ Health* 1999; 25(Suppl 2): 1–116.
23. Pollan M, Lopez-Abente G. Wood-related occupations and laryngeal cancer. *Cancer Detect Prev* 1995; 19: 250–257.

24. Wolf J, Schmezer P, Fengel D *et al*. The role of combination effects on the etiology of malignant tumours in the wood-working industry. *Acta Otolaryngol Suppl* 1998; 535: 1–16.

25. Boffetta P, Jourenkova N, Gustavsson P. Cancer risk from occupational and environmental exposure to polycyclic aromatic hydrocarbons. *Cancer Causes Control* 1997; 8: 444–472.

26. Nadon L, Siemiatycki J, Dewar R *et al*. Cancer risk due to occupational exposure to polycyclic aromatic hydrocarbons. *Am J Indust Med* 1995; 28: 303–324.

27. Hertzman C, Teschke K, Ostry A *et al*. Mortality and cancer incidence among sawmill workers exposed to chlorophenate wood preservatives. *Am J Public Health* 1997; 87: 71–79.

28. Kauppinen TP, Partanen TJ, Hernberg SG *et al*. Chemical exposures and respiratory cancer among Finnish woodworkers. *Br J Indust Med* 1993; 50: 143–148.

29. Wang QS, Boffetta P, Parkin DM, Kogevinas M. Occupational risk factors for lung cancer in Tianjn, China. *Am J Ind Med* 1995; 28: 353–362.

30. Gonzales CA, Agudo A. Occupational cancer in Spain. *Environ Health Perspect* 1999; 2: 273–277.

31. Matos E, Vilensky MV, Boffetta PB. Environmental and occupational cancer in Argentina: a case–control lung cancer study. *Cadernos de Saude Publica* 1998; 14(Suppl 3): 77–86.

32. Marshall SW, Kawachi I, Cryer PC *et al*. The epidemiology of forestry work-related injuries in New Zealand, 1975–88: fatalities and hospitalisations. *N Z Med J* 1994; 107: 434–437.

33. Malo JL, Cartier A, Desjardins A *et al*. Occupational asthma caused by oak wood. *Chest* 1995; 108: 856–858.

34. Lin FJ, Chen H, Chan-Yeung M. New method for an occupational dust challenge test. *Occup Environ Med* 1995; 52: 54–56.

35. Vandenplas O, Delwiche JP, Jamart J, Van de Weyer R. Increase in non-specific bronchial hyperresponsiveness as an early marker of bronchial response to occupational agents during specific inhalation challenges. *Thorax* 1996; 51: 472–478.

36. Lin FJ, Dimich-Ward H, Chan-Yeung M. Longitudinal decline in lung function in patients with occupational asthma due to western red cedar. *Occup Environ Med* 1996; 53: 753–756.

37. Hubbard R, Lewis S, Richards K *et al*. Occupational exposure to metal or wood dust and aetiology of cryptogenic fibrosing alveolitits. *Lancet* 1996; 347: 284–289.

38. Frew A, Chan H, Dryden P *et al*. Immunologic studies of the mechanisms of occupational asthma caused by western red cedar. *J Allergy Clin Immunol* 1993; 92: 466–478.

39. Malo JL, Cartier A, l'Archeveque J *et al*. Prevalence of occupational asthma among workers exposed to eastern white cedar. *Am J Respir Crit Care Med* 1994; 150: 1697–1701.

40. Malmberg PO, Rask-Andersen A, Larsson KA *et al*. Increased bronchial responsiveness in workers sawing Scots pine. *Am J Respir Crit Care Med* 1996; 153: 948–952.

41. Kauffman CA, Hajjeh R, Chapman SW. Practice guidelines for the management of patients with sporotrichosis. For the Mycosis Study Group; Infectious Diseases Society of America. *Clin Infect Dis* 2000; 30: 684–687.

42. Herbert FA, Hessel PA, Melenka LS *et al*. Pulmonary effects of simultaneous exposures to MDI, formaldehyde, and wood dust on workers in an oriented strand board plant. *J Occup Environ Med* 1995; 37: 461–5.

43. Rask-Andersen A, Land CJ, Enlund K, Lundin A. Inhalation fever and respiratory symptoms in the trimming department of Swedish sawmills. *Am J Indust Med* 1994; 25: 65–67.

44. Halpin DM, Graneek BJ, Turner-Warwick M, Newman Taylor AJ. Extrinsic allergic alveolitis and asthma in a sawmill worker: case report and review of the literature. *Occup Environ Med* 1994; 51: 160–164.

45. Mandryk J, Alwis KU, Hocking AD. Work-related symptoms and dose–response relationships for personal exposures and pulmonary function among woodworkers. *Am J Indust Med* 1999; 35: 481–490.

46. Alwis KU, Mandryk J, Hocking AD. Exposure to biohazards in wood dust: bacteria, fungi, endotoxins, and beta-D-glucans. *Appl Occup Environ Health* 1999; 14: 598–608.

47. Demers PA, Teschke K, Kennedy SSM. What to do about softwood: a review of respiratory effects and recommendations regarding exposure limits. *Am J Indust Med* 1997; 31: 385–398.

48. Woellner RC, Hall S, Greaves I, Schoenwetter WF. Epidemic of asthma in a wood products plant using methylene diphenyl diisocyanate. *Am J Indust Med* 1997; 31: 56–63.

49. Betchley C, Koenig JQ, van Belle G *et al*. Pulmonary function and respiratory symptoms in forest firefighters. *Am J Indust Med* 1997; 31: 503–509.

50. Perez-Padilla R, Regalado J, Vedal S *et al*. Exposure to biomass smoke and chronic airway disease in Mexican women. A case–control study. *Am J Respir Crit Care Med* 1996; 154: 701–706.

51. Sandoval J, Salas J, Martinez-Guerra ML *et al*. Pulmonary arterial hypertension and cor pulmonale associated with chronic domestic woodsmoke inhalation. *Chest* 1993; 103: 12–20.

52. Nakama H, Muramatsu K, Uchikama K, Yamagishi T. Possibility of Lyme disease as an occupational disease – seroepidemiological study of regional residents and forestry workers. *Asia Pac J Public Health* 1994; 7: 214–217.

53. Zhioua E, Rodhain F, Binet P, Perez-Eid C. Prevalence of antibodies to Borrelia burgdorferi in forestry workers of Ile de France. *Eur J Epidemiol* 1997; 13: 959–962.

54. Moll van Charante AW, Groen J, Mulder PG *et al*. Occupational risks of zoonotic infections in Dutch forestry workers and muskrat catchers. *Eur J Epidemiol* 1998; 14: 109–116.

55. Shimizu T, Hori T, Tokuyama K *et al*. Clinical and immunologic surveys of Hymenoptera hypersensitivity in Japanese forestry workers. *Ann Allergy Immunol* 1995; 74: 495–500.

56. Torén K, Blanc PD. The history of pulp and paper bleaching: respiratory-health effects. *Lancet* 1997; 349: 1316–1321.

57. Torén K, Jarvholm B, Morgan U. Mortality from asthma and chronic obstructive pulmonary disease among workers in a soft paper mill: a case–referent study. *Br J Indust Med* 1989; 46: 192–195.

58. Zuskin E, Mustajbegovic J, Schachter EN *et al*. Respiratory function and immunological status in paper-recycling workers. *J Occup Environ Med* 1998; 40: 986–993.

59. Rylander R, Thorn J, Attefors R. Airways inflammation among workers in a paper industry. *Eur Respir J* 1999; 13: 1151–1157.

60. Kennedy SM, Enarson DA, Janssen RG, Chan-Yeung M. Lung health consequences of reported accidental chlorine gas exposures among pulpmill workers. *Am Rev Respir Dis* 1991; 143: 74–79.

61. Henneberger PK, Ferris BG Jr, Sheehe PR. Accidental gassing incidents and the pulmonary function of pulp mill workers. *Am Rev Respir Dis* 1993; 148: 63–67.

62. Henneberger PK, Lax MB, Ferris BG Jr. Decrements in spirometry values associated with chlorine gassing events and pulp mill work. *Am J Respir Crit Care Med* 1996; 153: 225–231.

63. Schlueter DP, Fink JN, Henley GT. Wood pulp worker's disease: a hypersensitivity pneumonitis caused by *Alternaria. Ann Intern Med* 1972; 77: 907–914.

64. Torén K, Persson B, Wingren G. Health effects of working in pulp and paper mills: malignant diseases. *Am J Indust Med* 1996; 29: 123–130.

65. Langseth H, Andersen A. Cancer incidence among male pulp and paper workers in Norway. *Scand J Work Environ Health* 2000; 26: 99–105.

66. Rix BA, Villadsen E, Lynge E. Cancer incidence of sulfite pulp workers in Denmark. *Scand J Work Environ Health* 1997; 23: 458–461.

67. Rix BA, Villadsen E, Engholm G, Lynge E. Risk of cancer among paper recycling workers. *Occup Environ Med* 1997; 54: 729–733.

68. Henneberger PK, Ferris BG Jr, Monson RR. Mortality among pulp and paper workers in Berlin, New Hampshire. *Br J Indust Med* 1989; 46: 658–664.

69. Matanoski GM, Kanchanaraksa S, Lees PS *et al.* Industry-wide study of mortality of pulp and paper mill workers. *Am J Indust Med* 1998; 33: 354–365.

70. Wong O, Ragland DR, Marcero DH. An epidemiologic study of employees as seven pulp and paper mills. *Intern Arch Occup Environ Health* 1996; 68: 498–507.

71. Coggon D, Wield G, Pannett B *et al.* Mortality in employees of a Scottish paper mill. *Am J Indust Med* 1997; 32: 535–539.

72. Sala-Serra M, Sunyer J, Kogevinas M *et al.* Cohort study on cancer mortality among workers in the pulp and paper industry in Catalonia, Spain. *Am J Indust Med* 1996; 30: 87–92.

73. Henneberger PK, Lax MB. Lung cancer mortality in a cohort of older pulp and paper workers. *Intern J Occup Med Environ Health* 1998; 4: 147–154.

74. Solet D, Zoloth SR, Sullivan C *et al.* Patterns of mortality in pulp and paper workers. *J Occup Med* 1989; 31: 627–630.

75. Szadkowska-Stanczyk I, Szymczak W, Szeszenia-Dabrowska N, Wilczynska U. Cancer risk in workers of the pulp and paper industry in Poland. A continued follow-up. *Intern J Occup Med Environ Health* 1998; 11: 217–225.

76. Finnegan MJ, Little S, Gordon DJ *et al.* The effect of smoking on the development of allergic disease and specific immunological responses in a factory workforce exposed to humidifier contaminants. *Br J Indust Med* 1991; 48: 30–33.

77. Mamolen M, Lewis DM, Blanchet MA *et al.* Investigation of an outbreak of 'humidifier fever' in a print shop. *Am J Indust Med* 1993; 23: 483–490.

78. Robertson AS, Burge PS, Wieland GA, Carmalt MH. Extrinsic allergic alveolitis caused by a cold water humidifier. *Thorax* 1987; 42: 32–37.

79. Lee BW, Kelsey KT, Hashimoto D *et al.* The prevalence of pulmonary and upper respiratory tract symptoms and spirometric test findings among newspaper pressroom workers exposed to solvents. *J Occup Environ Med* 1997; 39: 960–969.

80. Leon DA. Mortality in the British printing industry: a historical cohort study of trade union members in Manchester. *Occup Environ Med* 1994; 51: 79–86.

81. Leon DA, Thomas P, Hutchings S. Lung cancer among newspaper printers exposed to ink mist: a study of trade union members in Manchester, England. *Occup Environ Med* 1994; 51: 87–94.

82. Lynge E, Rix BA, Villadsen E *et al.* Cancer in printing workers in Denmark. *Occup Environ Med* 1995; 52: 738–744.

83. Luce D, Landre MF, Clavel T *et al.* Cancer mortality among magazine printing workers. *Occup Environ Med* 1997; 54: 264–267.

84. Jahn I, Ahrens W, Bruske-Hohlfeld I *et al.* Occupational risk factors for lung cancer in women: results of a case–control study in Germany. *Am J Indust Med* 1999; 36: 90–100.

85. Hendrick DS, Walters EH, Bird AG. Occupational asthma. In: Raffle PAB, Lee WR, McCallum RI, Murray R, eds. *Hunter's Diseases of Occupations*, 7th edn, pp. 863–913. London: Hodder and Stoughton, 1987.

28 HEALTHCARE

P. Sherwood Burge and Alastair S. Robertson

INTRODUCTION

Respiratory diseases may be a hazard for health-care workers, and healthcare workers themselves may pose a risk of infection to their patients; both issues need to be taken into account in the occupational health setting. Respiratory diseases are much less common than back disorders, psychiatric illness, stress, and skin diseases as causes of ill health in healthcare workers and, apart from tuberculosis, have not received the attention that they deserve. Healthcare incorporates a range of jobs, some with specific hazards. Most workers have direct contact with potentially infectious patients; there are specific hazards in medical laboratories, building management services, and catering; and some hazards arise because of the building itself and its services.

In this chapter the focus is directed first to the hazards, and second to the adverse effects associated with them.

BUILDING-RELATED HAZARDS

'Sick' buildings

Sick building syndrome, which is discussed more fully in Chapter 15, is common amongst staff in hospitals [1,2]. High temperature, lack of control of the environment, sealed windows, and air conditioning are all risk factors in the office environment [3], and are common features of the hospital workplace. Sick building syndrome symptoms are more common in women than men, and in those with less control of their working time – again, common features of ward-based work. There are particular problems in some X-ray departments, which might relate partly to irritant or allergenic fumes (usually containing small amounts of glutaraldehyde amongst other materials) from radiograph chemistry [4]. X-ray departments often have other features that promote sick building syndrome such as poor lighting (to aid the examination of radiographs), no windows, and a hot environment.

A more certain cause of allergic respiratory disorders is microbial contamination of air-conditioning systems and humidifiers, and extrinsic allergic alveolitis (hypersensitivity pneumonitis) has occurred in hospitals (including operating theatres) as a consequence. A more exotic reported allergenic contaminant has been bat guano from bats nesting in hospital eaves; this has caused occupational asthma in a nurse [5].

Legionella and related hazards

There have been many outbreaks of *Legionella* pneumonia as a consequence of building contamination (not person-to-person spread), mainly affecting patients and visitors [6]. *Legionella* infection is more common in older age groups, particular heavy smokers and alcohol drinkers, and the immunosuppressed; this perhaps accounts for the relative sparing of staff during outbreaks affecting patients. Exposed staff do, however, commonly develop antibodies to *Legionella* during outbreaks [7], demonstrating that they have inhaled antigen. In one outbreak those with antibodies reported (in retrospect) influenza-like illnesses similar to Pontiac fever [8]. *Legionella* may be inhaled from air-conditioning systems, particularly when water drift from evaporative condensers has access to incoming air that enters the air-conditioning system [9]. Following a large outbreak in one hospital, one health region within the UK consequently removed all evaporative condensers from hospitals, and stopped recirculation of air from patient areas [10,11]. *Legionella* may also be inhaled via hot water (particularly shower) outlets [12,13]. Biocides are often added to cold water humidifiers to prevent *Legionella* growth [14]; they are a possible risk factor for sick building syndrome [15,16], and are a potential cause of asthma and rhinitis [17,18].

Cleaning and sterilizing agents

Cross-infection between humans is common in hospitals, which require cleaning with more than usual diligence. Many cleaning materials are sprayed on to floors and work surfaces, generating aerosols that can be inhaled. In addition, some floor cleaners leave a residue that can become airborne later. Simple detergent cleaners have been replaced in some hospitals with those containing biocides and other additives. The biocides, when inhaled, may lead to immediate eye, nose, and throat symptoms, and can result in occupational asthma. Other additives giving rise to occupational asthma include benzalkonium chloride (also a problem in swine confinement buildings) and colophony derivatives [19]. Occupational asthma of such origin can also occur in workers not present during the cleaning; one pharmacist developed severe occupational asthma due to benzalkonium chloride used to clean his department in the evenings. He relapsed when the same biocide was added to the final rinse during washing of nurses' uniforms in the hope of preventing the spread of methicillin-resistant staphylococci [20]. Some enclosures in sterile pharmacies have the airflow reversed, flowing from the cabinet over the worker, and cabinets are often sprayed with biocides. The use of chlorhexidine in this fashion has resulted in sensitization of a pharmacist and nurses [21,22].

Asbestos

Those maintaining buildings are additionally exposed to the common risks of all building maintenance workers, particularly asbestos which was widely used for boiler and hot water pipe insulation, and for fire proofing. Many hospital maintenance workers have developed asbestos-related pleural disease, although asbestosis is rare in this group. Carpenters are at risk from wood dusts; hard woods have been used in hospitals to a greater extent than in the domestic environment, particularly in laboratory benches and older fire-retardant doors. Several cases of occupational asthma and rhinitis have been recorded in this group.

THE CLINICAL ENVIRONMENT

The principal risk is from sensitization to latex, which can be measured in the air of all areas where latex gloves are used [23,24]. There has been a significant change in usage of latex gloves, particularly since the advent of human immunodeficiency virus (HIV) infection [25–27]. Latex gloves were previously used infrequently, and even washed and reused. Washing removes extractable latex and reduces the risks of sensitization. Latex binds to glove powder, significantly increasing airborne latex levels, and the substitution of talc with corn starch has increased the problem because latex binds better to corn starch [28]. Many healthcare workers now use more than 10 pairs of latex examination gloves per shift; they are used when changing bed linen, carrying excreta, and even going about office-type duties. There is some evidence that primary sensitization often occurs through the skin, with urticaria the first symptom. Asthma and rhinitis then develop as a consequence of antigen inhalation. There is an urgent need to replace latex with safer materials for general clinical use (such as vinyl or nitrile). The problems of latex allergy are described further in Chapter 4 (Asthma).

Glutaraldehyde is a common cold sterilizing agent in healthcare use. It is a common cause of asthma, rhinitis, and dermatitis in exposed workers, at levels well below current exposure standards [29,30]. Glutaraldehyde-containing sterilizing agents, such as Cidex, used to be found routinely in clinical areas for sterilizing common items such as auroscope ends, speculae, and lung function mouthpieces and airways until these problems became evident. Now these agents have generally been removed from clinical areas, but are still used for sterilizing endoscopes, where the need for total immersion has increased the amount of glutaraldehyde needed. Glutaraldehyde is also a common constituent of radiograph processing fluids, and its use has increased following the reduction of silver in radiograph film. Occupational asthma and rhinitis in those working with radiographic film is only sometimes due to glutaraldehyde; other chemical constituents are also involved [4,31].

THE LABORATORY ENVIRONMENT

Laboratory workers are exposed to infected specimens, latex, and glutaraldehyde in common with their clinical colleagues. In addition, some laboratory workers work with sensitizing chemicals, particularly enzymes added to microbiology and histopathology agents. Workers have developed occupational asthma in these situations [32–34].

PARTICULAR AGENTS

Pharmaceutical agents

Sensitization to drugs in powder form used to be common when these were dispensed from bulk containers, such as antibiotics (e.g. isoniazid [35]), psyllium (isphaghula) [36,37], and pancreatic enzymes sprinkled on to food [38]. Most are now used in non-inhalable preparations, transferring the hazards to pharmaceutical manufacturing workers [39–43]. The advent of nebulizer therapy, particularly with antibiotics and pentamidine (given for *Pneumocystis* prophylaxis in HIV infection), has caused occupation asthma and rhinitis in some with bystander exposures. Nebulizer output needs local exhaust extraction, similar to anaesthetic gases. Powdered alginates are used to pack pressure sores; they have caused asthma in those extracting the alginates from seaweed [44].

Infectious agents

Influenza, and other respiratory viruses, are often transmitted from patients to healthcare workers. The source of infection and consequences for staffing are often overlooked. Conversely, outbreaks of influenza in long-stay homes have been spread from healthcare workers to residents [45]. Vaccination of staff was shown to reduce deaths due to influenza in residents in one study from 22% to 13% [46]. The vaccination rate was 51% in the study population of staff, compared with 5% in staff of a control institution. Increasing staff vaccination rates from 26% to 38% did not, however, affect influenza rates amongst patients in one hospital study [47]. The development of specific vaccines and drugs for prophylaxis and treatment are likely to increase diagnostic precision and clinical interest for these diseases, which are often regarded as 'part of the job'.

Healthcare workers are at increased risk of developing tuberculosis, which proved fatal in 24% of healthcare workers in one African country [48]. The emergence of acquired immune deficiency syndrome (AIDS) and the development of multiple drug-resistant (MDR) tuberculosis has led to revised healthcare policies in more affluent countries. The subject is developed in more detail in Chapter 16 (Tuberculosis). There are major differences in the approach to the prevention of tuberculosis between countries. Clinical tuberculosis following exposure to an infectious patient is more common in those who are initially tuberculin skin test negative than in those who have a positive test following natural infection or bacille Calmette–Guérin (BCG) vaccination [49,50]. In many countries BCG vaccination is given to (or offered to) all healthcare workers who are tuberculin negative. There are differences in the results of individual studies of efficacy of BCG vaccination, a meta-analysis in adults showing more than 50% protection overall [51]. Protection is against both MDR and sensitive strains. Other countries rely on chemoprophylaxis if contact with an infectious patient leads to tuberculin conversion. After 6–12 months' treatment, the reduction in risk of progressive tuberculosis in roughly similar to that following BCG vaccination.

The number of healthcare workers who are themselves immunosuppressed has increased. Some with HIV infection and organ transplants remain well enough to perform normal clinical duties while remaining significantly immunosuppressed. They are at particular risk from tuberculosis (and non-respiratory infections such as herpes zoster). Healthcare workers with bronchiectasis (especially those with cystic fibrosis) are at risk from *Pseudomonas* infection from colonized patients, as are bronchiectatic patients from colonized healthcare workers.

Rare sensitizing agents

Methyl methacrylate used in bone cements, other acrylates used in dental prosthesis manufacture, and cyanoacrylates used to close skin wounds [52–54], are all occasional causes of occupational asthma and rhinitis. Isocyanates are sometimes present in support bandages and have caused asthma in plaster room staff, and a patient has been reported with acute bronchospasm following the application of coal tar bandages [55,56]. Asthma attributable to formaldehyde in operating theatre staff, dialysis staff, and pathology staff is an occasional problem [57,58]; there is a particular risk when inflating whole lungs with formaldehyde, where the exposures are potentially greater.

Occasional cases of asthma have resulted from ink sprayed onto recording paper [59]. Staff performing bronchial provocation tests have developed occupational asthma themselves [60].

DIFFICULT CASE

History

A 40-year-old ex-smoker had worked as a laboratory technician in a hospital histopathology department for 21 years and then began noticing wheeziness and episodic breathlessness. He had no previous history of respiratory illness, no history of atopic disorders, and no family history of either. He had been taking no medication and was generally well. Six months earlier his laboratory had started using an anhydrous powder preparation of the enzyme amylase. This was derived from pig pancreas and was used in histologic staining techniques for slide-mounted tissue samples. The 'powder technique' replaced his practice of using his saliva, which was considered 'unhygienic'. He would tap approximately 2 gm of the dry powder into a slide container from a height of 5–10 cm once a day, on most days of the week. The tapping action released a fine powder plume into the immediate atmosphere. His face would be about 20 cm from the slide container and he took no precautions against exposure. He wondered whether his respiratory symptoms were a consequence of this new procedure as there were occassions when he thought they began or worsened within a few minutes of it. However, they often persisted until late evening. He seemed to be untroubled at weekends or on holiday. After about 6 weeks he consulted a physician and was given salbutamol and beclomethasone metered-dose inhalers (200 μg as required and 200 μg twice daily respectively). These largely abolished his symptoms, and he continued to use the powder.

Issues

The obvious issues here are whether the amylase was indeed the cause of this man's apparent asthma, and whether the matter should have been investigated when he sought medical advice.

Comment

Asthma arising within 6–12 months of the onset of a new respiratory exposure at work should certainly provoke the question of whether it is occupational in origin. When the exposure involves an agent of recognized high asthmagenic potency, the balance of probabilities will lie in favour of occupational asthma. In this particular case, the history was additionally strongly suggestive of an occupational cause, but occupational asthma had not previously been reported in such a setting, and it may be that the history was, in fact, less convincing at the time of presentation.

Although symptoms were initially suppressed, they worsened after a few months and the technician sought the opinion of another physician. Occupational asthma was strongly suspected, but in view of the unusual circumstance he was referred for inhalation provocation tests. For 4 weeks prior to investigation he was asked to discontinue all medication and to avoid any possible exposure to the amylase. Analar lactose is similar in appearance to the amylase powder, and amylase was added to it to form mixtures containing 1%, 3.2%, 10%, or 32% by weight for potential sequential inhalation challenges on separate days. The challenge tests were conducted in a double-blind, 'placebo'-controlled fashion over 5 min at 1000 hours each day. The technician sat at a table and three times tipped 10 g of the lactose or lactose mixture back and forward between two aluminum containers in a fashion that simulated his exposure at work. He wore a nose-clip to disguise the odor of the amylase powder and remained seated for a period of 5 min, after which time there was no further exposure [34].

The first challenge, with lactose placebo, was not followed by symptoms or any significant change in FEV_1 (Fig. 28.1). The second challenge, using the 1% amylase mixture, failed to produce symptoms and was not accompanied by a late asthmatic reaction. There was a hint of an immediate asthmatic reaction (15% decrement in FEV_1). The third challenge, with the 3.2% mixture, produced a dramatic immediate asthmatic reaction with a decrement in FEV_1 of the order of 75%. This closely reproduced the symptoms and level of discomfort the man had experienced at work, and he remained surprisingly undistressed despite this apparent marked fall in FEV_1 (with such a rapid fall the measured minimum value may have been technically less accurate). Monitoring was therefore continued without bronchodilator intervention. He remained symptomatic but the FEV_1 improved steadily. However, it remained significantly decreased throughout the 2–12-hour post challenge surveillance period. This indicates that the immediate reaction was succeeded by a late reaction. It resolved within 24–48 hours. Methacholine tests before and after the test sequence demonstrated a significant increase in airway responsiveness i. e. the provoking dose responsible for a 20% decrement in FEV_1 (PD_{20}) decreased from 73 μg before to 19 μg after.

Following these investigations, which were considered to confirm occupational asthma attributable to porcine amylase, the enzyme was used in the form of an aqueous suspension, and the technician avoided any further exposure to the powder. His asthma remained mildly active, and he continued to use inhaled steroid and bronchodilator medication. A final methacholine test 15 months after the definitive investigations gave a PD_{20} value of 213 μg. This was much improved from the level measured initially, but airway responsiveness was still of a degree that is generally associated with active disease.

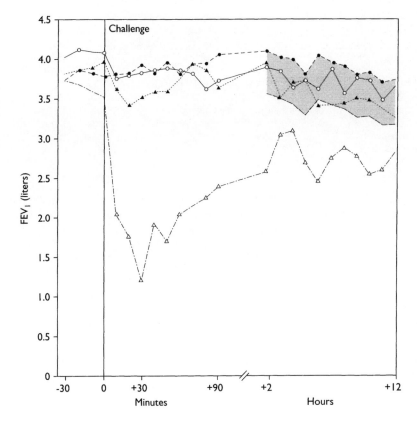

Fig. 28.1 Inhalation test results for the laboratory technician in the Difficult Case. ——●——, Control mean; – – – –, lower 95% CI; —○— amylase 0%; ---▲--- amylase 1%; ------△------ amylase 3.2%. Adapted from Aiken et al. [34].

SUMMARY POINTS

- Healthcare poses some risk of respiratory infection for healthcare workers from patients, and for patients from healthcare workers, particularly epidemic virus infections and tuberculosis.
- Additional respiratory hazards to healthcare workers may arise from the buildings in which they work, some being largely confined to certain occupational groups:
  - sick building syndrome (Chapter 15)
  - *Legionella* infection (Chapter 17)
  - allergic disorders from microorganisms or biocides in air conditioning and humidification systems, and certain cleaning and sterilizing agents (Chapter 4)
  - asbestos-induced disorders (Chapters 9,19,21,22) and allergy to wood dusts in maintenance workers and in carpenters and joiners (Chapters 4 and 14).

- In the clinical setting further allergenic hazards are related principally to the use of latex and glutaraldehyde.
- In the laboratory setting there are potential infectious, allergic, and toxic hazards.
- Agents with asthmagenic sensitizing potential of particular note include:
  - powdered or nebulized pharmaceutical agents (e.g. powdered isoniazid, psyllium, pancreatic enzymes, and nebulized pentamidine, gentamycin)
  - powdered alginates (bed sore management)
  - acrylates and cyanoacrylates (dental prostheses, skin wound closure)
  - special bandages and plasters (isocyanate, coal tar)
  - formaldehyde in pathology departments, operating theatres, renal dialysis units

REFERENCES

1. Nordstrom K, Norback D, Akselsson R. Influence of indoor air quality and personal factors on the sick building syndrome (SBS) in Swedish geriatric hospitals. *Occup Environ Med* 1995; 52(3): 170–176.
2. Fletcher AM, Niven RM, Pickering CAC. Prevalence of building sickness syndrome in hospital outpatient departments. *Thorax* 1990; 46: 313.

3. Burge PS, Hedge A, Wilson S *et al.* Sick building syndrome; a study of 4373 office workers. *Ann Occup Hyg* 1987; 31: 493–504.
4. Hewitt PJ. Occupational health problems in processing of X-ray photographic films. *Ann Occup Hyg* 1993; 37: 287–295.
5. El-Ansary EH, Tee BD, Gordon DJ, Newman Taylor AJ. Respiratory allergy to inhaled bat guano. *Lancet* 1987; i: 316–318.

6. Hart CA, Makin T. *Legionella* in hospitals: a review. *J Hosp Infect* 1991; 18(Suppl A): 481–498.

7. O'Mahony MC, Stanwell-Smith RE, Tillett HE *et al.* The Stafford outbreak of legionnaires' disease. *Epidemiol Infect* 1990; 104: 361–380.

8. Lloyd RS, Guest D, Fairfax AJ. Prolonged lethargy in hospital staff after legionella infection. *Thorax* 1991; 46: 285P.

9. Timbury MC, Donaldson JR, McCartney AC. Outbreak of legionnaires' disease in Glasgow Royal Infirmery: micobiological aspects. *J Hyg (Cambridge)* 1986; 97: 393–403.

10. Badenoch J. *First Report of the Committee of Enquiry into the Outbreak of Legionnaires' Disease in Stafford in April 1985.* London: HMSO, 1986.

11. Badenoch J. *Second Report of the Committee of Enquiry into the Outbreak of Legionnaires' Disease in Stafford in April 1985.* London: HMSO, 1987.

12. Niedeveld CJ, Pet FM, Meenhorst PL. Effect of rubbers and their constituents on proliferation of *Legionella pneumophila* in naturally contaminated hot water. *Lancet* 1986; ii: 180–183.

13. Muraca PW, Yu VL, Goetz A. Disinfection of water distribution systems for legionella: a review of application procedures and methodologies. *Infect Control Hosp Epidemiol* 1990; 11(2): 79–88.

14. Nagorka R, Rosskamp E, Seidel K. Air conditioning – assessment of humidification units. *Off Gesundheitswes* 1990; 52: 168–173.

15. Clark EG. Risk of isothiazolinones. *J Soc Occup Med* 1987; 37: 30–31.

16. von Rosskamp E. Raumlufttechnische Anlagen – ein gesundheitliches Problem. *Bundesgesundhbl* 1990; 117–121.

17. Moscato G, Omodeo P, Dellabianca A *et al.* Occupational asthma and rhinitis caused by 1,2-benzisothiazolin-3-one in a chemical worker. *Occup Med* 1997; 47(4): 249–251.

18. Bourke SJ, Convery RP, Stenton SC *et al.* Occupational asthma in an 5-isothiazolinone manufacturing plant. *Thorax* 1997; 52: 746–748.

19. McCoach JS, Robertson AS, Burge PS *et al.* Floor cleaning materials as a cause of occupational asthma. In: Raw G, Aizlewood C, Warren P, eds. *Indoor Air 1999*, Watford: Building Research Establishment, 1999.

20. Burge PS, Richardson MN. Occupational asthma due to indirect exposure to lauryl dimethyl benzyl ammonium chloride used in a floor cleaner. *Thorax* 1994; 49(8): 842–843.

21. Pham NH, Weiner JM, Reisner GS, Baldo BA. Anaphylaxis to chlorhexidine. Case report. Implication of immunoglobulin E antidodies and identification of an allergenic determinant. *Clin Exp Allergy* 2000; 30: 1001–1007.

22. Waclawski ER, McAlpine LG, Thomson NC. Occupational asthma in nurses due to chlorhexidine and alcohol aerosols. *BMJ* 1989; 298: 929–930.

23. Sri-Akajunt N, Sadra S, Jones M, Burge PS. Natural rubber latex aeroallergen exposure in rubber plantation workers and glove manufacturers in Thailand and health-care workers in a UK hospital. *Ann Occup Hyg* 2000; 44: 79–88.

24. Chaiear N, Foulds IS, Burge PS. Prevalence and risk factors for latex allergy. *Occup Environ Med* 2000; 57: 501.

25. Bubak ME, Reed CE, Fransway AF *et al.* Allergic reactions to latex among health-care workers. *Mayo Clin Proc* 1992; 67: 1075–1079.

26. Hunt LW, Fransway AF, Reed CE *et al.* An epidemic of occupational allergy to latex involving health care workers. *J Occup Environ Med* 1995; 37(10): 1204–1209.

27. Vandenplas O, Delwiche JP, Evard G *et al.* Prevalence of occupational asthma due to latex among hospital personnel. *Am J Respir Crit Care Med* 1995; 151(1): 54–60.

28. Jaeger D, Kleinhans D, Czuppon AB, Baur X. Latex-specific proteins causing immediate-type cutaneous, nasal, bronchial, and systemic reactions. *J Allergy Clin Immunol* 1992; 89: 759–768.

29. Gannon PFG, Bright P, Campbell M *et al.* Occupational asthma due to glutaraldehyde and formaldehyde in endoscopy and X-ray departments. *Thorax* 1995; 50: 156–159.

30. Di Stefano F, Siriruttanapruk S, McCoach J, Burge PS. Glutaraldehyde: an occupational hazard in the hospital setting. *Allergy* 1999; 54(10): 1105–1109.

31. Cullinan P, Hayes J, Cannon J *et al.* Occupational asthma in radiographers. *Lancet* 1992; 340: 1477.

32. Gailhofer G, Wilders-Truschnig M, Smolle J, Ludvan M. Asthma caused by bromelain: an occupational allergy. *Clin Allergy* 1988; 18: 445–450.

33. Bossert J, Fuchs E, Wahl R, Maasch HJ. Occupational sensitisation by inhalation of enzymes diaphorase and lipase. *Allergologie* 1988; 11: 179–181.

34. Aiken TC, Ward R, Peel ET, Hendrick DJ. Occupational asthma due to porcine pancreatic amylase. *Occup Environ Med* 1997; 54: 762–764.

35. Asai S, Shimoda T, Hara K, Fujiwara K. Occupational asthma caused by isonicotinic acid hydride (INH) inhalation. *J Allergy Clin Immunol* 1987; 80: 578–582.

36. Machado L, Stalenheim G. Respiratory symptoms in ispaghula-allergic nurses after oral challenge with ispaghula suspension. *Allergy* 1984; 39: 65–68.

37. Malo J-L, Cartier A, L'Archeveque J *et al.* Prevalence of occupational asthma and immunologic sensitisation to psyllium among health personnel in chronic care hospitals. *Am Rev Respir Dis* 1990; 142: 1359–1366.

38. Lipkin GW, Vickers DW. Allergy in cystic fibrosis nurses to pancreatic extract. *Lancet* 1987; i: 392.

39. Sastre J, Quirce S, Novalbos A *et al.* Occupational asthma induced by cephalosporins. *Eur Respir J* 1999; 13(5): 1189–1191.

40. Roberts EA. Occupational allergic reactions among workers in a penicillin-manufacturing plant. *Indust Hyg Occup Med* 1991; 00: 340–346.

41. Carlesi G, Ferrea E, Melino C *et al.* Aspects of occupational hygiene and epidemiology in a pharmaceutical company manufacturing amoxicillin. *Nuovi-Ann-Ig-Microbiol* 1979; 30: 185–196.

42. Coutts II, Dally MB, Newman Taylor AJ *et al.* Asthma in workers manufacturing cephalosporins. *BMJ* 1981; 283: 950.

43. Malo J-L, Cartier A. Occupational asthma in workers of a pharmaceutical company processing spiramycin. *Thorax* 1988; 43: 371–377.

44. Henderson AK, Ranger AF, Lloyd J *et al.* Pulmonary hypersensitivity in the alginate industry. *Scost Med J* 1984; 29: 90–95.

45. Coles FB, Balzano GJ, Morse DL. An outbreak of influenza A (H3N2) in a well immunized nursing home population. *J Am Geriatr Soc* 1992; 40(6): 589–592.

46. Carman WF, Elder AG, Wallace LA *et al.* Effects of influenza vaccination of health-care workers on mortality of elderly people in long-term care: a randomised controlled trial. *Lancet* 2000; 355: 93–97.

47. Adal KA, Flowers RH, Anglim AM *et al.* Prevention of nosocomial influenza. *Infect Control Hosp Epidemiol* 1996; 17(10): 641–648.

48. Harries AD, Nyirenda TE, Banerjee A *et al.* Tuberculosis in health care workers in Malawi. *Trans R Soc Trop Med Hyg* 1999; 93(1): 32–35.

49. Heimbeck J. Tuberculosis in hospital nurses. *Tubercle* 1936; 18: 97–99.

50. Fine PE, Ponnighaus JM, Maine N. The distribution and implications of BCG scars in northern Malawi. *Bull WHO* 1989; 67(1): 35–42.

51. Colditz GA, Brewer TF, Berkey CS *et al.* Efficacy of BCG vaccine in the prevention of tuberculosis. Meta-analysis of the published literature. *JAMA* 1994; 271(9): 698–702.

52. Burge PS. Single and serial measurements of lung function in the diagnosis of occupational asthma. *Eur J Respir Dis* 1982; 63(Suppl 123): 47–59.

53. Piirila P, Kanerva L, Keskinen H *et al.* Occupational respiratory hypersensitivity caused by preparations containing acrylates in dental personnel. *Clin Exp Allergy* 1998; 28(11): 1404–1411.

54. Pickering CAC, Bainbridge D, Birthwhistle IH, Griffiths DL. Occupational asthma due to methacrylate in an orthopaedic theatre sister. *Lancet* 1986; 292: 1362–1363.

55. Tanaka Y, Satoh F, Komatsu T *et al.* A case of suspected occupational asthma in an orthopedist, due to cast materials containing MDI. *Nippon Kyobu Shikkan Gakkai Zasshi* 1994; 32(6): 606–609.

56. Ibbotson SH, Stenton SC, Simpson N. Acute severe bronchoconstriction caused by exposure to coal tar bandages. *Clin Exp Dermatol* 1995; 20: 58–59.

57. Hendrick DJ, Rando RJ, Lane DJ, Morris MJ. Formaldehyde asthma; challenge exposure levels and fate after five years. *J Occup Med* 1982; 24: 893–897.

58. Salkie ML. Prevalence of atopy and hypersensitivity to formaldehyde in pathologists. *Arch Pathol Lab Med* 1991; 115: 614–616.

59. Keskinen H, Nordman H, Terho EO. ECG ink as a cause of asthma. *Allergy* 1981; 36: 275–276.

60. Hoeppner VH, Murdock KY, Kooner S, Cockcroft DW. Severe acute 'occupational asthma' caused by accidental allergen exposure in an allergen challenge laboratory. *Ann Allergy* 1985; 55: 36–37.

29 MINING

Robert L. Cowie

INTRODUCTION

The mine environment is complex and contains a wide variety of dusts, gases, fumes, bacteria and their products, fungi, and other organisms including amebae (Fig. 29.1). Well known and occupation-specific disorders such as silicosis, coal workers' pneumoconiosis, and asbestosis have become less common in working miners in the industrially developed world. Pneumoconiosis nevertheless remains an important indication of the degree of dust control in the mining industry and it remains prevalent outside industrially developed countries. In this chapter, consideration is given to other disorders of the lung associated with the occupation of mining.

GASES AND GASSING

A number of gases may be encountered in the underground mine environment, and there may be a variety of associated acute respiratory hazards.

Asphyxia

When organic matter is present (especially coal), slow oxidation is to be expected, causing oxygen to be replaced by carbon dioxide. The exothermic reaction is speeded by the heat it produces, leading to the additional possibility in coal mines of fire and the production of toxic gases with smoke. In practice, however, brisk ventilation has a useful cooling effect

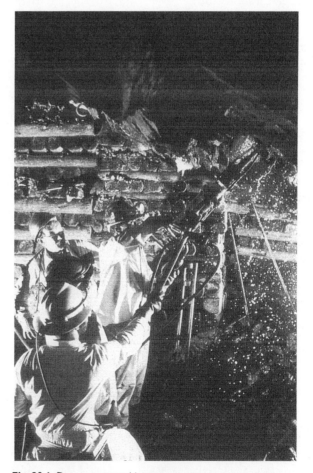

Fig. 29.1 Dust is generated by many processes in mines – most obviously drilling, controlled explosions, and harvesting. The figure shows 'machine workers' being trained to use a drill in a gold mine. Note the timber packs used to support the changing wall.

on the coal surfaces and helps to control this risk. With non-fossilized vegetable matter, microbial decay is the principal mechanism leading to the same effect. The resulting atmospheric mixture, deficient in oxygen and rich in carbon dioxide, is known as black damp, and poses a risk of asphyxia. When oxygen concentrations fall below 16% by volume, the atmosphere becomes immediately dangerous to life because of the risk of impaired cerebral function and loss of consciousness.

Explosion, fire, carbon monoxide poisoning

The decay of organic matter may also lead to the production of methane and carbon monoxide. Methane, too, will displace oxygen from mine air and so contribute to asphyxia, but a more dramatic risk is from explosion. Carbon monoxide, by contrast, may cause poisoning because of its very high affinity for hemoglobin. Both gases may contribute to the risk of fire, which carries in turn a risk of burn injuries to the respiratory tract in survivors. Fire and explosion are major risks in poorly ventilated coal mines, and are likely to increase further the risk of carbon monoxide poisoning and asphyxia. Canaries are usually much more susceptible than humans to carbon monoxide and were used historically (by their loss of consciousness) as an early warning of rising carbon monoxide levels. In modern mines the task is accomplished more reliably by continuous analytic monitoring.

Acute lung injury

Several gases and fumes that are encountered in the mining environment are capable of producing injury to the lung [1]. In general, the less soluble toxic gases, such as nitrogen oxides, are more likely to damage the lung parenchyma, and the more soluble toxic gases, such as ammonia, are more likely to damage the airway. Nitrogen oxides, notably nitrogen dioxide (NO_2), are released after blasting, and miners may be exposed when they enter areas of the mine where pockets of gas remain. Other sources of nitrogen oxides include welding in confined spaces. Miners encountering these gases may not be immediately aware of their exposure. Rarely, exposure can lead to sudden death; more commonly, symptoms (including a cough and dyspnea) develop within a few hours or may be delayed for as long as 24 hours after the exposure. Initially, the clinical picture may be unremarkable but progression to pulmonary edema and respiratory failure with a picture of acute respiratory distress syndrome

(ARDS) usually follows within 1–2 hours after the onset of symptoms if exposure is heavy. Death may occur if the patient is not treated with oxygen, and in some cases additional support is required (e.g. tracheal intubation and ventilation). The use of corticosteroid therapy in these cases is widespread, but no data exist for its efficacy.

A proportion of subjects, after recovery, develop new respiratory symptoms as a consequence of bronchiolitis obliterans. This is relatively uncommon but the diagnosis may be missed if it is not appreciated that features usually develop 3–6 weeks after apparent recovery from the acute lung injury. This pattern has resulted in the term 'third phase' being used to describe bronchiolitis obliterans in this setting, with the first phase being the acute presentation and the second the period of apparent recovery [2]. Treatment with oral corticosteroid, usually prednisone or prednisolone, appears to be effective in some cases. A dose of approximately 1 mg per kg bodyweight has been recommended. If effective, as assessed by repeated measurements of pulmonary function and chest radiography, it may be tapered after 3–6 weeks. There are no data to indicate an optimal period of treatment, but failure to demonstrate a response after 3 weeks of corticosteroid therapy suggests that the disease is likely to persist and progress.

Cadmium fumes, which may be generated when cadmium-coated metal objects in the mine are cut with a welding torch, produce a particularly intense and often fatal lung injury. The onset of respiratory symptoms may be preceded by a febrile illness similar to influenza or to metal fume fever. The picture of acute lung injury (ARDS) follows within hours and, depending upon the peak concentration of the cadmium fume exposure, may progress rapidly and cause death. Chronic exposure to cadmium fumes can lead to the development of emphysema, but such exposure would not be expected in the setting of a mine [1].

CHRONIC BRONCHITIS AND CHRONIC OBSTRUCTIVE PULMONARY DISEASE

These disorders probably affect a larger proportion of miners, both underground and surface, than any of the diseases conventionally regarded as being occupational. Chronic bronchitis or mucus hypersecretion is found in a large minority, or even a majority, of those exposed to dusty occupational environments including mining [3,4]. In the past it was thought that this disorder simply reflected the high prevalence of smoking in mine workers but it is now recognized that chronic bronchitis is found in miners who have never smoked. In one study of gold miners, 45% of the never-smokers had symptoms of chronic bronchitis [5]. The prevalence of chronic bronchitis correlated with the intensity of the dust exposure, ranging from 55% in workers (smokers and non-smokers) in occupations with a relatively low intensity to 71% in occupations with high intensity.

Chronic obstructive pulmonary disease (COPD) affects more miners than are affected by pneumoconiosis. In several studies of gold miners and one of granite crushers (suggesting that silica dust, rather than the general underground mine environment, is responsible) an annual loss of forced expiratory volume in 1s (FEV_1) of 8–13 ml has been attributable to workplace exposure, an amount similar to that attributable to a pack-year of tobacco smoking [4,6]. The association between coal mining and COPD has been debated, but the current evidence appears to support the association [7]. Gold and coal miners have been shown to have emphysema independent of any underlying pneumoconiosis [8,9]. In many reports the extent of the COPD has not been substantial, but it is important to appreciate that these are average data and, as with smoking, a significant minority may suffer from disabling disease induced by their occupation [10].

ASTHMA

Asthma has not been generally associated with the occupation of mining. A literature search linking mining and asthma produced only two reports that suggested an association [11,12], and another in which no association was found [13]. Nevertheless, exposure associated with mining (including contaminated humidifiers, isocyanates, epoxy resins, styrene, and other chemicals) are known to induce asthma in other settings [14,15]. The lack of reported asthma in miners could reflect the self-selection, by those with asthma, of less dirty and strenuous occupations, and the tendency of employers to exclude individuals with active asthma from underground work.

MYCOBACTERIAL DISEASES

In the industrialized world, tuberculosis is considered to be a disease of the past. However, many miners and others who are exposed to silica-containing dust live in regions of the world where tuberculosis remains the commonest infection. Studies from both the industrialized and industrializing world suggest that those exposed to silica but without silicosis have a 3-fold increased risk of developing tuberculosis above

that of the non-exposed general population [16,17]. Those with silicosis have a risk of tuberculosis that may exceed 20 times the rate in the general population. Tuberculosis in miners is most often pulmonary but, in those with silicosis, the rates of both pulmonary and extrapulmonary tuberculosis are increased [16]. The diagnostic procedures for tuberculosis in miners do not differ from those in non-miners. There should be an awareness of the disease and sputum should be sent for culture if there are any new radiologic features in miners with silicosis or coal workers' pneumoconiosis.

Since the inclusion of rifampicin in treatment protocols, the outcome of treated tuberculosis in miners with pneumoconiosis has been comparable to that in the general population [18]. However, one study of tuberculosis in miners with silicosis demonstrated a slightly increased risk of relapse; the authors proposed that the treatment regimen might be more effective if it were prolonged [19]. In other respects, treatment of tuberculosis in miners, including those with pneumoconiosis, does not differ from the standard regimens recommended nationally.

Miners, whether they reside in a community where the prevalence of tuberculosis is high or low, are at increased risk of developing disease caused by environmental mycobacteria (non-tuberculous mycobacteria; NTM). In many instances NTM are thought to be a contaminant of the mine environment. This seems to be true for *Mycobacterium kansasii* and *Mycobacterium scrofulaceum*, which cause disease in both miners and workers in other dusty occupations [20–22]. The organisms are thought to be delivered in the water used to control dust emission. The treatment regimens for disease caused by NTM will differ according to the organism and its drug susceptibility patterns. In general, disease caused by *M. kansasii* is responsive to rifampicin and ethambutol.

With the advent of human immunodeficiency virus (HIV) infection in mining populations, especially those who are migrant workers in southern Africa, the incidence of mycobacterial disease in miners has reached levels in the range of 2000 per 100 000 per year [23]. It appears, therefore, that there is an additive or even multiplicative effect between exposure to silica-containing dust and HIV in determining the risk for tuberculosis and NTM disease.

Chemoprophylaxis for tuberculosis is recommended for miners with silicosis and a positive tuberculin skin test [4]. In a crowded mining community with a high incidence of tuberculosis, chemoprophylaxis may not be effective because it is likely that postprimary tuberculosis is often caused by recently acquired exogenous infection rather than by reactivation of endogenous infection [24].

OTHER INFECTIONS

Pneumococcal pneumonia was a major cause of illness and death in the early days of gold mining in South Africa. The disease appeared to be more common in new miners and especially those who came from tropical areas such as Mozambique and Malawi. The reason for this high incidence (documented as being as high as 9% per year) is not known but may have had as much to do with the housing of large numbers of men in mine hostels as with the occupation of mining. The high incidence of the disease persists today and was utilized in recent times when the efficacy of pneumococcal vaccines was being tested in miners [25].

Acute histoplasmosis may occur in miners who have been occupied with the redevelopment of old mines, presumably when the area has been contaminated with *Histoplasma*-laden bat droppings. Symptoms may be dramatic and may be associated with widespread pulmonary opacities, and with mediastinal and hilar lymphadenopathy.

HUMIDIFIER FEVER AND HYPERSENSITIVITY PNEUMONITIS

Humidifier fever and hypersensitivity pneumonitis are immunologic disorders that may be induced by the inhalation of material from contaminated humidifiers. Although they have not been described in miners, they are well known to occur in industries where similar levels of humidity are maintained and where water sprays are used [14]. Humidification of mines is a crude operation and the water used is known to be often contaminated with sewage and mycobacteria; it is thus likely to have other contaminants including bacterial endotoxins, amoebae, and parasites, which have been implicated in humidifier fever and hypersensitivity pneumonitis.

CONNECTIVE TISSUE DISEASES

Rheumatoid disease associated with pulmonary fibrosis or with pulmonary nodules (Caplan syndrome) is a well documented concomitant of coal workers' pneumoconosis [9] and may also be associated with silicosis. The exact relationship between rheumatoid disease and these occupational diseases is uncertain. There are data suggesting that rheumatoid disease can aggravate silicosis [26]. Rheumatoid nodules in the lung may be mistaken for progressive massive fibrosis or for tumours. Histologically, a rheumatoid nodule may have features not dissimilar from those of tuberculosis or other granulomatous diseases such as histoplasmosis. There is no consistent association with other features of rheumatoid arthritis, apart from the frequent finding of circulating rheumatoid factor [9].

Systemic sclerosis (scleroderma) has long been known to be associated with exposure to silica-containing dust. Scleroderma with interstitial lung disease has been reported in gold miners and others exposed to silica-containing dust. Systemic sclerosis may occur with or without silicosis [4]. The disease is similar to that in a non-occupational setting. The associated interstitial lung disease, with its predominantly basal and reticular appearance, is easily distinguished from the upper zone and nodular opacification of silicosis. Pulmonary function tests show proportionately more restriction and a lower single breath diffusion for carbon monoxide than is usual for silicosis [27]. Management is similar to that offered in non-occupational scleroderma and has little impact on the pulmonary dysfunction.

LUNG CANCER

Silicosis and asbestosis are recognized to be associated with an increased risk of lung cancer [4,28]. There is a less certain relationship between silica or asbestos exposure and lung cancer. The risk of lung (and other) cancers may also be increased in underground miners because of exposure to the gas radon. This is especially, but not exclusively, true for uranium miners. Cigarette smoking has an additive and possibly a multiplicative effect with radon in relation to the risk of lung cancer. Radon is seven times heavier than air, and is colorless and odorless. It is the most important source of naturally occurring radiation. Radon gas diffuses from the rock into mine air and may also reach the mine environment from groundwater flowing into the mine. The α particles from radon and radon daughters penetrate tissue poorly and exert their greatest influence through inhalation and deposition on the bronchial epithelium. The highest levels of radon and radon daughters (which are the more significant source of α particles) are found in uranium mines or gold, hematite, and tin mines, presumably as a result of the presence of uranium-bearing rock. In the fluorspar mines of Newfoundland, high radon levels are attributed to the groundwater. Radon is not usually associated with coal mining and coal miners do not have an increased risk of lung cancer, although they may have an excess risk of gastric cancer [3].

Other exposures that may be related to an increased risk of lung cancer in miners include arsenic and diesel fumes. Tobacco smoking nevertheless remains the major risk factor for lung cancer in miners, and smoking cessation will substantially reduce the risk for those exposed to radon, asbestos, arsenic, and diesel fume in the mine environment. Occupational causes of lung cancer are discussed further in Chapter 19.

CHEST TRAUMA AND FAT EMBOLISM

Crushing injuries to the chest are common in rock falls in mines. Unfortunately, many of these injuries are associated with asphyxiation when the subject is trapped under rock with the chest compressed.

Contusion of the lung is common in those who survive the initial injury. The radiologic features and respiratory failure associated with lung contusion often progress over a period of 24–72 hours and the true extent of the injury may not be apparent on initial assessment [29]. The injury to the chest will be more obvious in those who have rib fractures, pneumothorax, or hemothorax.

The lungs may also be involved following injuries associated with fractures of the legs. Such injuries in a mine may occur in association with rock falls, which hinder access and may occur many kilometers from the main shaft. Suitable immobilization of the fracture may be difficult and transportation of the injured miner on a board over long distances and sometimes through narrow, steep tunnels may enhance the risks of fat embolism. Fat embolism with associated hypoxemia may be readily missed during efforts to attend to major orthopedic and other injuries.

DIFFICULT CASE

History

A 35-year-old man who worked as a welder in a gold mine, and who had previously been healthy, presented to his general practitioner complaining of fever, painful muscles, and a feeling of tightness of the chest. The doctor found no features to cause concern and sent the man home with the suggestion that he rest and take acetominophen (paracetamol) as required. Several hours later, he found that he was becoming short of breath and decided to visit the casualty/emergency department of his nearest hospital. Once again, no particular evidence of concern was noted and he was discharged home. He died during the following night. A postmortem examination revealed pulmonary edema. There was no evidence of heart disease, and no features to suggest aspiration were found.

Information obtained from the man's family and workplace revealed that he had been working underground in a box-hole during the equipping of a new shaft. The area was poorly ventilated. The tasks that he had performed during the morning before his death included the removal of two roof bolts using a welder's cutting torch. He had been alone during this operation. His first symptoms had developed 5 hours after completing the roof bolt cutting task. It was estimated that he had died 18 hours after first developing symptoms.

Issues

There are important diagnostic, management, and prognostic issues for this case. From the diagnostic viewpoint, what was the likely cause of death, what exposures are likely to have contributed to this outcome, and how might the opinions be tested? From the management viewpoint, what might have prevented his death? From the prognostic view-point, what residual pulmonary abnormalities might be expected had the man survived?

Comment

There was unanimous agreement among the book's contributors that death was attributable to toxic pneumonitis, possibly associated with ARDS. Most considered that oxides of nitrogen had probably played a contributory or primary role, but almost half recognized the possibility of cadmium being a component of the roof bolts, and of cadmium pneumonitis being the primary cause of death. To investigate the possibility of cadmium toxicity, it was suggested that an enquiry be made of the manufacturer concerning the components of the roof bolts, that the cadmium concentration be measured in autopsy material, and that the circumstances of exposure during the welding work be simulated so that atmospheric levels of any emissions could be analyzed. All contributors considered that adequate ventilation of the box-hole should have prevented the incident, and that close medical supervision following the initial presentation should have allowed appropriate treatment as necessary with supplemental oxygen, mechanical ventilation, corticosteroid medication, and other supportive measures. They were evenly divided between those who thought there would be no respiratory sequelae had the miner survived, and those who thought there would be bronchiolitis obliterans or a persistent reduction in gas transfer (T_LCO).

The nature of this man's actual exposure was later determined by simulating the work environment with an experimental chamber. The bolt cutting was done through sealed port holes while the atmosphere was collected through sampling ports. All the air samples contained amounts of NO, NO_2 and cadmium fumes far in excess of the permitted maximum levels. The level of NO_2 of 40 ppm was in the range expected to cause pulmonary edema after 60 min of exposure. The levels of cadmium fume varied during the experiment from 22 to 70 mg/m³, which vastly exceeded the maximum permitted ceiling level of 0.05 mg/m³ for instantaneous exposure. Levels of 0.5 to 2.5 mg/m³ cadmium have been associated with non-fatal pneumonitis, while levels such as those that developed during the experiment are associated with fatal pneumonitis.

It was thus concluded that the welder's death could be attributed to his exposure to exceedingly high levels of cadmium. His welding torch had also generated sufficiently high levels of nitrogen dioxide to have caused lung injury in the absence of cadmium exposure. (The Chamber of Mines of South Africa conducted this simulation and we thank them for providing the information and permitting its publication.)

SUMMARY POINTS

- Pneumoconioses, including silicosis, coal workers' pneumoconiosis, and asbestosis, are the best known lung diseases associated with mining.
- Oxygen-deficient air enriched with carbon dioxide (black damp) and/or methane may cause asphyxia.
- Fires and explosions may cause smoke injury, asphyxia, and carbon monoxide poisoning.
- Gases (typically nitrogen dioxide) and fumes (including cadmium) may cause acute and potentially fatal pneumonitis.
- Chronic bronchitis and COPD (including emphysema) are clearly attributable to working in the mine environment and may affect a large proportion of the workforce.
- COPD is known to occur in miners who have never smoked.

- Mycobacterial diseases, including tuberculosis, remain common in miners, especially those exposed to silica.
- Other mining-associated infections include pneumococcal pneumonia and histoplasmosis.
- Coal workers' pneumoconiosis and silicosis may be associated with connective tissue disorders such as rheumatoid pulmonary fibrosis, rheumatoid pulmonary nodules, and scleroderma.
- Miners are at excess risk of lung cancer if they develop silicosis or abestosis, and if they are exposed to radon, arsenic, or diesel fume.
- Trauma in the mine may cause direct lung injury, or involve the lung through fat embolism or ARDS.
- Agents known to be associated with asthma, humidifier fever, and hypersensitivity pneumonitis are common in the mine environment.

REFERENCES

1. International Labour Office. *Encyclopedia of Occupational Health and Safety*, 4th edn. Geneva: ILO, 1997.
2. Wright JL, Churg A. Diseases caused by gases and fumes. In: Churg A, Green FHY, eds. *Pathology of Occupational Lung Disease*, 2nd edn. Baltimore: Williams and Wilkins, 1998, pp. 57–75.
3. NIOSH. *Occupational Exposure to Respirable Coal Mine Dust*. Cincinnati, Ohio: US Department of Health and Human Services, Public Health Services, Centers for Disease Control and Prevention, 1995.
4. American Thoracic Society. Adverse effects of crystalline silica exposure. *Am J Respir Crit Care Med* 1997; 155: 761–765.
5. Cowie RL, Mabena SK. Silicosis, chronic airflow limitation, and chronic bronchitis in South African gold miners. *Am Rev Respir Dis* 1991; 143: 80–84.
6. Cowie RL. The influence of silicosis on deteriorating lung function in gold miners. *Chest* 1998; 113: 340–343.
7. Coggon D, Taylor AN. Coal mining and chronic obstructive pulmonary disease: a review of the evidence. *Thorax* 1998; 53: 398–407.
8. Leigh J, Driscoll TR, Cole BD *et al*. Quantitative relation between emphysema and lung mineral content in coalworkers. *Occup Environ Med* 1994; 51: 400–407.
9. Green FHY, Vallyathan V. Coal workers' pneumoconiosis and pneumoconiosis due to other carbonaceous dusts. In: Churg A, Green FHY, eds. *Pathology of Occupational Lung Disease*, 2nd edn, Baltimore: Williams and Wilkins, 1998; pp. 129–207.

10. Marine WM, Gurr D, Jacobsen M. Clinically important effects of dust exposure and smoking in British coal miners. *Am Rev Respir Dis* 1988; 137: 106–12.
11. Cowie RL, Mabena SK. Asthma in goldminers. *S Afr Med J* 1996; 86: 804–807.
12. Nemery B, Lenaerts L. Exposure to methylene diphenyl diisocyanate in coal mines. *Lancet* 1993; 341: 318.
13. Love RG, Miller BG, Groat SK *et al*. Respiratory health effects of opencast coalmining: a cross sectional study of current workers. *Occup Environ Med* 1997; 54: 416–423.
14. Pal TM, de Monchy JG, Groothoff JW, Post D. The clinical spectrum of humidifier disease in synthetic fiber plants. *Am J Ind Med* 1997; 31: 682–692.
15. Ulvestad B, Melbostad E, Fuglerud P. Asthma in tunnel workers exposed to synthetic resins. *Scand J Work Environ Health* 1999; 25: 335–341.
16. Cowie RL. The epidemiology of tuberculosis in gold miners with silicosis. *Am J Respir Crit Care Med* 1994; 150: 1460–1462.
17. Sherson D, Lander F. Morbidity of pulmonary tuberculosis among silicotic and nonsilicotic foundry workers in Denmark. *J Occup Med* 1990; 32: 110–113.
18. Jones FL. Rifampin-containing chemotherapy for pulmonary tuberculosis associated with coal workers' pneumoconiosis. *Am Rev Respir Dis* 1982; 125: 681–683.
19. Cowie RL. Silicotuberculosis: long-term outcome after short-course chemotherapy. *Tubercle Lung Dis* 1995; 76: 39–42.
20. Wolinsky E. Nontuberculous mycobacteria and associated diseases. *Am Rev Respir Dis* 1979; 119: 107–159.

21. Corbett EL, Hay M, Churchyard GJ *et al. Mycobacterium kansasii* and *M. scrofulaceum* isolates from HIV-negative South African gold miners: incidence, clinical significance and radiology. *Int J Tubercul Lung Dis* 1999; 3: 501–507.

22. Cowie RL. The mycobacteriology of pulmonary tuberculosis in South African gold miners. *Tubercle* 1990; 71: 39–42.

23. Churchyard GJ, Kleinschmidt I, Corbett EL *et al.* Mycobacterial disease in South African gold miners in the era of HIV infection. *Int J Tubercul Lung Dis* 1999; 3: 791–798.

24. van Rie A, Warren R, Richardson M *et al.* Exogenous reinfection as a cause of recurrent tuberculosis after curative treatment. *N Engl J Med* 1999; 341: 1174–1179.

25. Smit P, Oberholzer D, Hayden-Smith *et al.* Protective efficacy of pneumococcal polysaccharide vaccines. *JAMA* 1977; 238: 2613–2616.

26. Sluis-Cremer GK, Hessel PA, Hnizdo EH, Churchill AR. Relationship between silicosis and rheumatoid arthritis. *Thorax* 1986; 41: 596–601.

27. Cowie RL. Silica-dust-exposed mine workers with scleroderma (systemic sclerosis). *Chest* 1987; 92: 260–262.

28. Churg A. Neoplastic asbestos-induced disease. In: Churg A, Green FHY, eds. *Pathology of Occupational Lung Disease*, 2nd edn. Baltimore: Williams and Wilkins, 1998, pp. 339–391.

29. Cohn SM. Pulmonary contusion: review of the clinical entity. *J Trauma – Injury Inf Crit Care* 1997; 42: 973–979.

30 WELDING

Grant McMillan

INTRODUCTION

The emissions from welding processes may comprise ultraviolet (UV) and infrared radiations, visible light, and an airborne, dynamic, and often biologically active, mixture of particles and gases, termed 'welding fume'. This fume arises both directly from the processes and indirectly from the action of the UV and infrared emissions on gases and vapours in the adjacent atmosphere (Fig. 30.1). Given the potentially hazardous nature of some of the constituents of the fume, the ubiquitous nature of welding processes (with the work duties of an estimated 2–3 million people worldwide said to include some welding), and the extensive research literature on the health of welders, it would not be surprising for there to be a well-evidenced history of widespread acute and chronic adverse effects on respiratory health in welders and those in related trades.

This is, however, not the case. While there is general agreement on acute effects, wide variation is found between the conclusions of studies of long-term effects. This can be explained in large part by the range of welding processes, and the variations in the nature of fumes and level of exposure that may be experienced between, and even within, these processes. Moreover, many welders have been cigarette smokers and exposed to airborne asbestos fibers in addition to welding fumes.

It is cardinal rule that 'welders' cannot be regarded as a single homogeneous group. Welders are rarely employed at a single type of welding and over their working life use different welding processes on various metals. As will become apparent, this has a powerful influence on their potential exposure to metal fumes, gases and other pollutions. Moreover, national reporting schemes may contribute inadvertently to generating confusion by categorizing as 'welders' other craftsmen, such as braziers and solderers: they have a quite different potential for exposure to harmful agents (as described in the useful booklet 'Solder fume and you' published in 1997 by the UK Health and Safety Executive).

The uncertainty over health effects should not be fuel for complacency. There is a need for industry to take more proactive measures to recognize, evaluate, and control exposure to the emissions from welding processes and, through improved training and

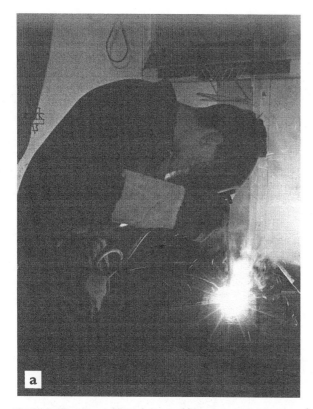 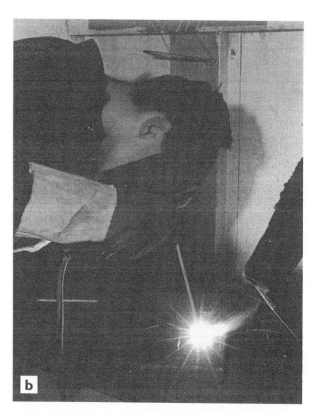

Fig. 30.1 The plume of fume from a welding process may rise towards the welder's breathing zone (a) but may be diverted from it and the risk of exposure reduced by using strategically placed local exhaust ventilation (b). (Courtesy of J H Dennis.)

education, to involve the welders more in protecting their health.

PRINCIPLES AND PROCESSES

Welding is the process whereby suitable materials are joined at points softened or liquefied by the application of heat, sometimes with associated application of pressure. In the welding of metals, the heat required may be derived in a variety of fashions including friction, electron beams, ultrasound, or the combustion of fuel gases such as a mixture of acetylene and oxygen, but by far the most common source is an electric arc struck between two conductors. Though much of this process is now automated, manual electric arc welding is still very common. Further consideration of the health hazards of welding will be restricted to joining metals by these manual electric arc processes, as there is the opportunity for so many workers to be harmed if fumes from these processes pose significant hazards to health and exposure to them is controlled inadequately.

In this book, interest in the adverse health effects of welding is concentrated on the respiratory system. It should, however, not be forgotten that absorbed welding fumes may affect other systems.

Moreover, inadequately controlled risks of fire, burns, or electric shock may each play an important part in the health of welders, as may high levels of noise, injury due to difficult access or egress, heavy lifting, and poor ergonomic design of the work process or workplace. Whereas a relatively recent study has found respiratory diseases to be the most common cause of medical wastage in shipyard welders [1], several other investigators have described injuries and chronically disabling diseases of the musculoskeletal system as the most common cause of morbidity and premature retirement from work in welders.

MANUAL ELECTRIC ARC WELDING

A basic appreciation of the principal electric arc welding processes is needed to understand the source and nature of the emissions and the potential that exists to control them. Fuller technical details are available in publications from the Welding Institute, Abington, Cambridge, UK, and the Job Knowledge section of its internet site at http://www.twi.co.uk/bestprac/.

The great heat generated by an electric arc, usually struck between an electrode held by the welder in a handpiece and the workpiece, melts the abutting surfaces of the pieces to be joined sufficiently for these to contribute molten metal to a common weld pool which, when cool, forms a solid joint. When the workpieces themselves cannot contribute sufficient metal to the pool, metal may be added from a filler wire held in the arc or weld pool. That wire may also act as the current-carrying electrode, in which case it is described as a 'consumable' electrode.

A gas shield is formed round the arc and weld pool to restrict access of oxygen and hydrogen and thus minimize reactions with these gases that could weaken the weld. This gas shield may be produced by combustion of the coating or core of the consumable, or may be provided directly as a flow of inert or active gas, such as argon or carbon dioxide respectively, forming a bubble-like stable and reproducible shielding microenvironment. The composition of the shield gas can be an important factor in controlling emissions.

There are significant general differences in the potential emission rate and composition of fume from each of the three main categories of electric arc welding processes. These are described below in increasing order of complexity and relative amount of emissions.

Tungsten inert gas (TIG) welding

The arc arises from a non-consumable electrode formed by a spike of tungsten (Fig. 30.2). The sharp configuration of this electrode must be maintained during arcing to ensure arc stability. This cannot be achieved with a pure tungsten electrode, and thus a tungsten alloy is used, most commonly with 0.5–4% thorium, an α particle emitter, which also gives other technical advantages. The electrode must be re-dressed as necessary to maintain the required contour, the grinding process typically occupying several minutes of the welder's time each day and producing dust of respirable particle size. The arc and weld pool is protected by a shroud of piped argon and/or helium as the inert shielding gas. If required, metal may be added from a handheld filler wire fed into the weld pool – as distinct from the higher temperature arc.

Metal inert gas (MIG) and metal active gas (MAG) welding

In these processes the electrode is a continuous consumable wire fed through the welding handpiece or 'gun' (Fig. 30.3). It is rendered molten by its own arc and contributes directly to the weld pool which, together with the electrode and arc, is shrouded by a shield of gas piped to the gun. This is inert gas in MIG welding and active gas such as carbon dioxide in MAG welding. A variation is 'flux core arc welding' in which the wire has a core of flux that burns to produce a gas shield, which may obviate the need for a piped gas supply.

Manual metal arc (MMA) welding

This is the most commonly used of the electric arc welding processes. The arc is struck between a short, consumable electrode, grasped stick-like in a handpiece, and the workpiece; indeed, it is commonly

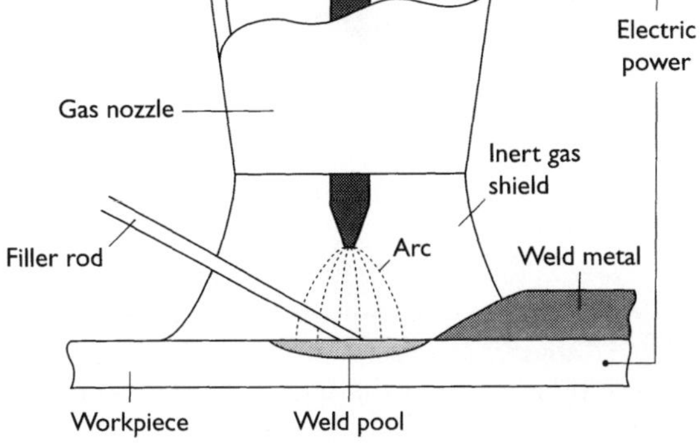

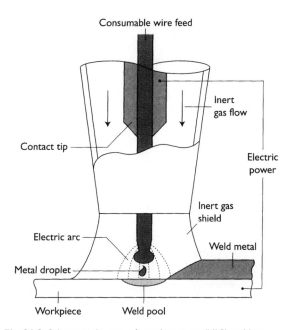

Fig. 30.2 Schematic diagram of tungsten inert gas (TIG) welding.

Fig. 30.3 Schematic diagram of metal inert gas (MIG) welding.

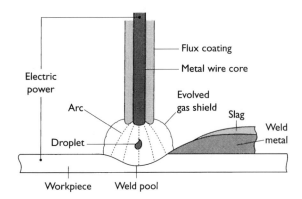

Fig. 30.4 Schematic diagram of manual metal arc (MMA) welding.

referred to as 'stick welding' (Fig. 30.4). The electrode is usually coated with a mixture of chemicals and alloying metals. In addition to forming a shield of combustion gases, this coating may contribute much to the properties of the weld and form a temporary residue (slag) over it to reduce oxidation and slow cooling.

A fourth process, 'electric resistance welding' (also called spot and/or seam welding), is also used widely. The two surfaces to be joined are held together very closely by pressure between highly conductive electrodes. When the high-current low-voltage pulse passes through the point of contact, the metal surfaces are fused.

WELDING EMISSIONS

Welding fume from open electric arc welding processes may pose a risk to health depending on its composition, concentration, and duration of exposure. In general, it is a mixture of airborne particles derived from the evaporation, condensation, and oxidation of metals, and with varying degrees of oxides of nitrogen, carbon monoxide, ozone, and other gases. Low melting point surface contaminants or coatings may also make a significant contribution.

The dynamic physical and chemical nature of welding fume presents challenges to meaningful sampling and analysis, and care must be taken to ensure that the results of analysis actually represent the hazard the welder is facing and have not been altered significantly by sampling methods. When assessing exposure, the fume should be sampled in the breathing zone, behind the welder's face shield. The amount of fume may be expressed as an emission rate (usually in milligrams per minute) to compare processes, or as an exposure in the units of the national occupational exposure limit for health risk assessment or surveillance.

Particulates

There are two principal types of particle. First, there is usually a high proportion of respirable fractionated and unfractionated mixed metal oxide particles, often in the form of chains and aggregates, reflecting the composition of the consumable electrode or filler wire (Table 30.1). Second, there are discrete, coarse, unfractionated particles of electrode called 'spatter', which are generally larger than the respirable range but, as they oxidize, are a secondary source of smaller, respirable, fume particles. When a coated or flux-cored electrode or filler wire is used, up to 95% of the particles derive from that coating or core. There are marked differences in size and physical properties of the particles arising from different processes [2]. These may be of biological significance but, apart from size, few of these properties have been explored in that context.

The constituents of welding fume are determined largely by the composition of the filler metal and, where used, the flux coating or core; the composition of the parent metal has a relatively minor effect. The constituents of these consumables should be available in technical data sheets provided by the supplier. Iron oxides are generated from filler and parent metal during the welding of iron and steels. Aluminum oxide is generated from filler and parent metals during welding of aluminum-based materials. Manganese oxides are common constituents of steel welding and are found in fume from any arc process using manganese-containing fillers, the concentration of manganese in the welding filler having a direct influence on the concentration of manganese oxide in the fume. Fluorides may be generated from the covering of manual metal arc welding electrodes or from the filling of flux-cored wires, and may reach 10–20% of the total fume. Barium compounds are generated during welding when barium is contained within the filler materials, the coating of electrodes, or the flux-cored wires. Potassium oxide, sodium oxide, and titanium dioxide may be generated from the coating of covered electrodes.

Trivalent and hexavalent chromium compounds are found in fume from welding using materials that contain chromium or chromates such as stainless steels, high chromium nickel alloys and low alloy steels, high alloy flux-covered wires, and materials coated with chromate paints or chromium plating. At present, only the hexavalent chromium compounds formed are a cause for concern with regard to respiratory health, principally because of their proven sensitizing, mutagenic, and carcinogenic actions in other occupational settings. The highest emissions of hexavalent chromium are associated with manual metal

Table 30.1 Welding fume composition related to welding processes, filler metals and consumables (Elemental components listed, including fluorine, are in the form of oxides). Source: Pooled experience from discussions between members of International Institute of Welding's Commission on Health and Safety, chaired by the author

Process	Filler metal	Shielding gases	Components of consumable	Key components analyzed in welding fume
Manual	Mild/low alloy steel	nil	Fe,Mn,Si,Na,F,K	Fe, Mn,Si,Na,F,K
	Stainless steel	nil	Fe,Mn,Si,F,K,Ni,Cr	Fe,Mn,Si,Na,F,K,Li,Ni,CrVI,Cr other
	Nickel, nickel alloy	nil	Fe,Ni,Ba,Cr,Ca,Cu,Si,Sr	Fe, Mn,Si,Na,F,K,Mg,Ni
	Hardfacing	nil	Fe,Mn,Si,K,F,Cr	Fe,Mn,Si,Na,F,K,Mg,Cr
Automatic and semi-automatic (flux core)	Mild/low alloy steel (self shielded)	nil	Fe,Mn,Ba,Si,F,Ca	Fe,Mn,Si,Na,F, K,Mg,Li,Ni, Sol Ba, InsolBa
	Mild/low alloy steel (gas shielded)	CO_2 Ar/CO_2	Fe,Mn,Si,F,Na,K,Cr	Fe,Mn,Si,Na,F,K,Mg,Li,Cr other
	Hardfacing	nil	Fe,Mn,Si,F,Cr	Fe,Mn,Si,Na,F,K,Mg,CrVI,Cr other
	Stainless steel (gas shielded)	CO_2 Ar/CO_2	Fe,Mn,Si,F,K,Cr	Fe,Mn,Si,Na,F,K,Mg, Ni,CrVI,Cr other
	Stainless steel (deep shielded)	nil	Fe,Mn,Si,F,K,Cr	Fe,Mn,Si,Na,F,K,Mg,Ni,CrVI,Cr other
Automatic and semi-automatic (solid wire)	Mild/low alloy steel (wire)	CO_2 Ar/CO_2	Fe,Mn,Si,Cu	Fe,Mn,Si
	Stainless wire	Ar/CO_2	Fe,Mn,Si,Ni,Cr	Fe,Mn,Ni,CrVI,Cr other

arc welding, and most notably MMA welding of stainless steel (a steel alloy containing chromium and mickel). The emission of hexavalent chromium from TIG welding of stainless steel is much lower. Welding mild steel (an alloy of iron, carbon, and silicon) should not produce exposure to hexavalent chromium, but in one study the urine and blood chromium levels in such welders who had never welded stainless steel were significantly higher than those in controls who had never welded at all. This suggests an alternative, but not positively identified, source of chromium [3]. One explanation offered is that construction mild steels may actually contain a very low concentration of chromium (less than 1%), which is increased in the resulting welding fume owing to preferential vaporization.

Nickel oxides are generated mainly by welding with pure nickel or nickel base alloys in the filler material. Air and biological sampling indicates that, in general, nickel compounds tend to constitute a very small proportion of welding fumes and are usually found in concentrations well below the existing UK regulatory limits (maximum allowable concentration of 0.1 mg/m³ for soluble compounds and 0.5 mg/m³ of insoluble compounds).

The contribution of surface coatings and contaminants or, during maintenance and repair, residues from production work, may be very significant (e.g. lead from lead-based paints).

Gases

Carbon monoxide is generated during metal active gas welding with carbon dioxide or mixed shield gases by thermal decomposition of carbon dioxide, and in all processes where there is combustion of carbon-containing materials in an inadequate oxygen supply. Nitrogen oxides are generated by oxidation of atmospheric nitrogen at the edge of the arc. Nitrogen monoxide is generated at temperatures exceeding 1000°C. It oxidizes to nitrogen dioxide at room temperature.

Ozone is generated by the photolysis of molecular oxygen in the ambient air by UV radiation emitted from the arc. It is formed both close to and a meter or more from the arc. The presence of other gases, fumes, or dust accelerates the decomposition of ozone to oxygen. Accordingly, ozone emission is higher in processes with low fume emission, relatively more being formed in TIG than in MIG welding, and much less than in MMA welding.

Phosgene and hydrogen chloride may be generated by heating or UV radiation of degreasing agents containing chlorinated hydrocarbons that are present on the welded metal. Gases will be generated by the action of the heat of welding on workpieces coated or contaminated by oil, paint, or other materials. Their nature and attendant risk to health will depend on the composition of the coating or contaminant. Examples include carbon monoxide, toluene diisocyanate, hydrogen cyanide, and hydrogen chloride.

Exposure determinants

The welder's skill and technique are powerful influences on emission, and the care he or she takes to avoid fume is a further important determinant of the cumulative level of exposure. Other influences include the materials to be welded and the materials in the filler wire or consumable, electric parameters and shield gases, and contaminants and surface coatings. Surface coatings and contaminants should be removed before welding whenever possible.

The effects on fume content and emission rate of adding reactive metals to the consumable or changing electric parameters and/or the shielding gas are complex. Much has been written about the scope of such variations and how they may be used to advantage to modify processes and thus reduce the risk of harm from their emissions [4–8], but much of this potential remains untapped.

Systemic absorption

The complexity of compounds and aggregations found in the respirable particles in welding fume makes it difficult to predict the absorption of their constituent parts from the lung by extrapolation from the behavior of pure elements or compounds. A start has been made to investigate this aspect of welding fume in current research sponsored by the American Welding Society.

ADVERSE EFFECTS

Over the years many studies of welders have been undertaken, the more recent refocusing concerns over the risks to respiratory health. A 40-year historical cohort study of shipyard welders [1] found medical wastage due to respiratory disease to be four times greater in welders than controls (shipwrights and engine fitters); this could not be explained by differential smoking habits alone.

While cause–effect relationships are seldom a matter of contention for the acute effects of welding fume inhalation on the respiratory system, the possibility and nature of chronic effects of exposure have long been the subjects of research. The results have not been at all consistent. Probable reasons for the wide variations among the conclusions include a statistical requirement for more subjects than have been available to give sufficient power to test the hypotheses satisfactorily; the variety in the nature of welding

work and thus of fume exposure between welders; failure to appreciate this variety when seeking to consolidate small, possibly disparate, groups of welders into larger and supposedly homogeneously exposed study groups; the absence of contemporaneous records of work or exposure from which some estimate of dose might be made; and failure or inability to take full account of confounding factors such as cigarette smoking and asbestos exposure in a group with a generally higher rate of smoking and greater chance of occupational exposure to asbestos than most. Moreover, many of the effects of metal fumes and gases on the respiratory system remain poorly understood. Debate continues on several topics.

Asphyxia

Asphyxia is a fortunately rare, sometimes fatal, acute condition suffered by welders through working in inadequately ventilated spaces where oxygen has been displaced by inert shielding gases, or depleted by combustion, or (most unusually) rusting of ferrous structures. Foolish measures taken to counter the risk of asphyxia by 'freshening the air' in such workplaces with oxygen, perhaps provided as a fuel gas in oxyacetylene welding or cutting, have led to fierce fires in the 'oxygen enriched' workplace – some with fatal consequences. There is merit in reducing the risk of such forbidden practices by odorizing the oxygen supplied as a fuel gas in workplaces so that increasing concentrations are easily and quickly detected.

Metal fume fever

One of the few ancient occupational diseases still encountered in modern industrial practice, metal fume fever is probably the most common acute harmful effect of electric arc welding on the respiratory system. When groups of welders have been asked specifically, up to 30% admit to having had an attack. It is also probably the most commonly occurring of the inhalation fevers – a group of acute, non-allergic, usually benign and self-limiting flu-like illnesses caused generally by heavy exposure to certain respirable environmental pollutants. They usually resolve within 1–3 days, with only supportive treatment required in the uncomplicated case. An important exception to the general rule is fume containing cadmium, as this may cause severe, even life-threatening, toxicity.

Metal fume fever is caused by a single exposure to freshly formed metal oxide fumes. The concentration need not be high; in a laboratory study inhalation of zinc oxide at 5 mg/m^3 (the prescribed 8-hour time-weighted occupational exposure limit in the UK) produced fever, symptoms and an increased plasma pyrogen interleukin 6 level after only 2 hours in initially healthy individuals [9], thus casting doubt on the adequacy of the standard.

Symptoms usually begin within a few hours of exposure onset, with bouts of intense shivering, muscle and joint pains, undulating low-grade fever (but sometimes high fever), and difficulty in keeping warm. In more severe cases there may also be chest pain, abdominal pain, and vomiting. Physical examination may reveal crackles and wheezes. Pulmonary function is commonly unaffected, or there may be transient acute impairment with reduced lung volumes and gas transfer, usually followed by complete recovery. Rarely, there is an asthma-like response. The chest radiograph is typically normal and there is a peripheral leucocytosis. If asked, the affected welder will usually admit to welding on material containing zinc (galvanized metal being most commonly involved), but the oxides of several other metals have been implicated.

While it is difficult to accept that there should be no long-term health penalty for repeated or severe attacks, long-term sequelae have been reported, but only rarely. The rapid and full recovery from metal fume fever leads to the illness often passing unreported; it is thus underestimated in studies based on recorded sickness absence.

Some welders believe that an attack early in the week confers temporary immunity or resistance, but it may be simply that the welder is more cautious of exposure in the days following such an unpleasant illness. Other inhalation fevers are also associated with such tolerance, however, most notably that associated with cotton dust exposure ('Monday fever'). Rarely, the welder may develop pneumonitis and pulmonary edema when the concentration of fumes has been particularly high, or when the illness is complicated by specific acute metal toxic damage, as in cadmium pneumonitis.

The pathogenesis of metal fume fever has not been established fully. Particles of freshly formed metal oxide can reach the alveoli. Taken together, the findings of various inhalation studies indicate that the lung itself plays a principal role in initiating metal fume fever rather than acting only as the point of absorption. This view is supported by observations that neither ingestion nor intravenous injection of toxic levels of zinc oxide in humans is associated with symptoms resembling those of metal fume fever.

The hypothesis for the initiating process that gains most favor currently is production of an endogenous pyrogen, possibly one or several proinflammatory cytokines released from pulmonary and blood cells some hours after exposure to the freshly formed oxide [10]. Human exposure studies indicate that zinc oxide fume inhalation, from welding and otherwise, results in marked pulmonary inflammation, especially at the periphery, with cytokine release in the lungs and raised levels of the pyrogen interleukin 6 in the subjects who develop symptoms [9,11]. In some evaluations, the data have shown a dose–response relationship. Blanc et al. [11] and others have suggested that tumor necrosis factor is a key mediator.

Pneumonitis

Many components of emissions from (or related to) welding processes have been associated with chemical (i.e. toxic) pneumonitis, including cadmium, manganese, oxides of nitrogen, ozone, and phosgene. Less commonly, hypersensitivity pneumonitis may occur. This is associated most with beryllium, which causes a sarcoidosis-like picture [12], but a case of recurrent bronchoalveolitis thought to be due to hypersensitivity pneumonitis has been described in a zinc smelter [13]. Both types of pneumonitis may produce symptoms 4–6 hours after exposure onset, but, whereas toxic pneumonitis may occur with the first exposure to such fumes, hypersensitivity pneumonitis requires one or more previous sensitizing exposures to the offending substance. Once sensitization has occurred, repeated episodes characteristically occur, often of increasing severity almost regardless of the level of exposure. A sensitized individual will typically develop symptoms and pulmonary infiltrates at levels of exposure that do not affect others similarly exposed in the same workplace. By contrast, the severity of repeated episodes of metal fume fever and toxic pneumonitis is closely related to the level of exposure, and similarly exposed individuals generally suffer symptoms of similar severity. While mild episodes of both types of pneumonitis are generally self-limiting without residual effect, severe episodes (particularly if repeated) may lead to the destruction of functional lung.

Chemical and hypersensitivity pneumonitis appears to be uncommon in welders. Welding on cadmium metal or its alloys (often unsuspectingly when it is present as a surface coating) is probably the most frequent cause, sometimes with a fatal outcome. Measuring the urinary cadmium concentration can be useful in differentiating between metal fume fever and cadmium pneumonitis early in the course of the illness, and may be lifesaving as survival from cadmium pneumonitis may require intensive care.

Pneumonia

Over several decades from 1959 to 1990, four successive surveys relating cause of death in England and Wales to occupation have shown there to be an excess risk of death from pneumonia in men of working age in the occupational group that contains welders [14]. Toxic pneumonitis was suspected as the explanation in the earlier surveys, but this has not proved to be the case [15]. The diversity of trades other than electric arc welding that may be included in the analysis group (others are gas, spot, and blacksmith welding) suggested that the cause was not specific to arc welding, and a similar pattern has been observed in coremakers and furnacemen. This has prompted the hypothesis that inhaled metal fume is the common factor and may have an immunotoxic effect, or that accumulated iron in the lung might facilitate infection. A controlled study to determine whether lobar pneumonia is an occupational disease of welders has been undertaken; preliminary indications are that there is an association between pneumonia and occupational exposure to metal fume (personal communication).

Asthma

Occupational asthma may follow the inhalation of irritant or sensitising agents, each often found in welding fumes. Yet, overall, reports of occupational

asthma in relation to welding fume are few in comparison with the other respiratory effects, suggesting an infrequent occurrence of the disease in association with welding.

The potential asthmagenic properties of fume from stainless steel welding have aroused particular interest as its constituents include nickel and hexavalent chromium, for which there is good evidence from other occupations for the induction of asthma, albeit uncommonly. While there are reports of asthma in stainless steel welders (Fig. 30.5), the number of reported cases is small: the disease has been reported only very rarely in individuals undertaking mild steel welding exclusively (and thus having no implied exposure to chromium or nickel) and evidence from bronchial challenge is conflicting. Whereas some epidemiological studies of welders in general have shown that exposure to welding fume may have been critical in causing asthma, others have failed to show any excess prevalence. Those studies which have focused on welders of stainless steel do not demonstrate an increased level of occupational asthma, but rather the symptoms of irritation found among all types of welders. In the author's opinion, the evidence to support the view that stainless steel welding fume

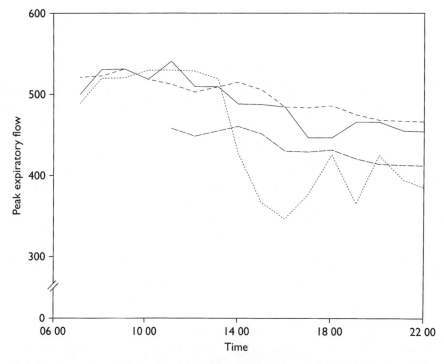

Fig. 30.5 Worksite inhalation provocation tests in a welder using mild steel and stainless steel. The subject was a 47-year-old shipyard welder who had worked intermittently with welding fumes since the age of 16 years. Over the 12 months preceding the investigation he had noted that work with stainless steel was associated with breathlessness and watering of the eyes. After 3 control days of hourly peak flow monitoring that followed an absence from work for 1 week, he spent day 1 with mild steel and day 2 with stainless steel (six to eight rods). Asthmatic symptoms began on day 2 several hours after he commenced work at 0815 hours. Serial measurements of airway responsiveness showed a significant improvement during the initial period away from work (PD_{20} 34.6 $\rightarrow$ 104 µg methacholine), followed by a deterioration of borderline significance after the challenge tests (PD_{20} 64 µg). ○---○, Mean of three control days; ————, lower boundary (95% confidence interval) to detect a late reaction; ▲——▲, work day 1 (mild steel); ▼--▼, work day 2 (stainless steel).

should be classified as a respiratory sensitiser is, at best, inconclusive.

Chronic obstructive pulmonary disease (COPD)

Many studies seeking an excess decline in pulmonary function in groups of welders over longer periods than a shift have been completed over the years. Almost all have been limited in value by their cross-sectional design. Even when account was taken of smoking habit, the results have been inconsistent. Most did not find evidence of significant adverse effects on pulmonary function attributable to employment as a welder. Some have shown a predominance of changes attributable to airway obstruction, others an excess number of welders with restrictive disease, and one an excess of welders with a mixture of patterns of diminished lung function. It was said that 'the lungs of the welders were physiologically 10–15 years older than those of the control group' [16].

Only three longitudinal studies designed to identify accelerated and chronic decline in lung function have been reported. The first confirmed the small level of bronchial obstruction that had been identified in excess in the same group of welders 5 years previously, but found that the disorder had not evolved more than in the control group in the intervening period [17], perhaps because exposures had been more adequately controlled in the intervening period. The second study [18], one of a series [19,20], showed that work in a group comprising welders, caulkers, and burners was associated with excess respiratory symptoms and changes in lung function suggestive of narrowing of all classes of airways, the effects being largely independent of smoking. The effects in caulkers and burners, but not the welders, were reversed after discontinuing exposure. Among the welders, the effect of the fumes was greatest in those who admitted to not using their exhaust ventilation at all times. The third study, also well designed, had yet to run long enough for there to be opportunities for optimal detection of such a change [21].

Chronic bronchitis

Studies reporting an excess of sputum expectoration in welders, especially cigarette smokers, some with evidence suggesting a dose–response relationship, have been almost matched in number by those that have reported no excess prevalence. That said, given the irritating nature of some of the most frequent constituents of welding fume, common sense suggests that if heavy exposure does not cause chronic bronchitis and related diseases, it is likely that it would at least aggravate them.

Siderosis and pulmonary fibrosis

Siderosis is a radiologically apparent pulmonary nodulation exhibited by varying proportions of electric arc welders as a result of inhaling iron oxide in welding fume. There can be considerable differences in the amount of retained lung dust in individuals in a group with apparently homogeneous exposure. It is unusual to find siderosis before 5 years' welding experience, but common after 15 years, with prevalence then increasing steadily with time. Iron clears from the lungs progressively after exposure to ferrous fume has ceased, and radiologic regression of opacities has been reported after exposure to welding fume has ceased – a phenomenon unlikely to be seen if the opacities were due to fibrosis. The majority of experimental, clinical, respiratory function, and histologic studies of welders with siderosis have revealed no significant abnormalities, supporting the general belief that siderosis is usually a benign condition without related fibrosis or pulmonary dysfunction.

There is, however, no doubt that siderosis and parenchymal fibrosis may coexist in the lungs of welders. Evidence supporting the hypothesis that siderosis is occasionally a fibrogenic condition comes largely from individual cases or small series, some with gross overexposure. Some investigators to have found siderosis and fibrosis coexisting in welders have postulated that an alternative single or mixed exposure was the true cause of the fibrosis, including oxides of nitrogen, zinc, silica, hexavalent chromium, nickel compounds, asbestos, aluminum, or an as yet unidentified fibrogenic agent in the welding fume. Alternatively the fibrogenic exposure may have been in another occupation. A further hypothesis is that occupational dusts may induce cryptogenic fibrosing alveolitis (idiopathic interstitial pulmonary fibrosis) non-specifically in susceptible individuals without necessarily having clear inherent fibrogenic properties.

Asbestos-related disorders

Welders are also at significant risk of developing mesothelioma and the other asbestos-related diseases consequent upon occupational exposure to asbestos dust (benign pleural disease, asbestosis, lung cancer) [22–24]. Especially at risk from asbestos are welders who have worked in shipyards, where many were exposed directly or indirectly to the dust arising from insulation materials. Welders also used asbestos matting to protect themselves from sparks, often tearing the cloth and thus releasing dust. The evidence in support of asbestos as the villain of the piece with regard to lung cancer excess in welders is growing convincingly (see below).

Mats and sheets made from glass or ceramic fiber are now used by welders to protect themselves from sparks and spatter. While research has shown that breathing zone fiber levels resulting from their use are acceptably low, the work did not include exposures during tearing or cutting when the welders' needs demanded that the cloth be 'tailored'. Even in the absence of convincing evidence of need, a ban on such practices should be enforced as it could obviate a risk that otherwise might not become apparent for years.

Lung cancer

The risk of lung cancer in those who are or have been employed as welders is about 30% greater than that of the general population. Compounds of nickel and chromium, proven carcinogens in other industrial circumstances, were initially thought to be the cause, and it was expected that the excess would be restricted to stainless steel welders who are most likely to be exposed to fume containing these compounds. Extensive research has shown that the excess is also found in those who reportedly have welded only mild steel and thus should have had no occupational exposure to chromium or nickel. As discussed earlier, however, some mild steel welders have been found to have significantly raised urinary and blood levels of chromium, the source remaining something of a mystery. It is conceivably a consequence of the welders not distinguishing low alloy steels (the alloy metal comprising less than 5%) from mild steel (with only carbon added to the iron). The International Agency for Research on Cancer (IARC) has classified welding fumes as being possibly carcinogenic to humans [22].

The excess of lung cancer in welders may be explained alternatively by unprotected occupational exposure to respirable asbestos dust and tobacco smoking; welders as a group have been found to have a higher proportion of cigarette smokers than many other occupational groups.

Some have thought that thorium in thoriated tungsten electrodes used in TIG welding might be the cause of the excess lung cancer. While thorium is a radioactive element and emits α rays, the electrodes emit only a negligible radiation compared with natural radiation because the thorium is enclosed in the tungsten matrix. It is, however, potentially dangerous, as dust that arises during grinding the electrode tip is respirable. There is, however, no evidence of a concentration of cases of lung cancer, nor indeed excess morbidity, among TIG welders. Nevertheless, it remains vitally important that these grinding wheels and bands are fitted with suitable extraction systems. A search has been made for technically satisfactory thorium-free electrodes, using alternatives additives, and several are now available commercially.

The electromagnetic fields created by welding apparatus have also come under suspicion as being carcinogenic, but the evidence weighs against this being the case.

RISK REDUCTION

There is a need for stricter application of currently available measures for controlling fume and ensuring the proper ventilation of workspaces. Pre-employment health scrutiny, accurate longitudinal environmental monitoring, in-employment health surveillance of respiratory symptoms and function, and possibly biologic monitoring, may all have a role to identify levels of risk and establish whether or not control is adequate. It is imperative that exposures should be minimized, at least to current national restriction levels. As exposure to welding fume and cigarette smoking appear to be synergistic for many adverse effects on respiratory health, smoking should be discouraged and welders assisted to give it up.

Training and education

Training and education are among the most powerful tools to reduce the risks of exposure to welding fumes and other harmful emissions. They need to extend to construction designers, welding engineers who specify the process, and the welders themselves, as experience has shown that the care taken to minimize the weld plume and keep the breathing zone clear of it can reduce exposure by a factor of 10. The potential health impact of excessive exposure to welding fumes, the proven role of cigarette smoking, and the potential for multiplicative interactions should be taught in the training package.

Good design

Good design of the work at the start can eliminate much that is dangerous during construction. It should extend to designing out the need for welders to work in awkward stances, perhaps with the head in the plume, or in confined spaces and other situations where it is difficult to achieve adequate exhaust ventilation, as such work is especially liable to result in heavy exposures.

Weld specification

Of the technically acceptable welding processes, that with the least hazard should be selected, together with the electric parameters and other factors that minimize fume emission. There may be an opportunity to modify a standard process to improve safety. Increasingly, it is technically possible to replace manual welding with an automated/robot method, or even with another method of joining. Adhesive bonding is an important alternative joining technique that is being used increasingly in engineering to replace welding (or at least to reduce the number of weld points required), though still in a relatively limited fashion.

Ventilation

Local exhaust ventilation is the most effective means to reduce further exposure to the welding plume. The opening of a negative pressure duct is placed adjacent to the weld site so that plume is drawn immediately away from the welder (and others working in the area) at source, while not significantly disturbing the gases shielding the arc and weld pool (Fig. 30.1b). Workplaces should also have adequate general ventilation, but this alone may not be adequate to draw welding fumes from the breathing zone.

Personal protective devices

A handheld protection device or helmet shield is required to protect the welder's face and eyes from the physical assaults of electric arc welding. They have the secondary advantage of acting as something of a barrier to fume entering the breathing zone, but should not be relied upon to contribute meaningfully to reducing exposure to acceptable levels as they have been shown to provide only marginal and highly variable reductions in fume exposure. Only when all other means of exposure reduction have proved insufficiently effective can the use of a personal respiratory protective device be justified. This should be incorporated in or fit snugly under the face shield and either simply filter ambient air or provide clean air by hose from a remote pressurized source. Good compliance in the use of such respiratory protection may be difficult to achieve, largely due to poor comfort factors, especially in warm conditions.

Surveys

Environmental exposure surveys should be carried out to monitor the use and effectiveness of all the control measures listed above, to detect breaches in the prescribed safe system of work, and (by way of air sampling) to identify excessive exposures before these can cause long-term harm.

HEALTH SURVEILLANCE

Pre-employment health screening

Screening of those who wish to be welders or work in allied trades should seek to identify those who are more likely than usual to be adversely affected by exposure to fumes at or below national occupational exposure levels so that they may make an informed choice about pursuing such an occupation and, if they choose to persist, may be specially protected. There will be some who cannot be accepted as welders where the work circumstances make it impossible for the employers to discharge their duty of care to them, no matter how they may try, because the candidates have a pre-existing health condition, such as severe asthma, which would be aggravated by exposure to welding fumes, even at a very low level. The reasons for arriving at this negative decision should be made clear to the candidate and recorded fully and carefully in the medical record.

The screening procedure should be designed to seek specific abnormalities. Nothing should be done unless the reasons for it have been defined and can be explained to employees and potential employees. As a minimum, the screening procedure should include a questionnaire based, for example, on that issued by the Medical Research Council for assessing respiratory symptoms, and measurement of FEV_1, FVC, and PEF as these indices measure different appropriate aspects of response [25]. Those with abnormalities should be seen by a doctor. There is no justification for chest radiography unless a specific clinical need is determined for individual examinees.

In-employment surveillance

This refers to specific measures carried out on a regular basis to detect biological indicators of excessive environmental exposures before more serious health outcomes result. Longitudinal monitoring should be a continuation of the pre-employment screening by questionnaire and monitoring of ventilatory function. The respiratory function equipment should be calibrated regularly and the technicians should be trained to the high standards required for longitudinal surveys. Biological monitoring for absorption of specific metals may be added.

DIFFICULT CASE

History

An electric arc welder spent his entire working life between 1947, when he was aged 17 years, and 1984 in shipyards. About 75% of his time was spent within confined spaces with poor fume extraction equipment. At an assessment for compensation in 1995 he reported having smoked up to five cigarettes per day from his mid teens, but earlier sequential medical records indicated daily consumption levels of 20, 15, 10, and 5. He developed undue breathlessness at about the age of 40 years. He could recall nighttime and early morning symptoms of cough and wheeziness from around this time, together with breathlessness on exertion, and cough when he was exposed to fumes at work. He could not recall any other periodicity to suggest occupational asthma. He was treated with a bronchodilator inhaler.

His disability was progressive and was the cause of his early retirement in 1984 at the age of 54 years. He had been able to undertake only light work during his last few years in the shipyard. His respiratory condition continued to deteriorate after he left work, although prebronchodilator measurements of FEV_1 (0.65 liters) were identical in 1987 and 1996. He died in 1999 from an unrelated illness at the age of 69 years.

Chest radiographs did not show evidence of any asbestos-related disorder, but showed overinflation of the lung fields. Spirometry measurements in 1966, 1972, 1979, 1987, and 1996 indicated an average annual FEV_1 loss of 38 ml, with an apparently steeper annual decline during the man's last 20 years at work (54 ml). The effect of an inhaled bronchodilator was evaluated on the last three occasions, when increments of 100–210 ml were noted. Measurements of lung volume and gas transfer were first made in 1979:

FEV_1	prebronchodilator	1.22	(42% predicted)
FEV_1	postbronchodilator	1.32	
FVC	prebronchodilator	2.57	(66% predicted)
FVC	post bronchodilator	3.20	
FEV_1/FVC	prebronchodilator	47%	
FEV_1/FVC	post bronchodilator	41%	
Total lung capacity		7.24	(117% predicted)
Residual volume		4.01	(187% predicted)
Transfer factor		11.05	(78% predicted)
Transfer coefficient		1.55	(109% predicted)

Issues

The primary issues in this case are whether the airway obstruction was a consequence of asthma or COPD (or both), and whether it was wholly or partly occupational in origin.

Comment

The book's contributors were agreed, almost uniformly, that the diagnosis was one of COPD, not asthma, although a small minority considered that both disorders had been present. All considered that occupational exposures had played a role, the majority assessing the occupational contribution at 25–49%. A few considered the occupational exposures to have played a greater role than cigarette smoking, and a few considered them to have exerted no more than a minor influence.

Neither the history nor the physiological tests provide convincing evidence of asthma, and the clinical picture is a reasonably typical one for COPD. The welder had worked in the shipyards of north-east England that were studied cross-sectionally and longitudinally by Cotes and colleagues [26,27]. They concluded that, on average, occupational exposure to welding fume and cigarette smoking contributed by approximately similar degrees to the development of COPD, and they found some evidence of an interaction so that the overall effect exceeded that to be expected from the two exposures separately.

The history suggests that this man had sustained a heavy cumulative level of welding fume exposure (although, as is commonly the case, there was no objective confirmatory evidence of this), but had probably consumed tobacco heavily also, and so both exposures are likely to have been relevant if the data of Cotes and colleagues are accepted. That the measured rate of annual decline in FEV_1 was greater during the years of occupational exposure than during the subsequent years of retirement does favor an occupational effect, but the reported levels of cigarette consumption were not reliable and it is possible that smoking also declined during retirement. Inescapable persisting difficulties are, therefore, the lack of critical objective data quantifying welding fume exposure and cigarette consumption, difficulties that occur frequently with assessments of this nature.

SUMMARY POINTS

- Published studies of the health of welders relate mainly to exposures in the past and are not necessarily relevant for present-day conditions.
- Prolonged occupational exposure to high concentrations of welding fume is likely to aggravate chronic bronchitis, however caused, and may be associated with a progressive excess decline in ventilatory function, especially in smokers.
- Welding fume may elicit symptoms of asthma in those who are already affected, and may prove to be a cause of occupational asthma – especially in welders working with stainless steel.
- Siderosis, usually a benign condition, may be found rarely in association with parenchymal fibrosis.
- Many welders are at risk of developing asbestos-related diseases, including mesothelioma.

- Welders are at excess risk of developing lung cancer, for which tobacco smoking and asbestos exposure are important contributory factors, although welding fume itself is classed as 'possibly carcinogenic to humans'.
- Other potential adverse respiratory effects of welding include asphyxia, metal fume fever, pneumonitis (toxic and hypersensitivity), and pneumonia.
- Risk reduction measures center on minimizing exposures as far as practicable, and should include improved training and education, thoughtful design and specification, process selection and modification, pre-employment health screening, longitudinal health surveillance, and environmental monitoring.

REFERENCES

1. Wanders SP, Zielhuis GQ, Vreuls HJH, Zielhuis RL. Medical wastage in shipyard welders: a forty-year historical cohort study. *Int Arch Occup Environ Health* 1992; 64: 281–291.
2. Hewett P. The particle size distribution, density, and specific surface area of fumes from SMAW and GMAW mild and stainless steel consumables. *Am Ind Hyg Assoc J* 1995; 56: 128–135.
3. Bonde JP, Christensen JM. Chromium in biological samples from low-level stainless steel and mild steel welders. *Arch Environ Health* 1991; 46(4): 225–229.
4. Hewitt PJ, Madden MG. The influence of gas composition and flow rate on fume formation in the micro and macro environments of welding arcs. *Proceedings of the Second Internation Symposium on Ventilation for Contaminant Control*, 20–23 September 1989, London, UK.
5. Hewitt PJ. Reducing fume emission through process parameter selections. *Occup Hyg* 1994; 1: 35–44.
6. Hewitt PJ. Occupational health in metal arc welding. *Indoor Built Environ* 1996; 5: 253–256.
7. Dennis JH, Mortazavi SB, French MJ et al. Reduction of hexavalent chromium concentration in fumes from metal cored arc welding by the addition of reactive metals. *Ann Occup Hyg* 1996; 40(3): 339–344.
8. Dennis JH, French MJ, Hewitt PJ et al. The effects of welding parameters on ultra-violet light emissions, ozone and Cr^{vi}, formation in MIG welding. *Ann Occup Hyg* 1997; 41(1): 95–104.
9. Fine JM, Gordon T, Chen LC et al. Metal fume fever. *J Occup Environ Med* 1997; 39(8): 722–726.
10. Kuschner WG, S'Alessandro A, Wong H, Blanc PD. Early pulmonary cytokine responses to zinc oxide fume formation. *Environ Res* 1997; 75(1): 7–11.
11. Blanc PD, Boushey HA, Wong H et al. Cytokines in metal fume fever. *Am Rev Respir Dis* 1993; 147(1): 134–138.
12. Newman LS. Beryllium disease and sarcoidosis: clinical and laboratory links. *Sarcoidosis* 1995; 12: 7–19.

13. Ameille J, Brechot JM, Brochard P et al. Occupational hypersensitivity pneumonitis in a smelter exposed to zinc fume. *Chest* 1992; 101: 862–863.
14. Coggon D, Inskip H, Winter P, Pannett B. Lobar pneumonia: an occupational disease in welders. *Lancet* 1994; 344: 41–43.
15. McMillan GHG, Pethybridge RJ. The health of welders in naval dockyards: proportional mortality study of welders and two control groups. *J Soc Occup Med* 1983; 33: 75–84.
16. Lyngenbo O, Groth S, Groth M et al. Occupational lung function impairment in never-smoking Danish welders. *Scand J Soc Med* 1989; 17: 157–164.
17. Mur JM, Teculescu D, Massin N et al. Arc welders, respiratory health evolution over 5 years. *Int Arch Occup Environ Health* 1989; 61: 321–327.
18. Chinn DJ, Cotes JE, EI Gamal FM, Wollaston JF. Respiratory health of young shipyard welders and other tradesmen studied cross sectionally and longitudinally. *Occup Environ Med* 1995; 55: 33–42.
19. Cotes JE, Feinmann EL, Male VJ et al. Respiratory symptoms and impairment in shipyard welders and caulker/burners. *Br J Indust Med* 1989; 46: 292–301.
20. Chinn DJ, Stevenson IC, Cotes JE. Longitudinal respiratory survey of shipyard workers: effect of trade and atopic status. *Br J Indust Med* 1990; 47: 83–90.
21. Beckett WS, Pace PE, Sferlazza SJ et al. Airway reactivity in welders; a controlled prospective cohort study. *J Occup Environ Med* 1996; 38(12): 1229–1238.
22. International Agency for Research on Cancer. *IARC Monographs on the Evaluation of Carcinogenic Risks to Humans. Chromium, Nickel and Welding*, vol 49. Lyons: IARC, 1990.
23. McMillan GHG. The risk of asbestos related diseases occurring in welders. *J Occup Med* 1983; 25: 727–730.
24. Becker N. Cancer mortality among arc welders exposed to fumes containing chromium and nickel. *J Occup Environ Med* 1999; 41(4): 294–303.
25. McMillan GHG. Welders' health examinations. *J Soc Occup Med* 1979; 29: 87–92.

SPECIALIZED DISCIPLINES

31 | IMAGING

Sue Copley and David M. Hansell

INTRODUCTION

Imaging strategies for the evaluation of a symptomatic individual, or large populations as part of a screening program, require the use of techniques that are sufficiently sensitive and specific. Ideally, these techniques should also be realistic and cost effective. Traditionally, the chest radiograph has been the mainstay of radiographic assessment of an individual with suspected occupational lung disease, as it is relatively simple to perform, cost effective, and readily available. A unique constraint of radiographic assessment is the issue of radiation dose. As with any investigation using ionizing radiation, the benefits to individuals and a population have to be weighed against the risks involved. Chest radiography remains the most widely used radiologic screening tool for the assessment of large populations of individuals with suspected occupationally induced lung disease, despite recent refinement of techniques such as high-resolution (i.e. thin section) computed tomography.

CHEST RADIOGRAPHY

With the exceptions of scanning equalization radiography and digital radiography, which are described below, the technique for obtaining plain chest radiographs has changed little in the century since its inception. The standard posteroanterior (PA) projection is obtained by standing the erect patient with hands on hips and elbows forward in order to abduct the scapulae away from the lungs. The patient is asked to take a full inspiration during the millisecond exposure and the X-ray beam traverses the thorax in a posterior–anterior direction to reach the X-ray film cassette positioned against the anterior chest wall.

- A PA radiograph of good technical quality and at adequate inspiration is required for the assessment of occupational lung disease.

- A lateral radiograph may be needed to clarify the position of an abnormality identified on the PA view.

- The need for special views, such as oblique or lordotic views to show pleural and apical lesions respectively, has diminished because computed tomography (CT) is now often used for such purposes.

The thorax consists of structures of widely varying densities from the bony skeleton through the soft tissue of the mediastinum to aerated lung; therefore perfect exposure to demonstrate all these structures optimally is difficult to achieve. The absorption of X-rays by different body tissues is to some extent dependent on the energy or kilovoltage of individual X-ray photons.

High- versus low-kilovoltage

High-kilovoltage (110–150 kVp) chest radiography is excellent for the demonstration of mediastinal structures and lung parenchyma due to enhanced penetration of overlying dense structures, particularly bone, which would otherwise obscure the image. Its inevitable disadvantage is the relatively poor demonstration of the bony thoracic cage.

Low-kilovoltage (80 kVp) chest radiography demonstrates the thoracic bony cage and other calcific densities (e.g. calcified pleural plaques) to greater advantage because of greater tissue contrast. It is less satisfactory for demonstrating subtle abnormalities of the lung parenchyma, particularly at the lung bases.

High- and low-kilovoltage chest radiography are comparable in terms of radiation and cost, after the initial capital outlay involved in purchasing a high-kilovoltage generator.

Advanced multiple beam equalization radiography (AMBER)

Scanning equalization radiography allows a continuous modulation of X-ray output in response to transmitted radiation in order to rectify the problems of incorrect regional exposure [1]. Further refinement of the technique was the division of the X-ray beam into small equal sections, each linked to a detector in a feedback loop; so-called advanced multiple beam equalization radiography (AMBER) [2]. A particular advantage of AMBER over conventional chest radiography is the detection of nodules obscured by the mediastinum, whereas no significant advantage has been demonstrated for the detection of diffuse lung disease [3]. The radiation dose from an AMBER chest radiograph is comparable to that from a conventional radiograph. After initial purchase of the equipment, the costs are also similar.

Digital radiography

The basic advantages of digital radiography are the linear dose–response curve of the image receptor (allowing satisfactory images over a wider range of exposures than a conventional film–screen combination) and transmission and storage of images in a digital format [4]. In practice, this allows images of sufficient diagnostic quality to be obtained from imperfect exposures, which may have resulted in a non-diagnostic conventional radiograph. More importantly, perhaps, images in digital form have the potential for further manipulation after processing to aid interpretation. Images can be stored and transmitted more readily which minimizes disruption caused by lost or misplaced radiographs, and facilitates cooperation between centers.

Phosphor plate technology is the most widely implemented form of digital radiography. This involves scanning the plate with a laser, and releasing light which is detected by a photomultiplier. The resultant signal is processed in digital form. More recently, solid-state image receptors have been developed [5].

The use of computer-aided diagnosis systems may also facilitate the detection and diagnosis of interstitial disease [6], but large-scale studies to confirm their efficacy in, for example, population screening have not been performed. Overall, radiation doses are reduced due to a decreased requirement for repeat radiographs following suboptimal exposures. However, the initial capital outlay is significantly greater than for conventional radiography.

ILO classification of pneumoconioses

The International Labour Office (ILO) (1980) classification of the pneumoconioses has been proposed as 'a means of recording systematically the radiographic abnormalities in the chest provoked by the inhalation of dusts' [7]. It represents the most recent modification of a series first introduced in 1930 with the main aims of standardizing the interpretation of posteroanterior radiographs in terms of the size and form of opacities, and profusion. Twenty-two radiographs showing various shapes and profusion of opacities are provided as a reference standard. The most recent classification additionally describes the extent and width of pleural thickening and pleural plaques. Sets of the standard films can be purchased in most countries (details from International Labour Office, CH-1211, Geneva 22, Switzerland).

Parenchymal abnormalities

Small opacities are defined by having maximum diameters less than 10 mm. They are assigned symbols p, q, or r, if they are rounded (nodular) (Fig. 31.1), and s, t or u if they are irregular (reticular) (Fig. 31.2). The rounded opacities are defined by the average diameter being <1.5 mm (p), 1.5–3 mm (q), and 3–10 mm (r); the irregular opacities necessarily being less precisely defined over the comparable range s–t–u as illustrated by the standard radiographs. Conventionally, two symbols are used to record whether opacities are of similar or different sizes and shapes, for instance p/p indicates

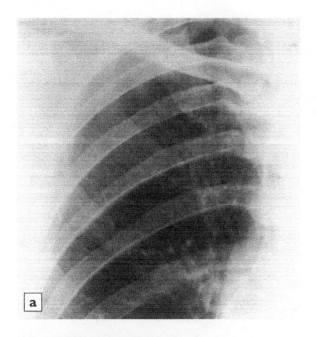

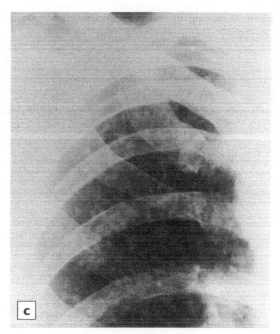

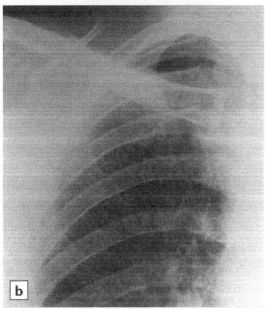

Fig. 31.1 Radiographs of rounded opacities: (a) *p* opacities; (b) *q* opacities; and (c) *r* opacities.

The use of two profusion categories in an expanded classification consequently permits a 12-point scale of increasing profusion which may be useful in epidemiological research:

Category 0   0/−, 0/0, 0/1
Category 1   1/0, 1/1, 1/2
Category 2   2/1, 2/2, 2/3
Category 3   3/2, 3/3, 3/4

The extreme classifications, 0/− and 3/4, indicate that the reviewed film showed, respectively, even less profusion of small opacities than the standard category 0 film, or even greater profusion than the category 3 film.

Large opacities, i.e. those with maximum diameters ≥10 mm, superimposed on a background of the small opacities define the condition of 'complicated' pneumoconiosis. This was formerly known as progressive massive fibrosis (PMF), and the term continues in common use. In the absence of PMF shadows, the small opacities define 'simple pneumoconiosis'. The large opacities are designated by the symbols A, B and C, and are defined in terms of the combined dimensions of all large opacities present. 'A' implies that the maximum diameter (or the total of maximum diameters) does not exceed 5 cm, whereas 'C' implies that an area more than that of the right upper zone is involved. 'B' is applied to the intermediate situation. Previous classification systems allowed a categorization of 'well defined' or 'ill defined', but this has been dropped from the current version.

that all (or almost all) opacities are round and less than 1.5 mm in diameter, and *p/s* denotes that *p* opacities are predominant but there are significant numbers of irregular *s* opacities.

Increasing profusion is classified in four categories (0–3) by comparison with the standard films, category 0 indicating that there is no excess of small opacities above normal. The symbols for two profusion categories may be used to categorize a profusion level which is intermediate between those of the standard films. Thus 1/2 indicates that overall category 1 comes closest to summarizing the observed profusion of the small opacities, but the reader has given serious consideration to choosing category 2.

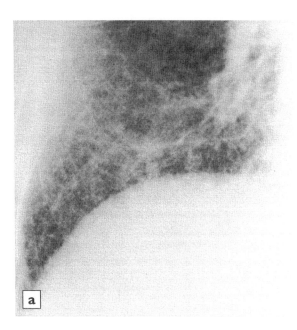

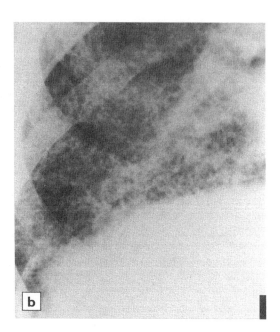

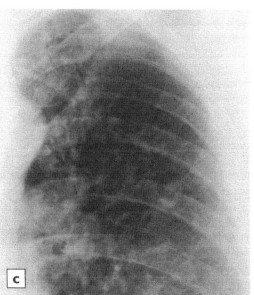

Fig. 31.2 Radiographs of irregular opacities: (a) s opacities; (b) t opacities ; and (c) u opacities.

The upper, mid, and lower zones on each side may be classified separately, but more commonly both lungs are classified together according to the dominant type (or two dominant types) of small opacity, the overall assessment of profusion, and the presence or absence of large opacities. In clinical practice, a Short Classification system is often used which simplifies the recording of profusion of small opacities as 0, 1, 2, or 3 (i.e. the first of the two figures in the expanded system); their shape and size by p–q–r and s–t–u; and the extent of large opacities by A, B or C. Thus, a classification of 'category $2q$B' indicates that the profusion of small opacities is 2 (though the reader may have given serious thought to 1 or 3); the dominant small opacity is q (nodular shadows 1.5–3 mm in diameter); and there is a large opacity (or opacities) implying complicated pneumoconiosis whose maximum diameter(s) exceeds 5 cm but whose total area does not exceed that of the right upper zone.

If the ILO classification is used, it should indicate that the reader has actually compared side by side the reported film with the standard films. The system was originally intended for epidemiological surveys and is therefore designed simply to provide a description of the radiographic appearances. Inferences regarding an individual patient's clinical symptoms and lung function abnormalities are deemed inappropriate. There are also strict criteria to ensure optimum radiographic technique.

Pleural abnormalities

The most recent version (1980) of the ILO classification recognizes two types of pleural involvement: diffuse pleural thickening and circumscribed pleural plaques. The right and left hemithoraces are evaluated separately according to the maximum width and the maximum length of chest wall involvement of both diffuse pleural thickening and circumscribed pleural plaques:

Width	a	up to 5 mm
	b	5–10 mm
	c	greater than 10 mm
Extent	1	$\frac{1}{4}$ of lateral chest wall involved
	2	$\frac{1}{4}$ to $\frac{1}{2}$
	3	greater than $\frac{1}{2}$

If pleural thickening can be seen only face on (that is, not in profile), the width cannot be recorded and only its presence or absence is stated. The presence or absence of costophrenic angle obliteration and of diaphragmatic plaques for each hemithorax is also recorded. Pleural calcification of the chest wall, diaphragm, and other sites including the mediastinal pleural and pericardial surfaces are recorded separately. The extent of pleural calcification is recorded on a scale of 1 to 3:

1 an area of pleural calcification with a greatest diameter of up to about 20 mm, or a number of areas the sum of whose greatest diameters does not exceed 20 mm
2 an area (or number of areas) with a greatest diameter of 20–100 mm
3 an area (or number of areas) with greatest diameter greater than 100 mm

Involvement of the minor fissure on the lateral radiograph occurs with sufficient frequency that a separate classification symbol 'pi' has been added to the ILO 1980 classification [7].

COMPUTED TOMOGRAPHY

CT relies on the differential absorption of X-rays by body tissues of varying densities, and in this respect is similar to conventional radiography. CT is more sensitive, however, for the detection of differing attenuation of the X-ray beam by different biologic materials, and a key advantage is that axial or transverse images can be obtained in sections (generally at 10-mm contiguous intervals) without superimposition of overlying structures. Thus the resulting two-dimensional image comes closer to representing a truly two-dimensional plane of the thorax, unlike the two-dimensional chest radiograph, which represents all three dimensions of the thorax.

Conventional CT

The technique uses a narrow X-ray beam to traverse the patient, and the emergent beam is detected by scintillation detectors. An image is produced by calculation of the absorption of the X-ray beam by the patient in a series of small cubes or voxels. A comparison is made between the intensity of the X-ray beam at source to the intensity of the X-ray beam attenuated by the patient, and a series of simultaneous equations is performed to determine the linear attenuation coefficient of X-rays in a given small volume (voxel). These data are then represented as a two-dimensional image or matrix of pixels and assigned a gray-scale value.

The attenuation value of water is arbitrarily assigned a Hounsfield unit (HU) of zero on a scale of −1000 to +1000 HU. Denser structures such as bone have a value of approximately +500 HU, whereas air has a value of −1000 HU [8]. The final CT image is usually displayed on a monitor and recorded on film, the CT numbers or Hounsfield Units being represented by a matrix containing up to 512 shades of gray. In order to produce images of tissues of interest of sufficient contrast, an appropriate 'window center' needs to be chosen: a window center of −500 HU is optimal for lung imaging, whereas for mediastinal structures or the chest wall a window center of +10 to −20 HU is appropriate. The 'window width' determines the number of gray-scale values displayed above and below the window center; values above the upper level of window width are displayed as white and those below as black. A narrow window width produces images of higher contrast, whereas a wide window width gives a lower contrast image as the gray scale is applied to a broader range of tissues. Standardization of window widths is important as too narrow a window width may result in the erroneous impression of ground glass attenuation, whereas too wide a window width may lead to insufficient contrast for the demonstration of subtle nodularity (Fig. 31.3).

Small structures, less than the width of a CT section, are susceptible to the effects of partial volume averaging in that they account for only a portion of the attenuation value of a voxel. Similarly, as the attenuation value of calcium is so much greater than water, even a small fleck of calcium in a voxel weights the average attenuation coefficient so the resultant pixel appears almost white. Therefore, the detection of small structures depends to a large extent on their density. The thinner the section width, the smaller the effect of partial volume averaging.

High-resolution CT

High-resolution CT (HRCT) is now used routinely to evaluate diffuse interstitial lung disease due to its increased sensitivity and specificity in comparison with chest radiography [9–11]. The technique of HRCT involves the use of thinly collimated 1–3 mm CT sections, to increase spatial resolution and provide detailed images of the lung parenchyma. There is no precise definition of collimation width which delineates an investigation as 'high resolution', but conventionally 1-mm or 1.5-mm sections are used. The use of thinner sections is constrained by unacceptable noise, whereas sections of 5 mm or greater do not improve spatial resolution [12]. The

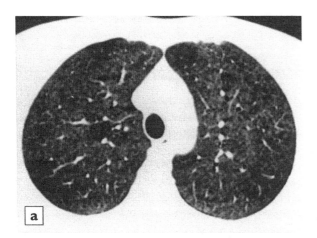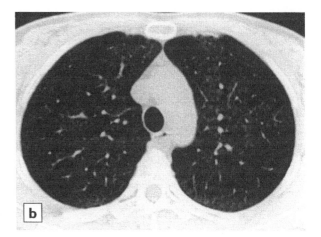

Fig. 31.3 The same HRCT image of a patient with subacute extrinsic allergic alveolitis (hypersensitivity pneumonitis) viewed with (a) narrow and (b) wide window settings. Notice how the ground glass attenuation and nodules are more apparent on the narrow window settings.

diagnostic yield may, however, be improved further by two additional procedures:

- Prone HRCT images are sometimes obtained to differentiate the subtle gravity-induced increase in attenuation seen in the dependent parts of the lung (the posterobasal segments) on supine sections from that due to interstitial lung disease which remains fixed on prone sections (Fig. 31.4).
- End-expiratory images, for which the patient is asked to suspend breathing at end expiration, can accentuate differences in parenchymal attenuation caused by air trapping. This is most valuable in diseases involving the small airways.

Air trapping has been defined as 'decreased attenuation of pulmonary parenchyma, especially manifest as less than normal increase in attenuation during expiration' [13] and is an HRCT feature of any disease with small airways involvement such as extrinsic allergic alveolitis (Fig. 31.5). A potential pitfall in the interpretation of expiratory HRCTs is the air trapping occasionally demonstrated in single pulmonary lobules in normal individuals [14], and in severe disease where there is a homogeneous decrease in attenuation of the lung parenchyma [15]. The sensitivity and interobserver agreement has been shown to be greater for expiratory images than for standard inspiratory images [16], but the actual diagnostic gain from the routine use of expiratory CT remains unknown [17].

There has been increasing interest in the use of image processing techniques to accentuate subtle

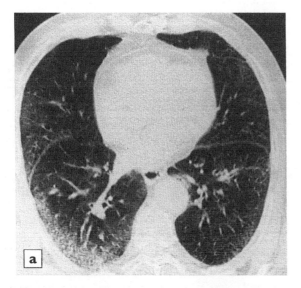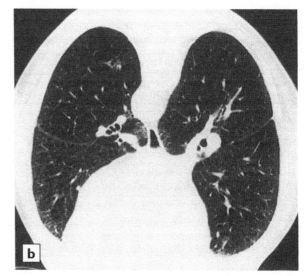

Fig. 31.4 Prone versus supine CT images in an individual with early asbestosis. The supine image (a) shows increased ground glass attenuation predominantly in dependent areas. The majority of these appearances resolve posteriorly on the prone image (b), apart from in the paraspinal regions, which remain fixed consistent with limited asbestosis.

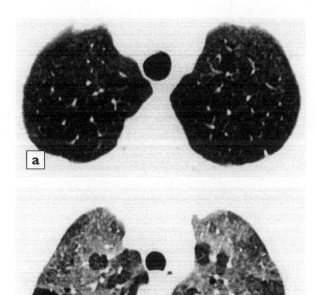

Fig. 31.5 (a) Inspiratory and (b) end-expiratory CT images in a patient with subacute extrinsic allergic alveolitis. The inspiratory image shows a subtle mosaic attenuation pattern of the lung parenchyma. The appearances are accentuated on the end-expiratory image with focal areas of air trapping (decreased attenuation).

regional inhomogeneity of the pulmonary parenchyma and for the detection of subtle micronodular patterns in diffuse interstitial lung disease [18,19]. Whether such sophisticated and time-consuming techniques substantially increase the diagnostic yield of clinically significant disease is yet to be determined.

Spiral (helical) CT

The advent of helical or spiral CT has led to reduced scan times and the entire thorax can be imaged in a single breath-hold. The principle of spiral CT involves continuous rotation of the X-ray beam and detectors around the patient while the table moves into the gantry. The technique also allows accurate timing of an intravenous injection of contrast medium for optimum opacification of the pulmonary arteries, enabling pulmonary emboli to be detected. Both conventional and spiral CT scanners can produce thin sections (HRCT), and the terms 'spiral CT' and 'HRCT' should not be confused.

Quantification of disease severity

In comparison with chest radiography, there have been few studies addressing the quantification of pneumoconioses with CT. Due to the lack of super-imposition of overlying structures, CT is useful for the quantification of different disease processes which sometimes coexist in individuals with occupationally induced lung disease, for example interstitial fibrosis and emphysema. Al Jarad *et al.* have modified the ILO radiographic scoring system for the pneumoconioses for CT in individuals exposed to asbestos, in order to account for the functional consequences of a combination of interstitial fibrosis, emphysema, and diffuse pleural thickening [20]. Better interobserver and intraobserver agreement was seen for interstitial fibrosis, emphysema, and diffuse pleural thickening using the HRCT score system compared with chest radiography, and HRCT was more accurate at detecting subtle disease in all three categories than chest radiography. Furthermore, HRCT morphology correlated well with physiologic indices of lung function.

Another approach for the CT quantification of the extent of parenchymal disease in the pneumoconioses is the objective measurement of lung density [21,22]. In early asbestosis, the CT density of the pulmonary parenchyma may be increased despite a normal chest radiograph [21,22]. Furthermore, Eterovic *et al.* found, in 22 patients with early or advanced asbestosis, that the CT density score correlated well with indices of pulmonary function [22].

In the future, despite the potential for a variable mixture of pathologic processes in patients with pneumoconioses, CT may have a role in quantifying the degree of functional impairment ascribable to individual pathologic processes, for instance smoking-related emphysema versus occupationally induced pulmonary fibrosis.

SCREENING, POPULATION STUDIES, RADIATION DOSE

Despite its relative lack of sensitivity and the substantial problem of interobserver variability, the chest radiograph remains the most widely used radiographic tool in surveillance programs and in screening individuals with suspected pneumoconioses [7,23,24]. The technique is widely available, quick to perform, and relatively cheap. Whilst the role of chest radiography in advanced parenchymal disease or isolated pleural disease is relatively straightforward, its value in detecting subtle parenchymal disease or in assessing the parenchyma accurately with coexisting pleural disease is clearly limited. Moreover, film quality and observer experience may also limit accurate interpretation of the chest radiograph in diffuse interstitial lung disease, although experienced observers are more able to compensate for radiographs of inferior quality [25].

A lack of experience with classification systems and a lack of familiarity with radiographic manifestations of the various pneumoconioses have also been identified by some authors as problem areas [26].

Several techniques, including AMBER and digital radiography, have sought to improve film quality, whilst the relatively recent introduction of image postprocessing and computer-aided models may redress some of the balance in terms of observer experience [6]. Although a large amount of information is obtainable from a single chest radiograph, it is often serial changes in appearances over time that are crucial in the assessment of an individual with suspected occupational lung disease.

The effective dose given by a conventional posteroanterior (PA) chest radiograph is approximately 0.03 millisieverts (mSv), and that for an AMBER PA chest radiograph is approximately 0.05 mSv (background radiation dose is approximately 2 mSv per annum). By comparison, other techniques such as an AP view of the lumbar spine and a barium enema give effective doses of 0.69 and 7.2 mSv respectively [27]. As with all procedures involving ionizing radiation, the benefits have to be weighed against the risks to the individual. It is often difficult to express risk in terms of development of malignancy from relatively small radiation doses, but data from analysis of the UK National Registry of Radiation Workers indicates that there is an excess relative risk of death from malignant neoplasms of 0.47 per sievert [28]. To put this in context, the risk of fatality from a chest radiograph is approximately the same as the risk of a 40-year-old person dying from natural causes in the next 6 hours.

Patient exposure is also an important constraint in CT imaging and the radiation dose from a conventional CT examination using 10-mm contiguous sections is approximately 100 times that of a standard PA chest radiograph [29]. Contiguous 10-mm sections result in a cumulative radiation dose due to X-ray beam scatter and, in comparison, the effective dose from an HRCT scan is less: approximately 12–15% that of a conventional CT [30]. Furthermore, an increase in the spacing of sections from 10 mm to 20 mm results in a decreased mean skin radiation dose of 50% [30]. In practice, it is possible to tailor an HRCT examination in a patient with suspected diffuse lung disease, so that the radiation dose is not much more than that of a few chest radiographs [31].

Zwirewich *et al.* found that by reducing the milliamperage from 200 mA to 20 mA for HRCT scans, there was no significant loss of spatial resolution or anatomic information, particularly for the demonstration of pulmonary vessels, bronchi, and secondary pulmonary lobules; but subtle emphysema

and ground glass attenuation were less well seen [32]. In a clinical setting, the use of low-dose HRCT does not result in significantly reduced observer confidence or diagnostic accuracy, in comparison with conventional dose HRCT or chest radiography for the diagnosis or diffuse infiltrative lung disease [33].

The combination of low-dose CT technique and single breath-hold CT scanning capabilities has led to interest in the use of CT as a screening method for patients with a high risk of developing lung cancer [34–36]. The technique may be particularly relevant in smokers with asbestosis (or heavy exposure to asbestos in the past), given the associated multiplicative increased risk of malignancy. Limited low-dose high-resolution tomography using five or six CT sections has been evaluated for the detection of benign asbestos-related disease, and although very low-dose images can detect pleural disease, subtle parenchymal abnormalities such as ground glass attenuation are better demonstrated on images of at least 80 mA [37].

Cost issues are also relevant. Although variations occur between centers, the cost for an HRCT examination is comparable to a four-view series of chest radiographs [38]. HRCT is less sensitive than histopathologic examination of biopsy material, but biopsy-proven pneumoconiosis (without radiological abnormality) is unlikely to pose any risk of physiologic impairment, relevant symptoms, or disability [39,40]. As yet the argument in favor of CT for screening of individuals for suspected pneumoconiosis is not compelling.

CHEST RADIOGRAPHY AND CT COMPARED

The relative advantages of chest radiography and CT in the assessment of individuals with occupational lung disease can be summarized as follows:

Chest radiography

- simple to perform and readily available
- cost effective
- relatively specific in certain conditions (e.g. advanced asbestosis)
- adequate for the assessment of benign pleural disease in the majority of cases
- less radiation dose than CT

CT scanning

- greater sensitivity for subtle interstitial lung disease than chest radiography
- greater specificity in certain conditions (e.g. extrinsic allergic alveolitis)

- superior intraobserver and interobserver agreement compared with chest radiography
- accurate evaluation of distinct coexisting disease (e.g. emphysema, diffuse pleural thickening, asbestosis)

ULTRASONOGRAPHY

The use of this technique in the chest is limited because high-frequency sound waves do not traverse air and are completely reflected at interfaces between soft tissue and normally aerated pulmonary parenchyma. However, fluid can be easily detected and ultrasonography is useful for the localization of small or loculated pleural effusions. Ultrasonography can also differentiate between pleural fluid and pleural thickening in cases in which radiography cannot make this distinction, and may demonstrate nodular pleural thickening in cases of pleural malignancy. Folded lung (synonymous with rounded atelectasis) has a characteristic ultrasonographic appearance consisting of a pleurally based mass with adjacent pleural thickening and a highly echogenic line extending into the mass [41]. These features may occasionally be helpful in differentiating between this benign entity and a bronchogenic carcinoma.

MAGNETIC RESONANCE IMAGING

The principles of magnetic resonance imaging (MRI) are very different to those of CT. An individual is placed in a strong magnetic field which polarizes some of the hydrogen protons (which behave like randomly oriented bar magnets) in the body so that they are aligned in the same orientation. Radiofrequency wave pulses of specified lengths and repetition (pulse sequences) displace the protons, and some of this transmitted energy is absorbed by them. With the cessation of the radiofrequency pulse, the protons return to their initial alignment and in so doing they emit some of the energy they have absorbed as a weak signal (induced electric current); this signal is received, amplified, and reconstructed into an image.

Compared with CT, MRI has a number of advantages and disadvantages:

Advantages

- ability to obtain sections in any plane (including axial, coronal, and sagittal)
- improved contrast resolution between different soft tissues

- use of special sequences which give functional information (e.g. the velocity of blood flow)
- lack of any risk from ionizing radiation

Disadvantages

- poor demonstration of normally aerated lung
- reduced spatial resolution
- inability to image calcium
- important contraindications, such as permanent cardiac pacemaker devices and ferromagnetic intraocular foreign bodies whose components may respond adversely to the magnetic field
- reduced acceptability to patients because of the claustrophobic narrow bore of the magnet

In many respects the imaging of the mediastinum by CT and MRI are comparable. However, MR images of the lungs are currently markedly inferior to CT images. This is because of the very low water (and therefore proton) content of the lungs; the signal produced by the normal lung is thus small and cannot be visualized adequately by conventional sequences.

At present, the role of MRI in the evaluation of pleural disease is limited, but MRI may be useful in the differentiation of benign from malignant pleural disease [42]. Although morphologic features on CT and MRI are similar, MRI signal intensity may be a useful discriminator, particularly as a reliable predictive sign of benign pleural disease [43]. Another potential advantage of MRI is its ability to characterize pleural fluid more accurately in comparison with CT [42], although this application is rarely used in clinical practice.

RADIONUCLIDE IMAGING

Ventilation/perfusion radionuclide scanning provides physiologic and, to a lesser extent, anatomic information about the lung. It is most frequently used to confirm or exclude the diagnosis of pulmonary embolism.

Regional pulmonary capillary perfusion can be assessed following the intravenous injection of a bolus of particles that have been labeled with ^{99m}Tc. These particles become temporarily lodged in a very small fraction (less than 0.5%) of the precapillary arterioles and capillaries of the lungs, the subsequent distribution of γ-ray emission from them being directly proportional to the regional pulmonary flow. A significant defect in perfusion is detected as a focal, wedge-shaped, photopenic area.

To improve the specificity of the diagnosis of pulmonary embolism, ventilation scintigraphy is usually performed at the same time as perfusion scanning.

The characteristic abnormality of pulmonary embolism, particularly if multiple, is the so-called mismatched defect in which a regional defect in perfusion is not matched by a defect in ventilation. Such mismatching reduces the likelihood of the perfusion defect being a consequence of some other respiratory disease, since most focal disease processes of the lung lead to a reduction of both perfusion and ventilation. Because of the importance of establishing a correct diagnosis of pulmonary embolism, ventilation/perfusion scans should always be interpreted in the light of current chest radiographs and clinical information; even so, a substantial proportion of ventilation/perfusion scans remain indeterminate, hence the increasing use of CT angiography and other tests in the diagnostic algorithm.

POSITRON EMISSION TOMOGRAPHY

Positron emission tomography relies on tissue uptake of radioisotopes which decay by positron emission. Detectors located around the patient map the site of origin of the two resultant photons emitted at 180° from each other. The most widely used isotope for the detection of pulmonary malignancy is ^{18}F-fluorodeoxyglucose (FDG), a D-glucose analog. The increased uptake and retention of glucose by malignant cells allows differentiation of benign from malignant pulmonary masses, detection of lymph node involvement by tumor, and identification of distant metastases. Limitations of the technique include false-positive results caused by granulomatous infection and acute inflammation, and false-negative results with certain tumors (e.g. bronchiolo-alveolar carcinomas and carcinoid tumors). The technique is also not widely available at present.

IMAGING IN SPECIFIC OCCUPATIONAL LUNG DISEASES

The following section discusses imaging in specific occupational lung diseases, starting with asbestos-induced pleural and parenchymal disease. Many of the considerations encountered with asbestos-related diseases also apply to other inorganic dust

diseases, and there is increasing use of imaging in this particular context. Leading from this, there is more radiologic literature on asbestos-related disease than for any other occupational lung diseases.

Asbestos-related pleural disease

The four types of asbestos-induced pleural disease encountered are pleural plaques, diffuse pleural thickening, benign asbestos-related pleural effusion, and malignant mesothelioma.

Pleural plaques

Pleural plaques are the commonest manifestation of asbestos exposure, and bilateral scattered calcified pleural plaques can be regarded as virtually pathognomonic of asbestos exposure [44]. According to radiographic studies, the characteristic sites for pleural plaques are the posterolateral chest wall between the seventh and tenth ribs, the lateral wall between sixth and ninth ribs, the dome of the diaphragm, and the mediastinal pleura particularly over the pericardium [45]. This distribution is largely borne out by CT studies, although on CT plaques seem to be more profuse beneath the anterior aspects of the upper ribs (an area poorly demonstrated by standard radiographic views) (Fig. 31.6). Plaques rarely arise from the visceral pleura but are occasionally found in the lower aspects of the interlobar fissures. CT is more sensitive than chest radiography for the detection of pleural plaques, particularly when non-calcified and located in the paravertebral area [46]. Asbestosis rarely occurs in the absence of pleural plaques [47];

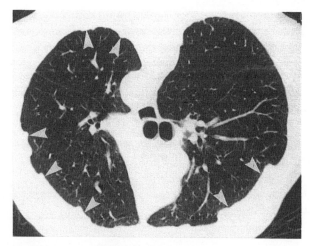

Fig. 31.6 Prone HRCT image at the level of the carina showing multiple, well-circumscribed plaques deep to the anterior ends of the ribs and in the paravertebral regions (arrow heads). These areas are poorly demonstrated on chest radiography. (Courtesy of Dr W Musk, Perth, W Australia.)

although there is a significant correlation between the severity of pleural disease and the presence and severity of asbestosis, most plaques usually occur in isolation [48,49].

Benign asbestos-induced pleural effusion

The development of a benign asbestos-related pleural effusion is probably the earliest manifestation of previous asbestos exposure. It usually occurs within 30 years of exposure onset and is the commonest complication of asbestos exposure for the initial 10 years after exposure. However, a benign asbestos pleural effusion can occur much later [50], at which time the important differential diagnosis is malignant mesothelioma. CT is often indicated to exclude an underlying pulmonary cause, or the presence of an obvious pleural soft tissue mass.

Diffuse pleural thickening

Diffuse pleural thickening is less specific to asbestos exposure than pleural plaques, given that many causes of exudative pleural effusion can give rise to diffuse pleural fibrosis. These include previous inflammatory episodes (such as a parapneumonic effusion), hemothorax, and connective tissue disease.

The revised edition of the ILO classification has partially addressed the issue of distinguishing plaques from diffuse pleural thickening [7]. However, there is still potential for confusion as the distinction is made solely on a single standard chest radiograph [51]. Radiographically, diffuse pleural thickening can be difficult to diagnose, but involvement of the interlobar fissures (by definition visceral pleural involvement) is the rule [52]. As with discrete pleural plaques, CT is more sensitive and specific for the detection of diffuse pleural thickening than chest radiography [48,53,54], in particular for differentiating extrapleural fat from pleural thickening (Fig. 31.7). Al Jarad *et al.* found that there was greater interobserver agreement regarding the type of pleural disease on CT compared with chest radiography [53]. On CT diffuse thickening appears continuous, commonly involving the posterior and lateral surfaces of the lower thorax [49,55]. Frequently there is a concomitant increase in extrapleural fat, presumably drawn inwards by pleural retraction [55]. Many studies have shown that diffuse pleural thickening, even in the absence of parenchymal fibrosis, results in a restrictive ventilatory defect [53,56–58]. CT may be particularly helpful in distinguishing malignant from benign pleural disease: the presence of pleural rind, pleural nodularity, pleural thickening greater than 1 cm, and mediastinal pleural involvement all being more frequent in malignant disease [59].

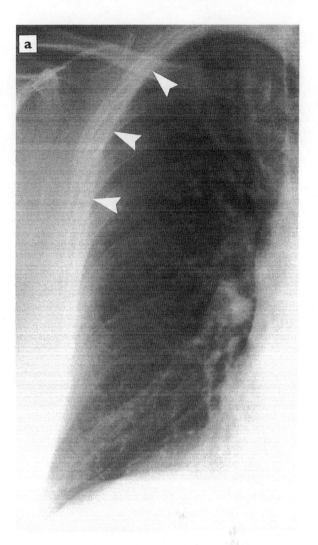

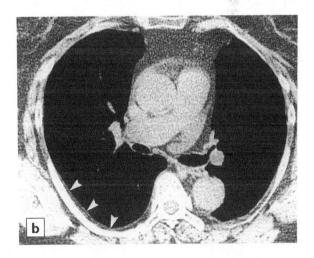

Fig. 31.7 Coned radiographic view of the right hemithorax of a patient with abundant extrapleural fat (arrowheads), which could be confused with diffuse pleural thickening (a). Note how the extrapleural fat extends over the apex but spares the costophrenic angle. The HRCT (b) is imaged on mediastinal windows showing extrapleural fat internal to the ribs on the right (arrowheads). The fat is of the same CT density as subcutaneous and mediastinal fat.

Folded lung refers to peripheral atelectatic lung adjacent to an area of pleural thickening with characteristic drawing in of the bronchi and vessels into the atelectatic segment [60]. Synonyms for folded lung include rounded atelectasis, pulmonary pseudotumor, and Blesovsky's syndrome. There is a strong association with previous asbestos exposure [61], but any cause of an organizing pleural exudate such as tuberculosis, histoplasmosis, Dressler's syndrome following cardiac surgery, and hemothorax may be responsible [41,62]. Conventional CT is most helpful in making the diagnosis and McHugh et al. described three major features:

1 rounded or oval mass (2.5–7 cm) abutting a peripheral pleural surface
2 the curving 'comet tail' of bronchovascular structures passing into the mass, resulting in a blurred central margin
3 thickening of the adjacent pleura with or without calcification, which is usually, but not always, thickest adjacent to the mass [60] (Fig. 31.8)

Lynch et al. included the further feature of evidence of volume loss in the adjacent lung [61].

Asbestosis

Chest radiography

Traditionally, the radiographic features of diffuse interstitial fibrosis have been regarded as a *sine qua non* for the diagnosis of asbestosis [63]. However, as with other causes of diffuse interstitial lung disease, the chest radiograph may be normal in individuals

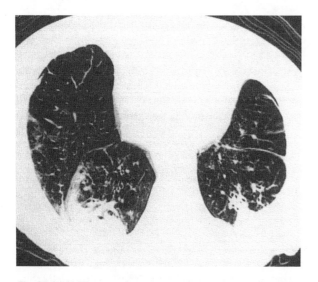

Fig. 31.8 HRCT image of a patient with bilateral areas of rounded atelectasis. The typical 'comet's tail' appearance is demonstrated on the right. Bilateral lower lobe volume loss is also seen. Mediastinal windows demonstrated extensive bilateral diffuse pleural thickening.

with mild disease [64,65]. Another disadvantage of the chest radiograph (including the ILO system) is the significant interobserver and intraobserver variability encountered for both parenchymal and pleural disease [66,67]. Technical factors such as X-ray exposure may also affect ILO interpretation: if a radiograph is overexposed, small discrete opacities tend to be classified in a lower category, whereas with underexposed films the reverse is true [25,68]. Despite these drawbacks, the classical radiographic findings of a combination of a bilateral reticulonodular pattern with coexisting calcified pleural plaques in an individual with an appropriate history of asbestos exposure is relatively specific for the condition [69]. In mild asbestosis, however, chest radiography may be insensitive, hence the increasing interest in techniques such as HRCT.

High-resolution computed tomography

HRCT is in many ways well suited to the task of early detection of asbestosis. In comparison with chest radiography, HRCT is more sensitive for the detection of parenchymal fibrosis, and therefore may show definite, but subtle, abnormalities despite a normal or equivocal chest radiograph [47,70]. HRCT, with supplementary prone images, is also more sensitive than conventional CT for the detection of parenchymal fibrosis despite limited 'sampling' of the lung parenchyma [48,71,72]. A small proportion of patients with normal or mildly abnormal HRCT images has been found to have histopathologic evidence of asbestosis, but in the same group of patients, not surprisingly, HRCT was still more sensitive than chest radiography [39].

The specificity of individual CT features for asbestosis is more controversial. Initially Yoshimura et al. proposed that the subpleural curvilinear line, representing fibrosing bronchioloalveolitis, was characteristic of asbestosis [73]. This feature was later described in a variety of patients without asbestos exposure and is no longer considered pathognomonic for asbestosis [74]. Furthermore, in a study evaluating the HRCT scans of patients investigated for a variety of indications, a significant proportion had individual features described in asbestosis, such as parenchymal bands, subpleural increased density, thickened interlobular septal lines, and honeycomb lung [74]. Most studies evaluating the specificity of HRCT for asbestosis are limited by the difficulty of obtaining pathologic specimens from the investigated individuals. No single CT feature is specific for asbestosis, but a constellation of features that are bilateral and multifocal with a coexisting appropriate occupational history is often diagnostic [39]. HRCT may also be useful in evaluating the lung parenchyma in the context of extensive pleural

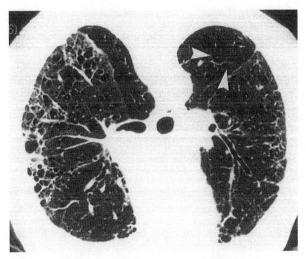

Fig. 31.9 Prone HRCT image of a patient with asbestosis and admixed centrilobular emphysema. The areas of emphysema are of decreased attenuation with vascular distortion. The arrowheads indicate an area of emphysema in the right lower lobe within relatively normal lung. (Courtesy of Dr W Musk, Perth, W Australia.)

disease. Further advantages are the potential to demonstrate coexisting non-pneumoconiotic lung disease, for example emphysema (Fig. 31.9).

Coal workers' pneumoconiosis and silicosis

The radiographic appearances of coal workers' pneumoconiosis and silicosis are similar: both conditions are characterized by a predominance of upper zone nodules which have the propensity to coalesce to form conglomerate masses, progressive massive fibrosis (Fig. 31.10). On HRCT the nodules may be centrilobular (adjacent to the structures in the center of the secondary pulmonary lobule) or subpleural and of varying size (Fig. 31.11) [75]. A small percentage of nodules calcify, increasing their conspicuity on HRCT. Gevenois *et al.* found that HRCT is more specific than chest radiography in early coal workers' pneumoconiosis as chest radiographic abnormalities may be shown to be due to emphysema or bronchiectasis by CT [76]. Rarely, a basal reticular or honeycomb pattern similar to that seen in cryptogenic fibrosing alveolitis is present [75].

CT studies have shown that emphysema develops in a significant proportion of never-smokers exposed to silica [77,78]. Furthermore, a study by Bergin *et al.* showed that, functionally, the most relevant finding is the extent of emphysema rather than the profusion of nodules in silicosis, even in never-smokers [79]. By contrast, Hnizdo *et al.*, in a study of never-smokers, found that impairment of pulmonary function was not related to emphysema, but to the extent of silicosis at autopsy, although the

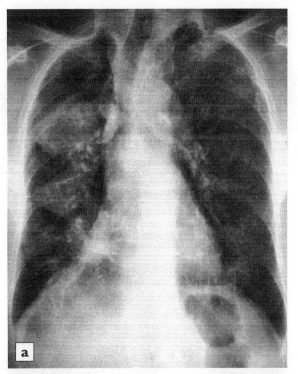

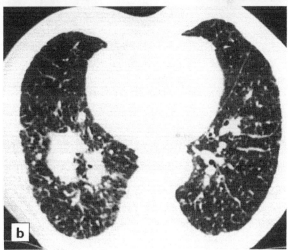

Fig. 31.10 (a) PA chest radiograph and (b) HRCT of a patient with coal workers' pneumoconiosis and progressive massive fibrosis. Typically the areas of confluent fibrosis are bilateral and symmetrical, but in this patient are predominantly right sided. The HRCT image shows confluent fibrosis in the right lower lobe and diffuse nodularity.

actual number of subjects with pathologically significant silicosis was small [80].

The main advantages of CT in individuals with suspected coal workers' pneumoconiosis and silicosis are therefore increased specificity in comparison with the chest radiograph and more accurate demonstration of complications or coincidental features (e.g. emphysema), which may be functionally significant.

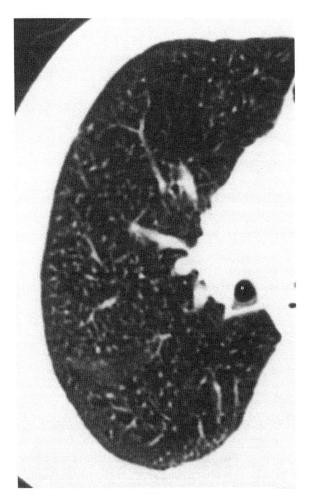

Fig. 31.11 HRCT image of the right lung in a patient with silicosis showing diffuse nodularity. Similar features are seen in simple coal workers' pneumoconiosis.

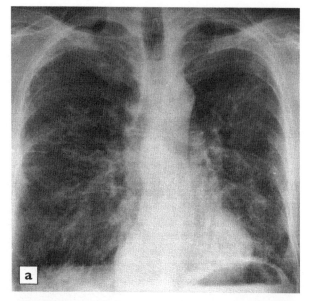

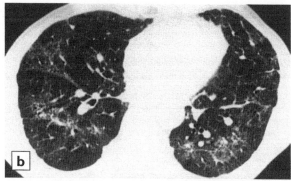

Fig. 31.12 (a) PA chest radiograph and (b) HRCT of a patient with chronic allergic alveolitis. The radiographic features are most apparent in the mid and lower zones bilaterally. The HRCT shows parenchymal distortion with traction bronchiectasis within areas of ground glass attenuation indicating an established interstitial fibrosis.

Extrinsic allergic alveolitis

Extrinsic allergic alveolitis (hypersensitivity pneumonitis) is an allergic granulomatous disorder caused by the inhalation of organic dust. It may occur as a result of an individual's occupation. Ground glass opacification or fine nodularity may be seen on the chest radiograph, but a substantial number of individuals with clinically significant disease have a normal radiograph [81]. CT and radiographic studies have shown that chronic extrinsic allergic alveolitis may result in fibrosis with a reticular pattern and honeycombing, which commonly has a widespread distribution or mid zone predominance (Fig. 31.12) [82]. These findings are contrary to earlier studies which reported an upper zone predominance based on chest radiographic findings alone [83,84].

Patients are rarely imaged during the acute phase of the disease, which is characterized by airspace consolidation [85]. More commonly, the HRCT features of the subacute phase are observed and

these consist typically of ill-defined centrilobular nodules on a background of widespread ground glass attenuation (Fig. 31.13) [85,86]. A mosaic attenuation pattern may also be observed with air trapping on end-expiratory images, reflecting the accompanying bronchiolitis [86]. This combination of HRCT features is relatively specific for the subacute phase of extrinsic allergic alveolitis [86], but in smokers the other possible differential diagnosis to consider is respiratory bronchiolitis–interstitial lung disease (RB-ILD), a relatively recently recognized form of interstitial lung disease thought to be a form of desquamative interstitial pneumonitis (DIP) associated with heavy cigarette smoking.

The HRCT features of chronic extrinsic allergic alveolitis consist of a reticular pattern with architectural distortion and honeycombing representative of established fibrosis (see Fig. 31.12) [82]. A lower zone and subpleural distribution of features may be

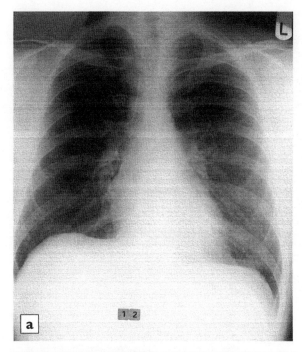

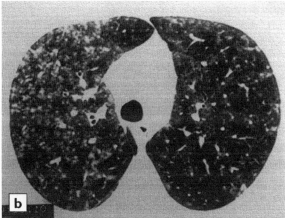

Fig. 31.13 (a) Chest radiograph and (b) HRCT image of a patient with subacute hypersensitivity pneumonitis due to hard metal exposure. The chest radiograph shows subtle nodularity and ground glass attenuation, most apparent in the mid and lower zones. The HRCT shows more extensive abnormality than the chest radiograph, consisting of ill-defined centrilobular nodules on a background of ground glass attenuation. There are also areas of decreased attenuation consistent with air trapping. These features are typical of subacute extrinsic allergic alveolitis. (Courtesy of Dr R J Butland.)

seen, making discrimination from cryptogenic fibrosing alveolitis difficult in some instances [87].

Obstructive lung disease

The radiographic features of chronic fixed obstructive lung disease (such as emphysema and small airways disease) are overinflation, decreased attenuation of the lung parenchyma, and pulmonary oligemia. Overinflation of the lungs results in flat-

tening of the normal diaphragmatic convexity, and an increase in the size of the retrosternal space on the lateral view. A specific, but relatively insensitive, sign for the presence of airflow obstruction on a PA radiograph is the level of the dome of the right hemidiaphragm at or below the anterior aspect of the seventh rib [88]. Depression and flattening of the diaphragm, particularly on the lateral view, is reportedly the most reliable sign of overinflation [89].

Whilst chest radiography is quite specific in moderate to severe emphysema, in mild disease its use is limited because of insensitivity [89,90]. Furthermore, the chest radiograph is even less reliable when coexisting chronic interstitial disease is present [90]. HRCT is more sensitive for the detection of mild disease than both chest radiography and pulmonary function testing [91,92]. There is good correlation between HRCT scores and histopathologic scores, but CT may not detect emphysema when the destructive foci are less than 0.5 mm in diameter, using histopathologic findings as the reference standard [93]. HRCT therefore allows earlier detection of emphysema than chest radiography and is particularly useful in demonstrating emphysema in individuals with coexisting interstitial lung disease.

Chest radiography is poor at demonstrating even advanced constrictive obliterative bronchiolitis (small airways disease); the indirect signs of areas of pulmonary vascular attenuation and increased transradiancy are non-specific and overlap with other causes of chronic airway obstruction [94]. The key HRCT findings described in constrictive obliterative bronchiolitis are: areas of parenchymal decreased attenuation giving rise to the so-called 'mosaic attenuation pattern', pulmonary vascular attenuation, bronchial wall thickening and dilatation and air trapping on expiratory CT (Fig. 31.14) [95,96]. The extent of decreased attenuation correlates most strongly with physiologic tests of small airway function and is therefore regarded as the cardinal HRCT sign of small airways disease [96]. The mosaic pattern of differing attenuation is due to shunting of blood away from underventilated to normally ventilated lung, resulting in increased attenuation in these relatively overperfused areas.

A recent study has confirmed that in acute airway obstruction hypoxic pulmonary vasoconstriction, rather than raised intraalveolar pressure, is responsible for the reduced perfusion [97]. Eventually vascular remodeling occurs and vasoconstriction becomes irreversible. The attenuated pulmonary vessels are not distorted, in contrast to the vascular distortion and disruption that characterizes emphysema.

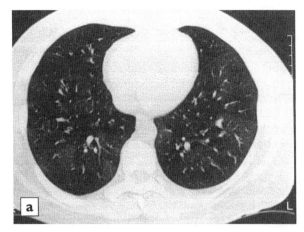
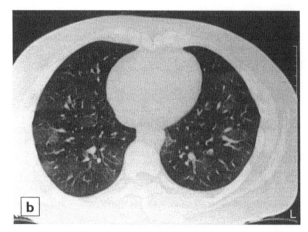

Fig. 31.14 (a) Inspiratory and (b) end-expiratory images of a patient with constrictive obliterative bronchiolitis. The inspiratory image shows a mosaic attenuation pattern (areas of black lung amongst lung parenchyma of increased attenuation). The large airways are also mildly thick-walled and dilated. End-expiratory images show air trapping (see text).

The sensitivity and specificity of the HRCT signs of constrictive obliterative bronchiolitis are difficult to determine accurately due to the absence of a diagnostic reference standard. The diagnosis is often made clinically; biopsy is rarely performed and may be insensitive because of the patchy nature of disease. However, the demonstration of air trapping by HRCT may permit detection of small airways obstruction in patients with clinically suspected disease, even when lung function tests are normal [98].

Miscellaneous

Berylliosis

Berylliosis typically results in small rounded opacities on the chest radiograph which may become irregular

as the disease progresses (Fig. 31.15a). The HRCT features are septal lines, bronchovascular nodules, and ground glass attenuation with a substantial proportion also demonstrating hilar and mediastinal lymphadenopathy which may be calcified (Fig. 31.15b) [99]. These features are indistinguishable from pulmonary sarcoidosis (Fig. 31.16) [99].

Hard metal disease

HRCT examinations of hard metal workers show areas of consolidation with traction bronchiectasis or well-demarcated ground glass attenuation with areas of air trapping (Fig. 31.17) [100]. Histopathologically these appearances correspond with an interstitial pneumonitis with fibrosis and a giant cell infiltrate [100].

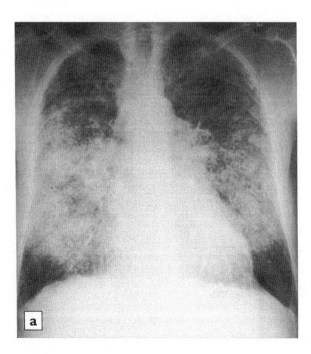

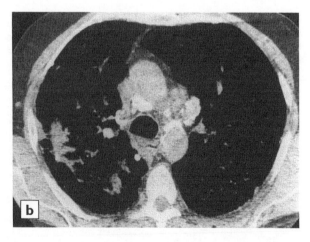

Fig. 31.15 (a) Chest radiograph and (b) HRCT of a patient with berylliosis. There is bilateral hilar lymphadenopathy which is partially obscured by predominantly mid zone nodularity, some of which has become confluent. The HRCT image on mediastinal window settings shows calcified mediastinal lymphadenopathy.

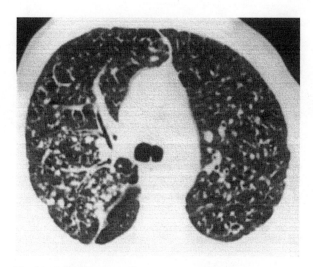

Fig. 31.16 HRCT of a patient with berylliosis. There is predominantly subpleural, fissural, and bronchovascular nodularity. Mediastinal and hilar lymphadenopathy were seen on mediastinal window settings. These HRCT features are identical to those of pulmonary sarcoidosis.

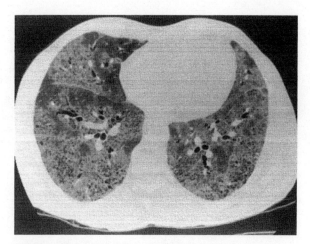

Fig. 31.17 HRCT image of a patient with hard metal-induced interstitial fibrosis. There is honeycombing and generalized increased attenuation, with dilated bronchi (traction bronchiectasis) indicating interstitial fibrosis. Histopathologically a granulomatous interstitial pneumonitis (GIP) was present.

REFERENCES

1. Plewes DB, Wandtke JC. A scanning equalization system for improved chest radiography. *Radiology* 1982; 142: 765–768.
2. Vlasbloem H, Schultze Kool LJ. AMBER: a scanning multiple-beam equalization system for chest radiography. *Radiology* 1988; 169: 29–34.
3. Hansell DM, Coleman R, du Bois RM *et al.* Advanced multiple beam equalization radiography (AMBER) in the detection of diffuse lung disease. *Clin Radiol* 1991; 44: 227–231.
4. Sonoda M, Takano M, Miyahara J, Kato H. Computed radiography utilizing scanning laser stimulated luminescence. *Radiology* 1983; 148: 833–838.
5. Chotas HG, Dobbins JT, Ravin CE. Principles of digital radiography with large-area, electronically readable detectors: a review of the basics. *Radiology* 1999; 210: 595–599.
6. Monnier-Cholley L, MacMahon H, Katsuragawa S *et al.* Computer-aided diagnosis for detection of interstitial opacities on chest radiographs. *Am J Roentgenol* 1998; 171: 1651–1656.
7. International Labour Office. *Guidelines for the use of the ILO International Classification of the Radiographs of Pneumoconioses,* revised edn 1980. International Labour Office Occupational Health and Safety Series, no 22 (rev 80) Geneva: ILO, 1980.
8. Curry TS, Dowdney JE, Murry RC. *Computed tomography. Christensen's Introduction to the Physics of Diagnostic Radiology,* 3rd edn, pp. 320–350. Philadelphia, PA: Lea & Febiger, 1984.
9. Mathieson J, Mayo JR, Staples CA, Müller NL. Chronic diffuse infiltrative lung disease: comparison of diagnostic accuracy of CT and chest radiography. *Radiology* 1989; 171: 111–116.
10. Grenier P, Valeyre D, Cluzel P *et al.* Chronic diffuse interstitial lung disease: diagnostic value of chest radiography and high-resolution CT. *Radiology* 1991; 179: 123–132.

11. Padley SP, Hansell DM, Flower CDR, Jennings P. Comparative accuracy of high resolution computed tomography and chest radiography in the diagnosis of chronic diffuse infiltrative lung disease. *Clin Radiol* 1991; 44: 222–226.
12. Webb WR, Müller NL, Naidich DP. *Technical aspects of HRCT. High-resolution CT of the Lung,* 2nd edn, pp. 1–21. Philadelphia: Lippincott-Raven, 1996.
13. Austin JHM, Müller NL, Friedman PJ *et al.* Glossary of terms for CT of the lungs: recommendations of the Nomenclature Committee of the Fleischner Society. *Radiology* 1996; 200: 327–331.
14. Webb WR, Stern EJ, Kanth N, Gamsu G. Dynamic pulmonary CT: findings in healthy adult men. *Radiology* 1993; 186: 117–124.
15. Yang CF, Wu MT, Chiang AA *et al.* Correlation of high-resolution CT and pulmonary function in bronchiolitis obliterans: a study based on 24 patients associated with consumption of *Sauropus androgynus. Am J Roentgenol* 1997; 168: 1045–1050.
16. Hansell DM, Wells AU, Rubens MB, Cole PJ. Bronchiectasis: functional significance of areas of decreased attenuation at expiratory CT. *Radiology* 1994; 193: 369–374.
17. Arakawa H, Webb WR, McCowin M *et al.* Inhomogeneous lung attenuation at thin-section CT: diagnostic value of expiratory scans. *Radiology* 1998; 206: 89–94.
18. Remy-Jardin M, Remy J, Artaud D *et al.* Diffuse infiltrative lung disease: clinical value of sliding-thin slab maximum intensity projection CT scans in the detection of mild micronodular patterns. *Radiology* 1996; 200: 333–339.
19. Bhalla M, Naidich DP, McGuinness G *et al.* Diffuse lung disease: assessment with helical CT – preliminary observations of the role of maximum and minimum intensity projection images. *Radiology* 1996; 200: 341–347.
20. Al Jarad N, Wilkinson P, Pearson MC, Rudd RM. A new high resolution computed tomography scoring system for pulmonary fibrosis, pleural disease, and

emphysema in patients with asbestos related disease. *Br J Ind Med* 1992; 49: 73–84.

21. Wollmer P, Jakobsson K, Albin M *et al.* Measurement of lung density by X-ray computed tomography: relation to lung mechanics in workers exposed to asbestos cement. *Chest* 1987; 91: 865–869.

22. Eterovic D, Dujic Z, Tocilj J, Capkun V. High resolution pulmonary computed tomography scans quantified by analysis of density distribution: application to asbestosis. *Br J Ind Med* 1993; 50: 514–519.

23. Fletcher CM, Oldham PD. Problems of consistent radiological diagnosis in coalminers' pneumoconiosis: experimental study. *Br J Ind Med* 1949; 6: 168–183.

24. Garland LH, Cochran AL. Results of an international test in chest roentgenogram interpretation. *JAMA* 1952; 149: 631–634.

25. Reger RB, Smith CA, Kibelstis JA. The effect of film quality and other factors on the roentgenographic categorization of coal worker's pneumoconiosis. *Am J Roentgenol* 1972; 115: 462–472.

26. Felson B, Morgan WKC, Bristol LJ *et al.* Observations on the results of multiple readings of chest films in coal miner's pneumoconiosis. *Radiology* 1973; 109: 19–23.

27. Hart D, Hillier MC, Wall BF *et al. Doses to patients from medical x-ray examinations in the UK–1995 review*, NRPB-289. National Radiological Protection Board. Chilton, England, 1995.

28. Kendall GM, Muirhead CR, MacGibbon BH *et al.* Mortality and occupational exposure to radiation: first analysis of the National Registry for Radiation Workers. *BMJ* 1992; 304: 220–225.

29. DiMarco AF, Briones B. Is chest CT performed too often? *Chest* 1993; 103: 985–986.

30. Mayo JR, Jackson SA, Müller NL. High-resolution CT of the chest: radiation dose.` *Am J Roentgenol* 1993; 160: 479–481.

31. van der Bruggen-Bogaarts BAHA, Broerse JJ, Lammers J-WJ *et al.* Radiation exposure in standard and high-resolution chest CT scans. *Chest* 1995; 107: 113–115.

32. Zwirewich CV, Mayo JR, Müller NL. Low-dose high-resolution CT of lung parenchyma. *Radiology* 1991; 180: 413–417.

33. Lee KS, Primack SL, Staples CA *et al.* Chronic infiltrative lung disease: comparison of diagnostic accuracies of radiography and low and conventional-dose thin-section CT. *Radiology* 1994; 191: 669–673.

34. Naidich DP, Marshall CH, Gribbin C *et al.* Low-dose CT of the lungs: preliminary observations. *Radiology* 1990; 175: 729–731.

35. Kaneko M, Eguchi K, Ohmatsu H *et al.* Peripheral lung cancer: screening and detection with low-dose spiral CT versus radiography. *Radiology* 1996; 201: 798–802.

36. Itoh S, Ikeda M, Isomura T *et al.* Screening helical CT for mass screening of lung cancer: application of low-dose and single-breath-hold scanning. *Radiat Med* 1998; 16: 75–83.

37. Majurin ML, Varpula M, Kurki T, Pakkala L. High-resolution CT of the lung in asbestos-exposed subjects. Comparison of low-dose and high-dose HRCT. *Acta Radiol* 1994; 35: 473–477.

38. Gamsu G. High-resolution CT in the diagnosis of asbestos-related pleuroparenchymal disease. *Am J Ind Med* 1989; 16: 115–117.

39. Gamsu G, Salmon CJ, Warnock ML, Blanc PD. CT quantification of interstitial fibrosis in patients with asbestosis: a comparison of two methods. *Am J Roentgenol* 1995; 164: 63–68.

40. Lynch DA, Rose CS, Way D, King TEJ. Hypersensitivity pneumonitis: sensitivity of high-resolution CT in a population-based study. *Am J Roentgenol* 1992; 159: 469–472.

41. Marchbank ND, Wilson AG, Joseph AE. Ultrasound features of folded lung. *Clin Radiol* 1996; 51: 433–437.

42. McLoud TC. CT and MR in pleural disease. *Clin Chest Med* 1998; 19: 261–276.

43. Falaschi F, Battolla L, Mascalchi M *et al.* Usefulness of MR signal intensity in distinguishing benign from malignant pleural disease. *Am J Roentgenol* 1996; 166: 963–968.

44. Hillerdal G, Lindgren A. Pleural plaques: correlation of autopsy findings to radiographic findings and occupational history. *Eur J Respir Dis* 1980; 61: 315–319.

45. Fletcher DE, Edge JR. The early radiological changes in pulmonary and pleural asbestosis. *Clin Radiol* 1970; 21: 355–365.

46. Aberle DR, Gamsu G, Ray CS. High-resolution CT of benign asbestos-related diseases: clinical and radiographic correlation. *Am J Roentgenol* 1988; 151: 883–891.

47. Gamsu G, Aberle DR, Lynch D. Computed tomography in the diagnosis of asbestos-related thoracic disease. *J Thorac Imaging* 1989; 4: 61–67.

48. Aberle DR, Gamsu G, Ray CS, Feuerstein IM. Asbestos-related pleural and parenchymal fibrosis: detection with high-resolution CT. *Radiology* 1988; 166: 729–734.

49. Solomon A. Radiological features of asbestos-related visceral pleural changes. *Am J Ind Med* 1991; 19: 339–355.

50. Fridriksson HV, Hedenstrom H, Hillerdal G, Malmberg P. Increased lung stiffness of persons with pleural plaques. *Eur J Respir Dis* 1981; 62: 412–424.

51. McCloud TC, Woods BO, Carrington CB *et al.* Diffuse pleural thickening in an asbestos-exposed population. *Am J Roentgenol* 1985; 144: 9–18.

52. Rockoff SD, Kagan E, Schwartz A *et al.* Visceral pleural thickening in asbestos exposure: the occurrence and implications of thickened interlobar fissures. *J Thorac Imaging* 1987; 2: 58–66.

53. Al Jarad N, Poulakis N, Pearson MC *et al.* Assessment of asbestos-induced pleural disease by computed tomography – correlation with chest radiograph and lung function. *Respir Med* 1991; 85: 203–208.

54. Friedman AC, Fiel SB, Fisher MS *et al.* Asbestos-related pleural disease and asbestosis: a comparison of CT and chest radiography. *Am J Roentgenol* 1988; 150: 269–275.

55. Aberle DR, Balmes JR. Computed tomography of asbestos-related pulmonary parenchymal and pleural diseases. *Clin Chest Med* 1991; 12: 115–131.

56. Cotes JE, King B. Relationship of lung function to radiographic reading (ILO) in patients with asbestos related lung disease. *Thorax* 1988; 43: 777–783.

57. Yates DH, Browne K, Stidolph PN, Neville E. Asbestos-related bilateral diffuse pleural thickening: natural history of radiographic and lung function abnormalities. *Am J Respir Crit Care Med* 1996; 153: 301–306.

58. Becklake MR. Asbestos and other fiber-related diseases of the lungs and pleura. Distribution and determinants in exposed populations. *Chest* 1991; 100: 248–254.

59. Leung AN, Müller NL, Miller RR. CT in differential diagnosis of diffuse pleural disease. *Am J Roentgenol* 1990; 154: 487–492.

60. McHugh K, Blaquiere RM. CT features of rounded atelectasis. *AJR Am J Roentgenol* 1989; 257–260.

61. Lynch DA, Gamsu G, Ray CS, Aberle DR. Asbestos-related focal lung masses: manifestations on conventional and high-resolution CT scans. *Radiology* 1988; 169: 603–607.

62. Hillerdal G. Rounded atelectasis. Clinical experience with 74 patients. *Chest* 1989; 95: 836–841.

63. Weill H. Diagnosis of asbestos-related disease. *Chest* 1987; 91: 802–803.

64. Epler GR, McLoud TC, Gaensler EA *et al*. Normal chest roentgenograms in chronic diffuse infiltrative lung disease. *N Engl J Med* 1978; 298: 934–939.

65. Kipen HM, Lilis R, Suzuki Y *et al*. Pulmonary fibrosis in asbestos insulation workers with lung cancer: a radiological and histopathological evaluation. *Br J Ind Med* 1987; 44: 96–100.

66. Bourbeau J, Ernst P. Between- and within-reader variability in the assessment of pleural abnormality using the ILO 1980 international classification of pneumoconioses. *Am J Ind Med* 1988; 14: 537–543.

67. Reger RB, Morgan WKC. On the factors influencing the consistency in the radiological diagnosis of pneumoconiosis. *Am Rev Respir Dis* 1970; 102: 905–915.

68. Wise ME, Oldham PO. Effect of radiographic technique on readings of categories of simple pneumoconioses. *Br J Ind Med* 1963; 10: 145–153.

69. American Thoracic Society. Medical Section of the American Lung Association: the diagnosis of nonmalignant diseases related to asbestos. *Am Rev Respir Dis* 1986; 134: 363–368.

70. Staples CA, Gamsu G, Ray CS, Webb WR. High resolution computed tomography and lung function in asbestos-exposed workers with normal chest radiographs. *Am Rev Respir Dis* 1989; 139: 1502–1508.

71. Bégin R, Ostiguy G, Filion R *et al*. Computed tomography in the early detection of asbestosis. *Br J Ind Med* 1993; 50: 689–698.

72. Gevenois PA, De Vuyst P, Dedeire S *et al*. Conventional and high-resolution CT in asymptomatic asbestos-exposed workers. *Acta Radiol* 1994; 35: 226–229.

73. Yoshimura H, Hatakeyama M, Otsuji H *et al*. Pulmonary asbestosis: CT study of subpleural curvilinear shadow. *Radiology* 1986; 158: 653–658.

74. Bergin C, Castellino RA, Blank N, Moses L. Specificity of high-resolution CT findings in pulmonary asbestosis. *Am J Roentgenol* 1994; 163: 551–555.

75. Remy-Jardin M, Degreef JM, Beuscart R *et al*. Coal workers' pneumoconiosis: CT assessment in exposed workers and correlation with radiographic findings. *Radiology* 1990; 177: 363–371.

76. Gevenois PA, Pichot E, Dargent F *et al*. Low grade coal workers' pneumoconiosis. Comparison of CT and chest radiography. *Acta Radiol* 1994; 35: 351–356.

77. Cowie RL, Hay M, Thomas RG. Association of silicosis, lung dysfunction, and emphysema in gold miners. *Thorax* 1993; 48: 746–749.

78. Bégin R, Filion R, Ostiguy G. Emphysema in silica- and asbestos-exposed workers seeking compensation. A CT scan study. *Chest* 1995; 108: 647–655.

79. Bergin CJ, Müller NL, Vedal S, Chan-Yeung M. CT in silicosis: correlation with plain films and pulmonary function tests. *Am J Roentgenol* 1986; 477–483.

80. Hnizdo E, Sluis-Cremer GK, Baskind E, Murray J. Emphysema and airway obstruction in non-smoking South African gold miners with long exposure to silica dust. *Occup Environ Med* 1994; 51: 557–563.

81. Hodgson MJ, Parkinson DK, Karpf M. Chest X-rays in hypersensitivity pneumonitis: a metaanalysis of secular trend. *Am J Ind Med* 1989; 16: 45–53.

82. Alder BD, Padley SP, Müller NL *et al*. Chronic hypersensitivity pneumonitis: high-resolution CT and radiographic features in 16 patients. *Radiology* 1992; 185: 91–95.

83. Hargreave F, Hinson KF, Reid L *et al*. The radiological appearances of allergic alveolitis due to bird sensitivity (bird fancier's lung). *Clin Radiol* 1972; 23: 1–10.

84. Cook PG, Wells IP, McGavin CR. The distribution of pulmonary shadowing in farmer's lung. *Clin Radiol* 1988; 39: 21–27.

85. Silver SF, Müller NL, Miller RR, Lefcoe MS. Hypersensitivity pneumonitis: evaluation with CT. *Radiology* 1989; 173: 441–445.

86. Hansell DM, Moskovic E. High-resolution computed tomography in extrinsic allergic alveolitis. *Clin Radiol* 1991; 43: 8–12.

87. Lynch DA, Newell JD, Logan PM *et al*. Can CT distinguish hypersensitivity pneumonitis from idiopathic pulmonary fibrosis? *AJR Am J Roentgenol* 1995; 165: 807–811.

88. Burki NK, Krumpelman JL. Correlation of pulmonary function with the chest roentgenogram in chronic airway obstruction. *Am Rev Respir Dis* 1980; 121: 217–223.

89. Nicklaus TM, Stowell DW, Christiansen WR, Renzetti ADJ. The accuracy of the roentgenologic diagnosis of chronic pulmonary emphysema. *Am Rev Respir Dis* 1966; 93: 889–899.

90. Thurlbeck WM, Simon G. Radiographic appearance of the chest in emphysema. *Am J Roentgenol* 1978; 130: 429–440.

91. Klein JS, Gamsu G, Webb WR *et al*. High-resolution CT diagnosis of emphysema in symptomatic patients with normal chest radiographs and isolated low diffusing capacity. *Radiology* 1992; 182: 817–821.

92. Gurney JW, Jones KK, Robbins RA *et al*. Regional distribution of emphysema: correlation of high-resolution CT with pulmonary function tests in unselected smokers. *Radiology* 1992; 183: 457–463.

93. Miller RR, Müller NL, Vedal S *et al*. Limitations of computed tomography in the assessment of emphysema. *Am Rev Respir Dis* 1989; 139: 980–983.

94. Geddes DM, Corrin B, Brewerton DA *et al*. Progressive airway obliteration in adults and its association with rheumatoid disease. *O J Med* 1977; 184: 427–444.

95. Müller NL, Miller RR. Diseases of the bronchioles: CT and histopathologic findings. *Radiology* 1995; 196: 3–12.

96. Hansell DM, Rubens MB, Padley SP, Wells AU. Obliterative bronchiolitis: individual CT signs of small airways disease and functional correlation. *Radiology* 1997; 203: 721–726.

97. Gückel C, Wells AU, Taylor D, *et al*. Mechanism of mosaic attenuation of the lungs on computed tomography. *J Appl Physiol* 1999; 86: 701–708.

98. Lucidarme O, Coche E, Cluzel P *et al*. Expiratory CT scans for chronic airway disease: correlation with pulmonary function test results. *Am J Roentgenol* 1998; 170: 301–307.

99. Newman LS, Buschman DL, Newell JD, Lynch DA. Beryllium disease: assessment with CT. *Radiology* 1994; 190: 835–840.

100. Akira M. Uncommon pneumoconioses: CT and pathologic findings. *Radiology* 1995; 197: 403–409.

32 LUNG FUNCTION MEASUREMENT

Jeremy Beach

INTRODUCTION

Lung function measurements provide an important tool in the diagnosis and management of occupational lung diseases. They provide objective evidence of the presence and type of respiratory disease, and its rate of progression, and they give insight to the probable degree of associated disability. As a consequence, some lung function measurements are used frequently in occupational health practice as a part of routine health assessment. Such assessments include apparently healthy individuals, as well as patients with suspected or confirmed respiratory disease.

Although measurements of lung function can give a great deal of useful information, it is necessary to ensure they are carried out rigorously and interpreted properly so as to maximize the information obtained. It is also important that they are carried out to a demonstrably verifiable standard. Improperly performed measurements, or measurements performed at the wrong time, may give misleading information and provide false reassurance about the absence of disease.

A large number of lung function measurements are available within specialized centres, but some are difficult and time consuming to perform. They remain largely the preserve of the respiratory specialist, and are encountered only infrequently in day-to-day occupational practice. The measurements most frequently used in practice are the forced expiratory volume in 1 s (FEV_1), forced vital capacity (FVC), and peak expiratory flow (PEF). The more complex measurements of lung function will be considered in less detail, though sufficient to allow meaningful interpretation of reported results. Full technical details of their performance should be sought elsewhere [1,2]; this chapter focuses on the particular needs of occupational physicians and their immediate colleagues.

For each test to be seen in perspective, an understanding of the various subdivisions of lung volume and their nomenclature (and abbreviations) is necessary. Fig. 32.1 provides an illustration.

Before lung function is measured the subject should rest, preferably for 15 min, although this is not always realistic, so that any exercise-induced reduction in expiratory flow or oxygen tension is reversed. The procedures that are subsequently required should be carefully explained and if necessary demonstrated. Use of a nose clip is mandatory for virtually all tests. The exception is for forced expiratory maneuvers, for which most people (but not all) are unable to exhale through the nose, even partly, if the mouth is open [1]. Subjects may sit or stand when performing maneuvers, although results are generally slightly lower when sitting [3].

TESTS OF VENTILATORY FUNCTION

The equipment conventionally used to measure dynamic gas volumes or timed inspiratory and expiratory

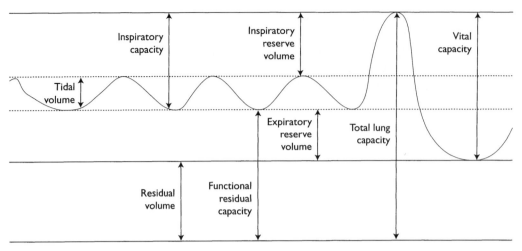

Fig. 32.1 Spirogram labeled to show static lung volumes.

volumes (flows) is a spirometer. The recording produced by this equipment is known as a spirogram. A number of different basic types exist but they fall into two broad categories.

Equipment

Volume displacement spirometers provide a direct measurement of respired gas by requiring the subject to breathe in and out of a sealed container. The container may be a water sealed bell, a piston with a 'rolling seal', or a bellows system, but its recommended volume is at least 8 liters, which inevitably makes this type of spirometer bulky and difficult to transport. They are usually very accurate when measuring volume provided they are appropriately calibrated, and they tend to be stable in performance as they are mechanically simple. The volume signal may be transformed mathematically to yield an estimate of flow in some spirometers, but because of the inertia of the equipment they usually respond relatively slowly to rapid changes in pressure and consequently give relatively inaccurate estimates of flow.

By contrast, flow sensing spirometers primarily measure flow using devices that respond rapidly during breathing maneuvers. Volume is then estimated by integration of the data obtained. Typically they quantify flow from the measured pressure drop across a resistance such as a mesh or bundle of parallel small tubes (pneumotachograph), from the measured cooling of a heated wire, or from the measured rotation of a turbine blade. As they do not need a large volume to contain respired gases they can be much smaller (often pocket size) than volume displacement spirometers, and yet by using microprocessors to perform the complex calculations required their use can be relatively straightforward. A disadvantage is their more complex function, and

a consequent proneness to volume measurement error. For example, a small error in calibrating zero flow can lead to a large error in estimating volume, as the error will be repeated in each of the component measurements used to generate the volume estimate. In addition, their responses to changes in flow may be non-linear, and affected by factors such as turbulence and gas viscosity. These cause difficulties in ensuring accurate calibration.

Standards of accuracy

The American Thoracic Society and the European Respiratory Society each publishes a series of similar minimum standards that spirometers should meet if they are to be used for clinical practice or research [1,2]. These cover properties such as volume range and accuracy, maximum driving pressure, and accuracy of timing. They are summarized in Table 32.1. Most modern spirometers will comply with all (or most) of these requirements, but there are some that do not. A good deal of caution is therefore necessary when choosing equipment so as to ensure that all spirometers do comply with these standards and allow lung function measurements to be interpreted meaningfully.

Calibration

Regular calibration using appropriate equipment is essential if a spirometer is to be accurate. Ideally calibration should be checked at the end of each test session as well as at the beginning to confirm that the spirometer has remained within the required functional parameters. For most purposes a calibration syringe is adequate to calibrate volumes, a 3-liter syringe being the volume recommended [1,2]. Regular checks for leaks, whether from the spirometer or the

Table 32.1 Summary of European Respiratory Society and American Thoracic Society minimum standards for spirometers

	European Respiratory Society	American Thoracic Society
Volume range	0–8 liters	0–8 liters
Volume accuracy	± 3% or 50 ml (whichever is the greater)	± 3% or 50 ml (whichever is the greater)
Volume resolution	25 ml	30 ml
Timing accuracy	± 1%	± 1%
Temperature	Measured in spirometer	Measured in spirometer
Calibration	Calibrated syringe (3 liters)	Calibrated syringe (3 liters)

tubing, should also be carried out. It is more difficult to check the calibration of flow measurements, and for this a pump capable of generating rapidly fluctuating as well as constant flow rates is required. Such equipment is costly and is generally available only in a few specialist centers. The American Thoracic Society produces a series of specimen flow curves that a spirometer should be able to reproduce with reasonable accuracy during initial calibration [2].

Volume displacement spirometers tend to be relatively stable. Although calibration should be checked frequently, adjustment is needed only rarely. Flow sensing spirometers, on the other hand, tend to be less stable in day-to-day use. A simple problem of condensation within the device can, for example, alter the pressure : flow characteristics sufficiently to introduce a large measurement error. In addition, estimates of volume from integrating flow rates may show considerable variability when the flow rate varies rapidly. This can be compounded by the effects of temperature change on the viscosity of exhaled gases. Ideally these spirometers should be calibrated using appropriate pumps over a range of temperatures, but the availability of such devices generally precludes this. The difficulty and expense of calibrating flow, and the frequent substitution of calibration by volume, is one of the problems inherent in flow sensing spirometers.

Correction for temperature, pressure, and humidity

One further difficulty that occurs in lung function measurement is that gases within the lungs are at body temperature and pressure, and are fully saturated with water vapor (BTPS). With exhalation they cool and contract, and water vapor condenses. They then conform to ambient conditions (ATPS). In normal use the volume of gas measured in the spirometer (i.e. at ATPS) is corrected to reflect that at BTPS, since it is the volume of gas standardized to conditions within the body that is of primary interest. This correction may be performed automatically by the spirometer using an integral thermometer to sense ambient temperature. In doing so it is assumed that almost instantaneous cooling of gases to ambient conditions occurs as they enter the spirometer, but this assumption may not always hold true, and errors can arise from this correction.

With flow sensing devices correction to BTPS is more difficult. They are usually sited only a short distance from the test subject, allowing little time for cooling of exhaled air to ambient conditions. The effects of temperature are more complex with these types of spirometer as temperature changes will affect both the volume and viscosity of exhaled gases. Alterations in viscosity will affect the pressure : flow characteristics of a gas in a tube such as a pneumotachograph, and will affect the response of a turbine at a given flow. Although correction to BTPS is still necessary, it may introduce errors if not carefully carried out.

Forced expiration

Probably the most commonly performed maneuver is forced expiration from full inspiration to full expiration, to provide the FVC. The subject is asked to inhale to total lung capacity (TLC), seal the mouth around the spirometer mouthpiece, and exhale as quickly and completely as possible to residual volume (RV). Alternatively, the subject has a period of quiet tidal breathing in and out of the spirometer before this forced expiratory maneuver is carried out. This allows measurement of inspiratory as well as expiratory flow rates and volumes, but is more complex to perform. It also has implications for infection control, requiring regular disinfection of the spirometer, and it increases carbon dioxide concentration in the closed breathing circuit. This requires the use of absorbing chemicals or regular flushing. A slow vital capacity (SVC) maneuver involves slow, not forced, expiration following full inhalation, and allows more accurate quantification of vital capacity in the presence of airway collapse. When none is present, FVC and SVC give similar values.

Spirometry

Results are conventionally displayed as a volume–time graph although they may sometimes be presented as a flow–volume graph (Figs 32.2 and 32.3).

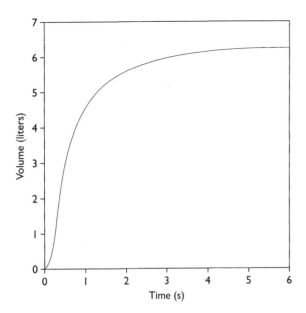

Fig. 32.2 Example of a volume–time graph.

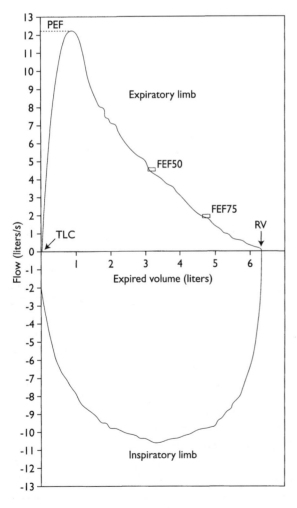

Fig. 32.3 Example of an inspiratory and expiratory flow – volume graph.

The volume–time graph is more easily interpreted, and the FEV_1, FVC, and a number of other indices can be directly read from it. A flow–volume curve relates the rate of flow to the level of lung inflation, and can be plotted for both inspiration and expiration. When both are obtained a closed flow–volume loop is produced. It can be useful in separating intrathoracic from extrathoracic airway obstruction, and in identifying obstruction in the smaller intrathoracic airways.

It is essential during an FVC maneuver that the subject does inhale fully, does not exhale prior to connecting to the mouthpiece, has a good seal on the mouthpiece, undertakes a maximal effort from the start of the maneuver, and completes a smooth, full, and rapid expiration without coughing. A small leak may be difficult to detect, but if there is any suspicion that a subject is leaking air through the nose a nose clip should be used. Occasionally subjects may abruptly terminate exhalation due either to glottic closure or obstruction of the disposable mouthpiece with the tongue. The latter problem can be overcome by cutting the proximal end of the mouthpiece at an angle, or by cutting a wedge out of it, so that the orifice is less easily obstructed.

A submaximal effort will inevitably distort the measurements. This can be identified best by a slow start on the volume–time graph, or by a large 'back extrapolated volume'. The 'back extrapolated volume' can be derived from the volume–time graph relatively easily, and many modern spirometers will estimate it automatically. It is customary to back extrapolate the volume–time curve from its steepest part to the time axis on the graph and use this point as zero time when estimating timed expiratory volumes such as FEV_1. This allows for the initial phase of rapid acceleration of gas flow as inertia in the subject's lungs and equipment is overcome. The 'back extrapolated volume' is the volume of gas exhaled during this acceleration phase and is usually only a relatively small volume. However, with submaximal effort this acceleration phase is prolonged, and the 'back extrapolated volume' consequently represents an unduly large proportion of vital capacity. There will also be increased variability when comparing the results from several expiratory maneuvres as it is difficult to reproduce closely a submaximal effort.

Because it can be difficult to identify these problems simply by observing the test subject, it is important to use a spirometer that displays the entire expiratory maneuver so that compliance with relevant standards can be ensured. The standards applied to assess the technical acceptability of forced expiratory maneuvers, and hence FVC and FEV_1 measurements, are shown in Table 32.2 [1].

Table 32.2 Summary of criteria used to assess validity of expiratory maneuvers [1]

Test feature	Criteria to be accepted as valid
Start of test	Back extrapolated volume < 5% or < 100 ml (whichever is the greater)
Number of 'blows'	Minimum of three technically satisfactory, maximum of eight without a rest
Duration of test	≥ 6 s, may be >18 s with significant obstruction
End of test	Plateau reached with flow < 25 ml in 0.5 s
Shape of curve	Smooth, with no abrupt changes suggesting obstruction by tongue, teeth, etc.
Reproducibility of FVC	Best two should be within 5% or 100 ml (whichever is greater)
Reproducibility of FEV_1	Best two should be within 5% or 100 ml (whichever is greater)

Subjects with underlying respiratory disease frequently have more trouble in producing a technically acceptable spirogram than a normal subject [4]. As a consequence, tests that do not meet acceptable standards should not simply be discarded but examined for evidence of underlying disease. With careful explanation and coaxing, the vast majority of subjects are able to perform spirometric measurements of lung function satisfactorily.

However the results are displayed, most modern spirometers can estimate a range of lung function measures. These usually comprise:

- Forced vital capacity (FVC). The volume of gas delivered during a full expiration made as forcefully and completely as possible starting from full inspiration.
- Forced expiratory volume in 1 s (FEV_1). The volume of gas exhaled in the first second of exhalation during a forced expiratory maneuvre starting from full inspiration. Other timed forced expiratory volumes are also sometimes measured (e.g. $FEV_{0.5}$, FEV_3).
- FEV_1 expressed as a percentage of FVC ($FEV_1/FVC\%$).
- Peak expiratory flow rate (PEFR), or simply peak expiratory flow (PEF). The maximal flow during a forced expiratory maneuver from a position of full inspiration.
- Maximal mid-expiratory flow (MMEF or Vmax 75–25). The mean forced expiratory flow in the middle part of an exhalation, i.e. between 75% and 25% of FVC. Also known as the FEF_{25-75} (i.e. forced expiratory flow from 25% to 75% of the expired volume).
- Maximal expiratory flow at a specified lung volume ($MEF_{x\%}$). The expiratory flow at the designated lung volume, the percentage representing the portion of FVC remaining to be exhaled. It is also known as the $FEF_{x\%}$ where the percentage represents the portion of FVC that has been exhaled.

Once technically acceptable results have been obtained they need to be interpreted as possible indicators of disease. They may, however, be influenced by a number of factors other than disease:

- Sex. Males generally have a larger FEV_1, FVC, and PEFR but a slightly lower $FEV_1/FVC\%$.
- Age. Lung function increases until early adulthood and then declines, peak values occurring at about the age of 25 years. The effect of ageing on FEV_1 has both linear and quadratic components, the rate of loss accelerating with increasing age. Most prediction equations assume a purely linear model, however, and so the predictions tend to underestimate the true values in middle life, but overestimate them in later life.
- Height. All dynamic lung volumes other than $FEV_1/FVC\%$ increase with standing height.
- Race. European and North American whites have a higher mean FEV_1 and FVC than individuals of Asian or African origin after allowing for other factors. In general, individuals of Asian origin have a FEV_1 and FVC approximately 10% lower than whites who are otherwise similar, while individuals of African origin have a FEV_1 or FVC lowered by approximately 13% [1]. There are also significant variations over smaller geographic areas, but the reasons are not clear. By contrast, there is little difference in PEFR between racial groups.

By including these four variables in regression analyses of lung function data from a 'normal' population, equations can be derived for each parameter of lung function which identify the expected levels (if the individual is average for the population) after adjusting for his/her sex, age, height, and race. The expected level so generated is generally known as the 'predicted' level, and the individual's measured level is often related to this as 'percentage of predicted', or simply %predicted [1]. This usefully allows ready comparison between individuals who show differences in sex, age, height, or race and as a result are not readily compared using the absolute level of measured lung function. A number of different prediction equations are in use, and so differences will arise according to which is adopted. These are largely a consequence of differences, usually minor, between the population samples used to generate the 'normal' data. Most do not currently incorporate measurements of weight and hence body mass index (weight/height²), which is increasingly recognized to influence FEV_1 and FVC, though lean body mass (reflecting muscle bulk) exerts its effect (a positive one) in the opposite direction to that of body fat. In addition, most do not model the effect of age adequately, as has been said, which leads to diminished reliability over the age of 70–80 years. Prediction equations are, nevertheless, extremely useful, despite this need to recognize their limitations.

Because the predicted value represents a mean from a sample of the reference population, a normal range can be calculated from this and the residual standard deviation. This varies among the various tests of lung function, and there is no simple rule of thumb that can be universally applied. A value of 80% of the predicted value is a useful approximation for the lower limit of normal for FEV_1 and FVC measurements. The data required for precise calculations are provided with most types of lung function equipment.

The values from prediction equations are derived from cross-sectional data, and are somewhat different from those which are derived longitudinally, especially estimates for the effect of age. The reasons are complex, but relate chiefly to the different principles involved. In cross-sectional studies the effect of increasing age is estimated from observed differences between older and younger participants, after appropriate adjustments have been made for recognized confounding and interacting variables. If full adjustments are not made (this may not be possible) some error is inevitable. If the true degrees of change in individuals over time are measured longitudinally, the contribution of ageing may again be confounded by other evolving variables (part of the decrement may be due to an unmeasured gain in weight, not increasing age) and those with the greatest loss may not survive to participate in the repeated measurements. In general, therefore, cross-sectional data overestimate the true average effect of ageing in the population as a whole, while longitudinal data underestimate it.

When available for an individual, longitudinal data have obvious advantages because they may allow a truly excessive loss to be detected despite measured values lying within the normal range. However, if the changes then observed are small, the relative importance of measurement error becomes greater. Inevitable changes in equipment and personnel supervising its use may provide additional sources of increased variability, thereby enhancing the difficulty in recognizing small but genuine changes in lung function. Strict adherence to technical standards

becomes critical in such circumstances.

Based on the lung function measurements described, abnormalities are conventionally classified by obstructive, restrictive, or mixed types. In obstructive ventilatory defects (e.g. from asthma, emphysema, obstructive bronchitis) the FEV_1 and other measures of airflow are reduced as the airways are significantly narrowed, but the vital capacity is less directly affected and may remain within the normal range. This leads to a reduction in the FEV_1/FVC%, which is diagnostic of airflow obstruction. With marked airflow obstruction the FVC may underestimate considerably the true vital capacity and it is necessary to measure SVC to obtain a more accurate estimate. With marked obstruction, however, there is air trapping, an increase in residual volume, and an inevitable reduction in vital capacity, since the two are confined within the limits of total lung capacity (see Fig. 32.1) despite the tendency for total lung capacity to increase in these circumstances.

With restrictive ventilatory defects (e.g. from interstitial lung disease, pleural disease, kyphoscoliosis) the FEV_1 and FVC are both reduced, the FEV_1/FVC% remains normal or is even increased, and lung volumes represented by total lung capacity (TLC) and residual volume (RV) are diminished also.

With a mixed defect there is a combination of the two, both FEV_1 and FVC being reduced, the FEV_1 proportionately more than the FVC so that the FEV_1/FVC% is also reduced. However, the latter is insufficiently reduced for the reduction in FVC to be a consequence solely of airflow obstruction.

Peak expiratory flow rate (PEFR)

Peak expiratory flow rate (or simply peak expiratory flow) is probably the easiest measurement of lung function to perform and can be measured using a simple and inexpensive peak flow meter. None the less, it may provide a great deal of valuable information in the context of occupational asthma, since asthma typically shows variation in airflow obstruction over short periods of time, to which PEFR is very sensitive [5]. PEFR is thought to be predominantly a measure of large rather than small airway caliber, but it is one of the measures of lung function that is most effort dependent [6]. This limits its usefulness. By using the peak flow meter on a number of occasions throughout the day, the diurnal variation typical of asthma can be identified. A change of 15% or more in PEFR is usually considered diagnostic [7]. An increase of similar magnitude following the inhalation of a bronchodilator is usually considered diagnostic of asthma also.

In performing a measurement of PEFR the subject inhales as fully as possible (to total lung capacity) and then exhales with maximal force into the measurement device. Dedicated peak flow meters generally use a vane, disk, or sphere, which is moved as the subject exhales. The movement pushes a marker along a scale and opens a vent, thereby allowing a progressively larger leak from the mechanism until the point where the leak is so large that the vane, disk, or sphere stops moving. Spirometers too may provide a measurement of PEFR, which is generally more accurate than that obtained from dedicated peak flow meters, but they are also more expensive and complex, and generally less convenient to use – especially repeatedly while at work.

A degree of care is necessary when interpreting PEFR results. A number of dedicated peak flow meter types exists, and measurements performed on one may differ considerably from those on another. There may be differences also between different instruments of the same type. This is a consequence of their relative crudity. They are most useful, therefore, in detecting change, not in quantifying measurement in an absolute sense. It is consequently important that the same meter is used throughout a recording period. There may also be problems of linearity concerning the measurement scale, so that change over one section may not reflect the same difference in PEFR as change over another. This can distort estimates of bronchodilator-induced reversibility, or occupationally induced bronchoconstriction [8]. Appropriate technical adjustments can be made but this increases expense and may detract from the simplicity of use, in turn diminishing usability.

A single PEFR reading may consequently give little useful information, having little sensitivity in identifying asthma [9]. The great value of PEFR measurements accrues from peak flow meters being so inexpensive and simple to use, that they can be given to patients to record variability in ventilatory function over prolonged periods. This is useful not only in identifying asthma and assessing its severity, but in demonstrating relationships between worsening values and relevant periods of exposure [10,11]. Perhaps the best described technique involves performing PEFR measurements every 2 hours during waking hours [10]. The results are then plotted to show the minimum, mean, and best values on each day (Fig. 32.4). Improvement in PEFR on days away from work and deterioration on days at work can often be identified with confidence when relevant exposures are encountered in the workplace. Computer software is now available to simplify much of the task of plotting and interpreting the results [12] and illustrations are provided in Chapter 4.

Forced inspiration

Many individuals find forced inspiratory maneuvers uncomfortable. In addition, they require hygiene precautions to ensure that the spirometer and its contents do not transmit infection, and they cannot be performed on all types of spirometers. They are used much less commonly than forced expiratory maneuvers.

Available measures include:

- Inspiratory vital capacity (IVC). The maximum volume of air which can be inhaled following a full expiration.

- Forced inspiratory vital capacity (FIVC). The maximum volume of air which can be inhaled following a full expiration during a forced inspiratory maneuver.

- Forced inspiratory volume in 1 s (FIV_1). The volume of air inhaled during the first second of a forced inspiratory maneuver starting from full

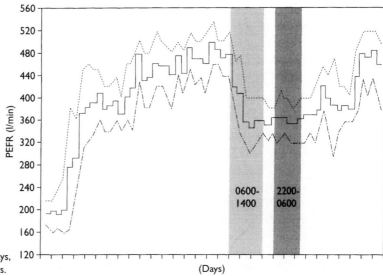

Fig. 32.4 Example of serial PEF recording from a subject exposed to diisocyanates. The maximum, minimum, and mean are plotted for each day, and periods at work are shown hatched. Surveilance starts immediately after the completion of a work period. Diminished PEF is associated with work days, but recovery away from work requires several days.

expiration. Other timed forced inspiratory volumes are also sometimes measured (e.g. $FIV_{0.5}$, FIV_3).

■ Peak inspiratory flow rate (PIFR). The maximal instantaneous flow achieved during an FIVC maneuver.

■ Maximal inspiratory flow at a specified lung volume ($MIF_{x\%}$). The maximal flow at the specified lung volume, when the given percentage of FIVC has been inhaled.

These measurements are of use principally in detecting obstruction of large extrathoracic airways and in discriminating between intrathoracic and extrathoracic airway obstruction. If the maximum inspiratory flow at 50% of IVC (MIF_{50}) is less than the maximum expiratory flow at 50% of FVC (MEF_{50}) extrathoracic obstruction is suggested, since inspiration in such circumstances exaggerates the usual decrease in extrathoracic airway caliber, as local pressure in the airway falls and external ambient air pressure remains unchanged. The ratio of MEF_{50} : MIF_{50} is normally about one. While an increase suggests extrathoracic obstruction, a decrease favors intrathoracic obstruction, since in such circumstances expiration exaggerates the usual decrease in intrathoracic airway caliber.

TESTS OF LUNG VOLUME

Lung volume is measured less frequently than forced expiratory flow. Not surprisingly volume measurements are most useful in detecting diseases characterized by altered lung volume, and in quantifying their severity. Principal examples are interstitial and pleural diseases, and musculoskeletal diseases which distort the thorax. Not all volume measurements can be performed using a spirometer as some include the volume of gas (residual volume) that cannot be exhaled as the lungs reach a minimum volume at end expiration. The various measurements are summarized in Fig. 32.1 and comprise [1]:

■ Vital capacity (VC). This is the volume change of the lungs between full inspiration and full expiration. As described above it can be measured as FVC, SVC, or even FIVC. It can also be calculated from its constituent subdivisions which comprise tidal volume, inspiratory reserve volume, and expiratory reserve volume.

■ Tidal volume. The volume of gas which is inhaled or exhaled during a normal respiratory cycle.

■ Inspiratory reserve volume (IRV). The maximal volume that can be inspired from the mean peak of inspiration during tidal breathing.

■ Expiratory reserve volume (ERV). The maximal volume that can be expired from the mean trough of expiration during tidal breathing.

■ Residual volume (RV). The volume of gas remaining in the lungs at the end of a full expiration. It is not possible to measure RV using a conventional spirometer. It is usually measured using a gas dilution method during 'steady state' breathing or by plethysmography. A full description of these techniques is beyond the scope of this text but can be found elsewhere [6].

■ Functional residual capacity (FRC). The volume of gas present in the lungs at the mean end expiratory level during tidal breathing at rest. It represents the state of equilibrium when the respiratory muscles are relaxed; the tendency of the lung to collapse because of its elasticity is balanced by the tendency of the chest wall to spring outwards. As FRC includes RV it can not be measured using a conventional spirometer.

■ Total lung capacity (TLC). The volume of gas in the lungs following full inspiration. It includes RV and so, again, cannot be measured using a conventional spirometer.

In restrictive diseases there is usually a reduction in TLC, VC, and RV, and the RV:TLC ratio is unchanged or reduced. The FRC and ERV are often markedly decreased in gross obesity whereas abnormalities of lung distensibility, such as pulmonary fibrosis, predominantly reduce the IRV.

Obstructive diseases tend to be associated with an increase in FRC and RV due to air trapping and consequent hyperinflation. The increase in RV may be sufficient to cause a reduction in VC, but there is usually some degree of compensatory increase in TLC (perhaps from the use of accessory muscles). A raised ratio of RV:TLC (RV/TLC) is nevertheless particularly characteristic of airway obstruction.

TESTS OF GAS EXCHANGE

In addition to inhaling and exhaling gas, the lungs must allow the exchange of oxygen and carbon dioxide with blood. Neither spirometry nor the measurement of static lung volumes allow this function to be adequately assessed. Rather the transfer factor (T_L), also known as the diffusing capacity (D_L), is measured. A number of different methods for measuring T_L exist but this type of test is usually available only in lung function laboratories as the equipment required is considerably more expensive to purchase and difficult to maintain than a spirometer.

The test is commonly performed using as a measure of the rate of gas transfer the uptake of a small amount of carbon monoxide (CO) from a single inhalation from RV. The rate for carbon monoxide is similar to that for oxygen though easier to quantify; hence the measurement is specifically described as the T_LCO. The results are quoted as the quantity of CO transferred per unit time per unit pressure difference (e.g. mmol min^{-1} kPa^{-1} or ml/min/mmHg). CO is particularly useful for this test as it should have a negligible tendency to diffuse back from red cell to alveoli, carboxyhemoglobin usually being found in only a low concentration in a normal individual's blood, and the CO being tightly bound to hemoglobin. Transfer is essentially in one direction only across the alveolar capillary membrane, and the tension of CO in pulmonary capillary blood can be assumed to be zero. This assumption may not be correct in smokers and individuals with occupational exposure to CO, for whom an appropriate adjustment can be made to the estimate for the back pressure of CO [13].

In addition to T_LCO, alveolar volume (V_A, the total volume into which the single inhalation is diluted, less dead space) is always measured at the same time. By adding a non-absorbed gas such as helium to the inhaled mixture that includes CO, the volume into which it is diluted can be estimated when the expired gases are analyzed. This should give a similar result to that obtained by adding the volume of inspired gas mixture to a previously measured value of RV, but if there is marked airway obstruction and poor mixing between inhaled and resident gases, the single breath method will underestimate the outcome derived from steady state RV measurements. The magnitude of the discrepancy consequently provides a measure of mixing inefficiency. An adjustment must then be made for estimated dead space in the measuring equipment and the anatomical dead space. The measurement of V_A allows a further variable to be estimated, T_LCO per unit volume of V_A. This variable is usually called the transfer coefficient (KCO) and is reported in units of mmol min^{-1} kPa^{-1} l^{-1} or ml/min/mmHg/L. It usefully compensates for variability in alveolar volume, by expressing gas transfer per unit of ventilated lung, Thus a patient with one lung resected and a normal remaining lung will have half the predicted T_LCO but a normal KCO.

A number of factors influence the interpretation of T_LCO and KCO measurements. Smoking or occupational exposure to CO have already been mentioned as potential problems. Anemia may additionally affect the uptake of CO into red cells and so lead to an underestimate (albeit adjustable) of T_LCO and KCO. Age, sex, race, stature, and habitual exercise may also affect gas transfer. Predicted or reference values should include terms for all these variables, but most include only sex, age, and height, and so are less well defined than those for spirometric measurements [13].

T_LCO and KCO may be reduced by a number of occupational lung diseases, but as the diffusion of gas from alveoli to red cells is a multistep process it may also be affected by a number of other factors. T_LCO and KCO are principally affected by:

- Loss of functioning lung units (e.g. bronchial obstruction and atelectasis)
- Alveolar enlargement with reduction in surface area available for gas exchange (e.g. emphysema)
- Alveolar capillary membrane thickening and ventilation/perfusion mismatch (e.g. pulmonary fibrosis)
- Reduction in CO binding by blood (e.g. anemia)
- Non-perfusion of ventilated alveoli (e.g. pulmonary emboli)

Generally T_LCO and KCO will both be reduced in the conditions mentioned above, but occasionally a discrepancy between T_LCO and KCO can give valuable additional information. Diseases that reduce lung volume without affecting the lung parenchyma, for example diffuse pleural thickening and respiratory muscle weakness, may cause a reduction in T_LCO (because there is less ventilated lung), while KCO remains unchanged or is increased (because parenchymal function is preserved and there is relatively more perfusion of ventilated regions). This situation generally arises when there is ventilatory restriction due to extra pulmonary not intrapulmonary disorders.

PATTERNS OF ABNORMALITY

Abnormalities in lung function are commonly divided into two broad categories, obstructive and restrictive. These reflect the two major functional components of the lungs: the conducting airways which cause an obstructive pattern when diseased, and the parenchyma (alveoli and interstitium) which causes a restrictive pattern. The latter is characteristically associated with impaired gas transfer, which helps to distinguish it from extrapulmonary disorders that additionally cause ventilatory restriction but do not impair gas transfer. A mixed pattern may be expected when different causes of impaired function coexist.

Obstructive

A reduction in FEV$_1$ and other measures of flow, such as PEFR and MMEF, is typical of obstructive defects in lung function. Inspiratory flow measurements may also be reduced although these tend to be less affected by intrathoracic abnormalities than expiratory flows.

A particularly useful and definitive measure of obstruction is the FEV_1 expressed as a percentage of the FVC (FEV_1/FVC%). It is typically 75–80%, although it does vary slightly with age. Values of 50% or less imply severe obstruction, with those around 30% or less indicating a significant threat to survival.

Obstructive abnormalities are reflected also in changes in static lung volumes, FRC and RV both being increased. The RV as a percentage of TLC (RV/TLC%) also increases, and may be a more sensitive measure of obstruction than measurements of flow or the FEV_1/FVC%. RV and RV/TLC may consequently allow early detection of obstructive diseases, before there is any other physiologic evidence [1].

Large airways

Measurements of flow at large lung volumes, such as FEV_1 and PEFR, are thought to reflect predominantly the function of large airways, such as the trachea and central bronchi. They tend to be affected in diseases causing acute changes in ventilatory function where the large central airways are the principal site of obstruction, such as asthma or acute bronchitis. They are relatively insensitive to diseases that predominantly affect small airways, but when these are severe abnormalities of FEV_1 and PEFR will be seen.

Small airways

Flow rates at low lung volumes are thought to reflect more closely the function of smaller intrathoracic airways. Such measures include the MMEF, MEF_{50}, MEF_{25}, and the forced late expiratory flow (FEF_{75-85}). These measures tend to be particularly affected in bronchiolitis, infection, and emphysema. Unfortunately these measurements are more variable than FEV_1 and PEFR, and normal values are less well characterized than those for FEV_1 and PEFR. Their interpretation is therefore more difficult and this limits their usefulness.

Reversibility

The characteristic physiologic abnormality of asthma is reversible airway obstruction, obstruction alone being consistent also with chronic obstructive pulmonary disease (COPD). Diagnostic tests of reversibility typically involve the measurement of FEV_1 or PEFR before and after an inhaled β-selective bronchodilator. Some individuals with asthma, especially those whose asthma is particularly severe at the time of testing, do not demonstrate an acute bronchodilator response until a short course of steroids has been given, and so this may be required over 1–2 weeks before asthmatic reversibility can be excluded. Furthermore, some subjects with long-

standing asthma develop fixed airway obstruction, which is not distinguishable from other causes of COPD by spirometric tests.

The method of quantifying the degree of reversibility and the amount that is considered significant is not adequately standardized. Many lung function laboratories express reversibility as a percentage of the prebronchodilator value, but this tends to produce high values in individuals with low initial lung function, which may involve change within the limits of measurement error. It may therefore be preferable to express the response in absolute terms, or as a percentage of the predicted or reference value after adjusting for age and height [1]. Thus a change in FEV_1 and FVC of > 200 ml and > 12%, respectively, would usually be accepted as clinically significant [1].

Restrictive

Restrictive abnormalities of lung function are typically characterized by a proportionate reduction in both FVC and FEV_1 and by reduction of TLC, VC, and other static lung volumes. Reduction in TLC is usually considered more definitive than reduction in VC, as the VC may be reduced in obstructive abnormalities due to gas trapping. However, TLC itself may not be very sensitive to mild changes, and so using a combination of measurements provides the best approach.

Interstitial disease

Restrictive defects due to interstitial diseases result from reduced distensibility (compliance) of the lung. This is associated with fibrosis, infiltration, or edema of the lung interstitial tissue. Typical causes include cryptogenic fibrosing alveolitis (idiopathic pulmonary fibrosis), sarcoidosis, fibrosis due to connective tissue disorders, and carcinomatous infiltration of the lung. In the occupational setting the most prominent causes include some types of pneumoconiosis, extrinsic allergic alveolitis, and exposure to toxic agents. Such disorders of the lung parenchyma also usually affect the diffusion of gases, and so T_Lco and Kco will be reduced. Because of the changes in the interstitial tissue of the lungs there also tends to be less dynamic compression of airways during exhalation and so FEV_1/FVC% is usually normal or may be increased. Occasionally the RV may be decreased because of a similar mechanism.

Extrapulmonary disease

Restrictive defects in lung function may arise not only due to changes in compliance of the lungs themselves but due to decreased compliance of surrounding tissue. Examples of diseases causing such effects include abnormalities of the pleura such as pleural effusions or visceral pleural thickening, and of the chest wall such as kyphoscoliosis, ankylosing spondylitis, and gross obesity. As the lungs themselves are essentially normal, diffusion of gases from alveoli to blood and *vice versa* is also essentially normal. Consequently $T_L\text{CO}$ is reduced but $K\text{CO}$ remains normal or is increased.

Muscle weakness

Diseases that cause systemic muscle weakness, or localized weakness of intercostal or diaphragmatic muscle, may also cause a restrictive extrapulmonary pattern of abnormality. Causes include myopathies, motor neuron disease, anticholinergic agents (such as organophosphates), and postinfective polyneuropathy (Guillain–Barré syndrome). These are characterized additionally by worsening reductions in VC and TLC when supine rather than standing, since the weak muscles have further difficulty in displacing the abdominal contents.

AIRWAY RESPONSIVENESS

Increasingly, measurements of airway responsiveness are used in identifying and quantifying the severity of asthma, including occupational asthma [14]. While such measurements have been made for more than 50 years [15], the methods remain poorly standardized, and the results from different methods are not readily compared. The principal use has been in research, but there is increasing interest in their use for diagnosis and health surveillance, and in guiding clinical care [16,17].

In principle, tests of airway responsiveness are uncomplicated. Increasing doses of a bronchoconstrictor are given at intervals by inhalation (generally by means of aerosols from solutions of increasing concentration) until the test subject develops significant bronchoconstriction, or a dose limited by the risk of adverse effects is reached. FEV_1, or another measure of airway caliber, is recorded after each dose to assess the effect. A 20% decrement in FEV_1 is usually taken to represent significant bronchoconstriction, being insufficient to cause much distress, but sufficient to exceed measurement error and most degrees of spontaneous variability. As soon as a decrement in FEV_1 of 20% or more has been achieved, or the maximum test dose has been given, the test is completed. The cumulative dose required to produce a given effect quantifies the level of airway responsiveness; the smaller the dose, the greater the level. A bronchodilator is usually given at this point to reverse any residual bronchoconstriction.

A number of agents have been used as bronchoconstrictors but the most common is methacholine (acetyl-β-methyl choline chloride). Histamine and hypertonic and hypotonic saline solutions have also been used extensively. In most protocols, methacholine is given in doubling cumulative doses at 5-min intervals, with FEV_1 being monitored after each dose [18,19]. It can take up to an hour to complete a measurement of airway responsiveness for a single subject, but the procedure may be shortened by omitting the lower and less relevant doses or by increasing the increment between each dose. Such devices imply some increase in risk for the development of an undue bronchoconstrictive response, and so require additional safeguards to ensure that abbreviated protocols are used only with subjects who are not likely to have high levels of responsiveness [16]. Furthermore, shortening protocols that use histamine rather than methacholine introduces inaccuracy, because the effect of the former (but not the latter) is not sufficiently cumulative over the time course of the test. As a result the outcomes from full and shortened protocols are different [20]. This problem does not occur with methacholine.

Three basic protocols are widely used for methacholine or histamine tests: the 'tidal breathing' method, the 'Yan' method, and the 'dosimeter' method [1,18,19,21,22].

When using pharmacologic agents, such as methacholine or histamine, the result is conventionally expressed as the dose of bronchoconstrictor estimated to cause a 20% decrement in FEV_1 ($PD_{20}.FEV_1$). PD_{20} is usually derived by linear interpolation from a plot of the log cumulative administered dose of methacholine or histamine against the decrement in FEV_1 (Fig. 32.5), or by using a simple formula [1,18]. It can be estimated for all subjects with a decrement in FEV_1 of 20%, and used as a quantitative measure of airway responsiveness ('asthmatic activity'). For some techniques, especially those based on the 'tidal breathing' method, the precise dose of administered bronchoconstrictor cannot be calculated, and so the concentrations of the aerosol generating solutions are used to estimate the concentration predicted to cause a 20% decrement in FEV_1 ($PC_{20}.FEV_1$) [14].

Alternatively, the dose estimated to produce a 15%, 10%, or other decrement in FEV_1 may be used (i.e. PD_{15}, PD_{10}, or PD_x), and, on occasion, measures of airway caliber other than FEV_1 are used (e.g. $PD_{20}.PEFR$, $PD_{40}.MMEF$). These measures can be particularly useful when quantifying airway responsiveness in subjects and populations without clinical asthma. A method by which all members of a study population can contribute a quantified measurement of airway responsiveness is to express the level from the dose–response slope [23].

This ability to quantify airway responsiveness in subjects without clinical evidence of asthma implies

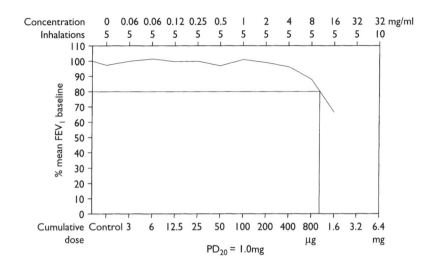

Fig. 32.5 Quantification of airway responsiveness as PD_{20} by interpolation.

limited specificity for the diagnosis of asthma. By using cumulative doses of inhaled methacholine up to 6.4 mg, PD_{20} can be quantified in approximately 40% of a normal adult population. This observation, together with other data (particularly from studies using the dose response slope to express airway responsiveness), suggests that airway responsiveness is distributed as a continuous variable in the population at large, those with asthma being found in the tail representing the high levels. There is some overlap between subjects with asthma, those with other respiratory diseases (particularly if airway caliber is diminished), and those who appear entirely healthy [17,23,24]. As a consequence, some caution is warranted in the interpretation of airway responsiveness measurements; they are best assessed by those familiar with the method of measurement used.

A high level of airway responsiveness is, nevertheless, very useful in confirming a diagnosis of asthma where doubt exists, especially if clearly defined limits are established for the measurement range which is associated with active disease [14,19]. Furthermore serial measurements, showing a clear relation between increasing levels of airway responsiveness and periods at work, provides valuable evidence of occupational asthma and of a causal asthma-inducing agent within the working environment. By contrast, a close relation between worsening measurements of PEFR and periods at work may simply be a consequence of non-specific bronchoconstriction attributable to irritants in the workplace, even physical exertion in cold air.

EXERCISE TESTS

Exercise can be useful in a number of settings to test lung function, although physical exertion of moder-

ate or severe degree inevitably carries some risk if there is a coincident risk of coronary artery disease. Less challenging exercise tests can be used outside the specialist laboratory as a general measure of fitness or exercise tolerance, or as a means to assess disablement from respiratory disease.

Well-established simple tests of general fitness include 12- and 6-min walk tests where the subject walks as far as possible, generally on the level indoors, in the given period. The distance covered provides a measure of fitness. Alternatively a step test can be performed. The 'Harvard' step test involves the subject stepping up to and down from a 50 cm (20 inches) high platform for a man and a 43 cm (17 inches) platform for a woman, at a rate of 30 step cycles per minute. This task is performed for 5 min, after which the subject rests for 1 min. The pulse is then counted over a period of 30 s to ascertain the subject's 'recovery' heart rate [6]. The 'recovery' heart rate can give an indication of fitness using the 'physical fitness index' (PFI) where:

$$PFI = \frac{\text{Duration of exercise (s)} \times 100}{5.5 \times \text{heart rate}}$$

A value of 80–50 is considered 'normal'; higher values place the subject in the 'fit' category, lower values in the 'unfit' category. Both of these tests depend on a number of factors besides lung function and fitness, but have the benefit of being simple to perform and requiring a minimum of equipment.

More specific to lung disease is the use of an oximeter during exercise to detect whether hypoxemia develops and the exertional level at which this occurs. Interstitial diseases of the lung are commonly associated with an inappropriately rapid increase in respiratory rate with exercise and with an undue degree of respiratory distress, and so the onset of breathlessness may prevent exercise continuing to the point when hypoxemia occurs.

More complex tests to quantify exercise tolerance or maximal oxygen uptake usually require a treadmill or a cycle ergometer, so that a subject can exercise while still remaining connected to test equipment. The subject exercises while breathing through a mouthpiece connected to 'real time' carbon dioxide and oxygen analyzers. Using this equipment the respiratory rate, tidal volume, oxygen uptake, and carbon dioxide output can be determined, thereby defining more accurately disease severity and the nature of any associated disability. While such investigations are invaluable in research focused on exercise physiology, they are rarely indicated in routine practice.

LUNG FUNCTION IN RESPIRATORY HEALTH SURVEILLANCE

The main use of respiratory health surveillance is to identify early the symptoms and signs of occupational lung disease among populations at risk. This encourages the introduction of appropriate measures of exposure reduction, so that disease progression can be prevented. Surveillance is particularly useful for workers exposed to respiratory sensitizers who are at risk of developing occupational asthma or extrinsic allergic alveolitis, or exposed to mineral dusts with the potential to cause pneumoconiosis. Surveillance of populations potentially exposed to respiratory carcinogens is less helpful as diagnostic tests rarely allow early enough intervention to prevent disease progression. However, it may be important at a population level to ensure there is no excess incidence of cancer, and hence no unrecognized exposure.

Most surveillance programs combine the reporting of respiratory illnesses with the regular administration of a respiratory symptom questionnaire and lung function measurement [25]. Surveillance programs for workers exposed to respiratory sensitizers are principally designed to detect asthma and usually incorporate spirometric measurements of FEV_1 and FVC. They should be repeated at intervals of 6–24 months depending on the perceived level of risk. Serial PEFR measurements may also be used once the suspicion of occupational asthma arises so that ventilatory function associated with days of work can be compared with that away from the workplace.

Regular spirometry is additionally of value as a screening tool for the evolution of COPD, but neither spirometry nor other tests of lung function have much value for the early detection of other occupationally induced disorders of the lung. Repeated measurements are essential if mild disease or disease progression is to be identified promptly, and the supervisor must be familiar with the basic principles and calibration requirements of the tests that are carried out. Otherwise there is very limited value in performing any lung function measurements within the workplace, and it may be preferable to refer individuals to a recognized lung function laboratory.

LUNG FUNCTION IN EPIDEMIOLOGY

Lung function measurements are frequently used in epidemiological studies where they are applied to detect respiratory disease in populations rather than individuals. The principles of measurement are, however, no different to those required in day-to-day clinical practice. It essential to use validated measurements, these must be performed on calibrated equipment by correctly trained operators, and the results must be properly adjusted for age, height, race, and sex. Weight, too, should be measured, although at present there is no standard method of adjustment for it.

Selecting validated tests that can be used in epidemiology can present a number of challenges. FEV_1 and FVC are probably the most suitable, and are widely used. MMEF and MEF_{50} are often used also, but their greater variability and the difficulty in adjusting for age, height, sex, and race pose difficulties in analysis. Practical considerations limit the application of tests of lung volume and gas transfer in epidemiology, particularly if measurements are required in a 'field' setting where calibration and maintenance pose additional difficulties.

Acknowledgements

I should like to thank Geraldine Metcalfe and the Medical Illustration Department of Bradford Hospitals NHS Trust for their assistance with a number of the figures.

REFERENCES

1. Working Party on Standardisation of Lung Function Tests. European Community for Steel and Coal. Standardized lung function testing. Official Statement of the European Respiratory Society. Lung volumes and forced ventilatory flows. *Eur Respir J* 1993; 6(Suppl 16): 1–40.

2. American Thoracic Society (ATS). Statement on Standardization of Spirometry – 1994 update. *Am J Respir Crit Care Med* 1995; 153: 1107–1136.

3. Townsend MC. Spirometric forced expiratory volumes measured in the standing versus the sitting posture. *Am Rev Respir Dis* 1984; 130: 123–124.

4. Humerfelt S, Eide GE, Kvale G, Gulsvik A. Predictors of spirometric test failure: a comparison of the 1983 and 1993 acceptability criteria from the European Community for Coal and Steel. *Occup Environ Med* 1995; 52: 547–553.

5. CIBA Guest symposium, September 24–26, 1958. Terminology, definitions, and classification of chronic pulmonary emphysema and related conditions. *Thorax* 1959; 14: 286–299.

6. Cotes JE. *Lung function: Assessment and Application in Medicine*, 5th edn. Oxford: Blackwell Scientific Publications, 1993.

7. National Heart, Lung, and Blood Institute. International Consensus Report on Diagnosis and Treatment of Asthma. Publication No 92–3091. *Eur Respir J* 1992; 5: 601–641.

8. Pedersen OF, Miller MR, Sigsgaard T *et al*. Peak flow meters: physical characteristics, influence of temperature, altitude, and humidity. *Eur Respir J* 1994; 7: 991–997.

9. Thiadens HA, De Bock GH, Van Houwelingen JC *et al*. Can peak expiratory flow measurements reliably identify the presence of airway obstruction and bronchodilator response as assessed by FEV_1 in primary care patients presenting with persistent cough? *Thorax* 1999; 54: 1055–1060.

10. Gannon PFG, Sherwood Burge P. Serial peak flow measurement in the diagnosis of occupational asthma. *Eur Respir J* 1997; 10(Suppl 24): 57s–63s.

11. Sherwood Burge P. The relationship between peak expiratory flow and respiratory symptoms. *Eur Respir J* 1997; 10(Suppl 24): 67s–68s.

12. Bright P, Sherwood Burge PS. The diagnosis of occupational asthma from serial measurements of lung function at and away from work. *Thorax* 1996; 51: 857–863.

13. Working Party on Standardisation of Lung Function Tests. European Community for Steel and Coal. Standardized lung function testing. Official Statement of the European Respiratory Society. Standardization of the measurement of transfer factor (diffusing capacity). *Eur Respir J* 1993; 6(Suppl 16): 41–52.

14. Cockcroft DW, Killian DN, Mellon JJA, Hargreave FE. Bronchial reactivity to inhaled histamine: a method and clinical survey. *Clin Allergy* 1977; 7: 235–243.

15. Curry JJ. Comparative action of acetyl-beta-methyl-choline-chloride and histamine in the respiratory tract in normals, patients with hay fever, and subjects with bronchial asthma. *J Clin Invest* 1947; 26: 430–438.

16. Hendrick DJ, Fabbri LM, Hughes JM *et al*. Modification of the methacholine inhalation test and its epidemiologic use in polyurethane workers. *Am Rev Respir Dis* 1986; 133: 600–604.

17. Beach JR, Dennis JH, Avery AJ *et al*. An epidemiologic investigation of asthma in welders. *Am J Respir Crit Care Med* 1996; 154: 1394–1400.

18. Working Party on Standardisation of Lung Function Tests. European Community for Steel and Coal. Standardized lung function testing. Official Statement of the European Respiratory Society. Airway responsiveness. Standardized challenge testing with pharmacological, physical, and sensitizing stimuli in adults. *Eur Respir J* 1993; 6(Suppl 16): 53–83.

19. Beach JR, Young CL, Stenton SC *et al*. Measurement of airway responsiveness to methacholine: relative importance of the precision of drug delivery and the method of assessing response. *Thorax* 1993; 48: 239–243.

20. Connolly MJ, Avery AJ, Walters EH, Hendrick DJ. The use of sequential doses of inhaled histamine in the measurement of bronchial responsiveness: cumulative effect and distortion caused by shortening the test protocol. *J Allergy Clin Immunol* 1988; 82: 863–8.

21. Yan K, Salome C, Woolcock AJ. Rapid method for the measurement of bronchial responsiveness. *Thorax* 1983; 38: 760–765.

22. Chai H, Farr RS, Froelich LA *et al*. Standardization of bronchial inhalation challenge procedures. *J Allergy Clin Immunol* 1975; 56: 323–327.

23. O'Connor G, Sparrow D, Taylor D *et al*. Analysis of dose–response curves to methacholine. An approach suitable for population studies. *Am Rev Respir Dis* 1997; 136: 1412–1417.

24. Cerveri I, Bruschi C, Zoia MC *et al*. Distribution of bronchial nonspecific reactivity in the general population. *Chest* 1988; 93: 26–30.

25. Health and Safety Executive. *Medical Aspects of Occupational Asthma*. Guidance note MS 25, 2nd edn. Sudbury: HSE Books, 1998.

33 | OCCUPATIONAL HYGIENE

Susan R. Woskie and Judy Sparer

INTRODUCTION

The goal of occupational hygiene, like other public health disciplines, is the prevention of disease before its initiation. In practice this is focused on:

■ Identification: Are there potentially harmful substances in the workplace?
■ Evaluation: Are such substances being used in a way that they are likely to cause harm?
■ Control: Elimination or reduction in exposure to a point where potential health hazards will not cause harm.

To achieve the goal of preventing occupational disease, occupational hygienists work in tandem with occupational and environmental health practitioners (Fig. 33.1). The prevention strategy illustrated in the figure requires knowledge of the workplace. This is most easily acquired if the hygienist and health practitioner are employees, or have contracts with the employer to provide on going healthcare or routine medical surveillance. Thus hygienist and physician may have the opportunity to study the workplace, review health and safety programs, examine the company's health and safety experience, and offer recommendations for improve-

ment. In addition, the need and/or sufficiency of any requested services can be assessed.

For physicians and hygienists not affiliated with a company, another opportunity for study of the worksite may come during the evaluation of a potential case of occupational disease. If evaluation leads to confirmation, the individual case can be considered a 'sentinel health event' (SHE). This prompts the need for a more extensive worksite evaluation to protect the index patient from further exposures and to prevent hazardous exposures to other workers at the site [1].

Working with employers

Ideally, an employer will be anxious to identify hazards within the worksite in order to eliminate them speedily. In practice, approaching the employer is generally most successful when initiated by an occupational physician who couches the discussion in the context of the health of the patients/employees. Nevertheless these discussions may require diplomatic skill, since there are often cost considerations, and management may resist the suggestion that the company's health and safety programs should be improved. If, in particular, the healthcare provider finds occupational disease during routine medical surveillance, the relationship with management may become strained if a

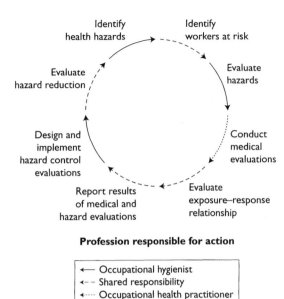

Identify health hazards → Identify workers at risk

Evaluate hazard reduction

Evaluate hazards

Design and implement hazard control evaluations

Conduct medical evaluations

Report results of medical and hazard evaluations

Evaluate exposure–response relationship

Profession responsible for action

← Occupational hygienist
←– Shared responsibility
←··· Occupational health practitioner

Fig. 33.1 Occupational safety and health professionals must collaborate in the process of identification, evaluation, and control of workplace hazards. Adapted from Dinardi [25].

preventive approach to occupational health and safety has not already been discussed and agreed upon. It is especially important that the procedures for following up possible cases of occupational disease or managing potential hazards be agreed upon at the start of any contractual relationship. Where labor unions and/or health and safety committees exist, representatives from these groups should participate in these planning discussions.

Perhaps the most difficult situation occurs when an occupational healthcare provider, with no prior relationship with an employer, diagnoses an occupational disease in a member of the workforce – a sentinel health event. To follow up the case with a worksite evaluation or intervention, the provider must gain the cooperation of the employer, since in most countries an inherent right of access is restricted to governmental agencies. Furthermore, the consent of the patient must be obtained before the employer is contacted, because of the possibility that his or her identification will lead to job loss or job change with diminished income. If the public health concern is sufficient, there may be situations when it is necessary to override a patient's reluctance, but this should not be done lightly and it requires anonymity. In the USA, the federal Occupational Safety and Health Administration (OSHA) has regulations that protect workers when exercising their rights regarding health and safety on the job, but in practice these regulations may not be sufficient to protect a worker from being fired.

If the employer is unwilling to cooperate directly with the healthcare provider, its management may

seek advice from the company's insurance carrier, and it may subsequently be willing to release the insurance company's report. This may provide useful information. Another option is for the employer to request help from a government consultation service. For example, in the USA, many states have programs funded jointly by the state government and the federal OSHA. Reports by these consultation groups are confidential, but the employer may be willing to share them with the independent occupational healthcare provider. Some employers prefer to hire their own private occupational hygiene consultants, or consult a university or other research organization, such as the National Institute for Occupational Safety and Health (NIOSH) in the USA.

For a resolutely uncooperative employer, it may be necessary to call a federal standards enforcement agency with jurisdiction at that workplace. In the USA, this would be OSHA. Some US states require reporting of sentinel or even suspected occupational illnesses to a public health or labor department within the state, but these state programs vary considerably over the extent of ensuing investigation. A call to the state or local public health department to discuss possible approaches to an unresponsive employer with a sentinel health event might nevertheless be helpful. Although many of these organizations can assist in the resolution of worksite health and safety problems, few have the resources to ensure that adequate follow-up is accomplished. Lack of employer cooperation may consequently result in delaying the identification and treatment of additional cases, and delaying the implementation of controls to prevent the development of new cases.

'Compliance' versus 'Public Health' approaches

The sentinel health event approach to occupational hygiene is based on a 'public health' model of using a case to identify additional cases, and to determine and control the hazardous exposure at the root of the problem. This approach is significantly different from a 'compliance' model, which generally presupposes that the short list of agents for which there are exposure standards includes all the potentially hazardous materials encountered in occupational settings. The compliance approach also assumes that the current standards are sufficient to protect workers from the initiation of occupational disease or the exacerbation of existing disease. Many occupational hygienists practice a compliance approach, relying on published standards to provide guidance as to what conditions are acceptable in the workplace. They do this in good faith, assuming that a workplace that is in compliance with these standards is a safe and healthy workplace.

However, there are now estimated to be over 68 000 chemicals in commerce in the USA [2]. Of these, only relatively few have standards for occupational exposures. Exposure limits are generally set by national governments, and terminology varies. For example: in the USA, the OSHA sets 'permissible exposure limits' (PELs); in the UK, the Health and Safety Executive sets 'occupational exposure limits' (OELs); in Germany, the Deutsch Forschungsgemeinschaft sets 'maximum allowable concentrations' (MACs).

Since 1942 a volunteer organization, the American Conference of Governmental Industrial Hygienists (ACGIH), has produced an independent annual listing of exposure limits called threshold limit values (TLVs), and in 1970 the OSHA PELs were established from the TLVs of 1968. The federal OSHA Act in the USA has provided for new standards to be adopted since 1970, but this process has not been applied sufficiently effectively to keep up with new chemicals and new health research. Since 1970 only 29 new or revised chemical standards have been added to the original PELs. The ACGIH TLV committee continues to update its TLVs at the rate of several a year, and these are widely used internationally as a basis for occupational health standards. However, the TLV process has come under considerable criticism, including charges of undue influence and conflict of interest among corporate consultants to the committee [3].

Thus, a public health approach using the sentinel health event model may often be more effective in protecting worker health because it does not depend exclusively on existing standards and air sampling results. Instead, in the sentinel health event model the occupational hygienist and physician work with the employer, the patient, and (if appropriate) the union or health and safety committee to identify potential hazardous exposures that may be associated with the sentinel patient's disease. The process is an interactive one where the occupational hygienist works with all the parties to develop interventions to control exposures, and then evaluates whether the interventions work [1]. In cases where the relevant exposure is easily identified and its relationship to health outcomes is well documented, this iterative process can work very well. When the hazard causing the occupational disorder is less clear, or when no specific outcome exists to indicate when efforts to reduce the hazard have been sufficient, this approach is more difficult to apply and may be less successful. A significant advantage of the public health approach is that it may be possible to bypass the costly and time-consuming need to make exposure measurements, moving directly to exposure control. This approach also allows for the improvement of worksite conditions in settings not previously associated with adverse health outcomes, or of exposures for which no standards exist.

Occupational safety and health programs

A good health and safety program in the workplace includes many components. Its breadth will reflect the overall importance the company places on the matter. Among regulatory agencies there is increasing emphasis on the creation of comprehensive programs tailored to individual worksites. Thus in the USA the OSHA, rather than issuing specification standards itself that require particular controls to be instituted, is taking an outcome-based approach which requires employers to set up effective programs to identify and control hazards. Similarly in the UK, there is now an obligation for employers to carry out a Control of Substances Hazardous to Health (COSHH) assessment within each workplace, and institute a suitable program of health protection that takes account of this. There is need for caution, however, if injury and illness statistics are the basis for judging program success, because this can encourage underreporting.

An example of this approach is the Voluntary Protection Program in which OSHA works with a company to ensure that a comprehensive health and safety program is incorporated into the management system. The key program areas can also be found in a number of voluntary Safety and Health Program Guidelines, published from 1989 (Table 33.1):

- Management Leadership and Employee Participation
- Workplace Hazard Analysis
- Accident and other Health and Safety Records Analysis
- Hazard Prevention and Control
- Emergency Response Planning
- Safety and Health Training

Use of these guidelines will help the employer to strengthen the overall health and safety plan, and thereby improve conditions for both the sentinel patient and all other workers at the facility. Companies operating in an international sphere are finding increasing benefit from obtaining certifications from the International Standards Organization

Table 33.1 Health and safety management guidelines

- Management Leadership and Employee Participation
  - management leadership (atmosphere, awareness, involvement and support for health and safety)
  - employee participation (atmosphere, awareness, involvement and support for health and safety)
  - joint labor and management health and safety committee
  - written health and safety program
  - implementation of health and safety program (adequate tools provided by management, including budget, information, personnel, assigned responsibility for actions, adequate expertise and authority, line accountability, and program review procedures)
  - outside contractor safety and health program review
- Workplace Hazard Analysis
  - regular survey and hazard analysis
  - inspection program
  - air sampling program
  - evaluation of new processes and new chemicals before used
  - results reported to individuals, health and safety committee, and responsible management
- Accident and Record Analysis
  - investigation of accidents and near-miss incidents
  - data analysis of injury and health records
  Hazard Prevention and Control
  - hazard control
  - maintenance of hazard control systems
  - medical surveillance program
- Emergency Response
  - emergency preparedness
  - first aid
- Safety and Health Training

(e.g. ISO 9000, Quality Management; ISO 14000, Environmental Management), and their desire for these may provide the occupational hygienist and the occupational health practitioner with useful leverage in building a strong health and safety program. A completely integrated health, safety, and environmental management system should become part of the total management system of the company.

Some occupational agents pose a need for specific health and safety programs. An example would be the relatively few identified by the US OSHA regulations since 1970 that have detailed specification standards. Thus benzene, lead, and asbestos, for example, require baseline exposure monitoring, which then determines the need for ongoing surveillance. If measured exposures are greater than a specified 'action level' (half of the occupational

exposure limit), then further exposure monitoring, medical monitoring, and training are required. If the measured exposures exceed the occupational exposure limit, all these program features, plus exposure reduction, are required.

Specific programs are required to deal with work in certain dangerous conditions, such as entry into hazardous spaces without easy egress. In the USA there are specific regulations under the OSHA for the use of respiratory protection, the training of workers, and the labeling of hazardous chemicals used in the workplace. All must be fully documented along with plans for implementation and review, and the documents should be reviewed by occupational health and hygiene practitioners responsible for worksite health and safety. However, a written program is only a first step, and for many employers, an easier one than actual implementation.

Unions and their role in health and safety

Perhaps the most important component of an effective health and safety program in the workplace is worker acceptance. A workforce that does not have a means to influence its conditions of employment is often cynical about health and safety programs, viewing them more as a basis for disciplinary action than worker well being. The best way to counteract this cynicism is to develop a program that demonstrates respect for worker input to the process. To this end, safety committees run jointly by management and labor can play a pivotal role. They are promoted by both the OSHA Voluntary Protection Program and the Safety and Health Program Management Guidelines, and in some US states their existence is required by law. Bracker and colleagues found that their existence correlated strongly with the actual implementation of control recommendations following a sentinel health event evaluation [1].

When investigating a sentinel health event it is important to work with representatives of labor to ensure optimal cooperation from the workforce. Not only may a trade union organization facilitate cooperation, but it may help contact members of the workforce absent through sickness. A number of unions exert wide influence through international offices, and their sophisticated health and safety departments may provide support at both local and national level on health and safety policy issues. However, in the USA, membership of trade unions has fallen from 38% of the national workforce in 1958 to 12% in 1990. Thus, many worksites do not have active unions, and lack of job security limits the role of workers on joint committees for health and safety.

IDENTIFICATION OF OCCUPATIONAL HAZARDS

Once a sentinel health event has been recognized, there is a need to identify the cause. This is best achieved by reviewing the relevant industrial processes undertaken in the patient's workplace, and by a qualitative evaluation of the workplace itself. For the latter a walk-through survey is invaluable.

Industrial processes

It is generally useful to interview the patient with the sentinel health event for details of the product(s) under manufacture, the raw materials, and the processes involved, although not all members of the workforce will have sufficiently comprehensive knowledge. The specific tasks of the affected patient, both usual and unusual (e.g. maintenance or clean-up), are of obvious and critical importance; and an enquiry should be made concerning any exposure controls already in place and the nature of any health and safety training. Workers can often provide useful information on the identity and quantity of specific chemicals in use, the frequency of potential exposure to them, the number of fellow workers at risk, and among them the prevalence of relevant symptoms or confirmed diagnoses.

The occupational hygienist or physician unfamiliar with the particular operations of the patient's workplace must then research the basic industrial processes in use from basic texts such as Burgess [4], Cralley and Cralley [5], and the International Labor Organization's encyclopedia [6]. Additional information about the plant's operations should be sought from management, including process flow diagrams, plant maps, and a list of materials used in the various processes. Material Safety Data Sheets (MSDSs) for chemicals used in the areas where the sentinel patient worked should also be obtained. The availability of MSDSs is regulated in the USA under the OSHA Hazard Communication standard. This requires that substances be labeled so that employees and their physicians can identify the constituents of every product. There must also be ready access to the MSDS of each end product. It must describe the potential adverse health effects, physical properties, and conditions of safe use and storage. Additionally, workers must be trained in the safe use of each material with which they work in a language that they understand (Table 33.2).

Any air sampling data collected by the company, their insurance carrier, or any compliance agency that pertain to the exposures of the sentinel case should also be requested. In the USA, such informa-tion is available to a treating physician under the OSHA regulations.

Qualitative worksite evaluation

The risk of illness is a function of the toxicity of the material in combination with the opportunity for exposure, the intensity of exposure, and the duration of exposure. The initial concern is qualitative – what exposures are likely to be occurring?

It is mainly through the walk-through survey that adequate information concerning the opportunity, intensity, and duration of any potential exposure can be acquired. It is only by observation or detailed interviews that the potential for worker contact with a hazardous agent can be evaluated. For example, processes that occur for 15 min once a month and use small quantities of moderately toxic substances at room temperature with good local exhaust ventilation may prove to be of less concern than a continuous, uncontrolled exposure to a less toxic chemical that is heated or used in some other way (e.g. aerosolized) that will increase the likelihood of a high airborne concentrations. Good preparation of what to expect of specific industries and particular operations is helpful, but plants vary. The walk-through provides an opportunity to note the various factors that impact exposure (Table 33.3).

The walk-through survey

For a person unfamiliar with a given worksite, the facility is most easily grasped if the tour begins at the start of a manufacturing process, where the raw materials are received; follows the flow of the manufacturing process though to the final product; and ends with its packaging and shipping. During this walk-through of the entire facility it is important to get as good an idea as possible of what is used where, how it is used, and how many people are exposed. Process parameters such as temperature, production rates, material usage rates, and the physical forms of the substances are all pertinent. Physical demands of the job and payment basis for the worker (salary or piece rate) should be noted. Local exhaust ventilation and any other engineering controls should also be noted. If personal protective equipment is used, note the specific type of protective respirator and cartridge, the glove, or other protective item. General housekeeping and maintenance should be evaluated.

At each process step, the qualitative evaluation should focus on identifying, locating, and observing sources of any chemicals (or other agents) that have potential health hazards. These sources could be process chemicals, process byproducts, process tooling, or some part of the building materials es-

Table 33.2 The Material Safety Data Sheet (MSDS)

Material Safety Data Sheets should be available for each material used in the workplace. In the USA, MSDSs are required under the federal OSHA regulation on Hazard Communication (29CFR 1910.1200). MSDSs contain much useful information, but it is important to bear in mind that not all of them are prepared completely and accurately. It may be necessary to contact the manufacturer to verify or update information. The following information should be available on an MSDS.

Section I: Product Identity
This section gives the name of the product as it appears on the label and the company's chemical inventory list; usually this is also the shop floor name. The manufacturer and a contact name and number should also be listed here.

Section II: Hazardous Ingredients
This section gives the chemical names and CAS (Chemical Abstract Service) number of every hazardous component that makes up more than 1% of the substance that has been deemed 'hazardous' (0.1% if that component is a carcinogen). This section also gives relevant exposure limits.

Section III: Physical Data
This section provides critical information about the properties of chemicals, such as vapor pressure, vapor density, boiling point, and evaporation rate. These factors enable an estimation of whether or not there is likely to be significant airborne exposure (those with high vapor pressure and evaporation rates).

Section IV: Fire and Explosion Hazard Data
This section contains basic information on fire prevention and control. The flashpoint is that temperature at which enough vapor is generated to sustain a fire if a spark is introduced. The lower the flashpoint, the greater the risk of fire.

Section V: Reactivity Data
This section gives information on how likely the chemical is to break down or to react with other substances, causing fires, explosions, or the release of other potentially dangerous chemicals. This section may also contain conditions relevant to storage (e.g. store apart from acids, store away from sunlight).

Section VI: Health Hazard Data
This section explains how the chemical may enter the body and how it may affect health. It is usually divided into acute and chronic health effects. Carcinogens must be identified. This section often does not contain the most recent toxicologic information on the components of the product, and may need updating.

Section VII: Precautions for Safe Handling and Use
This section should give information on what to do in case of spillage, and what to do in case of emergency. It should also give procedures for proper waste disposal.

Section VIII: Control Measures
This section provides information on ventilation and safe work practices. It should also describe very specifically what types of protective respirators and respirator cartridges should be used. It should also give details of what types of glove or clothing material are protective for the chemical components of the product.

caping into the workplace air. Examples include tungsten carbide from tool sharpening, flaking lead paint from overhead beams, or fiberglass (or microbial contaminants) from ventilation duct lining entering the ventilation system. Sometimes the most hazardous exposures can be a result of non-production operations such as cleaning or maintenance.

At each step where products are processed and potentially toxic materials are used, some assessment should be made of the possibility of worker contact. What are the possible routes of entry to the body for the hazardous agent (inhalation, ingestion, skin absorption, injection)? What is the intensity and duration of the potential exposure? Is it possible to envision a reasonable scenario in which the worker comes into sufficient contact with the agent to cause symptoms? Vapor pressure (the pressure exerted when the vapor of an agent is in equilibrium with its liquid or solid form) is an important characteristic to assess potential expo-

sure to volatile solvents. Vapors are the gaseous forms of substances that are normally in a liquid (or solid) state at room temperature and pressure. A liquid with a high vapor pressure will be found in the air in higher concentrations than a liquid with a low vapor pressure. However, vapor pressure increases with temperature, and any heating process will increase a chemical's vapor pressure and its concentration in air. It is helpful to spend as much time as possible in the area where the sentinel case occurred, observing. A case of oil folliculitis on the thighs may, for example, be caused by the storage of a wiping rag in a pocket, even when the outside of the pants does not appear to be contaminated. A worker with a skin allergy to rubber and a wrist rash may be using his/her wrists to store rubber bands, without being aware of either the action or the exposure.

Sometimes the potential for airborne exposure is reduced through the use of ventilation or other

Table 33.3 Guidelines for the worksite walk-through survey

The purpose of a walk-though survey is to identify potential health hazards based on the toxicity of the materials used in combination with the intensity and duration of potential exposures. Once identified, hazards are subject to further evaluation and control.

Before the Walk-through

■ Research the industry to gain an understanding of the processes used and any known hazards associated with the processes.

■ Obtain Material Safety Data Sheets (MSDSs) for chemicals used in the processes.

■ Use the MSDSs to research the toxicity of the chemical components of the raw materials used in the processes or the products of the processes.

■ Evaluate hazards of chemical intermediates or byproducts of a process.

■ Obtain reports of any occupational or environmental evaluations that may have been performed previously.

The Walk-through

■ Include members of the health and safety committee, as well as union and management representatives on your walk-through.

■ Start at the beginning, following the process flow.

■ Obtain or develop a diagram of the process.

■ Obtain a map with the facility floor plan.

■ Observe each process step and how workers do each task within the process step.

■ Note the following:

– usage of toxic materials previously identified

– process parameters including temperature, production rates, material usage rates, physical form of substances involved, anything that is likely to affect exposure

– observe proximity to chemicals used in process and potential for worker exposure by skin contact, ingestion, or inhalation

– evidence of gases, vapors, dusts, or mists (use your eyes, nose, and ears)

– note duration of potential exposure

– numbers of workers exposed

– observe work practices, especially those that may affect exposure such as any compressed air cleaning, contact with rag and solvent, any skin contact, awkward postures

– engineering controls such as local exhaust ventilation, enclosures, shielding, special tooling

– personal protective equipment used

– physical demands of job (workload may increase breathing rate and mouth breathing, increasing exposure)

– environment with excessive heat or cold (a physical stressor that may also alter chemical metabolism)

– housekeeping

– labeling of containers, pipes, piping systems, and waste containers

– general ventilation or other building conditions that may impact exposures.

■ Ask about processes not being done during the walk-through, such as cleaning, maintenance, unusual production processes.

The Report

■ *Summary*. Briefly summarize observations, list any major hazards identified, and recommend future controls or further evaluation needed.

■ *Introduction and background*

– include a brief description of who you are, why you are there, the purpose and the scope of your evaluation; do not discuss any individuals or medical records

– date and time of walk-through.

– description of facility, employees, and any health and safety committee

– description of processes and products

– plant layout

■ *Walk-through results*

– observations during walk-through, process step by process step

– discuss potential health hazards from process (include toxicity as well as degree of contact, intensity and duration)

– describe applicable regulations

– discuss the results of any testing that you may have done during the walk-through; note what you observed and what you were unable to observe

– report how walk-through results compare with any previous assessments you have obtained

■ *Recommendations for controls or further evaluations needed*

engineering controls. Many manufacturing facilities will have some form of local exhaust to extract hazardous emissions, and when high levels of exhaust ventilation are necessary high flow rates of fresh air have to be supplied. This sometimes results in discharged contaminants being entrained into the incoming air flow and returned to the building. Examination of the location of air intakes and exhausts is therefore an important step in most walk-through visits. It is also necessary to learn if there are any air filtering devices that may be removing contaminants before air is recirculated within the worksite. Recirculation may be necessary, for example, to limit the costs of heating or maintaining constant humidity. If so, maintenance and cleaning of the filtering devices can be highly hazardous procedures. If inadequately maintained, the filters may fail in their primary task and exhausted contaminants may be returned into the workplace air.

The qualitative walk-through evaluation is necessary to develop an effective strategy for quantitative evaluation. However, sometimes the qualitative evaluation is sufficient on its own to reveal the cause of a problem and so point to its solution without incurring the effort and cost of a thorough quantitative evaluation.

EVALUATION OF OCCUPATIONAL HAZARDS

Once hazardous agents have been identified, it may be desirable to quantify exposure levels. This can be a difficult task. The primary route of chemical exposure is through inhalation, and occupational standards for chemicals focus on this route. However, airborne exposure levels do not necessarily indicate the true dose sustained because there are variations in inhalation rate, absorption, clearance, and metabolism among individuals. In addition, there is increasing evidence that dermal exposures not only cause dermatitis but may also contribute to a variety of respiratory and systemic diseases. In addition to these difficulties, many chemicals have neither standard methods for sampling and analysis, nor any reference levels or standards for comparison. Finally, many workers are exposed to a mixture of chemicals, yet there are no standard ways to take account of these mixtures in exposure assessments. In fact, there has been very little toxicologic research on the health effects of mixed exposures.

Before recommending that air sampling be done, it is consequently important to be clear about the indication and the use that will be made of the results. How will sampling assist in reducing the hazards faced by the sentinel patient or fellow workers? How will the results be interpreted? When should exposure levels be considered too high or low enough? The answers to these questions will help determine what should be measured, as well as when, from where, and for how long the samples should be taken. The most common reasons include:

1. guidance for the design of engineering systems for exposure control
2. evaluation of their effect after introduction
3. baseline requirement as part of regulatory requirements
4. determination of compliance with regulations
5. development of an exposure database for research

Quantitative evaluations

In many cases, the choice of what chemicals to sample is driven by the compliance approach. In that case, the chemicals chosen for sampling will be those with the highest likelihood of exceeding their exposure standards. However, in the regulatory environment of the USA, only the 26 chemical standards developed since 1970 carry the specific requirement for initial or regular sampling to evaluate workplace exposures. For other hazardous occupational agents there is no obligation to prove compliance – the burden of proof remains with regulatory agencies to document that a standard has been exceeded. As the regulations stand there is little incentive for regular sampling by the employer [7].

If the purpose is to follow up a sentinel case, then the air sampling effort will focus on the chemical that has been identified as the probable causal agent. However, for occupational hygienists investigating a sentinel case there is often no specific chemical recognized to cause the disease in question. When complex mixtures are involved and no specific component stands out, it may be necessary to choose either a few key components or a single substance which acts as a marker for the whole mixture. The 'key components' approach usually targets chemicals present in the greatest quantity, those with high vapor pressures, or substances that are the most toxic. The latter may also be those with low occupational exposure limits. On the other hand, the approach to mixture evaluation that focuses on choosing a marker, will look for a chemical that is easy and inexpensive to sample, unique in its source generation, unaffected by other air contaminants, and proportional to the total mixture of interest [8]. Examples of marker sampling include measuring nicotine levels in air samples as a reflection of the passive cigarette smoke concentration or measuring elemental carbon in particulate samples as a marker of diesel exhaust.

Most occupational air sampling is achieved by workers wearing a small passive gas/vapor sampling badge or carrying a small battery operated pump connected to a particle or gas/vapor sampler. These 'personal samplers' are attached to the lapel of workers and provide the best estimate of exposure levels in their breathing zone (Fig. 33.2). Area samples, taken by placing the sampler in a stationary location, tend to underestimate the true exposures of the breathing zone. They can nevertheless be very useful in evaluating the effectiveness of newly installed exposure controls. Samples are usually collected over the length of the task of concern or for the whole workday, depending on the underlying purpose. For example, sampling to determine regulatory compliance usually requires a full workshift (8 hour) exposure to be measured.

In some situations it is desirable to sample for shorter periods. Short-term exposure limits (STELs) are 15 min averaged exposure standards developed to protect against irritation, narcosis, and irreversible tissue damage resulting from high short-term exposures [9]. The most biologically relevant sampling period depends on the toxicokinetics of the substance, its uptake, its half-life of elimination, and the nature of the potential adverse effect [10]. For developing control strategies it is often useful to sample during specific tasks or particular manufacturing procedures to determine whether they are major contributors to a worker's exposure, and to produce a baseline measure for postcontrol comparisons.

Physical state of air contaminants

In addition to the chemical composition of airborne exposures, their physical form is important in evaluating their hazard. Airborne chemicals can be in either a particulate (aerosol) form, including dusts, fumes, and mists, or a vapor/gaseous form. A chem-

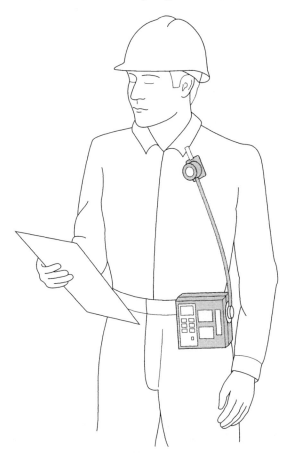

Fig. 33.2 A worker wearing a personal air sampler, which includes a small portable pump connected by tubing to a filter holder designed to collect the inhalable fraction of particulate matter. (Courtesy of SKC Inc.)

ical substance normally in the gaseous state at room temperature and pressure is called a gas. Vapors occur when a substance, that is normally a liquid (or solid) at room temperature and pressure, evaporates. In practice, substances that are normally liquid at normal temperature and pressure are often in equilibrium with their gaseous forms.

To an occupational hygienist, a dust consists of solid particles formed by mechanical processes. A fume is made up of very small particles produced when a solid that has been vaporized, condenses, as in welding. A mist consists of droplets of liquid dispersed into the air, as in spray painting. Biologic agents, such as bacteria, viruses, and fungi are treated as a special form of aerosol, especially if they are found in the airborne state as a component of a mist.

Quantitative sampling

Aerosol/particulate exposures

Aerosol quantification has come a long way since the 1950s and early 1960s when the transition was made from impinger sampling with microscopic particle counting to filter sampling with gravimetric analysis. The current movement is toward particle size-selective sampling and the development of particle size-selective standards for aerosols, since particle size is the chief determinant for the likely site of deposition and hence the likely site for adverse effects. The ACGIH in coordination with the International Standards Organization (ISO) and the European Standardization Committee (CEN) has developed a set of sampling criteria based on particle penetration into various regions of the respiratory tract (Fig. 33.3) [11]. These criteria will also be used to determine what type of size-selective standard should be applied to a chemical in liquid or solid particulate form.

'Inhalable' criteria are to be used with insoluble agents that can cause adverse health effects when deposited anywhere in the respiratory tract (i.e. the gas exchanging, tracheobronchial, or nasopharyngeal regions) (Fig. 33.3). The inhalable criteria should also be used with soluble materials that are absorbed across mucosal surfaces, resulting in systemic effects. These criteria specify a sampler that collects 50% of the particles with an aerodynamic diameter of 100 μm or greater, as well as smaller particles (Fig. 33.4) [11,12].

'Thoracic' (a subset of inhalable) criteria are to be used for agents whose adverse effects occur only when deposited within the tracheobronchial or the gas exchanging region of the lung (Fig. 33.3). These criteria specify a sampler that collects 50% of the particles with an aerodynamic diameter of 10 μm,

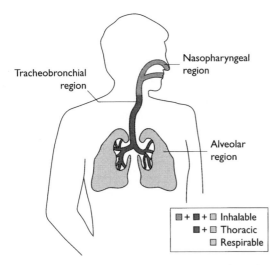

Fig. 33.3 Size-selective particulate standards are based on where particulates of various sizes can deposit in the respiratory tract. The inhalable fraction refers to particles that can deposit anywhere in the respiratory system. The thoracic fraction refers to particles that can deposit in the tracheobronchial or pulmonary region. The respirable fraction is for particles that can deposit in the alveolar region of the lung. (Courtesy of SKC Inc.)

as well as smaller particles and a few larger particles (Fig. 33.4) [11,12].

'Respirable' (a subset of thoracic) criteria are to be used for inhalation exposures to particles whose adverse effects occur only in the gas exchanging (alveolar) region of the lung (Fig. 33.3). These criteria specify a sampler that collects 50% of the particles with an aerodynamic diameter of 4 μm, as well as smaller particles and a few larger particles (Fig. 33.4) [11,12].

In the USA and the EU, personal aerosol sampling devices are available commercially that meet the size-selective sampling criteria (Fig. 33.4). The Environmental Protection Agency (EPA) in the USA has set up different sets of size-selective sampling criteria for par-

ticulate matter (PM). These are specified as PM 2.5 (50% collection of particles of aerodynamic diameter 2.5 μm) and PM 10 (50% collection of particles of aerodynamic diameter 10 μm) [13]. The PM 10 samples are similar in collection criteria to the 'thoracic' samplers, although they are, in most cases, large area samplers that are not suitable for use as personal samplers. The PM 2.5 sampler has no biologic basis. It was designed to collect small aerosols generated from combustion and its reaction byproducts. Samplers based on these EPA sampling criteria are primarily used for ambient environmental sampling rather than for occupational measurements.

Once aerosol samples have been collected, they are usually first analyzed gravimetrically. A number of specific additional analytical procedures may be carried out subsequently, which typically include atomic absorption for metals, X-ray diffraction for crystalline materials, microscopy for fibers, and high-pressure liquid chromatography for reactive organic compounds. Standard methods for sampling and analysis can be found in the NIOSH Manual of Analytical Methods, and are also available on the internet [14].

Gas/vapor exposures

Traditional integrated gas and vapor air samples are collected using personal sampling pumps connected to solid sorbent tubes containing activated charcoal or porous polymers, or by passive badges containing these same materials. The use of passive badges is expanding due to their convenient unobtrusive nature, low capital cost, and reports of good accuracy and precision for most applications [15]. However, only badges that have completed a thorough validation protocol, such as those proposed by NIOSH in the USA or by the Health and Safety Executive in the UK, should be used in workplace sampling. Analysis methods for gas/vapor samples

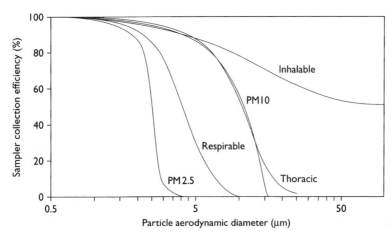

Fig. 33.4 Each size-selective particulate standard defines the mass fraction of each particle size that should be collected by the ideal air sampler. In addition to the occupational standards for inhalable, thoracic, and respirable fractions, there are environmental standards for the collection of particulate matter (PM 2.5 and PM 10).

typically include gas chromatography and high-pressure liquid chromatography. Standard methods for sampling and analysis can be found in the NIOSH Manual of Analytical Methods, and are also available on the internet [14].

If a hazard exists in both the aerosol and vapor phases, the occupational hygienist must account for the total exposure when planning a sampling strategy [16]. An example of this problem is often seen in evaluations of pesticide exposure or any spray application of a chemical mixture. Many pesticide and spray-painting operations represent both a vapor and aerosol hazard, yet often only one phase is collected.

Direct reading instruments

There is a wide variety of 'direct reading' instruments available for particulate or gas and vapor sampling [17]. The major advantage of these is that they give an immediate readout of concentration levels since they do not require laboratory analysis. They are a crucial part of the equipment used in confined space entry, emergency response, and the clean up of hazardous waste for this reason.

There are direct reading instruments that are very qualitative and others that are very quantitative. It is important to note that the quantitative instruments often have poorer precision and higher limits of detection than traditional methods of sampling and laboratory analysis. More important, in the real world, direct reading instruments are often non-specific in mixed chemical environments due to interference by chemicals of similar structure. This can result in incorrect estimation of the true concentration. It is easy for an inexperienced user to be overconfident with the readings produced by a direct reading instrument and to be unaware of how important maintenance and routine calibration are for proper functioning. When calibrated appropriately and used correctly, direct reading instruments with data logging and computer downloading capabilities can provide useful real-time methods for analysis of the contributions of various work activities to the exposure profile of an individual worker. When direct reading instruments are combined with videotaped exposure monitoring, they can also be quite useful in developing control strategies.

Interpretation of air sampling results

It is quite common to reference air sampling results to existing occupational health standards. As mentioned in the Introduction, many of the OSHA standards in the USA are now quite dated, having been based on a Threshold Limit Value (TLV) listing of 1968. In addition, one analysis of the data used to establish the TLV listings found that only a minority of the recommended TLVs were associated with no adverse health effects. The authors concluded that the TLVs 'may represent guides to levels that have been achieved (in industry) but they are certainly not thresholds' [18]. That air sampling results indicate compliance with published occupational exposure limits does not mean that the health condition identified is not related to workplace exposure.

The determination of compliance based on an air sampling result is, in reality, a complex task. A single sampling result can be compared with an occupational exposure limit or action level to determine whether the workplace was in compliance at the particular time and under the particular conditions when the sample was obtained. However, exposures vary tremendously from day to day, and even from worker to worker, due to variations in ventilation, season, weather, manufacturing process, production rate, work shift, individual work practices, and other factors. Thus much of the interpretation of sampling results comes from understanding how representative any given sample is of normal (or unusual) conditions.

When a sufficient number of samples are taken, analysis of the exposure levels usually shows them to follow a lognormal distribution. This skewed distribution is best described by a geometric mean (exponentiated mean of the logged exposure values) and a geometric standard deviation (GSD; exponentiated standard deviation of the logged exposure values). The geometric mean is always lower than the arithmetic mean, because the distribution is typically characterized by a tail of high exposures (Fig. 33.5). Of course, the more controlled the process, the smaller the tail of the distribution (lower GSD) and the more alike the arithmetic and geometric means will be. Because of the characteristic nature of the lognormal distribution, a few samples with relatively low concentrations cannot provide confidence that high levels of exposures do not occur.

In practice, the occupational hygienist and healthcare provider are often given a table showing results from a very few samples. The table will usually give the date and substance analyzed, the sampling times, and the results, accompanied by an occupational exposure limit. There is rarely any narrative describing why the samples were taken or what conditions existed during sampling. Little can be said based on results like these. Only with further sampling, and statistical analysis of the results after grouping workers with similar jobs, could the fraction of random samples likely to exceed the standard (or some health effect level) be estimated [19].

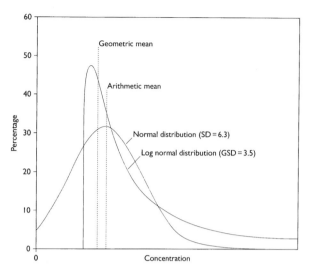

Fig. 33.5 The distribution of air sampling data is most often described as log normal. Such distributions are skewed to the right, compared to a normal distribution with the same arithmetic mean. The geometric mean is used to describe the central tendency of a log normal distribution. As a log normal distribution becomes less skewed (smaller geometric standard deviation), the arithmetic and geometric means become more similar.

Another common outcome among sampling results is that the particular agent was 'not detectable' (ND). This is commonly interpreted to mean that none was airborne. A 'ND' determination is made by the analytical laboratory when the sample accumulated on the collection media does not exceed the limit of detection (LOD) of the method. Such a result frequently occurs when short sampling periods are used, and the sample is inadequate. Depending on the sensitivity of the method and the sampling time, an ND result could even occur at exposures equal to the occupational exposure limit. If ND results are not to be misleading they should be reported as less than whatever concentration (mass/air volume) results from dividing the limit of detection for the method (mass/sample) by the volume of air collected for that sample (air volume/sample).

If air sampling results are to be compared to occupational standards, the duration of exposure (usually the working shift) has to be kept in mind. If it exceeds the standard period of 8 hours, a reduction factor can be applied to the occupational exposure limit so that the permissible cumulative level of exposure is not exceeded and account is taken of the decreased period for recovery. Several approaches are possible to provide a reduction factor (RF) which is multiplied by the exposure limit. Two such formulae were presented by Brief and Scala [20]:

RF = 8/sh × [(24 − sh)/16] for a 5-day working week, where sh is the shift length in hours

RF = 40/wh × [(168 − wh)/128] for a 7-day working week, where wh is the number of working hours per week

When exposure is to a mixture of compounds believed to have the same adverse effects (e.g. neurotoxicity from organic solvents), and each compound has an exposure limit, then the current compliance approach is to assume that the exposures are additive. Overexposure to the mixture can be evaluated using the following formula:

C1/OEL1 + C2/OEL2 ... Cn/OELn ≥ 1 indicates overexposure

where *C* is the measured concentration in air, and OEL is the occupational exposure limit for the compound.

The adequacy of this approach has not been determined by toxicologic research.

CONTROL OF OCCUPATIONAL HAZARDS

Recommendations based on worksite surveys

Since many workplaces have the same basic deficiencies, common industrial hygiene recommendations can be put into a standard checklist [21]. In the USA the health and safety regulation most commonly cited is a lack of or deficiency in the Hazard Communication Program (29 CFR 1910.1200). This standard requires training, labeling of hazardous chemicals, and onsite cataloging of MSDSs. Other commonly cited regulatory deficiencies include poor programs or program elements in the areas of personal protective equipment, respiratory protection, and hearing protection programs.

Training is a very important part of occupational health and one to which a healthcare provider can make a valuable contribution. Educational material can be provided to workers who come to an occupational health clinic. For example, there are excellent training materials on noise, noise reduction in the workplace, and hearing that can be used effectively in the context of annual audiometry. An occupational health practice might supply a series of fact sheets describing the components of a good health and safety system with specific information on the particular hazards within their contract companies. Many good fact sheets, relating to a wide variety of substances, are now available on the internet (see Internet Resources below).

For the occupational hygienist or physician who has made a workplace evaluation on behalf of a patient, a report is required for patient, physicians, and employer. It is always very important to keep all parties well informed of progress because the sentinel case may signify an outbreak of occupational disease. As a rule, the better the communication, the more cooperative all parties are and the more quickly and favorably the situation is resolved. A workplace evaluation report should describe the workplace and processes in a general way, and provide more detail about the processes carried out in the area of concern. This will give everyone an understanding of what was observed and how it was assessed (Fig. 33.6). Some discussion may be provided of the generic relationship of the potential hazards to the symptoms or disease suspected, but no individual's medical findings should be referred to in this report. Rules of patient confidentiality apply, and no medical information can be included in a report that is sent to an employer. The suggestions given in this report should be recommendations for improvements in safety in the workplace with an overall goal of producing a healthier work environment.

Recommendations may be general suggestions for improvement in programs or training, or specific steps to reduce exposures. Controls can be targeted at the emission source or the pathway of the exposures once emitted, or focused on the workers themselves. The most effective control is almost always at the source, so that emissions are reduced. The next most desirable step in the hierarchy is to intervene as early as possible in the pathway between source of contaminant and the worker. Interventions focused on the worker are, perhaps, the least desirable, since there is then no further line of defense if the intervention is unhelpful. Furthermore, personal protective equipment is far less effective under conditions of 'real world' use than in laboratory testing and certification situations. Personal protective equipment should only be used when all other attempts to control exposures have failed to be fully

satisfactory, or until other measures have been completed (Fig. 33.6). Several of the most important control strategies listed in Fig. 33.6 bear further discussion.

Toxic use reduction

Toxic use reduction (TUR) is a control strategy that evaluates the manufacturing process to determine whether the emission of hazardous agents can be controlled at their source (Fig. 33.6). Individual tactics include change (even elimination) in the manufacturing process, improvements in operations and maintenance, substitution of less toxic chemicals, product reformulation, use of wet for dry methods, and in-process recycling. A historical example of TUR occurred in 1941 in the USA, when the federal Public Health Service, the State of Connecticut Department of Public Health, industry, and labor unions agreed to replace mercuric nitrate with non-mercury compounds in the process of felt hat manufacture. The substitution worked, protecting workers from mercury toxicity and preserving the industry. Not all attempts at replacement are quite this successful. The difficulty lies in selecting an appropriate substitute. If a substitute does not work well, it will not be used. Some substances have been replaced with compounds of unstudied toxicity that have subsequently turned out to have hazards of their own. Substitution must be done with great care.

Many substitutions help the environment, as well as worker health and safety, if chosen after careful toxicologic review. Chlorinated hydrocarbons were a great innovation in the 1960s and 1970s, reducing substantially the fire hazard from previously used flammable solvents, but they are now known to be

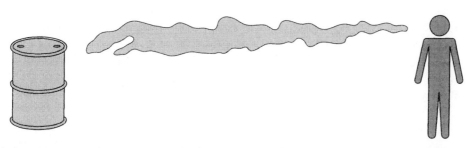

Emission source controls	Environmental (path) controls	Controls through worker
Substitution	Process enclosure	Training and education
Process change	Process Isolation	Limit duration of exposure
Process elimination	Local exhaust ventilation	(administrative rotation of workers)
Automation	Dilution ventilation	Personal protective equipment
Dry to wet methods	Housekeeping	(respirator, gloves, helmet, glasses
Preventive maintenance	Enclose worker	and clothing)
Product reformulation	(use remote control)	
In-process recycling		

Fig. 33.6 The control of workplace hazards can occur at the source, at the worker, or anywhere along the pathway between.

hazardous to both worker health and the environment (damage to the ozone layer). As a result, water-based cleaners are being substituted to remove oils from metals, and non-chlorinated compounds containing hydrofluorocarbons are being substituted in air conditioning. Other changes in the manufacturing process can also reduce ambient exposures. For example, the use of a cold process instead of a hot process could lower the vapor pressure of a toxic material and thus reduce the airborne concentration; a chemical could be added in slurry rather than powder form, reducing the release of dust. In paint-spraying operations, high-pressure sprays can be replaced with low-pressure spray guns, electrostatic painting, powder coating, or powder dipping to reduce the generation of aerosols.

Due to increasing costs for the disposal of toxic materials, source reduction through material conservation and in-process recycling has become ever more popular. These programs often translate into better housekeeping overall and lower ambient exposures.

Engineering controls

There are a variety of means of reducing worker exposures after hazardous agents have been emitted from a manufacturing process [22]. For example, an enclosure supplied with clean air could be built around the control panel which the worker operates. Perhaps a hazardous job could be automated. Automation, almost always done for speeding up production rather than increasing safety, sometimes benefits workers by allowing them to move further away from an emission source. Most often local exhaust ventilation for the process is recommended. This is used to remove contaminants from ambient air as close to the point of generation as possible.

Ancillary processes not directly involved in production may also cause or contribute to hazards in the workplace, and these too may be controlled by engineering modifications. In the USA, one successful modification was the reduction in the 1970s of pressure in compressed air lines from 100 to 30 pounds per square inch (psi). This reduced noise, injuries, and (when the compressed air lines were used for cleaning or spraying operations) exposure levels to chemicals.

Administrative controls

Reducing the time workers are scheduled to be present in contaminated areas will control duration, if not intensity of exposure, and so limit the cumulative exposure level. Such control is most often applied with radiation where workers (called 'jumpers') are used to repair nuclear reactors until they have received their maximum allowable dose of radiation. Risk of repetitive motion injuries may similarly be decreased by limiting the duration of repetitive tasks, varying the tasks within a given job, and by rotating workers from job to job. It can be difficult to maintain these administrative controls when production demands increase.

Personal protective equipment

Personal protective equipment (PPE) should be the method of last resort used when emission, engineering, and administrative controls are not able to provide sufficient reduction in exposure. PPE provides a final protective barrier between the exposure and the worker: gloves, laboratory coats, coveralls, ear plugs, face shields, glasses, goggles, hard hats, boots, respirators, etc. The key to selecting appropriate PPE is matching the device to the nature and intensity of the hazard, the task, and the comfort of the worker. If this is improperly done, exposure still occurs. For example, if gloves are breached, the barrier is compromised. If precision handling is required a heavy glove will not be used. If the respirator does not fit properly or has the wrong air purifying cartridge (or the worker takes it off), exposure occurs. Even hearing protection must be matched to the noise exposure profile.

It is commonly believed that PPE provides the easiest and most effective method of controlling worker exposure. It does not. PPE can be extremely uncomfortable, since it may be heavy and cumbersome, and often retains body heat. It usually impedes communication and may be almost impossible to tolerate for long periods. Therefore, worker compliance with PPE use is often poor. In order for properly selected PPE to provide effective protection each worker must accept the discomfort as a necessary trade-off for his or her health protection. Unless other means of exposure control have been attempted, the use of PPE is unlikely to gain acceptance.

It is important to remember that there are many costs to a PPE program that may not be initially apparent. They involve the initial equipment, as well as any initial or ongoing medical and environmental surveillance, worker and supervisor training, equipment maintenance, cleaning, and storage. The total true cost and the difficulty of ensuring compliance within the workforce, generally lead to the conclusion that PPE is not the solution of choice. In the USA, the law does not permit permanent reliance on respiratory protection in most situations.

Housekeeping and maintenance

The importance of good housekeeping and maintenance should need no emphasis. Dust that is not on the floor cannot be kicked up to become airborne again; unused chemicals that are properly disposed of cannot react to form dangerous byproducts. Faulty equipment can cause accidents, be noisy, overheat, and generate more dust and vapor. Metal working fluids that are not maintained properly grow bacteria and fungi, and are an increasingly recognized source of occupational respiratory disease.

Training

Training is now widely recognized as an important factor in improving health and safety practices in any workplace. Modern training programs use an active, skill based format that provides frequent feedback on progress. Evaluations of these programs have shown that they provide significant improvements in workplace health and safety [23].

Sustainable production

The term implies a proactive approach to industrial manufacture which aims to develop production systems that are non-polluting; economically efficient; safe and healthy for workers, neighbors, and consumers; socially and creatively rewarding for employees; and which conserve energy and natural resources [24]. Sustainable production is achieved by setting health, safety, and preservation of the environment as major parameters in the design and evaluation of new or existing production processes. It involves a systematic analysis of process hazards, checklists of sustainable production criteria for all plant personnel involved in the design or purchase of equipment or chemicals, and the development of standards for operating procedures, job requirements, and job training to make each job 'inherently safe'. Also covered under the rubric of sustainable production are the reduction of waste; diminished use of toxic substances; and development of products and packaging that maximize the product to raw materials ratio, conserve energy, and encourage recycling.

OUTCOMES OF SENTINEL CASES AND RECOMMENDATIONS

Very little work has been done in evaluating the effectiveness of sentinel case investigations. The exception is a study of 76 cases seen through an occupational medicine clinic [1]. Site visits were made to the patient's worksite and/or home, a written report including recommendations was sent to the employer, and health education materials were distributed at the worksite. The majority of recommended interventions involved engineering controls, followed by administrative controls, use of personal protective equipment, chemical or process substitution, and worker training.

Subsequent interviews found that 78% of the employers had implemented at least one of the recommended interventions. Employers were 3.7 times more likely to implement the priority intervention if they believed that the worker's illness was indeed work-related. However, this study found no relationship between the physician's view of the work-relatedness of the disease and the employer's view.

Employers with joint labor–management health and safety committees were 3.8 times more likely to implement the priority intervention. The sentinel patients were 10.4 times more likely to be still working if the employer had implemented any intervention. Those patients who left their original employer and found new work elsewhere suffered a median decrease in salary of 35%. The authors concluded that substantial improvements in patient health can be achieved through the sentinel health event model, even though most recommendations were not implemented [1].

Experience and research suggest that aggressive follow-up by the occupational hygienist and physician is the most effective way to bring about improvements in a worker's health and the general conditions of the worksite. This process may be iterative and may involve working closely with the employer over a period of years.

SUMMARY POINTS

- A public health approach to occupational hygiene focuses on the identification, evaluation, and control of potential hazards in the workplace, rather than on compliance with occupational exposure standards.
- The walk-through survey of a workplace is an important step in evaluating occupational health hazards, because it provides important information on the nature, intensity, and duration of potential exposures.
- Fundamental to any quantitative evaluation of exposures is the development of a comprehensive sampling strategy that is based on the reason for the sampling (compliance, baseline, epidemiological study, exposure control).
- The hierarchy of exposure control starts with the measures that are the most effective, i.e. those that

- target changes at the source of the exposure (process change, substitution, preventive maintenance).
- These are followed in the hierarchy by control measures which are implemented along the pathway between the source of the hazard and the worker (local exhaust ventilation, source enclosure, housekeeping).
- Generally, the least desirable methods of exposure control are those focused primarily on the worker (rotation to another location, use of personal protective equipment).
- Persistent and well-integrated follow-up of workplace surveys and sentinel cases, by the occupational hygienist and healthcare practitioner, is the most effective way to bring about improvement in worker health and worksite conditions.

INTERNET RESOURCES

http://www.cdc.gov/niosh/homepage.html
The National Institute for Occupational Safety and Health of the USA has the *NIOSH Analytical Methods, Guide to Chemical Hazards*, and a variety of other publications.

http://www.osha.gov
The Occupational Safety and Health Administration of the USA.

http://www.canoshweb.org/oshmainpage.html
The Canadian Occupational Safety and Health website.

http://www.open.gov.uk/hse/hsehome.htm
The Health and Safety Executive of the United Kingdom.

http://www.worksafe.gov.au/worksafe/home.htm
The National Occupational Safety and Health Commission of Australia (Worksafe Australia).

http://siri.uvm.edu/msds
A University of Vermont site with MSDS information and links to other MSDS sites.

http://www.state.nj.us/health/eoh/rtkweb/rtkhsfs.htm
The State of New Jersey (USA) site for right to know hazardous substance fact sheets.

REFERENCES

1. Bracker A, Blumberg J, Hodgson M, Storey E. Industrial hygiene recommendations as interventions: a collaborative model within occupational medicine. *Appl Occup Environ Hyg* 1999; 14: 85–96.
2. Environmental Protection Agency. *Toxic Substances Control Act, Chemical Substance Inventory: 1990 supplement.* US Government Printing Office, EPA 560/7-90-003, 1990.
3. Castleman BI, Ziem GE. Corporate Influence on Threshold Limit Values. *Am J Ind Med* 1988; 13: 531–559.
4. Burgess WA. *Recognition of Health Hazards in Industry: A Review of Materials Processes,* 2nd edn. New York: Wiley, 1995.
5. Cralley LV, Cralley LJ (eds). *Industrial Hygiene Aspects of Plant Operations.* New York: Macmillan, 1987.
6. International Labour Office. *Encyclopedia of Occupational Health and Safety,* 4th edn. Geneva: ILO, 1997.
7. Rappaport SM. The rules of the game: an analysis of OSHA's enforcement strategy. *Am J Ind Med* 1984; 6: 291–303.
8. Hammond SK. The use of markers to measure exposures to complex mixtures. In: Rappaport SM, Smith TJ eds.

Exposure Assessment for Epidemiology and Hazard Control. Chelsea, MI: Lewis, 1991.
9. American Conference of Governmental Industrial Hygienists. *TLVs and BEIs: Threshold Limit Values for Chemical Substances and Physical Agents.* Cincinnati, OH, 1999.
10. Roach SA. A most rational basis for air sampling programmes. *Ann Occup Hyg* 1997; 20: 65–84.
11. Phalen RF, Hinds WC, John W *et al.* Rationale and recommendations for particle size-selective sampling in the workplace. *Appl Ind Hyg* 1986; 1: 3–14.
12. Stuart BO, Lioy PJ, Phalen RE. Use of size-selection in establishing TLVs. *Ann Am Conf Ind Hyg* 1984; 11: 85–96.
13. Environmental Protection Agency. *Ambient Air Monitoring Reference and Equivalent Methods.* US Code of Federal Regulation (CFR) 40 CFR Part 53. Federal Register 52: 24724, 1987. 62: 38764, 1997
14. National Institute for Occupational Safety and Health (NIOSH). *Manual of Analytical Methods,* 4th edn. DHHS NIOSH Publication No. 94–113. Cincinnati, OH: NIOSH, 1994.
15. Perkins JL. Gases and vapors – passive monitoring. In: *Modern Industrial Hygiene: Recognition and Evaluation of*

Chemical Agents. pp. 480–506, New York, Van Nostrand Reinhold, 1997.

16. Perez C, Solderholm SC. Some chemicals requiring special consideration when deciding whether to sample the particle, vapor or both phases of an atmosphere. *Appl Occup Environ Hyg* 1991; 6(10): 859–864.

17. Gentry, SI. Instrument performance and standards. *Appl Occup Eny Hyg* 1993; 8: 260–266.

18. Roach SA, Rappaport SM. But they are not thresholds: a critical analysis of the documentation of threshold limit values. *Am J Ind Med* 1990; 17: 727–753.

19. Mulhausen JR, Damiano JA. *Strategy for Assessing and Managing Occupational Exposures,* 4th edn. Fairfax, VA: American Industrial Hygiene Association Press, 1998.

20. Brief RS, Scala RA. Occupational exposure limits for novel work schedules. *Am Ind Hyg Assoc J* 1975; 76: 467–476.

21. Tarlau ES. Playing industrial hygiene to win. *New Solutions* 1991; (14); 1(4): 72–81.

22. Rossi M, Ellenbecker M, Geiser K. Techniques in Toxics Use Reduction: from concept to action. *New Solutions* 1991; 2(2): 25–31.

23. National Institute for Occupational Safety and Health. *Assessing Occupational Safety and Health Training.* DHHS NIOSH Publication No. 98–145. Cincinnati, OH: NIOSH, 1998.

24. Quinn MM, Kriebel D, Geiser K, Moure-Eraso R. Sustainable production: a proposed strategy for the work environment. *Am J Ind Med* 1998; 34: 297–304.

25. Dinardi SR, ed. *The Occupational Environment – Its Evaluation and Control.* Fairfax, VA: American Industrial Hygiene Association Press, 1997.

FURTHER READING

Cohen BS, Hering SV eds. *Air Sampling Instruments for Evaluation of Atmospheric Contaminants.* Cincinnati, OH American Conference of Governmental Industrial Hygienists, 1995.

DiBerardinis LI. ed. *Handbook of Occupational Safety and Health.* New York, John Wiley, 1999.

Perkins JI. *Modern Industrial Hygiene: Recognition and Evaluation of Chemical Agents.* New York: Van Nostrand Reinhold, 1997.

34 MINERALOGIC ANALYSIS OF LUNG TISSUE

Andrew Churg

INTRODUCTION

In the correct setting, identification and/or quantification of the types, numbers, and (sometimes) sizes of mineral particles and fibers in lung tissue can be a useful adjunct in arriving at a diagnosis. This approach has been applied most commonly to evaluation of asbestos fiber and asbestos body content, and hence the techniques, overall, are often casually referred to as 'fiber burden analysis' or 'fiber counting'. Asbestos bodies are asbestos fibers coated in an iron-containing proteinaceous secretion of the lung, which gives them the alternative name of 'feruginous bodies'. However, mineralogic analysis can be applied to a number of other agents besides asbestos.

WHEN IS MINERALOGIC ANALYSIS USEFUL?

It is important to remember that mineralogic analysis is always an adjunct to diagnosis, and should be used only when the clinical, historic, or pathologic findings raise a very specific question. Equally important, the findings from mineralogic analysis need to be interpreted in conjunction with the other facts about the case (see Illustrative Cases 1–3); in and of itself, no concentration or number of particles, minerals, or elements establishes a diagnosis or constitutes a disease.

In the most common scenario, what mineralogic analysis does is provide an estimate of the amount of exposure to a specific substance. This may be a guide to the etiology of a particular disease if epidemiological or experimental data support the association. This point may appear simplistic but, unfortunately, some view the finding of an increased content of particles or fibers as proof of causation, no matter what the underlying disease might be. Some examples make this clear:

- Finding an increased tissue beryllium level in a patient with non-caseating granulomas on lung biopsy provides strong support for a diagnosis of berylliosis [1], but finding an increase in tissue beryllium concentration in a patient with some other histologic process merely establishes exposure to beryllium and does not indicate that beryllium caused the lesion in question.

- Similarly, finding a raised number of amosite asbestos fibers or asbestos bodies in a patient with a mesothelioma usually implicates asbestos as the cause of the tumor because of the strong and generally non-confounded association of commercial amphibole asbestos exposure and mesothelioma. But this is not true of carcinoma of the lung where the exact association with asbestos exposure (and the level of exposure required) is disputed and cigarette smoking is a significant confounder [2].

Mineralogic analysis can also be useful when the patient has what appears clinically to be an occupational lung disease, but the history of exposure is unclear or the patient is unaware of exposure. For example, in a patient with a mesothelioma but no

Table 34.1 Asbestos fiber burden in the lungs of the general population reported by two different laboratories

	Mean	Median	Upper 95th percentile
Vancouver (Churg) [6]			
Bodies/gm dry lung			
Asbestos			1 000
Fibers/gm dry lung > 0.5 μm			
Chrysotile	300 000	200 000	1 000 000
Tremolite	400 000	200 000	1 000 000
Amosite + Crocidolite	1 000	0	10 000
Montreal (McGill) [7]*			
Fibers/gm dry lung > 5 μm			
Chrysotile	62 000		
Tremolite	14 000		
Amosite + Crocidolite	10 000		

*Accident victims.

obvious exposure to asbestos, exposure can be shown or disproved by analyzing lung asbestos content (see Illustrative Cases 2 and 3). Similarly, the finding of particles of tungsten in the lungs of a patient with a histologic picture of giant cell interstitial pneumonia on biopsy but no history of hard metal exposure confirms the diagnosis of hard metal disease. This is because it establishes exposure to tungsten carbide, the causative agent of hard metal disease, in the presence of a classic morphologic picture of hard metal disease [1].

However, this approach is limited. A variety of attempts have been made to analyze cases of apparent idiopathic interstitial fibrosis by electron microscopy in the hope of finding raised levels of asbestos fibers (i.e. occult asbestosis) or of some other particle that might be claimed as the cause of the fibrosis. Virtually all such attempts have been futile. Empirically, if asbestos bodies or other particles are not visible by light microscopy, it is extremely unlikely that an (expensive) electron microscopic analysis will reveal an etiologic agent [3,4].

Mineralogic analysis may occasionally provide useful leads when a biopsy shows, unexpectedly, large amounts of dust or large amounts of crystalline material visible by polarization (see below). Thus the finding of brightly birefringent crystals in and around the small vessels is strongly suggestive of intravenous drug abuse, information that might have been hidden from the clinician. But care should be taken when imputing disease to crystalline material seen in tissue sections in the absence of a history of specific exposure, since artifacts abound, including crystals contaminating stain solutions. Physiologic crystals (calcium oxalate and carbonate) are commonly seen in granulomas, for example those of sarcoidosis [5].

QUANTIFICATION AND STANDARD REFERENCE VALUES

The words 'raised' and 'increased' are used above to describe tissue levels or particle numbers with very specific intent, because everyone in the population has in their lungs both asbestos fibers (Table 34.1) and non-fibrous particles derived from contamination of the air [2,8]. For this reason the mere qualitative demonstration of the presence of asbestos fibers or bodies in a tissue digest is usually of no value, and quantitative data are required to show that an exposure above that experienced by the general population has occurred. Exactly the same comment applies to most types of non-fibrous particulates, for example silica, talc, feldspars, metals (titanium, aluminum oxides), and mica, all of which are common in the lungs of the general population [8].

There are some exceptions to this rule. If a particle is not normally found in the lungs of the general population, then the finding of even one such particle probably indicates exposure. A good example is the finding of tungsten in a suspected case of hard metal disease, since tungsten particles are not present in the lungs of the general population when the analysis is carried out by tissue digestion and analytical electron microscope (but note that a different approach, such as atomic absorption spectroscopy, might reveal very low levels of tungsten – it is crucial to know the 'background' for the technique being used). A second exception is that, at least in North America, finding asbestos bodies in tissue sections almost always indicates significant occupational exposure to asbestos, because tissue sections are very insensitive detectors of asbestos bodies and the asbestos body burden of the general population is relatively low; i.e. a high pulmonary asbestos burden is required before asbestos bodies are visible in tissue sections. This, of course, is a crude variety of quantitative analysis.

A problem with mineralogic analysis is the frequent lack of standardization from laboratory to laboratory. This varies somewhat among different techniques. Pure bulk chemical analytical methods, such as atomic absorption spectroscopy, in theory provide numbers that might be compared directly from laboratory to laboratory if proper internal standards were used by the laboratory performing the test. Thus values for tissue beryllium in normal and exposed patients, based on chemical analysis, exist in the literature [1].

On the other hand, counting of particles, fibers, or asbestos bodies from lung digests or lavage fluid is not a standardized technique, and only a few laboratories perform this type of testing on a regular basis. For reasons that are not clear, but relate in part to use of different types of instruments (scanning or transmission electron microscopes), in part to different rules for the size of fibers that are counted, and in part to unknown factors, there are marked laboratory to laboratory differences in the asbestos body or fiber counts obtained, even when counting exactly the same specimen [9].

These differences are illustrated in Table 34.1 which shows background (i.e. reference) values for asbestos from my laboratory in Vancouver and one in Montreal. Vastly different counting rules are used (all fibers longer than 0.5 μm are counted in Vancouver, but only those longer than 5 μm are counted in Montreal) and there is a consequent marked disparity in the actual number of fibers each laboratory reports as 'background'. The same phenomenon appears in Table 34.2, where again there are marked discrepancies between the two laboratories in counts relating to specific diseases. While it can be argued that the cases contributing to the values in Table 34.1 and Table 34.2 from the two laboratories are completely different, the fact remains that all are derived from North America. It is highly unlikely that, for example, there is a 40-fold difference in the median fiber counts for asbestosis; the differences in Tables 34.1 and 34.2 in large measure reflect differences in counting technique alone.

This problem does not invalidate fiber or particle counting as a useful tool, because quite consistent correlations of fiber burden and disease are evident when each laboratory uses its own reference standards [10]. This can be seen from comparing Tables 34.1 and 34.2. Thus, every laboratory must provide its own data on the general population range (and preferably on the range of counts seen in specific diseases): a count from one laboratory cannot be interpreted in terms of background or disease values from another

Table 34.2 Relationship of amphibole (largely amosite) fiber burden and disease reported from two different laboratories (as fibers per g dry lung)

Disease	Vancouver[a] (Churg)	Durham, NC[b] (Roggli)
Asbestosis	10 000 000	253 000
Pleural plaque only	1 400 000	14 000
Exposed, no disease	700 000	4 990
General population	0	< 600

[a] Geometric mean values from 144 cases, all fibers > 0.5 μm, counted by transmission electron microscopy [11].
[b] Median values from 234 cases, all fibers > 5 μm, counted by scanning electron microscopy [12].

laboratory. The idea that some particular count, say '1 000 000 uncoated asbestos fibers per gram of dry tissue' or '1000 asbestos bodies per gram of dry tissue' is a number that, in and of itself, indicates some specific level of exposure, has no scientific basis and is extremely misleading. Such figures do, however, appear in the literature without adequate reference to the relevant standards.

It should additionally be noted that there are marked differences in the background levels for chrysotile, and the tremolite derived from chrysotile, compared with the commercial amphiboles, amosite and crocidolite (Table 34.1). This observation reinforces the idea that adoption of some arbitrary number of asbestos bodies or fibers, for example, 1 000 000 fibers per gram, as a general indicator of significant exposure, is misleading [13]. In an analysis done by my laboratory, a fiber concentration of 1 000 000 fibers of chrysotile per gram would be entirely consistent with background exposure, whereas 1 000 000 fibers of amosite per gram would indicate a very high occupational exposure (Tables 34.1, 34.2).

CHOICE OF SPECIMEN

Not all specimens are suitable for mineralogic analysis. In general, analyses should be performed only on lung tissue because lung tissue provides the most reliable estimate of exposure. There are some exceptions; for example, beryllium can be quantified in urine or mediastinal lymph nodes [1]. Inhaled particles tend to be very inhomogeneously distributed within the lung parenchyma, hence the smaller the specimen, the more likely that inhomogeneous distributions will create significant errors in quantitative analysis. For this reason transbronchial biopsies are far inferior to large open or thoracoscopic biopsies, or portions of resected lung or autopsy lung. As normal a portion of lung as possible should be used, and consolidated or tumor-bearing tissue avoided.

The value of analyzing bronchoalveolar lavage fluid or sputum is unclear. Finding specific particles in lavage may occasionally point to occult exposures, but the question of whether lavage asbestos fiber counts correlate adequately with levels of exposure, tissue burdens, or patterns of disease has provoked controversy (see Chapter 9 for another opinion) [14]. Even if fibers are detected, when the disease process itself is unclear the lavage burden of fibers is not a substitute for a tissue diagnosis [14]. Further comments about asbestos analyses are provided below.

TECHNICAL APPROACHES

A wide variety of techniques appears in the literature, but in practice many require very specialized equipment and relatively few are readily available [8].

Light microscopic examination

Simple light microscopic examination of histologic sections, with or without the aid of polarization, is by far the quickest, cheapest, and easiest method, and is often overlooked. Light microscopy has, however, distinct limitations: dusts must be colored and must be large enough, either as single particles or as aggregates, to be within the range of resolution of the light microscope. The presence of tissue also tends to mask particulates. As a practical rule individual particles must be greater than about 0.3 µm in diameter to be seen. Many substances of interest, such as ultrafine air pollution components and uncoated asbestos fibers, are below the level of resolution. Nevertheless, light microscopy is excellent at providing a crude estimate of the content of visible dusts such as coal, aggregated air pollution particles (visible in every urban lung to a greater or lesser extent), and asbestos in the form of asbestos bodies. Sheet silicates such as talc and mica may also be visible in ordinary sections. Iron staining of ordinary histologic sections is extremely useful for detecting and quantifying asbestos bodies with high sensitivity (see Table 34.4 and Section below on Analysis of Asbestos Content).

Polarization will often make visible transparent and colorless, or near colorless, particles. A mineralogic polarizing microscope is not necessary; all that is required is two sheets of plastic polaroid material. Table 34.3 shows particles and fibers that may be found by polarization. Again, a reference level is crucial, thus it is important for the pathologist doing the examination to have some (visual)

Table 34.3 Dusts visible by simple polarization of histologic sections

Strongly birefringent	Weakly birefringent	Not birefringent
Talc, mica Drug fillers (talc, mica, crystalline cellulose)	Crystalline silica	Asbestos Synthetic mineral fibers (fiberglass, etc.)

idea of the number of particles found by polarization in the normal lung before giving an opinion on an unknown case.

X-ray diffraction and atomic absorption spectroscopy

Instruments for these procedures are available in most universities, and atomic absorption spectrometers are found in some diagnostic clinical laboratories. X-ray diffraction can be used to identify elements, minerals, and polymorphs of minerals (e.g. quartz versus cristobalite, two different forms of crystalline silica), but is distinctly limited in sensitivity. Atomic absorption spectroscopy is very useful for identifying specific elements with high sensitivity (down to about 0.003 parts per million), and is thus the procedure of choice when elevations in the content of a specific element (beryllium, titanium, aluminum, cerium) are at issue.

Analytical electron microscopy

An analytical electron microscope is a scanning or transmission electron microscope equipped with an energy dispersive X-ray spectrometer. Transmission microscopes have the additional capability to perform electron diffraction. The analytical electron microscope allows specific, particle by particle, identification of particles or fibers extracted from lung tissue. The energy dispersive X-ray spectrometer, often casually referred to as an 'EDAX' or 'microprobe' machine, allows a microchemical analysis of any structure or particle that the electron microscope can resolve. The addition of electron diffraction along with particle morphology often permits species that are chemically similar, for example talc fibers and anthophyllite asbestos, to be distinguished from each other. Analytical electron microscopy is an excellent approach for providing quantitative data on the content of inhaled particulates, and has been particularly applied to the identification and counting of asbestos fibers (Tables 34.1, 34.2), ambient air particles [8], and other specific inhaled particles such as aluminum [15], tungsten from hard metal [1], and cerium [16].

A number of limitations apply to this technique. Transmission microscopes offer far higher resolution than scanning microscopes; both are suitable for detecting amphibole asbestos fibers (amosite and crocidolite) but scanning microscopes tend to miss the much finer chrysotile fibers. As well, most EDAX machines do not detect elements lighter than sodium, so that this technique is generally not suitable for detecting beryllium. The major disadvantage of this technique is that it is labor intensive and slow, and thus is relatively expensive.

ANALYSIS OF ASBESTOS CONTENT

Mineralogic analysis is an excellent method of assessing the role of asbestos in the causation of disease in a particular case, but the interpretation of such analyses is more complicated than that for most particulates since not all fibers are retained in lung to the same extent. Amphibole (amosite and crocidolite) asbestos fibers are cleared very slowly from lung tissue (estimated half-life of the order of decades), but chrysotile fibers are rapidly removed (estimated half-life of the order of months) [17]. Fiber burden studies can thus miss chrysotile exposure when that exposure is remote. As well, chrysotile forms asbestos bodies much less readily than amphibole asbestos. Because most chrysotile is naturally contaminated with the amphibole, tremolite, and this (like all amphiboles) is biopersistent, raised tremolite levels may be found in lungs in those with heavy exposure and can sometimes serve

as a surrogate for chrysotile. Unfortunately, the amount of tremolite in processed chrysotile products is quite variable, and the absence of both tremolite and chrysotile does not rule out a chrysotile exposure in the past. In this situation historic data are important in obtaining a coherent view of an individual case (see Illustrative Cases).

Fiber burden analyses should be restricted to lung tissue, because this is the only tissue for which reasonable standards of background level exist. Some authors believe, however, that bronchoalveolar lavage fluid may be useful also, as discussed above. Some asbestos appears to reach the pleura [18], but how much, if any, is translocated from the lung to other parts of the body is a disputed issue. In general asbestos-induced disease appears to relate better to the number of long compared to short fibers, although some exceptions have been reported. Most of the fibers that have been described outside the lung are very short fibers (< 2 μm, and usually < 1 μm) of chrysotile, fibers that, from chemical considerations, should have very short half-lives [19]. Given the apparent lack of pathogenicity of very short chrysotile fibers, the propensity of chrysotile to be rapidly removed from tissues, and the known contamination of air, water, and even paraffin blocks by short chrysotile fibers in some localities [20], the significance of finding only short chrysotile fibers in a fiber burden study is doubtful. Contamination of other organs during autopsies with fiber-containing fluid from the lung is a further problem.

Table 34.4 lists the various methods that can be applied to analyzing asbestos content. In many

Table 34.4 Approach to quantitative analysis of lung abestos content

Method	Uses	Advantages and disadvantages
Identification of asbestos bodies in 5-μm thick histologic sections (usually using iron stains)	Usually indicates high level exposure to asbestos (but, rarely, bodies are seen in lungs from the general population as a result of background exposure). Finding bodies in histologic sections is required for the pathologic diagnosis of asbestosis	Inexpensive. Relatively rapid Can be done by any laboratory Insensitive: significantly increased fiber burden may be present without asbestos bodies visible in sections. Bodies are largely a measure of amphibole exposure
Digesting tissue and counting asbestos bodies on a membrane filter by light microscopy	Provides quantitative data on amount of exposure	Inexpensive. Relatively rapid. No special equipment required (can be done in any laboratory, with practice). Standards for general population (i.e. background) values required. Largely detects amphiboles
Digesting tissue and counting and identifying uncoated asbestos fibers by electron microscopy	Provides quantitative data on amount of exposure. Identifies specific fiber types and sizes. May indicate source of exposure	Expensive and slow. Specialized equipment required. Few laboratories provide service. Standards for general population required. This technique can also identify other types of mineral

instances, demonstrating the presence of asbestos bodies in iron-stained sections is entirely adequate to establish an above background exposure; for example, counting asbestos bodies in tissue sections in one study provided just as good a discrimination between asbestosis and idiopathic pulmonary fibrosis as did electron microscopic analysis of the same cases [3]. Because ordinary 5-μm thick paraffin sections are such insensitive detectors of asbestos bodies, in most instances the finding of asbestos bodies in sections indicates a level of exposure in the range that can cause asbestosis. For actual quantification, counting of bodies or uncoated fibers in tissue digests should be used. The choice of technique depends on:

- cost and speed – electron microscopic analyses cost more and take much longer than counting asbestos bodies by light microscopy

- level of sensitivity required – electron microscopic counts are more sensitive and detect all types of fibers, whereas asbestos body counts are usually a surrogate for counts of relatively long amphibole (not chrysotile) fibers

Electron microscopic counts are the only way to determine that the asbestos burden is within the general population range, a finding that is sometimes useful in ruling out an asbestos etiology for a particular disease (see Illustrative Cases 2 and 3). As well, electron microscopic analysis is the only way to determine the level of chrysotile fibers present. Details of the methods used to prepare and count asbestos bodies or fibers in tissue digests are published elsewhere [2,21].

ILLUSTRATIVE CASES

CASE 1

History

A 37-year-old man was referred to a pulmonologist with a complaint of increasing shortness of breath of several months' duration. He had never smoked, and had no previous history of respiratory problems. He had been employed for the previous 15 years as a construction worker whose main job was make up cement from powder, and to cut concrete blocks. He claimed these processes were quite dusty and he apparently wore no respiratory protection. He had initially been seen by his family physician, who organized a chest radiography. This showed bilateral soft airspace infiltrates in the mid-lung fields. No nodular lesions were identified. Pulmonary function tests revealed a mild restrictive defect with a diffusing capacity ($D_{L}CO$) of 60% predicted.

The pulmonologist carried out a bronchoscopy, which was unremarkable, and a transbronchial biopsy. The latter provided a good sample of parenchyma and the alveoli were noted by the pathologist to be filled with granular pink material, consistent with alveolar proteinosis.

Analytical results

Polarization of the histologic sections showed a very small number of brightly birefringent crystals. A mineralogic examination performed in another laboratory using analytical electron microscopy was reported to show an approximately 2-fold increase in crystalline silica particles over maximum background. The remaining particles appeared to be ambient atmospheric particles in their usual concentrations. No uncommon dusts were found.

The patient brought a worker's compensation claim, specifically alleging that his disease was silicoproteinosis (acute silicosis) and that it was caused by exposure to silica dust from mixing and cutting of concrete.

Interpretation

Cement workers can be exposed to crystalline silica, and there are good data from clinical observation and from experimental animal studies that alveolar proteinosis can be caused by exposure to very high levels of finely divided dust, including crystalline silica. However, the development of silicoproteinosis requires an extremely high exposure, and such cases almost invariably show numerous fine particles of silica that are poorly birefringent on polarization. These particles were not present in this case; rather there were a few particles that appear to represent background atmospheric exposure to silicate minerals (the latter are brightly birefringent). The 2-fold increase in silica particle content by analytical electron microscopy may or not indicate a real increase, given measurement errors (particularly from a transbronchial biopsy) and individual retention variation, but in any event is far below the multi-fold increase expected in silicoproteinosis.

This case consequently appears to be one of spontaneous rather than dust-induced alveolar proteinosis. Of note, the patient was greatly improved after several bronchoalveolar lavage procedures, and both his chest radiograph and pulmonary function test results returned to normal.

Alveolar proteinosis has also been reported to follow the inhalation of aluminum dusts, but again only after very large levels of exposure [15].

CASE 2
History

A 60-year-old man presented with chest pain and weight loss, and was found to have a right pleural effusion. After draining the effusion, computed tomography showed irregular pleural thickening on the right, thought most likely to be a mesothelioma. At thoracoscopy multiple small tumor nodules were found over the parietal and visceral pleura, and a biopsy of one of them confirmed the diagnosis of mesothelioma. He died with extensive tumor 6 months after diagnosis.

Immediately after high school the patient had served in the US armed forces as an infantryman. On discharge he became an electrician and stayed in that career for his whole working life. He had worked almost entirely on residential construction, starting in the early 1960s. He had never handled asbestos himself, but claimed that he worked around roofers and wallboard installers who did handle asbestos or sanded asbestos-containing board. However, his job typically required him to complete his installations before wallboard was put in place. He was never at any job site where spray asbestos insulation was applied.

Analytical results

A portion of his autopsy lung was analyzed for asbestos content in an attempt to establish a cause for the mesothelioma. This analysis revealed that both chrysotile and tremolite fiber content were within background limits (300 000 fibers per gram of dry lung each; compare Table 34.1 for background values from the author's laboratory), but that the amosite content was raised 5-fold over the upper limit of background exposure (50 000 fibers per g dry lung).

Interpretation

The analytical findings suggest that this patient had modest but definite amosite exposure during the course of his career, and implicate amosite as the cause of the mesothelioma. The background levels of chrysotile and tremolite most likely indicate that the patient never had very high exposure to chrysotile. Thus the mineralogic analysis supports the historic data. Given that induction of mesothelioma by chrysotile requires a very high exposure, it is unlikely that chrysotile played any role in the genesis of this man's disease.

CASE 3

History

A 45-year-old man presented in 1998 with chest pain and pleural effusion. Investigation showed a left sided pleural-based tumor, and biopsy confirmed a diagnosis of mesothelioma. The patient had been a construction worker since leaving high school and claimed to have had occupational exposure to asbestos doing various aspects of this job, including residential construction, roofing, and cleanup at construction sites. However, further questioning suggested that he had never actually worked with asbestos-containing products, and had not worked at any location where pipe insulation was being applied or removed, or where asbestos spraying had taken place. Almost all of his time was actually spent outdoors.

Analytical results

The patient died from mesothelioma 18 months after diagnosis. A portion of autopsy lung was submitted for analytical electron microscopy and this showed no detectable amosite or crocidolite, no detectable chrysotile, and 80 000 fibers per g dry lung of tremolite (background upper 95th percentile value for tremolite in the author's laboratory is 1 000 000 fibers per g dry lung; Table 34.1). All the tremolite fibers detected were shorter than 5 μm.

Interpretation

Unlike Case 2, there is no evidence here for occupational exposure to asbestos on fiber analysis. The absence of amosite is important, as amosite is cleared very slowly and construction workers who have had asbestos exposure typically show an increase in amosite content in this region [11]. Some chrysotile exposure may have occurred, but nothing in the history suggests that there was a high level of exposure. The fact that the tremolite fibers were all shorter than 5 μm is also against significant chrysotile exposure, since it has been shown that occupational chrysotile exposure tends to be associated with the finding of fibers longer than 8 μm in the lung tissue [6]. This case consequently appears to be one of idiopathic mesothelioma.

REFERENCES

1. Churg A, Colby TV. Diseases caused by metals and related compounds. In: Churg A, Green FHY, eds. *Pathology of Occupational Lung Disease*, 2nd edn. Baltimore, MD: Williams and Wilkins, 1998. pp. 77–128.
2. Churg A. Nonneoplastic disease caused by asbestos. In: Churg A, Green FHY, eds. *Pathology of Occupational Lung Disease*, 2nd edn, pp. 277–338. Baltimore, MD: Williams and Wilkins, 1998.
3. Gaensler EA, Jederlinic PJ, Churg A. Idiopathic pulmonary fibrosis in asbestos-exposed workers. *Amer Rev Respir Dis* 1991; 144: 689–696.
4. Roggli VI. Scanning electron microscopic analysis of mineral fiber content of lung tissue in the evaluation of diffuse pulmonary fibrosis. *Scan Micros* 1991; 5: 71–83.
5. Visscher D, Churg A, Katzenstein A-LA. Significance of crystalline inclusions in lung granulomas. *Mod Pathol* 1988; 1: 415–419.
6. Churg A, Wiggs B. Fiber size and number in users of processed chrysotile ore, chrysotile miners, and members of the general population. *Am J Ind Med* 1986; 9: 143–152.
7. Case B, Sebastien P, McDonald JC. Lung fiber analysis in accident victims: a biological assessment of general environmental exposure. *Arch Environ Health* 1988; 43: 178–179.
8. Churg A, Green FHY. Analytical methods for identifying and quantifying mineral particles in lung tissue In: Churg A, Green FHY, eds. *Pathology of Occupational Lung Disease*, 2nd edn, pp. 45–56. Baltimore MD: Williams and Wilkins, 1998.
9. Gylseth B, Churg A, Davis JMG et al. Analysis of asbestos fibers and asbestos bodies in human lung tissue samples. An international laboratory trial. *Scand J Work Environ Health* 1985; 11: 107–110.
10. Mossman BT, Churg A. Mechanisms in the pathogenesis of asbestosis and silicosis. *Am J Respir Crit Care Med* 1998; 157: 1666–1680.

11. Churg A, Vedal S. Fiber burden and patterns of asbestos-related disease in workers with heavy mixed amosite and chrysotile exposure. *Am J Respir Crit Care Med* 1994; 150: 663–669.

12. Roggli VL, Sander LL. Asbestos content of lung tissue and carcinoma of the lung: a clinicopathologic correlation and mineral fiber analysis of 234 cases. *Ann Occup Hyg* 2000; 44: 109–117.

13. Asbestos, asbestosis, and cancer: the Helsinki criteria for diagnosis and attribution. *Scand J Work Environ Health.* 1997; 23(4): 311–316.

14. Schwartz DA, Galvin JR, Burmeister LF *et al.* The clinical utility and reliability of asbestos bodies in bronchoalveolar lavage fluid. *Am Rev Respir Dis* 1991; 144: 684–688.

15. Miller R, Churg A, Lam S. Pulmonary alveolar proteinosis and exposure to aluminum dust. *Am Rev Respir Dis* 1984; 130: 312–315.

16. McDonald JW, Ghio AJ, Sheehan CE *et al.* Rare earth (cerium oxide) pneumoconiosis: analytical scanning electron microscopy and literature review. *Mod Pathol* 1995; 8: 859–65.

17. Churg A. Deposition and clearance of chrysotile asbestos. *Ann Occup Hyg* 1994; 38: 625–634.

18. Boutin C, Dumortrier P, Rey F *et al.* Black spots concentrate oncogenic asbestos fibers in the parietal pleura. *Am J Respir Crit Care Med* 1996; 153: 444–449.

19. Hume LA, Rimstidt JD. The biodurability of chrysotile asbestos. *Am Mineral* 1992; 77: 1125–1128.

20. Lee RJ, Florida RG, Stewart IM. Asbestos contamination in paraffin tissue blocks. *Arch Pathol Lab Med* 1995; 119: 528–532.

21. Roggli VL, Greenberg SD, Pratt PC. *Pathology of Asbestos-Associated Diseases.* Boston, MA: Little Brown, 1992.

LEGISLATION

35 LEGISLATIVE CONTROLS AND COMPENSATION: NORTH AMERICA

Tee L. Guidotti

LEGISLATIVE CONTROLS

In Canada and the USA, the control of workplace hazards has been driven primarily by government regulation, and secondarily by the escalating insurance costs and third-party liability of employers. The general approach to regulation is similar in the two countries but the implementation has been different, reflecting constitutional differences in governance. Because so many workplace hazards are airborne chemical and dust exposures, the regulatory framework for these hazards is in the mainstream of occupational health and safety regulation and has defined many of its attributes.

US legislative structure

Occupational health and safety affairs in the USA are not centralized into one monolithic agency, such as the Environmental Protection Agency. Rather, it is intentionally fragmented among various agencies:

- National Institute for Occupational Safety and Health (NIOSH)
- Occupational Safety and Health Administration (OSHA)
- Occupational Health and Safety Review Commission (an appeals body)
- Mine Safety and Health Administration (MSHA)
- Mine Safety and Health Review Commission (the appeals body for the mining industry)

NIOSH

In addition to its role as the leading research and documentation agency recommending proposed standards, including those for respiratory hazards, to OSHA and MSHA, NIOSH tests the effectiveness of personal protective equipment against respiratory hazards. The Environmental Protection Agency regulates pesticide exposures. Other agencies have more limited roles with respect to occupational lung disorders.

OSHA

OSHA is responsible for most occupational health regulation in general industry, which constitutes employment outside mining, most agriculture, and other occupations covered under special legislation. OSHA maintains regional offices in the nine federal regions and directly supervizes occupational health and safety regulation in states that lack their own occupational health and safety agencies. However, OSHA primarily operates on the national level to ensure consistent standards and enforcement across the country in industries that do not fall under special regulatory authorities. OSHA compliance officers (inspectors), operate out of regional and local offices, conduct periodic inspections, and investigate hazards reported to them. OSHA provides limited consultation services to employers who request them, which are usually small enterprises that cannot afford commercial services.

Twenty-six states have workplace health and safety agencies ('State OSHAs') and conduct their own enforcement. State OSHAs sometimes adopt more stringent standards for hazards of local interest, but they are not permitted to adopt weaker standards. State OSHAs act primarily as state-level enforcement agencies for the national body of OSHA regulations.

MSHA

The Mine Safety and Health Administration is critically important in controlling occupational respiratory hazards. MSHA is similar to OSHA but its mandate under the Mine Safety and Health Act is specific to the mining industry. This Act has features that are more stringent than the OSH Act and that reflect the immediacy of hazards familiar in mine safety. For example, under the OSH Act an employer may appeal a citation and is not required to correct the situation until the appeal is decided, by which time the work or project may be over. Under the MSH Act, mine operators must correct the problem immediately even if they contest the citation. The MSH Act also empowers mine inspectors to evacuate an area of the mine subject to imminent danger and provides for full payment of wages during a closure or inspection, features absent from the OSH Act. Under the OSH Act, federal or state OSHA has discretion to inspect workplaces but under the MSH Act mines must be inspected regularly, on a strict schedule (four times a year for underground mines, twice for surface mines).

Review commissions

The Occupational Health and Safety Review Commission is an independent body established by the Occupational Health and Safety Act of 1970 (OSH Act). It functions as a system of administrative law courts run by administrative law judges under the oversight of a three-person commission. It has jurisdiction over disputes under the OSH Act related to inspections, usually pertaining to citations, penalties, and abatement. The Commission often uses an expedited trial format called an 'E-Z Trial' for simpler cases involving no fatalities, low fines, and small employers. The Commissioners themselves serve as the appeals body.

The Mine Safety and Health Review Commission is an independent body established by the Federal Mine Safety and Health Amendments Act of 1977 (Mine Act) to adjudicate disputes brought under the Mine Act. It operates as a system of courts presided over by administrative law judges, with the Commissioners themselves serving as a body of appeal. It has jurisdiction when there are disputes under the Act, usually related to violations, mine closures, discrimination on safety grounds and civil penalties.

Canadian legislative structure

In Canada, under the Constitution, occupational health is a provincial responsibility. The federal government is responsible only for federal workers and workers in federally regulated industries, including aviation, railways, and the nuclear industry. In practice, provincial occupational health and safety agencies across Canada have adopted a fairly consistent set of occupational exposure levels and other regulations. The federal government also established the Canadian Centre for Occupational Health and Safety, a reference and information agency (see Chapter 38, Information sources and investigation Centres: North America). There is no equivalent to either OSHA or NIOSH at the federal level in Canada.

Mexican legislative structure

In Mexico, occupational health and safety regulation is a federal responsibility. Standards as written are generally consistent with world benchmarks, including OSHA standards, but enforcement on the local level and the legal interpretation by state governments varies. Historically, occupational health and safety in Mexico has emphasized periodic health surveillance and the provision of health services to workers. Hazard control and compliance with worker protection have lagged behind. In this, Mexico is similar to other developing countries and to the USA and Canada in an earlier era.

The North American Free Trade Agreement (NAFTA), operating between the USA, Canada, and Mexico, is silent on occupational health matters, but side agreements on worker protection were concluded after the main treaty.

Regulatory standards

The interest of governments in regulating respiratory hazards, and occupational hazards in general, is 2-fold: to prevent the disorders that they cause and to provide a uniform regulatory framework so that the responsibility for compliance falls more or less evenly on all employers.

The prevention and control of occupational lung disorders is achieved by a variety of strategies, among them support of epidemiological and clinical research to characterize the problem, research on control of hazards, periodic health surveillance, compensation programs, training, and worker education. By far the most important is reduction of exposure to the inhaled hazard. Exposure standards govern the permissible levels of exposure to particular substances and are set individually for each hazard. Most of the examples in this section are from OSHA.

Engineering controls are preferred for reducing exposure to airborne hazards but the efficiency of exhaust ventilation, containment and dust suppression reaches diminishing returns and increasing costs the more efficiency is required. For a highly toxic substance used in the open, such as a solvent, or in working conditions that require free movement, engineering controls may be impractical. Personal protection is an important option when engineering controls to reduce or eliminate exposure are ineffective or not feasible. Modern regulations do not try to prescribe which control measures are used and how, realizing that innovation and ingenuity may solve exposure problems in new ways and that a prescribed technology may retard progress toward greater control.

Exposure limits

In both the USA and Canada, the standards for allowable exposure to respiratory hazards take the same general form although the terminology may differ. The enforceable standards for exposure in the workplace are called 'permissible exposure limits' (PELs) by OSHA and 'occupational exposure limits' (OELs) by federal and provincial occupational health and safety agencies in Canada.

OSHA PELs are developed by a laborious process. This process must be open to the public, must provide extensive periods during which there can be public comment and response from stakeholders, and is subject to legal challenge on procedural grounds at many points along the way. As a consequence, it is very difficult to introduce a new standard or to revise an old one. The original OSHA PELs reflected standards derived from 1969 American Conference of Governmental Industrial Hygienists (ACGIH) guidelines in effect when the OSH Act came into effect in 1970. OSHA was given the mandate of adopting those standards in current use by the federal government at the time and these standards were incorporated by reference because they applied to federal contractors. Since 1970, OSHA has succeeded in promulgating only about 25 new standards, far behind the many recommended exposure limits (RELs) presented to it by NIOSH. Most of the OSHA PELs now in force do not necessarily reflect current science or thinking in toxicology, as illustrated below. Efforts to streamline the process, as by regulating carcinogens as a group rather than individually, have not survived legal challenges because of the constraints placed on OSHA by the OSH Act.

Although they do not carry the force of law, a number of alternative, usually more protective, standards are used in practice by some employers to provide a wider margin of safety. Proposed standards that have been documented by NIOSH and presented to OSHA for consideration are called Recommended Exposure Limits and are often used by industry as operating standards in order to demonstrate due diligence. Another, highly influential set of voluntary standards that are also frequently used by industry are the 'threshold limit values' (TLVs) set by the ACGIH. The ACGIH is considered the leading private authority on chemical hazards in the workplace and their TLVs are often adopted or incorporated by reference in statutes and regulations in other countries, including Canada. In general, ACGIH and NIOSH recommendations are more or less in line (there is considerable variation for some chemical agents) and are lower than current OSHA PELs. These provisional standards are more easily and frequently updated than OSHA standards.

Protective equipment

Protection standards give specifications for the type, effectiveness, and proper use of personal protective equipment. The OSHA Cotton Dust Standard and the Mine Safety and Health Act, for example, govern many of the performance criteria for respiratory protection and provide a mandate and guidelines for NIOSH to evaluate personal protective equipment such as respirators. Personal respiratory protection is the use of equipment, such as respirators, to protect individuals in situations where it is not possible or practical to control the concentration of airborne exposures in the workplace environment. All respirators (respiratory protection devices) must be approved by NIOSH to be used legally in the workplace. OSHA mandates standards for respirators, which are evaluated by NIOSH, and requires fit testing to ensure that the respirator will perform for the individual worker as designed.

Engineering controls are always preferred to personal protection. Because the efficacy of personal protection is subject to individual cooperation and circumstances, personal protection is less reliable than engineering controls.

Compliance

Some OSHA regulations mandate that exposure be measured and periodically monitored to ensure that concentrations in the workplace are within the permissible exposure limit (e.g. acrylonitrile, asbestos, arsenic, benzene, coal dust, coke oven emissions, ethylene oxide, formaldehyde, lead, silica, and vinyl chloride monomer). This is not spelt out for most hazards.

Surveillance and reporting

Documentation standards, such as the OSHA 100 Log, govern the recording of acute occupational diseases and injuries or the discovery of a chronic condition. These documentation standards exist in parallel with the workers' compensation system and function separately from it because they are designed to record all non-trivial incidents. Workers' compensation reporting systems, on the other hand, are primarily designed to keep track of lost-time claims that require compensation or payment of medical expenses.

Surveillance standards mandate periodic health screening tests for workers exposed to respiratory hazards that may cause chronic disease. Surveillance programs are periodic health screening examinations provided by employers for the protection of workers. Surveillance is 'mandated', or required under the regulation for employers to provide to their employees, in many occupational health standards, such as the OSHA Asbestos Standard. Surveillance of occupational lung disease is important for many reasons. There is a possibility that early detection may lead to intervention that prevents progression of the disease. This is generally more applicable to benign disease than to lung cancer, which carries a similar prognosis despite early detection. At the very least, medical removal may prevent the progression of the disease, or, in the case of silicosis, progression beyond a certain point. Surveillance may also provide an indication that exposure control efforts in the workplace are inadequate. In general, surveillance is not itself an effective means of preventing occupational lung disease but is useful in combination with exposure controls.

COMPENSATION

Governmental programs

Immediate disability and expense

Workers' compensation is designed for uncomplicated problems that occur at work, such as injuries, and the system works well for these. By standardizing adjudication and case management, and following consistent guidelines for the evaluation of impairment, workers' compensation has expedited the handling of simple workplace injuries and reduced the cost to injured workers and employers. The system does not work as well for complicated cases and virtually all occupational disorders of the lung are complicated.

Workers' compensation is a no-fault insurance system, paid for by employers, that covers the medical treatment of injured workers and indemnifies them for lost earnings using a formula that takes into account impairment and earning potential. Workers' compensation does not require means

testing because benefits are earned and, in theory, based on assessments already paid.

In the USA, all 50 states, the Commonwealth of Puerto Rico, the District of Columbia, the territories of Guam and American Samoa and the US Virgin Islands, federal employees, coal miners, longshoremen, and workers in the nuclear industry have variations on the theme of workers' compensation. Merchant marine seamen and railroad workers engaged in interstate commerce are covered by federal legislation that makes recovery easier by litigation.

Excepting the federal systems, which are similar, workers' compensation legislation varies greatly from state to state. Most allow insurance companies to provide workers' compensation coverage to employers, or for employers to self-insure, under the supervision of a state board. Six states and all Canadian provinces have single, government-sponsored agencies that act as insurers and as regulatory boards. Coverage is mandatory for employers in all but three states (New Jersey, South Carolina, and Texas), and in those states employers who opt out lose the right to use customary common law defenses against lawsuits by employees.

The US federal government, through the Office of Workers' Compensation Programs, operates special workers' compensation programs for special populations. These include the Black Lung Program for coal miners, the Longshoreman and Harbor Workers' Compensation Program, the Federal Employees' Compensation Act system, and systems in the US Department of Energy for nuclear workers.

Federal legislation provides for more liberal grounds for indemnification for workers in two occupations that involve interstate commerce and therefore are poorly served by state compensation systems: railroad workers and seamen. The Federal Employers' Liability Act 1908, which covers railroad workers, and the Longshoreman and Harbor Workers' Act 1927, which covers seamen, both preceded the development of most workers' compensation systems in the USA. They make it easier for these groups to recover damages for job-related injuries and illness through legal action. However, there are no workers' compensation systems as such that provide coverage for these two occupations.

In Canada, all provinces and territories maintain workers' compensation boards, giving a total of 13. The federal government maintains a system for federal employees, under the Federal Government Employees Compensation Act, which is administered locally by the provincial or territorial boards. These are crown corporations (government sponsored but not controlled), with exclusive funds for the coverage of workers in their area of jurisdiction, and therefore tend to be large compared with American insurers.

Unlike the USA, few employers in Canada are self-insured, and those are mostly government agencies.

In the USA and Canada, the basic structure of workers' compensation is the same. A board or commission sets the rules, an insurer provides coverage on the basis of payroll for eligible workers, and cases are adjudicated in the first instance by the insurer and subsequently, if contested, by an appeals mechanism. Despite the early intent to eliminate litigation, the reality is that advocacy and even legal action remain part of the process in complicated or disputed cases at the appeals level, and sometimes even in the initial claim, especially in certain US states.

In Mexico, most relevant occupational health insurance coverage is provided through or in parallel with the requirements of the Instituto Mexicano del Seguro Social (IMSS; the Mexican Institute for Social Security), with a few health plans available, mostly in the banking industry. IMSS is financed by assessments on employers and functions as a single comprehensive agency for workers' compensation, personal sickness and injury coverage, and workplace inspection. A separate system exists for government employees. Historically, the development of insurance for workers in Mexico was influenced more strongly by France and by continental models than by the German model that prevailed in Canada and the United States.

In virtually all systems, occupational lung disorders represent a small but extremely expensive category of cases that are handled with difficulty. The problem is that the system is not well suited to difficult or complicated cases. Occupational lung disorders are often multifactorial, with contributions from preexisting disease (such as asthma) and cigarette smoking as well as multiple occupational exposures. Except for the pneumoconioses, they are not necessarily characteristic or easily diagnosed. Although occupational lung disorders often have a prolonged latency, sometimes appearing after retirement, many states have time limitations on the filing of claims after last exposure or first manifestation of the disease. It can be very difficult to reconstruct an accurate occupational history after substantial time has passed and comprehensive documentation is usually lacking.

Occupational lung disorder is a particularly difficult category of occupational disease in which to prove causation. Employers may contest claims and often do when they suspect that a disorder is unrelated to occupational exposures or is caused in part by personal lifestyle factors, such as cigarette smoking. Often, the worker is not able to know for certain and the claim is filed without detailed or sophisticated explanation. The path of least resistance on the part of an adjudicator or claims manager, is to reject the claim and to let the system sort it out on appeal, which is generally supervised by the state workers' compensation board. This forces the worker to bear the burden of proof and often to hire legal counsel to argue the claim in a quasi-legal, courtroom setting. The entire process can take many months, even years.

In cases for which the work-relationship or level of impairment is not clear or is disputed, workers' compensation boards may request independent medical examinations. These are evaluations in which the physician is acting as a neutral party, not as the treating physician, and is not deemed to have a physician–patient relationship with the claimant. The use of standardized impairment and disability guidelines is discussed below, in the section on Evaluation of Occupational Lung Disease.

Long-term disability and loss of earnings

Workers' compensation benefits are expected to meet the need in work-related disorders, and long-term disability (LTD) insurance or social security systems are intended to cover non-occupational disorders. Neither applies a means test because they are insurance-based indemnification programs, not welfare. However, because occupational lung disorders are difficult to identify and causation is often disputed, many workers fall through the cracks in the system. For this reason, it is important to understand the insurance regime covering non-occupational disability.

In general, LTD insurance and social security systems are reciprocal with workers' compensation. At best, they may be supplemental, providing partial payments to make up the difference between workers' compensation and the workers' full entitlement under the more generous program. Workers' compensation benefits are usually more generous than Social Security or Canada Pension, but less generous than some LTD policies, which may limit coverage to non-occupational injuries. The LTD insurance carrier may dispute a claim on the basis that the injury is work related, even after a claim has been rejected by the workers' compensation carrier. Some states have legislation in place to prevent this from happening. Even so, there is always a tendency for LTD carriers to question eligibility when short-term benefits end, especially if claims are under review by workers' compensation carriers, leading to frequent delays and interruptions in payments to workers who may be dependent on benefits for income.

Social Security Disability Insurance (SSDI) in the United States, and Canada Pension, allow medical treatment and partial income replacement benefits for claimants younger than 65 years of age if the claimants are permanently totally disabled, that is, unable to support themselves in any work, or blind.

Dependent survivors of deceased workers may also receive benefits from Social Security. Medicare provides medical care coverage to SSDI recipients after 2 years. Unlike retirement benefits, SSDI requires the states (through offices called 'Disability Determination Services') to develop medical evidence of impairment and to assess disability. To qualify, workers under 65 years of age must be covered by Social Security, must have worked recently and steadily by simple criteria, and must demonstrate 'disability', defined as 'the inability to engage in any substantial gainful activity' for a period expected to last at least a year. There is also a second program called the Supplemental Security Income Program (SSI) for qualified claimants with severe impairment who lack financial resources.

Medical practitioners provide input into the Disability Determination Services at the state level for their patients applying under Social Security programs. The criteria for impairment resulting in total disability are the same whether the disorder is occupational or non-occupational. Medical assessments are called 'consultative examinations' and are similar to independent medical examinations in workers' compensation. The information required to support a claim for SSDI for occupational lung disease includes a determination of maximal ventilatory volume (MVV) and complete spirometry, so these tests should always be included in the workup. The use of standardized impairment and disability guidelines is discussed below, in the section on Evaluation of occupational lung disorders.

Canada Pension Plan Disability Benefits and the Québec Pension Plan Disability Benefits are similar and set criteria for qualifying 'prolonged disability'. Return to work for those who can is encouraged and facilitated by the programs.

Appeal procedures

There is an appeal pathway open to Social Security claimants if the state makes an unfavorable decision: first an administrative review, then in sequence a hearing before an administrative law judge, review by an Appeals Council, and finally a civil suit in Federal District Court.

Civil litigation

Workers' compensation is an exclusive remedy in almost all jurisdictions in North America. In general, civil litigation is permitted only in disputes regarding the process of adjudicating claims and implementing the workers' compensation system. Notwithstanding this principle, it is common in many American states for lawyers and legal advocates (frequently associated with labor unions) to represent claimants.

Third party liability

The principal additional stimulus for civil action is the liability of third parties that are neither employees nor employers, such as the manufacturers of an allegedly harmful product used in the workplace. Third party liability is frequently the basis for class-action lawsuits, in which many plaintiffs with a similar complaint against the same defendant bring a shared legal action using the same legal counsel. The Federal Employees' Compensation Act lowers the bar of evidence required to award benefits to defendants in certain occupations who bring legal actions under the Act. This Act preceded and pre-empted state workers' compensation and was intended to make it easier to settle such cases fairly and in a uniform manner for workers who were employed in interstate commerce.

Insurance

The terms of private insurance vary, but most long-term disability policies are worded in some fashion to qualify workers if they are unable to perform the duties of any occupation. Only a few specify indemnification to disabled workers if they cannot engage in their usual occupation. This means that workers who can manage physically in lower-paying jobs may not qualify for LTD, even if their previous position had been highly remunerative or skilled. Some special insurance policies, such as disability insurance for physicians, are written for or carry riders that specify the patient's usual occupation but at a considerably greater premium than standard long-term disability coverage. The provisions of each policy can be subtly different and the criteria for what constitutes disability vary with each. It is worthwhile reading the actual language of the policy to determine what is being requested for before conducting an evaluation.

Unions, professional societies, and employers in highly paid, labor-dependent industries often provide short-term disability insurance plans. Five states (Rhode Island, California, New Jersey, New York, and Hawaii), Puerto Rico, and the railroad workers have state-operated or supervised temporary disability insurance systems ('cash sickness benefits').

Evaluation of occupational lung disorders

The recognition and diagnosis of an occupational lung disorder are part of a thorough integration of clinical information with the occupational history. Once the diagnosis is made, several steps are required beyond traditional diagnosis and management. This is why the treating physician's report is almost never sufficient in itself to support a workers' compensation claim. Additional information is required to assess causation, level of impairment, and estimates of duration of impairment.

Causation is the detective work of occupational lung disease. A careful review of the occupational history is the most essential step in assessing causation.

Impairment assessment is second only to causation in the evaluation of occupational lung disorders and is the first step in assessing disability. There are two elements in functional impairment assessment: assessing the loss of function and assessing the expected duration of impairment. The first is primarily a problem of assessing individual loss of function compared with either capacity before the injury, if this information is available, or to an estimate of normal function for a person of the same size (e.g. the familiar principle of predicted values in spirometry). The second is a judgment on whether or not the loss of function is permanent.

Impairment from respiratory disorders usually manifests itself as diminished lung function, symptoms interfering with normal activities, or exercise intolerance. The means used to assess occupational lung disorders include a detailed history of symptoms, including cough and dyspnea, chest film, spirometry, the maximal voluntary ventilation (MVV) test, diffusing capacity, arterial blood gases, and cardiopulmonary exercise testing. Chest films provide information on structural change but are poorly predictive of functional impairment; their primary role is to stage disease and to provide guidance in interpretation and estimation of duration or progression. The MVV test is used primarily in Social Security Disability insurance but is considered unreliable because it is effort dependent. Diffusing capacity is non-specific but corroborative, especially in cases of restrictive disease. Arterial blood gases are poorly predictive of performance but are administratively important as objective evidence of impairment in some systems, such as the Black Lung program. Cardiopulmonary exercise testing at maximal levels of exertion is a definitive and valuable test when there is doubt or the complaints of the claimant are disproportionate to the apparent impairment by other indicators, but is not usually necessary.

Respiratory impairment is usually rated in the USA by either of two systems: a comprehensive system developed by the American Thoracic Society and a more limited system developed by the American Medical Association and included in the authoritative *AMA Guides to the Evaluation of Permanent Impairment*. The two systems as they apply to permanent, fixed, obstructive or restrictive disease are summarized in Table 35.1. Some workers' compensation boards use their own systems, often incorporating parts of the *AMA Guides*. Most chronic occupational lung disorders, including the major pneumoconioses, may confer permanent or progressive impairment because their

Table 35.1 Classification of respiratory impairment recommended by the American Thoracic Society[a] and the American Medical Association[b]

Rating	Impairment of total person (%)	FVC (% predicted)	FEV$_1$ (% predicted)	FEV$_1$/FVC (ratio)	D$_L$CO (% predicted)	dV̇o$_2$ (ml O$_2$/ min/kg)	Criteria required
Class 1	0 (AMA)	≥80 ≥Lower limit of normal (AMA)	≥80 ≥Lower limit of normal (AMA)	≥0.70 (ATS) >Lower limit of normal (AMA)	≥Lower limit of normal (AMA) ≥80 (ATS)	>25	All
Class 2	10–25	60–79 60–Lower limit of normal (AMA)	60–79 60–Lower limit of normal (AMA)	0.60–0.70	60–69/79	20–25	One
Class 3	26–50	51–59	41–59	0.41–0.59	41–59	15–19	One
Class 4	51–100	≤50	≤40	≤0.40	<40	<15	One
Comments	AMA only	Predicted values from Crapo et al (1981)[c]	Predicted values from Crapo et al (1981)[c]	ATS only (except Class 1)	Predicted values from Crapo and Morris (1981)[d]	AMA only	Any one criterion Class 2–4

[a]American Thoracic Society. Guidelines for the evaluation of impairment/disability in patients with asthma. *Am Rev Respir Dis* 1993; 147: 1056–1061.
[b]American Medical Association. *Guides to the Evaluation of Permanent Impairment*, 5th edn, p. 107. Chicago: AMA, 2001.
[c]Crapo RO, Morris AH, Gardner PM. Reference spirometric values using techniques and equipment that meet ATS recommendations. *Am Rev Respir Dis* 1981; 123: 659–664.
[d]Crapo RO, Morris AH. Standardized single breath normal values for carbon monoxide diffusing capacity. *Am Rev Respir Dis* 1981; 123: 185–190.

Table 35.2 Scoring system for American Thoracic Society impairment rating classes for reactive airways disorders*

			Score
A Postbronchodilator FEV$_1$			
Within normal limits			0
70% predicted to lower limit of normal			1
60–69% predicted			2
50–59% predicted			3
< 50% predicted			4
B Reversibility of FEV$_1$	or	Airway hyperresponsiveness	
Change in FEV$_1$		PC$_{20}$ (mg/ml)	
< 10% predicted		> 8	0
10–19% predicted		> 0.5 to 8	1
20–29% predicted		> 0.125 to 0.5	2
≥30		≤ 0.125	3
Not applicable		Not applicable	4
C Minimum medication needed			
None			0
Occasional^a bronchodilator			1
Occasional^a cromolyn			
Daily bronchodilator, and/or			2
Daily cromolyn, and/or			
Daily low-dose^b inhaled steroid			
Bronchodilator on demand, and			3
Daily high-dose^c inhaled steroid, or			
Occasional^d course of systemic steroids			
Bronchodilator on demand, and			4
Daily high-dose^e inhaled steroid, and			
Daily systemic steroid			
D Summary classes for impairment rating			
Total score		Impairment class	
(A + B + C = D)			
0		0	
1–3		I	
4–6		II	
7–9		III	
10–12		IV	
Uncontrolled†		V	

^{a}Not daily; ^{b} <800 μg beclomethasone or equivalent; ^{c} > 800 μg beclomethasone or equivalent; ^{d} one to three times per year; ^{e} > 1000 μg beclomethasone or equivalent

†Asthma not controlled despite maximal treatment (FEV$_1$ ≥ 50% predicted value despite compliant use of 20 mg prednisone daily).

*American Thoracic Society. Guidelines for the evaluation of impairment/disability in patients with asthma. *Am Rev Respir Dis* 1993; 147: 1056–1061.

mechanism is fibrosis and thus irreversible. Reactive airways disorders are more difficult to assess because airflow is variable and the degree of impairment is variable. Table 35.2 summarizes the system developed by the American Thoracic Society to standardize and compare levels of impairment for asthma. The AMA system provides only general guidelines for evaluating impairment due to asthma.

The Federal Social Security Administration has its own system for purposes of administering SSDI and SSI. The Social Security system is based on physiologic parameters reflected in the degree of impair-

ment in relatively severe cases of chronic fixed obstructive pulmonary disease, asthma, restrictive pulmonary disease, and abnormalities of gas exchange. Physicians with patients who may qualify under this system should obtain particulars from the Federal Social Security Administration.

Often, the worker is disabled from a particular type of work but not others. For example, a worker with occupational asthma may need to avoid exposure to the offending antigen and non-specific respiratory irritants such as dusts. If the condition is permanent, is subject to reasonable accommodation, and does not otherwise interfere with the worker's ability to perform the work at an acceptable level of performance, the claimant may be covered under the Americans with Disabilities Act.

Temporary disability is another matter. An impairment assessment cannot be made for purposes of compensation while the subject's function is changing, although it can be monitored and followed. Duration of the impairment may be estimated to project a possible date for return to work. A useful guide to the duration of disability in common conditions is *The Official Disability Guidelines* issued annually by the Work-Loss Data Institute (500 N. Shoreline Blvd., Suite 1101 N, Corpus Christi, Texas 78471–9987). This resource also gives duration of disability associated with diagnosis and management by hospitalized or non-hospitalized patients, for occupational and non-occupational disorders. At the end of this period, however, there should be an assessment to evaluate fitness to work to ensure that the subject can work safely and to identify any accommodation that may be required to assist the transition.

36 LEGISLATIVE CONTROLS AND COMPENSATION: PACIFIC, FAR EAST AND AUSTRALASIA

Malcolm Sim and Wai-On Phoon

INTRODUCTION

This chapter outlines the legislative occupational health and safety (OHS) framework and workers' compensation systems in place in countries of the Pacific, Far East and Australasia. There is a major emphasis on the OHS systems in Australia and New Zealand, with shorter summaries of those in surrounding countries in the Asian and Pacific sections of the region. Legislative controls and compensation systems are related to occupational health in general, with specific comments when relevant to their application to occupational lung disease. As many of the countries in the region have been UK colonies at some stage in their history, the OHS legislation and systems in place have been heavily influenced by UK historical approaches. In addition, innovations of recent years owe much to the influence of the Robens report released in the UK in 1972. In almost all the countries of this region, OHS law has developed as a separate area of public health law due to the specific nature of work hazards, including those which affect the respiratory system.

Before looking at the OHS legislative frameworks in place in particular countries of this region, it is worthwhile making a few general points about the special characteristics of the region, which have influenced OHS law:

- The levels of industrialization between countries in the region encompass a wide spectrum. It is far greater than in North America or Western Europe. There are well-established industrialized countries which in recent years have moved away from primary industry and manufacturing into more service-related industries (e.g. Australia), newly industrialized countries (such as Korea, Singapore and Malaysia), and countries with little industrialization that remain subsistence or primary industry economies.

- The pace of industrialization has been very fast in many of the newly industrialized countries. This has brought a rapid increase in workplace hazards, which may have outpaced the introduction of legislation for their control.

- Most of the region is tropical, which has important implications for the types of industry, the nature of work hazards, and the spectrum of occupational lung disease. A hot climate additionally poses difficulty for the use of respiratory protective equipment. There is greater discomfort and inevitably a lower rate of compliance.

- Most countries in the region have been colonized by one or more European countries, such as the UK, France, and Holland, at some stage in their recent history. Therefore, OHS legal systems in these countries tend to have elements in common with the principles of the legal system in place in the colonizing country. This has caused some consistency in approach in those countries colonized by a common power, but wide variation between countries colonized by different powers.

- In many countries of the region there are limited resources to support the development and implementation of effective programs to control occupational lung disease. Where government infrastructure is limited also, the continuing and more immediate problems of infectious diseases (or other public health problems) may take priority over the control of occupational diseases, especially the common occupational lung diseases of long latency. Since accurate information on the extent of lung and other occupational diseases is often lacking, government awareness may be low, resulting in its attentions being focused elsewhere.

- Much of the industry in the majority of the region's countries is small. As a result there may be neither sufficient knowledge nor adequate resources at a workplace level to control respiratory hazards.

- Many of the countries in the region are poorly unionized, and this, coupled with the poverty associated with not having a job, can lead to ineffective grassroots pressure to control occupational diseases effectively.

LEGISLATIVE CONTROLS

This section outlines, in alphabetical order, the legislative framework for those countries in the region for which the authors were able to gain relevant information. As great changes in OHS legis-lation have been brought about in other parts of the world by the release in the UK of the Robens report in 1972, the legislative approach in each country is reviewed in terms of its similarity with the principles advocated by Robens. These princi-ples are discussed in detail only in the first listed country, Australia. Discussion about the subse-quent countries then refers to how each relates to this style of legislation. While Robens has been an important factor in the development of OHS leg-islative approaches in the region over the past 25 years or so, some countries have introduced changes in their legislative framework independent of the Robens report.

Australia

In Australia, control of workplace hazards is one of the three main aspects of OHS legislation. The other two are ensuring appropriate compensation is paid to employees who suffer occupational injury or disease, and the provision of effective rehabilita-tion programs. Compensation aspects of the OHS legislative framework are discussed later in the chapter.

Historically, occupational health preventive legislation in Australia has been heavily influenced by the UK models, based on the style of legislation contained in the UK Factories Acts. This resulted in a profusion of Acts introduced by the State Parliaments in Australia, supplemented by many regulations that were usually related to the pre-vention of illness or disease resulting from specific work hazards in particular industries. This legisla-tion tended to be very prescriptive, outlining very specific details for the preventive measures. The processes for enforcement of such legislation, usually through a factory inspectorate, were also heavily influenced by early UK OHS enforcement systems.

Up until the early 1980s much of the preventive occupational health legislation was fragmented, with a large number of Acts of Parliament and underlying Regulations to these Acts, which had been introduced in a piecemeal and *ad hoc* fashion. For example, mine safety was usually the subject of separate legislation under the auspices of a 'Mines Act' or similar. The main objective of such legisla-tion was to prevent and control occupational dis-eases, such as the pneumoconioses, which resulted from the inhalation of respirable airborne contami-nants, such as silica and coal dust. Mining has had an important historical role in industry in Australia. Fuller descriptions of the historical background and legislative framework can be found in the texts by Bohle and Quinlan [1] and Johnstone [2].

Preventive legislative structure

Occupational health and safety regulation in Australia is the responsibility of the six States and two Territories, with no overriding national legislative framework. Because many important workplace hazards are airborne chemical, dust, and gas exposures, the OHS regulatory framework has been designed around the control of these hazards.

The modern era of OHS legislation in the States and Territories of Australia began in the late 1970s and early 1980s. This was in response to the release of the Robens report in the UK, and the introduction of changes to UK OHS legislation. In the early 1980s, most States reviewed their OHS law and came to conclusions similar to those reached by Lord Robens:

- There were too many separate pieces of OHS law.
- There was too much focus on standard setting.
- There was too much prescription, rather than a set of guiding principles.
- Enforcement was often ineffective; there was a need for the primary responsibility to rest with employers, not government.
- There was too little involvement of major stakeholders, and a need for more effective consultation.
- Prevention legislation needed to be complemented by legislation concerned with appropriate compensation and rehabilitation.

Over the next few years, each Australian State enacted an overriding Occupational Health and Safety Act, which had a similar framework and outlined provisions relating to the above points and other aspects of disease and injury prevention. These included a general duty of care by employers, a requirement to achieve a level of health and safety that is 'reasonably practicable', an emphasis on the development of OHS policies, the establishment of OHS committees with representatives from all layers of the organization, the election of OHS representatives by workforces, and a requirement to monitor and protect the health and safety of employees. These Acts also imposed certain duties and responsibilities on employees to take all necessary steps to protect their own health at work. In addition, greater financial penalties for non-compliance with the provisions of the Act were introduced, as well as criminal sanctions for both corporations and individuals within corporations.

To administer this new legislation, most States also overhauled the government bodies responsible for administration and enforcement of the new Acts.

Where, in the past, government departments, usually in the areas of Health or Labor, had been responsible for the enforcement of OHS, new OHS commissions, or similar, were established. These were tripartite bodies, including representatives from government, industry, and trade unions. The role of these commissions has been to oversee the operation of the legislation, advise the relevant minister on matters of OHS policy, and advise on the development of regulations and codes of practice under the OHS Act.

The enforcement of the OHS legislation has also undergone substantial change in recent years. This has usually become the prime responsibility of state departments of labor, with a lesser involvement of departments of health, in line with the new philosophy that OHS is more an employment issue than a health issue. Whereas the OHS inspectorate had traditionally provided regular inspections of the workplace to see whether the specific provisions of the plethora of OHS regulations were being met, the role has changed to one of advice and assistance, so that the more general provisions of the new legislation are achieved. The change is appropriate to the new emphasis on the responsibility of the employer and employees, in consultation, to ensure that the workplace is safe, although inspectors can write infringement notices whenever they believe there is a failure to comply with an aspect of OHS legislation. As Australia has a large part of its workforce in small industry, which lacks the OHS resources of larger industry, the inspectorate tends to concentrate most of its effort there.

The aims of replacing all OHS legislation in a State under one overriding Act and of having one government department and enforcement agency responsible in a particular State have not been entirely achieved. In most States there are still other Acts dealing with particular aspects of OHS, such as mine safety, ionizing radiation, and infectious diseases. In many cases these areas are also administered by arms of government outside the main authority for OHS, such as departments of Health (for radiation) and Energy (for mine safety).

In parallel with the legislative changes occurring in each of the states, the Commonwealth of Australia introduced similar legislation for its own employees. As part of this, the Commonwealth established a tripartite National Occupational Health and Safety Commission (NOHSC). This body originally contained a National Institute for OHS which, like its US namesake, aimed to provide the Commission with high levels of technical and professional support for its regulation development role, and to conduct its own research, promote research outside NOHSC, and conduct training programs in

OHS. Unfortunately, these last three aims are no longer pursued. The roles of NOHSC now lie in regulation development, standards review, and compiling OHS statistics. The latter include data on compensation, which generally underestimate the true incidence of lung and other diseases of occupational origin.

As NOHSC has no direct responsibility for OHS regulation or administration outside Commonwealth of Australia employees, it can only partially fulfil its aim to develop national regulations. These are known as Model Regulations. To become law, they need to be passed by the State parliaments, which have the legislative role and power in the area of OHS. While this process is facilitated by having state representatives on NOHSC, not all States have implemented, without modification, the legislation developed by NOHSC, thereby undermining the goal of consistent national standards to prevent diseases from workplace respiratory and other hazards.

Bangladesh

Bangladesh has tended to follow the older style of UK legislation, rather than the principles of Robens, and its main OHS Act is the Factories Act (1965). In 1979 a set of rules, similar in principle to underlying OHS regulations, was introduced to supplement this act. The legislation operates nationally, and not at a state or provincial level. There is a specific government enforcement agency, the Department of Inspection for Factories and Establishments.

China

China has a complex mix of OHS legislation, which applies to various levels of government, including national, state, provincial, municipal, and district. Some of this legislation has a traditional basis, with a focus on specific prescriptive legislation in particular industry sectors. However, in some sections of the country, there have been moves towards a more Robens style of OHS legislation. This has occurred, for example, in the Shanghai Municipality where new legislation was enacted in 1996. There are specific government enforcement and compliance agencies, but again these operate at different levels and have a range of functions consistent with local provisions of the legislation.

Hong Kong is a separate administrative region of China, and has a different style of OHS legislation from the mainland. It enacted a Robens style Occupational Health and Safety Act in 1997, around the time of the handover from Britain. The legislation is administered by the Occupational Health and Safety Branch of the Labor Department. It has responsibility for enforcement of the OHS Act and associated regulations under the Factories and Industrial Undertakings Ordinance and Subsidiary Regulations.

India

Despite India's colonial history, it has not gone down the path of enacting Robens style OHS legislation. At the time of independence from Britain, it enacted the Indian Factories Act 1948, which remains the main OHS Act, but there are other smaller OHS Acts for specific industry sectors. This legislation has both state and national applications. The central government figure who has responsibility for administration of this legislation is the Director General of Factories. His department is responsible for advising on the administration of the Act and associated Acts and Regulations, and for training the factory inspectorate. At a regional level, there are Directorates of Industrial Safety and Health, which house officials of the inspectorate and administer the OHS legislation.

Indonesia

Although Indonesia enacted OHS legislation in 1970, 2 years before the Robens report was released, it has elements in common with the Robens approach. The legislation is enacted at a national level, and has a national Directorate General for Industrial Relations and Labor Standards within the Ministry of Manpower. The role of this government agency is to ensure compliance with the provisions of the OHS law and provisions, collect data on industrial accidents and disease, and provide reports to government evaluating the effect of the legislation.

Japan

Japan has an overriding Occupational Health and Safety Act, enacted in 1972. It covers the whole country, with a centralized national government administering body, the Labor Standards Bureau in the Ministry of Labor. This administering body has 347 local offices, which employ 'compliance officers' who have equivalent powers to the police under the legislation.

Malaysia

The situation in Malaysia is closer to that in Australia and New Zealand than that in surrounding countries, such as Singapore. Malaysia introduced in 1994 an Occupational Safety and Health

Act, with provisions along the lines of the Robens approach. In addition, Malaysia has kept its Factories and Machinery Act (1967), which relates to 'factories' defined specifically under this Act. The OHS Act relates to all other workplaces, except maritime and aviation facilities. The OHS legislation (both Acts) has national coverage. Although Malaysia has two main pieces of OHS legislation, it has one government department which administers both. This is the Department of Occupational Safety and Health (DOSH), which has a series of regional offices.

New Zealand

New Zealand is one of Australia's nearest neighbors and has many similarities in its history, including colonization by the UK and a legal system based on UK law. In common with Australia, the evolution of New Zealand OHS law has been heavily influenced by that in the UK: Australia and New Zealand also have strong trade and defense agreements, and there are many similarities in the structure of their respective societies. An important difference is that New Zealand, being much smaller in land area and population, does not have states. Its national OHS legislation consequently applies to the whole country, allowing for a greater degree of consistency across the country.

In 1992, New Zealand introduced into legislation the Health and Safety in Employment Act. It has the same general framework as that recommended by Robens, and is similar in style to that introduced into the states of Australia. As in Australia, the different aspects of OHS legislation had become complex, unwieldy, and fragmented, as it had been introduced over time in a piecemeal fashion. In 1980, for example, there were 31 different Acts covering different areas of OHS, administered by five different government departments. The new legislation has a strong emphasis on self-regulation, which has brought about a less interventionist approach from the government over the past 10 years. One major difference with the OHS legislation in the states of Australia is the lower emphasis on worker participation, health and safety committees, and health and safety representatives.

As well as simplifying the legislation, the introduction of the new Act brought into being a single administering government authority, the Occupational Safety and Health (OSH) Service of the Government Department of Labour. OSH has the task of monitoring compliance with the Act, collecting and monitoring OHS statistics, inspecting workplaces, issuing improvement notices, undertaking prosecutions, and requiring medical examinations to be performed. In recent years, OSH has introduced an occupational lung disease surveillance scheme, similar to SWORD in the UK, which encourages thoracic and occupational physicians throughout the country to notify voluntarily cases of several types of respiratory disease.

Philippines

The Philippines has Robens style OHS legislation, enacted in 1978. It has both a national and a state focus, and is administered by the Bureau of Working Conditions of the National Department of Labor and Employment. The role of the Bureau is to:

- formulate policies, rules, and regulations affecting working conditions in all places of employment
- develop standards relating to the administration and enforcement of wages, hours of work, and OHS
- conduct inspections for proper enforcement of statutory rules on working conditions

Singapore

Singapore has been one of the most rapidly industrializing countries in the region over the past two to three decades. Unlike Australia and New Zealand, Singapore has not introduced Robens style legislation. For many years it has had a Factories Act in place, but the definition of 'Factory' under this Act is very broad. As Singapore is a small country in area, there are no states and this piece of legislation is a national one. The specific government agency responsible for administering the Act is known as the Department of Industrial Health in the Ministry of Labor. The main role of this body is to set workplace exposure standards and enforce the provisions of the Act.

Sri Lanka

The main piece of OHS legislation in Sri Lanka is the Factories Ordinance of 1942. Therefore, Sri Lanka has many similarities with the legislative approach taken by its near neighbor, India. The Sri Lankan legislation is administered nationally by the Division of Industrial Safety, in the Department of Labor. This division is responsible for workplace inspections and prosecutions.

Taiwan

Taiwan has Robens style OHS legislation, which was enacted in 1974, the same year that the Health and

Safety at Work Act was enacted in the UK. This legislation has a national focus, and is administered by a single central government agency, the Council of Labor Affairs.

Thailand

Thailand enacted new national legislation in 1998, the Labor Protection Act, to provide a series of Occupational Health and Safety Regulations. It is administered and enforced by the Department of Social Welfare and Labor Protection of the Ministry of Labor and Social Welfare.

Vietnam

Vietnam is another country to enact a recent OHS Act in the Robens style, despite the country never having been colonized by Britain. It was enacted in 1995, has a national focus, and is administered by three main bodies. These comprise the Ministry of Labor, Invalids and Social Affairs, the Ministry of Health, and the Vietnam General Confederation of Labor. The first two bodies are responsible for making standards and enforcing the provisions in the legislation. All three bodies are involved in the development and circulation of OHS information and the management and coordination of OHS activities.

Summary

Several trends can be seen in this review of OHS legislation in countries of the Asia Pacific region:

- Almost all of the countries in the region have enacted new OHS legislation within the past 20–25 years.
- Much of this recent OHS legislation has been in the Robens style, similar in principle to the UK Health and Safety at Work Act of 1974. This demonstrates the widespread influence of the Robens report in the region, although similar approaches incorporating some of the themes have evolved in some countries independently of Robens. Australia, Indonesia, Japan, New Zealand, Philippines, Taiwan and Vietnam have broadly similar schemes; China and Malaysia have some similar components in some areas; while Bangladesh, India, Singapore, Sri Lanka and Thailand have not followed Robens principles to any great extent.
- In most of the countries in the region, the OHS legislation is enacted at a national level. One of the main exceptions is Australia, in which the states have the legislative power, despite this country having one of the smaller populations within the region. National legislation is the preferred model as it promotes a more consistent approach across the country.
- In almost all of the countries, the legislation is administered by one or more departments in a labor ministry rather than a health ministry. This reflects the view of OHS as an industrial relations issue, rather than a health issue.
- At the present time, there is no coordinated effort to achieve uniformity of legislation across the region, in contrast to Western Europe. This is probably a reflection of historical and cultural differences, and large differences between the various countries in their stages of development and industrialization.

REGULATORY EXPOSURE STANDARDS

One of the key tools used by governments in almost all countries to prevent occupational lung, and other, diseases is the setting of workplace exposure standards. This involves two stages; firstly the development of an appropriate exposure standard, and secondly widespread compliance with it within industry. It is important that there is a consistent framework for workplace exposure standards throughout a particular country, so that there can be no incentives to set up hazardous industries in those parts of the country where standards are less stringent. This same principle should ideally apply across geographic regions, indeed the whole world, but it is inevitable that exposure standards will be in different stages of development in different countries, and that some variation will result.

Occupational exposure standards are being introduced in an increasing number of countries in the Asia Pacific region, which is a sign of increasing OHS sophistication. The setting of such standards is a two-stage process. The first involves an examination of the available scientific evidence linking the particular workplace hazard to the development of the occupational disease, so that a health-based exposure limit can be developed. One example of this is reviewing the scientific data relating to crystalline silica as a cause of silicosis and lung cancer. Silica has long been known as a cause of silicosis, but it was designated in 1998 as a definite (Class 1) human carcinogen by the International Agency for Research on Cancer. It is important that exposure standards keep pace with such advances in scientific knowledge. For crystalline silica, this change of classification from a probable human carcinogen to a definite human carcinogen has necessitated a review of the silica standard in many countries. This change in carcinogenicity classification can have important implications for the exposure standard, as there is a strong argument that carcinogens should have more stringent exposure standards, due to the severity of the disease and the uncertainty about the shape of the dose–response curve at low exposure levels.

The second stage in the development of an exposure standard involves consideration of stakeholder (such as industry and trade unions) concerns and other non-health factors, such as technologic feasibility for control and monitoring, and economic factors. For example, a new technologic development in air contamination control may allow a lower workplace level to be achieved more practically and economically. This may then permit an exposure standard, set previously above the health-based limit for technologic reasons, to be lowered towards the health limit even if there is no new scientific information to justify such a reduction on health grounds.

Developing and maintaining currency of such workplace exposure standards is a very resource intensive exercise, both in terms of funding and the high level of scientific expertise required. In reality few, if any, countries in the Asia–Pacific region would have the resources available to develop, regularly review, and update where necessary, such OHS exposure standards. Therefore, they are likely to rely, to a greater or lesser extent, on exposure standards developed elsewhere [3,4], such as in the USA, by the Occupational Safety and Health Administration (OSHA) or the American Conference of Governmental Industrial Hygienists (ACGIH) [5]. Some modification may occur to satisfy local situations.

Many techniques may be used to achieve compliance with workplace exposure standards. These are described more fully in Chapter 33 on occupational hygiene. Sometimes exposure limits are referred to in specific legislation, such as regulations under an OHS Act. These usually set out what the exposure level should be, without dictating how it should be achieved. Sometimes codes of practice are developed in conjunction with a regulation, which do set out methods to achieve compliance. While employers are not usually bound to follow prescribed methods in codes of practice, under the legislation they may have to demonstrate that they have used methods which are equivalent to the suggested methods.

Almost all of the following countries have some exposure standards, which in most cases are the same as, or minor modifications of, exposure standards developed in another country. In developing countries in the region this may be problematic as

the technologic feasibility required to comply with these standards may not be available. Even if the standards are generally consistent with world benchmarks, enforcement at the local level may vary as may the legal interpretation by governments. In some developing countries in the region, there has been an emphasis on the provision of occupational health services, health surveillance, and treatment; while action on prevention, hazard control, and compliance with exposure standards has tended to lag behind the need to deal with the health consequences of poor control. Similar trends are evident in developing countries in other regions of the world.

In the following section is a description of the exposure standard setting process for each of the countries in the region for which information was available to the authors. In addition, to enable comparisons to be made between countries, current workplace exposure standards in each of these countries for two major respiratory hazards, asbestos (both chrysotile and crocidolite) and crystalline silica, are presented. A summary of this information is included in Table 36.1.

Australia

In Australia, the exposure standards for respiratory hazards take the same general form as exposure standards for workplace hazards causing other occupational diseases. The national framework for this is contained in the National Occupational Health and Safety Commission Act 1985. NOHSC does not have direct regulatory authority in the States for such exposure standards, and must rely on the individual states to enact these 'model regulations' into legally enforceable regulations. NOHSC has a tripartite committee structure which develops occupational exposure limits (OELs), with final recommendations being made by a Standards Development Standing Committee. Initially, background reviews would be prepared by NOHSC professional staff to inform the committee, but in more recent years this function has been contracted out to external consultants, primarily due to a reduction in NOHSC resources.

Historically, since exposure standards were first established after World War II, the Australian OELs have been based on the ACGIH TLV list, as a starting point. In more recent years, exposure standards from other countries have also been considered before deciding upon an appropriate OEL for Australia. NOHSC takes into account not only health information, but also technical feasibility and socioeconomic and political factors. There is a period of public comment on proposed new standards, or changes to existing standards.

Table 36.1 Occupational exposure limits for asbestos and silica

Country	Year of first enactment of asbestos legislation	OEL for asbestos (fibers/ml)		Year of first enactment of silica legislation	OEL for silica (mg/m³)
		Chrysotile	Crocidolite		
Australia	1978	1 f/ml	0.1 f/ml	1984	0.2 mg/m³
Bangladesh	NA	NA	NA	NA	NA
China mainland	1980s	0.5 f/ml	0.5 f/ml	1980s	2.0 mg/m³
Hong Kong	1987	0.5 f/ml (4 hours) 1.5 f/ml (10 min)	0.2 f/ml (4 hours) 0.6 f/ml (10 min)	1980s	0.1 mg/m³
India	1948	4 f/ml	4 f/ml	NA	NA
Indonesia	NA	2 f/ml	0.2 f/ml	NA	NA
Japan	1972	2 f/ml	Banned	1960	2.9/ (0.22 Q + 1) mg/m³
Malaysia	1986	1 f/ml	1 f/ml	1989	0.1 mg/m³
New Zealand	1993	1 f/ml	0.1 f/ml	1993	0.1–0.2 mg/m³
Philippines	NA	2 f/ml	2 f/ml	1978	Respirable: 10 mg/m³ Total: 30 mg/m³
Singapore	1980	0.1 f/ml	0.1 f/ml	NA	0.1 mg/m³
Sri Lanka	NA	NA	NA	NA	NA
Taiwan	1980s	1 f/ml	1 f/ml	1980s	Respirable: 10 mg/m³ Total: 30 mg/m³
Thailand	1977	5 f/ml	5 f/ml	1977	Respirable: 10 mg/m³ Total: 30 mg/m³
Vietnam	1992	1 f/ml (8 hours)	Banned	1992	0.3 mg/m³

NA, not applicable; Q, percentage of silica within measured dust.

Many regulations recommended by NOHSC are enacted with little change into state legislation. In addition, there may be an associated code of practice or guidance note, which documents measures to achieve the OEL. This may include recommendations on appropriate hazard control measures, respiratory protection use, and occupational hygiene monitoring. It is important to note that these codes of practice and guidance notes do not have the same legal status as regulations, are not legally binding, and aim to give advice and guidance on best practice only. Many substances, such as lead, asbestos, and silica, have their own set of regulations. However, cover for the full range of chemical hazards in industry would require a substantial number of such regulations – an unwieldy task. To rationalize this process, generic Hazardous Substances regulations have been developed by NOHSC, and are being introduced into the states. These outline general approaches for assessing, monitoring, and controlling different kinds of chemical hazards, including respiratory toxins, in Australian workplaces.

Sometimes these regulations or codes of practice include provisions for health surveillance, ie health screening tests that are required of workers exposed to respiratory and other hazards that may cause chronic disease. One example is the requirement for workers in the asbestos industry to have periodic medicals in order to detect lung changes consistent with pulmonary fibrosis at an early stage. The rationale for such surveillance is that early detection may lead to intervention that prevents further progression of the disease. This is generally more applicable to non-malignant disease than to cancers. Such medical surveillance also provides an indication of whether exposure control efforts in the workplace are adequate, but this is only really of use for respiratory and other diseases with short latent periods.

There are Australian OELs for the two respiratory hazards, asbestos and silica. For asbestos, there are separate OELs for chrysotile and crocidolite. For chrysotile the exposure limit is 1 fiber/ml, and for crocidolite it is 0.1 fiber/ml. For crystalline silica the OEL is 0.2 mg/m³, which was enacted in 1984. The silica standard is currently being reviewed in light of the recent IARC decision to define it as a Class 1 carcinogen (definitely carcinogenic to humans).

Bangladesh

At the present time, Bangladesh has no workplace exposure standards, and no regulations relating to these. This is an indication that other more immediately pressing public health problems, such as diarrheal diseases and inorganic arsenic in drinking water, are the main focus of government attention.

China

China first legislated for exposure standards, which are known as maximum allowable concentrations (MACs), in 1962, but time-weighted average (TWA) standards were also introduced in 1992. These exposure standards are part of the National Health standards for OHS. Unlike many of the other countries in the region, these MACs and TWAs are not based on the ACGIH TLVs. They were developed from an internal review of toxicologic and epidemiological studies, as well as from feasibility investigations. Approximately 250 chemical hazards are included.

Specific asbestos regulations were introduced in the 1980s. Under these regulations, the permissible exposure level for both chrysotile and crocidolite is 0.5 fiber/ml in Shanghai. There is some variation within the country at the provincial level. Silica exposure standards also come under the asbestos regulations. Under this regulation, the permissible exposure limit is 2.0 mg/m³.

In Hong Kong there are no occupational exposure limits for chemicals in the workplace, but there is a guidance note provided to industry called A Reference Note on Occupational Exposure Limits for Chemical Substances in the Work Environment. It is important to emphasize that this is only a guidance note and does not carry the legal status of regulation. The basis for the exposure limits is the ACGIH TLVs and approximately 400 chemicals come under this guidance note.

There is specific legislation dealing with asbestos in industry. This comes under the Factories and Industrial Undertaking (Asbestos Control Regulations), which was first enacted in Hong Kong in 1987, well before the handover to China. Under this regulation, the exposure limit for chrysotile is 0.5 fiber/ml (4 hours) and 1.5 fibers/ml (10 min). For crocidolite the corresponding limits are 0.2 fiber/ml (4 hours) and 0.6 fiber/ml (10 min). Hong Kong also has legislation specifically dealing with silica in the workplace. This comes under the Factories and Industrial Undertakings (Blasting by Abrasives) Special Regulations, which were first enacted in the early 1980s. The exposure limit for silica as quartz is 0.1 mg/m³.

India

India first enacted specific legislation relating to occupational exposure limits in the 1948 Factories Act of India and Mahrashgra Factories Rules of 1963. Under these rules there are some particular standards, codes of practice, and guidelines which govern exposure to chemicals in the workplace. The exposure limits are called standard permissible values and are published under the Central Pollution Control Board Series: PCL/4/1995–96. The exposure limits are not based on the ACGIH TLVs. Instead they have been developed by the Central Pollution Control Board using a range of data, including that obtained through national surveillance. Approximately 430 chemicals come under this specific legislation.

India does have an exposure standard for both chrysotile and crocidolite. It is 4 fibers/ml for each, which is considerably higher than the standard in most other countries in the region. There is no exposure limit for crystalline silica.

Indonesia

In Indonesia there are occupational exposure limits for workplace chemicals. These were first enacted in 1978 as the TLV of Indonesian Standard for Chemical Factors in the Workplace. They are based on the ACGIH TLVs. The regulation covers about 100 chemicals only. There are specific workplace exposure levels for the two types of asbestos mentioned. For the first of these, chrysotile, the exposure limit is 2 fibers/ml. For crocidolite, the exposure standard is 0.2 fiber/ml. For these asbestos exposure standards there are regulations, standards, codes of practice and guidance notes. The specific legislation is known as Occupational Safety and Health in the use of Asbestos 1995. Indonesia has no specific exposure limit for exposure to silica in the workplace.

Japan

Japan has had workplace exposure standards since 1972. They are known as The Work Environmental Control Limits. They are not based on the ACGIH TLVs, but were developed by the Japan Society for Occupational Health. Japan has an exposure limit for asbestos, but it is included in general regulations covering a range of chemical hazards. This is entitled the Regulation on Prevention of Health Hazards due to Specified Chemical Substances, which was first enacted in 1972. Under this regulation, there is an exposure limit for chrysotile asbestos of 2 fibers/ml. Crocidolite is a prohibited substance, so there is no exposure limit. There is specific legislation dealing with workplace exposure to silica, which is the Regulation on Prevention of Dust Hazards. This comes under the Pneumoconiosis Law, which was first enacted in 1960. The exposure standard is $2.9/(0.22Q + 1)$, where Q is the percentage content of silica in the dust.

Malaysia

Malaysia has several specific regulations for workplace exposures, and is currently introducing generic 'chemicals in workplace' regulations. The current specific regulations come under the Factories and Machinery Act and refer to permissible exposure levels. These have been based on the ACGIH TLVs, but also involved discussions with other agencies, university academics, and industry. It is anticipated that the new regulations will cover at least 500 chemical hazards.

There are specific asbestos regulations, which were introduced in 1986. Under these regulations, the permissible exposure level for both chrysotile and crocidolite is 0.1 fiber/ml, with an action level of 0.05 fiber/ml. Under these regulations, employees exposed to asbestos are required to have a medical examination every 2 years. Silica also has specific regulations, which were introduced in 1989. Under these, the permissible exposure limit is 0.1 mg/m^3 for quartz, and 0.05 mg/m^3 for cristobalite and for tridymite. As for asbestos, medical examinations for exposed employees are required every 2 years.

New Zealand

In New Zealand OELs are known as Workplace Exposure Standards, and the system for developing these has been in place for many years. They generally come under the respective regulations for particular substances, but most chemicals come under the Management of Substances Hazardous to Health (MOSHH) Regulations, which have a similar approach to the Hazardous Substances Regulations in Australia. These workplace exposure standards are generally based on the TLVs of the ACGIH and apply to all chemicals on the ACGIH list.

For chrysotile and crocidolite asbestos, the standards are the same as in Australia, 1.0 fiber/ml and 0.1 fiber/ml respectively. These standards are included in the 1998 Asbestos Regulations, and there is an accompanying code of practice. Crystalline silica comes under the MOSHH regulations and the OEL is 0.1–0.2 mg/m^3 depending upon the type. There is an associated guidance note under the MOSHH regulations, called 'Use of Crystalline Silica'.

Philippines

The Philippines has had legislation for occupational exposure limits (threshold limit values) for chemicals in the workplace since 1978. They were first adapted from the 1976 ACGIH TLVs, and come under the auspices of the Occupational Safety and Health Standards of the Department of Labor and Employment. Approximately 500 chemicals are included in this legislation. There are specific exposure limits for both chrysotile and crocidolite. All forms of asbestos have an exposure limit of 2 fibers/ml. There is also specific legislation related to silica exposure. This comes under rule 1070 (Occupational Health and Environmental Control) which was first enacted in 1978. The exposure limit for silica as respirable quartz is 10 mg/m^3.

Singapore

In Singapore, workplace exposure standards are known as 'Permissible Exposure Levels of Toxic Substances'. These were enacted in 1996, and are based upon the ACGIH TLVs. Approximately 600 chemicals come under the set of regulations responsible for these standards. Singapore has a specific regulation concerned with protection against lung diseases from asbestos exposure, called the Asbestos Regulation, which was enacted in 1980 under the Factories Act. The workplace standard for both chrysotile and crocidolite is 0.1 fiber/ml, which for chrysotile is an order of magnitude more stringent than the standard in both Australia and New Zealand. In addition to the asbestos regulation, there are guidance notes on the removal and handling of asbestos materials. While there is a standard for silica of 0.1 mg/m^3, there is no specific silica regulation or guidance note.

South Korea

South Korea first legislated for occupational exposure limits in 1986, using standards equivalent to the ACGIH TLVs and OSHA PELs. These levels were last revised in 1997 to align them with changes in the TLVs and PELs. In 1998 the Ministry of Labor announced the establishment of the first occupational exposure standard which did not follow the overseas standards previously used. This was for 2-bromopropane and was based on a review within South Korea of the relevant health data, mainly reproductive effects.

Sri Lanka

Sri Lanka does not currently have occupational exposure limits of any type. However, the Sri Lankan

Occupational Health and Safety Administration does refer to the ACGIH standards, which are used in an advisory role only. There is no legal backing to these standards. Consequently, in Sri Lanka there are no exposure limits related to asbestos or silica exposure.

Taiwan

Taiwan has workplace 'permissible exposure limits', mostly based on the ACGIH TLVs. Some are developed from other US limits, such as the OSHA permissible exposure limits. Only about 100 chemicals are included in this legislation. There is specific legislation dealing with asbestos exposure under the Workers Health Protection Act. This was first enacted in the 1980s. The exposure limit for both chrysotile and crocidolite is 1 fiber/ml. There is also special legislation for silica exposure and the exposure limit for respirable silica is 10 mg/m^3.

Thailand

Thailand has specific legislation related to occupational exposure limits, which was first enacted in 1977. This is the Environmental Working Safety Standard Related to Chemicals, and covers around 130 different workplace chemicals. They are based on the ACGIH TLVs. There are specific occupational exposure limits of 5 fibers/ml for several types of asbestos, including chrysotile and crocidolite. There is also a specific exposure limit for silica, which also comes under the Environmental Working Safety Standard Related to Chemicals enacted in 1977. The exposure limit for silica as quartz (respirable dust) is 10 mg/m^3.

Vietnam

Vietnam enacted occupational exposure limits for workplace chemicals in 1992. These are called Provisional Standards on Occupational Hygiene and the specific name is TLV for Toxic and Hazardous Chemicals at Workplaces. These have not been based on the ACGIH TLVs, but instead have been based on exposure limits used in Russia and other US standards. Only about 150 chemicals are covered by this legislation. The specific exposure standards for chrysotile are 1 fiber/ml for 8 hours and 2 fibers/ml for 1 hour. Crocidolite is prohibited for use in industry and does not have an exposure limit. Crystalline silica comes under the same set of regulations. The exposure limit is 0.3 mg/m^3 for the full work shift, and 0.5 mg/m^3 for a short time, the duration of which is not defined.

Summary

It can be seen that there is considerable variation in the approaches which have been taken in countries in the Asia–Pacific region in the setting of specific occupational exposure standards. Most countries have such standards and, of these, most have followed the ACGIH TLVs or similar OELs. However, these overseas standards have been developed in industrialized countries, such as the USA, which invariably have large differences in terms of social, economic, and technologic factors. These are important considerations in occupational standard setting in a particular country. Therefore, implementing such standards without considering local factors may not always be appropriate. Some countries have used ACGIH TLVs as a starting point, but have then modified them on the basis of local sources of information to establish their current workplace exposure limits.

Conversely, there are some countries in the region, such as Bangladesh and Sri Lanka, where occupational exposure limits have not been established in legislation, or have been set for only a small number of chemicals. This means that workers in those countries are working in unregulated environments at exposure levels that may be considered unacceptable in other countries of the region.

There is considerable variation between the countries in the exposure limits for the two respiratory hazards (asbestos and crystalline silica) used here as illustrations, and much more than in North America and Western Europe (Chapters 35 and 37). The exposure levels for some forms of asbestos in particular are considerably greater in some Asian countries than in Australia, western Europe, New Zealand, and the USA. This is likely to have important implications for the risks to respiratory health of employees in those countries.

Setting workplace exposure limits is only the first step in protecting the health of workers exposed to respiratory hazards. The effectiveness of such limits is very dependent upon the industries to which they apply, upon implementing control measures to comply with such limits, and upon carrying out appropriate and regular air monitoring of the actual levels of workplace exposures. It is also important that an effective enforcement agency exists to intervene where compliance with workplace exposure limits is poor, and that there exists an appropriately trained workforce to monitor and manage workplace exposures.

COMPENSATION

Preventive OHS legal structures and their enforcement processes are never completely effective and, as a result, workers are injured and develop diseases as a result of their occupations. There is, therefore, a need to have systems in place to compensate affected workers appropriately and, where possible, to provide rehabilitation for them. Compensation law, directed towards prevention, has had a long history of evolution in many parts of the world and current approaches necessarily differ from country to country. The systems in place in Australia and New Zealand are described to provide detailed illustrations, and an overview is provided for other countries in the region. The emphasis is on statutory compensation, rather than common law systems.

In many countries of the world, workers have two avenues available for gaining compensation for work related injury and disease:

- The first, in countries that have such a system, is under the provisions of common law. This requires the worker to prove negligence on the part of the employer or other parties (such as suppliers or designers of equipment), who are the defendants (and potential disbursers) in the civil law suit. For a claim to be successful, several points need to be demonstrated by the worker who is seeking compensation. These are: that the employer owed the worker a duty of care; that the employer's omissions breached this duty of care; that the breach caused the injury or illness for which the worker is claiming compensation; and that the worker suffered economic and/or non-economic loss as a result of this injury or disease. The burden of proof which is required is conventionally that of the balance of probabilities – not, as in a criminal court, 'beyond reasonable doubt'. The claimant (the plaintiff) has to demonstrate that it is more likely than not that the substance of the claim is true.

- The second is statutory compensation, operated by the government usually under a no-fault principle. Such systems had their origin in Europe. They came into being to provide compensation more quickly and effectively, by requiring a lower burden of proof than is usually required under a common law system. Such systems are usually funded by levies on employers, with built-in incentives and penalties based on performance. They tend to concentrate on the issue of whether the injury or disorder was truly occupational in origin, on the degree of any resulting disablement and/or loss of earnings, and the contribution of any non-occupational factors. The issues of responsibility and negligence are generally less critical to the claimant (though may determine who pays), and the procedures are supposed to be less adversarial.

These two approaches can and do coexist in many countries, although in others one may invalidate any use of the other.

With regard to compensation for occupational lung disease, claims under both systems are often more difficult to prove than claims for injury. There are several reasons for this. The disease may take many months or years to become clinically apparent (sometimes long after the worker has left the causal workplace), and it may occur also in non-occupational environments. Therefore, the link between the occupational exposure and the respiratory disease may not be readily made, especially if there has been a lengthy passage of time and confirmatory data concerning the relevant exposures are no longer available. Another problem may be the difficulty in teasing out the contribution of work exposure from that of other respiratory insults, such as cigarette smoking. For these reasons, it is generally accepted that compensation data do not provide an accurate measure of the epidemiology of occupational lung disease.

Clinical approaches to assessing disability associated with occupational lung disease are covered in Chapter 40.

Australia

As with preventive occupational health legislation, the responsibility for providing a workplace compensation scheme lies with the states. The federal government is responsible only for specific groups, such as its own employees and the military. In the early part of the 20th century, the states introduced workers' compensation legislation, which had several common features. These included one or more of: the principle of no-fault compensation, a broader coverage of conditions than would ordinarily be successful under common law, specified entitlements, mandatory coverage, and the right to appeal.

One important difference between Australia and many other industrialized countries was that common law rights were not abolished, at least initially. This enabled workers to sue their employer where there was clear evidence of negligence, and so gain a greater financial award than was available under the compensation schemes covered by state legislation. However, a series of reforms in all states and territories during the 1980s and 1990s has, in most cases, severely curtailed worker access to common law rights. Other reforms have included stricter definitions of conditions covered under the schemes and time limits on the duration of payment, in an effort to reduce costs.

LEGISLATIVE CONTROLS AND COMPENSATION: PACIFIC, FAR EAST AND AUSTRALASIA **567**

Occupational lung disease has generally not been well covered by these compensation schemes, because of difficulties in making accurate diagnoses, in linking disease with work exposure, the multifactorial nature of such diseases, the often long latent periods between exposure and disease, and the need to rely on epidemiological evidence to support a causal association. Such evidence is usually open to interpretation, and compensation authorities often have difficulty coping with this in the decision-making processes. This has been partly addressed in some schemes by the introduction of 'prescribed diseases' to supplement the definition of injury. These usually lag behind the current state of knowledge regarding occupational diseases and usually relate to traditional occupational poisonings, such as chrome ulceration of the nose. Occupational lung diseases tend not to feature in such lists of prescribed diseases.

One development in Australia which is of great relevance to the compensation of occupational lung disease was the establishment of the Dust Diseases Board in New South Wales. At first this Board was concerned mainly with the cases of pneumoconiosis in the state, due largely to the extensive mining industry. To assess the merits of claims for compensation from dust disease of occupational origin, the Board has established criteria that are more in line with the nature of occupational lung diseases than those of earlier compensation schemes that were focused almost entirely on injuries. As the incidence of the pneumoconioses has declined in recent years, this board is now dealing with a greater proportion of other occupational lung diseases, such as occupational asthma.

New Zealand

Developments in workplace injury and disease compensation in New Zealand have paralleled those in Australia, but have tended to occur earlier. By the Workers' Compensation for Accidents Act of 1900, New Zealand was one of the first countries in the world to introduce into legislation the principle of 'no-fault' compensation. After a review, this principle was extended in 1972 with the introduction of the Accident Compensation Act. This provided no-fault compensation for all types of injury, not just those occurring in occupational settings. The introduction of this compensation scheme brought with it the abolition of the common law right to sue to recover compensatory damages. The scheme was funded by an employer levy, based upon the number of compensatable accidents occurring in that company. This formula was criticized as most companies are too small to make a credible statistical

judgement on the amount of levy to be paid each year.

Over the following 20 years, a series of changes were made to the administration of the scheme by the Accident Compensation Commission, partly because of employer concerns over an escalation in cost. This culminated in the introduction of a replacement act in 1992, known as the Accident Rehabilitation Compensation Insurance Act. This aimed to reduce costs, largely through the introduction of more stringent definitions of 'injury', but also by some cost shifting to other sectors of the health system. In the new provisions, injuries and diseases of gradual onset were generally excluded, which has made it more difficult to gain compensation for many occupational lung diseases, and other diseases of slow onset. A further Act, the Accident Insurance Act, was introduced in 1998 in a further effort to shift costs away from the Government scheme. It required employers to obtain insurance cover through an insurance company. Despite these changes, which have come under some criticism, the costs and numbers of compensated injuries and fatalities have not significantly diminished.

Other countries

Of the other countries in the region covered by this review, almost all have some form of workers' compensation system in place. The systems are compulsory and are usually administered nationally, though administrative procedures differ markedly between the countries. Several have specific systems of compensation, including Japan (Employee State Insurance Scheme, Workman's Compensation Insurance), Singapore (Workman's Compensation Act), and Thailand (Workman's Compensation Fund).

China bases its compensation scheme in mainland China on a notified list of occupational diseases, while Hong Kong has employee compensation insurance for injuries, supplemented by the inclusion of 44 listed diseases. Hong Kong also has a Pneumoconiosis Compensation Fund for compensating cases of silicosis and asbestos-related disease.

Some countries have no specific workers' compensation scheme in place, but include compensation for occupational disorders under other health schemes. For example, Sri Lanka has some provisions for compensation under its general OHS legislation while Indonesia and Vietnam have provisions under their Social Security Schemes. Malaysia shares this responsibility under several areas of government, including the Social Security organization, Workman's Compensation Act, and Disability Pension scheme. The Philippines also has shared responsibilities between the Employees Compensation Commission, Social Security system, and government and private insurance schemes. While Taiwan has no specific compensation legislation or scheme, there are provisions for compensation in its general labor laws. Of the countries covered in this review, Bangladesh is the only country not to have a workers' compensation system.

In summary, workers' compensation legislation and administration in this region is very variable and is a rapidly evolving activity of government. While almost all countries have some type of compensation scheme in place, many rely upon provisions under other Acts, such as social security law or industrial law. Where specific compensation legislation is in place, this is usually directed at compensation for acute injury, and is not designed to meet the specific needs of occupational lung diseases. In some areas, such as Australia and Hong Kong, there are established Boards specifically dealing with compensation for lung diseases related to workplace exposures. This appears to be the most appropriate way to assess, compensate, and monitor such diseases.

REFERENCES

1. Bohle P, Quinlan M. *Managing Occupational Health and Safety: a Multidisciplinary Approach*, 2nd edn. Melbourne: Macmillan, 2000.
2. Johnstone R. *Occupational Health and Safety Law and Policy*. Sydney: LBC Information Services, 1997.
3. Hajssan S. *Setting the Limit: Occupational Health Standards and the Limits of Science*. New York: Oxford University Press, 1998.
4. Vincent J. International occupational exposure standards: a review and commentary. *Am Ind Hyg Assoc J* 1998; 59: 729–742.
5. American Conference of Governmental Industrial Hygienists. *Documentation of the Threshold Limit Values and Biological Exposure Indices*, Vols 1–3, 6th edn. Cincinnati: O, OH ACGIH, 1991.

37 LEGISLATIVE CONTROLS AND COMPENSATION: WESTERN EUROPE

Christophe Leroyer and Jean-Dominique Dewitte

INTRODUCTION

Legislation to control hazardous workplace exposures has evolved in different ways and at different speeds in the numerous countries of western Europe over the course of the last century. The mining industry in particular led to the recognition of pneumoconiosis as a potentially disabling, even life threatening, respiratory disease, and to major public concern. The first directives for compensating work-related diseases appeared at the beginning of the twentieth century, and in France, for example, some workers have been compensated since 1919 (for lead poisoning in relevant occupations). Each European country has necessarily developed its own policies over the years for occupational health and safety programs, and compensation, but more recently the European Union (EU) has been acquiring the power to direct health policy. This applies particularly to the promotion of health and safety at work.

This chapter consequently outlines the legislative occupational health and safety framework in the EU, which now encompasses 15 European countries. Legislative controls are discussed at the EU level, without special regard to individual member states, and the EU regulatory exposure standards are presented. By contrast, health insurance and compensation systems within member countries are not directed by EU legislation, and it is practical to do no more than illustrate the various mechanisms that are active in various parts of the western European region.

LEGISLATIVE CONTROLS

EU health institutions

The institutional system of the EU can be classified only with difficulty. Although the EU is a distinct entity, with its own parliament and extensive powers, it is not a federation to which national governments and parliaments are subordinated. As a result the extent of its powers is likely to be misunderstood by many, perhaps most, of its citizens. Since both its powers and its membership continue to evolve at rapid rates, we can attempt to describe only the general principles of its legislative program for preserving health among its workforce.

The concept of a European Union, from a historical perspective, was essentially political. The French writer Victor Hugo, chairman of the Paris Peace Congress held in 1848, advocated 'European friendship' based on universal suffrage, as a basis for the constitution of a 'United States of Europe'. However, in the foundation steps preceding the implementation of the current EU (namely, the European Coal and Steel Community in 1951, and the European Economic Community in 1958), trading concerns were predominant. Despite the wish of the participants of the Treaty of Rome in 1958 to promote health and safety at work, the economic perspective dominated the social perspective. It was the adoption of a single European Act in 1987 that gave new impetus to occupational health and safety proposals. This act allowed the Council of Ministers to adopt directives to protect health and safety at work. With the Treaty of Maastricht in December 1991, the EU assumed additional responsibility in the domain of public health, but this is restricted to the fields of prevention, information, and education.

At present, three European institutions share responsibility for health policy:

- The Council of Ministers convenes representatives of the member states (15 in 2000) and is the effective center for decision making. Social affairs are addressed by special boards and each member state takes turn acting as the chair. The board establishes community regulations, in particular by enacting directives, with the help of a permanent committee. Its business is brought to the Council of Ministers twice a year for approval or review.

- The European Parliament (626 delegates in 2000) provides incentive to health policy in Europe by way of resolutions. These are prepared by 'The environment, public health and consumer protection commission'. The parliament has an uncommitted budget of 'non-compulsory' expenses which is increasingly devoted to carrying out its health policy.

- The Commission of the EU has 20 members appointed by governments of member states for 5 years. With the assistance of more than 10 000 employees, the commission is the guardian of treaties. It ensures 'feedback' to member states and delivers recommendations in the case of non-compliance with EU policy. Several of the Commission's 24 directorates general are concerned with health problems but the fifth directorate, 'Health and Security', is the most influential. Under its direction, the major aspects of health and safety in the workplace and public health protection are managed.

Independent of these three EU institutions are a number of inter-governmental and international organizations, such as the World Health Organization (WHO) and the Council of Europe, which also work on major European health projects. The relevant regional office of WHO covers 31 countries from Greenland in the north to Malta in the south. It promotes the 'EUROHealth' program, which fosters increasing cooperation between the EU and eastern European countries. The Council of Europe was founded in 1949 with a head office in Strasbourg to organize cooperation between the governments of an even larger group of European countries (41 member states in April 1999). One of its major achievements has been the European Convention for Human Rights; included is the right of 'health for everyone'. It also convenes conferences of European health ministers that give policy direc-

tion in the domain of health. Principal actions to date have dealt with drug and alcohol abuse. Finally, non-governmental health organizations within Europe, such as the European Respiratory Society, play an increasing role in conducting major epidemiological surveys in the field of respiratory health, in promoting recommendations, and in influencing policy.

EU health legislation

The economic aims of the EU have been counterbalanced since 1958 by an expressed intention to provide extensive health and safety facilities in the workplace. At present legislation centers on the measures required to enforce the various health and safety framework directives:

- Measures that contain basic provisions for health and safety organization at the workplace; it outlines the separate responsibilities of employers and workers, and is supplemented by individual directives for specific groups of workers (e.g. pregnant women), specific workplaces (e.g. mineral extraction), or specific substances (e.g. carcinogens).

- Measures to protect the health and safety of workers against the risks arising from exposure to chemical, physical, and biologic agents at the workplace, supplemented by individual directives dealing with specific agents.

Unconnected to the framework directives are other measures that contain provisions for particular occupational activities or specific groups. It includes, for instance, measures related to young people, transport activities, physical agents, and explosive atmospheres.

Exposure standards

Principles

As in most countries, the setting of workplace exposure standards is the cornerstone of the EU occupational and safety program. Its main principles can be summarized as follows:

- health and safety are major objectives that overwhelm economic considerations
- adherence to regulatory exposure standards aims not only to protect workers against occupational hazards, but also to ensure uniformity throughout the member states to prevent any distortion of competitiveness
- the employer, not any external regulatory body, is responsible for the assessment of any

workplace hazard, as well as for the implementation of safety measures

- it is the responsibility of the employer to avoid the use of a harmful agent, if the nature of the manufacturing activity so permits, by replacing it with a less dangerous one

Interestingly, the principle of uniformity to prevent any competitive advantage illustrates a positive influence of EU market rules on health and safety at work. Of significant importance to the level of protection in individual member states is that adopted directives lay down minimum requirements concerning health and safety at work. Member states must raise their levels of protection if these are lower than the minimum requirements set by the directives. Beyond this, the adopted provisions do not prevent any member state from maintaining or introducing more stringent measures for the protection of its workers.

Following publication, the member states enact these EU recommendations in their national regulations. Member states then acquaint the EU institutions of all legislative measures taken at the national level that ensure proper application of the EU recommendations.

An EU commission, with the help of a scientific committee, is responsible for the elaboration of workplace exposure standards. An updated list of threshold limit values was published in June 2000. This extended two previously published versions, and took into account both relevant scientific data and technologic developments in air contamination control. For each substance, threshold limit values are given both as time-weighted average values over an 8-hour work period and as peak values over a maximum period of 15 min. Special mention is given if there is any risk of absorption into and/or through the skin. The published document with a list of agents, occupations at risk, and relevant information on scientific evidence is available on websites of the EU institutions:

'Protection of Health and Safety at Work; Exposure to chemical agents'

http://europa.eu.int/scadplus/leg/en/cha/c11140.htm

European agency for safety and health at work

The Agency's aim is to stimulate harmonization of health and safety measures at work throughout the EU. It provides recommendations to member states and it takes account of the legislative measures taken in each at a national level as a consequence. This interaction plays a key role in subsequent recommendations. In addition, the Agency is responsible for disseminating information to all rele-

vant institutions within the member states – a favored strategy within the EU to reinforce its policies and directives. The Agency thus provides the EU institutions, the member states, and those involved in health and safety at work with technical, scientific, and economic information of use in this field:

http://agency.osha.eu.int

A recent notable project of the Agency is 'The state of occupational safety and health in the EU – a pilot study'. It was published in September 2000 and provides a first step to the development of a uniform system for monitoring health and safety throughout the EU. Its purpose is to provide decision-makers with an overview of the current health and safety situation, and so support the identification of common challenges and priority areas for preventive action. Despite weaknesses in data collection from the diverse range of information sources throughout the EU, the pilot study presents a comprehensive summary of the current state of health and safety at work in the EU. Details of this pilot study are available on the webpage:

http://agency.osha.eu.int/publications/reports/stateofosh

In addition the study highlights possible needs for the development of specific preventive or compensation measures, for instance the possibility of recognizing that cancer of the larynx may be a consequence of occupational exposure to asbestos. The study also shows that almost all member states have organized, under ministries of labor or social affairs, councils on occupational risk prevention. As an example, the Institute for Occupational Safety and Health in Potsdam is coordinating occupational health and safety policy for the federal states of Germany. Organized under the Ministry of Labor, Social Affairs, Health, and Women, this institute provides an interdisciplinary group of scientists, physicians, psychologists, engineers, ergonomists, and social scientists. Its task is to develop proposals for focused campaigns, based on current data concerning work strain and health. Finally, at the international level, the institute functions as the coordinating body of the federal states of Germany, linked with the European Agency for Safety and Health at Work.

COMPENSATION

European Union

Despite extensive preventive measures, workers will continue to be injured through accidents and to develop disease as a result of their occupations. Even in the absence of accidents, two important mechanisms will cause an ongoing incidence of respiratory disorders. First, disorders attributable to hypersensitivity will inevitably occur in the few exposed individuals who happen to be the most susceptible. This will be so even when careful preventive measures have been followed and only low levels of exposure are encountered – levels that are generally without risk and can reasonably be considered acceptable. This applies especially to occupational asthma, which is unfortunately by far the most common type of occupational lung disease in western Europe.

Second, the latency period between exposure onset and disease onset may be long, implying that inadequate exposure standards of yesteryear will continue to contribute to today's burden of incident disease. This is unfortunately the case for the various disorders induced by asbestos, which collectively outnumber the current incident cases of occupational asthma in western Europe. Most incident asbestos-related cases, however, are of pleural plaques and so cause negligible disablement.

The issue of compensation will therefore remain a major concern throughout the EU. At present the compensation schemes of individual member states are independent, each having developed its own policy over periods of many years preceding European cooperation. There is consequently wide variation, and it is not practical to outline the details for each of the 15 member states. In this chapter we shall simply provide examples from two member states, France and the UK, to illustrate the differences that exist. However, all member states share a common rule of statutory state compensation. Unlike compensation suits in civil law, there is a 'no-fault' principle and the worker is not required to prove negligence on the part of the employer.

Table 37.1 lists information concerning state compensation within member states of the EU. Most compensation systems are administered by national agencies. Employers are generally responsible for funding through a general insurance system or taxation. Diagnoses are usually made by physicians employed by a national agency, though this often follows consultations with experts or boards of experts. Most member states rely on lists of 'accepted' agents and a compatible occupational and medical history. An advantage of such lists is transparency: employees, employers, and physicians alike are more easily aware of potentially harmful occupations and occupational agents, and this is believed to favor subsequent prevention.

This 'list system' does not necessarily exclude compensation for a disease that does not fall within the scope of the official list. However, the criteria for compensation awards are usually much more stringent in these circumstances. In some countries, such awards are made under the framework of a work accident, that is, a sudden onset of the disease closely following an unusual level of exposure. In others, the employee has to prove a relationship between his work and the onset of the disease.

France

In France, occupational diseases have been compensated since 1919. Two official legal lists exist of occupational diseases or causal agents (or both) – one for farmers and one for workers in other occupations. Each work-related disease has a schedule of defining characteristics for compensation purposes. These include symptoms, an indication of the workplaces where exposure may occur, and a minimum level of exposure. If a claimant develops a listed disease within the scope of an approved schedule, there is a strong assumption that compensation should be approved. Claims are made by workers to the local social security office, and are accompanied by a medical certificate indicating the type of occupational disease and the observed manifestations listed in the schedule. The social security office is then responsible for carrying out a medical and technical investigation, and a consulting physician employed by the social security office makes a decision on whether the claim should be approved or rejected.

If there is a doubt on the acceptability of the claim, the consulting physician can seek the expertise of a chest or other specialist physician working in a centre for occupational diseases. If the claim is accepted, a decision will also be made on any need to indemnify the claimant for a loss of income. If the claim is rejected, the worker can ask for an assessment by a medical expert.

Three recent modifications have been introduced to encourage greater harmonization within the EU:

- Separate procedures for compensating pneumoconiosis and related diseases were abolished in August 1999, thereby allowing a common procedural pathway for all occupationally induced disease.
- A surveillance program has been available since March 1995 for workers exposed occupationally to a listed carcinogen. This continues after the cessation of exposure and includes retired workers, although is not mandatory for the workers who qualify. The program is based on the assumption that early diagnosis may reduce the morbidity. It is run under the responsibility of Social Security Office physicians, and consists of appropriate clinical examinations and

Table 37.1 Systems of state compensation for occupational diseases in the EU

Member State	Trends in the number of exposed workers*	Who administers?	Who pays?	Who examines cases?	List of accepted diseases?	Permanent disability allocated?
Austria†	Decreased	?	?	?	?	?
Belgium	Decreased	National agency	Employers	Board of specialists	Yes	Yes
Denmark	Stable	National agency	Employers	Hospital-based occupational specialists	Yes	Yes
Finland	Decreased	?	?	?	?	?
France	Increased	Regional agencies	Employers	Social security practitioners	Yes	Yes
Germany	Decreased	Federal agencies	General taxation and employers	Labor practitioners	Yes	Yes
Greece	Decreased	National agency	Employers and employees	Social security practitioners	Yes	Yes
Ireland	Stable	Governmental agency	General taxation	?	Yes	Yes ('prescribed disease provisions')
Italy	Decreased	National agency	Employers	Decision made with specific expertise	Yes	Yes
Luxembourg		National agency	Employers	Board of physicians	Yes	Yes
The Netherlands		No specific system	Employers and employees	Board of physicians	No	No
Portugal	Increased	National agency	Employers	Social security practitioners	Yes	Yes
Spain	Increased	Governmental agency	Employers	Board of specialists	Yes	Yes
Sweden	Decreased	National agency	Employers	?	?	Yes
United Kingdom	Stable	Agency contracted to government ministry	General taxation	Board of government-employed physicians	Yes	Yes ('prescribed disease provisions')

Based mostly on 1996 data.
*Based on the pilot study of the European Agency for Safety and Health at Work.
†Further information for Austria is available at: http://at.osha.eu.int/

diagnostic tests at regular intervals (for instance, chest radiographs and spirometry at 2-year intervals following asbestos exposure).

- Because the listing system cannot always be fully comprehensive and cannot be updated immediately new knowledge becomes available, the EU has recommended the creation of regional committees to assess claims related to disorders that do not fall within the scope of an approved schedule (i.e. the official legal list in France). Such committees began operating in January 1993. They are composed of consulting physicians employed by the Social Security Office and an independent chest physician or occupational physician. In approving claims for compensation, the regional committees are likely to require a greater burden of proof that the disorder in the individual claimant is truly a consequence of occupational exposure than applies to claims assessed under the approved schedules.

United Kingdom

There are important differences in the administration of compensation in the UK compared with France. Most prominent is the facility of injured workers to seek compensation through civil litigation in courts of law as well as to obtain 'no fault' compensation from state resources. In many European countries state compensation precludes any further claims through civil proceedings, a situation which pertained also in the UK under earlier workers' compensation laws.

State compensation has both differences and similarities to that in France. It is covered at present under the provisions of the Social Security Act 1975 (Industrial Injuries), and is funded by taxation. Historically, compensation for injury resulting from accidents preceded more recent legislation for compensating lung disease that occurs without any demonstrable 'accident'. In consequence inhalation injuries that result from, for example, accidental spillages or the rupture of tanks or pipes, are compensated under the 'Accident Provisions' of the Act.

These would cover, in addition to toxic injury of the airways (bronchitis) and lung parenchyma (pneumonitis), most cases of the reactive airways dysfunction syndrome (RADS or 'irritant asthma') and may cover some cases of the organic dust toxic syndrome. They would also cover the rare cases of occupational asthma that are due to hypersensitivity, but arise because of an accident and a major 'toxic' exposure (e.g. to isocyanates).

The more common occupational disorders of the lung, those that arise from repeated everyday exposures rather than from a single identifiable incident, are covered by the 'Prescribed Diseases Regulations'. This legislative system is directly analogous to the 'list system' in France. Each listed disease and, where relevant, each listed causal agent, is identified in the pamphlet 'A guide to Industrial Injuries Scheme benefits' (DB1 1999) published by the Department of Social Security (Benefits Agency). The details are summarized in Table 37.2.

Table 37.2 Respiratory disorders 'prescribed' for state compensation in the UK

Number	Disease	Exposure
B6	Extrinsic allergic alveolitis	Moldy vegetable matter, edible fungi, birds
C15	Pneumonitis	Oxides of nitrogen
C17	Berylliosis	Beryllium
C18	Pneumonitis, emphysema	Cadmium
C22(b)	Lung cancer	Gaseous nickel compounds (Ni production)
D1	Pneumoconiosis	Mineral dust
D2	Byssinosis	Cotton or flax dust
D3	Mesothelioma	Asbestos
D7	Asthma	One of 22 'prescribed sensitizers'* or some other agent or environment for which there is persuasive evidence (e.g. bronchial challenge) of 'sensitization'
D8	Lung cancer	Asbestos (if there is asbestosis or asbestos-induced diffuse pleural thickening of defined degree)
D9	Diffuse pleural thickening of defined degree	Asbestos
D10	Lung cancer	Tin mine work, chloromethylethers, chromates
D11	Lung cancer	Silica (if there is silicosis)
D12	Chronic bronchitis or emphysema	Coal dust (if there has been underground work for $\geq$ 20 years, and if FEV_1 is $\geq$ 1 liter below the predicted value, or FEV_1 is < 1 Liter)

*Platinum salts, (di)isocyanates, epoxy resin curing systems, colophony fumes, proteolytic enzymes, laboratory animals and insects, flour and grain dust, castor bean dust, wood dust, antibiotics, cimetidine, psyllium, ipecacuanha, azodicarbonamide, glutaraldehyde, persulfates and henna, crustaceans and fish products, reactive dyes, soya bean dust, tea dust, green coffee bean dust, stainless steel welding fume.
A number of disorders that may affect the respiratory system, but do not necessarily do so, are also 'prescribed' if acquired occupationally. They comprise: disorders from changes in ambient pressure (dysbarism), and certain infections (anthrax, mellioidosis, spirochetal infection, ankylostomiasis, tuberculosis, brucellosis, chlamydial infection, Q fever, and hydatidosis).

Claims are submitted to the Disability Benefits Centre of the UK government's Benefits Agency (Department of Social Security), but medical evaluations are carried out by physicians of an independent subcontractor, Medical Services. Curiously, this organization is owned by a French company, SEMA, thereby providing a tenuous link between UK compensation procedures and those of mainland Europe. For the Medical Services evaluations, information and advice may be obtained from various sources – particularly regarding the nature of the occupational environment and the results of hospital investigations.

Claimants have the right to appeal against any adverse decisions, and appeals are heard by an independent body comprising a lawyer chair and one or two co-opted local respiratory physicians, who most commonly are employed by the UK National Health Service. The Appeals Service comes under the auspices of the government's Lord Chancellor, and so is entirely independent of the Benefits Agency and the Department of Social Security.

The state compensation system functions reasonably quickly and provides compensation within a national framework for disability incurred as a consequence of occupational disease or injury. It no longer provides compensation directly for loss of earnings, nor is it concerned with rehabilitation or retraining for alternative work. If a successful claimant is considered to be so disabled as to be totally incapable of gainful employment, disability is assessed at 100% and the maximum allowable benefit is paid. This maximum is of modest degree only, and takes no account of the claimant's previous earning capacity. Thus, low-paid manual workers may find that state compensation comes close to matching their former earnings, whereas white collar workers may suffer considerable losses in income. Redress for this may come from a civil action in the courts, the injured worker suing the relevant employer for whatever damages he or she has sustained as a consequence of the employer's negligence.

This parallel and independent system of compensation is therefore importantly different in two principles from that underlying the UK state system and the system in France. First, 'fault' is a critical issue, because the employer has to be proved negligent if he or she is to be liable over and above his or her tax contributions to the state compensation system. Proving negligence may not be straightforward, and it may be that a supplier of hazardous agents has acted negligently rather than the immediate employer. Second, the burden of proof lies with the claimant (the plaintiff in the civil action) to show that his or her illness is truly an effect of his or her work. This is not assumed simply because a 'listed' disease arose during a period of occupational exposure to a 'listed' causal agent, and in this respect an approved 'list' is irrelevant. The matter is, nevertheless, adjudicated by civil not criminal standards and the case is 'proved' if it is judged more likely than not.

The disadvantages to the claimant of pursuing compensation through civil proceedings are cost (often met by government grants) and complexity, and the inevitably long period (often years) before the matter is resolved. The advantages are that civil proceedings aim to provide indemnity for all the losses incurred (including lost potential income), together with appropriate compensation for the suffering involved. This implies, in turn, that any compensation received by way of state benefit awards is additional to a fair and comprehensive settlement, and in these circumstances the Benefits Agency may be entitled to recover some of its award or the civil settlement may be reduced to take account of the state benefit.

Future directions

Despite the considerable efforts of EU institutions and member states, a number of pitfalls remain.

First, occupational diseases in many individuals remain unrecognized and undiagnosed, and are thus undeclared. The magnitude of the problem is unclear and there is no registration of cases at an EU level. This is a consequence of the difficulty in compiling reliable data on trends in occupational diseases, and not all member states attempt this. The issue is discussed more fully in Chapter 2. There is consequently a major need for a standardized, accurate, and comprehensive procedure for registering lung (and other) diseases of occupational origin throughout the EU, so that emerging and continuing risks are properly identified.

Second, the widespread use of a 'list system' of accepted occupational hazards and diseases fails to provide proper compensation for disorders that are truly occupational in origin, but are not listed in the statutory schedules. The regional committees recommended by the EU redress this problem to some degree, but any regional system is likely to create discrepancies between regions, and at present not all member states within the EC have adopted this recommendation. Since different member states currently have independent mechanisms for compensating occupational disease, the possibilities for discrepancy throughout the EU are already formidable.

Finally, any 'list system' needs to be updated regularly. There is possibly a need for an EU expert committee to advise on new relevant knowledge, and for standard recommendations to be made at EU level for consideration within the member states. The European Agency for Safety and Health at Work could play a key role in administering this.

WEBSITES

Information centre of European Union:
http://europa.eu.int
http://europa.eu.int/eur-lex/fr/index.html
http://europa.eu.int/eur-lex/fr/lif/dat/1998/
fr_398L0098.html
http://europa.eu.int/eur-lex/fr/consleg/pdf/1987/
fr_1987L0217_do_001.pdf

The European Agency for Safety and Health at work:
http://agency.osha.eu.int/publications/reports/
stateofosh

Information sites of the Institut de Santé et Sécurité
au Travail (INRS, France):
http://www.inrs.fr/indexnosdoss.html

REFERENCES

1. Mebazaa A. *Guide to Health in Europe*. Paris: Impact Médecin, 1992.
2. Hen C, Léonard J. *L'Union Européenne*, Paris: La Découverte, 2000.
3. Dewitte JD, Chan-Yeung M, Malo J-L. Medicolegal and compensation aspects of occupational asthma. *Eur Respir J* 1994; 7: 969–980.
4. Institut National de Recherche et de Sécurité. *Les Maladies Professionnelles*. Paris: INRS, 1999.
5. Scott Newman L. Occupational illness. *N Engl J Med* 1995; 333: 1128–1134.

INFORMATION TECHNOLOGY

38 INFORMATION SOURCES AND INVESTIGATION CENTERS: NORTH AMERICA

Akshay Sood

INTRODUCTION

Chapters 38–40 identify sources of information and centers of investigation for three global regions. Included are clinical, research, and professional organizations, laboratories, governmental and non-governmental bodies, and regulatory offices. All may contribute to the management and control of occupational disorders of the lung. While many offer advice or information at an international level, most are focused to local needs. This chapter addresses specifically the separate geographical region of North America.

The internet is the single most useful tool for accessing sources of information. It has generated a virtual revolution in accessing and disseminating data in the field of occupational safety and health. Web resources are dynamic, constantly expanding and changing, and not all those of possible relevance can be reviewed here. The reader must exercise his or her own judgment as these resources are explored, and what follows should not be construed as an endorsement of any particular website.

Every single resource on the internet has its own unique address called the 'Uniform Resource Locator'. Many of the most useful are included below under the sections on sources of informa-

tion. Some software programs require specific web browsers to enable the reader to retrieve and display information resources on the web. Many 'search engines' (software that conducts searches of the internet according to the user's instructions) are available, so that resources can be identified without knowledge of the Uniform Resource Locator. Search engines identify websites related to a specified topic. 'Yahoo!' (http://www.yahoo.com) is an example of a search engine, and is one of several good ones for beginners.

Hyperlinked websites are sites that organize and list a number of other topically related websites. In the USA and Canada, for example, hyperlinks allow easy access to numerous federal governmental and non-governmental agencies.

Mail-lists are automated systems by which messages can be sent to, or received from, all subscribers. A reply from the organization can be sent privately to the enquirer, or to the whole list of subscribers. Communication may use either postal or email services.

A final common means of disseminating information in many countries is through telephone enquiry services. These may be active only during normal working hours or, for emergency situations, throughout each 24-hour period.

INFORMATION TECHNOLOGY

Internet

Listed in Table 38.1 are three hyperlinked websites that may be useful when physicians and industrial managers are faced with questions of diagnosis and management. These websites are not specific for lung disease, but may contain information useful for pulmonary specialists. One of the most useful and comprehensive websites is the Duke University Occupational and Environmental Medicine WWW Resource Index. The National Institute for Occupational Safety and Health (NIOSH) has provided grant support for this web page. Internet Learning Center, another such hyperlinked website, also lists Spanish language links. This website was established at the 1998 American Occupational Health Conference, and is refined annually. Occupational and Environmental Resources is a similar site that is further listed by specialty area, including a disability and impairment section, a medical surveillance section (which includes respiratory protection), and an occupational injury and illness section (which includes occupational asthma).

Mail-lists

The most well known are the 'Occ-Env-Med-L Internet Mail List' and the 'Medical Center Occupational Health Mail-List' which are available at the Duke University's Occupational and Environmental Medicine WWW Resource Index, and the 'Occupational and Environmental Resources' home pages, respectively (see Table 38.1). Subscription to both these lists is free. While not 'lung-specific', these mail-lists provide interactive spots to unofficial email contributions on topics of occupational and environmental health, and a way to participate in informal discussions without the expense of conference travel.

Telephone information lines

Several sources of direct telephone consultation regarding occupational lung diseases are now available. The National Jewish Center for Immunology and Respiratory Medicine (Denver, Colorado USA [1] provides information on lung diseases caused by chemical exposure through the 'Lungline' at 1 800 222 LUNG (5864). The Canadian Centre for Occupational Health and Safety maintains an inquiry phone line at 1 800 668 4284 that is toll-free in Canada and the USA [2]. The National Institute for Occupational Safety and Health offers a toll-free technical information service that provides convenient public access to its information resources [3]. This service is available in the USA at 1 800 35 NIOSH (1 800 356 4674). The callers may reach a technical information specialist during business hours. In addition, an automated voice-mail system operates for 24 hours a day at the same number. Outside the USA, the commercial toll numbers are (513) 533 8328 for technical information and (513) 533 8471 for publication requests. However, these telephone lines are not meant for emergencies.

For managing chemical emergencies, there are two lines available: the Chemical Spills Emergency Hotline at 1 800 535 0202 and the Environmental Protection Agency (EPA) Hazardous Waste Hotline at 1 800 535 0202. Local Poison Control Centers can also provide useful help in such situations.

SOURCES OF INFORMATION

National Institute for Occupational Safety and Health (NIOSH)

NIOSH is a very useful place to begin when confronted with an occupational pulmonary problem. It is part of the Centers for Disease Control and Prevention (CDC) of the Department of Health and Human Services in the USA. It is the only US federal agency that conducts research, trains professionals, and develops innovative solutions to occupational health and safety problems. Members of the general public may obtain information about NIOSH activities, order NIOSH publications, or request information about any aspect of occupational safety and health by telephone (above), by mail [3], or by the internet (below).

Table 38.1 Three most useful hyperlinked internet sites for occupational pulmonary physicians to access resources available on the internet

Resource	Internet site
Duke's Occupational and Environmental Medicine WWW Resource Index	http://occ-env-med.mc.duke.edu/oem/index2.htm
Internet Learning Center	http://www.occhealth.org/medsites.html
Occupational and Environmental Resources	http://www.occenvmed.net/

NIOSH publishes criteria documents that outline the health hazards of specific occupational exposures, for example asbestos (Publications Catalog # 77–169). These provide the basis for comprehensive occupational safety and health standards in the USA. A listing of all NIOSH publications (Publications Catalog # 98–110), and the various types of publications themselves can be obtained without charge by sending a request by email, mail, telephone, or fax. Some are also available on a CD-ROM for purchase. The publications relevant to lung disease include the NIOSH *Pocket Guide to Chemical Hazards*, December 1998 (NTIS No: PB 99–500–449); *Guide to Industrial Respiratory Protection* (Publications Catalog # 87–116); Information about the NIOSH B Reader certification program (Publications Catalog # 97–104, 'To B or not to B a NIOSH B Reader'); *Building Indoor Air Quality* (a manual for building owners with air quality problems, Publications Catalog # 91–114); and numerous other publications relating to respiratory hazards in the mining industry.

NIOSH now has a home page on the internet at this address: http://www.cdc.gov/niosh/homepage.html. Its publications are also accessible through this home page and single copies of many of these can be directly downloaded, or ordered at no cost. Some of these files require an Adobe Acrobat Reader for viewing which can also be downloaded without charge at that site. The NIOSH home page also includes access to the International Chemical Safety Cards (ICSC) that summarize health and safety information on chemicals for 'lay' individuals. The usefulness of the ICSC and Material Safety Data Sheets (MSDS) during the evaluation of an occupational pulmonary problem is further discussed in the section on MSDS below.

NIOSH Technical Information Center (NIOSHTIC) is a bibliographic database containing references to workplace safety and health literature (abstracts and citations of journal articles). Many of the key references in occupational respiratory disease are included, and these can be searched by topic, substance, author, journal, etc. One of the unusual advantages of the NIOSHTIC database is that it includes references published in medical and scientific journals predating the start of MEDLINE in 1966. Several commercial vendors provide NIOSHTIC on CD-ROM [2,4] and on the internet databases [5–7] for a fee.

NIOSH has also established 15 Education and Research Centers in the USA (Table 38.2). These are academic programs that are designed to enhance the knowledge of the professional and paraprofessional workforce in this field. These centers also conduct research, training, and technical assistance programs to identify and reduce hazardous working conditions. For physicians interested in formal training in occupational lung disease issues, most Education and Research Centers conduct short continuing medical education courses throughout the year, which include pulmonary topics.

Websites for NIOSH and other relevant US and Canadian government bodies are listed in Table 38.3.

Table 38.2 NIOSH Education and Research Centers

Alabama ERC, Birmingham, AL [8]
California ERC (Northern), Berkeley, CA [9]
California ERC (Southern), Los Angeles, CA [10]
Cincinnati ERC, Cincinnati, OH [11]
Harvard ERC, Boston, MA [12]
Illinois ERC, Chicago, IL [13]
Johns Hopkins ERC, Baltimore, MD [14]
Michigan ERC, Ann Arbor, MI [15]
Minnesota ERC, Minneapolis, MN [16]
New York/New Jersey ERC, New York, NY [17]
North Carolina ERC, Chapel Hill, NC [18]
South Florida ERC, Tampa, FL [19]
Texas ERC, Houston, TX [20]
Utah ERC, Salt Lake City, UT [21]
Washington ERC, Seattle, WA [22]

Complete address and contact information for these centers is included at the end of the chapter.

Table 38.3 Internet addresses for occupational and environmental bodies of the US and Canadian governments

	Internet site
Centers for Disease Prevention and Control (CDC)	http://www.cdc.gov/
Occupational Safety and Health Administration (OSHA) [9]	http://www.osha.gov/
USA Environmental Protection Agency (EPA)	http://www.epa.gov/
Agency for Toxic Substances and Disease Registry (ATSDR)	http://atsdr1.atsdr.cdc.gov/
National Institute of Occupational Safety and Health (NIOSH) [3]	http://www.cdc.gov/niosh/homepage.html
Canadian Centre for Occupational Health and Safety (CCOHS) [2]	http://www.ccohs.ca/

Canadian Centre for Occupational Health and Safety (CCOHS)

The Canadian Centre for Occupational Health and Safety (CCOHS) is Canada's national center for occupational safety and health information [2]. Its documents are available as CCINFOWeb on the internet on the website, http://www.ccohs.ca (Table 38.3). It also maintains an inquiry phone line at (800) 668 4284 that is toll-free from Canada and the USA. The inquiries service is available both in English and French. It issues CCINFOdisc, a CD-ROM series that contains databases, publications, full-text Canadian safety and environmental legislation, and multimedia training packages. Both the CCINFOWeb and the CCINFOdisc databases include the NIOSHTIC database, at a lower cost than commercial vendors.

MEDLINE

MEDLINE (MEDlars onLINE) is the US National Library of Medicine's bibliographic medical database, containing approximately nine million records dating back to 1966 (see Table 38.4 for internet access). This database is available at no charge. The PRE-MEDLINE database provides basic citation information and abstracts for recent publications before the full records are prepared and added to MEDLINE. Toxicology Information On-line (TOXLINE), created by the National Library of Medicine, can also be accessed at no charge on the internet. It offers comprehensive bibliographic coverage of toxicology information. These databases provide easy and useful sources of occupational pulmonary information.

Online material safety data sheets

Often the physician is faced with patients exposed to substances with unfamiliar trade names. In such a situation, it is important to request from the employer the Material Safety Data Sheets (MSDS) of the substance. Should the MSDS not be available from the employer, the internet is a useful alternative source. MSDS include such information as physical data, toxicity, health effects, first aid, reactivity, disposal, protective equipment, and spill/leak procedures regarding that substance. The section on health effects usually contains information on pulmonary effects of inhaled substances. Unfortunately, this information is often meager.

The information can be supplemented by using the MSDS to identify the specific chemical constituents of the commercial product. The potential adverse respiratory effects of each constituent can then be identified by searching the index of various databases available over the internet (see below in the section on 'Other databases'). MSDS usually identify chemical constituents by a Chemical Abstracts Service (CAS) number, a unique identifier for every chemical substance that may have multiple chemical names; for example, crystalline silicon dioxide, CAS 14808-60-7, is known as silica, quartz, onyx, agate, and silicon dioxide.

The internet has a wide range of free resources that offer MSDS information. A useful place to begin is Interactive Learning Paradigms web page (http://www.ilpi.com/msds/index.html) which provides links to other websites that serve MSDS. Some of the sites on this hyperlinked web page are shown in Table 38.5. The CCINFOWeb provides MSDS data in French as well. In addition, the NIOSH home page includes access to the International Chemical Safety Cards (ICSCs) which summarize health and safety information on chemicals for 'lay' individuals. These are easier for the shopfloor and can be used instead of the Material Safety Data Sheets (MSDSs), which are technically more complex and more extensive.

Online services for physicians

There are a number of online services directed at physicians. Once registration is complete, most provide a basic service, which includes a MEDLINE search. The most prominent among them are Medscape and the SilverPlatter Physicians' home page.

Medscape

Medscape (http://www.medscape.com) [23] is a service without charge. It also offers access to Toxline.

SilverPlatter physicians' home page

SilverPlatter physicians' home page (http://www. silverplatter.com) [4] provides access to various

Table 38.4 Internet access to MEDLINE without charge

MEDLINE connection	Website address	Comment
PubMed by the National Library of Medicine	http://www.ncbi.nlm.nih.gov/PubMed/	Also provides links to any online journals available
Grateful Med on Internet by the National Library of Medicine	http://igm.nlm.nih.gov/	Also has Toxline

Table 38.5 Some useful internet websites for information on material safety data sheets (MSDSs)

Types of data	Comments
General MSDS sites	
Cornell University	A keyword-searchable MSDS database with 325 000 MSDSs
CCINFOWeb: MSDS and FTSS databases by the Canadian Centre for Occupational Health and Safety (CCOHS)	Over 150 000 MSDSs in English and French, supplied by North American manufacturers
Vermont SIRI	A keyword-searchable database with 180 000 MSDSs
Less technical data	
CDC, NIOSH, and WHO International Chemical Safety Cards	Good for basic understanding of 869 chemicals, not MSDSs
New Jersey Hazardous Chemical Fact sheets	Plain English descriptions of common household, workplace, and environmental chemicals (great for non-chemists)
Data on carcinogenic potential	
International Agency for Research on Cancer (IARC)	Reports on cancer risks to humans by 800+ chemicals, not MSDSs

These sites can be accessed on the hyperlinked web page of Interactive Learning Paradigms (http://www.ilpi.com/msds/index.html).

databases, both online and on CD-ROM, for a fee. Useful databases include OSH-ROM, and CHEMBANK.

Other databases

Most physicians outside research institutions will have little need for the additional databases listed below. They provide a wealth of information on occupational health and safety, including pulmonary topics. As mentioned previously, one of the most useful is NIOSHTIC, which is available both as part of the OSH-ROM and CCINFOWeb/CCINFOdisc databases below.

- The OSH-ROM database (Table 38.6) brings together six databases covering critical international occupational health and safety information from 1960 to the present. OSH-ROM is marketed by a commercial firm, SilverPlatter [4], either online or on a CD-ROM, on a paid subscription basis.

- HAZDAT is a database for hazardous substances by the Agency for Toxic Substances and Disease Registry (ATSDR). It is available on the internet without charge at http://www.atsdr.cdc.gov/hazdat.html. It provides information on the release of hazardous substances into the environment and their ill-effects on humans.

Table 38.6 Constituents of OSH-ROM database

Database name	Description
NIOSHTIC, from the National Institute for Occupational Safety and Health	Bibliographic database of literature in field of occupational safety and health
Health and Safety Executive Line (HSELINE) produced by HSE, the arm of the UK government responsible for occupational safety and health	Covers all UK Health and Safety Commission and Health and Safety Executive publications in addition to bibliographic database of literature in field of occupational safety and health
CISDOC produced by the International Labor Organization	Bibliographic database of literature in field of occupational safety and health
Major Hazard Incident Data Service (MHIDAS) produced by the Atomic Energy Authority of the UK	Information on more than 4000 worldwide incidents involving release of hazardous substances that caused or had the potential of causing a major public impact
Ryerson International Labor Occupational Safety and Health (RILOSH)	Bibliographic database of literature in field of occupational safety and health
MEDL-OEM by the National Library of Medicine	MEDLINE's Occupational and Environmental Medicine subset

▫ Toxicology Data Network (TOXNET), developed by the National Library of Medicine, is a particulary useful computerized system of files oriented towards toxicology. It can be accessed without charge on the internet at the following address: http://toxnet.nlm.nih.gov/. Some of the files included in TOXNET are shown in Table 38.7.

▫ CCINFOWeb allows internet access to the information services of the Canadian Centre for Occupational Health and Safety (CCOHS) [2] at the following address: http://ccinfoweb.ccohs.ca/aboutCCINFOWeb.html. In addition to free access to the CHEMINDEX database, CCINFOWeb provides subscription to seven other databases (see Table 38.8). Most of this information is also available as a CD-ROM series called the CCINFOdisc.

Professional organizations

Several North American professional organizations have specific interest sections or special assemblies on occupational and environmental lung diseases. Some of these are listed in Table 38.9.

Regulatory organizations

The Occupational Safety and Health Administration (OSHA) [24] is the US governmental regulatory body that sets and enforces workplace standards. OSHA

Table 38.7 Constituents of TOXNET database

Database	Details
Hazardous Substance Data Bank (HSDB)	A factual database of more than 4200 chemicals
Registry of Toxic Effects of Chemical Substances (RTECS)	Toxicology exposure limits and regulatory information on over 140 000 chemicals
Toxic Chemical Release Inventory (TRI)	Database from the US Environmental Protection Agency (EPA) containing data on estimated quantities of chemicals released into the environment
Integrated Risk Information System (IRIS)	Database from the US Environmental Protection Agency (EPA) containing information on estimated releases to the environment of more than 300 toxic chemicals reported by industries

Table 38.8 Database access provided by CCINFOWeb

Database	Details
MSDS (Material Safety Data Sheet)	Over 150 000 MSDSs, in English, contributed by North American manufacturers and suppliers
FTSS (Fiche technique sur la sécurité des substances)	Over 150 000 MSDSs, in French, contributed by North American manufacturers and suppliers
CHEMINFO	Practical summarized occupational health and safety information on over 1200 chemicals
Canadian enviroOSH legislation	The complete text of all Canadian health, safety, and environmental legislation, as well as critical guidelines and standards
Registry for Toxic Effects of Chemical Substances (RTECS)	Toxicology exposure limits and regulatory information on over 140 000 chemicals
NIOSHTIC from the National Institute of Occupational Safety and Health	Bibliographic database on occupational safety and health
Health and Safety Executive Line (HSELine)	Covers all UK Health and Safety Commission and Health and Safety Executive publications in addition to bibliographic database of literature in field of occupational safety and health
CHEMINDEX	Free access provided. Convenient guide to over 20 CCINFO databases containing information on chemicals

Table 38.9 Prominent professional occupational and environmental medicine organizations, with specific emphasis on occupational pulmonary disorders

Organization	Details
American Thoracic Society (ATS) [25]	Scientific Assembly on Environmental and Occupational Health has a special emphasis on epidemiological and laboratory approaches
American College of Chest Physicians (ACCP) [26]	Section on Occupational and Environmental Health
American College of Occupational and Environmental Medicine (ACOEM) [27]	Lists board-certified occupational medicine physicians
Association of Occupational and Environmental clinics (AOEC) [28]	Network of 63 clinics specializing in clinical diagnosis of occupational hazardous substance exposures. Three Pediatric Environmental Health Specialty Units (PEHSUs) [29–31] recently set up
American Conference of Governmental Industrial Hygienists (ACGIH) [32]	Offers high-quality technical publications on occupational health and safety, including the TLV® booklet

also provides technical information and assistance about health hazards and interpretation of occupational health standards. OSHA can be easily accessed on the web at http://www.osha.gov. OSHA Regulations and Compliance Links on this website provides comprehensive and easy-to-obtain current OSHA standards and compliance-related information. In addition, several states have their own OSHA programs. Regional OSHA offices can be found in the governmental section of the telephone book (blue pages) under US Department of Labor, and on the internet. Free OSHA consultation services are available to employers to find out potential hazards at their worksite. Physicians may also, on behalf of their patients, make an online to request to OSHA through its homepage to investigate an occupational lung hazard. There is no federal equivalent to OSHA in Canada.

The Workers' Compensation system is designed to ensure that employees who are injured or disabled because of their work are provided with fixed monetary awards to compensate lost work time, medical costs, and permanent disability, thereby eliminating the need for litigation. The state laws regarding workers' compensation vary, and physicians in both the USA and Canada are advised to obtain more information from the Workers' Compensation agency in their respective states or provinces. US federal employees and certain other employed groups (railroad workers, longshoremen) are covered by separate compensation programs. A useful website about US workers' compensation is maintained by Cornell University (http://www.law.cornell.edu/topics/workers_compensation.html).

For further details, see Chapter 35 on Legislative Controls and Compensation for North America.

INVESTIGATION CENTERS

Specific diseases

Investigation centers for specific disease include numerous institutions, of which local hospitals and universities will generally suffice. They, the professional bodies identified in Table 38.9, and the sources of information identified in Tables 38.1–3 are best consulted for advice concerning diagnostic or management problems of particular cases. Listed here are additional institutions for which special interest, expertize, and facilities are recognized.

Rhinitis

Facilities are available for nasal lavage, acoustic rhinometery, and rhinomanometry at the Gage Occupational and Environmental Health Unit, University of Toronto [33] and at Penn State's Milton S. Hershey Medical Center [34]. These tests are used primarily for clinical research and have little role to play in the diagnosis and management of occupational rhinitis for a clinician.

Asthma

A patient with occupational asthma may require specific inhalation challenge testing in the rare situation when the diagnosis of occupational asthma or the specific causal exposure is in doubt. The purpose is to assess specific responsiveness to 'sensitizing' substances. This contrasts with non-specific inhalation challenge testing to determine the level of airway responsiveness to such non-specific stimuli as pharmacological agents (like histamine and methacholine), cold air, and exercise, and hence to assess whether asthma itself exists and whether particular exposures cause the level of asthmatic activity to increase.

Inhalation tests for non-specific airway responsiveness are available in many hospital-based pulmonary function laboratories. Specific inhalation challenge tests can be conducted in either the workplace (where the exposure cannot be controlled experimentally) or in a carefully controlled laboratory environment offered by a select few specialized centers (see Fig. 38.1). Specific challenge testing is time consuming – often involving two or more days of testing, and not devoid of danger – and may require in-patient hospitalization (see Chapter 4). Furthermore, a negative test does not necessarily exclude a diagnosis of occupational asthma. Many of the centers offer only a limited number of specific agents for challenge testing, so detailed discussion of the individual case prior to referral is essential. Most of these centers use such tests primarily for clinical research. Centers where specific challenge is available for clinical purposes include:

- Occupational and Environmental Medicine Program at Yale University School of Medicine, New Haven, Connecticut. This is a research-oriented inhalation challenge chamber currently geared towards isocyanate testing [35].
- Gage Occupational and Environmental Health Unit, University of Toronto, Toronto, Ontario [33].
- Université de Montréal and Hôpital du Sacré-Coeur, Montréal, Québec [36].
- Occupational and Environmental Medicine Division at the National Jewish Center for Immunology and Respiratory Medicine, Denver, Colorado [1].
- Environmental and Occupational Medicine Consultative Clinic at the Emory Clinic, Atlanta, Georgia [37].

- Occupational and Environmental Medicine Program, University of Washington Harborview Medical Center, Seattle, Washington [38].
- Royal University Hospital, University of Saskatchewan, Saskatchewan, Canada [39].
- Respiratory Division, Vancouver General Hospital, University of British Columbia, Canada [40].
- Pulmonary Diseases, Critical Care, and Environmental Medicine, Tulane University, New Orleans, Louisiana [41].

The Canadian sites offer services for Canadian provinces but usually refrain from offering services to patients residing in the USA. Contact information for these centers is listed at the end of the chapter.

In addition to specific inhalation tests, demonstration of specific immunoglobulin E (IgE) antibodies to various occupational allergens by enzyme-linked immunosorbent assay (ELISA) testing or radioallergosorbent test (RAST) may be useful to corroborate a diagnosis of occupational asthma. Tests for IgE and IgG antibodies against isocyanates, phthalic anhydride, and trimellitic anhydride are available at Northwestern University, Chicago [42]. It should be borne in mind that the presence of specific IgE antibodies merely indicates immunological sensitization; this may occur in exposed workers without asthma.

Hypersensitivity pneumonitis

Serum precipitins to specific substances can be useful in the diagnosis of extrinsic allergic alveolitis (hypersensitivity pneumonitis). The National Jewish Medical and Research Center [1], Specialty Laboratories, Santa Monica, California [43], Mayo Medical Laboratories, Northwestern University at Chicago [42], and several other reference laboratories across North America offer these tests for occupational and environmental antigens that cause extrinsic allergic alveolitis. Some of these tests are listed in Table 38.10. If the desired antigen is not on the list, the laboratory should be contacted to see whether it can be obtained. Some laboratories can also prepare extracts of antigens from the patient's environment and test for specific precipitins in the patient's serum against these antigens, or use it as a skin test reagent. Dust can also be analyzed by measuring the amount of antigens from house dust mite, cat, dog, and cockroach. ELISA tests for IgE and IgG antibodies against isocyanates and trimellitic anhydride are available at Northwestern University, Chicago [42]. Again, the presence of specific antibodies indicates sensitization, and may occur in exposed workers without disease.

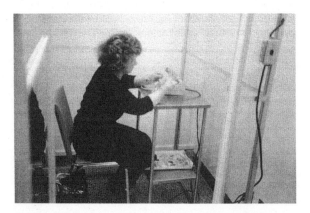

Fig. 38.1 A patient undergoing specific inhalation challenge testing for colophony in soldering flux in a special exposure chamber. (Courtesy of Dr Susan M Tarlo, Occupational Lung Disease Clinic, The Toronto Hospital, Toronto.)

Table 38.10 Some serum precipitin tests currently available for the diagnosis of hypersensitivity pneumonitis

Occupational lung disease	Precipitins to antigens
Bagassosis	Thermoactinomyces vulgaris
Farmer's lung	Micropolyspora faeni
Bird breeder's lung	Avian sera and droppings
Humidifier lung/sauna-taker's disease	Aureobasidium pullulans
Malt worker's lung	Aspergillus clavatus
Animal handler's lung	Urine, serum, and pelts of animals
Hot-tub hypersensitivity pneumonitis	Cladosporium species
Suberosis	Penicillium frequentans
Wood pulp worker's lung	Alternaria species

Berylliosis

Beryllium lymphocyte transformation testing can be done on blood and bronchoalveolar lavage fluid to evaluate sensitization to beryllium in suspected cases of chronic beryllium lung disease. It also helps to detect sensitization to beryllium exposure in the past or the present; and demonstrates the effectiveness of exposure control efforts. The centers with this capability include:

- National Jewish Medical and Research Center at Denver, Colorado [1]
- Hospital of the University of Pennsylvania, Philadelphia, Pennsylvania [44]
- Specialty Laboratories, Inc., Santa Monica, California [43]
- The Cleveland Clinic Foundation, Cleveland, Ohio [45]
- Vanderbilt University Medical Center, Nashville, Tennessee [46]

The first three centers listed above have most experience. In addition, Los Alamos National Laboratories (LANL), New Mexico, and Oak Ridge Institute of Science and Education (ORISE), Tennessee are conducting some experimental testing for the US Department of Energy facilities. Contact information for these centers is listed at the end of the chapter.

PARTICLE ANALYSIS

In occasional patients with pneumoconiosis, lung particle analysis by light or analytical electron microscopy can be useful in documenting the level of exposure to an inorganic dust, or in proving exposure when the clinical history is unclear. Light microscopic analysis for asbestos body content is a useful way of documenting asbestos exposure, but light microscopic analysis is generally not useful for other types of dust. Analytic electron microscopy provides much higher sensitivity and can be used to document the presence of many inorganic dusts (see Fig. 38.2), although most analytic systems cannot detect very light elements such as beryllium.

Several laboratories in North America provide analytical electron microscopy services for documenting inorganic dust content:

- Duke University Department of Pathology, Durham, NC (Dr Victor Roggli) [47]
- University of British Columbia Department of Pathology, Vancouver, BC (Dr Andrew Churg) [48]
- State University of New York Department of Pathology, Syracuse, NY (Dr Jerrold Abraham) [49]
- McGill University Department of Pathology, Montreal, Quebec (Dr B Case) [50]

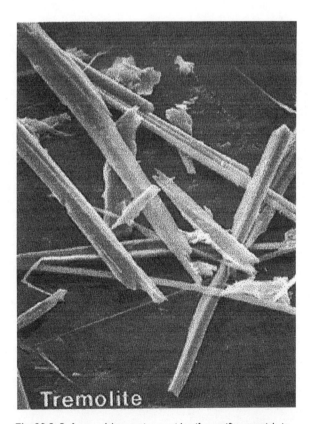

Tremolite

Fig. 38.2 Reference laboratories can identify specific materials in lung tissue specimens. The asbestos mineral, tremolite, crystallizes as characteristic long thin fibers as seen under the scanning electron microscope. (Courtesy of Dr Jerrold L Abraham, Department of Pathology, College of Medicine, SUNY Health Science Center, Syracuse, NY.)

REFERENCES
(Contact information)

Current addresses and contact information for all the organizations listed above are as follows. While these were accurate at the time of writing, changes may have occurred since.

1. National Jewish Medical and Research Center
   Pulmonary Division and
   Occupational/Environmental Medicine Division
   1400 Jackson Street
   Denver, CO 80206
   Tel: LUNG LINE (800) 222 LUNG (5864)
   Beryllium laboratory under Dr Lee
   Newman/Tom Lane: (303) 398 1974
   Complement laboratory: (303) 398 1343
   Web: http://www.njc.org/Diagnostic_Services/
   Email: lungline@njc.org

2. Canadian Centre for Occupational Health and Safety (CCOHS)
   250 Main Street East
   Hamilton, Ontario
   Canada
   L8N 1H6
   Tel: (800) 668 4284 (toll-free in Canada and USA), (905) 570 8094
   Fax: (905) 572 2206
   Email: custserv@ccohs.ca
   Web: http://www.ccohs.ca

3. NIOSH Publications
   4676 Columbia Parkway, Mail-stop C-13
   Cincinnati, OH 45226-1998
   Tel: (800) 35 NIOSH
   Fax: (513) 533 8573
   Web: http://www.cdc.gov/niosh/inquiry.html
   Email: pubstaft@cdc.gov

4. SilverPlatter Information, Inc.
   100 River Ridge Drive
   Norwood, MA 02062-5043
   Tel: (781) 769 2599
   Toll-free: 800 343 0064 (USA and Canada)
   Fax: (781) 769 8763
   Web: http://www.silverplatter.com

5. NTIS Subscriptions Department ATTN: GRC
   5285 Port Royal Road
   Springfield, VA 22161
   Tel: (800) 363 2068, (703) 605 6060
   Fax: (703) 605 6880
   Email: subscriptions@ntis.fedworld.gov

6. DIALOG Information Services, Inc.
   Marketing Department
   3460 Hillview Avenue
   Palo Alto, CA 94304
   Tel: (415) 858 3785
   Tel: (800) 334 2564

7. STN International
   c/o Chemical Abstracts Service
   2540 Olentangy River Road
   PO Box 3012
   Columbus, OH 43210-0012
   Tel: (614) 447 3600
   Fax: (614) 447 3798
   Email: help@cas.org

8. Alabama Education and Research Center
   University of Alabama at Birmingham
   School of Public Health
   Birmingham, AL 35294-2010
   Tel: (205) 934 7178
   Email: dsc@uab.edu
   Director: Dr Kent Oestenstad

9. California Education and Research Center – Northern
   University of California at Berkeley
   School of Public Health
   140 Warren
   Berkeley, CA 94720-7360
   Tel: (510) 642 0761
   Email: spear@uclink2.berkeley.edu
   Director: Dr Robert C Spear

10. California Education and Research Center – Southern University of Southern California
    School of Medicine
    Department of Preventive Medicine
    1540 Alcazar Street
    Suite 236
    Los Angeles, CA 90033
    Tel: (213) 342 1096
    Email: jpeters@hsc.usc.edu
    Director: Dr John M Peters

11. Cincinnati Education and Research Center
    University of Cincinnati
    Department of Environmental Health
    PO Box 670056
    Cincinnati, Ohio 45267-0056
    Tel: (513) 558 1749
    Email: clarkcs@ucbeh.san.uc.edu
    Director: Dr C Scott Clark

12. Harvard Education and Research Center
    Harvard School of Public Health

Department of Environmental Health
665 Huntington Avenue
Boston, MA 02115
Tel: (617) 432 3323
Email: dchris@hohp.harvard.edu
Director: Dr David C Christiani

13. Illinois Education and Research Center
University of Illinois at Chicago
School of Public Health
2121 West Taylor Street
M/C 922
Chicago, IL 60612-7260
Tel: (312) 996 7887
Email: Inickels@uic.edu
Director: Dr Daniel O Hryhorczuk

14. Johns Hopkins Education and Research Center
Johns Hopkins University
School of Hygiene and Public Health
615 North Wolfe Street
Baltimore, MD 21205
Tel: (410) 955 4082
Email: jagnew@jhsph.edu
Director: Dr Jacqueline Agnew

15. Michigan Education and Research Center
University of Michigan
College of Engineering
Department of Industrial and Operations
Engineering Building
1205 Beal Avenue
Ann Arbor, MI 48109
Tel: (313) 763 0563
Email: wmkeyser@umich.edu
Director: Dr W Monroe Keyserling

16. Minnesota Education and Research Center
University of Minnesota
School of Public Health
Minneapolis, MN 55455
Tel: (612) 626 0900
Email: igreaves@cccs.umn.edu
Director: Dr Ian A Greaves

17. New York/New Jersey Education and Research
Center
Department of Community Medicine
Mt Sinai School of Medicine
PO Box 1057
One Gustave L Levy Place
New York, NY 10029-6574
Tel: (212) 241 4804
Email: p_landrigan@smtplink.mssm.edu
Director: Dr Philip J Landrigan

18. North Carolina Education and Research Center
University of North Carolina
School of Public Health
Rosenau Hall, CB# 7400
Chapel Hill, NC 27599-7400
Tel: (919) 966 3473
Email: mflynn@sophia.sph.unc.edu
Director: Dr Michael R Flynn

19. South Florida Education and Research Center
University of South Florida
College of Public Health
13201 Bruce B Downs Blvd, MDC Box 56
Tampa, FL 33612-3805
Tel: (813) 974 6626
Email: sbrooks@com1.med.usf.edu
Director: Dr Stuart M Brooks

20. Texas Education and Research Center
The University of Texas Health Science
Center at Houston
School of Public Health
PO Box 20186
Houston, TX 77225-0186
Tel: (713) 500 9459
Email: gdelclos@utsph.sph.uth.tmc.edu
Director: Dr George L Delclos

21. Utah Education and Research Center
University of Utah
Rocky Mountain Center for Occupational
and Environmental Health
Bldg 512, Salt Lake City
UT 84112
Tel: (801) 581 8719
Email: rmoser@rmcoeh.utah.edu
Director: Dr Royce Moser Jr

22. Washington Education and Research Center
University of Washington
Department of Environmental Health
PO Box 357234
Seattle, WA 98195-7234
Tel: (206) 543 6991
Email: vanbelle@u.washington.edu
Director: Dr Gerald van Belle

23. Medscape
134 W. 29th Street
New York, NY 10001-5399
Tel: (212) 760 3100
Web: http://www.medscape.com/

24. US Department of Labor
Occupational Safety and Health Administration
Office of Public Affairs – Room N3647
200 Constitution Avenue

Washington, DC 20210
Tel: (202) 693 1999
Web: http://www.osha.gov/

25. American Thoracic Society
1740 Broadway, New York,
NY 10019
Tel: (212) 315 8700
Fax: (212) 315 6498
Web: http://www.thoracic.org/

26. American College of Chest Physicians
3300 Dundee Road
Northbrook
IL 60062-2348
Tel: (847) 498 1400, (800) 343 2227 (toll
free in the USA)
Fax: (847) 498 5460
Email: accp@chestnet.org
Web: http://www.chestnet.org/

27. American College of Occupational and
Environmental Medicine
1114 N. Arlington Heights Road
Arlington Heights, IL 60004
Tel: (847) 818 1800
Fax: (847) 818 9266
Web: http://www.acoem.org/

28. Association of Occupational and
Environmental Clinics
1010 Vermont Avenue, NW #513,
Washington, DC 20005
Tel: (202) 347 4976
Email: aoec@DGS.dgsys.com
Web: http://152.3.65.120/oem/aoec.htm

29. Pediatric Environmental Health Center at
Children's Hospital
Occupational and Environmental Health
Center at Cambridge Hospital
1493 Cambridge Street Clinic
Cambridge, MA 02139
Tel: (888)-CHILD14 (888 244 5314), (617)
498 1580
Fax: (617) 498 1671
Web: http://gilligan.mc.duke.edu/oem/
clin-d.htm#Cambridge

30. Children's Environmental Health Center
University of Washington Occupational and
Environmental Medicine Program
325 Ninth Ave. #359739 Clinic
Seattle, WA 98104-2499
Tel: (877)-KID-CHEM (877 543 2436) The

(877) phone number is restricted to west of
the Mississippi River (206) 731 3005
Fax: (206) 731 8247
Web: http://occ-env-
med.mc.duke.edu/oem/clin-i.htm#Washington

31. Mt Sinai Pediatric Environmental Health Unit
Mt Sinai–Irving J Selikoff Center for
Occupational and Environmental Medicine
Box 1058
One Gustave L Levy Place
New York, NY 10029
Tel: (212) 241 6173, (212) 241 0176
Fax: (212) 996 0407
Web: http://occ-env-
med.mc.duke.edu/oem/clin-f.htm#Mt Sinai

32. American Conference of Governmental
Industrial Hygienists
1330 Kemper Meadow Drive, Suite 600,
Cincinnati, OH 45240;
Tel: (513) 742 2020
Fax: (513) 742 3355
Email: mail@acgih.org
Web: http://www.acgih.org/

33. The GAGE Occupational and Environmental
Health Unit – Toronto
1 King's College Circle
Toronto, Ontario
Canada M5S 1A8
Tel: (416) 978 6585
Fax: (416) 978 1774
Email: medicine.web@utoronto.ca
Web: http://www.utoronto.ca/occmed/index.htm

34. Milton S Hershey Medical Center (Dr Rebecca
Bascom)
Penn State Geisinger Health Care System
Mailcode HO 39,
PO Box 850
Hershey
PA 17033
Tel: (717) 531 6525
Fax: (717) 5315785
Email: rbascom@medhmc.pshgs.edu

35. Occupational and Environmental Medicine
Program (Dr Carrie Redlich)
Yale University School Of Medicine
135 College Street, 3rd floor
New Haven, CT 06510
Tel: (203) 785 7202
Fax: (203) 785 7391
Email: carrie@revco.med.yale.edu

36. Hôspital du Sacré-Coeur de Montréal
    Université de Montréal
    5400 Boulevard Goulin Quest
    Montreal, Quebec
    Canada H4J 1C5

37. Environmental and Occupational Medicine
    Consultative Clinic
    The Emory Clinic
    1525 Clifton Road

38. Occupational and Environmental Medicine
    Program
    University of Washington Harborview Medical
    Center
    325 Ninth Avenue, # 359739
    Seattle, WA 98104
    Tel: (206) 731 3005
    Fax: (206) 731 8247

39. Department of Medicine
    Royal University Hospital
    103 Hospital Drive
    University of Saskatchewan
    Saskatoon, Saskatchewan
    Canada S7N OW8
    Tel: (306) 966 7947
    Fax: (306) 966 8021
    Web: www.usask.ca/medicine/medicine/
    division.htm

40. Respiratory Division
    Department of Medicine
    Vancouver General Hospital
    2775 Heather Street
    Vancouver, BC
    Canada V5Z 3J5
    Tel: (604) 875 4122
    Fax: (604) 875 4695

41. Pulmonary Diseases, Critical Care and
    Enviromental Medicine
    Tulane University
    1430 Tulane Ave, Box SL-9
    New Orleans, LA 70112
    Tel: (504) 588 2250
    Fax: (504) 587 2144
    E-mail: rnjones@tulane.edu.

42. Northwestern University (Dr Leslie Grammer)
    303 East Chicago Avenue,
    Tarry Building, 3rd floor
    Chicago, IL 60611
    Tel: (312) 908 8171
    Email: L_Grammer@nwu.edu

43. Specialty Laboratories, Inc.
    OncQuest
    2211 Michigan Avenue
    Santa Monica, CA 90404-3900
    Tel: (310) 828 6543, (800) 421 4449
    Web: http://www.specialtylabs.com/

44. Hospital of the University of Pennsylvania
    Pulmonary Immunology Laboratory
    815 East Gates Building
    4300 Spruce Street
    Philadelphia, PA 19104-4283
    Tel: (215) 349 5172
    Fax: (215) 349 5172
    Web: http://www.upenn.edu/

45. Division of Pulmonary and Critical Care
    Medicine (Dr Reid Dweik)
    The Cleveland Clinic Foundation
    9500 Euclid Avenue
    Cleveland, OH 44195-0001
    Tel: (216) 444 8355
    Fax: (216) 445 8160
    Web: http://www.ccf.org

46. Vanderbilt University Medical Center
    Web: http//www.mc.vanderbilt.edu/

47. Department of Pathology
    Duke University Medical Center
    Box 3712
    Durham, NC 27710
    Tel: (919) 286 0411
    Fax: (919) 286 6818

48. Department of Pathology
    University of British Columbia
    2211 Westbrook Mall
    Vancouver, BC
    Canada V6T 2B5
    Tel: (604) 822 7775
    Fax: (604) 802 7635

49. Environmental and Occupational Pathology
    Division
    Department of Pathology
    College of Medicine
    SUNY Health Science Center
    Syracuse, NY 13210
    Director: Dr Jerold L Abraham
    Web: http://www.hscsyr.edu/~pathenvi/

50. Department of Pathology
    McGill University
    3775 University Street
    Montreal,
    Canada PQ H3A 2B4

39 INFORMATION SOURCES, AND INVESTIGATION CENTERS: PACIFIC, FAR EAST, AND AUSTRALASIA

Wai-On Phoon and Malcolm Sim

INTRODUCTION

This chapter identifies information and investigation resources in the Asia–Pacific region. There are special characteristics concerning the occupational health resources of this region, in which two-thirds of the population of the world live. They are as follows:

- There has been quite significant progress in occupational health and safety (OHS) in the Asia–Pacific Region, especially in the past 20 years. Information technology has also made rapid strides in countries such as Japan, Australia, Singapore, and Korea. Taiwan and Hong Kong are, moreover, in the vanguard of world centers developing, manufacturing, and using electronic communications in commerce, finance, and government. However, the use of electronic technology in the collation, storage, and retrieval of OHS information has generally lagged behind that in North American and western Europe.

- Although English underlies the 'lingua franca' of the region, it is not (except in Australia and New Zealand) the mother tongue of most of the countries. Almost everyone in the Philippines and Singapore is fluent in English, but this is not necessarily true in the other countries except for intellectuals and business elites. Up to now, many databases and periodicals in OHS in those countries are mostly in their national languages and therefore not readily useful to the international community. We have therefore concentrated on sources of information that are in English, even if only in summary.

- There are very few OHS sources of information that are dedicated to the investigation, management, research, control, or epidemiology of occupational lung diseases. We have therefore been able, by and large, to give details only of institutions (largely research) and information sources that cover the whole spectrum of OHS conditions. However, we have tried to identify those resources that put emphasis on pulmonary problems.

- The quantity of available information varies very much from industrially developed countries, such as Japan and Australia, to less developed countries or smaller states. Moreover, we have not been able to obtain any relevant information from certain countries, despite repeated attempts to do so. This may indicate that few, if any, information sources or investigation centers exist in them.

Readers are also advised to consult Chapter 38 for information regarding internet information sources. As these electronic resources are available globally, and are not specific to a geographic region, they have not been duplicated here.

MAJOR RESOURCE CENTERS

This section contains details about large national OHS bodies in several countries in the region, which have major responsibilities for many aspects of OHS, including occupational lung disease. Such activities may include a combination of research, statistical collation, teaching, regulation development, workplace investigation, or information provision. This is followed by a section containing the contact details for a range of smaller organizations, usually responsible for a particular aspect of either information and/or investigation in relation to occupational lung disease. These listings are not exhaustive; the contact details given are current at the time of writing and may change over time.

National Occupational Health and Safety Commission (NOHSC), Australia

NOHSC is a statutory body of the Commonwealth of Australia. In 1996–1997 NOHSC identified its core functions as follows:

- The development of national standards for occupational health and safety
- Provision of a tripartite (i.e. government, employers, and employees) national forum
- Collection of national statistics
- Facilitation and dissemination of OHS information and resource material
- Conduct of an extramural and small intramural research program that supports the national standards function
- Chemical assessment, including industrial, agricultural, and veterinary chemicals

NOHSC publications include national standards, codes of practice, guidance notes, exposure standards, statistical reports, research reports, and full public and summary reports on new chemical assessments. NOHSC's website includes full-text versions of its publications (http://www.worksafe.gov.au).

In recent years, the research functions have declined substantially, but one continuing research activity at NOHSC is maintaining the Australian Mesothelioma Register (Australia has one of the highest incidences of mesothelioma in the world; see Chapter 22).

Australian mesothelioma register

The Australian Mesothelioma Register developed from the Australian Mesothelioma Surveillance Programme in 1980. Cases are notified from all the six states and two territories of Australia. The notification network includes state cancer registries, pathologists, thoracic physicians, occupational physicians, hospitals, and government divisions of occupational health to ensure as complete an ascertainment of cases as possible.

Registrar: NOHSC, GPO Box 58, Sydney NSW 2001, Australia

Japan chemical industry ecology–toxicology and information center (JETOC)

JETOC conducts a number of seminars on chemical safety in Japan and other countries in the Asia–Pacific Region. It also publishes information sheets relating to laws, regulations, results of toxicity testing, and toxicologic data on chemicals. Much of the information is in Japanese, but information sheets and some summaries of toxicity testing are published in English.

JETOC was established by members of the Japan Chemical Industry Association in 1978. In 1980 JETOC was officially recognized as a non-profit and independent organization by the Ministry of Health and Welfare, the Ministry of International Trade and Industry, and the Ministry of Labor in Japan.

Japan Industrial Safety and Health Association (JISHA)

JISHA was founded in 1964 and is a non-profit organization with associations of business owners as members. The main programs are:

- Promotion of the efforts to prevent occupational accidents
- Establishment and operation of facilities to support educational and technical programs
- Training and assistance relating to technical matters

- Collection and dissemination of information and resource materials
- Research and public relations
- Surveys on chemical toxicity, programs to create comfortable working environments, and other activities commissioned by the government
- International collaboration (e.g. joint research with US National Safety Council)
- The Japan Advanced Information Center of Safety and Health opened in January 2000; most of its publications are in Japanese only

World Health Organization regional offices

The Asia–Pacific region contains two regional World Health Organization (WHO) offices and a wide network of collaborating centers in occupational health in several countries in the region. Their responsibilities include occupational health.

Regional office for South-East Asia (SEARO)

World Health House
Indraprastha Estate
Mahatma Gandhi Road
New Delhi 110002
India
Tel: (0091) 11 331 7804 or 11 331 7823
Fax: (0091) 11 331 8607 or 11 332 7972
Email: postmaster@whosea.org
Web: http://www.whosea.org

Regional office for the Western Pacific (WPRO)

PO Box 2932
1000 Manilla
Philippines
Tel: (00632) 528 8001
Fax: (00632) 521 1036 or 536 0279
Email: postmaster@who.org.ph
Web: http://www.wpro.who.int

World Health Organization collaborating centers

These are listed by country in alphabetical order.

Australia

National Occupational Health and Safety Commission
GPO Box 58
Sydney NSW 2001
Australia
Tel: +612 9577 9303
Fax: +612 9577 9300

China

Institute of Occupational Medicine
Chinese Academy of Preventive Medicine
Director of the WHO Collaborating Center in Occupational Health (Beijing)
Professor Fengsheng He
29 Nan Wei Road
Beijing 100050
The People's Republic Of China
Tel: +8610 6381 5751
Fax: +8610 6301 4323
Email: HEFS@40p.capm.ac.cn

Shanghai Medical University
School of Public Health
Professor Liang You-xin, Director
138 Yi Xue Yuan Road
Shanghai 200032
The People's Republic of China
Tel: +8621 6404 1900 (ext) 2196
Fax: +8621 6417 8160
Email: yxliang@shmu.edu.cn

India

National Institute of Occupational Health
Dr HN Saiyed
Meghani Nagar
Ahmedabad 380016
India
Tel: +91 79 2865 5174 or 2866842
Fax: +91 79 2866630
Email: niohahd@ad1.vsnl.net.in

Japan

Institute of Industrial Ecological Sciences
University of Occupational and Environmental Health (UOEH), Japan
Professor Takesumi Yoshimra, Acting Director
1-1 Iseigaoka Yahatanishi
Kiakyushu 807–8555
Japan
Tel: +81 93 6917403
Fax: +81 93 6030158

National Institute of Industrial Health
Ministry of Labor
Dr Sohie Yamamoto, Director
21-1, Nagao 6 chome, Tama-ku
Kawasaki 214–8585
Japan
Tel: +81 44 8656111
Fax: +81 44 8656116
Web: http://www.niih.go.jp

Singapore

Department of Community, Occupational and
Family Medicine
Faculty of Medicine
National University of Singapore
Professor Kee-seng Chia, Director
WHO Collaborating Center
Lower Kent Ridge Road
Singapore 119260
Tel: +65 8744 988
Fax: +65 7791 489
Email: cofsec@nus.edu.sg

Department of Industrial Health
Ministry of Manpower
Director
18 Havelock Rd #05–01
Singapore 059764
Tel: +65 5395 366
Fax: +65 5395 140

Thailand

Division of Occupational Health
Department of Health
Ministry of Public Health
Dr Rathavuth Sukme, Director
Tivanont Road
Nonthabury 11000
Thailand
Tel: +66 2 5918 173, 5904 381
Fax: +66 2 5904 388

Vietnam

National Institute of Occupational and
Environmental Health
Professor Le Van Trung, Director
1B ho Yec Xanh
Hanoi
Vietnam
Tel: +2 63649
Fax: +2 42 12894
Email: letrung@hn.vnn.vn

OTHER DATA SOURCES AND INVESTIGATION CENTERS

Addresses and contact information for other, smaller, sources of information in the countries of the region are listed below, according to the most up-to-date information available to the authors of this chapter. They are often, additionally, investigation centers and comprise a mix of academic units, government departments, hospital units, and others. These bodies usually have one or more functions related to occupational lung disease, including compilation of statistics, train-ing, regulation enforcement, workplace assessments, and clinical management of cases. For example, regulatory bodies provide information and undertake investigations, although for the latter usually only on a regional basis. The listing is not exhaustive, and is intended to provide starting points for accessing information and/or services in each country. The contact details are listed by country, alphabetically.

Australia

Australian Centre for International and Tropical
Health and Nutrition
Mayne Medical School
Herston Road
Herston
Queensland 4006
Tel: +61 7 3365 5393
Fax: +61 7 3365 5599
Email: enquiries@acithn.uq.edu.au
Director: Professor Ian Riley

Australian Chamber of Commerce and Industry
Level 4, 55 Exhibition Street
Melbourne, Victoria 3000
Tel: (03) 9289 5289
Fax: (03) 9289 5250
Web: http://www.acci.asn.au

Australian Council of Trade Unions
Trades Hall, 54 Victoria Street
Carlton South, Victoria 3053
Tel: OHS Unit (03) 9664 7310
Fax: (03) 9663 8220
Web: http://www.actu.asn.au

Dust Diseases Board
2/82 Elizabeth Street
Sydney, New South Wales 2000
Tel: +61 2 8223 660
Fax: +61 2 8223 6699

National Industrial Chemicals Notification and
Assessment Scheme (NICNAS)
92/94 Parramatta Road
Camperdown, New South Wales 2050
GPO Box 58
Sydney, New South Wales 2001
Tel: +61 2 9577 9578

Occupational Hygiene Unit
Faculty of Biological Sciences
Deakin University
Waurn Ponds, Victoria
Respiratory Medicine Unit
Sir Charles Gairdner Hospital
Perth, Western Australia

Royal Prince Alfred Hospital
Missenden Road
Camperdown, New South Wales 2050
(a) Institute of Respiratory Medicine
(b) Division of Respiratory Medicine (Occupational
Respiratory Diseases)
Tel: +61 2 9515 6111

Surveillance of Australian Workplace-Based
Respiratory Events (SABRE program)
Unit of Occupational and Environmental Health
Department of Epidemiology and Preventive
Medicine
Monash University
Commercial Road
Prahran, Victoria 3181
Tel: +61 3 9903 0582
Fax: +61 3 9903 0556
Email: malcolm.sim@med.monash.edu.au

Australian Regulatory Authorities

In Australia, each of the six states and two territories
has general control of occupational health and safety
in its own jurisdiction. Each publishes a large volume
of literature on many subjects relevant to occupational lung disease. Their contact addresses, following
that of the federal OHS Agency, are as follows.

Australian Public Service OHS Agency

COMCARE
CFM Building
12 Moore Street
Canberra, ACT 2601
Tel: (02) 6275 0000; 1300 366 979
Fax: (02) 6257 5634
http://www.comcare.gov.au

New South Wales

WorkCover NSW
400 Kent Street
Sydney, New South Wales 2000
Tel: (02) 9370 5000; 1800 451 462
Fax: (02) 9370 6120
Web: http://www.workcover.nsw.gov.au

Queensland

Division of Workplace Health and Safety
Department of Employment, Training and Industrial
Relations
75 William Street
Brisbane, QLD 4000
Tel: (07) 3247 4711; 1800 177 717
Fax: (07) 3220 0143
Web: http:/www.detir.qld.gov.au

South Australia

WorkCover Corporation
100 Weymouth Street
Adelaide, SA 5000
Tel: (08) 8233 2222; 1800 888 508 (all states);
1800 188 000 (SA only)
Fax: (08) 8233 2466
Web: http://www.workcover.sa.gov.au

Tasmania

Workplace Standards Tasmania, Department of
Infrastructure, Energy and Resources
30 Gordons Hill Road
Rosny Park, Tasmania 7018
Tel: (03) 6233 7657; 1300 366 322 (Tas only)
Fax: (03) 6233 8338
Web: http://www.wsa.tas.gov.au

Victoria

Victorian WorkCover Authority
222 Exhibition Street
Melbourne, Victoria 3000
Tel: (03) 9628 8111; 1800 136 089 (Vic only)
Fax: (03) 9641 1222
Web: http://www.workcover.vic.gov.au

Western Australia

WorkSafe Western Australia
1260 Hay Street
West Perth, WA 6005
Tel: (08) 9327 8777
Fax: (08) 9321 8973
Web: http://www.safetyline.wa.gov.au

Australian Capital Territory

ACT WorkCover
3rd Floor, FAI House
197 London Circuit
Civic, ACT 2601
Tel: (02) 6205 0200
Fax: (02) 6205 0797
Web: http://www.act.gov.au

Northern Territory

Department of Industries and Business Work
Health Branch
Minerals House
66 The Esplanade
Darwin, NT 0800
Tel: (08) 8999 5010; 1800 019 115
Fax: (08) 8999 5141
Web: http://www.nt.gov.au/wha

China

Institute of Occupational Medicine
Academy of Preventive Medicine
29 Nan Wei Road, Beijing 100050
Email: dehong@263.net

Occupational Medicine Division, Labor Department
15/F Harbour Building
38 Pier Road
Central
Tel: 852 3852 4041

India

National Institute of Occupational Health
Meghaninagar
Ahmedabad
Gujarat State 380016
Tel: 91 79 786 6630
Fax: 91 79 786 6630
Email: nohahd@ad.1.rsn.net.in

Ramazzini Research Institute and Occupational
Health Services
577 Shukrawar Peth
Subhashnagar
Pune 41 1002

Indonesia

Ergonomic Program
Department of Physiology
Udayana University
Jalan Serma Gede
18 Denpasar 800114, Bali
Tel: 62 361 237 614
Fax: 62 361 237 614
Email: adman@denpasar.wasantara.net.id

Japan

Institute for Science of Labor
2–8–14 Sugao
Miyamae-ku
Kawasaki 216–8501
Tel: 81 44 977 2121
Fax: 81 44 976 8659

Japan Chemical Industry Ecology–Toxicology and
Information Center, JETOC
NANBA Building
2F, 19–4, 1-chome
Nishishinbashi
Minato-ku
Tokyo 105–0003
Tel: 81 3 3593 1190
Fax: 81 3 3593 1116

Japan Industrial Safety and Health Association
(ILO-CIS National Center in Japan)
5–351–1, Shiba
Minato-ku
Tokyo 108–100 14
Tel: 81 3 3452 6841
Fax: 81 3 3451 4596
Email: kokusai@jisha.or.jp
Web: http://www.jisha.or.jp

National Institute of Industrial Health
6–21–1 Nagao
Tamaku
Kawasaki 214–8585
Tel: 81 44 865 6111
Fax: 81 44 865 6116
Email: sakurai@niih.go.jp

University of Occupational and Environmental
Health
1–1 Iseigaoka Yahatanishi-ku
Kitakyusha
Tel: 81 93 691 7462
Fax: 81 93 692 4590

Korea

Department of Preventive Medicine
The Catholic University of Korea
505 Banpo-dong
Socho-ku
Seoul 137–701
Tel: 82 2 590 1236
Fax: 82 2 532 3820
Email: cmcpm@challian.dacom.co.kr

New Zealand

New Zealand Occupational and Environmental
Health Research Centre
Private Bag 92019
Auckland
Tel: 64 9 373 7599
Fax: 64 9 373 7503
Email: mchtkjellstrom@mednovl.auckland.ac.nz

Occupational Safety and Health, Department of
Labour,
62–66 The Terrace
Wellington
Tel: 64 4 495 4431

Philippines

Philippines College of Occupational Medicine
Room 106 PMA Building
North Avenue

Quezon City
Tel: 455 2410/524 2703/455 2410
Fax: 929 7741 521 1394/929 7745
Email: pcom@netasia.net

Singapore

Department of Community, Occupational and
Family Medicine
National University of Singapore
Singapore 119074
Tel: 65 874 4985
Fax: 65 779 1489
Email: cofjeya@leonis.nus.edu.sg

Department of Industrial Health
Ministry of Manpower
18 Havelock Road,
05–01, Singapore 059764
Tel: 65 539 5135
Fax: 65 539 5140
Email: momdih@cs.gov.sg
Director: Dr WH Phoon

Taiwan

Institute of Occupational Medicine and Industrial
Hygiene
National Taiwan University College of Public
Health
Tel: 886 2 2356 2224
Fax: 886 2 2322 4660
Email: lionluck@hotmail.com

Institute of Occupational Medicine and Industrial
Hygiene
No. 1 Sec. 1, Jen-Ai Road
Taipei 10016
Tel: 886 2 2356 2224
Fax: 886 2 2322 4660
Email: jdwang@ha.mc.ntu.edu.fw
Director: Professor Jung-Der Wang
Tel: 8610 6301 6891
Fax: 8610 6301 4323
Email: dehong@263.net

Thailand

Division of Occupational Health
Department of Health
Ministry of Public Health,
Tivanont Road
Nonthaburi 11000

National Institute for the Improvement of Working
Conditions and Environment
Department of Labor
Bangkok

Occupational Health Unit, Department of Health
Ministry of Public Health
Nonthburi 11000
Tel: 662 5904230
Fax: 662 965 9245
Email: wilawan@anamai.morph.go.th

Vietnam

Department of Preventive Medicine
Ministry of Health
138A Jiang Vo Street
Hanoi
Tel: 84 4 8460 347
Fax: 84 4 8460 507
Email: hongtu@netnam.org.vn
Dr Thi Hong Tu Nguyen

OCCUPATIONAL HEALTH JOURNALS

Occupational health journals published within
countries in the region can be an invaluable source
of information about local activities in occupational
lung disease, as well as providing recent information
about individuals active in the field and their contact
details. The journals listed below are published in
English.

Indian Journal of Industrial Medicine
(published by the Indian Association of
Occupational Health)
c/o Hindustan Lever Ltd
Mumbai 400–020
India

Journal of Human Ergology
(published by the Human Ergology Society and the
South-East Asian Ergonomics Society)
Business
Center of Academics Societies Japan
4–16 Yayoi 2-chome,
Bunkyo-ku
Tokyo 113
Japan

Journal of Occupational Health
(publication of the Japan Society for
Occupational Health)
Public Health Building
1–29–8 Shinjuku
Tokyo 160
Japan

*Journal of Occupational Health and Safety,
Australia and New Zealand*
CCH Australia Ltd
GPO 4072
Sydney 2001
Australia
Tel: +61 2 9857 1845

Journal of Occupational Medicine
(published by the Society of Occupational Medicine,
Singapore)
Level 2, Alumni Medical Centre
2 College Road
Singapore 169850

*Journal of the University of Occupational and
Environmental Health*
University of Occupational and Environmental
Health Japan
Kitakyushu 807
Japan
Tel: 093 603 1611
(in English and Japanese)

Safety and Health in Japan
(newsletter of the Japan Industrial Safety and
Health Association; JISHA) (ILO/CIS National
Center)
5–35–1 Shiba
Minato-ku
Tokyo 108–1004
Japan
Tel: 81 3 3452 6841
Fax: 81 3 3451 4596
Email: kokusai@jisha.or.jp
Web: http://www.jisha.or.jp

*Southeast Asian Journal of Tropical Medicine and Public
Health*
420/6 Rajvathi Road
Bangkok 10400
Thailand
Tel: and Fax: +66 2 247 7721
Email: tmseamed@diamond.mahidol.ac.th

Worksafe News
(publication of the National Occupational Health
and Safety Commission)
GPO Box 58
Sydney 2001
Australia
Fax:(612) 9577 9207

PROFESSIONAL ORGANIZATIONS

Some of the following organizations undertake
research for governments and international bodies,
and publish papers and reports on their findings.
They are listed alphabetically:

Asian Association of Occupational Health (AAOH)
c/o PhilamCare Health Systems
7/F Philamlife Building
United Nations Avenue
Ermita
Manila
Philippines
(The AAOH has run triennial Asian Conferences on
Occupational Health since 1954 and publishes pro-
ceedings of such conferences.)

Australasian Faculty of Occupational Medicine
Royal Australasian College of Physicians
145 Macquarie Street
Sydney, NSW 2000
Australia
Tel: +61 2 9256 5400
Fax: +61 2 9247 8082
Email: afom@racp.edu.au
Web: www.racp.edu.au/afom/index.htm
President: Dr Ian Gardner

Australian College of Occupational Health Nurses
80 Stephensons Rd
Mount Waverley
Victoria 3149
Australia
Tel: +61 3 9886 5795

Australian Institute Of Occupational Hygienists
34 Carrick Drive
Tullamarine
Victoria 3043
Australia
Tel: +61 3 9335 2577
Fax: +61 3 9335 3454

Australian Lung Foundation
Level 3
454 Upper Edward Street
Spring Hill
Queensland 4000
Australia

Australian and New Zealand Society of
Occupational Medicine
c/o PO Box 1044,
South Melbourne
Victoria 3205
Australia

Indian Association of Occupational Health
c/o Medical Advisor
Siemens Ltd
130 Pandurang Budkhar Marg
Morli
Mumbai 400018
India
Tel: 91 22 493 6251
Fax: 91 22 495 0552

Indonesia Medical Association for
Occupational Health
Gedung Mochtar
Jalan Pegangsaan
Timur No. 16
Jakarta
Indonesia

Japan Association of Industrial Health
c/o Public Health Building
1–29–8 Shinjuka Shinjuku-ku,
Tokyo 160
Japan

Japan Industrial Safety and Health Association
5–35–1 Shiba
Minato-ku 108–0014
Tel: 03 3452 6841

Occupational Medicine Association of Thailand
c/o Department of Preventive Medicine
Faculty of Medicine
Srinakharinwirot University
681 Samsen Road
Susit
Bangkok 10300
Thailand

Philippine College of Occupational Medicine
Room 106, Philippine Medical Association Building
North Avenue
Quezon City
Philippines

Safety Institute of Australia
51 City Road
South Melbourne 3205
Tel: +61 3 9645 9166

Singapore Medical Association
Level 2, Alumni Medical Center
2 College Rd
Singapore 169850

Society of Occupational Medicine Singapore
Singapore Medical Association
Level 2, Alumni Medical Center
2 College Road
Singapore 169850

Thoracic Society of Australia and New Zealand
145 Macquarie Street
Sydney, NSW 2000
Australia
Tel: 61 2 9256 5457
Fax: +61 2 9241 4162
Web: www.thoracic.org.au

40 INFORMATION SOURCES AND INVESTIGATION CENTERS: WESTERN EUROPE

Henrik Nordman

INTRODUCTION

Europe is changing as the European Union (EU) expands and becomes increasingly influential, and so this chapter on the western European region focuses on the EU itself. It has many sources of information, and they are widely dispersed. It may consequently be difficult to find the most appropriate source for a specific problem and to retrieve the information required. The large number of languages may pose a further problem, and this sometimes hampers accessibility of information. However, for the vast majority of information exchanges, English may be used.

The major European medical associations and their journals are particularly valuable sources of information, as are international organizations such as the United Nations or the EU. Their publications can be ordered directly or from their affiliated organizations in individual countries, and are often available for subscribers over the internet as online services. Criteria documents for harmful substances are produced by several European Expert Groups, some of which are published and accessible over the net. Others are available through the administration of the Expert Group.

Much additional information is available from respiratory medicine clinics, research groups, or individual clinicians. Research institutes and regulatory bodies generally produce publications that can be purchased, and some may be found on the Internet. At a domestic level most institutes offer services over the telephone, and many have websites in English. The information that is offered is not always fully up-to-date, as it can change over short periods of time.

INFORMATION TECHNOLOGY

The internet provides an increasingly useful and accessible means of communicating and disseminating information, but at present data are often unstructured and difficult to retrieve, and a multitude of websites are still in the process of being developed. Nevertheless, some websites provide excellent information, and several organizations and journals offer their products over the net. Bibliographies are accessible with particular ease. Many of the institutes and clinics listed below have websites, and it is likely that the internet will shortly be one of the most, if not the most, important source of information. It certainly provides the most rapid way of exchanging information, for instance the swift notification of a new occupational hazard.

AsmaWork

http://www.remcomp.com/asmanet/asmapro/
asmawork.htm

This is an excellent website on occupational asthma. It is administered by the Clinic for Lung Diseases at the Hôpital Arnaud de Villeneuve in Montpellier, France. It gives information about causative agents and occupations, and provides a bibliography.

North America

Europeans, like residents of other regions, additionally have ready and invaluable access to much of the information technology (IT) of North America, details of which are presented in Chapter 38.

SOURCES OF INFORMATION

European Commission (EC)

http://europa.eu.int/eur-lex/en/search.html.

The European Commission has activities that relate in various ways to occupational pulmonary medicine. All official directives adopted by the Commission can be found on the website. However, annexes of respective directives are not available on the net; they have to be ordered separately.

The Directorate General for Health and Consumer Protection is responsible for classifying and labeling substances and preparations (Council Directive 92/32/EEC). Substances that may be irritant to the respiratory system receive the assignment R37. These substances normally cause reversible irritation to the upper respiratory tract.

Substances that cause sensitization by inhalation are assigned the symbol ('Xn') indicating harmfulness, and the risk designation R42. Labeling a substance as a sensitizer does not require that an immunologic mechanism has been demonstrated, and this is stated in the corresponding Annex VI (General classification and labeling requirements for dangerous substances and preparations; 3.2.7). Thus, isocyanates are labeled as sensitizers because of their recognized high potency in a generic sense to cause sensitization, unless there is evidence that an individual isocyanate compound does not cause respiratory hypersensitivity. With individual organic acid anhydrides, however, the R42 label is applied only if specific sensitizing properties are evident for the particular compound; so far only a couple have been labeled R42. The present labeling practice does not concern preparations where the sensitizing substance is present in a concentration below 1%. This may allow Safety Data Cards to ignore the sensitizing property of such 'trace' agents, and so have an adverse effect on the quality of the information displayed.

Scientific Committée for Occupational Exposure Limits (SCOEL)

http://www.europa.eu.int/en/comm/dg05/hs/
mainhs/htm

SCOEL was made an official committee of the EC in 1995 (Commission decision 95/320/EC) to review and recommend occupational exposure limits for substances. The recommendations are published as a summary containing substance identification, use and occurrence, health significance, recommendation (including the critical effect, key studies, uncertainty factors, proposed occupational limit), and a bibliography. Further information on the publications may be obtained from:

European Commission
Directorate-General V
Employment, Industrial Relations and Social Affairs
Directorate V/F-Public Health and Safety at Work
Unit V/F/5
Euroforum Building, L-2920 Luxembourg
Tel: + 352 430 13 49 88

European Agency for Safety and Health at Work (EASHW)

http://europe.osha.eu.int/

EASHW was set up in Bilbao, Spain, in 1997 by the EU to serve the information needs within the field of occupational safety and health. The Agency coordinates a network of Focal Points in each member state. Information is provided on legislation and statistics of member states.

International Programme on Chemical Safety (IPCS)

http://www.unep.org/unep/partners/un/ipcs/

IPCS is a joint program of three cooperating organizations, the International Labour Office (ILO), the United Nations and the World Health Organization (WHO) which is also the executing agency. IPCS is a scientifically based program implementing activities related to chemical safety that offers a vast amount of information on chemicals and related hazards. Its areas of activity include evaluation of chemical risks to human health and the environment, methodologies for evaluation of hazards and risks, prevention and management of toxic exposures and chemical emergencies, and development of the human resources required in the above areas. Some of the most useful products of the IPCS are:

Evaluation of chemical risks to human health and the environment

- Risk evaluation of priority chemicals
- Environmental health criteria documents (a list of chemicals for which documents have been published is on the website)
- Health and safety guides (a list of items is on the website)
- Concise international chemical assessment documents abstracted in English, French and Spanish
- Health and environment based guidelines for exposure

Joint UN Food and Agriculture Organization (FAO)

- WHO Expert committee on food additives
- WHO Drinking water quality guidelines
- WHO Air quality guidelines for Europe (WHO Regional Office for Europe)
- WHO Recommended classification of pesticides by hazard and guidelines to classification 1998–1999

Chemical risk communication

- International Chemical Safety Cards (about 1250 cards available in several languages) http://www.cdc.gov/niosh/ipcs/icstart.html
- Pesticide data sheets (a published list of pesticides by WHO/FAO may be ordered from WHO:sta
- Technical information for professionals
- IPCS INCHEM CD-ROM
- Global information network on chemicals
- Public education and awareness campaigns

International Agency for Research on Cancer (IARC)

http://www.iarc.fr

IARC is the best source of information on the carcinogenicity of specific substances. Databases and other resources at IARC include the Monographs Database which contains a complete list of agents, mixtures, and exposures, all evaluated with their classifications; the Cancer Epidemiology Database which provides access to information on the occur-

rence of cancer worldwide; IARC's P53 Database; and other useful resources. The following resources are among those available at the IARC website:

IARC Monographs database on carcinogenic risks to humans

- Preamble to the Monographs series
- Complete list of agents, mixtures, and exposures evaluated and their classification
- Complete list of all Monographs and supplements published to date
- SEARCH IARC Agents and summary evaluations
- Monographs recently published and in press, and ordering information
- IARC Monographs on CD-ROM and online
- Agents evaluated most recently
- Agents scheduled for evaluation at future meetings
- Recent advisory group recommendations
- Directory of agents being tested for carcinogenicity
- EPA/IARC Genetic activity profiles (GAP) database and software
- IARC Scientific publications and IARC technical reports related to IARC Monographs evaluations
- About the unit of carcinogen identification and evaluation

IARC Cancer epidemiology database

- Information on annual cancer incidence, mortality and survival
- Resources for researchers and cancer registries

Carex

Carex is an international source of information on worker exposure to carcinogens. The international data have been compiled by the Finnish Institute of Occupational Health in collaboration with IARC. Carex is a Microsoft® Access database which contains estimates of the numbers of workers occupationally exposed to carcinogens in the 15 countries of the EU and provides descriptive reports and data tables on carcinogen exposure. Carex also contains information on industrial distribution of the employed, summarized exposure data, numbers exposed by occupation, definitions of carcinogenic exposure, descriptions of the estimation procedures, and bibliographic references.

International Labour Office (ILO)

ILO has published guidelines since 1980 for the radiographic classification of pneumoconioses. The classification includes a series of pulmonary radiographs with instructions for classification. The ninth impression is from 1995. The *Guidelines for the use of ILO international classification of radiographs of pneumoconioses* are also available in French. The guidelines and the model radiographs can be obtained via ILO local offices or direct from ILO Publications, International Labour Office, CH-1211 Geneva, Switzerland. The classification itself is described in Chapter 31.

Professional organizations and journals

Information on occupational and environmental lung disorders may be obtained from professional organizations and medical associations, and their journals. The most relevant European organizations are the European Respiratory Society and the European Academy of Allergy and Clinical Immunology. Both publish journals as do a number of national societies of EU countries:

European Respiratory Society (ERS)

Email: info@ersnet.org
1 Bd de Grancy
1006 Lausanne
Switzerland
Tel: (41) 21 613 0202
Fax: (41) 21 617 2865

The ERS is responsible for the publication of several periodicals. The most important is the official publication of the ERS, the *European Respiratory Journal*, with 12 issues per year. The journal is available online. ERS also publishes the *European Respiratory Review*, which appears 6–8 times annually. The *ERS Respiratory Topic* is a quarterly digest of articles on respiratory medicine with topical reviews of current respiratory literature. ERS Monographs is a series of clinical monographs intended for practising physicians and pulmonologists. The *ERS Newsletter* is prepared for society members about society events and news.

European Academy of Allergology and Clinical Immunology (EAACI)

http://www.eaaci.org/
PO Box 24 140
SE-104 51 Stockholm
Tel: +46 8 459 66 23
Email: executive.office@eaaci.org
The executive office is situated in Stockholm, Sweden. The association publishes the journal *Allergy*, which is also available on the Internet as an online service for subscribers and members.

Thorax

http://www.thoraxjnl.com

Thorax is the official journal of the British Thoracic Society. The journal is published monthly. It may be ordered from the Subscription Manager, Thorax, BMJ Publishing Group, BMA House, Tavistock Square, London WC1H 9JR, UK.

Scandinavian Journal of Work, Environment and Health

http://www.occuphealth.fi/sjweh

This journal is published by the Finnish Institute of Occupational Health in Helsinki. It frequently includes articles pertaining to occupational and environmental lung disorders. The subscription address is Topeliuksenkatu 41 aA, FIN-00250, Helsinki, Finland. The journal has been available on line for subscribers since the beginning of 2001.

Occupational and environmental medicine

http://oem.bmjjournals.com

Occupational and Environmental Medicine contains articles bearing on occupational and environmental pulmonary issues. It is available online for subscribers.

International archives of occupational and environmental health

http://link.springer.de/link/service/journals/forum.htm

This is a journal for subscribers published by Springer. Subscribers can obtain the journal online.

Occupational medicine

http://occmed.oupjournals.org

Occupational Medicine is the journal of the UK Society of Occupational Medicine. It is not yet accessible on the internet. The Society can be contacted at:

6 St Andrew's Place
London NW1 4LB
Tel: +44 (0)20 7486 2641
Fax: +44 (0)20 7486 0028
Email som@sococcmed.demon.co.uk

Expert groups

There are national expert groups producing criteria documents for regulatory bodies and the setting of occupational exposure limits. These documents contain extremely valuable data on toxicokinetics, toxicity, and health effects of reviewed substances.

Some documents are produced, and the risk assessments made, by international groups such as the EU Committe SCOEL (see above) and the Nordic Expert Group: http://www.nordicexpertgroup.org

The criteria documents produced by the Nordic Expert Group are published in English in the scientific series 'Arbete och Hälsa' by the National Institute for Working Life, Förlagstjänst, S-112 79 Stockholm, Sweden; Tel: +46 8 619 69 00; http://www.niwl.se/ah/

At a national level, invaluable criteria documents are produced by the German MAK Commission. Its recommendations are published annually as the 'List of MAK and BAT Values' in German and English by Wiley VCH, Weinheim. Full documentation of the proposals in the list is published in German as 'Toxikologisch-arbeitsmedizinische Begründungen von MAK-Werten', and in English as 'Occupational Toxicants' by the same publisher (Wiley-VCH, D-69451 Weinheim, Germany).

The Dutch Expert Committee on Occupational Standards (DECOS), or the DECOS-Committee, is part of the Health Council of the Netherlands. The committee derives health-based recommended limits for occupational exposure to toxic substances. The well-written DECOS documents are published by the Health Council and can be ordered from: http://www.gr.nl/engels/Interactive/general/main. htm

Gesondheidsraad
Health Council of the Netherlands
Postbus 1236
2280 CE Rijswijk
The Netherlands
Fax: 31 70 3407523

Information on disease frequency

Registers on incidence of occupational pulmonary diseases are uncommon. Statutory sources of information have been proven grossly to underestimate the true occurrence of disease. The information from existing registers is often inconsistent because data may be collected in different and not comparable ways. There are thus compulsory reporting systems (e.g. Finland) and systems based on voluntary self-reporting by the affected employee (e.g. Sweden).

The Finnish Register on Occupational Diseases (FROD) was established in 1964. It is maintained by the Finnish Institute of Occupational Health. Since 1974, physicians have been obliged by law to report all ascertained or suspected cases of occupational disease. Finnish legislation requires the demonstration of a causal relationship between disease and exposure. The compensation system is comparatively liberal acting as an incentive for workers to report any work-related symptoms. Finnish workers must be insured, whereas the self-employed often have voluntary insurance; thus, the coverage of the register is reasonably good. The FROD appears to be the most accurate register available on occupational diseases. Statistics are published annually in Finnish and, every fifth year, in English.

Since 1989, two voluntary reporting systems have existed in the UK. The Surveillance of Work-related and Occupational Respiratory Disease (SWORD) receives reports on new occupational lung diseases from specialists in occupational or respiratory medicine all over the UK. It is part of the Occupational Disease Information Network (ODIN). SWORD produces annual reports which have been published in the journal *Occupational Medicine*. More information about SWORD may be obtained from:

Centre for Occupational and Environmental Health
Stopford Building
Oxford Road
Manchester M13 9PT
Tel: +44 161 275 7103
Fax: +44 161 275 5506.

The other voluntary UK reporting system, SHIELD, covers the West Midlands. Reports are obtained from specialists in occupational and respiratory medicine and also from local Medical Boarding Centers for state compensation. SHIELD has a somewhat better coverage locally, whereas SWORD gives the overall picture from the UK. Information in a synopsis form on SHIELD can be obtained as follows:

Tel: +44 121 424 2745
Fax: +44 121 772 0292
Email: Occupationalasthma.com

INVESTIGATION CENTERS

Several European countries have strong traditions in occupational respiratory medicine, and there are numerous institutes and clinics for occupational medicine. Some are both research centers as well as diagnostic clinics. The majority of diagnostic clinics are sited in universities or specialized clinics of respiratory medicine, and most cooperate with (or are situated in) local hospitals. A complete list of investigation centers is impractical, and the author and editors are anxious to avoid any implication that some centers are to be endorsed rather than others. Furthermore, the expertize and knowledge within a particular field in a particular institution may be linked to the activities and interests of only a few (or even a single) scientists or clinicians. A list may therefore become obsolete over a rather short period of time, and contain inaccuracies of both omission and commission. The following are simply some centers within western Europe where assistance and advice may be obtained.

Belgium

Department of Chest Medicine:
Service de Pneumologie
Clinique Universitaire de Mont-Godinne
Université Catholique de Louvain
B-5530 Yvoir
Tel: +32 81 42 33 51
Fax: +32 81 42 33 52

Institute of Hygiene and Epidemiology:
Institut Scientifique de la Santé Publique–Louis Pasteur
14 Rue J Wytsman
1050 Bruxelles

Laboratory of Pneumonology:
Laboratorium voor Long Toxicologie
(Unit of Lung Toxicology)
Katholieke Universiteit Leuven
Herestraat 49
B-3000 Leuven
Tel: +32 16 34 71 21
Fax: +32 16 34 71 24

Occupational Diseases Fund:
Fonds voor de Beroepsziekten–Fonds des Maladie Professionnelles
Sterrenkundelaan
1 Avenue de l'Astronomie
B-1210 Bruxelles

Research Unit on the Toxicity of Mineral Particles:
Service de Pneumologie
Université Libre de Bruxelles
Hôpital Erasme
808 Route de Lennik
Bruxelles 1070

Denmark

Department of Occupational Medicine
Aalborg Regional Hospitalt
PO Box 561
DK-9100 Aalborg
Tel: +45 96313400
Fax: +45 96313401

Departments of Respiratory Disease and Occupational and Environmental medicine
Århus Universitetshospital
University of Aarhus
Norregrogade 44
DK-8000 Aarhus
Tel: +45 89 33 33
Fax: +45 89 49 21 10

Department of Occupational Medicine
National Institute of Occupational Health
Lersö Parkallé 105
DK-2100 Copenhagen
Tel: +45 39 165214
Fax: +45 39 165201

Department of Occupational and Environmental Medicine
Odense University Hospital
Södra Boulevard 29
DK-5000 Odense C
Tel: +45 65414990
Fax: +45 65414988

Finland

Finnish Institute of Occupational Health
Topeliuksenkatu 41 aA
00250 Helsinki
Tel: +358 9 47471
Fax: +358 9 4587 092
Web: http://www.occuphealth.fi

Kuopio Regional Institute of Occupational health
PL 93
Neulaniementie 4
70701 Kuopio
Tel: +358 17 201211
Fax: +358 17 201 474
Email: @occuphealth.fi

Lappeenranta Regional Institute of Occupational Health
Laserkatu 6
53850 Lappeenranta
Tel: +358 5 62411
Fax: +358 5 6243230

National Public Health Institute
PL 95
Neulaniementie 4
70701 Kuopio
Tel: +358 17 201211
Email: @ktl.fi

Uusimaa Regional Institute of Occupational Health
Arinatie 3 A
00370 Helsinki
Tel: +358 9 47471
Fax: +358 9 5061087
Web: http://www.occuphealth.fi/e/dept/u

France

Clinique de Maladies Respiratoires
Hôpital Arnaud de Villenuve
371 Avenue Doyen Gaston Giraud
34295 Montpellier Cedex 5
Tel: +33 04 67336102
Web: http://www.remcomp.com/asmanet/asmapro/
asmawork.htm

Clinique des Maladies Respiratoires
Service de Pneumologie et Immuno-allergologie
Hôpital A Calmette
Boulevard J Leclerc
59037 Lille Cedex
Tel: 03 20 44 50 36
Fax: 03 20 44 66 93

Department of Internal Medicine and Chest Diseses
Hôpital de la Cavale Blanche
29609 Brest Cedex
Tel: +33 2 98 34 73 48
Fax: +33 2 98 34 79 44

Department of Occupational Diseases
Hôpital Morvan
29609 Brest Cedex
Tel: +33 2 98 22 35 09
Fax: +33 2 98 23 39 59

Inserm Unit 169
Rech en Epidemiologie
16 Avenue Paul-Vaillant-Couturier
Fn-94807 Villejuis Cedex
Tel: +33 1 45 59 50 72
Fax: +33 1 45 59 51 69

Institut National de Recherche et de Sécurité (INRS)
30 Rue Olivier-Noyer
75680 Paris Cedex 14
Tel: +33 1 40 44 30 00
Web: http://www.inrs.fr

Observatoire National des Asthmes Professionnels
(ONAP)
SPLF-ONAP
66 Boulevard Saint Michel
75006 Paris
Tel: +33 1 88 11 58 33
Fax: +33 1 46 34 58 27
Web: http://www.splf.org

Réseau National de Santé Publique (RNSP)
Unité Santé et Environnement
11 Rue du Val d'Oise
94415. Saint Maurice Cedex
Tel: +33 1 41 79 67 00
Fax: +33 1 41 79 67 67
Web: http://www.rnsp-sante.fr/

Service de Pneumologie et Allergie
Hôpital Nord
S-13915
Marseille Cedex 20
Tel: +33 4 91 96 86 31
Fax: +33 4 91 09 09 94
Email: dcharpin@ap_hm.fr

Germany

Berufsgenossenschaftlihes Forschungsinstitut für
Arbeitsmedizin!
Ruhr-Universität Bochum
Bochum

Institut für Arbeitsphysiologie
Universität Dortmund
Ardeystrasse 67
D-44139 Dortmund
Tel: +49 231 1084348
Fax: +49 231 1084403

Institut und Poliklinik für Arbeits-, Social- ind
Unweltmedizin
Schillerstrasse 25 u 29
D-91054 Erlangen
Tel: +49 9131 856112
Fax: +49 9131 852317

Institute & Outpatient Clinic for Occupational and
Environmental Medicine
Luwig-Maximilians University
Ziemensstrasse 1
D-80336 Muenchen
Tel: +49 89 5160 2301
Fax: +49 89 5160 4445
Web: http://www.med.uni-muenchen.de/arbmed

Italy

Department of Allergy and Clinical Immunology
Fondazione Clinica del Lavore
Via S Boezio 26
27 100 Pavia
Tel: +39 382 592281
Fax: +39 382 20114

Dipartimento di Medicina Ambientale e Sanità
Pubblica
Medicina del Lavoro
Università di Padova
Via Giustiniani 2
35128 Padova
Tel: +39 49 8212540
Fax: +39 49 8212542

Dipartimento di Traumatologia, Ortopedia e Medicina
del Lavoro dell'Università
Ospedale CTO
Via Zuretti 29
10126 Torino
Tel: +39 011 6933500 (secretary)
     +39 011 6933461 (allergy and respiratory unit)
Fax: +39 011 6963662
Web: www.cto.unito.it

Fondazione Salvatore Maugeri, IRCCS
Clinica del Lavoro e della Riabilitazione
Via Ferrata 4
27 100 Pavia
Tel: +39 382 592941
Web: www.fsm.it

Institute of Occupational Health
University of Milan
Via San Barnaba, 8
I-201122 Milano
Tel: +39 02 55181723
Fax: +39 02 5456025

Instituto di Medicina del Lavoro
University of Padova
Via Facciolati 71
35127 Padova
Tel: +39 49 8216632
Fax: +39 49 8216631

Research Center on Asthma and COPD
University of Ferrara
Sezione di Fisiopatologia
Istituto di Patologia Gene
Via L Borsari 46
1-44100 Ferrara
Tel: +39 53 2 210420
Fax: +39 53 2 210297

Norway

National Institute of Occupational Health
P.b 8149 Dep
NO-0033 Oslo
Tel: +47 23195100
Web: www.stami.no

Center for Occupational and Environmental
Respiratory Medicine
Department of Respiratory Medicine
The National Hospital
N-0027 Oslo
Tel: +47 23070000
Fax: +47 23073917

Haukeland Hospital
Department of Occupational Medicine
N-5021 Bergen
Tel: +47 55 973899
Fax: +47 55 975137
University Hospital of Trondheim
Department of Occupational Medicine
N-7006 Trondheim
Tel: +47 73867315
Fax: +47 73868970

Spain

Environmental and Respiratory Health Research Unit
Institut Municipal d'Investigació Mèdica
Dr Aiguader 80
08003 Barcelona
Tel: +34 93 221 1009
Fax: +34 93 221 3237
www.imim.es

Instituto Nacional de Seguridad e Higiene en el
Trabajo (CNNT)
Jefe de Area de Higiene y Medicina
C/Torrelaguna 73
E-28027 Madrid
Tel: +34 91 4037000
Fax: +34 91 4030050

Centro Nacional de Conditiones de Trabajo
Instituto Nacional de Seguridad e Hygiene en el
Trabajo (INSHT)
Dolcet, 2–10
08034 Barcelona
Tel: +34 93 2800102
Fax: +34 93 2803642
www.mtas.es/insht/principal/orgacnct.htm

European Agency for Safety and Health at Work
Gran Via 33
48009 Bilbao
Tel: +34 94 479 4360
Fax: +34 94 479 4383
www.osha.eu.int

Pneumology Service
Hospital Vall d'Hebron
Passeig de la Vall d'Hebron 119–129

08035 Barcelona
Tel: +34 93 274 6100
www.vhebron.es

Sweden

Department of Experimental Research on Asthma
and Allergy
Institute of Environmental Medicine
Karolinska Institute
S-171 77 Stockholm
Tel: +46 8 728 7203
Web: www.ki.se

Department of Medical Sciences/Occupational and
Environmental Medicine
University Hospital
S-753 31 Uppsala
Tel: +46 18 6113655
Web: www.occmed.uu.se

Department of Occupational and Evironmental
Medicine
Faculty of Medicine
University Hospital
S-581 85 Linköping
Tel: +46 13 221447
Fax: +46 13 145831

Department of Occupational and Environmental
Health
Karolinska Hospital
Norrbacka 3rd floor
S-171 76 Stockholm
Tel: +46 8 5177 7901
Web: www.sll.se/miliomedicin

Department of Occupational and Environmental
Medicine
Regional Hospital
S-701 85 Örebro
Tel: +46 19 152469
Fax: +46 19 120404

Department of Occupational and Environmental
Medicine
University Hospital
SE-221 85 Lund
Tel: +46 46 173185
Web: www.ymed.lu.se

Department of Occupational Medicine
University of Göteborg
S:t Sigfridsgatan 85
SE-412 66 Göteborg
Tel: +46 31 3354872
Fax: +46 31 409728

National Institute for Working Life
Ekelundsvägen 16
Solna
112 79 Stockholm
Tel: +46 8 309601
Fax: +46 8 7309897
Web: www.niwl.se

Nordic School of Public Health
PO Box 12133
SE-402 42 Göteborg
Tel: +46 31 693980
Fax: +46 31 691777

The Netherlands

Department of Environmental Sciences
Environmental and Occupational Health Group
University of Wageningen
Post Box 238
NL-6700 AE Wageningen

Coronel Institute for Occupational and Environmental
Health
Division of Occupational Health
University of Amsterdam
PO Box 22700
NL-1100 DE Amsterdam
Tel: +31 20 5665325
Fax: +31 20 6977161

Netherlands Expertise
Centre for Occupational and Pulmonary Diseases
PO Box 9001
NL-6560 GB Groesbeek
Tel: +31 246859582
Fax: +31 246859290

United Kingdom

Department of Environmental and Occupational
Medicine
University of Aberdeen
Forester Hill Road
Aberdeen
AB21 22P
Tel: +44 1224 558 188
Fax: +44 1224 662 990
Email: oem050@abdn.ac.uk
Web: www.abdn.ac.uk/deom

Department of Occupational and Environmental
Medicine
Royal Brompton National Heart and Lung Institute
16 Manresa Road
London SW3 6LR
Tel: +44 20 7351 8328
Fax: +44 20 7351 8328

Health Effects Section (Immunologic Studies)
Health and Safety Laboratory
Broad Lane
Sheffield S3 7HQ
Tel: +44 114 289 2716
Fax: +44 114 289 2768
E-mail: andrew.curran@hsl.gov.uk
Web: www.hsl.gov.uk

Health and Safety Commission
HSE Information Services
Caerphilly Business Park
Caerphilly
Mid Glamorgan
CF83 3GG
Tel: +44 8701 545500
Web: www.hse.gov.uk

Institute of Occupational Health
University of Birmingham
University Road West
Edgbaston
PO Box 363
Birmingham B15 2TT
Tel: +44 121 414 6673
Fax: +44 121 414 6217

Institute of Occupational Medicine
8 Roxburgh Place
Edinburgh EH8 9SU
Tel: +44 131 667 5131
Fax: +44 131 667 0136

North West Lung Centre
Wythenshawe Hospital
Southmoor Road
Manchester M23 9LT
Tel: +44 161 291 7070
Fax: +44 161 9462603

Occupational Lung Diseases Unit
Birmingham Heartlands Hospital
Bordersley Green East
Birmingham B9 5SS
Tel: +44 121 242 4000
Fax: +44 121 772 0292

Regional Unit for Occupational Lung Disease
Department of Respiratory Medicine
Royal Victoria Infirmary
University of Newcastle upon Tyne
Tel: +44 191 282 0143
Fax: +44 191 227 5224

Particle analysis: ERS Working Group

A working group of the European Respiratory Society, with participation from nine laboratories, has recently published guidelines [1] for microscopic techniques for analysing asbestos fibers in lung tissue and bronchoalveolar lavage fluid. Such analyses are increasingly applied for clinical work and medicolegal matters. Differences in sampling, preparation and counting techniques, definitions of reference populations, and expression of results have caused major difficulties in comparing results from different laboratories, and so it appeared necessary to harmonize these analyzes between the European laboratories active in this field. The published article touched upon five main issues:

1. Definitions of control populations and reference levels
2. Sampling, preparation and analytical techniques
3. Asbestos fibres in lung tissues in different pathologies
4. Asbestos bodies in lung tissue, bronchoalveolar lavage, and sputum
5. The basis for the interpretation of fibers and asbestos bodies in biological samples.

The guidelines emphasize the crucial importance of several factors for the interpretation of the results; namely, adequate sampling, comparable analytical procedures and expression of the results, the use of well-defined reference populations, and a comprehensive understanding of the factors affecting the fiber retention and the dose-responses associated with the different asbestos-related diseases. Contact details for the collaborating centers which remain active are as follows:

Belgium

Prof. P. De Vuyst
Dr. P. Dumortier
Laboratory of Mineralogy – Chest Department
Erasme Hospital
Route de Lennik, 808
B1070 Brussels
Tel: +32 2 555 42 55
Fax: +32 2 555 42 55 or 44 11
E-mail: pdumorti@ulb.ac.be
        pdevuyst@ulb.ac.be

Finland

Dr A. Tossavainen
Finnish Institute of Occupational Health
Aerosol Laboratory
Topeliuksenkatu 41
00250 Helsinki
Tel: + 358 9 474 72233
Fax: + 358 9 474 72208
E-mail: atos@occuphealth.fi

France

Mme M. A. Billion-Galland
Laboratoire d'étude des particules inhalées
Rue Georges Eastman 11
F 75043 Paris
France
Tel: + 33 1 44 97 88 46
fax: + 32 1 44 97 88 45
E-mail: marie-annick.billion-galland@mairie-paris.fr

Germany

Dr K. Rödelsperger
Institute and Outpatient Clinic for Occupational
and Social Medicine
Justus Liebig Universität
Aulweg 129/III
D 35392 Giessen
Germany
Tel: + 49 641 99 41330
Fax: + 49 641 99 41339
E-mail: Klaus.Roedelsperger@arbmed.med.
uni-giessen.de

Dr M. Fischer
Institut für Pathologie und Mesotheliomregister
Berufsgenossenschaftliche Kliniken Bergmannsheil
Brükle-de-la-Camp Platz 1
D 44789 Bochum
Germany
Tel: + 49 234 302 9701
Fax: + 49 234 302 6671

Italy

Prof. F. Mollo
Dr P. Burlo
Dipartimento di Scienze Biomediche e Oncologia
Umana – Sezione di Anatomica Patologica
Università di Torino
via Santena 7
10126 Torino
Italy
Tel: + 39 011 6706509
Fax: + 39 011 6635267
E-mail: franco.mollo@unito.it

Spain

Dr E. Monsó
Servei de Pneumologia
Hospital Germans Trias i Pujol
Carretera de Canyet s/n.
08916 Badalona
Catalonia
Spain
Tel: + 34 934978920
Fax: + 34 934978843
E-mail: emonso@ns.hugtip.scs.es

United Kingdom

Dr. A.R. Gibbs
Department of Histopathology
Llandough Hospital
Penlan Road
Penarth
Vale of Glamorgan CF64 2XX
UK
Tel: + 44 29 20715283
Fax: + 44 29 20712979
E-mail: allen.gibbs@lhct-tr.wales.nhs.uk

REFERENCES

1. De Vuyst P, Karjalainen A, Dumortier P, Pairon JC, Monso E, Brochard P, et al. Guidelines for mineral fibre analyses in biological samples: report of the ERS Working Group. European Respiratory Society. Eur Respir J 1998; 11: 1416–26.

Abbreviations

AAOH	Asian Association of Occupational Health	CFK	Coburn–Forster–Kane (equation)
ABG	Arterial blood gas	CFR	Code of Federal Regulation
ACGIH	American Conference of Governmental Industrial Hygienists	cfu	Colony forming units (microbial culture)
		CH_4	Methane
ACTH	Adrenocorticotrophic hormone	CH_3COOH	Acetic acid
AD	Area decrement (FEV_1 plot, usually 2-12 hours)	CI	Confidence interval
		CK	Cytokeratin
AFB	Acid-fast bacilli	CLA	Chemiluminescent assay
AGE	Arterial gas embolism	cm	Centimetre
AIDS	Acquired immunodeficiency syndrome	CMME	Chloromethyl methyl ether
		CN	Cyanide
AMA	American Medical Association	CN gas	w-chloroacetophenone (tear gas)
AMBER	Advanced multiple beam radiography	CNS	Central nervous system
		CO	Carbon monoxide
AMS	Acute mountain sickness	CO_2	Carbon dioxide
AR	Airway responsiveness	$COCl_2$	Phosgene
ARDS	Adult respiratory distress syndrome	COHb	Carboxyhemoglobin
		COP	Cryptogenic organizing pneumonia
ata	Atmospheres absolute (pressure)		
ATPS	Ambient temperature and pressure standardized	COPD	Chronic obstructive pulmonary disease
ATS	American Thoracic Society	COSHH	Control of Substances Hazardous to Health
ATSDR	Agency for Toxic Substances and Disease Registry	Cr	Chromium
		CRP	C reactive protein
B_{12}	Hydroxocobalamin	CS gas	ortho-chlorobenzylidene malononitrile (tear gas)
BAL	Bronchoalveolar lavage		
BCG	Bacille Calmette-Guérin	CT	Computed tomogram
BCME	Bis(chloromethyl) ether	CWP	Coal workers' pneumoconiosis
BID	Twice daily	DAN	Divers Alert Network
BOOP	Bronchiolitis obliterans organizing pneumonia	DCI	Decompression illness
		DCS	Decompression sickness
BTPS	Body temperature and pressure standardized	DECOS	Dutch Expert Committee on Occupational Standards
C	Centigrade (temperature)	*D. farinae/ pteronyssinus*	Dermatophagoides (mite species)
CAVH	Chronic ateriovenous hemofiltration		
		DFR	Doctor's First Report
CCOHS	Canadian Centre for Occupational Health and Safety	DIP	Desquamative interstitial pneumonitis
CDC	Centers for Disease Prevention and Control	dl	Deci-litre
		D_LCO (or T_LCO)	Gas transfer factor for carbon monoxide
CD4/CD8	Ratio of helper to suppressor T lymphocyte numbers		
		DMAP	Dimethylaminophenol
CdO	Cadmium oxide	DNA	Deoxyribonucleic acid
CEA	Carcinoembryonic antigen	dVO_2	Oxygen consumption
CEN	European Standardization Committee	EAACI	European Academy of Allergology and Clinical Immunology
CFA	Cryptogenic fibrosing alveolitis		

EASHW	European Agency for Safety and Health at Work	HRCT	High resolution computed tomography
EC	European Commission	H_2S	Hydrogen sulfide
ECG	Electrocardiogram	HSA	Human serum albumin
EDAX	Energy dispersive x-ray spectrometer	HSE	Health and Safety Executive
		HU	Hounsfield unit
EDTA	Ethylenediaminetetraacetic acid (edetic acid)	HVAC	Heating, ventilation, and air-conditioning systems
EHAE	Epithelioid hemangioendothelioma	IARC	International Agency for Research on Cancer
ELISA	Enzyme-linked immunosorbent assay	ICAM1	Intracellular adhesion molecule-1
EMA	Epithelial membrane antigen	ICD	International Classification of Diseases
EPA	Environmental Protection Agency	ICSC	International Chemical Safety Cards
ERC	Education and Research Center (NIOSH)	IgE	Immunoglobulin E
		IGF	Insulin-like growth factor
ERS	European Respiratory Society	IgG	Immunoglobulin G
ERV	Expiratory reserve volume	IL	Interleukin
ESR	Erythrocyte sedimentation rate	ILO	International Labour Office
ETS	Environmental tobacco smoke	IMSS	Mexican Institute for Social Security
EU	European Union		
F	Farenheit (temperature)	IPCS	International Program on Chemical Safety
FDG	Fluorodeoxyglucose (PET scanning)	IPDI	Isophorone diisocyanate
FEF	Forced expiratory flow	IPF	Idiopathic pulmonary fibrosis
FEV_1	Forced expired volume in one second	IPPV	Intermittent positive pressure ventilation
FGF	Fibroblast growth factor	IRV	Inspiratory reserve volume
FiO_2	Concentration of inspired oxygen	ISO	International Standards Organization
FIV_1	Forced inspiratory volume in one second	IT	Information technology
FIVC	Forced inspiratory vital capacity	IV	Intravenous
f/ml	Fiber concentration in fibers/ml	IVC	Inspiratory vital capacity
FRC	Functional residual capacity	JETOC	Japan Chemical Industry Ecology-Toxicology and Information Center
FROD	Finnish Register on Occupational Diseases		
FVC	Forced vital capacity	JISHA	Japan Industrial Safety and Health Association
g	Gram		
GIP	Giant cell interstitial pneumonia	Kco	Gas transfer coefficient (T_LCO/V_a)
gm	Gram	kg	Kilogram
GSD	Geometric standard deviation	km	Kilometer
HACE	High altitude cerebral edema	kPa	Kilopascal
HAPE	High altitude pulmonary edema	kVp	Kilovoltage
HBME	Mesothelial cell antibody	L or l	Liter
HBO	Hyperbaric oxygen	LOD	Limit of detection
HCHO	Formaldehyde	LTD	Longterm disability
HCl	Hydrogen chloride	m	Meter
HCN	Hydrogen cyanide	*M.*	Mycobacterium
HDI	Hexamethylene diisocyanate	mA	Milliamperage
HEPA	High-efficiency particulate air filter	MAC	Maximum allowable concentration
Hg	Mercury	MAG	Metal active gas (welding)
HIV	Human immunodeficiency virus	MDI	Diphenylmethane diisocyanate
HP	Hypersensitivity pneumonitis	MDR	Multiple drug resistant (tuberculosis)
hr	Hour		

MEDLINE	MEDlars onLINE	ODIN	Occupational Disease Information Network
MEF	Maximum expiratory flow	ODTS	Organic dust toxic syndrome
MEL	Maximum exposure limit	OEL	Occupational exposure limit
MetHb	Methemoglobin	$OH^{\cdot}$	Hydroxyl radical
mg	Milligram	OHS	Occupational Health and Safety
MIF	Maximal inspiratory flow	OR	Odds ratio
MIG	Metal inert gas (welding)	OSH	Occupational Safety and Health
min	Minute	OSHA	Occupational Safety and Health Administration
MIP1a	Macrophage inflammatory protein 1a	PA	Phthallic anhydride / Plicatic acid / Postero-anterior (chest radiograph projection) / Pulmonary artery
ml	Milliliter		
mm	Millimetre		
MMA	Manual metal arc (welding)		
MMEF	Maximal mid expiratory flow		
mmol	Millimole	$Paco_2$ (or Pco_2)	Arterial carbon dioxide tension
MMVF	Manmade vitreous fibers	PAHs	Polycyclic aromatic hydrocarbons
Mn	Manganese	Pao_2 (or Po_2)	Arterial oxygen tension
mol	Molecule	PAP	Pulmonary alveolar proteinosis
MOSHH	Management of Substances Hazardous to Health	PAS	Periodic acid-Schiff
		PC_{20}	Provoking concentration causing a 20% decrement in FEV_1
mppcf	Millions of particles per cubic foot		
		PCNA	Proliferating cell nuclear antigen
MRC	Medical Research Council	Pco_2 (or $Paco_2$)	Arterial carbon dioxide tension
MRI	Magnetic resonance imaging	PCOM	Phase contrast optical microscopy
MSDS	Material Safety Data Sheet		
MSHA	Mine Safety and Health Administration	PCR	Polymerized chain reaction
		PD_{20}	Provoking dose causing a 20% decrement in FEV_1
mSv	Millisieverts		
MTBE	Methyl tertiary butyl ether	PDGF	Platelet-derived growth factor
mth	Month	PEF	Peak expiratory flow
MTHPA	Methyl-tetrahydrophthalic anhydride	PEFR	Peak expiratory flow rate
		PEL	Permissible exposure limit
MVV	Maximal ventilatory volume	PET	Positron emission tomography
MWF	Metal working fluid	PFI	Physical fitness index
N_2	Nitrogen	pH	Hydrogen ion concentration (log 1/[H^+])
NA	Not applicable		
NAFTA	North American Free Trade Agreement	PIFR	Peak inspiratory flow rate
		PM_{10}	Particles <10 μm in diameter
NBO	Normobaric oxygen	PMF	Progressive massive fibrosis
ND	Not detectable	pmn	Polymorphonuclear cells (leucocytes)
NDI	Naphthylene diisocyanate		
NH_3	Ammonia	PMR	Proportionate mortality ratio
NHS	National Health Service	Po_2 (or Pao_2)	Arterial oxygen tension
NIOSH	National Institute for Occupational Safety and Health	ppb	Parts per billion
		PPE	Personal protective equipment
NO	Nitric oxide	PPI	Polymethylene polyphenylisocyanate
NO_2	Nitrogen dioxide		
NOHSC	National Occupational Health and Safety Commission	psi	Pounds per square inch
		PTFE	Polytetrafluoroethylene (Teflon)
NOx	Oxides of nitrogen	PVC	Polyvinyl chloride
NRL	Natural rubber latex	RADS	Reactive airways dysfunction syndrome
NTM	Non-tuberculous mycobacteria		
O_2	Oxygen	RAST	Radioallergosorbent test
O_2^-	Superoxide anion	Raw	Airway resistance
O_3	Ozone	RB-ILD	Respiratory bronchiolitis-interstitial lung disease
OASYS	Occupational asthma system		

RCF	Refractory ceramic fiber	TCPA	Tetrachlorophthalic anhydride
REL	Recommended exposure limit	TDI	Toluene diisocyanate
RF	Reduction factor	TGFβ	Transforming growth factor-β
RFLP	Restriction fragment length polymorphism	TGIC	Triglycidyl-isocyanurate
RIDDOR	Reporting on Injuries, Disease, and Dangerous Occurrences Regulations	TIG	Tungsten inert gas (welding)
		TLC	Total lung capacity
		T_LCO (or D_LCO)	Gas transfer factor for carbon monoxide
RNA	Ribonucleic acid	TLV	Threshold limit value
RPE	Respiratory protection equipment	TMA	Trimellitic anhydride
		TNFα	Tumour necrosis factor alpha
RV	Residual volume	TNM	Tumour-Node-Metastasis
Rx	Treatment	torr	Pressure measured in mm Hg
s (or sec)	Second	T4/T8	Ratio of helper to suppressor T lymphocyte numbers
SaO_2	Arterial oxygen saturation		
sBPT	Specific bronchial provocation tests	TVOC	Total volatile organic compounds (VOC)
SBS	Sick building syndrome	TWA	Time weighted average
SCBA	Self-contained breathing apparatus	UICC	International Union against Cancer
SCN	Thiocyanate	UIP	Usual interstitial pneumonia
SCOEL	Scientific Committee for Occupational Exposure Limits (EU)	UK	United Kingdom
		US	United States
		USA	United States of America
SDS	Safety data sheet	UV	Ultraviolet
sec (or s)	Second	V_a	Alveolar volume
SEM	Scanning electron microscopy	VAT	Video-assisted thoracoscopy
SHE	Sentinel health event	VC	Vital capacity
SINOS	Sodium nonanoyloxybenzene sulphonate	VOCs	Volatile organic compounds
		WBC	White blood cell (count)
SMR	Standardized mortality ratio	WHO	World Health Organisation
SO_2	Sulphur dioxide	WRC	Western red cedar
SORDSA	Surveillance of Occupational Respiratory Diseases in South Africa	yr	Year
		ZnO	Zinc oxide
SPT	Skin prick test	μ	Micro
SSDI	Social Security Disability Insurance	μg	Microgram
		μm	Micrometer
SSI	Supplemental Security Income	μmol	Micromolecule
STEL	Short-term exposure limit		
SV40	Simian virus 40	1mmHg	0.133kPa
SVC	Slow vital capacity	1kPa	7.519mmHg
SWORD	Surveillance of Work-related and Occupational Respiratory Disease	1 lb	0.45 kg
		1 kg	2.2 lb
TAG	T antigen	long ton (UK)	2240 lb
TB	Tuberculosis	short ton (US)	2000 lb
TCDD	Tetrachlorodibenzo-para-dioxin	metric ton (tonne)	1000 kg (2204.6 lb)

Index